PREHOSPITAL SYST
MEDICAL OVERSIGHT

Third Edition

National Association of EMS Physicians

Edited by

Alexander E. Kuehl, MD, MPH, FACS, FACEP

Director of Public Health
  St. Lawrence County (NY)

Medical Director
  E.J. Noble Hospital, Gouverneur, NY

Robert Wood Johnson Clinical Scholar
  Johns Hopkins Medical Institutions (1974–1978)

Director of Medical Affairs
  Maryland Institute for EMS Systems (1979–1981)

Medical Director and CEO
  New York City EMS (1981–1989)

Associate Professor of Surgery and Public Health
  Cornell University Medical College (1985–2001)

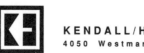

KENDALL/HUNT PUBLISHING COMPANY
4050 Westmark Drive   Dubuque, Iowa 52002

DEDICATION

*To those teachers, colleagues and students
who are no longer with us—thank you;
we will not forget your efforts.*

Contents

Foreword V
Preface VII
Contributors xi

SECTION ONE SYSTEMS

INTRODUCTION 1
1   HISTORY 3
2   MODELS AND LEGISLATION 20
3   URBAN 33
4   RURAL 41
5   WILDERNESS 51
6   FIRE 68
7   PRIVATE 75
8   MILITARY 81
9   INTERNATIONAL 90

SECTION TWO ELEMENTS

INTRODUCTION 97
10   RESPONSE PHASES 99
11   LEVELS OF PROVIDERS 106
12   SYSTEM DESIGN 114
13   FUNDING 132
14   REIMBURSEMENT TRENDS 139
15   MEDICAL INTERVENTIONS 143
16   COMMUNICATIONS 162
17   EMERGENCY MEDICAL DISPATCH 172
18   PRIORITY DISPATCH RESPONSE 208
19   RESPONSE CHOICES 229
20   FIRST RESPONDERS 236
21   RESUSCITATION ISSUES 245
22   INFORMATION SYSTEMS 261
23   EVALUATION 276
24   RESEARCH 288

SECTION THREE MEDICAL OVERSIGHT

INTRODUCTION 299
25   MEDICAL OVERSIGHT 301
26   INDIRECT MEDICAL OVERSIGHT 308

27   DIRECT MEDICAL OVERSIGHT 318
28   ON-SCENE SUPERVISION 330
29   EDUCATION 340
30   QUALITY MANAGEMENT 355
31   RISK MANAGEMENT 388
32   LEGAL ISSUES 395
33   ETHICAL ISSUES 420
34   POLITICAL REALITIES 431
35   AUTHORIZATION AND EMPOWERMENT 439

SECTION FOUR PERSPECTIVES

INTRODUCTION 447
36   ED INTERACTION WITH PREHOSPITAL PROVIDERS 449
37   NURSES 452
38   VOLUNTEERS 460
39   SPOUSES 466
40   STATE OFFICE 468
41   FEDERAL 472
42   LEADERSHIP AND TEAM BUILDING 477
43   MEDIA 481
     SECTION FOUR APPENDIX 493

SECTION FIVE MEDICAL OPERATIONS

INTRODUCTION 505
44   REFUSAL OF MEDICAL ASSISTANCE 507
45   PHYSICIANS AT THE SCENE 519
46   THE PNEUMATIC ANTI-SHOCK GARMENT 525
47   AUTOMATED DEFIBRILLATORS 530
48   PEDIATRIC 539
49   GERIATRIC 556
50   AIR SERVICES 567
51   INTERFACILITY TRANSPORT 576
52   PREHOSPITAL PROVIDERS IN THE EMERGENCY DEPARTMENT 584
53   INAPPROPRIATE USE AND UNMET NEED 590

Section Six Medical Protocols

54 Procedures 607

55 Pharmacotherapy 639

56 Analgesia 659

57 Shortness of Breath 665

58 Chest Pain 672

59 Dysrhythmias 683

60 Cardiac Arrest 693

61 Hypotension and Shock 704

62 Trauma 713

63 Obstetric and Gynecologic 719

64 Pediatric 728

65 Poisoning and Overdose 741

66 Behavioral 762

67 Altered Level of Consciousness 774

Section Seven Administrative Operations

68 Due Process 785

69 Communicable Diseases 798

70 Hazardous Materials 811

71 Multiple Casualty Incidents 821

72 Catastrophic Events 828

73 Terrorism and Weapons of
Mass Destruction 840

74 Tactical Emergency Medical Support 860

75 Diversion and Bypass 871

76 Regionalization and Designation of
Medical Facilities 886

77 Mass Gathering Medical Care 894

78 Critical Incident Stress Management 914

Section Eight Futures

79 EMS Agenda for the Future 923

80 Public Health 935

81 Injury Prevention 941

82 Managed Care 946

Epilogue 959

Intro to Glossary 967

Glossary 969

Index 983

Foreword

This is an extremely exciting time in the growth and development of emergency medical services, not only in the United States, but internationally. Although released several years ago, the NHTSA *EMS Agenda for the Future* is still focusing and pushing forward our vision for the future of EMS activities. The *EMS Education Agenda* has recently been published and is starting to exert its influence on EMS Education. The *EMS Research Agenda* project is just completed; we anxiously look forward to the impact that this document will have. The EMS community is beginning to work more closely with public health organizations to improve the health of our communities. The tragic events that began on the morning of September 11, 2001 have focused us on the need for further activities in appropriate planning and response for catastrophic disaster events. Within the context of all of these activities, we present the 3rd Edition of Prehospital Systems and Medical Oversight.

An integral component of the activities of the EMS community involves the medical oversight of all aspects of out-of-hospital medical care. Note that there is a transition here from what we have viewed in the past as "prehospital care" to a broader vision of "out-of-hospital" care. EMS is increasingly being seen as an integral part of the overall healthcare system, and that perspective will continue to grow. All of the activities that currently exist, and will occur in the future, involve medical care provided by various levels of out-of-hospital personnel operating under the supervision of dedicated, knowledgeable physicians. As the level and scope of these activities performed by those personnel become better matched to the need of the out-of-hospital patient, so must the knowledge of the physicians working with them. The physicians must continue to lead those activities. There truly is a "unique body of knowledge" that allows physicians to function effectively as EMS physicians.

The National Association of EMS Physicians (NAEMSP) is committed to the support and growth of EMS physicians, EMS medical directors, and those non-physicians involved in supporting medical oversight activities. Through this text, we strive to provide that solid base of knowledge for EMS physicians as we continue to grow and mature in our special area of medical practice. Under the direction of Alexander Kuehl, M.D., Editor in Chief of this text, a group of dedicated section editors and authors have provided you with an extremely valuable resource to use in your daily practice of out-of-hospital medicine.

The material presented here is contemporary, functional, and applicable. It is designed to be a resource for medical students interested in EMS, physicians in training as residents or fellows, new EMS physicians as well as experienced EMS physicians, and non-physicians responsible for out-of-hospital activities. Although most of the information presented is based on the "North American" model, much of the information is applicable in other parts of the world. We must also realize that we have much to learn from the out-of-hospital experiences of those outside of North America.

The NAEMSP is very proud of the contribution to medical care of the community that is provided by EMS systems, and of the role that the Association has been able to play in providing leadership in the growth and development of EMS. We appreciate the interaction we have had with other organizations supporting that development, and look forward to continuing to contribute to that development.

The collective knowledge imparted by EMS physician experts in this text serves as a foundation to further the NAEMSP's mission "to provide leadership and foster excellence in out-of-hospital emergency medical services."

We trust that you will find this text useful in your practice.

Richard C. Hunt, MD
President

Jon R. Krohmer, MD
Immediate Past President

Preface

Alexander E. Kuehl, MD, MPH

At its 1986 annual meeting, the National Association of EMS Physicians (NAEMSP) clearly and forcefully articulated the need for a textbook that would address the medical aspects of designing, implementing, and operating EMS systems. Those medical aspects of EMS systems are defined broadly by both NAEMSP and by the editor. *Prehospital Systems and Medical Oversight* represents the product of a continuing, interdisciplinary effort to collate the thoughts, recommendations, and predictions of many EMS professionals, not all of whom are physicians.

The entire text is crafted to be read from cover to cover, although it may be used as a definitive reference on specific issues. Some concepts and topics are discussed repeatedly in the text, and each additional citation should add another dimension to the issue. If, after completing the text, the neophyte EMS medical director feels simultaneously stimulated, concerned, and confident, the authors have accomplished what they set out to do. Parenthetically, students will find the text to be a useful companion reference to NAEMSP's National EMS Medical Directors' Course and Practicum.

Although every attempt has been made to provide a broad and varied array of solutions to the most common problems that the EMS physician is likely to encounter during the various phases of EMS system development, no two EMS systems are exactly alike; solutions that are successful in one jurisdiction may not be practical, possible, or even legal in another. The reader is cautioned to use the ideas and approaches described herein as suggestions for guiding the evolution of a system, rather than as absolute templates for local system design. Of course, a number of problems still defy solution.

As the science of prehospital and disaster medicine has matured, so has the terminology used to describe it. Terms such as "medical control," "advanced life support (ALS)," and "disaster" originally were used to describe relatively uncomplicated concepts which, with time, have become increasingly sophisticated. In addition, regional variations in usage gradually developed. "ALS" in Montana was different from "ALS" in Maryland; "disasters" in New York were different from "disasters" in Arkansas; and "medical control" was defined differently by every state legislature. As the authors of the individual chapters of the first edition described the past, analyzed the present, and predicted the future, it became painfully apparent to the editor that new terms needed to be invented, and that old terms required more precise definitions. For example, to continue to differentiate arbitrarily between "basic" and "advanced" life support no longer made sense, because all prehospital care requires medical oversight; the scope of prehospital medicine is a continuum from fundamental first aid through the most sophisticated clinical intervention. Unfortunately, the federal government regulations continue to reimburse providers through a two-tiered system that uses the outmoded and somewhat confusing terminology.

Since the 1960s EMS administrators, philosophers, and educators have attempted to define more precisely "medical control," "medical direction," and "medical command." In the first edition of this text, the authors recognized both that "on-line" and "off-line" "medical control" had come to mean many different things, and that modern prehospital medicine required standard national terms. Specifically, neither "off-line" nor "on-line" ever adequately described the hands-on patient care provided by EMS medical directors. Therefore, the term "direct" was chosen to describe all activities in which the physician was contemporaneously providing *or* supervising patient care, that is, all the functions that were the traditional practice of medicine with a clear duty to the patient. The term "indirect" was then reserved for those activities that were removed by time or function from the immediate care of the patient. Both of those activities could be delegated to others by the physician who was ultimately and finally responsible. The term for the ultimate medical, legal, and moral responsibility for the medical aspects of prehospital care is "medical oversight."

In this edition, we have abandoned "medical control" altogether and use our previously coined term of "medical oversight" to describe all of the medical aspects of EMS, from the ultimate authority to the smallest task.

In the sections of this text addressing catastrophic events and multiple casualty incidents, the authors have adopted the more encompassing and descriptive lexicon of "potential injury-causing event" (PICE). Undoubtedly, terminology will evolve further with both time and experience; that is as it should be.

Before 1981, no physicians exclusively devoted their practices or their careers to EMS medical oversight. Although a slowly expanding number of jurisdictions have established full-time EMS medical director positions, most local and regional EMS systems rely on either dedicated practicing physicians or the chairpersons of regional EMS medical advisory groups as their medical directors. For the foreseeable future, most EMS physicians will continue to provide medical oversight as an adjunct to their other practices of medicine. Although it is the expressed intent of the editorial leadership to promote the concept of full-time EMS medical directors, we recognize that most readers have significant professional and personal responsibilities beyond prehospital and disaster medicine.

Nevertheless, the number of physicians in full-time EMS medical director positions continues to grow, as do the variations in EMS system administrative and medical structure. At one extreme the physician director is responsible for all of the medical and operational aspects of EMS; at the other, the physician is simply an informal advisor to the EMS administrator, the fire chief, the board of directors, or the regional medical advisory committee. The degree of actual authority of the physician over medical matters also varies. Occasionally the medical authority of the physician is absolute; more commonly, medical oversight policies and protocols are implemented only with the advice and consent of local physicians and administrators.

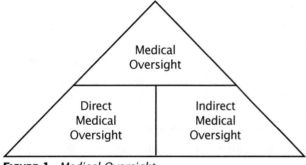

FIGURE 1. *Medical Oversight*

Undeniably the practices of prehospital and disaster medicine are becoming more complicated, more standardized, and more formalized; appropriately, the medically and legally responsible physicians are exercising greater authority over the entire range of medical oversight issues. There are occasionally heated debates over whether issues such as response time targets, length of duty shifts, and dispatch policies fall in the jurisdiction of medical oversight. Physicians who wish to expand the scope of medical oversight often do not appreciate that with additional authority and responsibility also come increased accountability and liability.

Over the last decade, the general community of emergency physicians has grown significantly more comfortable with its responsibility to include prehospital medical oversight as an integral part of both the residency curricula and the American Board of Emergency Medicine certification criteria. In addition, physicians have begun to recognize that the simple acts of receiving and caring for ambulance patients should not and do not empower them to publicly criticize the medical practice of those physicians charged with prehospital medical oversight. With time, recognition of prehospital and disaster medicine as a subspecialty of emergency medicine, or perhaps even as a separate specialty of medicine, will likely emerge. We trust that this text both expands and defines the knowledge base that helps frame that evolving medical practice.

This textbook is divided into eight discrete sections. Section One presents the reader with a broad overview of EMS systems, focusing particularly on the historical background, legislative underpinnings, and those basic structural issues that must be addressed relatively early in the planning and developmental process.

Section Two describes the various crucial elements of an EMS system that must be specifically structurally addressed for a service or system to actually function.

Section Three introduces and develops the concept of medical oversight, presenting first an historical perspective and then the varied philosophies and mechanisms for the provision of medical oversight. This section challenges the reader to expand widely the horizons of medical involvement in EMS, and admittedly emphasizes a philosophy of public health rather than one of public safety or of emergency medicine.

Section Four merges the perspectives of those involved in prehospital medicine into a loose credo that will be of assistance to even the most experienced medical director in creating the shared paradigm necessary for a truly successful system.

Section Five addresses the specific broad medical policy issues that a medical director must understand before developing individual medical protocols.

Section Six is the result of the confluence of the updated clinical portions of the text *Prehospital Medicine* (edited by Paris, Roth, and Verdile), and of this text. Only after most of the issues raised in the first five sections are addressed can clinical protocols logically be developed. It is expected that there will be regional differences; however, evidence-based medicine should prevail.

Section Seven addresses specific administrative operational challenges that virtually every EMS physician will be expected to quickly identify, intelligently evaluate, and adeptly solve. In many cases the rubric is embarrassingly thin; the limited references and lack of scientific basis reflect the immaturity of our specialty, rather than any shortcomings on the part of the Section editor or the individual authors.

Section Eight attempts to capture as accurate a vision of the immediate future of EMS as can be determined from where we currently stand.

The text ends with a unique and comprehensive glossary that has already been recognized as a driving force in the standardization of the diverse terminology used to describe EMS operations throughout the world. After understanding the terms, the novice medical director should be able to speak and understand our new and evolving language; however, some regional dialects are not included, and a few of the definitions are perilously close to being arbitrary. Before starting to read the text, the reader should peruse the glossary so that both student and teacher are familiar with the vocabulary.

The Epilogue is painfully introspective, marginally optimistic, and somewhat vague; it simply encourages the reader to view broadly and openly the more distant future of EMS medical oversight from the vantage point of the present, tempered moderately by the accumulated wisdom of the past.

Finally, on a personal note, I wish to continue the analogy between the growth of my daughter, Kendall, and the evolution of EMS that I first addressed in the previous editions. Ten years ago she was barely out of adolescence; today she has fully merged her family, education, and aspirations with those of her husband, Rick, and two new members of the next generation. And like most citizens of the world on September 11, those two new parents found their priorities shifted and their view of the world altered, perhaps permanently. One day my grandchildren may ask Kendall why her father and a few other individuals were eventually joined by so many others in tilting at windmills, forming NAEMSP, creating the National EMS Medical Directors' Course, and struggling with the various editions of this book. The following anonymous verse, brought to my attention by Jay Fitch, continues to best express what I hope she can explain.

The Bridge Builder

An old man going a lone highway
Came at the evening cold and grey
To a chasm vast and wide and steep
With waters rolling cold and deep.
The old man crossed in the twilight dim—
The sullen stream held no fear for him—
But he turned when safe on the other side
And built a bridge to span the tide.
"Old man," said a fellow pilgrim near,
"You're wasting your strength with building here.
Your journey will end with the ending day,
You'll never again cross this way,
You've crossed the chasm deep and wide.
Why build this bridge at eventide?"
The builder lifted his old grey head.
"Good friend, on the path I have come," he said,
"There followeth after me today
A youth whose feet must pass this way.
The chasm that was naught to me
To that fairhead youth may a pitfall be.
He, too, must cross in the twilight dim.
Good friend, I am building this bridge for him."

Anonymous

Contributors

The following individuals have been individually noted by one or more of the authors for their significant contributions toward the successful completion of this text, including authoring chapters in previous editions.

Juanita N. Abston
Adrian Anast, PhD
Terese Arena
R. Jack Ayers, Jr.
Susan Barcus, MD
Stacie M. Beckwith, CMP
Kristen Bensen
Nicholas Bensten, MD, MBA
Russel B. Biezick, MD
Wendy Birmbaun, BSN
Leo Bosner, MSW
George Boolukas, MD
Allan Braslow, PhD
Odelia Braun, MD
John F. Brown, MD
Marie Brown, MD
William Brown, RN, EMT-P
Brenda Bruns, MD
Richard Carmona, MD
Christine Carroll
Charles Conole, FACHE
Richard T. Cook, MD
Michael K. Copass, MD
Christina Coughlin, RPA
Wendy Cruz
Daniel Culhane, MD
Jack Delaney, EMT-P
Gayle Dunsmore
Terry V. Fotre, MD
Serena Fox, MD
Suzanne Fry, MD
Deidre Gish-Panjada, MBA
Ross Goldberg
John K. Green
Jinnette Grimes, RN
William Hathaway, MS
Mary Alice Helikisen, MD

Elizabeth Heywood, MSN
Lenard Hudson, MD
Richard C. Hunt, MD
Thomas Judge, CCT-P
Kevin Kelly
Jennifer Kimzey
Theodor Klaudt, MD
Barbara Knight
Robert Knopp, MD
Kim Kourofsky
Ronald L. Krome, MD
Marion Lyver, MD
Robert R. Maisel, MD
Dan Mayer, MD
John McMahen, MD
Nina Meher-Homji
James J. Menegazzi, PhD
Claire Merrick
William Metcalf, EMT-P
Suzanne Michael, PhD
Laura Michalowicz, BSN
Gregory Michels
Barbara A. Mikulski, MSW
Iris Morales
Virginia G. Mork, MD
Karol Louise Murov, BSN, MA
Anthony Mustalish, MD
Georgia O'Gilvie-Rose
Maria Ongsiako, MD
Laurie Otto, MD
Beth Panther
Jeanne Payett
Lenora Payne
Ernest Pretto, MD
Kathy L. Price
Howard David Reines, MD
Matthew M. Rice, MD, JD
Steven Rottman, MD
William R. Roush, MD
Susan Schnall, BSN
Jane Elizabeth Scott
Roger Sergel
G. Tom Shires, MD
John Skiendzielewski, MD

Carol W. Smith
JoAnn Smith, RRT
John Spoor, MD
Kathleen M. Stage-Kern
Ronald D. Stewart, MD
Thomas Talbert

Marilee Tremlett
Thomas W. Turbiak, MD
Charles Weigel, MD
Kenneth A. Williams, MD
Stanley M. Zydlo, MD, JD

CONTENTS

Section Editors

Robert R. Bass, MD, FACEP
Executive Director,
Maryland Institute for Emergency Medical
    Services Systems;
Associate Professor of Surgery
    (Emergency Medicine),
University of Maryland, Baltimore,
Baltimore, MD

David C. Cone, MD, FACEP
Chief, Division of EMS,
Section of Emergency Medicine,
Yale School of Medicine,
New Haven, CT

Michael R. Gunderson
Executive Vice President,
Health Analytics, LLC,
Lakeland, FL;
Distance Education Faculty,
Emergency Health Services,
University of Maryland, Baltimore County,
    Baltimore, Maryland

Mark C. Henry, MD, FACEP
Professor and Chairman,
Department of Emergency Medicine,
    State University of New York, Stony Brook,
Stony Brook, NY;
Medical Director,
EMS Program, New York State Dept. of Health
Troy, NY

Jon R. Krohmer, MD, FACEP
Medical Director
Kent County EMS
Grand Rapids, MI

Robert E. O'Connor, MD, MPH, FACEP
Professor of Emergency Medicine,
Thomas Jefferson University,
Philadelphia, PA;
Director of Education and Research,
Department of Emergency Medicine,
Christiana Care Health System,
Newark, DE

Ronald Roth, MD, FACEP
Associate Professor,
Department of Emergency Medicine,
University of Pittsburgh School of Medicine,
Pittsburgh, PA

Sandra Schneider, MD, FACEP
Professor and Chair,
Department of Emergency Medicine,
University of Rochester,
Rochester, NY

Robert Swor, DO
Clinical Instructor,
Department of Surgery,
University of Michigan,
Ann Arbor, MI;
EMS Coordinator, Department of
    Emergency Medicine,
William Beaumont Hospital,
Royal Oak, MI

Authors

Beth Adams, MA, RN, NREMT-P
ALS-CME Coordinator, EMS Program,
Assistant Professor of Emergency Medicine,
George Washington University School
    of Medicine and Health Science,
Washington, DC

James G. Adams, MD, FACEP
Professor and Chairman,
Division of Emergency Medicine,
Feinberg School of Medicine,
Northwestern University,
Chicago, IL

Richard C. Alcorta, MD, FACEP
Maryland State EMS Director,
University of Maryland Medical School,
Baltimore, MD

Hector Alonso-Serra, MD, MPH, FACEP
Medical Director, Commonwealth of
    Puerto Rico EMS,
San Juan, Puerto Rico

William J. Angelos, MD, FACEP
Chairman, Department of Emergency Medicine
Southern Ohio Medical Center
Portsmouth, OH

Jeffery Arnold, MD, FACEP, FAAEM
Assistant Professor of Emergency Medicine
Tufts University School of Medicine
Springfield, MA

James Atkins, MD, FACP
Director of Emergency Medicine Education,
Professor of Internal Medicine,
Southwestern Medical Center,
University of Texas,
Dallas, TX

James J. Augustine, MD, FACEP
Medical Director, Atlanta Fire Department;
Vice Chairman for Clinical Operations,
Department of Emergency Medicine,
Emory University School of Medicine,
Atlanta, GA

Bob Bailey, MA
Executive Director, Clinical Assistant Professor,
Injury Control Center,
Department of Emergency Medicine,
Upstate Medical University,
State University of New York
Syracuse, NY

Eileen F. Baker, MD, FACEP
EMS Medical Director
Union Hospital
Dover, OH

Paul W. Beck, MD, FACEP
Instructor, Department of Emergency Medicine,
University of Pittsburgh School of Medicine,
Pittsburgh, PA

Fernando L. Benitez, MD, FACEP
Assistant Professor of Surgery,
Southwestern Medical Center,
University of Texas,
Dallas, TX

Michael Casner, MD
EMS Fellow,
University of Chicago,
Chicago, IL

Michael Cassara, DO, FACEP
Attending Physician,
Department of Emergency Medicine,
North Shore University Hospital,
Manhasset, NY

C. Gene Cayten, MD, MPH
Director of Surgery,
Our Lady of Mercy Medical Center,
Bronx, NY;
Consultant, Surgery,
Westchester County Medical Center,
Valhalla, NY

Jeffery J. Clawson, MD
Council of Standards, College of Fellows,
National Academy of Emergency Dispatch,
Salt Lake City, UT

Daniel J. Cobaugh, PharmD, DABAT
Associate Director, American Association of
   Poison Control Centers;
Department of Emergency Medicine,
George Washington University,
Washington, D.C.

Alisdair Keith Thurburn Conn, MD, FACS
Chief, Emergency Services,
Massachusetts General Hospital,
Assistant Professor of Surgery,
   Harvard Medical School
Boston, MA

Keith Conover, MD, FACEP
Medical Director,
Wilderness EMS Institute;
Clinical Assistant Professor,
Department of Emergency Medicine,
University of Pittsburgh,
Pittsburgh, PA

Arthur Cooper, MD, FACS, FAAP, FCCM
Associate Professor of Clinical Surgery,
College of Physicians and Surgeons of Columbia
   University,
Division of Pediatric Surgery
Harlem Hospital Center,
New York, NY

Lynne Susan Cooper, JD
Attorney-At-Law,
New York, NY

Bethaney A. Cummings, DO
Department of Emergency Medicine,
University of Rochester,
Rochester, NY

Adrian D'Amico, MD, FACEP
Chairman, Emergency Medicine
Suburban General Hospital
Pittsburgh, PA

Eric Davis, MD, FACEP
Assistant Professor,
Department of Emergency Medicine,
Strong Memorial Hospital,
Rochester, NY

Robert Davis
Medical Writer, USA Today;
Kaiser Media Fellow,
Arlington, VA

Ted Delbridge, MD, MPH, FACEP
Department of Emergency Medicine,
University of Pittsburgh,
Pittsburgh, PA

Robert Delorenzo, MD, FACEP
Lt. Col. Medical Corps,
Brooke Army Medical Center,
United States Army,
Fort Sam Houston, TX

Norman Dinerman, MD, FACEP
Medical Director, Life Flight of Maine;
Eastern Maine Medical Center,
Bangor, ME

Susan Dunmire, MD, FACEP
Associate Professor,
Department of Emergency Medicine,
University of Pittsburgh School of Medicine,
Pittsburgh, PA

Eelco H. Dykstra, MD
Professor (visiting) in International Emergency
   Management,
Faculty of Social Sciences,
Department of Health Policy and Management,
University of Kuopio,
Kuopio, Finland

Gina Eckstein, BA
Los Angeles, CA

Marc Eckstein, MD, FACEP
Medical Director,
Los Angeles Fire Department,
Assistant Professor of Emergency Medicine,
University of Southern California School of
   Medicine
Los Angeles, CA

Richard D. Elliott, NREMT-P
Griffin, GA

Susan Elliott, MD, FACEP
Department of Emergency Medicine,
University of Vermont,
Burlington, VT

Joseph J. Fitch, PhD
President, Fitch and Associates, Inc.,
Kansas City, MO

Douglas J. Floccare, MD, MPH, FACEP
Maryland State Aeromedical Medical Director,
MIEMSS,
Baltimore, MD

George L. Foltin, MD, FAAP, FACEP
Director, Pediatric Emergency Services,
Bellevue Hospital Center;
Associate Professor of Pediatrics,
New York University School of Medicine,
New York, NY

Raymond L. Fowler, MD, FACEP
Assistant Professor of Emergency Medicine,
Southwestern Medical Center,
University of Texas,
Dallas, TX

Thomas D. Fowlkes, MD, FACEP
Chief Medical Officer, Priority EMS,
Oxford Emergency Group,
Oxford, MS

Susan M. Fuchs, MD, FAAP, FACEP
Associate Professor of Pediatrics,
Northwestern University Medical School,
Chicago, IL

Lorraine Maria Giordano, MD, FACEP
(Former) Medical Director, EMS,
New York Health and Hospitals,
New York, NY

Cai Glushak, MD, FACEP
Associate Professor of Clinical Medicine,
University of Chicago Hospitals Cooperation;
EMS Medical Director,
Chicago South EMS Systems,
Chicago, IL

Mark Greenwood, DO, JD
EMS Fellow,
University of Chicago,
Chicago, IL

Spencer Hall, MD, JD, FCLM
EMS Medical Director,
Lincoln, NM

Daniel Grant Hankins, MD, FACEP
Consultant, Department of Emergency
    Medicine,
Mayo Clinic;
Co-Medical Director, Mayo Medical Transport,
Rochester, MN

Russell W. Hartung, DO
Associate Director, Emergency Care Center,
EMS Medical Director,
Champlain Valley Physician Hospital,
Plattsburgh, NY

Theresa S. Hatcher, DO
EMS Medical Director,
Omaha Fire Department,
Bellevere, NE

Joseph Heck, DO, FACEP
Medical Director
Casualty Care Research Center
Bethesda, MD

Christine Houser, MD, FACEP, FACOEP
Clinical Assistant Professor,
Department of Emergency Medicine,
University of Texas Health Science Center,
Houston, TX

Alexander P. Isakov, MD, MPH, FACEP
Assistant Professor of Emergency Medicine,
Emergency Medical School,
Medical Director Emory Flight,
Atlanta, GA

David Jaslow, MD, MPH, FAAEM
Assistant Professor,
Director Operational EMS,
Department of Emergency Medicine,
Temple University,
Philadelphia, PA

Mark Johnson, MPA
Chief, Emergency Medical Services Section,
Alaska Department of Health and Social Services,
Juneau, AK;
Chairman, EMS Communications Committee,
National Association of State EMS Directors,
Carlsbad, CA

Alan A. Katz, MD, FACEP
Associate Chairman, Department of Emergency
    Medicine,
South Nassau Community Hospital,
Oceanside, NY

Kristi L. Koenig, MD, FACEP
National Director, Emergency Management
    Strategic Healthcare Group,
Department of Veterans Affairs;
Clinical Professor of Emergency Medicine,
George Washington University School of
    Medicine and Health Sciences
Washington, DC

Douglas F. Kupas, MD, FACEP
EMS Medical Director,
Geisinger Medical Center,
Danville, PA

G. Patrick Lilja, MD, FACEP
Medical Director, Emergency and
  Trauma Services,
North Memorial Medicine Center;
Clinical Associate Professor of Family Practice
  and Community Health,
University of Minnesota Medical School,
Minneapolis, MN

Ronald B. Low, MD, MS, FACEP
Associate Chairman of Emergency Medicine,
SUNY Health Sciences Center,
Kings County Medical Center,
Brooklyn, NY

Michael Madsen, DO
Department of Emergency Medicine,
Tutality Community Hospital,
Hillsboro, OR

Thomas McGuire, EMT-P
Alameda County EMS,
Oakland, CA

Norman E. McSwain, Jr., MD, FACS
Professor of Surgery,
Department of Surgery School of Medicine
Tulane University
New Orleans, Louisiana

Barbara A. McIntosh, MD, FACEP
St. John's Queens Hospital Center,
  Catholic Medical Center,
Elmhurst, NY

Juan March, MD, FACEP
Associate Professor,
Department of Emergency Medicine,
Chief, Division of EMS,
Brody School of Medicine,
East Carolina University,
Greenville, NC

Steven A. Meador, MD, FACEP
Assistant Professor of Medicine,
Director of Emergency Medical Services,
The Milton S. Hershey Medical Center,
The Pennsylvania State University,
Hershey, PA

Greg Mears, MD, FACEP
Associate Professor,
Department of Emergency Medicine,
University of North Carolina,
Chapel Hill, NC

Jeffrey P. Michaels, PhD
Chief, EMS Division,
National Highway Traffic Safety Administration
Department of Transportation,
Washington, DC

Jeffrey T. Mitchell, PhD
Clinical Associate Professor,
Baltimore County Emergency Health Services,
University of Maryland,
Baltimore, MD

David L. Morgan, MD, FACEP
Assistant Professor,
Division of Emergency Medicine,
Southwestern Medical Center,
University of Texas,
Dallas, TX

Vincent N. Mosesso, MD, FACEP
Assistant Professor of Emergency Medicine,
Department of Emergency Medicine,
University of Pittsburgh School of Medicine,
Pittsburgh, PA

Jerry Mothershead, MD, FACEP
Commander, Medical Corps, United States
  Navy;
Senior Medical Consultant, Navy Medicine
  Office of Homeland Security,
Bureau of Medicine and Surgery,
Washington, DC

John Lawrence Mottley, MD, MHSA
Associate Professor, Emergency Medicine,
Boston University School of Medicine;
Former Executive Director, Boston Emergency
  Medical Services,
Boston, MA

Jerry Overton, MBA
Executive Director,
Richmond Ambulance Authority;
Associate Professor,
Medical College of Virginia,
Richmond, VA

James O. Page, JD
President, JEMS Communications,
Carlsbad, CA

Paul M. Paris, MD, FACEP
Professor and Chairman,
Department of Emergency Medicine,
University of Pittsburgh School of Medicine,
Pittsburgh, PA

Linda L. Pepe
Former Television News Producer
Dallas, TX

Paul E. Pepe, MD, MPH, FACP, FACEP, FCCP,
    FCCM
Professor of Medicine and Surgery,
Department of Emergency Medicine,
Southwestern Medical Center,
University of Texas,
Dallas, TX

David E. Persse, MD, FACEP
Medical Director,
City of Houston EMS;
Associate Professor of Emergency Medicine,
University of Texas Medical School,
Houston, TX

James Pointer, MD, FACEP
Medical Director,
Alameda County EMS,
Oakland, CA

Carl Joseph Post, BA, MA, PhD, EMT-D
Associate Director, Graduate EMS Program,
School of Health Sciences,
New York Medical College,
Valhalla, NY;
Associate Professor at Large, Graduate School,
School of Humanities,
Hahnemann University,
Philadelphia, PA

Franklin D. Pratt, MD, FACEP
Medical Director,
Los Angeles County Fire Department,
Los Angeles, CA

Edward M. Racht, MD, FACEP
Medical Director,
City of Austin, Travis County EMS System,
Austin, TX

Jay H. Reich, MD, FACEP
Instructor,
Department of Emergency Medicine,
University of Pittsburgh School of Medicine,
Pittsburgh, PA

Joseph L. Ryan, MD, FACEP
Medical Director, Regional EMS Authority,
Reno, NV;
Medical Director,
North Lake Tahoe Fire Protection District,
Incline Village, NV;
Clinical Assistant Professor,
Division of Emergency Medicine,
Department of Surgery, Stanford University,
Palo Alto, CA

Angelo A. Salvucci, MD
EMS Medical Director,
Ventura and Santa Barbara Counties,
Santa Barbara, CA

Brian Schwartz, MD
Director, Division of Prehospital Care,
Sunnybrooke and Womens Health Science
    Center,
Toronto, ON

Jack L. Stout, BA
The Fourth Party, Incorporated,
West River, MD

Michael A. Sucher, MD
Acting Medical Director,
Bureau of EMS, State of Arizona;
Former Medical Director,
Rural Metro Corporation,
Scottsdale, AZ

James Syrett, MD
Strong Memorial Hospital,
University of Rochester Medical School,
Rochester, NY

Michael A. Taigman, EMT-P
Director of Quality Improvement, Med-Trans
San Francisco, CA

Margaret Trimble, BSN, MA
Pennsylvania State EMS Director,
Harrisburg, PA

Marsha Treiber, MPS
Executive Director,
Center for Pediatric Emergency Medicine;
Assistant Research Scientist,
New York University School of Medicine,
New York, NY

David P. Thomson, MD, FACEP
Associate Professor,
Director of Transport Medicine,
SUNY Upstate Medical Center,
Syracuse, NY

Michael P. Wainscott, MD, FACEP
Assistant Professor and Director of Medical
    Education,
Division of Emergency Medicine,
Southwestern Medical Center,
University of Texas;
Dallas, TX

Bruce John Walz, PhD
Assistant Professor,
Department of Emergency Health Services,
University of Maryland—Baltimore County,
Catonsville, MD

Katherine H. West, BSN, MSEd
Assistant Professor,
Department of Emergency Medicine,
George Washington University School of
    Medicine,
Washington, DC;
President, Infection Control/
    Emerging Concepts, Inc.,
Springfield, VA

Jane G. Wigginton, MD
Assistant Professor of Surgery,
Southwestern Medical Center,
University of Texas,
Dallas, TX

Richard C. Wuerz, MD, FACEP
Assistant Professor of Emergency Medicine,
The Pennsylvania State University College of
    Medicine,
Associate Director, Prehospital and
    Flight Services,
The Milton Hershey Medical Center,
Hershey, PA

Arthur M. Yancey, MD, MPH, FACEP
Assistant Professor,
Department of Emergency Medicine,
Emory University School of Medicine,
Medical Director,
Fulton County EMS,
Atlanta, GA

Donald M. Yealy, MD, FACEP
Professor and Vice Chair of Emergency
    Medicine,
University of Pittsburgh School of Medicine,
Pittsburgh, PA

Joseph Zalkin
Assistant Director,
Wake County EMS,
Raleigh, NC

AUTHORS

Section One

David C. Cone, MD

S Y S T E M S

This section describes the history and development of EMS, and the various system models used to implement modern EMS in a variety of settings. Moreso than most fields of medicine, EMS relies on the concept of systems. While individual components such as ambulances, defibrillators, and providers are of course important, these components cannot and do not operate in a vacuum, regardless of how well they perform their individual tasks. Rather, the entire EMS system functions well when the components are brought together in a rational and effective manner. A well implemented and operated system can likely function quite nicely despite flaws in a few of its components, but a poorly designed or implemented system likely cannot function well even with the best of components.

"System design" is almost an oxymoron: few systems have actually been designed from scratch. Rather, most systems have evolved consequent to local resources, interests, and politics. This history of EMS brings many patterns, restrictions, and traditions. Attempts to modify the design of systems are often met with resistance from the vested political, financial, legal, and historical forces. Despite these forces of inertia, and despite many regional and local variations in everything from provider training standards to allowed medications, certain commonalities have emerged, not only among systems within the same generic type (e.g., large urban fire-based systems in different states), but among systems in different types (e.g., a large urban fire-based system and a small rural volunteer system).

Many of these commonalities have developed as the result of the work of interdisciplinary teams. Some have said that EMS is the practice of public health, in the public safety environment, with the technology of emergency medicine. Themes have been drawn from these three arenas (as well as others), and applied in a variety of ways to a variety of practice settings. Many of these themes are reflected in the chapters of this section, and readers wishing to maximize their understanding of each environment may wish to seek out the public health, public safety, and emergency medicine aspects of each.

It may appear that each chapter has an overriding flavor. The "Urban Systems" chapter stresses the labor issues particular to city unions, while the Rural chapter focuses largely on issues related to volunteer providers. The Wilderness chapter stresses the challenges of providing prolonged care in an environment where medical oversight is more remote. The Fire chapter focuses on the integration of EMS into a previously established emergency response system, and the Military chapter highlights the unique organizational and logistical structure of the armed services. Finally, the International chapter broadens our perspective, to examine models of EMS delivery that are completely different from those found in the United States. But it will be quickly clear to the reader that each chapter covers all three features of the public health/public safety/ emergency medicine Venn diagram, since no practice environment or EMS system functions in only one of these three arenas. With the History and Models and Legislation chapters serving to introduce ideas of how we got to where we are, this section neatly summarizes what EMS delivery is all about. While at times certain biases of the authors come through, these biases simply reflect the passions they feel for their systems and their unique environments. These passions should, in my opinion, be regarded as a strength, not a weakness. While EMS is full of controversy, each of these systems ultimately has the best interests of patient care as its mission. Whether after completing this section you feel that the differences among system environments are trivial or overwhelming, you will no doubt understand the concept that EMS is about systems.

CHAPTER 1

History

Carl Post, PhD, EMT-D
Marsha Treiber, MPS

Over the last four decades, EMS in the United States has undergone major expansion, development, and change. The object of neglect before 1966, EMS has progressed and improved since receiving emphasis by public and private agencies, resulting in the development of innovative systems, multiple levels of providers, and a new specialty in medicine. Although the events were partially due to the application of a systematic approach, the adoption of clinical breakthroughs, the integration of the hospital and prehospital phases of emergency medical care, and heightened political and public awareness, in a real sense the advances evolved naturally. Sadly, a clear definition or mechanism for reimbursement for day-to-day EMS operations did not manifest itself during this development.

This chapter analyzes the historical development of EMS, discusses philosophical and social events that fueled change, and reviews major trends. It focuses on key events and concepts from the 1960s onward. Additional details regarding the history of the development of EMS from the military perspective are given in chapter 7, Military.

Pre-1966: Background

Early hunters and warriors provided care for the injured. Although the methods used to stanch bleeding, stabilize fractures, and provide nourishment were primitive, the need for treatment was undoubtedly recognized. The basic elements of prehistoric response to injury still guide contemporary EMS programs. Recognition of the need for action led to the development of medical and surgical emergency treatment techniques. These techniques in turn made way for systems of communication, treatment, and transport, all geared toward reducing morbidity and mortality.

The *Edwin Smith Papyrus*, written in 1500 B.C., vividly describes triage and treatment protocols.[1] Reference to emergency care is also found in the *Babylonian Code of Hammurabi* where a detailed protocol for treatment of the injured is described.[2] In the Old Testament, Elisha breathed into the mouth of a dead child and brought the child back to life.[3] The Good Samaritan not only treated the injured traveler but also instructed others to do likewise.[4] Greeks and Romans had surgeons present during battle to treat the wounded.

The most direct root of modern prehospital systems is found in the efforts of Jean Dominique Larrey, Napoleon's chief military physician. Larrey developed a prehospital system in which the injured were treated on the battlefield and horse-drawn wagons were used to carry them away.[5] In 1797 Larrey built "ambulance volantes" of two or four wheels to rescue the wounded. Larrey had introduced a new concept in military surgery: early transport from the battlefield to the aid stations and then to the frontline hospital. This method is comparable to the way that modern physicians modified the military use of helicopters in Korea and Vietnam. Larrey also initiated detailed treatment protocols, such as the early amputation of shattered limbs to prevent gangrene.

The Civil War is the starting point for EMS systems in the United States.[6] Learning from the lessons of the Napoleonic and Crimean Wars, military physicians led by Joseph Barnes and Jonathan Letterman established an extensive system of prehospital care. The Union Army trained medical corpsmen to provide treatment in the field; a transportation system, which included railroads, was developed to bring the wounded to medical facilities. The wounded received suboptimal care in these facilities, stirring Clara Barton's crusade for better care.[7]

The medical experiences of the Civil War stimulated the beginning of civilian urban ambulance services, the first being established in cities such as Cincinnati, New York, London, and Paris. Edward Dalton, Sanitary Superintendent of the Board of

Health in New York City, established a city ambulance program in 1869. Dalton, a former surgeon in the Union Army, spearheaded the development of urban civilian ambulances to permit greater speed, enhance comfort, and increase maneuverability on city streets.[8] His ambulances carried medical equipment such as splints, bandages, strait-jackets, and a stomach pump, as well as a medicine chest of antidotes, anesthetics, brandy, and morphine. By the turn of the century, interns accompanied the ambulance. Care was rendered and the patient left at home. Ambulance drivers had virtually no medical training. Our knowledge of turn-of-the-century urban ambulance service comes from the writings of Emily Barringer, the first woman ambulance surgeon in New York City.[9]

Further development of urban ambulance services continued in the years before World War I. Electric, steam, and gasoline-powered carriages were used as ambulances. Calls for service were generally processed and dispatched by the individual hospital, although improved telegraph and telephone systems with signal boxes throughout New York City were developed to connect the police department and the hospitals.

During World War I, the introduction of the traction splint by Thomas, for the stabilization of patients with leg fractures, led to a decrease in morbidity and mortality. Between the two world wars, ambulances began to be dispatched by mobile radios. In the 1920s, in Roanoke, Virginia, the first volunteer rescue squad model was begun, and in many areas volunteer rescue or ambulance squads gradually provided an alternate to the local fire department or undertaker. After the American entry into World War II, the military demand for physicians pulled the interns from ambulances, never to return, resulting in badly staffed units and nonstandardized prehospital care. Postwar ambulances were poorly equipped hearses and similar vehicles, staffed by untrained personnel. Half of the ambulances were operated by mortuary attendants, most of whom had never taken even a first-aid course.[10]

Throughout the 1950s and 1960s, two geographic patterns of ambulance service evolved. In cities, hospital-based ambulances gradually coalesced into more centrally coordinated citywide programs, usually administered and staffed by the municipal hospital or fire department. In rural areas, funeral home hearses were sporadically replaced by a variety of units operated by the local fire department or a newly formed rescue squad. Additionally, in both urban and rural areas, a few profit-making providers delivered transport services and occasionally contracted with local government to provide emergency prehospital services and transport. Before 1966 very little legislation and regulation applicable to ambulance services existed. Providers had relatively little formal training, and physician involvement at all levels was minimal.

A number of factors combined in the mid-1960s to stimulate a revolution in prehospital care. Advances in medical treatments led to a perception that decreases in mortality and morbidity were possible. Closed-chest cardiopulmonary resuscitation (CPR), reported as successful in 1960 by W.B. Kouwenhoven,[11] was quickly adopted as the medical standard for cardiac arrest in the prehospital setting. New evidence that CPR, pharmaceuticals, and defibrillation could save lives immediately created a demand for physician providers of those interventions in both the hospital and the prehospital environments. Throughout the 1960s, fundamental understanding of the pathophysiology of potentially fatal dysrhythmias expanded significantly. Rescue breathing and what we now call defibrillation were refined by Peter Safar, Leonard Cobb, Herbert Loon, and Eugene Nagel.[12] Safar persuaded many others that defibrillation and resuscitation were viable areas of medical research and clinical intervention.

In 1966 Pantridge and Geddes pioneered and documented the use of a mobile coronary care unit ambulance for prehospital resuscitation of patients in Belfast, Ireland. Their treatment protocols, originally developed for the treatment of myocardial infarction in intensive-care units, were moved into the field.[13] Because the medical team was often with the patient at the time of cardiac arrest, the resuscitation rate was an unheard-of 20%. His flying squads added a dimension of heroic excitement to the job of being an ambulance driver, and his performance data helped convince American city health officials and physicians that a more medically sophisticated prehospital Advanced Life Support (ALS) system was possible.

1966: The NAS-NRC Report

The modern era of prehospital care in the United States began in 1966. In that year, the recognition of an urgent need, the crucial element necessary for development of prehospital systems nationwide, was heralded by a report generated by the National Academy of Sciences-National Research Council (NAS-

NRC), a private organization chartered by Congress to provide scientific advice to the federal government. *Accidental Death and Disability: The Neglected Disease of Modern Society* documented the enormous failure of the U.S. health care system to provide even minimal care for the emergency patient. The NAS-NRC report identified key issues and problems facing the United States in providing emergency care (fig. 1). Its summary report listed 24 proposed recommendations that would serve as a blueprint for EMS development, including such things as first-aid training for the lay public, state-level regulation of ambulance services, emergency department improvements, development of trauma registries, and disaster planning.[14] This document established a benchmark to measure subsequent progress and change.

The 1966 NAS-NRC document described both prehospital services and hospital emergency departments as being woefully inadequate. In the prehospital arena, treatment protocols, trained medical personnel, rapid transportation, and modern communications concepts such as two-way radios and emergency call numbers were all identified as necessities, but were simply not available to civilians. Although there were more than 7,000 accredited hospitals in the country at the time, very few were prepared to meet the increased demand that developed between 1945 and 1965. From 1958 to 1970, the number of emergency department visits increased from 18 million to more than 49 million.[14] In addition, emergency departments were staffed by the least experienced personnel, who had little education in the treatment of multiple injuries or critical medical emergencies. Early efforts of the American College of Surgeons (ACS) and the American Academy of Orthopedic Surgeons (AAOS) to improve emergency care were largely unsuccessful because medical interest was essentially nonexistent.[15,16,17,18]

The 1966 NAS-NRC document was the first to recommend that emergency facilities be categorized. It also emphasized aggressive clinical management of trauma, suggesting that local trauma systems develop databases, and that studies be instituted to designate select injuries to be incorporated in the epidemiological reports of the Public Health Service. Changes were also recommended concerning legal problems, autopsies, and disaster response reviews. Trauma research was especially emphasized, with the ultimate goal of establishing a National Institute of Trauma.[14] Another problem identified in the report was the broad gap between existing knowledge and operational activity.

Inadequacies of Prehospital Care in 1966

1. The general public is insensitive to the magnitude of the problem of accidental death and injury.
2. Millions lack instruction in basic first aid.
3. Few are adequately trained in the advanced techniques of cardiopulmonary resuscitation, childbirth, or other life-saving measures, yet every ambulance and rescue squad attendant, policeman, fire fighter, paramedical worker, and worker in high-risk industry should be trained.
4. Local political authorities have neglected their responsibility to provide optimum emergency medical services.
5. Research on trauma has not been supported or identified at the National Institutes of Health on a level consistent with its importance as the fourth leading cause of death and a primary cause of disability.
6. The potentials of the U.S. Public Health Service Program in accident prevention and emergency medical services have not been fully exploited.
7. Data are lacking on how to determine the number of individuals whose lives are lost through injuries compounded by misguided attempts at rescue and first aid, absence of physicians at the scene of the injury, unsuitable ambulances with inadequate equipment and untrained attendants, lack of traffic control, or the lack of voice communication facilities.
8. Helicopter ambulances have not been adapted to civilian peacetime needs.
9. Emergency departments of hospitals are overcrowded, some are archaic, and there are no systematic surveys on which to base requirements for space, equipment, or staffing for present, let alone future, needs.
10. Fundamental research on shock and trauma is inadequately supported; medical and health-related organizations have failed to join forces to apply knowledge already available to advanced treatment of trauma, or educate the public and inform Congress.[20]

From *Accidental death and disability: The neglected disease of modern society,* National Academy of Sciences, Washington, D.C., 1966. National Academy Press.

FIGURE 1

The NAS-NRC report did not appear out of thin air. The President's Commission on Highway Safety[19] had previously published a report entitled *Health, Medical Care, and Transportation of Injured,* which recommended a national program to reduce deaths and injuries caused by highway accidents. Its findings were complemented by and consistent with the NAS-NRC report. The recommendations in both documents were used when the Highway Safety Act of 1966 was drafted. This law established the cabinet-level Department of Transportation (DOT) and gave it legislative and financial authority to improve EMS. Specific emphasis was placed on developing a highway safety program, including standards and activities for improving both ambulance service and provider training.[20]

The Highway Safety Act also authorized funds to develop EMS standards and implement programs that would improve ambulance services. Matching funds were provided for EMS demonstration projects and studies. All states were required to have highway safety programs in accordance with the regulatory standards promulgated by the DOT. The standard on EMS required each state to develop regional EMS systems that could handle prehospital emergency medical needs. Ambulances, equipment, personnel, and administration costs were funded by the highway safety program. Regional financing, as opposed to county or state funding, was a new concept that would be echoed in federal health legislation throughout the remainder of the decade.[20]

With the Highway Safety Act as a catalyst, the DOT contributed more than $142 million to regional EMS systems between 1968 and 1979. A total of roughly $10 million was spent on research alone, including $4.9 million for EMS demonstration projects. A number of other federal EMS initiatives in the late 1960s and early 1970s poured additional funds into EMS, including $16 million in funding from the Health Services and Mental Health Administration, which had been designated as the lead EMS agency of the Department of Health, Education, and Welfare (DHEW), to areas of Arkansas, California, Florida, Illinois, and Ohio for the development of model regional EMS systems.[21]

In 1969 the Airlie House Conference proposed a hospital categorization scheme.[22] The AMA Commission on EMS urged facility categorization and published its own scheme, which identified staffing, equipment, services, and personnel types.[23] This became known as "horizontal categorization." Al-

though it was supported by professional and hospital associations, many hospitals and physicians feared hospitals in lower categories would suffer a loss of prestige, patients, or reimbursement. The demonstration projects developed a categorization scheme based on hospital-wide care of specific disease processes. Known as "vertical categorization," this concept was ultimately embraced by many regional programs as a major theme in the development of EMS systems.

By the late 1960s, drugs, defibrillation, and personnel were available to improve prehospital care. Space-age telemetric technology was also available, so responders with limited medical training did not have to interpret rhythm strips. As early as 1967, the first physician responder mobile programs metamorphosed into "paramedic" programs using physician-monitored telemetry as a modification of the approach by Pantrige in Belfast.

The "Heartmobile" program, begun in 1969 in Columbus, Ohio, initially involved a physician and three EMTs. Within two years, 22 highly trained (2,000 hours) paramedics provided the field care, and the physician role had become supervisory. Similarly, in Seattle, physicians supervised highly trained paramedics, increasing the survival rate from 10% to 30% for prehospital cardiac arrest patients whose presenting rhythm was ventricular fibrillation. The Seattle story was also one in which fire department first responders played a crucial role in building what we now call a chain of survival. In Dade County, Florida, rapid response of mobile paramedic units was combined with hospital physician direction via radio and telemetry for the first time.[24] In Brighton, England, non-physician personnel provided field care without direct medical oversight. Electrocardiographic data were recorded continuously to permit retrospective review by a physician.[25]

National professional organizations such as the American College of Surgeons (ACS), the American Academy of Orthopaedic Surgeons (AAOS), the American Heart Association (AHA), and the American Society of Anesthesiologists (ASA), in concert with other groups, provided extensive medical input into the early development of EMS. New organizations were formed to focus on EMS, including the American Medical Association's Commission on EMS, the American Hospital Association's Committee on Community Emergency Health Services, the American Trauma Society, the Emergency Nurses Association, the Society of Critical Care Medicine, the National Registry of Emergency Medical Technicians, and the American College of Emergency Physicians. In the years prior to 1973, such groups exerted significant but uncoordinated efforts toward the reorganization, restructure, improvement, expansion, and politicization of EMS.[22,23,26,27]

In 1972 the NAS-NRC published *Roles and Resources of Federal Agencies in Support of Comprehensive Emergency Medical Services,* which asserted that the federal government had not kept pace with efforts by professional and lay health organizations to upgrade EMS. The document endorsed a vigorous federal government role in the provision and upgrading of EMS. It recommended that President Nixon acknowledge the magnitude of the accidental death and disability problem by proposing action by the legislative and executive branches to ensure optimum universal emergency care. It urged the integration of all federal resources for delivery of emergency services under the direction of a single division of DHEW, which would have primary responsibility for the entire emergency medical program. It also recommended that the focal point for local emergency medical care be at the state level, and that all federal efforts be coordinated through regional EMS programs.[28] This recommendation set the stage for new EMS regional programs to directly conflict with both the counties and the states.

1973: The Emergency Medical Services System Act

By 1973 several major lessons had emerged from the demonstration projects and the various studies undertaken during the preceding seven years. Although the federal initiative had been limited to the five 1968 DHEW regional demonstration projects mentioned above, significant progress had been made toward clearly defining a potential program goal. The projects proved that a regional EMS system approach could work; however, they did not prove that a regional approach was necessarily the best.

By early 1973 many national organizations supported further federal involvement, both in establishing EMS program goals and in providing direct financial support. The first efforts at passing federal EMS legislation were defeated, but a later modified EMS bill passed with support from numerous public and professional groups. President Nixon vetoed this bill in August 1973. The standard conservative philosophy was that EMS was a service that should be provided by local government, and the federal government should neither underwrite operations nor purchase equipment. Additional congressional hearings led to the reintroduction of a bill proposing an extensive federal EMS program, based on the rationale that individual communities would not be able to develop regional systems without federal encouragement, guidelines, and funding. Finally, in November 1973, the Emergency Medical Services System Act was passed and signed. It was added as Title XII to the Public Health Service Act, wherein it addressed EMS systems, research grants, and contracts. It also added a new section to the existing Title VII concerning EMS training grants.[29]

Although the law was amended to re-authorize expenditures in 1976, 1978, and again in 1979, its goal remained to encourage development of comprehensive regional EMS systems throughout the country. The available grant funds were divided among the four major portions of the EMS System Act: Section 1202—Feasibility studies and planning; Section 1203—Initial operations; Section 1204—Expansion and improvement; Section 1205—Research. Applicants were encouraged to use existing health resources, facilities, and personnel. The EMS regions were ultimately expected to become financially self-sufficient; therefore, a phase-out of all federal funding was targeted for 1979, but later extended to 1982. The program was administered in the DHEW through the Division of Emergency Medical Services (DEMS), with David Boyd, the medical director of the Illinois demonstration project, named as director. The law and subsequent regulations emphasized a regional systems approach, a trauma orientation, and a requirement that each funded system address the 15 "essential components" (fig. 2). It should be noted that medical oversight not emphasized. Although the EMS Systems Act and its subsequent regulations encouraged a degree of medical oversight, the focus was on the project medical director who, in retrospect at least, seems far removed from the practice of prehospital medicine.

1973–1978: Growth, Scrutiny, and Belief

In 1974 the Robert Wood Johnson Foundation (RWJF) allocated $15 million for EMS-related activities, the largest single contribution for the development of health systems ever made in the United States by a nonprofit foundation. Forty-four areas

The Fifteen Essential EMS Components (1973)

1. Manpower
2. Training
3. Communications
4. Transportation
5. Facilities
6. Critical care units
7. Public safety agencies
8. Consumer participation
9. Access to care
10. Patient transfer
11. Coordinated patient record-keeping
12. Public information and education
13. Review and evaluation
14. Disaster plan
15. Mutual aid

FIGURE 2

received grants of up to $400,000 to develop EMS systems.[30] This money was intended to encourage communities to build regional EMS systems, emphasizing the overall goal of improving access to general medical care. The money was provided over a two-year period to establish new demonstration projects and develop regional emergency medical communications systems.[31]

In early 1974 a newly reorganized DHEW-DEMS began implementing the legislative mandate. Adopted from earlier experiences, the basic principles were that (1) an effective and comprehensive system must have resources sufficient in quality and quantity to meet a wide variety of demands, and (2) the discrete geographic regions established must have sufficient populations and resources to enable them eventually to become self-sufficient. The 15 essential EMS components may have been flawed, but the concept that an EMS chain of survival was only as strong as its weakest link was correct.

Each state was to designate a coordinating agency for statewide EMS efforts. Ultimately, 304 EMS regions were established nationwide. By 1979, 17 regions were fully functional and independent of federal money. However, of the 304 geographic areas, there were 22 that had no activity and 96 that were still in the planning phase.[32] Testimony was given before the congressional committee considering extension of funding, and an additional year of funding was authorized as the 1202b program for planning.

In the regulations, David Boyd strictly interpreted the congressional legislative intent of the EMS Systems Act to mandate that all communities adopt the 15 essential components. Regions were limited to five grants, and with each year of funding, progress toward more sophisticated operational levels was expected. By the end of the third year of funding, regions were expected to have basic life support (BLS) capabilities, which required no physician involvement. Advanced life support (ALS) capability, which was expected to perform traditional physician activities, was expected at the end of the fifth year. The use of BLS and ALS terminology in the regulations spread widely. However, the original definitions that corresponded directly to the EMT-A and paramedic levels of training quickly became elusive as variations in the EMT-A and paramedic levels emerged. The EMT-A level required no medical input, but some states such as Kentucky did extend medical oversight to BLS because of dubious insurance laws—laws making medical care and transportation across a county line virtually impossible without a physician's approval over the radio.

Developing the geographic regions required to secure federal funding through the EMS Systems Act usually required new EMS legislation at the state level. The state laws that developed throughout the 1970s varied markedly in regard to the issues of medial oversight, overall operational authority, and financing. In some states, physician involvement was required. In others, medical oversight was not even mentioned. Often, the responsibility for coordinating activities was assigned to a regional EMS council of physicians, prehospital providers, insurance companies, and consumers who often had interests to protect; commonly, physician input was somewhat removed from the medical mainstream.

Personnel

Lack of appropriately trained emergency personnel at every level of care had been identified in the NAS-NRC document.[14] After 1973, extensive effort and money was directed at correcting this educational deficiency, and serendipity played a role. A large number of medical corpsmen, physicians, and nurses, who understood that trained non-physicians could perform lifesaving tasks in the field, were returning from Vietnam. Many argued that rapid transport and early surgery could improve civilian trauma practice.

PHYSICIANS. In 1966 the NAS-NRC document stated: "No longer can responsibility be assigned to the least experienced member of the medical staff, or solely to specialists, who, by the nature of their training and experience, cannot render adequate care without the support of other staff members."[14] Thus the importance of physician leadership and training in EMS was identified early. During the 25 years following World War II, increasing demands for care were placed on hospital emergency departments. Not surprisingly, a branch of medicine evolved with its focus on the critically ill. The academic discipline and scientific rigor necessary to define a separate medical specialty began to develop.

In 1968 the American College of Emergency Physicians (ACEP) was founded by physicians interested in the organization and delivery of emergency medical care. In 1970 the first emergency medicine residency was established at the University of Cincinnati, and the first academic Department of Emergency Medicine in a medical school was formed at the University of Southern California. Soon the directors of medical school hospital emergency departments founded the University Association for Emergency Medical Services. Between 1972 and 1980 more than 740 residents completed training programs in 51 emergency medicine residencies throughout the country.[33,34,35] The first major step toward certification as a specialty occurred in 1973 when the AMA authorized a provisional Section of Emergency Medicine. In 1974 a Committee on Board Establishment was appointed, and a liaison Residency Endorsement Committee was formed.[35] Further impetus toward expansion of residency programs in emergency medicine occurred with the formation of the American Board of Emergency Medicine in 1976.[36] Before that time there was some hesitancy to create residency programs that might not lead to board certification.

In September 1979, emergency medicine was formally recognized as a specialty by the AMA Committee on Medical Education and the American Board of Medical Specialties. One of the strongest arguments in favor of the new specialty was that emergency physicians had a unique role in the oversight of prehospital medicine. ABEM gave its first certifying examination in 1980, which incidentally did not touch on any areas of prehospital care.

While emergency medicine, emergency nursing, and prehospital care were all nourished by the funds distributed between 1973 and 1982, the interest of ACEP in EMS activities lagged, perhaps because individual physician interest lagged. The first full-time EMS medical director was not appointed until April 1981; previously all had been part-time, and some had simply been functionaries. Shortly thereafter, cities like Salt Lake City and Houston followed New York's lead, and appointed full-time EMS medical directors. Even then, EMS as a physician career choice was perceived by many as limited and perhaps threatening.

PREHOSPITAL PROVIDERS. The Highway Safety Act of 1966 funded Emergency Medical Technician-Ambulance (EMT-A) training and curriculum development. By 1982, there were approximately 100,000 providers trained at the EMT-A level. They were trained to provide elementary, non-invasive emergency care at the scene and during transport, including such skills as CPR, control of bleeding, ventilation, oxygen administration, fracture management, extrication, obstetric delivery, and transport of the patient. The educational requirements, which began as a 70-hour curriculum published by AAOS in 1969, soon grew to 81 hours of didactic lectures, skills training, and hospital observation, with most of the increase in hours being due to the addition of training in the use of pneumatic antishock garments. After working six months, graduates were allowed to take a national certifying examination administered by the National Registry of Emergency Medical Technicians (NREMT). Founded in 1970, the National Registry developed a standardized examination for EMT-A personnel as one requirement for maintaining registration. Many states recognized National Registry registration for purposes of reciprocity, but most still required additional state certification.[27]

While the EMT-A quickly became a nationally recognized standard, the development of national consensus at the paramedic level lagged behind, with marked difference in training from locality to locality. Paramedic practices became somewhat formalized with the adoption of the DOT EMT-P curriculum. By 1982, EMT-P training ranged from a few hundred to 2000 hours of educational and clinical experience. Typical clinical skills included cardiac defibrillation, endotracheal intubation, venipuncture, and the administration of a variety of drugs. The use of these skills was based on interpretation of history, clinical signs, and rhythm strips. Telemetric and voice communications with physicians were usually required. In the early days of paramedicine, extensive "on-line" medical oversight was mandatory for all calls in most systems. With time, this requirement was modified by the introduction of protocols allowing for greater use of standing orders.[37] However, a great deal of variation in the use of direct medical oversight remained. As early as 1980, paramedics in decentralized systems such as New York's used many clinical protocols, most of which had few indications for mandatory direct medical oversight. On the other hand, as late as 1992, centralized systems like the Houston Fire Department's had only one protocol (for cardiac arrest) that did not require contemporaneous instruction from direct medical oversight.

The concept of the EMT-Intermediate (EMT-I) evolved as a provider level located somewhere between EMT-A and EMT-P. Airway management, IV therapy, fluid replacement, rhythm recognition, and defibrillation were the most common "advanced" skills included in the EMT-I curriculum, though significant variation existed (and still does) from state to state. Many states developed several levels of EMT-I, often in a modular progression with formal bridge courses; by 1979, formally recognized prehospital providers existed at dozens of levels, with highly variable requirements for medical oversight.

With the evolution of the EMT-A into the EMT-Basic (EMT-B) in the early 1990s, with a new DOT national standard curriculum, it became obvious that there needed to be a logical development of tasks, skills, teaching objectives, curricula, and levels. The *Blueprint for Education* was a start in that direction.

Public Education

CPR training gradually became more widely accepted, as evidenced by participation in training programs throughout the country. As early as 1977 a Gallup poll reported that 12 million Americans had taken a CPR course and another 80 million were familiar with the technique and wanted formal training.[6] The success of public training was documented by many studies.[38,39] The issues of whom to train and how to improve skill retention continue to be explored, as reflected in the American Heart Association/International Liaison Committee on Resuscitation's "Guidelines 2000" document, which contains significant changes in how the techniques of CPR and emergency cardiac care are taught to laypersons.[40]

Communications

Before 1973 there were few communication systems available for emergency medical care. Only one in 20 ambulances had voice communications with a hospital, a universal telephone number was not operational, and telephones were not available on highways and rural roads. Centralized dispatch was uncommon and there were problems in communications because of community resistance, cost, and insufficient technology. With DOT funding, major steps were taken toward overcoming these communication problems. National conferences, seminars, and public awareness programs advocated diverse methodologies for EMS communication systems. A communications manual published in 1972 provided technical systems information.[41] In 1973 the 9-1-1 universal emergency number was advocated as a national standard by the DOT and the White House Office of Telecommunications. The Federal Communications Commission (FCC) established rules and regulations for EMS communication and dedicated a limited number of radio frequencies for emergency systems. In 1977 the DHEW issued guidelines for a model EMS communications plan.[42]

EMS medical directors gradually began to appreciate the importance of more structured call receiving, patient prioritizing, and vehicle dispatching. Physicians were forced to look seriously at EMS operational issues that had previously been seen as neither critical nor medical.[43] On the other hand, telemetry as it had been pioneered by Nagel in Florida was generally seen to be impractical, expensive, and unnecessary, and has essentially disappeared, to be replaced only recently in some systems by transmission of 12-lead electrocardiograms from the field to the ED for patients with chest pain.

Transportation

Transportation of the critically ill or injured patient rapidly improved after 1973. Although national standards for ambulance equipment were developed in the early 1960s, a 1965 survey of 900 cities reported that fewer than 23% had an ordinance regulating ambulance services. An even smaller percentage required an attendant other than the driver, and only 72 cities reported training at the level of an American Red Cross advanced first-aid course, the nearest thing to a standard ambulance attendant course before the advent of EMT-A in 1969.[44]

The hearses and station wagons used in the 1960s did not allow personnel room to provide CPR or other treatments to critically ill patients. The vehicles were designed to carry coffins and horizontal loads, not a medical team and a sick patient. In the 1960s, two reports focused national attention on the hazardous conditions of the nation's ambulances.[14,45] In addition to inadequate policies, staff training, and communications, ambulance design was faulty and equipment absent or inadequate. Morticians ran 50% of the ambulance services because they owned the only vehicles capable of carrying patients horizontally. No U.S. manufacturer built a vehicle that could be termed an ambulance.

As early as 1970 the DOT and the ACS had developed ambulance design and equipment recommendations.[46,47] In 1973 the DHEW released the comprehensive article, "Medical Requirements for Ambulance Design and Equipment," and a year later the General Services Administration issued federal specifications KKK-A 1822 for ambulances.[48] Although the KKK specifications were originally developed for government procurement contracts, local EMS agencies were often politically obligated to meet or exceed the specifications when ordering new ambulances. A 1978 study of 183 EMS regions described the status of ambulance services within 151 of the regions. Only 65% of the 13,790 ambulances in those regions met the federal KKK standards. Eighty-one regions used paramedics and 72 had some type of air ambulance capability. Response time was often longer than 10 minutes in urban areas and as much as 30 minutes in rural areas.[49]

Hospitals

When awarding grants for EMS under the EMS Systems Act, the DHEW required regions to develop standards and guidelines for categorization of emergency departments in the following eight critical clinical groups: trauma, burns, spinal cord injuries, poisoning, cardiac, high-risk infants, alcohol and drug abuse, and behavioral emergencies. Regions were required to identify the most appropriate hospital for each of these clinical problems.

In reality, only a small portion of emergency facilities was functionally categorized and in many cases the system did not work as described on paper. Hospital administrators resisted losing control, physicians feared surrendering clinical judgment, and both feared losing patient revenues. Despite this resistance, the DHEW used EMS hospital categorization fairly effectively to restructure acute patient distribution along the lines of clinical capability rather than market share.

1978–1981: EMS at Midpassage

By 1978 many of the original problems and questions had come into focus. Most of the deficiencies identified in the 1966 NAS-NRC report had been attacked, and progress was being made in many areas. Economic resources and political support were being contributed by local and state governments, private foundations, nonprofit organizations, and professional groups. However, there was still tremendous geographic variability regarding distribution of services, access, accessibility, quality, and quantity of EMS resources. Basic questions concerning the effectiveness of the various components, system designs, and relationships still existed, and future funding was uncertain.

In 1978 NAS-NRC released a report called "Emergency Medical Services at Midpassage," which stated, "EMS in the United States in midpassage [is] urgently in need of midcourse corrections but uncertain as to the best direction and degree." The report was sharply critical of how the EMS System Act had been implemented by DHEW, and recommended "research and evaluation directed both to questions of immediate importance to EMS system development and to long-range questions. Without adequate investment in both types of research, EMS in the United States will be in the same position of uncertainty a generation hence as it is today."[50] The report documented coordination problems among various governmental agencies, focusing particular concern on the multiple standards promulgated as a condition of funding. Some of the standards were conflicting; often they had never been evaluated.[50]

Between 1974 and 1981 there were various sources of federal and private funds, and each grant often came with a new set of requirements. DOT established standards for ambulance design, provider training, and other transportation elements, while DHEW announced seven critical care areas as the basis for a systems approach and 15 components as modular elements for EMS design. A variety of private organizations also produced standards. For example, with regard to the technique of CPR, the American Red Cross and the AHA established slightly different standards, criteria, and training requirements.

By 1978 some states still had not enacted EMS legislation, whereas others had legislated exactly what prehospital providers could do, potentially hampering the flexibility needed for successful local development. Lack of national conformity or agreement precluded the development of universally accepted national standards in most areas of EMS.

On October 26, 1978, a memorandum of understanding was signed by DOT and DHEW describing each organization's responsibilities relating to development of EMS systems.[47] The agreement was an attempt to coordinate government activities and assign national-level responsibility for EMS development and direction. DOT, in coordination with DHEW, was to "develop uniform standards and procedures for the transportation phases of emergency care and response." DHEW was responsible, in coordination with DOT, for developing "medical standards and procedures for initial, supportive, and definitive care phases of EMS systems." Research and technical assistance were to be performed cooperatively, and both agencies agreed to exchange information and "establish joint working arrangements from time to time."[51]

Because the roots, constituencies, and operating philosophies of the agencies were markedly different, the 1978 agreement quickly failed. Over the four subsequent years an intense civil war was fought. Critical care medicine was shunted aside, and prehospital providers were standardized by highway engineers.[52]

In 1980 the EMS directors from each state banded together to form the National Association of State EMS Directors (NASEMSD). With membership from all 50 states and the territories, they attempted to take a leadership role with regard to national EMS policy, and to collaborate on the development of effective, integrated, community-based, consistent EMS systems. Their current strategy is to "achieve our mission by the participation of all the states and territories, by being a strong national voice for EMS, an acknowledged key resource for EMS information and policy, and a leader in developing and disseminating evidence-based decisions and policy."[53]

Financing

By 1978 termination of federal funding in most regions was imminent, and the potential impact on operations and future development began to raise concerns. The 1976 and 1979 amendments to the EMS System Act reflected concerns about future funding and had consequently demanded evidence of financial self-sufficiency as one basis for further support. Significant disagreement in describing financial self-sufficiency was apparent in the testimony and documents provided by the various agencies. The DOT estimates of nonfederal monies spent annually between 1968 and 1980 ranged up to $800 million.

In 1979 DHEW officials estimated in testimony that 90% of regions with paramedic service had achieved financial self-sufficiency by 1978.[42] However, the comptroller general, in a 1976 report entitled "Progress in Developing Emergency Medical Services Systems," cited considerable inconsistency in the degree and duration of support provided by community resources.[54] A few years later, in 1979, the comptroller general testified on the financial status of the EMS regions after analyzing grant applications under the 1976 amendments. Regions were required to document commitment by local governments to continue financial support after federal funds were terminated under Title XII. By the 1980s, the discrepancy between DHEW and the comptroller general's estimates of financial self-sufficiency of EMS systems suggested serious unrecognized difficulties in the continued underwriting of EMS systems.

The financial demands on an EMS system were considerable, related to four major elements: prehospital care, hospital care, communications, and management. The specific costs varied by community. The original 1966 NAS-NRC report estimated that ambulance services account for about one fourth of total EMS system costs, with 75% of that amount for personnel. Communications costs varied from 7% of total cost when there was integration with existing public services, to 35% when completely new systems needed to be established. Although management costs were high during the development phases, they were originally expected to account for less than 2% of the total cost during the operational phase.[50]

Health insurance reimbursement did not keep pace with EMS costs, which presented a real problem for EMS providers. Healthcare benefits were often limited to hospital care and had maximum fixed reimbursements. For example, 20% of Blue Cross patients were not covered for emergency transport and of those covered, one-third were only covered after an accident. By 1982 the NAS-NRC wrote, "Availability of advanced emergency care throughout the nation is a worthy objective, but the cost of such services may prohibit communities from obtaining them."[50]

Research

A total of $22 million was appropriated between 1974 and 1979 for EMS research. The National Center for Health Services Research (NCHSR), in coordination with the DHEW, funded various clinical and systems research projects. During the 1979 legislative hearings, testimony from the DHEW and the leadership of academic research centers stressed the need for continued EMS research. Annual reports from the DHEW detailed the type of research underway, questions being studied, and the scope of long-term and short-term research projects funded under Section 1205 of Title XII.[49] These projects included "methods to measure the performance of EMS personnel, evaluate the benefits and the costs of advanced life support systems, examine the impact of categorization efforts, determine the clinical significance of response time, and explore the consequences of alternative system configurations and procedures."[55] Other projects focused on "developing systems of quality assurance, designing and testing clinical algorithms, and examining the relationships between Emergency Departments and their parent hospitals (including rural-urban differences)."[55]

In early 1979 the Center for the Study of Emergency Health Services at the University of Pennsylvania urged continued support of EMS research: "Dollars spent in EMS research have great potential to help control rising health care costs, [and can] have a significant and visible effect in preventing death and enhancing the quality of patient life following emergency events."[56] The Center suggested research identifying EMS cost control potentials because the phasing out of federal funds, coupled with the effects of local tax revolts, would certainly reduce financing. As the 1980s progressed, the demand for more efficient, effective systems would become universal. Managers of EMS systems, just like their counterparts elsewhere, needed to know which components of the system were crucial and which could be deleted if funding were limited. The answers to those questions were anything but clear.

1981: The Omnibus Budget Reconciliation Act

Late in the summer of 1981 President Reagan signed comprehensive cost containment legislation that converted 25 Department of Health and Human Services (DHHS) funding programs into seven consolidated block grants.[57] EMS was included in the Preventive Health Block Grant, along with seven other programs such as rodent control and water fluoridation. In effect, individual states were left to determine how much money from the block grants would be distributed locally. Although existing EMS programs were temporarily guaranteed minimal support, a state could later decide to withdraw all block grant money from one or more regional EMS programs. This concept, simply a fundamental premise of conservative federal government, evolved quite differently in each of the states. As with decisions regarding how to implement provider levels and assure competence, the funding process was generally quite political, with little direct input from the public or the medical community.

The 1976 "Forward Plan for the Health Services Administration" made it clear that by 1982, all federal EMS System financial support would end, and regional EMS programs would be the responsibility of the regional agencies. The federal role was to be "one of technical assistance and coordination."[58]

1982 to the Present: A New Path

The public health initiative for developing a national EMS system came to a gradual, quiet, and unceremonious demise after 1981. In most regions the remnants of the old DHEW program were left to die off slowly under the cloud of confusion occasioned by Preventive Health Block Grants formula. In most, but not all, states EMS regional programs were lost in the shuffle of competing health programs while the Reagan administration was systematically eliminating federal support for all such programs. In fact, in most jurisdictions the regional EMS momentum present throughout the 1970s simply evaporated. Paradoxically, some individuals involved in EMS saw the end of the DHEW era as cause for rejoicing, because escape from the excessive, capricious, and special regulations might allow the development and implementation of alternative innovative approaches.[59] Unfortunately, freedom to explore new methodologies was often akin to being disinherited and cast out into the world at a fragile age.

Organizations such as the National Registry, NAEMT, and NASEMSD tried to preserve some semblance of an infrastructure. While attendance lagged and membership sagged, national EMS organizations struggled to survive and keep EMS alive as a discrete cause. Some state EMS agencies managed to keep the momentum by sponsoring well-attended statewide provider conferences.

In 1984, the Emergency Services Bureau of NHTSA was instrumental in creating the American Society for Testing and Materials (ASTM) Committee F-30. Through ASTM, NHTSA sought to legitimize the promulgation of standards in many areas of EMS. The standards branch of ASTM was based in Philadelphia, and through a complex consensus process, technical standards were arrived at in many different industries, including construction and building. As of 1993, over 7000 assorted standards had been developed through the ASTM process. Although these standards have no federal mandate, they were often enforced at the local level, for example, in building codes. Since a confusing but enthusiastic beginning in 1984, more than 30 EMS-related standards have been developed, including those for the EMT-A curriculum, rotary and fixed-wing medical aircraft, and EMS system organization. This last document outlines the roles and responsibilities of state, regional, and local EMS agencies. The resultant standards, although mandated by no authority, were considered by several state legislatures when state EMS laws or guidelines, written to obtain federal funding in the mid-1970s, required updating.

The F-30 Committee prospered as long as physician involvement was evident and decisive, but it was clearly NHTSA's decision what standard to expedite and when. The National Registry, NAEMT, and other interest groups joined the physicians, each to protect themselves. Although many physicians and physician groups eventually tired of the F-30 exercise, NHTSA preserved some semblance of a central authority. However, the real significance of the standards remains unclear.

As early as 1983, NHTSA began trying to wear the mantle associated with the old DHEW program. Many of the original evaluation staff were hired on a part-time basis to promote use of EMS management information systems. Management conferences were arranged for regional EMS system grantees. Saddled with growing financial problems under block grants, few could attend. In 1988, NHTSA tried to organize electronic exchange of information among surviving EMS clearinghouses. Three years of posturing came to nothing when hopes of private-public cooperation in EMS were shattered by withdrawal of the largest private clearinghouse. Because NHTSA had no mandate to promote specific programs on a nationwide basis, that was left to the states, often falling victim to the political process.

Training was not much different. Physician organizations backed one brand of trauma life support, but provider groups supported another. The American Red Cross, the National Safety Council, and a number of local EMS organizations prospered in the citizen CPR and first-aid responder business. Most states developed their own "home-grown" provider curricula, even when provider levels were similar or identical to those in neighboring states.

In 1986 NHTSA's newest and least likely role was that of standard bearer for trauma EMS system research. From 1982 to 1992, outcome measurement gradually lost relevance. Many jurisdictions and providers simply refused to underwrite the cost for "knife and gun club" specialty centers. Proofs that the system might work were supplanted by more palatable concepts. Faced with economic dislocation and cost shifting, traumatologists found themselves studying quality assurance, population-based research, and the statistical nuances of an outcome study conducted at a large number of hospitals nationwide. NHTSA evolved into the handmaiden of the CDC, awarding grants to researchers defining the structure of EMS and trauma care in the 1990s. On the bright side, the passage of the Trauma Care Systems Planning and Development Act in 1990 (Public Law 101-590) raised EMS, once again a subset of trauma, to a greater level of national awareness.

It would be incorrect to view the period since 1982 as simply stagnant. It might be better characterized as a time when centrifugal forces played havoc with attempts by the federal government and national organizations to define and standardize EMS. Managers, visionaries, and guardians of disciplinary parochialism were kept off balance by the fact that neither an operational consensus nor a discrete EMS development philosophy emerged. Across the country, local activists battled others in pursuit of diminishing funds. Zealous idealism metamorphosed into an earnest and businesslike focus transforming EMS leaders and providers into hardened idealists with a passion for survival. By 1992 patients had clearly emerged as customers, and by the beginning of the Clinton administration, EMS was just as conceptually unified, standardized, efficient, expensive, and confused as the rest of American healthcare. The Clinton healthcare plan of 1993 barely mentioned ambulance services, and did not address EMS systems at all.

The Emergency Medical Services for Children (EMSC) program was first authorized and funded by the U.S. Congress in 1984 as a demonstration program under Public Law 98-555. Administration of the EMSC program is jointly shared by the Health Resources and Services Administration's Maternal and Child Health Bureau (MCHB) and NHTSA. This program is a national initiative designed to reduce child and youth disability and death caused by severe illness or injury,[60] and serves as an example of a successful collaboration between government and academic forces.

In the late 1970s the Hawaii Medical Association laid the groundwork for the EMSC Program. It urged members of the American Academy of Pediatrics (AAP) to develop multifaceted EMS programs that would decrease morbidity and mortality in children. It worked with Senator Daniel Inouye (D-HI) and his staff to write legislation for a pediatric emergency medical services initiative.

In 1983 a particular incident demonstrated the need for these services. One of Senator Inouye's senior staff members had an infant daughter who became critically ill. Her treatment showed the serious shortcomings of an average emergency department when caring for a child in crisis. A year later, Senators Orrin Hatch (R-UT) and Lowell Weicker (R-CT), backed by staff members with disturbing experiences of their own, joined Senator Inouye in sponsoring the first EMSC legislation. The federal EMSC Program was established in 1984.

Initial funding from the EMSC program supported four state demonstration projects. These state projects developed some of the first strategies for addressing important pediatric emergency care issues, such as disseminating educational programs for prehospital and hospital-based providers, establishing data collection processes to identify significant pediatric issues in the EMS system, and developing tools for assessing critically ill and injured children. In later years, additional states were funded to develop other strategies and to implement programs developed by their predecessors. This work progressed through the 1990s when all fifty states and the territories received funding to improve EMSC and integrate it into their existing EMS systems. In response to the available money, in many areas prehospital care of children became the focus of all EMS innovation.

After several years, with projects developing many useful and innovative approaches to taking care of children in the prehospital setting, a mechanism was needed to make these ideas and products more easily accessible to interested states. In 1991 two national

resource centers were funded to provide technical assistance to states and to manage the dissemination of information and EMSC products. In 1995 the EMSC National Resource Center in Washington, D.C. was designated the single such center for the nation. Additionally, with the recognition for the dire need for research and the lack of qualified individuals in each state to perform it, a new center was funded, the National EMSC Data Analysis Resource Center (NEDARC), located at the University of Utah School of Medicine. Created through a cooperative agreement with the Maternal and Child Health Bureau, NEDARC was established to "help states accelerate adoption of common EMS data definitions, and to enhance data collection and analysis throughout the country."[61]

As the 1980s ended, members of Congress requested information that justified continued funding of the EMSC Program. The Institute of Medicine (IOM) of the National Academy of Sciences was commissioned in 1991 to conduct a study of the status of pediatric emergency medicine in the nation. A panel of experts was convened to review existing data and model systems of care, and to make recommendations as appropriate. The findings from this national study revealed continuing deficiencies in pediatric emergency care for many areas of the country and listed 22 recommendations for the improvement of pediatric emergency care nationwide.[62] These recommendations fell into the following categories: education and training, equipment and supplies, categorization and regionalization of hospital resources, communication and 9-1-1 systems, data collection, research, federal and state agencies and advisory groups, and federal funding. These findings convinced Congress to raise funding for the EMSC program.

In response to the IOM report, the EMSC program developed a strategic plan. With the assistance of multiple professionals, including physicians, nurses, and prehospital providers, major goals and objectives were identified. The *EMSC 5 Year Plan, 1995–2000* served as a guideline for further development of the program.[63] The plan had 13 goals and 48 objectives. Each objective had a specific plan with national needs, suggested activities, mechanisms to achieve the objective, and potential partners. In 1998 the plan was updated with baseline data, refined objectives, and progress in completing activities.[64]

EMS Physicians

Throughout the 1970s, emergency physicians and the fledgling American College of Emergency Physicians (ACEP) supported the visibility and strength federal money gave regional EMS programs. Unfortunately, by 1983, emergency physicians and the embryonic state chapters of ACEP, like most everyone else, had evolved into competitors for the same resources and recognition. Local physicians, EMS medical directors, and provider agencies were often at odds with each other. The new breed of EMS medical directors needed a forum to exchange ideas and ACEP, unfortunately, had not been receptive. In 1982 and 1983 the last unrestricted vestiges of block grant funding allowed the New York City EMS agency to gather a few proponents of strong EMS medical oversight to better define the emerging field of prehospital medicine, especially in the complicated urban environment. The brotherhood of these few individuals responsible for the medical stewardship of their respective systems was immediately self-evident. After a series of organizational meetings, the National Association of EMS Physicians (NAEMSP) was created in 1985, with Dr. Ron Stewart as its first president. As the importance of EMS to local government grew and NAEMSP focused attention, existing groups like ACEP and the Society for Academic Emergency Medicine (SAEM) once again emphasized and encouraged EMS activities among their members.

Training

DOT began the 1980s urging EMS agencies to adopt EMT-I as a less expensive alternative to EMT-P. In the middle of the decade, some administrators began advocating greater use of First Responders to obviate the need for expensive EMT-A (soon to become EMT-B) refresher training. If volunteers did not have time to refresh their skills, then it made sense to some to require less skill. Something was literally better than nothing. New Jersey experimentally grandfathered roughly half its 20,000 first-aid providers to the EMT-A level, totally missing the point that provider tasks, teaching objectives, curricula, and appropriate classroom hours must be determined in a logical, rational progression.[52]

An alternative approach developed between 1988 and 1992. Although the EMT-P could continue approximating the level of a physician extender in the field, a new EMT-B curriculum stole the spotlight,

emphasizing treatment algorithms over presumptive diagnosis. During the first three years of the 1990s, NHTSA struggled to reframe the old EMT-A curriculum. Without knowing how this "new" provider level would fit into the larger system or individual states, the process was flawed; many say it was yet another overt attempt to encumber local options with overly precise national standards. Although it was clear no one knew exactly how much EMS was enough, the National EMS Blueprint Project Task Force (sponsored by the National Registry and chaired by Drew Dawson) began the definition process early in 1993.[65]

The new EMT-B curriculum was a qualified success, and most states adopted it. However, after 20 years it had finally become logically, if not scientifically, clear that early defibrillation saved a proportion of people in cardiac arrest. Simply getting the newly developed automated external defibrillators to the right patients with a fast provider became a goal. The Guidelines 2000 document now places tremendous emphasis on rapid defibrillation as a function of EMS, and on the new concept of public access defibrillation.[40]

Transportation

Laissez-faire and voluntary standards served as hallmarks for EMS transportation from 1983 to 1990. Because ambulances were expensive and difficult to replace, more than half of EMS providers remained fire department-based. During that period, EMS began to become both professional and rational. Partly an outgrowth of priority dispatch came the need and ability to analyze how quickly and in what mode EMS vehicle response was required. Once again, medical input was key. By 1990 issues of ambulance operations, safety, and optimal mode of response were starting to be important medical and risk-management concerns.

By 1990 medical evacuation helicopters were available to most trauma centers and many rural rescue units. Care delayed was no longer care denied, but it cost millions to run even a modest air medical operation. EMS systems operating on a regional basis worked out the best possible local arrangements, but relatively few air medical ventures were financially successful, and a number of services have since shut down for financial reasons. Often, differences in state law and insurance reimbursement were key to the success or failure of a specific program. Like land ambulances, the air ambulances sometimes crashed. With as many as 44 such crashes in one year, the scope and longevity of the programs involved were seriously diminished.

Facilities

Researchers tried predicting outcomes and defining severity to justify enormous medical bills. By 1990 the trauma center designation criteria of the 1980s were being challenged and undermined. In most systems, every reasonably sized hospital with the desire to be a trauma center was designated as such. Urban blight and crime waves tied to inexpensive drugs like crack ensured unreimbursed health expenses. Hospital administrators often had to shift costs throughout the hospital to pay for trauma centers. Federal cutbacks in funding for teaching for trauma residents served only to amplify the problem. The hospital came to resent the trauma service, through which vast amounts of money were lost.

A related problem for EMS providers was the passage of the 1985 COBRA/EMTALA legislation aimed at penalizing emergency departments for refusing patients, either overtly or through diversions tied to the classic wallet biopsy.[66] It appeared that in some jurisdictions the poor were legally diverted by ambulance to the public hospitals.

Tactical EMS

In the last decade of the twentieth century, government officials became aware of very new roles for EMS personnel. The 1993 World Trade Center bombing punctuated the need for coherent emergency response to terrorist activity. Special precautions were required for the safety of personnel involved; burns, puncture wounds, and infectious disease elements are all intrinsically involved in EMS planning and response. The public had already been aroused because of the Oklahoma City bombing disaster prior to terrorist destruction of the World Trade Center. The importance of public safety was reorganized as a component of American life.

The EMS Agenda for the Future

In 1996, NHTSA and the Health Resources and Services Administration (HRSA) published the "EMS Agenda for the Future." This document was the culmination of a year-long process to develop a common vision for the future of EMS. The federally funded project was coordinated by NAEMSP and NASEMSD, but involved hundreds of other organizations and EMS-interested individuals who provided input to the spirit and the content of the Agenda. In addition to describing a vision for the future of EMS, the document discusses 14 attributes of the EMS system and outlines steps that will create progress toward realizing that vision. Shortly after its initial publication, thousands of copies of the EMS Agenda for the Future had been distributed for use by government and private organizations at national, state, and local levels to help guide EMS system-related planning, policy creation, and decision making.

Summary

During the last 20 years of the twentieth century, EMS providers experienced a sudden and at times brutal evolutionary process. Once a popular community resource, EMS was now asked to justify its very existence, usually resulting in service cutbacks, capital reductions, reconfiguration of vehicle fleets, and revisions of provider levels.

If the first few years of the 1990s were a dark age for EMS, then there were also isolated points of light portending a future renaissance. EMS physicians increasingly joined other EMS professionals in the quest to redefine and reframe EMS. This expanding physician involvement in clinical prehospital medical research, as well as in the planning and operating of prehospitals systems, was a hopeful sign. Professional organizations established guidelines and fostered discipline in research methodologies.

These actions are already resulting in change, increased medical accountability, and better assessment of prehospital therapy. Prehospital professionals jointly evaluate protocols, procedures, and practices, perhaps to discard some and enhance others. Financial constraints, legal issues, and community expectations are also forcing reassessment and refinement of how and what EMS is doing. Federal legislation and case law are mandating accountability of all medical practices; therefore, a sound scientific and medical basis is being demanded for the clinical practice of prehospital care. Research establishing this medical basis is now emerging as a major priority.

The financial considerations of the first years of the new century, especially changes in medical reimbursment continue to be major factors in EMS development and operations. Public policy and opinion influence decisions affecting staffing, coverage, equipment, and operations. However, spending more money does not always result in better care. Operational and basic research assist in making decisions that result in more efficient and higher quality systems. Those responsible for EMS system financing must understand the rising operational costs brought about by higher wages, increased personnel, greater demand, and expanding technology. For EMS to be accessible, new financing mechanisms, perhaps tied to a national health program or a variety of managed care programs, must be developed quickly.

After more than 25 years of rapid growth, change and progress, the key issues of concern as EMS enters the new millennium are system design, management economics, and effectiveness. System analysis and evaluation are still necessary and underfunded. EMS researchers and evaluators must continue investigating system problems to answer questions being asked by EMS managers, medical directors, and legislatures as they develop and mandate the EMS systems of the future.

The destruction of the twin towers of the World Trade Center focused national and global attention on the prehospital systems and disaster response in the United States. Our world will clearly be different, the question is how.

The irony is that most of the newly invented tools can be used by any EMS provider, yet few providers can independently supply all the operational components required in a given system. Our society still has not yet learned that the cost of EMS failure is significantly greater than the cost of EMS success. Unlike the past, the future of EMS belongs to the efficient and the innovative. Supporting evidence and a shared paradigm are required.

References

1. Breasted JH. *Bull Hist Med.* 1923;3:58–78.
2. Major RH. *A history of medicine,* Vol. 1, Springfield IL, 1984, Charles C. Thomas.
3. 1 Kings 17: 17-24.
4. Luke 10:25-37.
5. Garrison FH: *An introduction to the history of medicine,* Philadelphia, 1929, WB Saunders Co.
6. The Gallup Poll, *Field Newspaper Syndicate,* June 30, 1977.
7. Post CJ, Red Crossader, *EMS* Jan 1997, 64.
8. Haller JR, John S. *J Emer Med* 8:743–755, 1990.
9. Barringer ED. *Bowery to Bellevue.* New York: 1950, WW Norton & Co.
10. Barkley KT: The history of the ambulance. *Proceedings, International Congress of the History of Medicine.* 1974;23:456-466.
11. Kouwenhoven WB, Jude JR, Knickerbocker GB: Closed chest cardiac massage, *JAMA* 173:1064, 1960.
12. Eisenberg MS, *Life in the Balance: emergency medicine and the quest to reverse sudden death,* New York, 1997, Oxford University Press.
13. Pantridge JF, Geddes JS. A mobile intensive care unit in the management of myocardial infarction, *Lancet* 1:807–808, 1966.
14. Committee on Trauma and Committee on Shock: *Accidental death and disability: the neglected disease of modern society,* September 1966, Washington DC, Fifth printing by the Commission on Emergency Medical Services, January 1970, American Medical Association.
15. Committee on Trauma: Minimal equipment for ambulances, *BullColl Surgeons* 136, July–August 1961.
16. Committee on Trauma: Minimal equipment for ambulances, *Bull Am Coll Surgeons* 92–96, March–April 1967.
17. Hampton OP: The systematic approach to emergency medical services, *Bull Am Coll Surgeons* September–October 1968.
18. Hampton OP: Transportation of the injured: a report, *Bull Am Coll Surgeons* 55, January–February 1960.
19. President's Commission on Highway Safety: *Health, medical care and transportation of injured,* US Government Printing Office, 1965.
20. *National Highway Safety Act of 1966:* Public Law 89-564, Washington DC, 1966.
21. Jelenko, Frey CF. Emergency medical services: an overview, Bowie MD, 1976, The Brady Company.
22. Committee on Trauma: *Recommendations for an approach to an urgent national problem:* Proceedings of the Airlie Conference on Emergency Medical Services, Airlie House, Warrenton, VA, May 5–6, 1969, Chicago, 1969, American College of Surgeons, American Academy of Orthopedic Surgeons.
23. Commission of Emergency Medical Services. *Recommendations of the conference on the guidelines for the categorization of hospital emergency capabilities,* 1971, American Medical Association.
24. Nagel E et al. Telemetry medical command in coronary and other mobile emergency care systems, *JAMA* 214: 333–338, 1970.
25. Lewis R et al: Effectiveness of advanced paramedics in a mobile coronary care system, *JAMA* 241:1902–1904, 1979.
26. American Heart Association, National Academy of Sciences, National Research Council. Cardiopulmonary resuscitation. *JAMA.* 1966;198:372–379.
27. Boyd DR, Edlich RF, Micik S. *Systems approach to emergency care.* Norwalk CT: Appleton-Century-Crofts; 1983.
28. Committee on Emergency Medical Services: *Roles and resources of federal agencies in support of comprehensive emergency medical services,* Washington DC, 1972, National Research Council.
29. *EMS System Act of 1973,* Public Law 93-154, Washington DC, 1973.
30. The Robert Wood Johnson Foundation: *Special report,* Number 2, 1977.

31. The Robert Wood Johnson Foundation, National Competitive Program Grants for Regional Emergency Medical Communications Systems Administered in Cooperation with National Academy of Sciences: *Program guidelines,* 1973.

32. Lythcott GI. Statement before the Subcommittee on Health and Scientific Research Committee on Labor and Human Resources, In: *United States Senate Hearing Report.* 24, Feb 28, 1979.

33. Anwar AH, Hogan MH. Residency-trained physicians: where have all the flowers gone? *JACEP.* 1979;8(2):85.

34. Emergency Medicine Residents Association: *A survey by EMRA,* May 1980.

35. Liaison Residency Endorsement Committee: American College of Emergency Physicians, Information supplied, June 5, 1980.

36. American Board of Emergency Medicine. *Eligibility requirements.* Adopted June 27, 1976.

37. *Essentials and guidelines of an accredited educational program for the emergency medical technician-paramedic,* Essentials adopted 1978, guidelines approved 1979, Joint Review Committee on Educational Programs for EMT-Paramedics.

38. Eisenberg MS, Berger L, Hallstrom A: Epidemiology of cardiac arrest and resuscitation in a suburban community, *JACEP,* 1979.

39. McElroy CR. Citizen CPR: the role of the layperson in prehospital care, *Topics in Emergency Medicine* 1(4):37, 1980.

40. American Heart Association. Guidelines 2000 for cardiopulmonary resuscitation and emergency cardiovascular care. Circulation 2000; 102(suppl 1).

41. National Highway Traffic Safety Administration: *Communication: guidelines for emergency medical services,* September 1972, US Department of Transportation.

42. Emergency Medical Services Division, Department of Health, Education, and Welfare: HAS 77-2036, March 1977.

43. Kuehl AE, Kerr JT: Urban EMS systems, *Am J Emerg Med* 5:217, 1984.

44. Hampton OP: Present status of ambulance services in the United States, *Bull Am Coll Surgeons* 177–178, July-August 1965.

45. Summary report of the task force on ambulance services, Washington DC, April 1967, National Academy of Sciences, National Research Council.

46. Essential equipment for ambulances, *Bull Am Coll Surgeons* 55(5):7–13, 1970.

47. National Highway Traffic Safety Administration: *Ambulance design criteria,* Washington DC, May 1971, US Government Printing Office.

48. Roemer R, Kramer C, Frink JE. *Planning urban health services: jungle to system,* New York, 1975, Springer Publishing Co Inc.

49. Answers to questions submitted by members of Subcommittee on Health and Scientific Research of the Committee on Labor and Human Resources. In: *United States Senate hearing report,* 98-100, Feb 28, 1979.

50. *Emergency medical services at midpassage,* Washington DC, 1978, National Research Council.

51. Memorandum of understanding between the US Department of Transportation and the US Department of Health, Education, and Welfare: *Procedures relating to Emergency Medical Services systems,* Washington DC, Oct 26, 1978.

52. Post CJ. *Omaha orange: a popular history of EMS in America,* Boston, 1992, Jones and Bartlett.

53. National Association of State EMS Directors website: http://www.nasemsd.org, June 20, 2000.

54. Comptroller General of the United States. Progress in developing emergency medical services systems. HRD 76–150, 13 July 1976.

55. Boyd DR. *Emergency medical services systems evaluation.* Statement submitted to the Subcommittee on Health and Scientific Research, Committee on Labor and Human Resources. In: *United States Senate hearing report,* 47-57, Feb 28, 1979.

56. Cayten GC. Testimony to the Subcommittee on Health and Scientific Research of the Committee on Labor and Human Resources. In: *United States Senate hearing report.* 156–166, Feb 28, 1979.

57. *The Omnibus Budget Reconciliation Act of 1981,* Public Law 97-35, Washington DC, 1981.

58. US Department of Health, Education and Welfare: *The forward plan for the health services administration,* 1976, US Government Printing Office.

59. Page J. *History and Legislation Panel,* EMS medical directors' course, Phoenix, March 25, 1993.

60. Ball J. Emergency medical services for children. In: Foltin G, Tunik M, Cooper A, Markenson D, Treiber M, Karpeles T. *Teaching Resource for Instructors in Prehospital Pediatrics,* 2000.

61. "Getting Help from NEDARC," *CPEM Bare Facts,* News You Can Use, Volume 2, Number 3, Spring 2000, http://www.cpem.org/newsletter.

62. Durch, JS, and Lohr, KN. *Emergency medical services for children.* Washington, DC, 1993, National Academy Press.

63. US Department of Health and Human Services, Health Resources and Services Administration, Maternal and Child Health Bureau, *5 Year Plan: Emergency Medical Services for Children, 1995–2000.* Washington, DC, 1995, Emergency Medical Services for Children National Resource Center.

64. US. Department of Health and Human Services, Health Resources and Services Administration, Maternal and Child Health Bureau, *5 Year Plan: Midcourse Review, Emergency Medical Services for Children, 1995–2000.* Washington, DC, 1998, Emergency Medical Services for Children National Resource Center.

65. National EMS Training Blueprint (working draft) Columbus OH, 1993, National Registry.

66. *Consolidated Omnibus Budget Reconciliation Act of 1985,* Public Law 99-1, Washington DC, 1985.

Models & Legislation

Ray Fowler, MD

Emergency Medical Services is the provision of patient evaluation and management through the use of out-of-hospital medical providers. Excellence in out-of-hospital emergency medical management requires careful attention to EMS system structure and design at state, regional, and local levels. In some systems, on-scene physician attention is a dynamic portion of patient care; however, for the most part, field personnel provide patient assessment and management in the absence of physicians. Previous parlance has suggested that the skills of the providers are generally considered extensions of the medical oversight physician. With enhanced education programs nationwide, more and more of these professionals are becoming respected members of the professional patient care team.

EMS providers are rarely authorized to function as independent practitioners. They are trained in specific skills and have quite rigid descriptions of clinical conditions for which they may render patient care. EMS providers are permitted to carry out their various medical duties and responsibilities as "dependent practitioners." Though they possess specific skills and are allowed by law to perform certain procedures, they can apply these skills only through authorization by physicians either by pre-arranged protocol (indirect medical oversight) or real-time physician order (direct medical oversight). All EMS providers have a specific "scope of practice." This means that they may perform only those skills delineated either written in statute or in regulations. Therefore, independence to "practice medicine and surgery" is not a privilege of these providers, who are limited to the skills mentioned.

This chapter describes how EMS providers become authorized to perform skills in the out-of-hospital environment. Mention will be made as to how legislation and regulation provide a legal framework for the development of EMS systems. Sample legislation that may be examined as a model for the design and implementation of EMS systems is also offered at the conclusion of the chapter.

General Concepts

The fundamental element of an EMS system is medicine. Its basic purpose is to offer relief for public cries of distress caused by acute medical conditions. The fundamental parameters required to operate a system such as hiring educating personnel, providing equipment, managing finances, maintaining supervision, solving problems, and managing paperwork can easily relegate the "medicine" of EMS as secondary to "operations." System design and structure must revolve around the concept of the total quality management of the medical services that are provided.

EMS systems, like most medical provider systems, provide most of the hands-on medical care given through technical support; EMS medical care is generally practiced in the physical absence of the physician. Initially in the history of EMS legislation and practice, various assessment and management skills were felt to be "physician" skills that were being extended through the legislation to non-physician providers. With the increasing responsibility and training of EMS professionals, these skills are becoming part of the scope of practice.

Some EMS legislation places other individuals between the physician and the patient. For example, in California the mobile intensive care nurse (MICN) provides out-of-hospital care and instructs EMS personnel. The MICN is a registered nurse who is functioning pursuant to section 2725-2742 of the Business and Professions Code, which lays out general nursing training duties. The code also defines who has been authorized by the medical director of the local EMS agency as qualified to provide out-of-hospital advanced life support or to issue instructions to out-of-hospital emergency medical care personnel, all within an EMS system according to standardized procedures developed by the local EMS agency consistent with statewide guidelines established by the EMS authority.[1,2]

In the emergency department, the physician can maintain a direct relationship with a patient; there is no distance between them. If the physician gives an order to the nurse caring for the patient, some distance develops between the physician and the patient as the nurse performs the duty. It is the physician's responsibility to maintain the relationship with the patient. In the field the care is a direct extension of the physician and must be maintained in accordance with the contract between the physician and the patient. When the physician's role in the monitoring of patient care falls to zero, the physician's relationship with the patient is breached.

History and Development

Independent physician practice acts have been in existence in the United States for generations. Patient encounters, including the diagnosis, disposition, treatment, and release of patients, are limited to physician authority, except in states where independent practitioners such as nurse practitioners and physician assistants are authorized to initiate and conclude patient encounters. In many of these instances the non-physicians practice under some form of blanket authority extended to them by licensed physicians. It should be emphasized that this discussion is essentially limited to the Unites States and "westernized" nations in general. Many countries, including France, Russia and China, utilize physicians as part of routine care in the field. While in many developing countries, non-physician personnel commonly provide assessment and management skills for patients with a wide range of acute and chronic illnesses. Some countries require field "rotation" as a part of a physician's routine duties under a national or local medicine provision program.

EMS is relatively new in the long history of medical practice. The lack of physicians to respond to the scene of accidents and illnesses, the growing sophistication of extrication and transport techniques, the general lack of familiarity by physicians of field conditions, and the growing need for secondary transport to alternative levels of care led to the increased demand for and subsequent provision of out-of-hospital medical providers who are not actually independent practitioners, yet seem to function in that manner.

Provision of initial patient evaluation and treatment by non-physician technicians, especially when advanced skills such as endotracheal intubation and intravenous medications are used, generally requires the enactment of a state law "enabling" these non-physicians to assume certain medical skills with physician oversight. Laws enacted for this purpose are deemed "enabling legislation." Other aspects of such laws enable the state, region, or locality to develop regulations to fulfill legislative goals and intent.

Enabling legislation allows non-physicians to utilize specific diagnosis and treatment skills. Although all states provide some sort of enabling legislation, many do not view their statutes as providing specific extension of a physician's license to the out-of-hospital arena. This is due in part to the development of extensive medical oversight, often long after the original statutes were set in place. Only later did EMS physicians realize that field providers were practicing medical skills requiring physician authorization, skill, time, risk, and judgment, and that the subsequent medicolegal risk was directly extended to the physicians themselves. In the 1980s revised statutes began to reflect that the medical oversight physician was extending his medical license and authority to the non-physician technician.

One reason for the recent formal licensure extension was the need to assure the quality of medical care through physician review and direction. Whether by clear and concise mandate or inferential statutory construction, the role of the physician's quality and risk management processes is generally acknowledged as the central element of medical oversight.

Another reason for licensure extension has been the merger of the "traditional" terms "advanced life support" (ALS) and "basic life support" (BLS). The differences between ALS and BLS skills have essentially disappeared. Initially, any invasive procedure requiring medical oversight was considered ALS; however, in most jurisdictions all prehospital care requires medical oversight. Suctioning an airway, traditionally a BLS skill, incurs great risk to the patient if inappropriately performed. Medical oversight physicians bear the ultimate responsibility for assuring that a satisfactory performance level is maintained for all out-of-hospital skills. Thus, the medical oversight physician is responsible for all assessment and management skills practiced by all levels of out-of-hospital providers.

Rule-making

Newcomers to the legislative process may not be familiar with the concepts of legislative mandate and departmental rule-making. The state legislature is the collective voice of the citizens of a given state. Federal issue generally supersedes state legislative issue. The legislative voice of the state, through discussions and votes, provides laws or statutes. After the initial generation and subsequent modification of a particular statute, further definition and explanation are required. State executive departments promulgate regulations in fulfillment of their own operational roles which provide further definition, explanation, and process statements. The formation of rules and regulations is an important method by which a state significantly shapes policy to modify the general instructions given under a statute.

A statute may contain only a few sentences, but the rules and regulations addressing the statute may run to reams. For example, the Georgia EMS statute states that " to enhance the provision of medical care, each ambulance service shall be required to have a medical advisor [and] the duties of the medical advisor shall be to provide medical direction and training for the ambulance service personnel in concordance with acceptable emergency medical practices and procedures." The Georgia Department of Human Resources rules and regulations list many headings by which the medical advisor is to perform these duties, including formulation of policy and procedures affecting patient care; the formulation, development, and evaluation of training objectives; the establishment of quality control methods; and the performance of liaison roles in the medical community.[3,4]

It is critical that the EMS physician be knowledgable of the statutes and the regulations relative to EMS in the state in which he is working. Meaningful input is essential when statutes or rules and regulations are being created or changed by government.

Approaches to the creation of statutes and rules differ from state to state. What is written in law and what is left to rules and regulations vary significantly; however the statute and subsequent regulations carry the same authority. Penalties may exist for violations of either statutes or rules. Finally, it is far easier to modify a regulation than to amend a statute, given that passing a new statute or modifying an old one requires the complex law-making process. Changing a rule may often be accomplished through the hearing process of a state agency, provided that changes are consistent with statute.

Components of EMS Law

EMS statutes contain many elements. This section discusses in some detail the concepts of selected elements that may be found in a state EMS statute.

Title

Each EMS statute has a title indicative of the content that will follow. Typical titles include such phrases as "Emergency Medical Services"[5] and "Emergency Medical Care Personnel."

EMS is a service provided to the public similar to fire and police protection. The titles of EMS statutes make it clear that medicine is the service. There may be a medical act separate from the legislative act establishing the state medical board. The public can demand and the state can provide that service irrespective of existing medical acts. The entirety of the EMS statute could be covered under the rules established by the state medical board; however, the complexity of EMS, including personnel, management, certification, and ambulance licensure, necessitates detail that often cannot be included solely in the state medical board purview. Thus, EMS statutes usually provide direction to a department that can manage such administrative details.

The provision of EMS is rooted in many different resources such as fire departments, other public safety agencies, and hospitals. There are private providers in the business of providing EMS. In addition, public providers were established by many counties, fire districts, rescue agencies, and municipalities. Ideally, the EMS statutes create the framework for out-of-hospital medicine to be provided by well trained personnel, staffing carefully maintained vehicles, dispatching through controlled communications systems, ultimately providing an equitable distribution of patient calls.

Rationale

In the "rationale" section of an EMS statute, a statement is made as to why the state legislature approved the statute. Typically it states that the legislature finds it in the public interest to assure that emergency medical services are readily available and coordinated. Occasionally the need for quality in the provision of these services is included. The complex nature of EMS makes coordination essential; it is not a given that such services are in fact coordinated. In general, if something is important to the good of the people

---

but becomes something that cannot take care of itself, the government will usually step in and ascertain the need for a law that provides regulation of that entity. This is an important justification for EMS laws. It is equally important, of course, to allow extension of physician practice to non-physician providers in the out-of-hospital environment: that EMS is important to the public is most commonly the driving force behind legislation.

The state is responsible for protecting the public interest and has broad power through the legislative and regulatory process to carry out this duty. In general, a state can regulate anything considered in the public interest or presenting a risk to citizens. EMS is viewed by many legislatures as just such an entity that should be broadly regulated to protect the public interest. Matters relative to EMS that are typically regulated include how emergency calls are distributed, the number of EMS providers permitted to function in an area (which is usually established in the interest of economy and efficiency), the regulation of the flow of patients to trauma centers, the provision of immunity from civil liability and the description of which individuals are allowed to carry out EMS duties.[4]

State and Local Administration

Typically, EMS statutes address the various official positions required for the administration of the system.

STATE EMS DIRECTOR. Statewide direction of the EMS system is generally under the guidance of a state EMS director. There is a national organization of these directors (the National Association of State EMS Directors, *www.nasemsd.org*). The state EMS director is usually not a physician, although this varies from state to state. For example, the State of California mandates, "The Emergency Medical Services Authority shall be headed by the Director of the Emergency Medical Services Authority who shall be appointed by the Governor upon nomination of the Secretary of the Health and Welfare Agency. The Director shall be a physician and a surgeon licensed in California pursuant to the provisions of Chapter 5 of Division 2 of the business of professions code, and who has substantial experience in the practice of emergency medicine" (1979.101). The Texas statute states that the bureau shall be under the direction of a bureau chief with proven ability as an administrator

and organizer and with direct experience in emergency medical services; in filling this position, per statute, preference is given to any applicant who is a physician.

The state EMS director functions both as the manager of the office that generates the state EMS regulations, and as the enforcer of those regulations. Other duties include direction of the licensure process, certification of ambulance services and personnel, recertification of the same, and provision of investigative and disciplinary processes. Typically, the appointment is made by the governor of the state, by the director of the state health or by the public safety agency. Responsibilities include total management of the state EMS system, but the management of medical matters that rise to the state level is generally given over to a state advisory body composed of medical agents such as EMS physicians and EMS professionals. The state EMS director is generally not considered a medical authority, and in the absence of medical training, the state EMS director generally does not give medical opinions nor make quality management judgments regarding medical care. Indeed, the need for a person with a medical background to make such judgments cannot be overemphasized; quality medical oversight remains a vital component to EMS systems at all levels.

STATE EMS COMMITTEE, COUNCIL, OR COMMISSION. Many state statutes provide for the appointment of a state EMS governing or advisory committee, council, or commission. The responsibilities, compositions, authority, and appointments of the members of these groups vary significantly. Progressive statutes provide for appointment of a representative group from the community including physicians, EMS professionals, fire chiefs, administrators, county commissioners, and laypersons. In California, the law provides for appointment of a Commission on Emergency Medical Services consisting of 16 members: one physician whose primary practice is emergency medicine, one trauma surgeon, one physician representative from the California Medical Association, a county health officer, a registered nurse, a full-time paramedic, a private provider, a representative of fire protection, an emergency physician who is knowledgeable in state emergency medical services programs and issues, a hospital administrator of a base hospital, a peace officer, two public members who have experience in local EMS policy issues and an active member of one of the firefighting associations. This commission has the direct responsibility to review and approve regulations, standards, and guidelines to be developed by the EMS Authority; to advise the Authority on the development of emergency medical data collections system; to advise state health facilities; and to make recommendations for further developments. The commission may use technical advisory panels. Although the EMS Board of Trustees in Tennessee is similarly structured, this centralization of power is uncommon. The Tennessee statute provides for a board of 13 members similar to California although with fewer mandated physician members. This Tennessee board approves EMS schools and curricula; promulgates regulations for the issuance of licenses and certificates of personnel, services, and vehicles; provides for hearings; and establishes standards for the amounts and types of insurance coverage required for ambulance services. It also regulates the development and operation of telecommunications systems, and regulates fees. The Board's rulings are advisory to the Tennessee Board of Health. Alabama has a state EMS medical control board consisting of physician representatives from the state's six EMS regions. Advisory in nature, this board makes recommendations directly to the Alabama Board of Health. In New York, recommendations of the state EMS medical board are made to the state EMS council for final approval.

The direct authority of the California EMS Commission should be contrasted with states such as Georgia, where no reference to an "Emergency Medical Services Advisory Council" is made in the statute. The Georgia council is appointed by the state EMS director and has no direct authority.[6] As in many other states, recommendations are made by the state council to the regulatory agency (in this case the Georgia Department of Human Resources), which can act either positively or negatively on those recommendations. In practice, the opinions of this body are accepted as authoritative, although they require review and final approval by the Department of Human Resources, the Composite Board of Medical Examiners, or both.

Georgia recently added a State EMS Medical Directors Advisory Council, by which the many issues of medical oversight of EMS systems in Georgia are reviewed for consideration. This council was added at the pleasure of the Department, not being required either in statute or regulation. Highly politicized attempts to codify this physician medical direction council were defeated.

FORMATION OF RULES AND REGULATIONS. EMS statutes generally provide an element that allows state governments to make rules and regulations that "carry out the purposes and intent of this part and to enable the authority to exercise the powers and perform the duties conferred upon it by this part not inconsistent with any of the provisions of any statute of the state."[7] It is neither practical nor logical for the statute to contain all necessary policy and procedure for the provision of EMS.

One area of great variability among EMS statutes is the amount of detail. In the California statute the specific duties of EMS personnel are enumerated, but the certification and recertification standards are left to the regulatory agency approved by the EMS Commission; however, in the Georgia law the specific matters of the scope of practice for EMT-Basics are actually delineated in the statute.[8] Specific national standards have bearing on this statute, with the use of the United States Department of Transportation's (DOT) training course for EMT-B being codified as the training program for this provider level.

Rules and regulations become the living organ of the provision and administration of EMS, and the statute is the guiding force for the formation of the rules. Therefore, if the law states that the regulatory agency should determine certification requirements for EMS providers, then the rules should provide for these requirements, generally after consultation with EMS experts and the public.

Less flexible statutes provide significant operational detail in the language of the law. Changes in the scope of practice for prehospital providers then require changes in the law through the legislative process. In Georgia, for example, all duties of EMS personnel are spelled out in the statute because the DOT curriculum is named as the approved training program. Thus, under Georgia law, what the DOT program teaches is what the EMT-B is allowed to do; the wording and detail in the writing of EMS law are critical to the progress and growth of systems. Changes in regulation are much easier to make than changes in statute, because rules changes can be made without the mobilization of the state legislature. A well constructed statute will need very little modification.

REGIONAL EMS COUNCILS AND COORDINATING ENTITIES. The impact of the 1973 EMS System Act may be traced across the country by the development of regional EMS councils.[9] These councils dramatically influenced the training of personnel, the purchasing of equipment, and the initial design and direction of systems. Fiery politics raged when state legislators addressed the issue of regional EMS councils. Many private and public providers had a stake, some of them financial, in the channeling of patients within the system. Regional councils in many states were authorized to make determinations of need and award emergency response zones to various providers.

The Georgia EMS law delineates a bureaucratic process for patient routing through a "local coordinating entity." This entity operates at the regional level in the stead of the controlling board of the state regulatory agency or its designee, the Director of Public Health.[10] Thus, the regional level receives guidance and policy mandates from the state through the conduit of the local coordinating entity. The membership of these local coordinating entities is not spelled out in Georgia law. This portion of the statute is quoted in the references in its entirety, so as to allow the reader the opportunity to view this statutory process of awarding of ambulance response zones. This is a direct, persisting, vestigial remnant in Georgia of the original "regions" of the EMS Systems Act. Moreover, the rising strength of "home rule" has provided conflicting relations between these entities and local jurisdictions.

The Pennsylvania EMS law details the membership, terms, quorums, and duties of the regional body; carrying out "the emergency medical services plan" of the state and region is included in the duties. The Texas statute provides for regional EMS councils, but it also allows local providers to make their cases with the county commission or local municipalities regarding zoning. An appeal to the state is also available. A distinct flavor of the initial organization of a state EMS structure can be gained from analyzing the establishment of regional EMS councils.

LOCAL EMS PLANNING. Many EMS statutes address the need for comprehensive planning by local EMS systems. The complex and sophisticated nature of EMS is exemplified in the delineations of how local level issues should be handled. Such issues include awarding calls and response zones to various providers, handling complaints, managing the communications system locally, coordinating with state emergency preparedness agencies and providing for mutual aid, approving new EMS providers, initiating contracts, providing for local hearings, appointing EMS medical directors, developing mechanisms for quality improvement, and assigning responsibilities to a local EMS office.

This section of EMS law is vitally important in areas where personnel cannot carry out the medical acts unless employed. Since "local-level certification" is provided in such areas, these personnel are allowed to perform their duties only when employed by an approved service in the geographical area. Lack of employment means inability to perform out-of-hospital skills professionally. Local-level medical oversight and system design become prominent parts of the provision of EMS in these settings.

Ambulance Services

EMS statutes provide for methods to approve vehicles that may be utilized and to licensure of the services themselves. The extent to which methods are covered varies. While some statutes go as far as establishing local certificate of need (CON) procedures similar to those required for hospitals, others leave the determination of approval to the state agency or to local EMS systems.

The Georgia statute includes specifics on the application for licensure, the description and location of ambulances, the duties of the license officer, the requirements of insurance coverage, the ambulance standards specifications, and the procedures for renewal, suspension, and revocation.[11] The Tennessee law requires a state EMS board to form standards for ambulance vehicles and equipment, but licensure, permit, and certification criteria are in another section of the law.[12]

In general, EMS statutes provide for the licensure of ground, air, and water vehicles and the systems that operate them. Performance standards are often defined either in law or rules. Inspections typically must be conducted by a state or local governmental entity. An inclusion common in statute or rule is a provision for the revocation of system or vehicle licenses, including allowable reasons for revocation, and a method for appeal. Whether the ambulance license revocation process is directly in the law or indirectly assigned to some portion of the system varies.

Medical Oversight

Authorization of EMS personnel to carry out medical activities varies in EMS laws across the country.

Typically the need for EMS and its coordinated provision is stated in the opening rationale statement. Statutory descriptions of EMS as the provision of physician medical care through others are unusual and becoming relics of the history of EMS. In the past, EMS physicians in many states lacked statutory authority for medical oversight and performance review. Fortunately, modern statutes provide for specific authorization of medical oversight.

The Georgia statute is a good example of the medical oversight problem. Although EMS systems are required to have a medical director to "enhance the provision of emergency medical care," this physician must simply be licensed to practice medicine in the state. If a medical director cannot be obtained, the district health director should fill the role, either directly or through a subordinate. According to the statute, the enumerated duties of the medical director should include providing medical oversight and training for the ambulance service personnel "in conformance with acceptable emergency medical practices and procedures." Notably and commendably, the rules and regulations use that statement to lay out "acceptable emergency medical practices and procedures" of the medical director.[13] Georgia Senate Bill 320 (passed in 1989 and now Code Chapter 31-11-60.1) provided for a name change from EMS medical "advisor" to "director" and provided for the first time sufficient authority for the medical director to perform quality management duties. Interestingly, this bill did not go into effect until 1991; small municipalities that operate EMS services are not required by Georgia law to provide medical oversight for those services.[13]

Since EMS laws in many areas may not instruct the responsible agency to draw up medical oversight regulations, it has been argued that the agency does not have the authority to address and expand the medical oversight portion of the statute by issuing rules and regulations; broad interpretation of the state EMS agency's responsibilities allows for such authority. In Georgia, rules and regulations have been established for trauma systems despite the absence of specific authorization;[14] over the years statutory modification has provided for greater specificity in medical oversight and authorization for these rules.

A striking contrast is the California law, which provides for medical oversight of EMS systems through policy and procedure, concurrent review, direct management, and retrospective audit.[15] It further states that these are minimum standards for any system

implemented in the state. Such statutory declaration sculpts a mandatory performance standard that carries the influence of law.

A good EMS law should provide direct physician authority to provide qualified physician oversight for the medicine that is being practiced in the field. A medicolegal environment that holds the physician liable for the practice of medicine in the field should provide authority for design, implementation, maintenance, and quality improvement, with the statute as the final arbiter. EMS physicians must determine, in joint counsel with the providers, how out-of-hospital medicine will be practiced and monitored. Otherwise, the medical care delivered may not have quality control and risk management. Difficulty establishing medical oversight at the state level often is caused by the absence of national standards for the EMS medical director education and responsibility. Fortunately, the National Association of EMS Physicians has produced substantial information and guidance for the provision of medical oversight; national acceptance of uniform guidelines of EMS system medical quality management is a work in progress.

Patient Care Reports

The requirement for record-keeping is highly variable in EMS statutes. The Georgia law states, "Records of each ambulance trip shall be made by the ambulance service in a manner and on such forms as may be described through the Department through regulations. Such records shall be available for inspection by the Department at any time, and a summary of ambulance service activities shall be prepared on specific cases and furnished to the Department upon request." The rules and regulations of Georgia detail what should be included in the documentation and in the summary that must be submitted to the state upon request.

While the need for medical record confidentiality is mentioned in many statutes, the subject of medical records is mentioned neither in the Tennessee statute or rules nor in the California and Texas statutes. In Tennessee, there exists a general requirement for record-keeping in a policy statement issued under authority of regulation. In California, there is regulation providing for record-keeping under statutory authority.

The new federal Health Insurance Portability and Accountability Act (HIPAA) regulations addressing medical record confidentiality will adversely impact record-keeping requirements for EMS systems, placing increased responsibility on services to protect the privacy of records while at the same time being confronted with increasingly difficult data collection and billing issues.

Communications

The federal effort to bolster EMS through the 1977 legislation focused heavily on providing communication equipment for municipalities. Consequently, state statutes usually included methods of system design and regulation for such equipment, including the regulation of frequencies and occasionally the licensing of users. The term "communications" usually included handling public calls, such as through 9-1-1 systems, and operating radio and telephone response equipment. Advancing communications technology has caused a gradual metamorphosis of EMS statutes. Cellular equipment and satellite communications are current targets for local legislation and regulation.

An important part of communications addressed in the state statutes is the provision of care in the absence of radio communication with direct medical oversight. The California statute addresses this point extensively.[16] Some states require the completion of a special report, similar to a hospital incident report, if direct medical oversight contact cannot be made and advanced procedures are used. Georgia requires such a report; however its use is rare.

Providers

A fundamental area of EMS law is the provision for the training and certification of personnel. Some state laws mention provider levels, but assign state or local authorities to define these levels. California allows for modification of the paramedic scope of practice by local medical directors. Local medical directors may petition a committee of EMS medical directors named by the Emergency Medical Directors Association of California for additions to their local paramedic scope of practice. The Georgia statute meticulously defines all levels of providers through the use of the DOT curricula as the defining training program. Such statutory delineation presents difficulties within the modern EMS world; changing the duties of personnel is difficult when specifics are written into statute. Defibrillation could not be added as an EMT-B skill in Georgia until the law was changed. In New York, emergency medical technician-defibrillation (EMT-D) was implemented across the state, but only under the guise of an experimental trial. Examples abound regarding the changing of the scope of practice due to statutory specifics.

The Texas Code of 1983, as an example of a progressive statute, provides minimum skill levels for providers, but allows the state agency to determine precisely what skills they can perform. Other states allow localities to define the care provided at a given provider level.

Standards commonly found in EMS statutes regarding EMS provider issues include certification, recertification, continuing education, active practice requirements, services by providers working in hospitals, methods for obtaining medications, disciplinary procedures, and guidelines for the use of standing orders.

The inclusion of certain items in statute may make later educational change cumbersome. For example, in Georgia, state-level recertification materials had been minutely delineated for many years, including the previous requirement that five "different and discrete" modules be covered over five years; as a consequence it became very difficult to annually cover skills such as patient assessment and endotracheal intubation without conflicting with the statute. Later iterations of the recertification requirement did allow input by the local medical director as to the retraining requirements.[17]

The Indiana EMS law is extremely progressive and should be read when contemplating a change in law. A state agency is responsible for drawing up recertification requirements and the result is an excellent model.[18]

Many states now "license" paramedics. The meaning of this licensure varies from state to state. The usual interpretation is that the licensed paramedic may carry out certain skills and procedures without direct medical oversight. This "dependent licensure," however, requires various system components such as indirect medical oversight to allow for the use of standing orders. However, many states that allow advanced providers to use standing orders simply call this process "certification."

Specifics to Individual States

The local flavor of various state EMS statutes is reflected in the details included in the language of the statute. For example, "invalid cars," vehicles used for convalescent calls, are often mentioned. In the New York and Georgia laws, these vehicles are specifically not regulated by the EMS statutes.[19] Apparently in the development of EMS law in these states, political forces were able to influence legislators to protect these types of vehicles as a separate class of care not subject to regulation.

Small counties are often excluded from law for economic reasons. The Georgia law excuses counties with populations less than 12,000 specifically from the regulations implied by the statute.[20] The Tennessee statute excludes counties with populations less than 50,000.[21]

Good Samaritan laws and other liability limitations are included in many EMS statutes; however, in some states, such as Colorado, the limitations are elsewhere in law. Liability for simple negligence is usually excused; however, Good Samaritan laws generally do not provide immunity from gross negligence or willful and wanton misconduct.

An immunity statute in no way protects the provider from litigation. Rather, it excuses the provider from liability if the individual is not guilty of gross negligence or willful and wanton misconduct; liability is generally absent if the provider acts competently within the standard of care. For example, in California the liability limitation extends to providers who are actually on the job, and not found guilty of gross negligence.[22] Occasionally, similar provisions are made for EMS medical directors or council members who serve without remuneration.

The standard of care for medical oversight is far more complex than it was a few years ago. To avoid being guilty of willful and wanton negligence physicians must demonstrate that they have provided reasonable direct and indirect medical oversight. Litigation against a medical oversight physician might include claims of "failure to appropriately train and supervise EMS personnel."[23]

Regional trauma systems and other programs are allowed to divert patients to "appropriate facilities" in many statutes. The Georgia law was amended recently to allow agencies to route out-of-hospital patients to trauma centers. The California law includes a section entitled "Regional Trauma Systems." Statutory expansion of the "regionalization" of patients with specific medical conditions is likely in the future. Regionalization in the era of shrinking medical dollars, requirements of patient choice and pressures from managed care make destination policies vital elements of EMS systems.

Indemnification is a new concept in some statutes; providers of public services may be offered a settlement for injuries or death resulting from their work. It is debatable at this time whether private providers and EMS medical directors shall be included in such indemnification.

Local Ordinances

One of the most vital areas of legal control of EMS is the development of local ordinances. Municipalities and counties establish local ordinances as part of standard operating procedure. These decrees set rationales and structures for the performance and regulation of various matters.

If a city declares, for example, that it is in the interest of the populace to forbid the sale of alcoholic beverages within certain distances of churches, then this issue is a "local law," with various penalties for infractions thereof. Likewise, if a county determines that standards must be met by road contractors building thoroughfares within the county, then such roadways can only be built according to such specifications. Local ordinance cannot conflict with state statute or federal regulation. Furthermore, local ordinance often requires a complex hearing process before adoption. Local jurisdictions may issue ordinances concerning EMS. Such standards are powerful tools for medical directors and should be carefully studied and pursued. Topics that can be addressed locally include the following:

1. Direct medical oversight training standards
2. Indirect medical oversight requirements and contractual arrangements
3. Specifications for vehicles
4. Minimum response times
5. Minimum equipment standards for vehicles
6. Minimum training standards for providers
7. Quality management requirements

The medical oversight physician must carefully review the existing local ordinances in the community; the most significant impact of the medical director can be the creation of a lasting, local ordinance that provides for physician medical oversight of EMS activities.

California law enumerates the specific issues that must be addressed by local agencies that provide EMS services.[24] If the state statute is specific as to how the local area (in this case, the county) will address EMS, extensive locally adopted ordinances may be obviated.

A Model EMS State Legislation Outline

I. Title of the EMS act and rationale for EMS provision

II. State administration
- A. State professional director of EMS
  1. Qualifications
  2. Powers
  3. Duties
- B. State medical director of EMS (if state director is a non-physician)
  1. Qualifications
  2. Powers
  3. Duties
- C. State EMS commission
  1. Appointments
  2. Responsibilities
  3. Authority, both direct and indirect
- D. EMS state department
  1. Allowance for formation of rules and regulations
  2. EMS department duties

III. Regional administration
- A. Regional EMS councils
- B. Regional EMS medical director
- C. Regional EMS coordinator
- D. Provision for regional patient flow guidance

IV. Provision for county or municipality EMS administration
- A. Local EMS councils
- B. Local EMS system directors
- C. Local EMS medical directors

V. Ambulance services (specifics may be controlled by the Commission and/or the EMS State Department)
- A. Licensure of ground, air, and water vehicles
- B. Standards for ambulances
- C. Inspections
- D. Revocation of licenses
- E. Penalties

VI. Medical oversight
- A. Authorization for physician authority and medical direction
- B. General statement on EMS physician qualifications
- C. General statement on EMS physician responsibilities to EMS systems

VII. Indemnification

VIII. Limitations on liability

IX. Medical records keeping

X. Communications
- A. Rationale: The responsibility to respond to the public cry for distress
- B. Confidentiality

XI. EMS technicians (specifics may be relegated to the Department or to the Commission)
- A. Certification
- B. Recertification
- C. Services provided by technicians
- D. Continuing education
- E. Active practice requirements
- F. Hospital services
- G. Obtaining pharmaceuticals for EMS services
- H. Revocation of certificates
- I. Penalties
- J. Standing orders

XII. Specific to states
- A. "Invalid cars"
- B. Special provisions for small counties or large cities
- C. DNR provisions in the field
- D. Consent for care
- E. Management of multi-casualty incidents
- F. Provisions for mutual or automatic aid
- G. Funding (such as through speeding fines, license fees, or subscriptions)
- H. Data collection

FIGURE 1. *A Model EMS State Legislation Outline*

Summary

The proper formation of statutes, regulations and ordinances is critical to the continued maturation of EMS systems. Many aspects of EMS practice are found outside the enabling legislation, making the search for medical oversight authority mandatory; in some states the specifics of medical oversight are not found in the statute but in the activities of a state medical board.

EMS statutes should limit inclusion of matters such as criteria for the training of personnel, continuing education requirements, and medical scope of practice. Authoritative bodies of physicians, providers, administrators, and other qualified personnel can then determine the responsibilities and training providers through the regulatory process.

A state-level EMS commission, including qualified physicians practicing within the state EMS system, is essential. This commission must have statutory authority and must be more than advisory. When regional systems were established the medical oversight necessary for the proper monitoring and functioning of EMS was largely absent. Medical oversight is necessary for all EMS providers, as is statutory authority for the carrying-out of the duties and responsibilities of medical oversight physicians.

All physicians responsible for aspects of medical oversight should assume a dynamic, committed role in the review, monitoring, and creation of their EMS statutes so as to facilitate excellence in EMS practice and to allow for future maturation. They must assume, in addition, that liability limitation laws do not protect them unless they can demonstrate and document active participation in the design and management of their EMS systems.

References

1. California Codes, Business and Professions Code, Section 2725–2742, amended.
2. 1797.56. California Codes, Health and Safety Code Section 1797.50–1797.97: " 'Authorized registered nurse,' 'mobile intensive care nurse,' or 'MICN' means a registered nurse who is functioning pursuant to Section 2725 of the Business and Professions Code and who has been authorized by the medical director of the local EMS agency as qualified to provide prehospital advanced life support or to issue instructions to prehospital emergency medical care personnel within an EMS system according to standardized procedures developed by the local EMS agency consistent with statewide guidelines established by the authority. Nothing in this section shall be deemed to abridge or restrict the duties or functions of a registered nurse or mobile intensive care nurse as otherwise provided by law."
3. Georgia EMS Code Section 31-11-1.
   "(a) The General Assembly finds and determines:
      (1) That the furnishing of emergency medical services is a matter of substantial importance to the people of this state;
      (2) That the cost and quality of emergency medical services are matters within the public interest;
      (3) That it is highly desirable for the state to participate in emergency medical systems communications programs established pursuant to Public Law 93-154, entitled the Emergency Medical Services Systems Act of 1973;
      (4) That the administration of an emergency medical systems communications program should be the responsibility of the Department of Human Resources, acting upon the recommendations of the local entity which coordinates the program; all ambulance services shall be a part of this system even if this system is the '911' emergency telephone number;
      (5) That an emergency medical systems communications program in a health district should be operated as economically and efficiently as possible to serve the public welfare and, to achieve this goal, should involve the designation of geographical territories to be serviced by participating ambulance providers and should involve an economic and efficient procedure to distribute emergency calls among participating ambulance providers serving the same health district; and
      (6) Any first responder falls under the department's rules and regulations governing ambulances and can transport only in life-threatening situations or by orders of a licensed physician or when a licensed ambulance cannot respond.
   (b) The General Assembly therefore declares that, in the exercise of the sovereign powers of the state to safeguard and protect the public health and general well-being of its citizens, it is the public policy of this state to encourage, foster, and promote emergency medical systems communications programs and that such programs shall be accomplished in a manner that is coordinated, orderly, economical, and without unnecessary duplication of services and facilities."
4. Georgia Department of Human Resources Regulations: "Under the authority of the O.C.G.A. Chapter 31-11, these rules establish standards for ambulance services, medical first responder services, neonatal transport services, designation of trauma centers and base station facilities, training and certification requirements for medics, instructor certification and approval requirements for emergency medical technician, cardiac technician and paramedic training programs, and others as may be related to O.C.G.A. Chapter 31-11. Authority O.C.G.A. Secs. 31-2-4, 31-11-1, 31-11-2, 31-11-5."
5. Colorado Emergency Medical Services Act, Title 25, Article 3.5, Emergency Medical Services.
6. Georgia 290-5-30-.03 EMSAC (Emergency Medical Services Advisory Council)

General Provisions

"1. Council recommendations are advisory and are not binding to the department or agencies under contract to the department.
2. The council shall be composed of not more than 25 members who are knowledgeable in the field of emergency medical services, who represent a broad section of Georgia's citizens, including consumers of services, providers of services, and recognized experts in the field."
7. California EMS Code 1797.107: Rules and regulations. (Note that the EMS Commission in California must approve all regulations promulgated by the EMS Authority.)
8. Georgia EMS Code 31-11-53. Services which may be rendered by certified emergency medical technicians and trainees.
   "(a) Upon certification by the department, emergency medical technicians may do any of the following:

(1) Render first-aid and resuscitation services as taught in the United States Department of Transportation basic training courses for emergency medical technicians or an equivalent course approved by the department; and

(2) Upon the order of a duly licensed physician, administer approved intravenous solutions.

(b) While in training preparatory to becoming certified, emergency medical technician trainees may perform any of the functions specified in this Code section under the direct supervision of a duly licensed physician or a registered nurse."

9. Public Law 93-154, Emergency Medical Services Systems Act of 1973, Title XII of the Public Health Service Act.

10. Georgia EMS Code 31-11-3. Recommendations by local coordinating entity as to administration of EMSC Program; hearing and appeal.

"(a) The Board of Human Resources shall have the authority on behalf of the state to designate and contract with a public or nonprofit local entity to coordinate and administer the EMSC Program for each health district designated by the Department of Human Resources. The local coordinating entity thus designated shall be responsible for recommending to the board or its designee the manner in which the EMS Program is to be conducted. In making its recommendations, the local coordinating entity shall give the priority to making the EMSC Program function as efficiently and economically as possible. Each licensed ambulance provider in the health district shall have the opportunity to participate in the EMSC Program.

(b) The local coordinating entity shall request from each licensed ambulance provider in its health district a written description of the territory in which it can respond to emergency calls, based upon the provider's average response time from its base location within such territory; and such written description shall be due within ten days of the request by the local coordinating entity.

(c) After receipt of the written descriptions of territory in which the ambulance providers propose to respond to emergency calls, the local coordinating entity shall within ten days recommend in writing to the board or its designee the territories within the health district to be serviced by the ambulance providers; and at this same time the local coordinating entity shall also recommend the method of distributing emergency calls among the providers, based primarily on considerations of economy, efficiency, and benefit to the public welfare. The recommendation of the local coordinating entity shall be forwarded immediately to the board or its designee for approval or modification of the territorial zones and method of distributing calls among the ambulance providers participating in the EMSC Program in the health district.

(d) The board, or its designee, is empowered to conduct a hearing into the recommendations made by the local coordinating entity, and such hearing shall be conducted according to the procedures set forth in Code Section 31-5-2.

(e) The recommendations of the local coordinating entity shall not be modified unless the board or its designee shall find, after a hearing, that the determination of the district health director is not consistent with the operation of the EMSC Program in an efficient, economical manner that benefits the public welfare. The decision of the board or its designee shall be rendered as soon as possible and shall be final and conclusive concerning the operation of the EMSC Program; and appeal from such decision shall be pursuant to Code Section 31-5-3.

(f) The local coordinating entity shall begin administering the EMSC Program in accord with the decision by the board or its designee immediately after the decision by the board or it designee regarding approval or modification of the recommendations made by the local coordinating entity; and the EMSC Program shall be operated in such manner pending the resolution of any appeals filed pursuant to Code Section 31-5-3."

11. Georgia EMS Code 31-11-30 through 31-11-36.

12. Tennessee EMS Statutes 68-140-506: "Standards for the design, construction, equipment, sanitation, operation, and maintenance of vehicles, invalid vehicles, and for the operations and minimum emergency care equipment for emergency response vehicles shall be promulgated by the EMS board. The EMS board may authorize standards for licensure of air ambulance services to provide for such personnel equipment operation and activities as may be necessary. Permits shall not be required for individual aircraft."

13. Georgia EMS Code 31-11-50: Medical adviser.

"(a) To enhance the provision of emergency medical care, each ambulance service shall be required to have a medical adviser. The adviser shall be a physician licensed to practice medicine in this state and subject to approval by the medical consultant of the Emergency Health Section (in the Division of Physical Health of the Department of Human Resources). Ambulance services unable to obtain a medical adviser, due to unavailability or refusal of physicians to act as medical advisers, may request the district health director or his designee to act as medical adviser until the services of a physician are available.

(b) The duties of the medical adviser shall be to provide medical direction and training for the ambulance service personnel in conformance with acceptable emergency medical practices and procedures.

(c) This Code section shall not apply to any county having a population under 12,000 according to the United States decennial census of 1970 or any such future census."

14. Georgia Trauma System Policy Manual Standards

"1. The designation of trauma centers must comply with the Rules and Regulations as adopted by the Board of Human Resources. (See Appendix A.)

Trauma centers designated by the Board of Human Resources must comply with the most recent American College of Surgeons document, Resources for Optimal Care of the Injured Patient."

15. California EMS Act, 1798.(a).: "The medical direction and management of an emergency medical services system shall be under the medical control of the medical director of the local EMS agency." [Note: In 1990, the California EMS statute was changed (1797.202) to require that each local EMS agency have a medical director. This medical director must be a physician who has substantial experience in the practice of emergency medicine.]

16. California Code of Regulations Title 22, Social Security, Division 9, Pre-Hospital Emergency Medical Services, Chapter 4, EMT-Paramedic, Section 100144, Scope of Practice. "When an EMT-P who, at the scene of an emergency, reasonably determines that voice contact or telemetered electrocardiogram for monitoring by a physician or authorized registered nurse cannot be established or maintained and that delaying treatment may jeopardize the life of a patient, and when authorized by policies and procedures approved by local EMS authority, the EMT-P may initiate any paramedic procedure specified in this section in which such EMT-P has received training until such direct communication may be established or maintained or until the patient is brought to a general acute care hospital."

17. Georgia 290-5-30-.13 Recertification of Emergency Medical Technician.
   "(b) Continuing education that meets the requirements of this section must be approved in writing by either the department, a regional medical director, an ambulance service medical director, a medical first responder medical director or a neonatal transport service medical director. The local medical director may approve continuing education for the emergency medical technicians within the ambulance service for which he/she is responsible. If approved by the local medical director, a description of the training shall be filed with the regional EMS office prior to the beginning of the continuing education on a form approved by the department."

18. State of Indiana Official Rules and Regulations for the Operation and Administration of Advanced Life Support, revised September 1984, 836 IAC 2-6-4 Continuing Education Reporting Requirements.

19. Georgia EMS Code 31-11-11(4). "This chapter shall not apply to an invalid car or the operator thereof."

20. Georgia EMS Code 31-11-50(c). "This Code section shall not apply to any county having a population of under 12,000."

21. Tennessee EMS Statutes 68-140-516(c).

22. California Liability Limitation 1799.108. "Any person who has a certificate issued pursuant to this division from a certifying agency to provide prehospital emergency field care treatment at the scene of an emergency, as defined in Section 1799.102, shall be liable for civil damages only for acts or omissions performed in a grossly negligent manner or acts or omissions not performed in good faith."

23. Georgia EMS Code 31-11-8(b). "A physician shall not be civilly liable for damages resulting from that physician's acting as medical advisor to an ambulance service if those dangers are not a result of that physician's willful and wanton negligence."

24. California Codes, Health and Safety Code, Sections 1797.200–1797.226, 1797.200. "Each county may develop an emergency medical services program. Each county developing such a program shall designate a local EMS agency which shall be the county health department, an agency established and operated by the county, an entity with which the county contracts for the purposes of local emergency medical services administration, or a joint powers agency created for the administration of emergency medical services by agreement between counties or cities and counties pursuant to the provisions of Chapter 5 (commencing with Section 6500) of Division 7 of Title 1 of the Government."

CHAPTER 3

Urban

Lorraine Maria Giordano, MD
Nicholas Vincent Cagliuso, Sr., MPH, EMT-D

Recent strategies for promoting health and preventing disease in cities have included increasing the access to and the quality of health services, reducing behaviors associated with increased risk of poor health, and improving social and environmental conditions, all of which have been linked to the health status of cities.[1,2,3] The key to successful integration of these initiatives is the formation of a targeted effort to support the entire spectrum of health care. Public health strategies such as the New York City EMT-B asthma program, which brings potentially life-saving medications to the patient, and the public access defibrillation initiative, which has made defibrillators readily available in public places (such as airports and casinos), have intertwined long-term public health programs with short-term EMS response capabilities. This has resulted in a unique op-portunity for EMS to interface with both the com-munity and the healthcare system in the urban environment.

More than 80% of the U.S. population currently lives in metropolitan areas, which are defined as including both cities and their surrounding suburbs.[4] Over the past quarter century, the boundaries between the suburbs and their urban areas have blurred, so that the demographic and health profiles that were historically found solely in urban areas are now experienced in both "edge cities" and the underserved suburbs. Because of these changes it has been difficult for EMS administrators to codify their EMS, public health, and public safety systems with rules and regulations that would be universally applicable.

In the rural United States, EMS generally developed as a volunteer activity; however, in most cities, EMS began as hospital-based ambulance services staffed by full-time career personnel. Over the last 30 years, most hospital-based ambulances have given way to municipally sponsored fire department or third-service programs, though a few hospital-based or hybrid urban services still exist.[5,6] The concept of full-time professionals, or at least a mixture of paid and volunteer personnel, is also spreading to suburban areas and will probably develop in all but the most sparsely populated rural regions. The challenges facing urban medical directors differ from those of their rural or suburban counterparts, and the most significant differences are addressed in this chapter.

Higher Call Volume

Throughout the country, medically underserved individuals have increasingly turned to 9-1-1 and EMS systems as their entry point to healthcare services due to multiple social issues and higher population densities. Urban EMS total call volume is higher and units are generally busier. Consequently, urban ambulances are generally used more efficiently with less downtime than their rural counterparts. Operationally, the result is an effectively lower reserve capacity to draw from when call volume increases, and patients wait for ambulances more often than ambulances wait for patients. Therefore, as call volume increases, response times also increase, and the utilization of system status management becomes more critical as a time-series analytical tool.[7]

Assuming that no overcrowding occurs at the receiving hospitals (an assumption that is not always true in many urban emergency departments), efficient urban EMS units can process approximately one call every hour. This rate can be translated into a staffing pattern, depending on time of day and usage patterns, requiring on average one ambulance for every 40,000 people. As a general rule, early evening (1700 to 2100 hours) requires nearly twice as many units as early morning (0200 to 0600 hours), while other time periods fall between the two extremes. Depending on citizen use characteristics, some areas require more ambulances, while others require fewer.[8] Analysis of usage patterns must be combined with continual monitoring of call volume so that a fluid system of staffing adjustment and unit redeployment meets local needs. Demographics of the population served must also be factored into the planning process; for example, the cardiac arrest rate is known to be higher in lower-income areas.[9]

The increased call volume of urban areas presents a unique opportunity for research and evaluation of innovations. However, it also creates more wear and tear on the vehicles and probably more stress for the personnel. The street life of an urban ambulance is shorter than its rural counterpart, resulting in proportionally higher capital costs for ambulance replacement. Additionally, the constant stress has deleterious short- and long-term effects on the personnel and their families. Surveys have indicated that stress levels of EMS personnel are high and manifested as both somatic and organizational distress, as demonstrated by overall job dissatisfaction.[10,11] Furthermore, morale issues, which frequently affect job turnover rates, should be of concern to the urban medical director. In all-paramedic systems, paramedics may feel that their level of work is not consistent with their training. In tiered systems, EMTs may resent always being assigned to routine tasks.[12] In a fire department-based system, it may be possible to rotate EMTs and paramedics through fire service duties and EMS roles to help alleviate this stress.[12]

Recent advances increasing the efficiency of the high-volume urban system, but also contributing to increased cost, are the Global Positioning System (GPS), Geographic Information System (GIS), automatic vehicle locator (AVL) system, Enhanced 9-1-1 (E-911), priority dispatch, and computer-aided dispatch terminals for printouts of calls in field units. Implementation and maintenance of a computerized data collection system that may interface with hospitals also have a significant cost factor attached, especially if ambulance call reports that become part of the patient's medical record are to be printed at the receiving facility.

More Paid Full-Time Employees

In urban systems, the prehospital care providers are usually paid full-time fire department or third-service employees; however, there are EMS systems in a significant number of municipalities that provide services through contracted commercial ambulance operators. Having multiple types of providers within the same service may result in recruitment and retention problems due to variation in salaries and employee benefits packages. Full-time personnel acquire more field experience, require less refresher training, and burn out more rapidly than volunteer providers in relatively low-volume environments. Effective stress management programs, occupational health monitoring, vaccination programs, and blood-borne pathogen programs are increasingly important.[13,14,15] Employed providers present a myriad of labor management issues, all of which complicate the job of the medical director. Political relationships, religious observance considerations, and equal opportunity issues are likely to have a greater effect on staffing and planning.

There is also a higher probability that a union will represent urban EMS employees, creating additional considerations that must be addressed. Unions may demand that skill upgrades be accompanied by contract negotiations and an increased salary. The larger the number of employees, the higher the absolute cost to management for salary and benefit increases. There is also greater potential for labor relation and arbitration cases in a paid urban system. Issues of infection control, homelessness, drug-related violence, and domestic disputes necessitate a strong employee health service and employee assistance program. These employee health services should work closely with the police department as well as the infection control departments of hospitals to which patients are transported to ensure safety for personnel. An effective urban medical director should also develop crisis intervention teams that can meet the physical and emotional needs of EMS personnel and their families.[16]

Utilization of a Tiered System

A tiered response usually makes sense in an urban EMS system. Many urban programs are dual tiered, with the advanced tier and the basic tier occasionally working for different agencies. The relatively constant stream of calls in high-volume urban systems coupled with modern priority dispatch allows for more efficient use of the more expensive and relatively scarce paramedic personnel. With an effective priority dispatch system, the routine dispatch of both components is not necessary except for the most serious calls or when the paramedic unit lacks transport capabilities. Although a minimum of one ambulance is generally required for every 40,000 people, a single paramedic unit with state-of-the-art priority dispatch may be adequate for up to 200,000 people if sufficient basic level transport is available.[17]

Despite arguments by some for all-paramedic systems, a two-tiered system allows a given number of paramedic units to serve a larger population while maintaining a rapid response time if EMT-B level providers are appropriately dispatched.[18] Particularly in large urban centers, the tiered system can be employed to reduce response intervals to critical calls, primarily through the use of sophisticated dispatch protocols.[12] This tactic obviates the need for more paramedics and appears, in some systems, to provide medical care advantages through higher volume of skills utilization for individual ALS providers as well as a greater focus for medical oversight.[12] A recent meta-analysis also suggests that two-tier EMS systems have a higher survival after out-of-hospital cardiac arrest than one-tiered systems.[19]

Nontransporting first responder or emergency medical technician-defibrillator (EMT-D) programs, which have automated external defibrillation (AED) capability, are proliferating and add another potential tier in many urban environments. While these programs can improve survival statistics, they must be tightly linked with both an ambulance transport service and more advanced medical backup. If AED programs are not integrated into an EMS system, a lack of coordinated protocols, program management, medical oversight, and contracts may occur.

As previously stated, the use of a tiered system of units offers opportunity to improve both skills and paramedic response intervals for the critical calls in which they are needed.[20,21] Clearly, factors influencing local service demands, such as catchment population served, statutory and jurisdictional issues, funding availability, accessibility of receiving facilities, and quality of care concerns, must be taken into consideration in determining the most applicable type of deployment systems. Given these issues, expert medical oversight and sophisticated management and technological tools are warranted.[12]

Nontransport Vehicles

Responses by personnel in nontransport vehicles require the availability of secondary transport capability. Where adequate capability exists, system efficiency may be improved by using relatively inexpensive vehicles (costing a third of the price of an ambulance) for the nontransporting responder.

It is logical to use medically sophisticated personnel in nontransport vehicles and to dispatch them to cases in which an advanced intervention is most likely necessary. The use of basic personnel in nontransport vehicles makes little sense, except when ambulances are in short supply. Of course, if fire or police personnel with basic first aid, first responder, or EMT-B training are available, the urban system should seriously consider using them as the initial tier, responding in fire apparatus or police cars, which traditionally have shorter response times. Given effective training programs, triage protocols, and medical oversight, police officers may even become authorized transporters of sexual assault survivors without seriously compromising patient care.[22]

Response Time Factors

Ambulance cycle times of about one hour are usual in both rural and urban systems; however, system variables differ. Whereas cycle times are often extended in rural systems because of scattered population and long travel times (which may result in the utilization of different therapeutic interventions such as thrombolysis), in urban areas they may be prolonged by vertical access requirements, traffic congestion, or the lack of immediately available ambulances because of call volume surges or extended turnaround times in overcrowded emergency departments.[23] Operational and treatment protocols must acknowledge these differences.

In cities with high-rise buildings, actual response times to the patient may be significantly greater than recorded response times to the address, because of difficulties in vertical access from street level. For the urban medical director to develop medically optimal response-time goals, the high-rise factor and other similar patient access issues (e.g., the prison environment) must be considered in system and treatment protocol development.[23,24]

Because of the higher utilization rates, adding ambulance resources usually has a greater positive effect on response time in an urban system than in a rural area. However, in densely populated cities, traffic congestion related to rush hours, lunchtime pedestrians, construction, more frequent mass-media events and demonstrations, and public and political figure appearances may limit the expected benefits of adding these units.

In busy systems, dispatchers hold calls while waiting for an available ambulance more often than in relatively low-volume systems. Delayed response outliers are not only significant patient-care issues, but political and media time bombs for the urban medical director. As a result, potential liability and political environments often underpin the transportation system. The medical director must be cognizant of the political environment, finances, and the risks public officials are willing to take. For example, does public policy allow withholding the last available paramedic ambulance from a BLS call? Does the projected response time allowed by the budget support quality medical care?

Need for Standardization of Quality Management and Education

The large number of providers in urban systems requires highly structured medical oversight and quality management (QM). Ideally, a single urban medical director should provide direction for no more than thirty to fifty providers. Because urban prehospital providers use numerous receiving hospitals, there may be a tendency for medical oversight to be fragmented in large systems. Although this is not necessarily inappropriate, effectiveness may be compromised if the same level of providers in a single system have different protocols, educational backgrounds, or direct medical oversight physicians. If state or regional protocols and education requirements are not mandated, the medical directors in urban areas should voluntarily work together to develop standardized approaches to medical treatment, and work with legislators to develop minimum local standards to ensure the uniformity of patient-care delivered.

Because an urban medical director may be required to supervise a large number of personnel, he or she may lack personal contact with the individual providers, which results in the increased need for routine clinical observation by field supervisors. These field supervisors should be charged with identifying system problems, and also identifying problematic providers who should be entered into a more intense education and monitoring program. Assuming no cohesive regional quality management program is in place, an individual providing poor patient-care can get lost in the volume of a large urban service. If the solution is developing multiple "surrogate" medical directors at a number of medical facilities rather than utilizing field supervisors, a confusing variability of patient-care can result unless there is a predetermined consensus on training, treatment, and operational protocols.

Quality management programs must be proactive and ubiquitous. They must reinforce positive behaviors, and reeducate and sometimes discipline the negative. All sectors, whether municipal, hospital-based, volunteer, or commercial, must be brought into the system. Both emergent and interfacility transports must be evaluated on a regular basis. There is an even greater need in the more densely populated urban system than in rural areas for individual services to actively interface quality management activities with receiving hospital facilities so that compliance with protocols and skill performance can be effectively evaluated against patient outcome.

Because coordination among organizations is often more difficult in the urban system, voluntary cooperation efforts, external planning agencies, and/or regulatory control over system participants become even more critical.[21] Organizational autonomy can conflict with an organized response. This must be addressed to ensure the successful management of a multiple casualty incident. Daily interactions with police, fire, and receiving facilities become crucial, since all affect system performance.

Need for Complex Organization and Supervision Structure

As the number of personnel increases, the supervisory and support staff requirements expand both within the agency and systemwide. Financial issues require a physician's expertise in areas such as budget, payroll, contract negotiation, and bid processing. A separate materials management section may be necessary to coordinate purchasing and inventory. A unit may be needed just to process ambulance call reports and other paperwork. As the call volume increases, so do insurance claims and legal exposure, necessitating an expanded risk management unit and perhaps even on-site legal counsel. Not surprisingly, an unwieldy bureaucracy may develop both within the agency and among the various providers. It can become more difficult to conduct investigations and harder to develop consensus. In the urban EMS system, care must be taken so that neither a multitude of uncoordinated small fragmented systems nor a truly unmanageable colossus evolves. "How big is too big" for the efficient provision of quality prehospital emergency medical care by a system remains an issue that requires further research.

Availability of More Medical Facilities

There are usually more hospitals, both general and specialized, in an urban system. Consequently, greater consideration should be given in choosing the most appropriate ambulance destination for a prehospital patient. This not only means that field personnel must be taught to be more discriminating in facility choices but also that the local system must take the lead in evaluating the emergency facilities of the receiving institutions and ensuring that they meet minimum benchmark guidelines.[8,25] As more and more institutions are merging, regionalization of services within hospital systems must be acknowledged in triage, treatment, and transportation protocols. Medical insurance coverage provided by managed care organizations represents another destination determinant, which may result in the need for expansion of an interfacility transfer system.

Increased institutional competition may lead to excessive political interference in site selection, direct medical oversight, and post locations of active units. The urban medical director must interface with all interested parties during the development of the system and ambulance-destination protocols.

Less Medical Consensus

In urban environments there are often diverse and divergent medical opinions concerning appropriate medical care in the field. Ideally, a single physician director with medical oversight responsibility should have the ultimate authority for approving medical protocols and supervising prehospital care. The greater the number of physicians involved in protocol development, the less likelihood of consensus. A formal, interdisciplinary, area-wide medical advisory committee is critical to assist in developing prehospital medical policies and protocols. Strong negotiating skills are useful in bringing these diverse opinions to a compromise position. There are few situations more demoralizing to a system and to its medical director than retrospective criticism and "Monday morning quarterbacking" by the medical community.

Increased Physician On-Scene Presence

In many urban areas, there is an increased likelihood of a physician unknown to the prehospital providers being present at the scene of an emergency. These physicians may not be licensed in the jurisdiction nor capable of dealing with the medical situation at hand. Therefore, it is essential to have a structured procedure for dealing with unsolicited physician intervention at the scene.

Direct Medical Oversight

Although all system medical directors must have working familiarity with the histories of their systems, the varying capabilities of their systems and personnel, the political environments of their communities, and the current relevant biomedical science impacting prehospital care, are of these all critical in the urban environment.[26] As one aspect of medical oversight, direct medical oversight must incorporate the clinical and operational aspects of each component of the system to ensure the timely and appropriate delivery of patient care.[27] Direct medical oversight should be centralized in a large city to ensure uniformity of patient care, but this may be more difficult to achieve in a system with multiple physician involvement.

There are numerous benefits to direct voice contact among the patient, the prehospital care providers, and the on-line physician, particularly in urban areas. Given the growing populations of geriatric patients residing in cities, specific policies that deal with older persons who wish to refuse medical aid and/or transport to a medical facility should be in place.[28] Many geriatric patients often resist transport to a medical facility even though it is in their best interest to be further evaluated and treated in a hospital. By having these patients speak directly to a physician, the likelihood of their accepting transportation will rise, and untoward medical outcomes, time to definitive care, and legal ramifications will decrease.[28]

Increased Numbers of Non-English Speaking Patients

Individuals who do not speak English are often concentrated in urban areas; therefore, the likelihood of non-English speaking patients accessing urban systems is significant. Recent immigrants who not only have minimal English skills but who are also unfamiliar with the appropriate use of the emergency healthcare system can accentuate problems for the system. They may have their own cultural biases regarding utilization and the expectation of services to be provided. Some may come from a culture where physicians staff ambulances, and may expect medical treatment on scene; others may believe that ambulances are for the one-way transport of dying patients to hospitals and hence may be unwilling to accept transport. The urban system communication center must have a large language bank of translators readily available to deal with administrative as well as medical issues during triage and treatment.

Increased Nonemergent Use

Most residents of rural and suburban areas, regardless of financial status, have access to private vehicles and use them for the transportation of non-urgent problems as well as emergencies. In the urban setting, demand for transport to hospitals is higher and is greatest in the more disadvantaged communities. Because private and public transportation systems are often bypassed due to inaccessibility (e.g., financial or disability), urban systems experience a much higher percentage of nonemergent requests for ambulances and a greater per-capita usage rate than in suburban and rural systems. Patients with chronic conditions are more prone to recurrent EMS use.[29] These patients may also represent the population least likely to pay, thereby imposing further financial burden on the ambulance system. The percentage of nonemergent calls in New York City's system, for example, is estimated to be between 20% and 50%, depending on the local definition and circumstances. Given the association between socioeconomic status and health status in U.S. cities, urban medical directors must be cognizant of these outcomes and guide system policies to reflect and address the wide disparity of resource needs in their jurisdictions.

From an economic standpoint, some authors have suggested that EMS systems are a business with high fixed and low variable costs.[30] Most expenses are in the EMTs' and paramedics' salaries as well as ambulances, medical equipment, and communications gear. The variable costs, those associated with each run, are very small by comparison; they include fuel, paperwork, and the supplies used on the patient.[30] The marginal cost, the cost of making one additional

run, is rather small since some of the variable costs have already been incurred.[30] That said, it has been argued that it makes little economic, not to mention medicolegal, sense to refuse transportation.[43] Although nonemergent use is on the decline, it is still one of the most vexing problems for urban systems.[31]

Limited Requirement for Aeromedical Capability

The safety and efficacy of air medical transportation in large metropolitan areas is under debate. Studies have reported national accident rates ranging from 20 per 100,000 flight hours in the 1980s to 2.0 per 100,000 flight hours in the 1990s.[32,33,34]

Medical helicopters are usually less important and more rarely accessed on a per-capita basis in urban areas. However, their use still may be necessary to overcome difficulties of geographic access or congested traffic rather than extended travel distances. Even in dense metropolitan areas, there will be an occasional medically appropriate need for the helicopter transport. Thus, a degree of aeromedical capability should be developed in all systems, with triage, dispatch, and quality improvement mandates. In urban areas, competing hospitals may attempt to develop air medical programs; however, all such programs should be locally approved, and must be coordinated by the regional EMS system.[35]

In many urban systems, once the helicopter has been activated, the patient must be taken to the landing zone by the initial ambulance, loaded onto the helicopter, flown to a pre-designated landing zone at the hospital (some of which are not within walking distance of the hospital), and often reloaded and transported to the medical facility by a second waiting ground ambulance.[36] Thus, given the short ground transport times and higher numbers of receiving facilities usually found in cities, the general efficacy of aeromedical transport is doubtful in urban environments.[36]

Testing Disaster Plans

Although disaster planning is no less important in the rural setting, the more common occurrences of multiple casualty incidents and even disasters in urban systems allow for the use and evaluation of disaster response procedures on a more frequent basis. This fact underscores the need for urban systems to follow standard incident command system procedures when dealing with all serious incidents so that the operational procedures are familiar and routine when providers face major disasters and minimal disruption occurs.[37,38]

A region-specific disaster plan is essential in every EMS system, but because the spectrum and consequences of possible disasters (natural and planned) are more varied in the urban environment, urban medical directors should spend a larger percentage of time than their rural counterparts with liaisons from other agencies, developing plans for the range of potential disaster scenarios possible by locale. Additionally, because of the increased volume of the urban system's quality monitoring of the frequency of call types and clinical patient presentations by well trained providers can lead to earlier identification of infectious disease events in urban communities. This surveillance technique represents a new tool for identifying epidemics and potential bioterrorism threats.

Political Reality and Inter-agency Coordination

Political influence and interagency relations are arguably the two most difficult barriers to effective action in EMS systems. Since most urban EMS services reside within complex bureaucracies, converting the scientific, evidence-based approach to operational and patient care protocols can often be overshadowed by political factions with vested interests.

Moreover, the level of importance allocated to EMS is often less than that accorded older public safety services. In many cities, EMS systems have become sub-units of the fire or police departments, often to the detriment of the EMS leader's influence on policy development. Consequently, the public, and particularly the voters, may perceive EMS as a less vital service, until an event such as an extended response to an emergency or a shift in unit placement occurs within their area. Then, the all-too-often-seen reactive approach to policymaking is set into motion.

Since system design is often a product of local government policy, elected officials may address or ignore the question of value, depending on competition for local tax dollars. Where funding is scarce, a choice must be made: either impose budgetary restrictions and compromise service or employ a more resourceful system.[12]

In many systems, EMS services are provided by an amalgamation of municipal, private, hospital-based, and volunteer agencies, each with varying levels of resources and capabilities. These variables create tensions from the perspective of EMS physicians, administrators, labor unions, and politicians, each of which depends on the next move of the other to plan their own course of action. Since EMS is a relatively young service competing for funding with more established public service entities, it is incumbent upon the medical director to educate both politicians and the public in early recognition of medical disease and emergencies, as well as the functioning and proper utilization of the system.

Summary

Although every jurisdiction requires development of a "tailored" EMS system, differences do exist between urban and rural systems. It should be noted that around the country and around the world, urban systems are becoming remarkably similar in design and operation. While both rural and urban medical directors are involved in quality improvement and educational activities, the urban medical director faces greater challenges on a more frequent basis, has a greater opportunity for research analysis, and is more involved in administrative and executive functions than his rural counterpart.[39]

Higher call volumes, larger systems, and wider variations in personnel, training programs, patient populations, and call characteristics are just a few of the variables that make the job of the urban EMS medical director a unique and challenging one. Medical directors should educate citizens, interest groups, and policymakers about the impact of EMS systems on the overall health of urban populations. By engaging a broad spectrum of stakeholders in the decision-making process, EMS administrators can better allocate resources necessary to improve the prehospital health care provided to the urban communities that they serve. Given the myriad social, political, and economic issues faced by urban EMS administrators, EMS physicians with advanced education and experience in public health, public policy, and law will be among the best prepared and most effective in managing these complex systems.

References

1. Andrulis DP. Community, service, and policy strategies to improve health care access in the changing urban environment. *Am J Public Health*. 2000;90:858–862.

2. Geronimus A. To mitigate, resist or undo: addressing structural influences on the health of urban populations. *Am J Public Health*. 2000;90:867–872.

3. Leviton LC, Snell E, McGinnis M. Urban issues in health promotion strategies. *Am J Public Health*. 2000;90:863–866.

4. Freudenberg N. Time for a national agenda to improve the health of urban populations. *Am J Public Health*. 2000;90:837–840.

5. Cady G. EMS in the United States: a survey of providers in the 200 most populous cities. *JEMS*. 1992;17:75–92.

6. Mayfield T, Lindstrom AM. 1999 200-city survey: EMS trends in America's most populous cities. *JEMS*. 2000;25:54–70.

7. Tandberg D, Tibbetts J, Sklar DP. Time series forecasts of ambulance run volume. *Am J Emerg Med*. 1998;16:232–237.

8. Cayten CG, Longmore W. Prolongation of scene time by advanced life support in an urban setting. *J Trauma*. 1985;25:679.

9. Ferro S, Hedges JR, Stevens P. Demographics of cardiac arrest: association with residence in a low-income area. *Acad Emerg Med*. 1995;2:11–16.

10. Boudreaux E, Mandry C, Brantley PJ. Stress, job satisfaction, coping, and psychological distress among emergency medical technicians. *Prehospital Disaster Med*. 1997;12:242–249.

11. Cydulka RK, Emerman CL, Shade B, Kubincanek J. Stress levels in EMS personnel: a national survey. *Prehospital Disaster Med*. 1997;12:136–140.

12. Stout J, Pepe PE, Mosesso VN. All-advanced life support vs. tiered-response ambulance systems. *Prehosp Emerg Care*. 2000;4:1–6.

13. Lee DJ, Carillo L, Fleming L. Epidemiology of hepatitis B vaccine acceptance among urban paramedics and emergency medical technicians. *Am J Infect Control*. 1997;25:421–423.

14. Weidner BL, Gotsch AR, Delmevo CD, et al. Worker health and safety training: assessing impact among responders. *Am J Ind Med*. 1998;33:241–246.

15. Werman HA, Gwinn R. Seroprevalence of hepatitis B and hepatitis C among rural emergency medical care personnel. *Am J Emerg Med*. 1997;15:248–251.

16. Rodgers LM. A five year study comparing early retirements on medical grounds in ambulance personnel with those in other groups of health service staff: Part 1, Incidences of retirements. *Occ Med* (Lond, Eng). 1998;48:7–16.

17. Kuehl AE, Kerr JT. Urban EMS systems. *Am J Emerg Med*. 1984;2:13.

18. Braun O, McCallion R, Fazackerley J. Characteristics of mid-sized urban EMS systems. *Ann Emerg Med*. 1990;19:536–546.

19. Nichol G, Detsky AS, Steill IG, et al. Effectiveness of emergency medical services for victims of out-of-hospital cardiac arrest: a meta-analysis. *Ann Emerg Med*. 1996;27:700–710.

20. Curka PA, Pepe PE, Ginger VF, et al. Emergency medical services priority dispatch. *Ann Emerg Med*. 1993;22:45–52.

21. Narad RA. Coordination of the EMS system: an organizational theory approach. *Prehosp Emerg Care*. 1998;2:145–152.

22. Branas CC, Sing RF, Davidson SJ. Urban trauma transport of assaulted patients using nonmedical personnel. *Acad Emerg Med*. 1995;2:486–493.

23. Lombardi G, Gallagher J, Gennis P. Outcome of out-of-hospital cardiac arrest in New York City. *JAMA*. 1994;271:678–683.

24. Lumpe D. Focuses on prehospital care. *JEMS*. 1992;17:21–27.

25. Goldfrank L, Henneman PL, Ling LJ, Prescott JE, Rosen C, Sama A. Emergency center categorization standards. *Acad Emerg Med*. 1999;6:638–655.

26. Delbridge TR, Verdile VP, Sullivan MP. Contemporary medical direction. In Paris P, Roth R, Verdile VP, eds. *Prehospital Medicine: The Art of On-line Medical Command*. St. Louis: Mosby-Lifeline; 1996:15–17.

27. Cherson AW, Cagliuso NV Sr, Giordano LM, Mulqueen T. On-line medical control in an urban EMS system: clinical vs. operational contacts. *JEMS*. 2000;25:S-23.

28. Cagliuso NV. *Outcome of patients 65 and over who initially refuse prehospital medical aid and transport, but whose decision is reversed as a result of on-line medical control contact* [master's thesis]. Valhalla, NY: New York Medical College; 1998.

29. Brokaw J, Olson L, Fullerton L, et al. Repeated ambulance use by patients with acute alcohol intoxication, seizure disorder, and respiratory illness. *Am J Emerg Med*. 1998;16:1–4.

30. Zachariah BS. The problem of ambulance misuse: whose problem is it anyway? *Acad Emerg Med*. 1999;6:2–5.

31. Kuehl AE, Kerr JT. Issues in urban EMS. *Urban Health*. 1987;13:24.

32. DeLorenzo RA, Freid RL, Villarin AR. Army aeromedical crash rates. *Milit Med*. 1999;164:116–118.

33. Frazer R. Air medical accidents: a 20-year search for information. *Air Med*. Sep/Oct 1999;34–39.

34. Low RB, Dunne MJ, Blumer IJ, Tagney G. Factors associated with the safety of EMS helicopters. *Am J Emerg Med*. 1991;9:103–106.

35. Kuehl A, Kerr JT, Fenwick J. The second international urban EMS conference. *Am J Emerg Med*. 1985;3:564–567.

36. Asaeda G, Cherson A, Giordano L, Kusick M. Utilization of air medical transport in a large urban environment: a retrospective analysis. *Prehosp Emerg Care*. 2001;5:36–39.

37. Kerr JT, Weiman E. The planned disaster strategy for the masses. *JEMS*. 1982;7:22–23.

38. Kerr JT, Weiman E. NYC-EMS: disaster planning pays off. *JEMS*. 1984;9:13–14.

39. Tortella BJ, Lavery RF, Cody RP, Doran J. Physician medical direction and advanced life support in the United States. *Acad Emerg Med*. 1995;2:274–279.

Rural

Greg Mears, MD
Bethany Cummings, DO

Introduction

I t is contested whether rural EMS is truly different from EMS in the urban and suburban sectors. While there are obviously shared bottom-line concerns of quality and affordable expedient health care, the rural venue also entails unique challenges and issues, among which are dependence on the recruitment and retention of volunteers; medical direction, also often volunteer; extended transport times; and distance, both responding to and transporting patients. The challenge of operating standard-of-care services with limited "chicken dinner" fundraising budgets and the continual challenge of disseminating current practices and clinical care standards in a reliable and reproducible manner is immense. While wilderness/frontier areas often have an exotic appeal that helps to attract providers, rural systems have the challenge of creating an environment that will stimulate and entice involvement for the community, by the community.

Creativity often abounds in the EMS ranks and is shared in the rural setting. Calls involving muddy fields, uneven terrain, and environmental obstacles are not rare and often require the imagination and inventiveness of the field provider. The Farmedic program is an example of a program created for rural EMS providers to instruct them on the machinations and dangers of farm equipment for unique situations encountered in rural environments such as silo rescues, disengaging tractor power take-offs, and the like.

Rapid response is also often a challenge in a system where providers may respond from their homes, as opposed to a fixed EMS base or station. The use of various EMS delivery systems has been developed to allow rural EMS providers to respond in non-traditional ways as first responders prior to the arrival of a formal transport ambulance.

There are certain advantages to be found in rural EMS, as the patient is often known to the EMS provider as friend, family, or neighbor. This condition creates an increased desire to provide quality care, but can also create an environment of increased stress on caring with objectivity.

Change is inevitable in any environment, and the rural environment is changing more rapidly than most other subsets of EMS; there is a solidness that creates a community spirit, but also can create an obstacle to change.

Definitions

"Rural" can be described in many ways using terms such as area, size, population density, geography, lifestyle, values, and behavioral patterns. The federal government has defined "rural" through documents published by three agencies that describe urban settings. All remaining areas are then, through the process of exclusion, classified as "rural."

The Bureau of Census defines an "urbanized area" as a central city with any surrounding densely settled territory, which together has a population of at least 50,000 and a population density of at least 1,000 people per square mile. In addition, all persons living in areas such as cities, towns, and villages with a population of 2,500 or more outside of these urbanized areas are considered "urban." All other areas are considered "rural." The Bureau of Census definition does not consider county lines in its definition.

The Office of Management and Budget uses metropolitan statistical areas (MSAs). An MSA is defined as at least one city with at least 50,000 people or an "urbanized area" (defined by the Bureau of Census) with at least 50,000 people and a total MSA population of at least 100,000 (75,000 in New England). The MSA definition must include the entire county in which the central city is located and may include adjacent counties if they are economically or socially integrated with the central county. As with the Bureau of Census, all areas that do not meet this definition are considered "rural."

The United States Department of Agriculture (USDA) uses rural-urban continuum codes to distinguish metropolitan counties by size and non-metropolitan counties by their degree of urbanization or proximity to metropolitan areas. USDA codes 0 through 3 are considered metropolitan, and 4 through 9 are considered non-metropolitan. Code 4, for example, represents an urban population of 20,000 or more, adjacent to a metropolitan area. Code 9 represents a completely rural area with a population of less than 2,500, not adjacent to a metropolitan area.

The Public Health Service has further subdivided rural into more isolated rural areas known as "frontier" areas. Frontier areas have a population density of six or fewer people per square mile. Frontier areas are much more common in the western half of the United States and Alaska, but small frontier areas exist in most states.

The Committee on Trauma of the American College of Surgeons defines "rural" as an area where geography, population density, weather, distance, or availability of professional or institutional resources combine to isolate the trauma victim in an environment where access to definitive care is limited. Although this definition seems to be a very reasonable description of "rural" from a trauma perspective, it is not reproducible and makes detailed research and evaluation of rural areas difficult. Rogers and colleagues suggest that a rural trauma area should combine ecological, operational, and socio-cultural attributes. Using this method, rural trauma regions would be areas that have fewer than 2,500 people with a population density of less than 50 per square mile, have only basic life support capabilities with prehospital transport times that exceed 30 minutes, and are lacking in subspecialty coverage at local hospitals.

Formal EMS system development has progressed in the urban setting, with such principles as System Status Management.[1] Research has been done in large urban settings regarding the efficiency of various EMS system models. This approach has led to the development of tiered response systems, formal response time standards, and formal definitions of EMS service delivery. These principles have predicted that the most efficient EMS system delivery requires a population of just over 1 million. Stout also states that these principles and methods are unproven in EMS systems that serve populations of less than 250,000.[1] Rural EMS systems must closely evaluate the impact that urban-based EMS system research and design may have on system resources and service delivery.

Demographics

Rural populations are in many ways different from urban populations, and are often different even from other rural populations. It is important to consider the number, type, and frequency of medical and traumatic problems along with the demographics of each community when developing or managing a rural EMS system. Although little research has been done in rural settings, there is a generally higher demand for ambulance services in rural areas for medical conditions.[2] There is also an older age distribution among rural residents. Ambulance calls have been found to be more likely to be "urgent or critical" in rural areas of Texas and South Carolina than in urban settings, and admission rates for EMS arrivals have been found to be greater in rural settings.[2]

Rural residents are almost 50% more likely to die from trauma than their urban counterparts.[3] Motor vehicle crashes are the single greatest cause of mortality for both urban and rural trauma victims, but the rural rate (29.5 per 100,000) is almost twice the urban rate (16.3 per 100,000).[3] Suicide, homicide, and falls are the second, third, and fourth most common causes of traumatic death in both rural and urban populations. In each of these categories, rural populations are at a greater risk of death (1.21, 1.25, and 1.50 relative risk, respectively).[3]

Pediatric trauma death rates have also been shown to be twice as high in rural areas. In one study, 87% of fatally injured children never reached a hospital.[4]

History

The development of EMS can be tied formally to two specific clinical problems: trauma and cardiac arrest. While the principles of patient care involved are of course applicable to rural EMS systems, the roots of EMS were primarily military and urban.

The first civilian EMS systems grew from the need to transport patients. The only business that had the resources to provide transportation was typically the community funeral home. Rescue squads began to rise in number and popularity in the 1950s and 1960s as motor vehicles, and the need to extricate patients from traumatic crashes, became more prevalent. These rescue squads were typically community-based and volunteer. Fire services at this point had been around for years and were the other birthplace for rural EMS. Most every rural community had a fire district that often picked up the rescue responsibilities. Fire services had an advantage over freestanding rescue squads in that they were more entrenched in the community and physically resided in districts, which generally provided for improved response capabilities.

While the 1973 Emergency Medical Services Act provided funds for system development in rural areas as well as urban and suburban areas, these funds have disappeared and no federal funding for rural system development has been available since the early 1990s.

In 1996 the EMS Agenda for the Future document was published jointly by the National Highway Traffic Safety Administration and the Health Resources and Service Administration.[5] The Agenda proposed a community-based EMS system that is fully integrated with the healthcare system, with EMS systems providing acute care, injury prevention, and community health monitoring. Most rural systems are in a position to excel in a community-based healthcare environment based on their longstanding integration into the community.

Components

The EMS Agenda for the Future describes a system based on 14 components.[5] Each of the components will be discussed here from a rural perspective.

Human Resources

The bedrock foundation of rural EMS has been volunteer providers of basic and advanced prehospital care. The nature of the rural environment, with a sparse population and few ambulance calls per 24-hour period, coupled with a higher average of uninsured patients, creates an environment of financial challenges for survival.[3] Few proprietary ambulance companies find the rural setting financially viable, and therefore care goes to a voluntary mode of helping one's neighbors. The psychology of volunteerism is diverse and the demographics are intriguing, reflecting some of the basic human needs for a sense of belonging and a desire for recognition. In order to

recruit and retain volunteer prehospital providers successfully it is helpful to understand some basic concepts.

Webster's Dictionary defines the verb "volunteer" as: "to give freely of one's time or services," and perhaps in EMS the key word is time. Average time of duty for an EMS provider varies, but 16 to 24 hours weekly is not unusual. This time is divided into actual duty call, training, meetings, fundraising, and "chores," including maintenance and cleaning of the equipment. This time typically reflects one's spare time spent outside of the typical work hours from the provider's primary career or source of income. This is also time spent away from family and friends. Self-employment may increase the provider's flexibility by allowing response to calls during work hours. Some employers willingly support their volunteer EMS employees by allowing them to leave work at a moment's notice for calls, creating an environment of coverage and allotment. However, this is not universally so. Many systems have developed formal agreements and contracts with each of their members. These contracts formalize time commitments and help the volunteer to better understand what time commitments exist and how they can participate based on their primary job or career. Time constraints are often cited as reasons for leaving a volunteer EMS squad.

Age is often skewed toward the early adult years, particularly the 20s and 30s, which has given EMS a reputation as being a young person's profession. However, the older the existence of the organization, the more likely there will be participants with longevity, particularly in the administrative roles. Gender is nearly equal and the race of volunteers tends to reflect the different ethnic and racial composition of the rural area. Preexisting education varies from area to area, but in general the EMS volunteer has a higher accrued level of education than the average citizen.[6]

After considering the time requirements, training expectations, and job stresses of working in sometimes dangerous and unpredictable conditions, one might wonder why people volunteer at all for these positions. Additionally, the current economic environment often requires two incomes in a family, making spare time a very valuable commodity. When volunteer EMS providers are asked why they do it, often the answer is altruistic. A chance to give back to one's community, to insure and take part in the health care of family, neighbors, and friends, and the ability to belong and make a difference are the most common answers.[6] This is perhaps best illustrated in a study of volunteers queried on possible incentives to facilitate and increase recruitment and retention. Continuing education, financial assistance, tax credits, and health benefits were the most popular options expressed ranging from 60–64%, with "cash awards" trailing at the bottom at 34% (see table 4.1).[7]

Systems have applied this information to successful recruitment and retention programs. While early adulthood is the most common age group in volunteer EMS services, there are other age groups to be considered. Youth, teens, and the retired elderly share increased amounts of available free time. Cadet programs such as those in the fire service and the civil air patrol can utilize young providers in roles appropriate for their maturity and abilities. These roles could include babysitting services (for members who would otherwise be excluded from availability due to lack of child care resources, particularly with limited time notice), and lifting help, which is sometimes needed for certain patients and situations. Including youth in a rural EMS system creates a natural progression into full active service, which is encouraged through exposure to EMS daily activities and calls, mock drills, and so on. The older volunteer can bring years of experience and sometimes a calming influence to certain circumstances. As it takes a village to raise a child, it takes a team to effectively provide prehospital care, particularly in the rural environment.

Volunteer services also encourage and promote community involvement by the honor, respect, and tradition they bestow on the community. By displaying the service or squad patch, the volunteers are showing daily their allegiance and commitment to the community. The pride with which these are worn is reflected in the faces of volunteers, and is a good advertisement for initial discussion of recruitment. These are not without cost, and financial assistance in the form of the provision of jackets or uniform shirts can be an added incentive to join or stay with an organization.

Volunteerism remains the cornerstone of rural EMS, although current economic restraints sometimes require paid-volunteer assistance for shifts that remain uncovered. To retain volunteers, one must address and attempt to meet the needs of the volunteer as best as possible. An informal or formal needs assessment of what keeps people on and common reasons for leaving can go a long way. Community-based need, admission criteria, high visibility, strong medical oversight, interagency cooperation, a formal organizational structure, sound business operation, personal success, and a cohesive community environment have been found as characteristics and attributes of successful rural systems.[6] Creativity, ingenuity, enthusiasm, and persistence have always been the hallmarks of EMS, and are necessary factors for continued survival in the changing healthcare arena.

State and the federal government should work with local systems to provide leadership and technical support, through financial assistance with training, supplies, and equipment, or through health and retirement benefits. Leadership training, critical incident stress management services, safety training, and general information dissemination regarding successful programs are of value to rural EMS systems, and are often difficult for local systems to provide on their own.

Educational Systems

Educational issues can be divided into two broad categories with respect to rural EMS. The first involves a discussion of what level of technician is most appropriate and the second involves training and maintaining technicians to a standard level of education and performance.

Rural systems are typically dependent on volunteers or a mixture of paid and volunteer providers. Most rural EMS systems provide services based on the EMT-Basic level or below. The scope of practice of the level of technician is typically set by the state. Most states allow EMT-Basic to defibrillate and treat medical and traumatic conditions with basic life support maneuvers. In some rural areas these basic-level

TABLE 4.1			
Perceived Effectiveness of Incentives			
INCENTIVES	VERY EFFECTIVE	MODERATELY EFFECTIVE	NOT EFFECTIVE
Cash Awards	34%	35%	31%
Community Awards	46%	48%	6%
Continuing Education	64%	28%	8%
Health Benefits	60%	32%	8%
Tax Credits	64%	26%	10%
Pension Plan	50%	31%	19%
Life Insurance	32%	44%	24%

technicians are backed up by providers at the EMT-Intermediate or Paramedic level. These advanced technicians are uncommon in rural settings, due to the increased educational and training requirements.

Currently there is much debate on what level of provider is needed in rural environments and what skills and training are realistic for rural environments given the constraints placed on volunteer providers. From a cardiac arrest perspective, the most important link for initial EMS response and treatment is based on early activation, early CPR, and early defibrillation. Many rural EMS systems can never achieve recommended response times due to geographical limitations. From a trauma perspective, basic level care can have a positive impact on patient outcome, but there are still issues of response times and facility resources required for the critically injured.

Triage and appropriate transport of patients can significantly influence the availability of rural EMS resources. Systems are often required to transport patients who may not need urgent or emergent medical care; the inability to determine this status at the scene leaves the community uncovered while the nonemergent patient is transported to receive a formal medical evaluation. The Red River Project in New Mexico is an example of how a rural EMS system uses paramedics with advanced decision-making and technical skills to provide a higher level of service within a rural community, decreasing the number of long transports.[8] Urban systems typically do not transport 20 to 40% of their patients, and therefore more advanced decision-making skills of paramedics may be justified in rural settings. However, the advanced procedural skills that these paramedics possess will be infrequently used in the rural setting, and over time are difficult to maintain.

The Department of Transportation (DOT) national standard curricula contain the suggested initial training requirements of the various EMS technician levels. These requirements are typically formalized at the state level, with many states adopting the DOT standards verbatim. Education takes place at various locations and institutions; many states provide initial education through the community college system, while others provide courses at the community level. Many rural communities do not have access to postsecondary educational institutions at all. Initial training for many provider levels also requires a significant amount of training within a hospital or clinic setting. Rural communities often do not have these resources,

thus forcing students to travel significant distances to complete clinical precepting requirements.

Rural technicians who do receive training at the more advanced levels are less likely to stay in rural areas, due to financial constraints, they often find opportunities are much more prevalent in urban settings.

Continuing education is another serious issue in rural EMS systems, as more requirements are being placed on EMS systems by federal and state agencies. Additionally, the trend is for more advanced care to be provided at lower technician levels. For example, EMT-Bs now defibrillate with automated defibrillators and this skill requires ongoing education in addition to the normal EMT-B continuing education program. Other requirements, such as blood-borne pathogen training and vehicle safety, require more time and commitment.

Access to continuing education is a significant problem for many rural systems. Both the quality and content of continuing education programs are dependent on the quality of the teachers and the availability of teaching resources. Technology is beginning to improve this problem Internet or video educational packages are still in their infancy and many rural EMS systems do not yet have internet access. Montana and South Dakota have developed internet-based continuing education programs for their rural systems. The TENKIDS project provides every local EMS system in Montana with a multimedia computer plus access to an electronic bulletin board and CD-ROM training programs.[9]

The FARMEDIC program was created in 1981 in New York State to train fire, rescue, and EMS providers in planning for agricultural emergencies. The course is now offered nationally, teaching providers how to assist patients who have been exposed to farm-related trauma due to machinery, confined spaces, chemicals, animals, electricity, and weather. Providers are trained in the management of tractor injuries, power take-off entanglements, pesticide toxicities, and silo fires. Other programs have been developed with rural EMS in mind: the Basic Trauma Life Support and PreHospital Trauma Life Support courses provide trauma care training to EMT-Bs.[10]

In summary, rural EMS systems require innovative approaches to education that address quality, content, and accessibility for both initial training and continuing education. Problems that must be addressed include a limited student pool with a lower level of formal education, training scheduled around the full-time careers of volunteers, a small number of qualified instructors, insufficient educational materials and resources, limited access to healthcare facilities for clinical experience, limited exposure to clinical conditions and patient presentations, difficulties in skill maintenance due to low volumes (especially relating to children), limited physician supervision, and limited quality management of educational programs. The federal and state governments must work with rural agencies to develop strategies to address these issues. Distance learning can significantly assist rural systems if the financial resources are provided.

Communication Systems and Public Access

Communications systems within rural communities related to EMS services are often lacking. While currently about 85% of the U.S. population is covered by 9-1-1 and 95% of all 9-1-1 services by population are E-9-1-1, only about 50% of the geography has 9-1-1 services and only 25% of the geography has E-9-1-1 service. This means that much of the nation's rural territory does not have 9-1-1 service, and many rural dispatchers lack the ability to automatically locate a caller. Systems without 9-1-1 often do have a single seven-digit EMS access number, but the correct number must be dialed.

Dispatch capabilities are generally less developed in rural communities. Very few rural EMS agencies use emergency medical dispatch systems that allows dispatchers to define the emergency and provide the appropriate EMS response and prearrival instructions based on the problem. This situation could significantly impact systems when response times are very long. The ability to determine the appropriate level of care will significantly improve rural system resource utilization and prolong the life of the volunteer labor force.

Rural EMS is also much less developed with respect to internal communications capabilities. The ability to talk between the dispatch center and the crew is often limited due to dated technology; and the ability to transmit data, such as a 12-lead ECG, is typically nonexistent in rural settings. A survey in 1999 by the National Association of State EMS Directors identified the communications infrastructure as the area of greatest need financially for rural systems.[11] Innovative communication approaches using satellite and internet-based technology can provide telemedicine services, distance learning and an environment for improved information exchange and educational opportunities.

Integration of Health Services and Prevention

Integration in the health services refers to the linkage of EMS services to other community health and public health initiatives. The goal is to provide a higher degrees of continuity of services and efficiency. Historically EMS has been linked to the public safety sector along with law enforcement and the fire service. EMS must be more formally linked to the healthcare system to ensure that patients are referred or transported to the most appropriate facility. Healthcare initiatives, including injury prevention, must incorporate EMS services. In many states, EMS injury prevention and public health initiatives are already ongoing. Rural systems have a greater potential for success in this arena than urban systems due to the relatively low call volume and their integration within the community. As an example the Red River Project in New Mexico successfully included an immunization program into its service.[8] The Welcome to the World Project in Orange County, North Carolina involved visits to the homes of newborns incorporating a home safety check with the distribution of public health educational materials about injuries to newborns and toddlers.[12] It should be pointed out that these initiatives should not interfere with the services that systems primarily provide; research is needed to better define potential in this arena.

At the federal level, there are existing initiatives to promote innovative hospital conversions, such as essential access community hospitals, rural primary care hospitals, limited service hospitals, and medical assistance facilities, which recognize the importance of integrating EMS as part of the overall system of care in rural areas.

Information Systems, Evaluation, and Research

From a scientific perspective, there is very little objective information describing rural EMS systems from an evaluation or quality-management perspective. Urban systems are just now beginning to capture data using standard elements and definitions. EMS quality management is in its infancy, with neither real definitions yet established for outcomes nor defined evaluation tools.

Rural EMS compounds these problem due to limited personnel, equipment, and expertise. Rural EMS providers generally have limited training regarding

EMS quality management methods. Most rural providers are volunteers who participate for social and community-based objectives. There is an importance placed on the quality of care, but typically not on documentation. Many rural EMS services do not bill patients for their services, further decreasing the incentives to document. All EMS systems should have a formalized record-keeping system that allows system and patient information to be captured in a defined, standardized way. The NHTSA Pre-Hospital Dataset identifies and defines what information local systems should be collecting.[13]

Even as information is being collected by rural systems, it typically resides in paper form only. Resources and skills required for computerized data entry and analysis are typically not available. Federally, NHTSA and the EMS-C program have promoted the use of data and quality management within EMS. Many states have developed, or are in the process of developing, statewide information systems from which rural EMS systems can benefit. As with any other component of the healthcare system, EMS must continually evaluate and measure itself through quality-improvement initiatives that are data driven.

Public Education

All community and public health initiatives, including injury prevention, require the public to have an understanding of a concept and be willing to act in a positive manner. Examples include knowing when and how to call 9-1-1, when and how to do CPR, how to properly install a child car seat, and how to provide safety protection in the home a toddler. EMS is in a unique setting to contribute positively to these initiatives, since EMS agencies and providers are typically well known and respected in the community. It has also been shown that the public has very little understanding of the capabilities and services provided by EMS. Because of the low call volumes most rural EMS systems experience, the opportunity to work within the community to promote itself and improve community health can be invaluable. This exposure can also lead to increased community awareness, improved fundraising capabilities, and improved membership recruitment and retention.

Legislation and Regulation

National agencies, federal and state government, and jurisdictional statutes and regulations all affect rural systems. At the federal level, provider curricula and system requirements define EMS systems and their personnel. National organizations define the sizes and shapes of ambulances, the equipment they carry, and methods of communication. State governments promulgate the EMS laws that each system and provider must follow. County and city ordinances and franchise agreements define the service areas and functions of many systems. Governmental entities and national organizations also provide resources to rural systems either in the form of information or services.

Rural systems are often at odds with urban systems regarding many of these requirements, laws, and regulations. As the EMS scope of practice expands, rural systems are often placed in difficult positions. Educational and equipment requirements may be increased when rural systems are already stretched to their limits. In most rural settings, the ability to provide advanced-level care is dependent upon educational and equipment requirements set in standards or regulations. As urban systems become more complex, many rural systems are negatively affected. Although rural systems have gradually moved to more advanced level providers as the system matures, increased regulatory requirements have forced some rural systems to move back to less advanced levels of care due to increased federal and state regulations.[14] EMS lead agencies at the federal and state level must understand the needs and unique qualities of rural systems when law and policy are drafted.

System Finance

Rural EMS was born as, and to a great degree still exists as, a community resource often provided at no cost to the individual patient; since the early 1990s, EMS systems have had no federal support outside of rare grant opportunities. Urban systems have migrated to a fee-based structure, and that transition is now taking place in rural systems. Historically, EMS has been unable to obtain cost-based reimbursement for services. First, EMS must provide significantly more resources than are needed at any one time to have an acceptable response time within the community. Even urban systems are rarely busy more than 40% of the time because of this preparedness model.[1] Second, federal reimbursement through Medicare has always taken into account issues such as prevailing historic rates and other factors that negatively affect most rural EMS systems. Rural systems typically have high operational costs to maintain reasonable response times. Transport times are considerably longer than urban settings and utilization rates of the personnel and equipment are typically much lower than in urban systems.

In the past, financial issues have been addressed through barbeques, chicken dinners, or other fundraising events. Over the past several years, the cost and complexity of prehospital systems in terms of equipment, training, and care expectations have increased exponentially, leading to many creative finance strategies. As personnel requirements increase and as the ability of a volunteer to leave his primary job to respond decreases, many rural systems have been subsidized by the local governmental entity. For example, a county may hire paid staff to cover daytime, weekday hours for a volunteer service so that its membership can work at their primary occupations. Hospitals in rural northern New York State hire providers to work in the facilities and respond in the field during daytime working hours. From a cost perspective, rural systems have been very creative in supplementing their fundraisers. Subscription programs are successful in many areas. A subscription program allows citizens or families within the community to pay a small amount of money to the rural system in return for service they would need during the year. Subscription programs require that the EMS system bill those who are not subscribers. Other systems receive tax subsidies from the local government either at the county or city level. Finally, many systems are billing for services directly to customers and/or healthcare providers. Despite these efforts, the reimbursement rural systems receive is typically inadequate, and most operate in extreme financial duress.

Recent rulemaking activity by the Center for Medicare and Medicaid Services (CMS) regarding ambulance reimbursement has attempted to address these issues. The new payment plan for Medicare participants provides EMS reimbursement regardless of prevailing or historic rates. In the past, billing Medicare often provided little or no reimbursement since prevailing and historic rates were very low (due to volunteer, no-fee services) and inadequately measured the costs associated with long transport distances. Implementation of the new reimbursement method may begin as early as 2002; while this new reimbursement strategy is an improvement for most rural EMS systems, it is still not based on a cost-based valuation of services.

Medical Oversight

Medical oversight is one of the most significant issues facing rural EMS. Rural systems are typically isolated from healthcare facilities and from physicians experienced or interested in EMS. It has only been since the 1996 publication of the EMS Agenda for the Future that the importance of medical oversight has been documented and institutionalized. Medical oversight for rural EMS systems is often done with little, if any, compensation, since the system is typically volunteer-based. Medical oversight is needed in all aspects of EMS: initial training, protocol development, quality assurance, resource planning and utilization, continuing education, community relations, and clinical care. Each of the attributes described in the EMS Agenda for the Future and in this chapter can benefit from physician oversight. Shortages of physicians in rural areas are a significant barrier, and many rural systems must look for alternatives to local medical oversight, through regional or statewide oversight systems, physician extenders such as Physician Assistants or Nurse Practitioners, or a combination of both.[15] These physician extenders can perform a variety of medical oversight functions, including case reviews, continuing education, and quality management, either in conjunction with physicians, or as medical directors.

The National Association of EMS Physicians (NAEMSP), the National Association of State EMS Directors (NASEMSD) and the American College of Emergency Physicians (ACEP) have developed documents to assist rural systems in the recruitment and training of medical directors.[2] NAEMSP has developed a four-day medical director course designed to prepare a physician for EMS oversight. This course is designed both for urban and rural medical directors. NHTSA, in conjunction with NAEMSP, has also completed the curriculum for a one-day medical oversight course which can be tailored to rural EMS issues. A few states currently provide courses as well.

Clinical Care

EMS is beginning to evolve as a business model within the healthcare system. Defining "who is the customer" and "what is the product" are key to the future of rural EMS. The customer could be defined as the community or, more important, the individual patient. The product could be a service such as transportation or public safety, but more important is clinical care. To provide a quality product (clinical care), each of the attributes discussed in this chapter must intertwine and work as a system. Clinical care must be defined, and in a rural setting this can be difficult, since rural EMS has been defined typically as transportation. Clinical care could be defined in this manner, but quality clinical care may not require transportation and the system may actually be negatively affected if every patient is transported. EMS systems must work with the community, the medical director, the state EMS agency, and their patients to identify what services are of most benefit and how best to provide those. This process, which should be data driven through accepted quality-management principles, requires resources that rural systems seldom possess. State and federal agencies must provide tools and resources for rural EMS quality management and evaluation.

System Issues

Several system issues are important with respect to rural EMS. Traditional EMS delivery models have been proposed and implemented, based on two EMS encounter types: trauma and cardiac arrest. Based on these encounters, the need for a rapid response is delineated and the needed skills, equipment, and personnel are defined. Current guidelines for response times of less than five minutes for early defibrillation in cardiac arrest and eight-minute response times for advanced medical care are unrealistic for rural EMS environments and are not scientifically proven. EMS must make system-based decisions that take into account the entire patient population and the spectrum of complaint categories they will experience, while considering the overall financial picture of the system. There are national guidelines that describe the ideal EMS response to trauma, stroke, cardiac arrest, pediatric emergencies, seizures, and head injuries; these are guidelines and not standards of care. All EMS systems must evaluate themselves to assure that essential components are in place and functioning adequately, before less essential components are added. An example would be the addition of 12-lead ECG capabilities before all first responders have automated external defibrillators. By improving the overall system performance, each of these targeted issues can be addressed. Federal and state agencies should assist rural EMS in making these decisions and promote a systems approach to quality patient care.

Many rural systems have developed creative implementation schemes to address rural issues. The Red River Project trained paramedics with community health skills who respond into their community and often transport the patient back to the EMS station for further evaluation and treatment rather than to a distant hospital.[8] Orange County, North Carolina created an EMS structure where paramedic level care was separated from transport. Using Emergency Medical Dispatch criteria, paramedics are often sent to calls in nontransport vehicles without an ambulance. On scene, the paramedics evaluate the patient through protocols and direct medical oversight to determine if the patient should be transported by the paramedics, transported by less advanced personnel, transported by private vehicle, or treated and released to medical follow-up. It is important to note that both of these examples were implemented with great detail to training, education, quality management, and medical oversight.

Rural systems should not consider themselves islands, but should instead have mutual aid agreements with other adjacent systems, public safety agencies, search-and-rescue teams, air-transport services, and special rescue teams. The limited resources of a rural system may be easily overwhelmed by a single motor vehicle crash. It is better to activate mutual aid plans early and then cancel responding resources if they are not needed, than to activate too late.

Rural EMS must also consider the resources that exist at the hospital level. Rural hospitals may not have the necessary resources and services for the entire gamut of emergencies expected in a rural environment. Neighboring rural hospitals, air medical services, and other community resources should be identified and incorporated into operational procedures as needed to account for local deficiencies.

Finally, many rural areas are impacted by tourists, festivals, and other special events and mass gatherings. Rural EMS systems should identify and anticipate these situations and create a mass gathering plan that can be implemented as needed.

Summary

The goal of each rural EMS system is to provide the best service delivery model and the best clinical care to its customers, who are its patients and its community. Each rural EMS system is unique, based on hundreds of variables, and is further complicated by the fact that these variables can change often and without warning. Whether the issues are based on resources, patient volumes, geography, technology challenges, volunteer or providers issues, medical oversight, politics, education, communications, or financial concerns, each system can use the innovation EMS was born with, to create and provide patient care. EMS is alive and well despite some current weaknesses, and will be there when other areas of health care fail. EMS is the true safety net of the health care system, even in the rural environment.

References

1. Stout JL. System status management: the strategy of ambulance placement. *JEMS*. 1983;8(5):22–32.
2. National Association of State EMS Directors. Challenges of Rural Emergency Medical Services: Opinion Survey of State EMS Directors. 2000. Available at http://www.nasemed.org
3. Rogers FB, Shackford SR, Osler RM, Vane DW, Davis JH. Rural trauma: the challenge for the next decade. *J Trauma*. 1999;47:802–821.
4. Vane DW, Shedd FG, Grosfeld JK, et al. An analysis of pediatric trauma deaths in Indiana. *J Ped Surg*. 1990;25:955–960.
5. *Emergency Medical Services: Agenda for the Future.* Washington, DC: National Highway Traffic Safety Administration; 1996.
6. Reich J. The rural route to success: comparing EMS in three Alabama counties. *JEMS*. 1991;16(2):53–56.
7. Thompson A. Rural emergency volunteers and their communities: a demographic comparison. *J Comm Health*. 1993;18:379–392.
8. Shoup S. Red River project: expanded scope program for New Mexico medics. *JEMS*. 1995;20(12):43–47.
9. Anonymous. TENKIDS: a virtual EMS community. *JEMS*. 1999;24(12):44–51, 78.
10. Hill DE. FARMEDIC: a systematic approach to train rural EMS, fire, and rescue personnel at the grassroots level. *J Agromed*. 1994;1:57–64.
11. Mears G. New insight into rural EMS. *NAEMSP News*. 2000;9(4):8–9.
12. Overby B, Mears G, Christian L. Implementation of an EMS expanded scope project for injury prevention: welcome to the world [abstract]. *J Emerg Nursing*. Dec 1999;25:461–462.
13. *Uniform Pre-Hospital Emergency Medical Services (EMS) Data Conference: Final Report.* Washington, DC: National Highway Traffic Safety Administration; 1994.
14. Ott JS. The Wyoming experiment: rural EMS issues, needs, problems and actions. *JEMS*. 1993;18(2):46–52.
15. Johnson R. The PA's role in rural EMS education. *J Am Acad Physician Assistants*. 1990;3:429–432.

Additional Readings:
1. Brown LH, Prasad H, Grimmer K. Public perceptions of a rural emergency medical services system. *Prehospital Disaster Med*. 1994;9:257–259.
2. Garrison HG, Foltin G, Becker L, et al: Consensus statement: the role of out-of-hospital emergency medical services in primary injury prevention. *Consensus Workshop on the Role of EMS in Injury Prevention. Final Report.* Arlington, VA; August 25–26, 1995.
3. Johnson JC. Prehospital care: the future of emergency medical services. *Ann Emerg Med*. 1991;20:426–430.
4. Pullum JD, Nels D, Sanddal MS, Obbink K. Training for rural prehospital providers: a retrospective analysis from Montana. *Prehosp Emerg Care*. 1999;3:231–238.
5. Anonymous. Rural ambulance teams may not get enough practice to maintain sophisticated lifesaving skills. *Research Activities*. 1996;10:194.
6. *Rural and Frontier Emergency Medical Services Toward the Year 2000.* Washington, D.C.: National Rural Health Association; 1997.
7. US General Accounting Office. *Rural Development: Profile of Rural Areas.* Washington, DC: Congressional Office of Technology Assessment; 1989. Publication OTA-H-445.
8. US Congress, Office of Technology Assessment. *Rural Emergency Medical Services.* Special Report, Stock No. 052-033-011735. Washington, DC: US Government Printing Office; 1989.

Wilderness

Keith Conover, MD

Introduction

In the 1960s, prehospital care in the U.S. was in its infancy. The idea of taking the hospital to the patient was not yet well accepted by the public or by the medical community, and neither were the practitioners of this new discipline, both field providers and their physician supervisors, sure of the best way forward.

This early and fragmented EMS system was a hotbed of experimentation and innovation. EMS was carving out a new niche for itself—starting as a tiny new concept, wedged in the cracks between the existing medical system and public safety sectors. At the beginning, neither medicine, as practiced in offices and hospitals, nor the established public safety system, as carried out by fire and police services, recognized EMS as a significant partner in their day-to-day business. EMS practitioners at all levels deeply felt the need for more professionalism, more standards, more universal availability, and above all, more respect for the idea of EMS.

As the bulk of this text confirms, forty years later, all has changed. But even in the early part of the 21st century, wilderness EMS is much like "street" EMS in the 1960s—neither well accepted nor well understood, full of experiments and inventions, but lacking standardization, a universal presence, and respect. Indeed, some have argued that wilderness EMS really doesn't exist, as the "street" EMS system is adequate to meet all of a wilderness patient's needs. A central goal of this chapter is to lay out and describe the discipline of wilderness EMS, and to argue that, indeed, there *is* a discipline of wilderness EMS, and that it is, to a degree, separate and distinct from "street" EMS. This is not to say that practitioners of "street" EMS cannot or should not also practice wilderness EMS—

only that delivering high-quality prehospital care in the backcountry often requires slightly different planning, equipment, guidelines, protocols, and medical oversight than "street" EMS.

Wilderness EMS in the Interstices

In the 1960s, EMS fit between the medical and public safety sectors. In the opening years of the 21st century, wilderness EMS fits between the search-and-rescue, wilderness medicine, and EMS sectors (fig. 5.1, table 5.1). While most readers of this text are familiar with the discipline of EMS, search-and-rescue

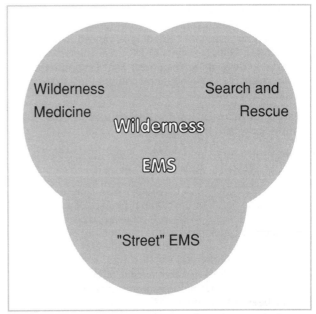

FIGURE 5.1. *Wilderness EMS, as a discipline, includes aspects of medicine, prehospital emergency medical services, and search-and-rescue. Contacts for lead organizations in each field are listed in Table 5.1.*

---

*Portions of this chapter have been adapted, with permission, from copyrighted materials of The Wilderness EMS Institute

TABLE 5.1

Selected lead organizations in disciplines related to wilderness EMS (listed alphabetically)

ASTM Committee F-30 on Emergency Medical Services
100 Barr Harbor Drive
West Conshohocken, PA 19428-2959
(610) 832-9500
http://www.astm.org/COMMIT/F30.htm

ASTM, originally the American Society for Testing and Materials, is an international standards-setting organization. Within the field of wilderness EMS, ASTM has developed documents that specify the scope of practice and training for the Wilderness First Responder. Committee F-30 has also considered such standards for the Wilderness EMT level.

Maryland Institute for Emergency Medical Services Systems (MIEMSS)
653 W. Pratt Street, Baltimore, MD 21201-1536
410-706-5074
http://miemss.umaryland.edu/Home.htm

Maryland is one of several states that are incorporating wilderness EMS into the state EMS system. The Maryland Wilderness EMS protocols are available on-line.

Mountain Rescue Association
P.O. Box 501
Poway, CA 92074-0501
http://www.mra.org

The teams and regions of the Mountain Rescue Association, generally regarded as the elite of the wilderness search-and-rescue community in the U.S., have a long history of providing advanced medical care in the field. Members of MRA teams were instrumental in developing Wilderness First Responder and Wilderness EMT training, and continue this tradition today.

National Association for Search and Rescue
4500 Southgate Place, Suite 100
Chantilly, VA 20151-1714
(703) 222-6277
http://www.nasar.org/

In the 1970s, NASAR's Emergency Medicine Committee was instrumental in developing the idea of a (then-called) Wilderness Medical Technician course. Later curriculum development efforts moved to other organizations, such as independent WEMT training schools, the Wilderness EMS Institute, and the Wilderness Medical Society. Later, NASAR offered proprietary Wilderness EMT training programs; however, these have been discontinued.

National Cave Rescue Commission
National Speleological Society
2813 Cave Avenue
Huntsville, AL 35810-4431
256-852-1300
http://www.caves.org/~ncrc/

The National Cave Rescue Commission, and particularly its Eastern Region, has long been a proponent of advanced medical care in the field. NCRC cave rescue physicians and other NCRC professionals have had significant input into the content of wilderness prehospital training, including WEMSI and other WEMT curricula.

Wilderness EMS Institute
Department of Emergency Medicine
Mercy Hospital of Pittsburgh
Pittsburgh, PA 15219-5166
http://www.wemsi.org

WEMSI started with the goal of developing a detailed, peer-reviewed medical curriculum for SAR team EMTs and paramedics, carrying on the work started by the Emergency Medicine Committee of NASAR. WEMSI has since expanded this mission to include promoting model wilderness EMS systems design, research, and development of a curriculum for physicians who provide medical direction for SAR team EMTs and paramedics. The WEMSI curriculum is currently used by SAR and EMS organizations in several countries for their training. WEMSI's curricula, although still in development, are available to organizations who wish to use them to run Wilderness EMT and Wilderness Command Physician training courses. The 130-page Wilderness EMT Course Guide and Lesson Plans may be downloaded free of charge from the WEMSI web site.

Wilderness Medical Society
3595 E. Fountain Blvd., Suite A-1
Colorado Springs, CO 80910
(719) 572-9255
http://www.wms.org

The WMS is described above in some detail. It is primarily an organization of physicians, and for the most part, most are not active in EMS locally or at a national level. However, a focus of the WMS is on the first-aid and medical training of trip leaders and SAR team members, and the WMS has been active particularly in trying to standardize Wilderness First Responder training throughout the 1990s.

and wilderness medicine are also disciplines in their own right, each with an accumulated body of expertise, standards, training, and national organizations.

The term "search-and-rescue" (SAR) encompasses many activities: searching for ships or aircraft lost at sea, kayaks overturned in a whitewater river, or miners trapped after an explosion; hostage rescue; rescue during battle; rescue from sunken submarines; rescue from buildings that have collapsed or are on fire; or rescue from crushed vehicles. Each has its own domain of expert knowledge and resources, and through its close association with fire-rescue, EMS providers generally have or can get training in fire, building, and vehicle rescue. The National Association for Search and Rescue (NASAR) is a central resource for further information about all such types of SAR.

Many EMS providers become involved in SAR in a much prosaic setting, with hikers, hunters, children, or the demented elderly who become lost or injured in the woods or hills. Many rural and suburban areas have dedicated search-and-rescue teams that deal with such situations. Some are affiliated with EMS agencies, some are part of police or sheriff's departments, and some are independent. Some such teams subspecialize in particular situations, such as mountain rescue, cliff rescue, cave rescue, and whitewater rescue. But the general art and science of searching for and rescuing people in the outdoors, as with the other types of SAR listed above, have become a specific domain of expertise. There are universally accepted core principles and practices, and national and state standards, training, and certification. In many ways, the "SAR system" for inland ground search-and-rescue parallels the EMS system.

One outstanding example is the SAR system in Virginia, which has state standards and training for SAR personnel.[1] Over the past 20 years, improved SAR in Virginia has cut the time to find and rescue those lost or injured in the backcountry, with a corresponding decrease in mortality and morbidity.

Wilderness Medicine

With the founding of the Wilderness Medical Society in 1983, wilderness medicine became a recognized medical domain of expertise, with the *Journal of Wilderness Medicine*, later renamed *The Journal of Wilderness and Environmental Medicine* as its core scholarly journal. To quote the Wilderness Medical Society's web site: "Wilderness medicine focuses on medical problems and treatment in remote environments. It includes aspects of physiology, clinical medicine, preventive medicine, and public health. While wilderness medicine shares many interests and methods with other specialties such as sports medicine and emergency medicine, it incorporates a unique spectrum of topics and distinctive perspective that validate it as an individual field of study."

• • •

"Search and rescue are essential components of wilderness medicine. Heroism must be tempered by reality and the need to avoid creating more victims. Helicopters are frequently overrated in their ability to fly in any conditions, and, thus, dangerously overused. Search and rescue involves coordination and close interaction between emergency medical technicians (EMTs and paramedics), guides, and those with technical skills such as climbers, pilots, and physicians. Evacuation may take extended periods of time (hours to days), during which clinical problems must be actively managed, not merely stabilized as in urban protocols. This reliance on paramedical and non-medical personnel creates interesting problems in training and medical control. As a result, Wilderness EMT programs have developed with new treatment protocols that allow more advanced intervention than urban protocols designed for short transport times. These proposed treatment standards can also be useful in remote rural areas that experience longer transport times."[2]

As one of the main organizations seeing wilderness EMS as part of its purview, the Wilderness Medical Society has been active in developing both the intellectual domain of wilderness EMS and standards for training out-of-hospital providers. The *Practice Guidelines for Wilderness Emergency Care*, now in its second edition, is arguably the definitive clinical standard of care for backcountry care.[3]

Traditions

No person hoping for success or understanding can ignore tradition, even within a relatively new discipline like EMS. WEMS, now that we grace it with its own acronym, is melding the institutional traditions of EMS, SAR, and wilderness medicine into its own unique institutional traditions.

EMS has a tradition that providers must follow rigid protocols, because they aren't smart enough, well trained enough, or in possession of enough clinical judgment to make decisions on their own. While this is a gross characterization that belies the experience and expertise of many out-of-hospital providers, this tradition has grown such that development of "protocols" is a critical part of the oversight of EMS. A focus on time-critical illness and injury, short transport times, and general assurance of communication with a physician help perpetuate this protocol-driven EMS tradition. EMS also has a tradition of concern with law and regulation related to what can and cannot be done by out-of-hospital providers.

The tradition in wilderness medicine and first aid is the precise opposite. Wilderness trip leaders and expedition medics expect to be presented with a variety of medical complaints, from time-critical to downright chronic, to have to care for their patients for many hours or days, and, until the recent spread of cellular telephones, to never being able to speak with a physician. The wilderness medicine community isn't particularly concerned about scope of practice or EMS regulations, although they are indeed concerned about tort liability under common law.

As wilderness EMS matures, it, as with EMS before it, is starting to develop its own traditions—a blending of the traditions of EMS and wilderness medicine. While still fluid and evolving, and always at odds with some EMS, SAR, or wilderness medicine traditions, some of the central ones seem to be as follows:

- **Patient care is central**—Do not let worries about scope of practice regulations, state laws, or common-law liability principles result in bad patient care. "If you deliver bad care, or withhold good care, because of some supposed law or regulation, you're at great legal risk." (Personal communication: Earl W. Maxwell, WV State Prosecuting Attorney.)

- **Work with the system**—Coordinate as closely as possible with the existing EMS and SAR systems, and work to change them as needed to allow good patient care in the wilderness context.

- **Preventing delayed morbidity is our job**— "Street" EMS providers seldom have to worry about their patients' developing dehydration, starvation, hypothermia, renal failure, decubitus ulcers, or deep venous thrombi during transport. But these considerations are central to caring for patients in the wilderness context, which can last for hours or days. In some ways,

wilderness EMS is more like intensive-care-unit nursing than like street EMS or even Emergency Department care.

- **Physician oversight is key**—If wilderness EMS providers are expected to be able to deal with difficult and critical decision-making in the field, they need the best information they can get. For non-physician providers, this means they need help from physicians. Physicians should be integral to wilderness EMS providers' training, and should interact regularly with providers in reviewing cases and providing continuing education. Whenever possible—and this is increasingly possible as we enter the 21st century—wilderness EMS providers should have access to real-time physician advice. Physicians involved with wilderness EMS providers must, however, be familiar with the providers' training, weather and terrain constraints, and limitations of the search-and-rescue environment. Advice need not be limited to EMS physicians; it is reasonable (and now fairly common), especially during a many-hour evacuation, for an EMS physician to get a specialty physician, such as a neurosurgeon, trauma surgeon, or ophthalmologist on-line to provide additional advice to the provider.

- **Use common sense**—It used to be the tradition that EMS providers were supposed to leave their common-sense judgment at the door of the classroom, and to follow books and protocols. "We aren't here to make you into mini-doctors" was the opening remark at one of the first EMT classes ever conducted. (Personal communication, Richard F. Edlich, M.D., Ph.D., Charlottesville VA, February 1975.) Wilderness providers, however, are expected to marshal whatever knowledge and skills that they have, from whatever sources, to make the best patient-care decisions they can, often without physician support or oversight. "Personnel providing medical care should follow their first-aid or emergency medical training except in those specific situations covered in these protocols. In situations not covered by these protocols or by previous training, personnel must use their best judgment."[4]

- **Be flexible**—In EMS texts and in EMS classes, and to a lesser extent in "street" EMS practice, there is an official way to manage almost any situation, often embedded in written protocols. In the wilderness context, that is not so. Decision-making is more complex, and often requires picking the least of several evils. An example would be due to the danger to the patient and the team from an approaching cold front and storm, deciding to "clear" a cervical spine and move a trauma patient without waiting hours for immobilization gear to arrive, despite some mild midline neck tenderness and a mildly diminished mental status due to hypothermia.

The wilderness chapter in the first edition of this text detailed the various roots of what is now a true, if young, wilderness EMS discipline and tradition— mountaineering medicine, wilderness first-aid, early developments in mountain and cave rescue medicine, and the early development of a Wilderness Medical Technician curriculum by the later-defunct Emergency Medicine Committee of NASAR, and later development of the Wilderness EMT curricula by SOLO (North Conway, NH—formerly Stonehearth Open Learning Opportunities), the Wilderness EMS Institute, and others. In the interim, the field has developed enough of a consensus that such a survey is no longer needed, and those interested in historical roots of wilderness EMS are referred to that first edition chapter.

Wilderness EMS Protocols

Wilderness EMS is neither EMS, nor SAR, nor wilderness medicine, but rather the intersection of EMS, SAR, and wilderness medicine. If one is pressed to define it briefly, one might say that wilderness EMS is emergency backcountry medical care, following recognized standards established by the wilderness medicine community, provided by members of SAR teams, and EMS physician oversight of this care. While not all-encompassing, this definition does capture the major WEMS contributions of each of the three communities.

Wilderness EMS includes management of patients over extended periods, and treatment of exposure, trauma, shock, and infections, and can include the use of drugs, intravenous lines, and other invasive procedures. As with "street" EMS, wilderness EMS can be divided into different phases (see fig. 5.2). At the citizen first-aid level, at the first-responder level, and at the EMT-Basic/EMT-Paramedic level, proper

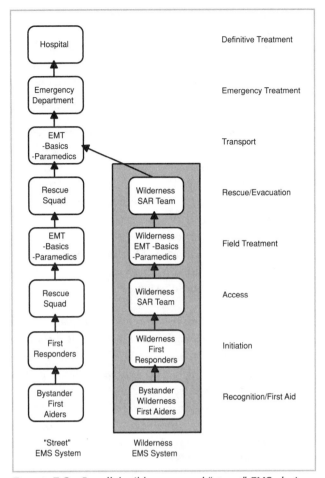

FIGURE 5.2. *Parallel wilderness and "street" EMS chains.*

backcountry care is for the most part similar to that on the street, though there are significant differences that can change patient outcome. Patients may cross over from the wilderness chain to the "street" chain at any point, but the ideal is to have those trained for the wilderness context caring for patients in the backcountry.

The operational necessities of wilderness EMS require different protocols and procedures than "street" EMS and, as described above, wide latitude for decision-making by wilderness EMS providers, with physician oversight whenever possible.

Central issues to be covered in wilderness EMS protocols include:

1. **Authority**—Who is authorizing wilderness EMS providers to care for patients? Under what physician's oversight and state laws or regulations?
2. **Scope**—Who can use these procedures and protocols? What kind of training do they need?

When can they use the procedures and protocols, and who decides?

3. **Dealing with Conflict**—What do wilderness EMS providers do when there are several different "street" and wilderness EMS providers at the scene, with different medical protocols?

The state of Maryland has recently instituted Wilderness EMS protocols that may provide some insight into an approach to these issues, as do the initial sections of the Wilderness EMS Institute (WEMSI) protocols.[5,6] The Operations Manual of the Wilderness EMS Institute, designed to serve a pilot program, outlines some systems issues for wilderness EMS and potential solutions.[4] This quotation from the WEMSI Operations Manual can serve as a focus for thinking about these issues:

1. *When faced with a patient care situation in the wilderness context, WEMSI-accredited Field Providers shall attempt to establish Medical Communication with, and obtain patient-specific medical control from, a WEMSI-accredited Wilderness Command Physician. If the delay in making such an attempt will adversely affect the patient, Field Providers may start acting on the basis of the WEMSI Protocols and Standing Orders. WEMSI Field Providers may accept patient-specific medical direction from a WEMSI Wilderness Command Physician only when there is Medical Communication between the Field Providers and the Wilderness Command Physician.*

2. *As used in this policy, Medical Communication is a specific and circumscribed term defined in the WEMSI Medical Communication Policy.*

3. *If unable to establish or maintain Medical Communication, WEMSI Field Providers shall use the WEMSI Protocols and WEMSI Standing Orders to guide their patient care; if the Protocols or Standing Orders do not address the problem at hand, Field Providers shall provide patient care in accordance with their training, their best judgment, and the patient's best interests, and shall continue attempting to establish Medical Communication.*

4. *WEMSI personnel are not authorized to act under remote or direct medical control of physicians who are not WEMSI-accredited Wilderness Command Physicians.*

5. *When in the wilderness context, WEMSI Field Providers shall turn patient care over to a licensed but non-WEMSI physician at the patient's side, if and only if said physician (a) identifies self by name and by state license number in writing, and (b) signs a statement accepting all responsibility for the patient's care on a continuing basis.*

6. *Once a patient is out of the wilderness context, WEMSI Field Providers are authorized to transfer patient care responsibility to (1) the physician directing a "street" EMS agency's (ground, air or water) ambulance crew, (2) a licensed physician in a health care facility, or (3) directly to a WEMS Wilderness Command Physician. A WEMSI Field Provider should continue to attend the patient and provide advice to the "street" EMS agency's physician and ambulance crew, except (1) when safety concerns dictate otherwise (e.g., aircraft payload limitations), or (2) the WEMSI Field Provider, preferably in consultation with a WEMSI Wilderness Command Physician, believes that the patient is stable, and that the WEMSI Field Provider's special training is unlikely to be needed during transportation to a health care facility.[4]*

The "Wilderness Context"

It may seem odd that a definition for the wilderness context appears so late in this chapter, but this is by design. Defining the wilderness context is not at all easy. Random House *Webster's Unabridged Dictionary* defines "wilderness" as follows:

1. a wild and uncultivated region, as of forest or desert, uninhabited or inhabited only by wild animals; a tract of wasteland.
2. a tract of land officially designated as such and protected by the U.S. government.
3. any desolate tract, as of open sea.

For those planning for wilderness EMS operations and training, this is not all that helpful. The Operations Policy Manual of the Wilderness EMS Institute suggests the following as a more workable definition:

Wilderness context for EMS: situations in which EMS delivery is complicated by one or more of the following four factors:

- *remoteness as far as logistics and access;*
- *a significant delay in the delivery of care to the patient;*
- *an environment that is stressful to both patients and rescuers; or*
- *lack of equipment and supplies.*

Certainly, one can look at EMS calls and pick out ones that almost anyone would agree are "wilderness calls," and then try to pick out the aspects that make them "wilderness-ish." Using this approach, one arrives at a list something like the following:

1. **Time**—Wilderness EMS operations take a long time.
2. **Distance**—Wilderness EMS is a long way from a road or helicopter landing zone (LZ).
3. **Limited Equipment**—Wilderness EMS providers have to make do, often for a long time, with what they can carry on their backs.
4. **Environment**—Wilderness EMS providers and their patients are exposed to a potentially hostile environment for significant periods.
5. **Terrain**—Wilderness EMS has to take place while a patient is evacuated across, or (in the case of a cave rescue) under and through, significantly rough terrain to a helicopter landing zone or roadhead. (SAR teams use the term "evacuation" for the process of getting a patient to the road or LZ, and "transportation" thereafter, a tradition that wilderness EMS has adopted.)

Wilderness vs. "Street" Protocols: Critical Decisions

Over the past five years or so, the definition of the "wilderness context" has changed significantly; a unique definition of "wilderness context" is really not necessary. Instead, what the system needs are good decisions about whether to follow "street" protocols and procedures, or wilderness EMS protocols and procedures. The EMS system procedures should require that this decision is made in the best interests of the patient—not necessarily an easy thing to do. Procedures are more likely to facilitate good decisions and good patient care if they embody the following principles:

1. *The decision should be made by a provider at the scene.* Those at the scene will have more and better information than someone on the other end of a cellular phone or radio.

2. *The decision should be made by the provider with the best understanding of the situation.* It is difficult, if not impossible, to decide ahead of time who is going to be the best decision-maker, but in line with the principle of allowing local decision-making at the scene, protocols can outline the principles of selecting a local decision-maker and allow those at the scene to use these principles to pick a decision-maker. The following principles apply:

   a. *Training and Certification Level*—The best decision-maker is generally the provider with the highest level of medical training. This doesn't necessarily mean the highest certification, or local EMS authorization; for the best decisions, a wilderness-trained EMS physician from outside the local area should outrank a local EMS agency EMT-Basic.

   b. *Wilderness-Specific Expertise*—Another concern is whether wilderness-specific training confers expertise beyond the training or certification level. For example, a wilderness-trained EMT-B might know more about hypothermia management than an EMT-P with no wilderness training or expertise.

   c. *SAR Expertise*—Decisions about wilderness vs. "street" protocols will often involve questions about the length of the evacuation, and hazards to team and patient; expertise in SAR is critical to such decisions.

3. *The decision should be made in consultation with a physician.* Ideally, this would be a wilderness-EMS and SAR-trained physician at the scene. An alternative is an on-line physician with wilderness expertise, or if necessary, an on-line physician with no wilderness expertise, who then should defer significantly to the domain expertise of those at the scene and act primarily as an advisor.

The decision about which protocols to follow—wilderness or "street"—must be made based on many different considerations. It is a clinical, medical decision, although requiring input about weather, terrain, resources, and other search-and-rescue factors. A few real examples will "bracket" the possibilities and make this more concrete:

1. On a fine summer day, a young man is riding a motorcycle on a backcountry trail about a half-mile from a major interstate highway, and sustains a leg injury. Local EMS personnel, including a wilderness EMT-P who is also a member of the local Mountain Rescue Association team, respond. The EMS crew determines that the patient has no injury except for a patella dislocation. "Street" EMS protocols require splinting and transporting, but wilderness protocols recommend an attempt at reduction. The wilderness EMT-P decides that calling out the entire Mountain Rescue Association team is unnecessary, even though it would allow him to work under wilderness protocols. However, reducing the patellar dislocation is easy, without significant risk, and will make the evacuation much easier on the patient. The wilderness EMT-P calls his (non-wilderness) EMS direct medical oversight physician, explains the situation, and requests that the physician consult with his Wilderness Command Physician and allow him to reduce the patellar dislocation to facilitate the evacuation. The EMS physician says, "We don't need to call your Wilderness Command Physician; since you're trained to reduce the dislocation, you can just take it as an order from me. Let me know if you have any problems."

2. A man, winter backpacking at dusk along a steep canyon, falls about 20 feet, landing on his right knee and developing severe pain in his right hip. Local SAR team WEMTs arrive, and diagnose a posterior hip dislocation with a fairly high reliability. They have been trained to reduce hip dislocations, but also have been taught how difficult the procedure can be. They discuss the case with their EMS on-line physician, and explain that the evacuation of about 30 to 45 minutes to a good helicopter LZ should be fairly easy. With the direct medical control physician, they jointly determine it would be best to provide analgesia, immobilize the hip (they have a full-body vacuum mattress instead of a backboard, which makes the process easier) and evacuate to the helicopter LZ, with an expected arrival at the hospital ED in about 1 to 2 hours.

3. An experienced caver is in a deep but very narrow canyon (about 1–3 feet wide) about a mile into a fairly difficult limestone cave. He starts ascending a rope but attaches one of his ascend-ers incorrectly. He falls backward about 5 to 10 feet, cracks his helmet, and sustains an injury to his left shoulder. EMTs with very basic cave rescue training (but not WEMT training) from the local EMS agency arrive, travel into the cave, immobilize the shoulder, provide some acetaminophen, food, water, and insulation, and await arrival of a cave rescue team. The cave rescue team includes an emergency physician, an orthopedic surgeon, and a variety of other EMS providers with cave rescue and WEMT training. Examination is difficult as the WEMT has to hang upside down from a seat harness in the narrow crevice to evaluate the patient. Using methods including army-surplus field phones for communication, the physicians and WEMTs decide that, despite the mechanism of injury and a potential distracting injury, the likelihood of an unstable cervical spine injury is low. Further, looking at the narrow, wet crevice and other passages leading out and up to the entrance, they realize that spinal immobilization could turn a 12- to 24-hour evacuation into a multi-day operation, with great risk to rescuers and patient alike from hypothermia, exhaustion, and subsequent injury in a hazardous environment. After due consideration, they decide to omit cervical immobilization. Once the patient has been moved gradually through the crevice for about 10 hours (in a seat harness), they reach an area large enough to perform a proper assessment, determine the patient has a shoulder dislocation, and reduce it without an x-ray. (Subsequent x-rays revealed only a clinically insignificant chip fracture, and the patient had no subsequent symptoms of neck injury.) They then (carefully) walk the patient out, cutting the entire rescue to 11 hours.

As can be seen from the above examples, wilderness/"street" protocol decision-making balances the environment, the patient's particular injury or illness, the certainty of the diagnoses, the expected length of the evacuation, and other factors to provide maximal benefit for the patient and minimal risk for the patient and rescuers. If close to the road, a simple and quick minimal-risk wilderness intervention is appropriate, but a difficult high-risk intervention may not be, and the question of "how close to the road?" is a clinical one.

Wilderness EMS Protocols

The wilderness EMS community would argue that almost all systems should have wilderness protocols available. Although the need is most obvious in rural and suburban systems with significantly wild areas, even some urban systems have the potential for "wilderness" situations. As described above, the wilderness context is really more of a situational decision to deal with delays in access to definitive care, and changes in weather (e.g., an ice storm) have turned many a city into a "wilderness context."

Most EMS traditions and protocols were developed for urban systems, and some make a compelling argument that rural and wilderness EMS are more similar to each other than to urban EMS. Certainly, many of the treatment variations appropriate for the wilderness context are also appropriate for rural EMS systems with many-hour transports. However, rural EMS do not have the same constraints of limited resources and a stressful environment that characterize wilderness EMS.

Wilderness EMS and Catastrophic Disasters

A catastrophic disaster is very similar to a wilderness search-and-rescue operation.

There is no shelter, and exposure to environmental extremes is important to victims and rescuers alike. There is neither potable water nor food. WEMTs need overland evacuation skills since the roads and streets may be impassable. WEMTs must be ready to care for patients for a long time. The local hospitals may be destroyed or overwhelmed, and many local doctors and nurses may be dead or injured themselves. Transportation of the sick or injured out of the area may be delayed for days; it may take a day or more for a field disaster hospital to set up in the area. Although victims may be entrapped in ways that require special urban rescue skills, many may simply need evacuation by simple mountain/cave rescue techniques. As in the wilderness, EMTs must be self-sufficient in terms of food, water, and shelter. Since, during the first hours to days, all medical resources will be aimed at the critically ill, WEMTs will be called upon to care for minor injuries.

For all these reasons, WEMTs represent a major asset for any catastrophic disaster, and should be included in any disaster plan.

Wilderness Epidemiology

Most of the data available on the subject of wilderness trauma have come from the mountaineering and caving journals. Unfortunately, very little has been published about injuries that occur on the trail. The statistical data that is available, though far from comprehensive, indicate that trauma is the most common emergency that presents in the wilderness. Not surprisingly, the vast majority of wilderness trauma is the result of a fall. In addition, due to significant time factors inherent in the wilderness incident, patients frequently develop secondary complications such as hypothermia, infection, and dehydration, which are immediate concerns in wilderness trauma management.

The periodicals *Accidents in North American Mountaineering* and *American Caving Accidents* offer compelling information regarding how wilderness accidents occur. Critiques of mountaineering accidents during the past 40 years show many have a primary cause of human error, often with hypothermia and exhaustion as contributing factors. This includes climbing without a helmet, misuse of equipment, inexperience, and surpassing one's abilities.

Compared with these climbing injury statistics, information gathered by the Appalachian Search and Rescue Conference regarding SAR subjects from 25 years of experience across several central Appalachian states represents a more general SAR patient population. Because many of these search subjects have not sustained major trauma, dehydration and hypothermia assume larger dimensions. Diabetic hypoglycemia, psychiatric problems, and epilepsy are also disproportionately represented. Trauma and burns from light aircraft crashes, and gunshot wounds from hunting accidents, are the major sources of trauma in their data.

Wilderness Trauma Implications

Most EMS providers divide trauma patients into three classes: dead, immediately life-threatening, or not life-threatening. At least as far as trauma is concerned, the patients that wilderness SAR teams find alive almost always fall into the third category since if the injury is immediately life-threatening, the patient will not be alive when found. The focus of urban trauma care is to save those who are in danger of dying in a matter of minutes, and it is generally accepted that "scoop and run" is the appropriate treatment for urban trauma patients. All measures are geared to rapid treatment and rapid transport to the operating theater. In the wilderness, however, those with such severe injuries are already dead when found, or will die long before evacuation is completed. This is simply a function of time. As an example, in the special case of aircraft crashes, if the SAR teams do not find patients within the first 24 hours, they are not likely to find them alive. This is called the "Golden Day"; the U.S. Air Force Rescue Coordination Center maintains a constantly updated database of air crashes, which shows a large jump in mortality after the first 24 hours. For these and other wilderness traumas, it takes too long for someone to walk out for help, and too long for a team to respond. Therefore, the procedures taught in courses like Basic Trauma Life Support (BTLS) and PreHospital Trauma Life Support (PHTLS) have little relevance for wilderness EMS.

Wilderness patients differ from urban trauma patients in other ways as well. First, they almost always have multiple problems. For example, cold exposure and dehydration are common. Urban providers do not have to worry about these problems, since transport times are generally relatively short. Second, they require long evacuations, and things happen during long evacuations. Patients develop the delayed trauma complications that urban providers never see, such as compartment syndrome, deep venous thrombosis, acute renal failure, or adult respiratory distress syndrome. All trauma patients are in danger from such problems, but on the street, EMTs can usually outrun them. Third, they all have normal human metabolism. For long evacuations, providers must ensure nutrition and hydration, and provide for elimination.

For the most part, urban providers can legitimately dump these long-term problems on the Emergency Department or trauma staff. Wilderness providers, on the other hand, must recognize and deal with these problems; they simply have no choice if they want to keep their patients alive and relatively well, and not have them die of complications days or weeks later. Preventing the intermediate-term complications of trauma and illness is the meat and potatoes of wilderness EMS training.

Equipment for Wilderness EMS

The goals of equipment used in wilderness EMS are the same as for the equipment used on an ambulance: the delivery of quality prehospital care. However, much of the equipment used on an ambulance is inappropriate for a wilderness setting. For instance, a standard ambulance cot is not well suited for cliff or cave rescue. However, the underlying reasons for ambulance equipment requirements may, after consideration, give clues about the equipment one should use for wilderness EMS.

Consider what makes up a wilderness "ambulance." The litter team members' booted feet are its "tires." Blistered feet or slippery shoes on a rescue team may be just as hazardous as bald tires on an ambulance. Training in good foot care and proper personal equipment are essential parts of the wilderness "ambulance." One might argue that the rescue team's equipment can serve all team members, with no need for personal equipment, but a quick thought about boots will belie this notion. A five-mile hike in standard, not-broken-in boots would make any rescuer into a casualty.

The headlamps are the wilderness ambulance headlights. Night-time wilderness rescuers trying to carry and care for a patient using hand-held flashlights are probably worse off than providers in an ambulance with no headlights and no interior lighting. These analogies can, of course, be carried to extremes, but are a useful starting place for examining the equipment needs of a wilderness rescue team.

Wilderness Training and Scope of Practice

Originally, a very limited scope of practice was considered essential to any EMS legislation, to assure passage despite the potential opposition of an entrenched medical establishment with a jealously guarded medical practice license from the state. In some cases this opposition was real, more often theoretical, but when restricted to the prehospital domain, seldom does the idea of a restrictive prehospital scope of practice serve a useful political purpose for EMS today. Indeed, the *EMS Education Agenda for the Future* states: "Curricula become synonymous with scope of practice in many states. . . . In many states, the scope of practice was still driven by the national standard curricula, thus politicizing and complicating the writing of national standard curricula. . . . Many states have not changed their current provider levels to comply with the National EMS Education and Practice Blueprint, and many state laws and regulations continue to refer to the national standard curricula when defining EMS provider scope of practice."[8]

While this confusion between scope and curriculum was identified as a problem for the future of EMS in general, it is a particular problem for the wilderness EMS community. The original EMT-A program was developed by the Department of Transportation (DOT). Understandably, there was a bias toward motor vehicle accidents. At the time, motor vehicles were recognized as a major source of injury and death, and to assure funding, the DOT needed to make sure its new program reflected transportation. Although the EMT-A and later the EMT-P programs gradually broadened their horizons to include medical and other emergency problems, they still remain closely tied to ambulances. Indeed, the attorney responsible for EMS in one state has opined that the state law, by a strict reading, only allows the state EMS office to regulate care by prehospital providers when operating in or near an ambulance, leaving SAR teams without an ambulance entirely outside the EMS system (personal communication, Kenneth Brody, Asst. Counsel, Pennsylvania Department of Health, 7 March 1994).

For this and other reasons, early efforts to develop medical training for SAR teams in the 1970s focused on a training track entirely separate from the ambulance-centric EMT and then paramedic curricula. By 1980, however, the increasing availability of EMT and paramedic training persuaded the nascent wilderness EMS community that it made more sense to "piggyback" wilderness EMS training on traditional EMS training.

By 1986 a model for wilderness EMT training, developed for the most part by the wilderness EMS Institute (previously the Wilderness Emergency Medicine Curriculum Development Project), became the dominant tradition in the wilderness EMS community. This model was developed after WEMSI undertook a national survey of SAR teams to determine their medical needs and recommendations.

There are four essential parts of this model. First, field providers and their physician supervisors can be classified along a two-dimensional spectrum of training levels and professional duty/responsibility levels (fig. 5.3). Second, the wilderness EMT training module consists of a relatively small module that adds to existing EMS training. Third, wilderness EMS providers should be trained and certified in SAR by SAR organizations, not by EMS or wilderness medicine organizations. SAR should not be part of the WEMT training module. Figure 5.4 graphically shows how

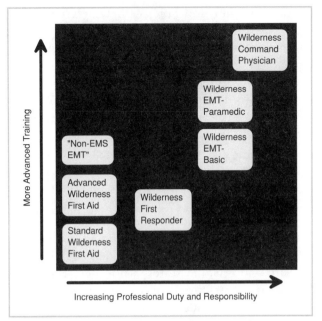

FIGURE 5.3. *Training, responsibility, and wilderness EMS provider types.*

this model works, using a wilderness EMT module to bind together EMS training and SAR training. Fourth, the same WEMT training module is appropriate for wilderness EMS providers from EMT-Basic through EMT-Paramedic to physician.

The reasons for this fourth portion of the model are as follows.

Most wilderness material is new to providers of all levels. Wilderness operations require no invasive skills beyond those of a paramedic. Some skills such as

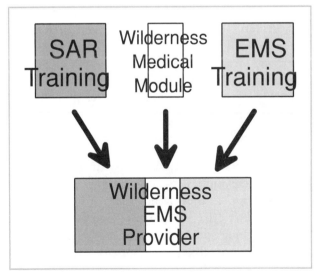

FIGURE 5.4. *Building the wilderness EMT.*

nasogastric tube and Foley catheter placement are rarely used in urban EMS, but are within the scope of practice of paramedics in many jurisdictions. Paramedics can easily learn these clinical skills during an ED rotation. Interaction between EMT-Basics and EMT-Paramedics in class is educationally sound, and mimics the situation during wilderness rescues, where large medical teams, with members of widely varying skill levels, often have to work together to provide patient care.

From a wilderness perspective, there are three scopes of practice for prehospital providers. Wilderness first-aiders, Wilderness First Responders, and some wilderness EMT-Bs operate with no medications or invasive procedures. Providers at various levels (including some states' wilderness EMT-Bs), nurses, nurse practitioners, and physician assistants provide a limited subset of advanced medical care, including some medications and some invasive procedures. Physicians can employ the full armamentarium of appropriate medical procedures. Let us now look at the various training levels in the wilderness EMS.

Wilderness First Aid

An early Wilderness Medical Society document defined wilderness first aid:

Backcountry First Aid can be defined as first aid rendered under conditions where immediate, definitive medical care is unavailable because of distance, adverse travel conditions, or difficulties in communications. The term "backcountry first aid," therefore, can be applied to first aid rendered at high and low altitudes, from arctic ice and subarctic tundra to forests, deserts, seashores, the tropics, and even under the seas. Small boat sailors, inhabitants of isolated villages, and victims of disasters where medical facilities and communications have been destroyed may all require "backcountry first aid." Backcountry first aid differs from the usual type of first aid and EMT training in three major ways:

(a) The need to learn new procedures in order to handle injuries and illnesses in which a delay of more than a few hours or days will likely cause adverse effects which outweigh the dangers of teaching such new procedures to lay persons. Standard urban protocols for these illnesses and injuries are not adequate for the backcountry setting.

(b) The need to deal with entirely new illnesses and injuries not seen in the urban setting.

(c) The need to learn basic care of an injured or ill person so that ordinary day-to-day requirements of the body will be met until definitive care is secured. These requirements include temperature control, shelter, water, food, cleanliness, psychological support, and the management of excretory functions. . .

Several wilderness first-aid courses are now available nationally, including the National Safety Council *Wilderness First Aid* course, with a textbook co-sponsored by the Wilderness Medical Society, the National Ski Patrol *Outdoor Emergency Care* program, and the American Red Cross *When Help Is Delayed* module, which can be used in conjunction with any of the Red Cross first aid courses.[9,10,11] Although there are differences in coverage, all offer high-quality education, and to a high degree represent the consensus position of the wilderness medicine community.

The Wilderness First Responder

Assume that a day-hiker in a local state park breaks a leg, and one of his companions hikes out to call for help. A state park ranger hikes in to the patient. The local wilderness SAR team responds eventually to evacuate the patient, who is by now hypothermic, and then the local ambulance service brings the patient to the hospital. What sort of wilderness first-aid/medical training should the park ranger have? Rangers are wilderness first responders, and since they will see major injuries much more often than the occasional day-hiker, they should have training in the care of major problems (to a greater extent than in wilderness first-aid courses). However, unlike the wilderness first-aider who needs to care for minor problems in self and friends, rangers do not have as much need for training in the use of over-the-counter and prescription medications for common minor problems.

The standard DOT Emergency Care—First Responder curriculum does not address many needs of the wilderness first responder: improvised equipment; environmental illnesses, injuries, and hazards; and the care of patients for extended periods.[12] Many commercial providers offer wilderness-oriented First Responder courses that include the standard DOT curriculum.

In the 1990s, wilderness First Responder training became more standardized. The American Society for Testing and Materials (ASTM) developed standards for the scope of performance of, and the training of, the Wilderness First Responder.[13,14]

The Wilderness Medical Society also developed an overview curriculum of topics for training providers in wilderness emergency care, termed the Wilderness Prehospital Emergency Care Curriculum. This seven-page document, while broad and general, represents a consensus overview of topics to be taught in WEMT and Wilderness First Responder classes.[15] More recently, the WMS has developed a more detailed set of recommended minimum course topics for Wilderness First Responder programs.[16]

The Wilderness EMT

The wilderness SAR team that evacuates the victim needs wilderness first-aid/medical training similar to and if possible, even more extensive than that of the park ranger. Because the problems are different in the wilderness, and standards of prehospital care are different for wilderness rescues, EMTs working in the wilderness context need specialized training. The term "wilderness EMT" refers to an EMT—of any level, from EMT-B to EMT-P—who has had additional wilderness-specific training. Some problems are more common in the wilderness than on the street, and WEMTs must be trained to deal with them routinely, particularly environmental problems such as hypothermia. Wilderness patients often need longer evacuations, monitoring the urine output by a Foley catheter or Texas drain. Infections, atelectasis, and deep venous thrombosis may become problems during an extended wilderness evacuation.

Wilderness emergency medical equipment is limited by what the team members can carry on their backs or improvise. Some special procedures (such as reducing dislocations) may require special licensing by the state. Wilderness EMTs need special training for the wilderness environment and for search-and-rescue. The WEMT must carry out emergency medical tasks despite severe environmental stresses and to keep the operation moving smoothly. The WEMT must interface smoothly into a large SAR operation even if not actually assisting with SAR tasks.

When a SAR team is out for a day or more, and especially when the team is out of contact with a physician, the EMT is the medical expert for whatever problems arise. Wilderness EMTs will be asked to provide incidental medical care for team members' minor injuries and illnesses. Management of some problems common to the wilderness, such as plant contact dermatitis or friction blisters on the heel, are not taught to most EMTs. Although they may seem minor in another environment, these problems may cause severe illness or be temporarily disabling in the wilderness. During a long rescue, sending a team member back to the base camp for medical care might be disastrous; a team member or two must accompany the victim, and the depletion of the team might delay an evacuation for hours, perhaps even resulting in the patient's death. Since wilderness rescue often stresses team members to the limit, injuries and illnesses that might be minor at home loom much larger in the wilderness. While direct medical oversight is ideal, the limited radio and cellular phone coverage in remote mountains and in caves requires WEMTs to be able to operate independently at need.

Wilderness EMTs need not be physician assistants or nurse practitioners capable of providing all routine primary care services. However, they should be able to care for minor injuries and medical problems common in the wilderness, at least to the extent of recommending and dispensing simple oral over-the-counter and a limited number of prescription medications. Even if the WEMT is not specifically authorized to provide such care, team members who do carry such medications in their packs will come to the WEMT for advice, and so the use of common medications for common problems must be a part of the training. Physicians serving as medical advisors to wilderness EMS agencies should take this into account in training prehospital personnel, and when providing protocols to wilderness providers.

Many organizations offer "Wilderness First Responder" or "Wilderness EMT" training, but more in the wilderness medicine than in the EMS tradition. For the most part, those completing such courses operate not as part of a physician-supervised SAR team or EMS agency, but as a backcountry trip leader or expedition medic. There is a need for such training, and better patient care will result if trip leaders and expedition medics are well trained. Based on job description rather than training, they are really advanced first-aiders. But with wide availability of EMT programs, wide availability of WEMT training programs, and the cachet of the WEMT title, this is not likely to change. The majority of those graduating from WEMT programs will not be working as what EMS professionals would view as even a part-time volunteer EMT. Indeed, some EMS professionals would view SAR team WEMTs the same way—but a goal of this chapter is to change that perception.

The Wilderness EMS Institute specifically oriented their Wilderness EMT curriculum development toward the needs of physician-supervised SAR team EMTs, and away from the needs of trip leaders. WEMSI-WEMT courses are primarily offered by SAR organizations and EMS agencies rather than by outdoor training schools, although some of the latter use the WEMSI-WEMT curriculum.

Wilderness Medical Oversight

The ideal oversight physician for Wilderness EMTs is likely a residency-trained, board-certified, full-time emergency physician who is also a Mountain Rescue Association-certified member of a wilderness SAR team, and who has completed a Wilderness Command Physician class. (Use of the term "Wilderness Command Physician" originated in Pennsylvania, where the course began. State regulations use the term "command physician" to describe physicians providing direct medical oversight.) Since such physicians are rare, one should accept compromises. For instance, an understanding of the field problems of WEMTs is necessary, but the ability to serve in the field is not. Therefore, one would be happy to have an oversight physician with an outdoor background (winter backpacking would be ideal) who has been through a realistic rescue orientation such as a Wilderness Command Physician course. If cave rescue or whitewater rescue were to be part of the Wilderness EMS System that the command physician will supervise, physicians should participate in cave rescue or whitewater simulations as part of their training. The oversight physician must have a broad base of knowledge about the prehospital aspects of emergency medicine, and have experience giving direct medical oversight to paramedics, but employment as a full-time emergency physician might not be a requirement. Many physicians have had experience "moonlighting" in emergency departments, and perhaps a minimum number of hours of ED experience would be acceptable in lieu of full-time ED staff status. If one accepts this, perhaps one should require that each Wilderness Command Physician have completed the National Association of EMS Physicians Medical Directors Course.[17]

Wilderness rescue operations take many hours, sometimes lasting a day or more. Thus, a wilderness rescue might easily run through several shifts of ED physicians. Oversight of wilderness EMT-P will thus be much different from most prehospital direct medical oversight situations, and one might even argue that wilderness rescue entails an extended physician-patient relationship through the paramedic. For continuity of care, one would prefer a single physician providing oversight for the entire rescue. Since the condition of the patient will be known well before arrival in the ED, the Wilderness Command Physician will have ample opportunity to discuss the case with the primary physician and specialists who will care for the patient once admitted. This allows the Wilderness Command Physician to obtain specialists help in the prehospital management of the patient. Therefore, the Wilderness Command Physician should be well educated about both the prehospital and in-hospital management of wilderness problems.

Since present communications technology will permit us to connect the wilderness paramedic to the Wilderness Command Physician in different ways, the physician could provide direct medical oversight from a home telephone, from a radio in the emergency department, or from a telephone in the office. During a long evacuation, a command physician at one ED could pass direct oversight of the wilderness rescue to a physician at another ED across town, then to an internist or surgeon at the office, and then to a physician at home. Or, if continuity of care were thought to be important enough, the same Wilderness Command Physician could follow the case through, even if not on duty in the ED the entire time.

Certification and Licensure of Wilderness Prehospital Providers

Choosing the term "license" for simplicity, recognizing that some states license prehospital personnel while others certify them, the following questions arise. If someone is licensed to practice as an EMT, does that person need an additional license to practice as a wilderness EMT? The knowledge and skills required of wilderness EMTs are slightly different from those of more urban providers, but is the difference enough to require a different license? Since wilderness and non-wilderness EMTs are doing the same job but in different environments, can one just certify WEMTs without separate licenses?

There is no need for wilderness licenses beyond the "standard" EMT license. Wilderness EMTs will be performing the same level of skills as their non-wilderness counterparts, as adapted for the wilderness; basic WEMTs will be restricted to non-invasive therapy, for example, leaving IVs and drugs for the Wilderness EMT-Intermediate and Wilderness EMT-Paramedic. Thus, there should be little concern for licensing WEMTs, provided they hold proper EMT certificates or licenses.

Let us closely examine an example: dealing with shoulder dislocations in the wilderness. The current teaching for most providers: "Never, however, should you attempt to reduce a dislocated shoulder. This maneuver should only be done in the hospital after x-rays have been taken."[18] However, the standard street treatment of a knee dislocation without a pulse is to attempt reduction: "Gently straighten the deformity by applying gentle longitudinal traction in the axis of the limb."[18]

Even with a good distal pulse, reducing an anterior shoulder dislocation in the wilderness makes good sense. At a minimum, it will reduce pain and suffering, and it may well avoid the need for reduction under general anesthesia at the hospital (when spasm has been intensifying for many hours, reduction may be impossible without general anesthesia). The 1989 Wilderness Medical Society position statement (which preceded the current Practice Guidelines[1]) said: "The common anterior shoulder dislocation can usually be reduced without too much difficulty and the sooner this is attempted, the easier it will be."[19]

EMT-B have been trained to use axial traction to straighten angulated limbs. The very first EMT textbook said: ". . . a severely angulated fracture should be straightened prior to splinting, for this may lessen the chance of permanent damage to blood vessels and nerves around the fracture site. . . . Straightening an angulated fracture may cause the patient momentary pain, but this should lessen when the fracture is straightened and splinted. If the straightening can be performed immediately after the fracture occurs, the patient may experience little or no pain; frequently there is numbness around the site for several minutes following a severe fracture. . . . Gently but firmly grasp the extremity with both hands. Place one hand just below the site of fracture and the other hand farther down the extremity. If possible, have someone provide countertraction. . . ."[20]

The logical argument can be summarized: EMTs are told to use axial traction to straighten fractures, and EMTs are told to reduce certain dislocations when medically appropriate, AND the standard for care of the anterior shoulder dislocation in the wilderness is reduction; THEREFORE, EMTs who have been trained by a physician to reduce anterior shoulder dislocations should be able to do so within the scope of their EMT licenses.

An interesting and very close analogy to WEMT certification is with the EMT continuing education courses (BTLS) Basic Trauma Life Support and (PHTLS) PreHospital Trauma Life Support. These courses teach EMTs new ways to perform basic-level skills in an acute urban trauma setting, and offer certification. The states do not see this training as needing a new level of licensure. BTLS and PHTLS, however, concentrate on a specific type of patient already covered in EMT-B and EMT-P training, while WEMT training focuses on patients and problems not covered in regular EMT training, and thus may appropriately be licensed as a new level of EMT.

To return to the original question: Does WEMT training require a new license? The answer will depend on the state. If state laws or EMS regulations specifically prohibit EMTs from reducing shoulder dislocations or performing other skills of a WEMT, then separate WEMT licensure would be needed.

Standard of Care

As described at the outset of this chapter, wilderness EMS is developing its own traditions, and one of the most important traditions is something that can be called a standard of care. Many different organizations teach wilderness first-aid, Wilderness First Responder, WEMT, or similar classes, and there is a general consensus among them about the correct way to manage trauma and illness in the wilderness context. In many cases, this is different from "street" EMS protocols—a ripe setting for a court decision when an EMS provider is sued for following "street" protocols rather than the established "standard of care" for the backcountry. Luckily, EMS physicians and EMS system administrators have two sets of authoritative guidelines to look to in this regard.

First are a series of four position statements by the National Association of EMS Physicians, published in *Prehospital and Disaster Medicine* in the early 1990s. These cover four major situations where there are critical differences between "street" and wilderness EMS care. They cover CPR, dislocations, clearing the cervical spine, and wounds and open fractures.[21-24] Although parts of the CPR guideline have been superseded by a more detailed and up-to-date position paper on termination of resuscitation in the prehospital setting for adult patients suffering non-traumatic cardiac arrest, the original guideline still contains valuable guidance for wilderness providers that does not appear in the more recent paper.[25] The guideline on clearing the cervical spine in the back-country, however, has been completely overtaken by events in "street" EMS. More recent research has led to an NAEMSP position paper essentially recommending that the wilderness approach, using examination rather than just mechanism of injury, should be used on the street as well.[26] But as pointed out above, and described in a 1992 editorial, decision-making about cervical spine injury can become more complex, requiring balancing of risks, so there is still a significant difference between urban and back-country management of suspected spinal injuries.[27] The most definitive and recent guidelines are the Wilderness Medical Society Practice Guidelines. This document, now in its second edition, represents the reasoned consensus of the wilderness medicine community, and covers a great variety of topics.[1]

Conclusion

Wilderness EMS is complex, and perhaps difficult to approach because it seems so different from traditional EMS. This chapter will help physicians and system administrators feel more comfortable approaching the topic. There are also many resources available to help develop a wilderness component to EMS systems. EMS systems should not be caught unprepared when the next wide-body aircraft crashes far from the road.

References

1. Virginia Dept. of Emergency Services. *Search and Rescue Resource Guide*. Available at http://www.vdem.state.va.us/library/sarguide.cfm
2. Wilderness Medical Society. *What is wilderness medicine?* Available at http://www.wms.org.about_fr.htm
3. Forgey WW. *Wilderness Medical Society: Practice Guidelines for Wilderness Emergency Care*. Guilford, CT: Globe Pequot Press; 2001:109.
4. WEMSI Protocols. Available at http://www.wemsi.org/opp.html
5. Maryland Institute for EMS Systems. miemss.umaryland.edu/protocols2000.pdf
6. Wilderness EMS Institute. www.wemsi.org/protocol.html
7. Wilderness EMS Institute. www.wemsi.org/opsman10.pdf
8. National Highway Traffic Safety Administration. *EMS Education Agenda for the Future*. Washington, DC: NHTSA; 2000.
9. Paton BC. Wilderness first aid: emergency care for remote locations (National Safety Council—Wilderness Medical Society). Sudbury, MA: Jones and Bartlett; 1998:350.
10. Bowman WD. Outdoor emergency care: comprehensive first aid for nonurban settings. *National Ski Patrol*. 1998:636.
11. American Red Cross—Health and Safety Services. *First Aid: When Help Is Delayed*. St. Louis, MO: Mosby Lifeline; 1998:23.
12. U.S. Department of Transportation NHTSA. *Emergency Medical Services: First Responder Training Course* (course guide, instructor's lesson plans, student study guide). Washington, DC: U.S. Government Printing Office; 1994.
13. ASTM Committee F-30 on Emergency Medical Services. *F 1616-95: Standard Guide for Scope of Performance of First Responders Who Practice in the Wilderness, Delayed or Prolonged Transport Settings*. West Conshohocken, PA: ASTM; 1995.
14. ASTM Committee F-30 on Emergency Medical Services. *F 1655-95: Standard Guide for Training First Responders Who Practice in the Wilderness, Delayed or Prolonged Transport Settings*. West Conshohocken, PA: ASTM; 1995.
15. Prehospital Committee WMS. Wilderness prehospital emergency care (WPHEC) curriculum. *J Wild Med*. 1991;2:80–87.
16. Wilderness Medical Society www.wms.org/education/WFR%20Topics.pdf
17. Dickinson E, Grunow J, Grandey J, Carlson E. *Base Station Course: A Product of the NAEMSP Education Committee*. Lenexa, KS: National Association of EMS Physicians; 2000.
18. Heckman JD. *Emergency Care and Transportation of the Sick and Injured*. Park Ridge, IL: American Academy of Orthopedic Surgeons; 1992.
19. Iserson KV. *Wilderness Medical Society Position Statement: Orthopedic Injuries in the Wilderness*. Point Reyes Station, CA: Wilderness Medical Society; 1989.
20. American Academy of Orthopaedic Surgeons. *Emergency Care and Transportation of the Sick and Injured*. 1971. AAUS Chicago.
21. Goth P, Garnett G, Rural Affairs Committee, National Association of EMS Physicians. Clinical guidelines for delayed/prolonged transport. I. Cardiorespiratory arrest. *Prehosp Disaster Med*. 1991;6:335–340.
22. Goth P, Garnett G, Rural Affairs Committee, National Association of EMS Physicians. Clinical guidelines for delayed or prolonged transport. II. Dislocations. *Prehosp Disaster Med*. 1993;8:77–80.
23. Goth P, Garnett G, Rural Affairs Committee, National Association of EMS Physicians. Clinical guidelines for delayed or prolonged transport. III. Spine injury. *Prehosp Disaster Med*. 1993;8:369–371.

24. Goth P, Garnett G, Rural Affairs Committee, National Association of EMS Physicians. Clinical guidelines for delayed or prolonged transport. IV. Wounds. *Prehosp Disaster Med*. 1993;8:253–255.

25. Bailey ED, Wydro GC, Cone DC, for the National Association of EMS Physicians Standards and Clinical Practice Committee. Termination of resuscitation in the prehospital setting for adult patients suffering non-traumatic cardiac arrest. *Prehosp Emerg Care*. 2000;4:190–195.

26. Domeier RM, for the National Association of EMS Physicians Standards and Clinical Practice Committee. Indications for prehospital spinal immobilization. *Prehosp Emerg Care*. 1999;3:251–253.

27. Conover K. EMTs should be able to clear the cervical spine in the wilderness [editorial]. *J Wild Med*. 1992;3:339–343.

CHAPTER 6

Fire

Marc Eckstein, MD
Franklin D. Pratt, MD

Introduction

There are a number of different configurations for prehospital emergency medical services (EMS) systems across the United States, with fire departments serving as the largest single group of providers.[1] In its mission to preserve life and property, the fire service has assumed an ever-increasing role in every aspect of EMS.

As the community role of the fire service has expanded considerably over the past few decades, EMS has assumed a greater role within the fire service. Fire suppression activity now represents a small percentage of the emergency workload for most fire departments, and a number of other functions of the fire service have evolved, including fire prevention, hazardous materials incident management, disaster preparedness, swift water rescue, urban search-and-rescue (USAR), and preparedness for weapons of mass destruction. Even with the increasingly diverse response types, for most fire departments that deliver EMS it comprises the majority of emergency activity.

Historical Perspective

Firefighters across North America have provided oxygen and first-aid for colleagues since the early 1900s. Treating community members was a natural outgrowth of fire scene medical care. The first paramedics in the United States were certified in 1967. Miami firefighters, under the supervision of Dr. Eugene Nagel, expanded the concept of "bringing the CCU to the field" with prehospital defibrillation and advanced airway management. Soon a number of cities and counties, including Los Angeles, California; King County, Washington; and Cincinnati, Ohio trained groups of firefighters as paramedics.

While relatively small numbers of firefighters from these fire departments were trained as paramedics, the majority of firefighters received higher levels of EMS training than they previously had, initially to the level of a first responder, and later progressing to the emergency medical technician-basic (EMT-B) level. As more research on cardiac arrest was completed, the importance of early defibrillation was validated. With response times for paramedics typically around ten minutes from receipt of the 9-1-1 call, the concept of providing EMT-B with defibrillators was developed; in 1984 firefighters in King County, Washington became the first to use semi-automated external defibrillators (AEDs).

The concept of fire-based EMS continued to expand during the 1990s. Government officials from many different types and sizes of municipalities realized that their fire departments already had sufficient equipment and personnel to provide first response medical care. Since strict time lines were already in place for responses to structure fires, these resources were uniquely positioned to provide timely response to all types of medical emergencies. This need for timely response for certain types of medical emergencies was reinforced by the American Heart Association in 1991 when it published the cardiac arrest "chain of survival" response intervals.[2] These guidelines recommended a four-minute response from the time of collapse until arrival of basic life support (BLS) and an eight-minute response for advanced life support (ALS). These published guidelines, albeit flawed, provided a response-time benchmark for EMS systems. Many systems that utilized either municipal third services or private ambulance-based services could not meet these response-time goals. Because preexisting geographic location helped the fire service approach the time goals, movement of service into the fire EMS was a natural occurrence.

Within the political structure of the fire service, there was an increasing recognition of the benefits provided to the community by fire-based EMS. This culminated in the creation of a section of EMS within both the International Association of Firefighters

(IAFF) and the International Association of Fire Chiefs (IAFC). These organizations urged fire services to expand their role in the provision of EMS.[3] As of 1999, 96% of U.S. fire departments provide first responder EMS service.[1]

Attributes of a Fire-Based EMS System

Since the inception of EMS systems, the need for timely response of emergency personnel and equipment has been paramount. Fire departments have some unique attributes that make them ideally suited to provide EMS. Short response times are particularly critical for appropriately treating victims of sudden cardiac death and major trauma. Due to the requirements already in place for fire departments to respond to structure fires within minutes, fire departments across the country, particularly paid departments in larger cities, already have the infrastructure in place to get emergency personnel on scene within a few minutes of call receipt. Fire stations are in place throughout each jurisdiction, and in most urban and suburban municipalities, personnel are on duty at all times, ready to respond quickly to emergencies. Furthermore, sophisticated communications systems are already in place, along with dispatch centers. Thus, incorporating EMS into the preexisting duties of the fire service primarily requires adding additional equipment, training, and supervision to a standing emergency response system.

The training of some firefighters as paramedics, and later the training of paramedics as firefighters, solidified the concept of cross-trained or dual-function firefighter/paramedics (FF/PMs). FF/PMs are trained in fire suppression and rescue activities and are licensed or certified paramedics. These personnel give fire departments tremendous flexibility in staffing their resources, which has led to the creation of a number of different EMS staffing configurations for fire apparatus.

From an economic perspective, the dual-function FF/PM provides a fire department with "two employees for the price of one." This versatility allows these departments to utilize these cross-trained dual-function personnel on both fire suppression and EMS resources. In addition, many departments have turned what were once apparatus used solely for fire suppression into combined fire suppression and EMS resources. An existing model uses an engine company originally staffed by four firefighters trained to the level of certified first responder (CFR) or more commonly emergency medical technician-defibrillator (EMT-D), with one or two positions now to be staffed by FF/PMs. This model elevates the medical capability of that resource to a "paramedic assessment engine." These personnel can perform an advanced level of patient assessment and perform cardiac monitoring, administer medications, and establish an advanced airway.

These personnel can also integrate medical care into rescue operations. At the scene of a complex rescue, medical care can be initiated while the patients are being disentangled, physically stabilized, or moved. The physical, mental, and philosophical integration of medical services into the emergency incident environment is one of the most compelling benefits of fire based EMS.

Many fire departments had not previously included the transport aspect of EMS, but this too has changed over the last few years due to a number of factors, not least of which is the competition for the ever-shrinking healthcare dollar. Under current rules set by the Center for Medicare and Medicaid Services (CMS), patient transport is the only EMS service that is billable.[4] Thus, providing transport capability enables fire departments to offset some of the costs of providing EMS, particularly the high costs of providing paramedic responses.

Dispatching and Communications

Fire-based EMS systems typically have an established, technologically advanced communications system in place. Enhanced 9-1-1 systems, which automatically provide the location and callback number to the dispatch center, have become an integral component in most systems. These systems, utilizing computer-aided dispatch (CAD), provide fast, accurate assignment of response units to the incident. Most systems, particularly those in high-density population areas, also employ some type of tiered dispatch system that matches responses to the request with the probable type of medical intervention needed.

Fire-based EMS systems have embraced the incident command system (ICS) since its inception over thirty years ago. The need for a coordinated chain of command with uniform standards, roles, responsibilities, and communications became apparent after the large wildfires in Southern California in the 1970s. With multiple agencies responding to these large incidents, each with its own supervisors, standard operating procedures, and communications channels, the confusion and dangers to personnel readily became apparent. ICS provides a clear chain of command with specifically designated roles and responsibilities for each responder.[5] ICS has been incorporated into every aspect of the fire service and is employed on every incident, from the single patient encounter to the mass casualty incident.

Training

Firefighters are accustomed to rigorous training and physical fitness standards. Drilling and mock scenarios have always been integral parts of the fire service. Integrating EMS into these drills has been accomplished successfully in most fire departments that provide EMS. In addition, many EMS incidents also involve the mitigation of other life and safety hazards, usually requiring the actions of fire suppression personnel. Such incidents are not limited to structure or brush fires, but also include hazardous materials incidents, swift-water rescues, physical extrications, structural collapses, and terrorist actions. Since the fire service has already incorporated training and expertise in these types of incidents, the provision of EMS is a natural progression. Furthermore, the need for discipline and strict regard for the chain of command within the ICS is paramount when these types of incidents can pose significant risks to the emergency personnel. Teaching when to "hold back" and not become a victim has become a major part of training within most fire departments.[6] The need to don personal protective equipment (PPE), possibly including self-contained breathing apparatus (SCBA), is a basic part of fire suppression training and drilling.

Job Satisfaction and Attrition

Firefighters typically enjoy high job satisfaction and have low attrition rates. This is particularly true of dual-function FF/PMs, who have the greatest number of career and promotional opportunities within the fire service. Since EMS comprises the majority of most fire department emergency workload, the need for paramedic-trained officers has increased. Dual-function FF/PMs have a tremendous variety of work assignments, which may minimize burnout and therefore decrease attrition. The opposite is true for single-function paramedics, who have fairly limited career options. With the exception of dispatching, quality improvement assignments, or special duty work, fire-based EMS personnel who are not trained in fire suppression must usually remain working on an ambulance. In busy EMS systems, working full time on an ambulance for many years can lead to significant physical and emotional stress, which contributes to attrition.[7]

Cost Effectiveness

Firefighters, including dual function FF/PMs, often work 24-hour shifts. According to the Fair Labor Standards Act (FLSA), which was amended in 1999, personnel certified in fire suppression are not paid overtime until they have worked over 53 hours per week. In contrast, EMS personnel who are not fire-suppression certified must be paid overtime after they have worked 40 hours in a seven-day period. This so-called "7(k) exemption" of the FLSA is in effect for fire department personnel who are fire-suppression certified, regardless of the percentage of time spent in fire suppression/prevention versus EMS activity.[8] In a large system with significant numbers of single-function paramedics, this provision of the FLSA can have a significant negative fiscal impact.

Role of the Private Provider

As reimbursement for EMS continues to decline, fire departments have begun to bid competitively against private ambulance companies for the authority to provide ambulance transport within a particular jurisdiction. According to reimbursement rules set forth by the CMS, only those prehospital care services that involve transport of the patient to the hospital are billable.[4] Thus, even though a fire department may provide paramedic intervention, if a private ambulance provides transport, only the private ambulance company may bill the patient or the insurance company. While reimbursement for EMS in most jurisdictions typically does not approach the "break even" level (due to a high percentage of uninsured or under-insured patients), the provision of billable ambulance transport does offset a percentage of the costs associated with the provision of EMS.

In some systems such as the Los Angeles County Fire Department, the use of a private provider, even with the potential negative financial impact, is preferred because of the flexibility provided. A patient with only basic medical needs can be transported to the hospital by the private ambulance while fire department resources are released for other use.

Conversely, fire departments that also provide transport such as the Los Angeles City Fire Department have the benefit of uniformity and autonomy over all of their personnel. There are no potential problems resulting from private ambulance personnel being unfamiliar with fire department policies or procedures. This uniformity ensures that everyone can be held accountable to the same standards.

Role of the Medical Director

Regardless of the amount of time the medical director commits in a fire-based EMS system, there are certain attributes that are required and certain activities that are necessary in order to be effective. Fire departments are often paramilitary organizations with very strict rules, regulations, and policies. Following the "chain of command" is one of the basic tenets of any large fire department. Since the medical director typically is not a "sworn" uniformed personnel, fitting into the existing chain of command as a civilian poses unique challenges. In the hospital setting, physicians are accustomed to being in charge. On the fire ground or on the scene of an emergency, a fire officer is typically in charge as the incident commander (IC). The medical director serves as a technical advisor to the IC, and may on rare occasion step in to render hands-on patient care. However, while the medical director can make recommendations to the IC, he is not ultimately in command of the incident, even though he may ultimately be responsible for patient care. This sometimes difficult understanding is paramount for the medical director to function successfully in a fire-based EMS system.

The medical director should have at least a rudimentary understanding of the fire ground operation, ICS, and fire department field procedures. This understanding enables the medical director to be part of the team and ultimately to be more effective. Maintaining clinical excellence typically requires continued clinical work in the emergency department setting, which is also important for credibility. Conversely, it is important to "get out in the field" whenever possible in order to have a better grasp of the system strengths and weaknesses, to be seen as someone willing to "get their hands dirty," and not be perceived as a bureaucrat.

Many jurisdictions have a medical director who provides medical oversight for a regulatory agency, often on a regional basis. This position typically involves creating policies and guidelines for patient treatment and transport to which provider agencies must adhere. The fire department medical director may be obligated to work within these parameters, acting as an advisor and recommending internal policies for the department.

The medical director role in a fire-based EMS system varies widely among different departments, as does the reporting structure and number of work hours. Both of these areas may have significant implications in terms about the director's impact on a number of areas. In order to illustrate some of these differences, three fire-based EMS departments are examined.

Los Angeles City Fire Department

The Los Angeles City Fire Department (LAFD) created the position of Medical Director in 1981. This was a half-time position where the physician served under a personal-services contract to the Fire Chief. The medical director role was primarily to advise the fire chief on EMS-related issues, particularly paramedic equipment (AEDs), policies, and dispatch. With the deployment of semi-automatic external defibrillators to all fire companies in 1988, a major portion of the medical director's responsibilities were to oversee the implementation of AEPs and to perform quality improvement on AED use and effectiveness.

With the expansion of the EMS role, and medical calls approaching 80% of all emergency responses, the need for increased medical oversight became more apparent. The medical director of LAFD is now actively involved in the department continuing education program for its EMS providers, the quality improvement program, the dispatch system, field resource deployment, new equipment evaluation and acquisition, field policies and procedures, risk management, and research; he also serves as liaison between the fire department and the medical community. In addition, the medical director has become more involved with field activities in terms of emergency response for on-scene evaluation and assistance, as well as participating as medical team manager for the department USAR team. Finally, the medical director assists fire department members who are seriously ill or injured to ensure that they receive optimal care, and helps to relay medical information from the treating physicians to the family and to the department.

Originally, the medical director's arrangement was a year-to-year contract, whereby the medical director could be terminated without cause. This position has recently evolved to a city employee position rather than an independent contractor. Although the reporting structure remains that he still reports to the fire chief, the role of the medical director of LAFD has expanded greatly whereby he is now involved with virtually every aspect of the department's EMS delivery system.

A number of programs and improvements to the EMS system have been accomplished. These include the development and implementation of standing field treatment protocols, the introduction of paramedic assessment engines, the use of end-tidal CO_2 detectors and bulb syringes to confirm endotracheal tube placement, the introduction of field digital glucometers, the overhaul of the dispatch system with national accreditation of all dispatchers to the national emergency medical dispatcher level, and expansion of EMS field supervision and quality improvement.[9]

Houston Fire Department

When the medical director position at the Houston Fire Department was created the potential conflict of interest if the medical director reported to the fire chief was recognized. If the medical director disagreed with the fire chief's policies and positions, he could be terminated. Thus the medical director reported directly to the mayor. While this arrangement keeps the position a political one, it enables medical oversight to remain focused on patient-care issues without needing to be overly concerned with potential conflicts with the fire chief. The goal was to have the fire chief and medical director work in concert; and this reporting structure automatically elevated the level of the position within the organization. The impact of a full-time dedicated physician was felt to have led to a significantly improved cardiac arrest survival rate.[10]

Los Angeles County Fire Department

The medical director of the Los Angeles County Fire Department is a half-time position, working as an independent contractor who reports directly to the fire chief. The position was created in 1988. The success of the position is dependent upon the relationship between the fire chief and the medical director. The autonomy of the medical director is always a concern, but to date has not been a barrier to implementation of several significant programs. The first AED program in L.A. County, the implementation of a department-wide oversight process staffed by eleven registered nurses, and the implementation of an extensive data management program have emerged. The sensitive relationship between the fire chief and the medical director requires both parties to evaluate medical services carefully as an integrated part of the fire department's mission. The medical director also is involved with the department's occupational medicine programs, hazardous materials and USAR medical programs, and medical risk management issues for the department. The medical director also directly addresses concerns from the physician community and handles patient-care complaints from residents.

Deployment

Fire-based EMS systems often utilize a fixed deployment model with constant staffing, meaning that the same complement of emergency resources is available at all times in known, fixed locations. By contrast, many private providers as well as some non-fire department-based EMS systems utilize system status management (SSM).

SSM uses statistical models to predict the need for EMS.[11] Using retrospective data, the demand for EMS follows a fairly predictable curve, with increased levels of demand at certain hours of the day and on certain days of the week. By using this predictive model, these providers can have the minimum level of staffing during the usually light workload hours, such as between midnight and six in the morning, with increased levels of staffing during the peak demand periods, such as between noon and midnight. This model allows a system to be much more cost-effective than having constant staffing.

One potential problem with SSM is that while historically EMS demand is fairly predictable, the nature of EMS is inherently unpredictable. This is particularly true for natural disasters. One example was the Northridge, California earthquake of 1994. This earthquake struck at 0430 hours on a holiday morning. If fire departments in the area had employed SSM, they would have been woefully unprepared to handle the incredible number of calls for service that flooded the dispatch center immediately after the earthquake struck. During the first 24 hours after the earthquake, LAFD's dispatch center received 3,358 emergency calls for service, compared to their daily average during that time of just over 1,000 calls.[12]

Benefits to the Fire Service

While the provision of EMS by a fire department provides that department with many training, morale, administrative, logistical, and financial challenges, there are several benefits for the fire service as well. Fire suppression activity has decreased substantially over the past thirty years. This is largely the result of successful fire prevention efforts. Legislation created through the lobbying efforts of the fire service has made smoke detectors, building codes, occupancy laws, and sprinklers mandatory in most jurisdictions. Over the past thirty years, the annual number of structure fires in the United States has decreased by 70%, and the number of civilian fatalities from structure fires has also declined precipitously.[13,14,15] This reduction in demand for fire suppression services has required the fire service to adapt itself to its new environment.

Demand for EMS services has accelerated as overall fire activity has declined. Fire departments not providing EMS services have seen their overall activity decrease, and many of these departments have struggled to maintain their staffing and equipment levels. This condition has led some fire departments to begin to respond to EMS incidents and to train their firefighters to the CFR or EMT-B levels.

The provision of EMS also helps maintain the positive image of the fire service in the community, particularly evident for fire departments that have performed community outreach programs such as CPR training, emergency-response disaster training, and injury prevention. Positive public relations may translate into the successful passage of voter-approved propositions for bond monies to upgrade the various aspects of a particular fire department, such as building new stations or expanding older ones.

Challenges for Fire-Based EMS

The integration of the fire service with EMS has not come without some significant challenges. Perhaps the most fundamental one is whether firefighters possess the desire to provide EMS. Many of the larger fire departments, such as New York, Chicago, and Los Angeles, are steeped in a tradition historically based upon the physical tasks needed to fight fires in residential and commercial structures located in densely populated areas. These departments pride themselves on their abilities to fight structure fires, and have embraced a very paramilitary firehouse culture. The physical demands of the job are rooted in this fire-suppression culture, and rescuing a live victim from a fire- and smoke-filled structure is the pinnacle of a firefighter's job. Moments of terror in extinguishing or "knocking down" a fire are followed by what may be hours of tedious overhaul in order to make certain that the fire does not flare up later.

Contrast this with a typical EMS call, where providers must display compassion, a "soft touch," careful patient assessment, adherence to written EMS policies, and maintenance of a "good bedside manner." Upon initial analysis, many of these skills would seem to run counter to the requisite skills for effective, safe fire suppression. One can question whether success in this environment is compatible with success in providing EMS.

Most firefighters entered the fire service to fight fire, and in the past the delivery of EMS was generally not a primary incentive for a career in the fire service. It would be shortsighted to assume that an experienced firefighter in a traditional, busy urban fire department would easily adapt to the integration of EMS. Significant change in any traditional organization comes only with time. Integration of these two disciplines requires considerable effort, and has successfully been accomplished when the leadership and culture of the fire department emphasizes the goals of service and protection of life and property. EMS and fire suppression are both means to that end. The longer the history of fire and EMS integration within a department, the more the integration of the two seems to be accepted.

EMS accounts for the majority of emergency calls. Fire departments must have supervisors and administrative personnel with EMS expertise as well as field credibility. The greater the number of emergency medical personnel, the greater the need for effective medical oversight within the organization. Positive attitudes toward EMS and high quality patient-care must be reinforced at every level. Having a strong medical director with high standing within the organization is a vital component toward achieving that goal.

Examples of Fire-Based EMS Systems

Los Angeles

The Los Angeles City Fire Department (LAFD) is an extremely busy urban fire department that provides all levels of fire prevention, fire suppression, EMS, and rescue for almost four million people living in

Los Angeles. Founded in 1889, it has always prided itself as one of the best in terms of fighting structure fires. The first fire department ambulance was placed into service in 1927. In 1934, the ambulance service was transferred out of the fire department under the auspices of a city hospital, only to be transferred back to the LAFD in 1970. All fire companies began to carry AEDs in 1988.

LAFD hired single-function paramedics from 1970 to 1991, after which time all new recruits had to first complete fire-suppression training. Firefighters were encouraged to train as paramedics and existing single-function paramedics were encouraged to cross-train as firefighters. LAFD currently has 2565 FF/EMTs and 600 paramedics, of whom 400 are dual-function FF/PMs. It has one paramedic air ambulance, 60 paramedic ambulances, 30 EMT-B ambulances, 74 EMT-B engines, 9 paramedic engines, 20 paramedic assessment engines, and 48 EMT-B truck companies, which respond to approximately 250,000 incidents annually.

Los Angeles County

The Los Angeles County Fire Department initiated dual-function FF/PM services in 1969 with six paramedics who functioned in the field with the presence of a registered nurse. In 1979 the department required all uniformed personnel to be certified to the EMT-B level. As the population of the county grew, additional nontransporting paramedic squads were added. Paramedic helicopters were put into service in 1978. AEDs were first placed on engine companies in 1988, the first of any agency in L.A. County. Transportation is provided by private ambulance companies. Currently the department has 3,200 EMT-Ds, 750 EMT-Ps, 84 paramedic units, and 175 EMT-D units.

New York City

Since 1970 the hospital based municipal ambulance service (NYC*EMS) and the fire department (FDNY) struggled for funding, recognition and patients. In 1993, the Mayoral Health Transition Team under the leadership of Dr. Alexander Kuehl, recommended the merging of the two entities. It took eight years, a television show *(Third Watch)*, and ultimately the response to the terrorist attacks on the World Trade Center to fuse the two organizations into a resource that could take advantage of the firefighters'

availability and lifesaving tradition, and the EMT's medical expertise and innovation. Some pundits had predicted that the successful integration of the two services would take decades.

Summary

Fire-based EMS provides our communities with a great potential to integrate EMS with the many other life, safety, and property-preserving services provided by the fire service. Integration of these complex tasks requires diligence, integrated medical oversight, and an unwavering commitment to the people and communities we serve.

References

1. Mayfield T. EMS in the nation's most populous cities. *JEMS*. 2000;23:50–69.
2. Cummins RO, Ornato JP, Thies WH, et al. Improving survival from sudden cardiac arrest: the "chain of survival" concept. *Circulation*. 1991;83:1833–1847.
3. International Association of Firefighters. *Mission Statement from its Department of Emergency Medical Services.* Washington, DC; 1998.
4. *Ambulance Fee Schedule.* Health Care Financing Administration, Washington, DC; 1999.
5. *Incident Command System National Training Curriculum.* Boise, ID: National Interagency Fire Center; 1994.
6. Eckstein M, Hutson R. Street gangs: save yourself while saving a life. *Emerg Med Services.* 1994;23:18–22.
7. Streeter K. An SOS from Los Angeles' lifesavers. *Los Angeles Times,* Dec. 17, 2000;1.
8. United States Department of Labor, 29 CFR 553.201 Sec 7(k), Amended in statute §203(y), December 1999.
9. Eckstein M, Cardillo A. Implementation of standing field treatment protocols (SFTPs) in an urban EMS system. *Am J Emerg Med.* May, 2001 (in press).
10. Pepe PE, Mattox KL, Duke JH, et al. Effect of full-time, specialized physician supervision on the success of a large, urban emergency medical services system. *Crit Care Med.* 1993;21:1279–1286.
11. Stout JL. System status management. *JEMS.* 1983;8:22–23.
12. *Historical Overview Report of the January 17, 1994 Northridge Earthquake.* Los Angeles City Fire Department, Los Angeles, California. 1994.
13. Leovy J. No longer a burning issue. *Los Angeles Times,* October 8, 1998.
14. Karter MJ. 1999 US fire loss report. *NFPA Journal.* Sept/Oct 2000.
15. McCarthy R. 1999 catastrophic multiple death fires. *NFPA Journal.* Sept/Oct 2000.

CHAPTER 7

Private

Michel A. Sucher, MD

The Origins of Private Ambulance Services

The private ambulance and EMS industry originated in a very diverse and fragmented manner. Prior to the development of modern EMS, ambulance services were quite provincial and unorganized. Earlier last century, health care was local, with much less care provided in the hospital. Integrated delivery systems did not exist.

When ambulance service was necessary, the local funeral home or taxi service was asked to provide the service. In many communities the hearse that transported a deceased person to the funeral home was the same vehicle that had transported him to the hospital; ambulance attendants were untrained drivers with rudimentary knowledge of first aid. There was no prehospital medical care, only transportation. Also, some hospitals developed ambulance services when the local need was not otherwise met. Some of these companies grew significantly in later years.

Therefore, services that provided transportation evolved into the early ambulance service from the private sector. Most of these early ambulance services were supplemental business for the funeral or taxi services. Additionally, there were a few small private fire protection companies. In some cases the community being served recognized a need for ambulance service, and some of these companies also expanded into ambulance transportation. Many of these added services became quite significant over time, even though they had begun as sideline activiites.

While private ambulance services were beginning to develop, the fire departments of most cities were expanding into an increasing role in rescue and transport services. Also, volunteer services were being asked to assume this role in many rural communities.

Virtually all of these early private ambulance services were individually or family-owned businesses. There was no formal organization or collegiality among the services. The services were not professional or medically oriented, and only provided transportation services. This all began to change and evolve with the advent of modern EMS systems.

The Advent and Evolution of Modern EMS Systems

The major catalyst for the development and implementation of modern EMS systems came directly from the passage of major federal legislation known as the EMS Act of 1973. This was preceded by the development of modern emergency medicine with the establishment of the American College of Emergency Physicians in 1968. Prior to the mid-1960s there was very little career emergency medicine. The late 1960s saw the beginning of emergency medicine's evolution into a true medical specialty. Along with that evolution was an interest in prehospital medicine by those physicians who received patients in the emergency department.

Those early emergency physicians were a major force behind the EMS Act of 1973. That act defined and created standards for prehospital providers. It established the funding for training and oversight of prehospital care, and was the beginning of modern EMS system development. For the first time, trained emergency medical technicians and paramedics responded to emergency situations and provided medically directed care in the field before and during transport to the hospital.

Soon, state, county and local oversight agencies were put in place to define each community's standards for the operation of EMS systems. The local involvement of emergency physicians and nurses was also quite high, and provided much energy and enthusiasm to take the emergency department to the home and field.

This involvement heralded the transformation of the ambulance industry from being merely transportation to being mobile medical care. Since many community fire departments were focused on firefighting, and were either unwilling or afraid to get into this new "prehospital medicine," many of the private ambulance companies were the logical party to fill this role, themselves or in combination with the local fire department. Also, some of the hospital-based ambulance services filled this void.

In the early days many of the small private ambulance operators were overwhelmed by the expansion of prehospital medicine and the additional responsibilities and liabilities that it entailed. They were ill-equipped to hire and manage the modern prehospital provider. They did not easily see themselves as being in the healthcare business nor recognize that they were practicing medicine. One consequence of the EMS Act of 1973 was the establishment of the medical director. Many of these private ambulance companies were extremely uncomfortable having physicians involved in their business; they did not know how to manage physicians and were threatened by their presence. Often the physician would demand purchase of expensive equipment and/or medications that the budget-minded owner did not understand.

Other ambulance service owners simply saw the medical director as a necessary evil to be used only as a required signatory. Often this made relationships difficult. Many owners simply hired their personal physician, who was usually a general practitioner with no knowledge of emergency medicine.

Needless to say, these early ambulance service owners were challenged to make the transformation from unsophisticated transportation services to professional providers of mobile health care. However, many of them rose to the challenge, providing high-quality medical care while utilizing professional emergency physicians in an active medical director role. Again, this practice was very fragmented, and varied extensively from community to community.

In many communities the private ambulance service became the contracted emergency response and transport service independently or in combination with the local fire department. Since public fire department EMS was evolving simultaneously, many communities already had fire-based EMS. Other communities established public EMS services which were separate from the fire department. Furthermore, some hospital-based ambulance services became the local EMS agency.

In those early days of professional EMS, standards for EMS system design, performance, and response times were either undeveloped or in early development. There was no national standard and often no local standard. While today there are generally regional or local performance standards, there is still no national standard, which is probably the result of the separate origin of EMS (private and fire-based) from the rest of organized medicine. With the further evolution of modern EMS came the development of the modern EMS system, which included dispatch, communication, training, quality improvement, transportation, and medical oversight.

In 30 to 40% of American communities the private ambulance service actively participated in the delivery of prehospital care. As EMS systems developed there was continuing evolution in the remainder of the healthcare industry, including the development or expansion of hospital systems, home health, nursing homes, and other extended care facilities. This development dramatically increased the need for ambulance service in the nonemergency sector.

Nonemergency ambulance transportation fueled significant growth in the private ambulance world and also subsidized the EMS charity/indigent services. As the Medicare and Medicaid programs expanded throughout the country and the utilization of these payors dramatically increased, ambulance companies had a ready source of revenue. While there were definitions of what constituted medical necessity for ambulance transportation, these standards were rather loosely interpreted and enforced. As a result, many patients were transported by ambulance with good reimbursement being obtained for these services.

With the increased demand for and utilization of nonemergency ambulance service, private ambulance companies thrived in the 1970s and early 1980s. Many companies now saw this side line become the primary growth business for them, which led to the early consolidation movement in the private ambulance world.

Consolidation of the Private Ambulance Industry

The very first consolidation of ambulance services occurred in the early 1980s. Two companies were the primary parties involved in this initial consolidation phase; both went on to become major consolidators in the early 1990s when the larger consolidation of the private ambulance industry began.

Rural/Metro Corporation, which had begun as a private fire service in the late 1940s entered the ambulance business in 1969 when the small retirement community of Green Valley, Arizona asked it to provide ambulance transportation to Tucson. It quickly found that the ambulance business was profitable and much easier to expand than the private municipal fire department business with its local political and public fire department resistance. Rural/Metro then started acquiring ambulance companies in the Phoenix, Tucson and Yuma, Arizona areas as well as in parts of Texas, New Mexico, and Florida. It also had a private fire business in Knoxville, Tennessee, and was the successful bidder on an EMS contract for Knox County in 1985. They quickly followed with a purchase of the local provider, thereby consolidating that market as well.

At the same time, a company with Japanese ownership, named SecoAmerica began purchasing ambulance companies, primarily in Florida. It later evolved into LifeFleet and subsequently Careline which was briefly a public company.

These early consolidators expanded rapidly, but quickly outgrew their existing management and operational capabilities. They became fairly large businesses managed by small businessmen and, in the case of Rural/Metro, career firefighters with little business or management backgound. They hired more professional management but were unable to capitalize on the potential economies of scale or to generate operating efficiencies. Rural/Metro Corporation courted bankruptcy in the late 1980s as a result of their rapid expansion. With a new professional management, however, it was able to refocus and consolidate the company in preparation for the true consolidation phase which followed.

The second and larger period of consolidation began in 1992 with the formation of American Medical Response. AMR was formed by the merger of four independent ambulance companies with the purpose of establishing a truly consolidated ambulance business. AMR quickly went public under the symbol EMT on the New York Stock Exchange and experienced rapid growth. Around the same time, Rural/Metro Corporation was preparing to launch its Initial Public Offering (IPO), which occurred in mid 1993. MedTrans, which was a division of the Canadian corporation Laidlaw, also began a rapid acquisition campaign, as did CareLine.

During the early and mid 1990s all four companies acquired local ambulance companies. The annual American Ambulance Association meetings in 1993, 1994, and 1995 were feeding frenzies for the "big four." There was intense competition for acquisition candidates, often ending in bidding wars with significantly escalated purchase prices. They also targeted hospital-based ambulance companies for acquisition. Many hospital-based services were developed to bring in patients to the hospital system, which did not always occur due to EMS triage protocols specifying the closest appropriate facility. Also, hospitals often did not have the expertise to run an ambulance service profitably, and were willing to sell the service to a private provider for needed cash. The four companies had currency with their corporate stock and plenty of cash funded by the IPO and secondary offerings.

From 1992–1996 hundreds of companies were acquired by the four consolidators who generated significant revenue growth and became the darlings of Wall Street. During this period there were similar acquisitions and consolidations going on in the hospital arena (Columbia Healthcare) and in the physician practice management arena (FPA, PhyCor, MedPartners, EmCare, Coastal, InPhyNet). They experienced the same type of popularity and growth in the investment community, and many former owners of ambulance companies and group practices became instant millionaires.

The premise behind consolidation was that large size would bring economy of scale and more efficient infrastructure, which would result in higher profit margins and excellent shareholder value. This was touted as a more effective way to deal with managed care companies and insurers, thereby giving the previously small provider much more leverage in dealing with the bigger insurance companies. Also, many of the ambulance providers felt they could, through consolidation, work more closely with emergency medicine groups, hospitals/integrated delivery systems, and nurse triage companies to consolidate what was called "episodic care."

The Integrated Episodic Care Movement

One of the most intriguing elements of consolidation was the origination of Integrated Episodic Care. Nurse triage call centers became the vogue for managed-care contractors to better deal with patient questions and concerns in a cost-effective manner and to save costly 9-1-1 calls and emergency department visits that were felt to be unnecessary. Many nurse triage companies, such as Access Health, Informed Access, and National Health Enhancements, grew quickly and opened multiple call centers to handle the influx of business.

Forward-thinking ambulance providers, particularly MedTrans, AMR, and Rural/Metro, became intrigued with working with the Call Center companies and emergency groups to integrate, manage and capitate episodic care services through the dispatch/nurse triage center. This service was package priced and marketed to many managed-care companies, some of whom were interested but most were not. They had difficulty understanding the concept and believing it would work and produce savings. Also, managed care was focused on the big dollars in hospital and physician costs, not the 1 or 2% of the healthcare dollar represented by ambulance and emergency physician fees.

AMR committed millions of dollars and much time and energy to American Medical Pathways. They developed a separate corporation, a call center, and a marketing arm. They had a large contract with Kaiser Permanente, which appeared quite promising for the industry. Similarly, Rural/Metro Corporation developed a partnership with National Health Enhancements (NHES) by purchasing 10% of their company and opening a joint call center in Arizona. Unfortunately the Kaiser deal didn't work as planned, and National Health Enhancements was sold to HBOC, which also acquired Access Health and did not share the same belief in the project. The Rural/Metro-NHES center was closed and the deal unfolded.

During this period AMR and Rural/Metro Corporation contemplated becoming involved in the emergency medicine contract management business. Rural/Metro Corporation did significant due diligence regarding acquisition of emergency groups, but AMR stunned Wall Street with its unanticipated acquisition of a small Texas emergency provider. This move caused AMR stock to drop 25% in a few weeks, which in turn caused Rural/Metro Corporation to abandon its foray into this area.

One of the more successful projects to come from consolidation was the public private partnership. In this model the private provider partnered with the local municipal fire service to develop a joint venture to provide 9-1-1 response and transport. The most notable and successful model occurred in San Diego, where Rural/Metro Corporation and the City of San Diego Life Safety Service (the Fire Department) joined in an equal partnership to bid on and win the contract. Through this system the fire department provided initial 9-1-1 response and transport, with Rural/Metro providing 9-1-1 backup and general transport utilizing a shared infrastructure of communications, dispatch, fleet maintenance, and billing. This model now has been in effect for nearly five years and has been successful for both partners and for the citizens of San Diego. The contract was recently renewed for an additional five-year term. Other similar joint ventures have also been developed and implemented around the country; and the model provides opportunities for others blending the best of the private and public sectors.

The Failure of the Consolidation Movement

The consolidation movement continued with the merger of the consolidators. MedTrans acquired CareLine and then, in 1997, Laidlaw acquired American Medical Response. AMR became the surviving entity in that merger by managing the MedTrans business under the Laidlaw umbrella. Rural/Metro Corporation had been involved in numerous merger talks with Laidlaw and AMR but was never able to consummate a deal, and thus remained independent. In addition to Laidlaw acquiring AMR they also purchased EmCare, a large provider of emergency medicine contract management services, to further emphasize integrated episodic care.

As the consolidation movement moved into 1998 these providers had exhausted most of the desirable acquisitions and were focusing on integrating what they had bought. This proved to be much more difficult than anticipated and the projected economy of scale did not materialize. AMR had much to digest with MedTrans and CareLine. Rural/Metro had to integrate its 90 or so acquisitions, including an early 1998 acquisition of a large ambulance service in Argentina.

As the consolidation phase of health care in general waned, the hospital and practice management companies also experienced similar difficulties. Stock prices fell precipitously and some companies even declared bankruptcy.

Both Rural/Metro Corporation and AMR had borrowed large sums of money to finance acquisitions, build infrastructure, and purchase ambulances. Servicing this debt became an enormous burden for companies in a low-margin business with the additional pressures of declining reimbursement, managed care discounts, and the disastrous effects of the Balanced Budget Act of 1997 on Medicare payments. These companies also experienced a large increase in Medicare and Medicaid compliance audit activity.

In Argentina, the collapse of the peso in January, 2002 led to the closure of several of the recently purchased ambulance companies.

Another consequence of this consolidation and acquisition activity was the departure or termination of many prior owners after the acquisition, because they could not "fit into the corporate world" of big business. These former owners, who had built successful businesses and the community relationships, were disenfranchised and had expiring non-compete agreements. They could now compete against their acquirers or buy back their business at a substantial discount from the purchase price. This has, in fact, occurred in many cases, much to the consternation of AMR and Rural/Metro Corporation.

During 2000 and 2001 the ambulance industry has been under severe pressure. There has been a decreasing volume of ambulance transport in most markets, mostly due to a shift to lower levels of transport, which are not covered by health insurance. The continuing impact of the Balanced Budget Act of 1997 puts downward pressure on Medicare ambulance reimbursement. Managed-care companies continue to deny coverage, discount fees, and delay payment.

The two remaining consolidators have experienced tremendous financial strain. Laidlaw, the parent of AMR, has been trying to sell AMR for over a year, with no takers. Laidlaw now considers AMR and its other healthcare businesses as discontinued operations; in fact, Laidlaw filed for bankruptcy protection earlier this year. Rural/Metro has experienced similar problems, with declining transport numbers and revenues. In the fiscal year completed in June, 2001, ambulance revenue made up less than 80% of the company's revenue, reversing a multi-year trend in the opposite direction. Although Rural/Metro has not sought bankruptcy protection because of the largesse of its lenders, the operating environment remains difficult and the company's future is far from certain. Both consolidators have closed underperforming operations and significantly downsized their non-clinical workforce. Small private ambulance companies are also stressed by the difficult reimbursement climate and decreasing ambulance transports.

The Future of Private EMS

The future of the private ambulance is positive but it will be unlike the past and present. The ambulance industry must more efficiently handle operations and manage overhead. It must partner with public EMS and fire departments in a manner similar to the successful model in San Diego. Similarly, it must partner with integrated delivery systems, hospital systems, and payors to continue to provide the nonemergency transportation as well. With the ageing of the population, the advances in medicine, and the evolution of integrated healthcare delivery systems, the need to transport patients will increase significantly. It will be incumbent on those companies that wish to be successful in the new millennium to truly understand the direction of health care and its needs, and to learn how to partner with the other stakeholders in health care.

There are significant threats. Reimbursement will continue to be a challenge. Medicare has been planning a national ambulance fee schedule for some time. It has been repeatedly delayed in its implementation, although 2002 should see it actually come to fruition. Successful ambulance companies will need to understand the new fee schedule and how it will affect service delivery, level of service, documentation requirements, and reimbursement. During the negotiated rule-making process a subgroup of physicians, nurses, and paramedics developed a condition coding system that would make medical necessity documentation and reimbursement much more appropriate and simple. If implemented with the fee schedule, it would ease reimbursement and decrease audit risk. There has not yet been a final determination regarding inclusion of the condition codes, but it would be a strong positive for ambulance providers.

There is also opportunity in expanding the spectrum of services offered. Transportation, from the very simple and nonmedical (taxi, van) through the more complex forms of critical care, specialty care, and air ambulance, need to be offered, coordinated, and managed. The private sector is in the optimal position to assume this management role, enabling one-stop shopping for customers of transportation services and putting the incentive for efficiency on the operators of private EMS Services. The large consolidators would be in a very good position to benefit from the upcoming opportunities if they can shed their debt, learn to provide lower-level services in a more profitable manner, and partner with the municipal fire departments, municipal EMS services, insurance payors, and integrated delivery systems.

Physician medical directors can play a very effective role in assisting the management of ambulance companies to benefit from the opportunities and to minimize the threats and risks. For medical directors who understand the business of medical transportation and who are networked in their medical, healthcare, and public safety communities, the opportunity to succeed and assist their employers has never been greater.

Military

Maj. Robert A. De Lorenzo, MC, USA
Cmdr. Jerry Mothershead, MC, USN

Introduction

"Necessity is the mother of invention" is an apt maxim for the early development of military EMS. A structured and organized system of early medical care and evacuation has developed over the centuries to deal with the high numbers of casualties in armed conflicts. Interestingly, many of the earliest innovations in modern civilian EMS came as a result of information and expertise gathered through medical support of military operations.

Throughout much of history, the care of wounded soldiers was neglected or poorly administered. Military commanders were more concerned with tactics, troop movements, and supply. Before the eighteenth century, surgeons accompanying armies served only the nobility. The troops had to depend on comrades or family. Queen Isabella of Spain was the first monarch to organize help for wounded soldiers. In 1487 at the siege of Malaga, her armies carried wounded soldiers in bedded wagons to large tent hospitals in safe areas. These ambulances were cumbersome, requiring up to 40 horses to pull them, and were stationed miles from the battlefield. Surgeons waited hours to provide what little care was possible. Progressive military leaders recognized that poor medical care wasted military manpower and was demoralizing to the soldier.[1]

Systematic collection of the wounded from the battlefield began during the Napoleonic Wars. Recognizing that battlefield casualty care approached chaos, Napoleon appointed Jean Larrey to develop what became known as the "ambulance volantes" or flying field hospitals. These lightweight carriages and hospital facilities moved quickly to collect, transport, and care for the injured even as the fighting continued.[2]

The first major test of U.S. military emergency medical care came during the Civil War. More than 300,000 soldiers died on the Union side alone. The first major battle of the war, Bull Run in 1861, was a disaster by most military and medical standards. The Union Army entered the battle with few ambulances or medical personnel. Litter bearers were untrained bandsmen who laid down their instruments and picked up litters. Civilian ambulance drivers drank the alcohol in their medicine chest and stayed near the battlefield only long enough to rob the wounded. Nonwounded, panicking Union soldiers often used ambulances that had not broken down or been commandeered by officers for their personal use. In the Union Army's retreat, not a single wounded person was transported to safety. Three days after the battle, 3000 wounded men still lay on the battlefield without food, water, or protection from the summer sun and rain. Some were without care for 6 to 7 days. Many died from lack of food, water, and basic medical care.[3]

As a result of the Bull Run fiasco, the Union Army restructured its haphazard wartime emergency care services. William Hammond, Surgeon General of the Union Army, and Jonathan Letterman, medical director of the Army of the Potomac, were the primary agents of change. Letterman is credited with developing the first Army-wide ambulance service in 1862.[4] In 1887 the Hospital Corps was established, which is the forerunner of the modern enlisted medical corps. Men who volunteered from line units were given training in first-aid and litter bearing. After a one-year apprenticeship, candidates could take an examination for selection as privates in the Hospital Corps. Following one year of probationary training and passage of another examination, they could be appointed Hospital Stewards.[5]

The military EMS system relies on the training of individual nonmedical soldiers in basic preventive medicine and first-aid, pre-positioned care providers, adequate numbers of appropriate ambulances, and a system of graduated care. Rapid transport and early hospitalization and surgery made a tremendous impact on military preparedness by preventing disease, boosting morale, and conserving manpower. Through evolving technology and individual creativity, the military medical system has continually improved wartime military casualty survival rate (table 8.1). An estimated 22,000 lives were saved in Vietnam as a result of advances developed as a result of, or after, the Korean War.[6]

Lessons learned and innovations developed in Vietnam were brought to the United States by returning military care providers. Elements of the systems approach to emergency medical care were integrated into the civilian community. Contributing to civilian EMS improvements were military influences such as aeromedical evacuation, centers specializing in the care of trauma victims, provision of advanced life support care, and multiple levels of providers.[7,8] Civilian EMS services enjoyed tremendous growth during the 1960s and 1970s, in part due to the role the military played in laying the groundwork for prehospital care.

Current Military EMS

The modern military EMS system exists as a result of military wartime and peacetime requirements. The goal of each is to accomplish a mission. The military medical system's specific mission is to conserve the fighting strength.[9] During peacetime the mission is accomplished much as it is in the civilian EMS community, but it is drastically modified during conflict. The wartime medical system can best be understood by describing its personnel, organization, transportation, equipment, communications, and control.

Personnel

The military services provide medical assistance through a spectrum of trained personnel. From frontline medics with basic skills to sophisticated nursing, physician, administrative, and logistical support, individuals are assigned a specific job with associated training and skills that are divided into different levels of care provider.

All nonmedical personnel receive basic first-aid training in such procedures as bleeding control and simple splinting. The military uses the terms "self-aid" and "buddy-aid" to describe this first line of emergency medical defense. In the Army, selected *nonmedical* soldiers (usually one per vehicle crew or operating team) are given an additional 40 hours of training to include intravenous insertion, advanced splinting, and other more advanced first-aid measures. This level is termed "combat lifesaver" and approximates the civilian certified first responder program, with an expanded scope of practice.[9]

The Army Military Occupational Specialty (MOS) 91B Medical Specialist (combat medic) receives ten weeks of training that roughly correlates to basic emergency medical technician (EMT-B) training. Additional training is provided in intravenous insertion and the care of patients with military-related problems such as nuclear, biological, and chemical warfare injuries.[5] Medical noncommissioned officers (sergeants) receive ten weeks of additional training, roughly equivalent to EMT Intermediate (EMT-I). Skills include intubations, intravenous access, and advanced cardiac life support (ACLS). Beginning in 2001, the Army embarks on a major overhaul of the combat medic program that includes increased initial training (to 16 weeks), expansion of skills, and increased emphasis on preventive medicine and weapons of mass destruction casualty management. Increased medical oversight, clinical practicums in initial training, and a minimum requirement for EMT-B certification by the National Registry of EMTs will become standard.[10,11] Because there are nearly 38,000 combat medics in the active Army, Army Reserve, and National Guard, this massive re-engineering will take approximately six to eight years to fully accomplish. These individuals will be assigned the MOS of 91W.

The Air Force's version of the Army identification system is the Air Force Specialty Code (AFSC). The 90230 medical technician receives 16 weeks of training including an EMT-B curriculum and additional training similar to that given to Army counterparts. Medical technicians progress to the 90250 level by completing self-study Career Development Courses (CDC) while enrolled in on-the-job training. The 90270 level is achieved by completing one year in upgrade training time and additional CDCs.

TABLE 8.1	
Mortality of Battle Casualties Reaching Treatment Facilities[19]	
WAR	**MORTALITY (%)**
World War I	8.0
World War II	4.5
Korea	2.5
Vietnam	2.0

Navy enlisted hospital corps personnel provide the vast majority of the manpower for prehospital emergency care. Prior to 2000, hospital corpsmen received all didactic material and practical skills training in accordance with the EMT-B National Standard Curriculum, as part of Hospital Corpsman Basic "A" School. Some of this material has since been removed, but the majority of the information is still provided. Following completion of "A" School, corpsmen are classified as general duty, or 0000. Corpsmen assigned to deployable Fleet Marine Force Units are provided further training as Field Medical Technicians (8404). This training, approximately 12 weeks in length, includes the equivalent of Prehospital Trauma Life Support, treatment of chemical, biological, and nuclear agent casualties, and other medical skills. Additional training for shipboard hospital corpsmen is primarily "on-the-job," but includes those skills necessary to assist shipboard medical officers or Independent Duty Hospital Corpsmen (see below). There is no Navy equivalent to the Army 91W.

The military sports another level of provider with no real counterpart in the civilian system. This is the "independent duty medic" and is represented by the Navy Independent Duty Hospital Corpsman, Air Force Independent Duty Technician, and Army Special Operations Medic. Although their training is slightly different, each shares the common experience of extensive (1000–2000 hours) training in limited primary care to include diagnosis and treatment of minor ailments, and limited laboratory and radiographic interpretation.[12,13] Individuals assigned duty with special operations forces are additionally registered with the National Registry of EMTs as paramedics. Independent duty medics exist in limited numbers and have a practice generally restricted to active-duty service members. Most serve in locations such as on ships or at remote bases where an on-site physician would be impractical. They have the training, skills, and a scope of practice somewhat equivalent to a physician assistant.

The branch medical corps provides medical oversight. Military physicians are required to be state licensed, and the majority are specialty board eligible or certified. Unique military requirements necessitate that physicians be proficient in medical problems specific to their patient populations. Physician assistants also play an important role in bridging the gap between physicians and the ever-mobile and widely dispersed soldiers, sailors, and airmen.

Many nurses in the Air Force, and a more limited number in the Navy, are trained as Flight Nurses. These personnel are provided additional training to allow them to serve, independent of direct medical oversight, during fixed-wing air evacuations. All are certified in Advanced Cardiac Life Support and receive additional training in advanced life-support procedures, as well as specific training in the physiological effects of flight on patients.

All providers receive training in emergency care specific to military needs, including treatment of chemical and radiation casualties and handling mass casualty incidents. Military hospitals and EMS systems are mandated to exercise their mass casualty capabilities several times a year; deployable assets such as ships and special support facilities have these exercises on an even more frequent and mission-specific basis.

Organization

The military Levels of Care (formerly referred to as "Echelons of Care") system describes a graduated hierarchy of combat medical care and facilities (table 8.2).[14,15] Treatment capabilities are roughly standardized for each level of care across the services, in compliance with Joint Chief of Staff doctrinal directives.

Level I is located closest to the fighting, and thus, Level I care is austere and its elements are light and mobile. It includes four levels of care: (1) self- and buddy-aid, (2) combat lifesaving, (3) combat medic care, and (4) "aid station care." The first three of these have previously been discussed. For the U.S. Army and Marines, the battalion aid station is the first medical "facility" casualties will encounter, and may be staffed by physicians or physician assistants. It is austere and highly mobile, with advanced trauma life support capabilities, including endotracheal intubation, tube thoracostomy, intravenous medication and other physician-directed medical care. Navy ships have a rough equivalent in various satellite "battle dressing stations" located remotely from the primary shipboard medical department.

Level II is a divisional level "clearing station" that is staffed by a medical company of physicians, nurses, and medics. Casualties are examined to determine treatment needs and evacuation precedence. Emergency medical treatment, including initial comprehensive resuscitation, is provided, and is supported by limited radiographic, dental, and laboratory services with whole-blood capacity. It provides limited dura-

TABLE 8.2
Levels of Military Medical Care

LEVEL	MILITARY HIERARCHY	PERSONNEL/FACILITY	TYPE OF CARE
I	Unit	Self/Buddy Aid	First Aid
		Combat Lifesaver	First Aid, beginning Emergency Treatment
		Combat Medic	Emergency Medical Treatment
		Battalion Aid Station	Advanced Trauma and Medical Management
II	Division	Medical Company (Clearing Station)	Initial Resuscitation
		Field Surgical Support Group	
III	Corps	Combat Support Hospital	Resuscitative Surgery and Medical Care
		Fleet Hospitals	
		Augmented Amphibious Ships	
IV	Echelons above Corps	Combat Support Hospital	Definitive Care
		Host Nation Hospitals	
		Hospital Ships	
V	Out of Theater Continental US	Fixed Medical Facilities	Restorative and Rehabilitative Care

tion patient-holding capability for personnel, roughly at the general ward level. Ship medical departments approximate this capability, as do the Marine Fleet Surgical Support Groups. In the case of casualties generated by a shipboard incident, response by the ship's medical department is usually rapid and effective. Patients with injuries or illnesses beyond the capabilities of the ship's sick bay are evacuated to a rear-area facility or major hospital ship.

Level III is the first true medical facility a casualty will encounter on the battlefield. Presently, this will be a U.S. Army combat support hospital, the Air Force air transportable hospitals, the Navy fleet hospitals, and the major amphibious assault ships, if augmented by surgical support teams. These amphibious vessels are capable of converting several hundred marine berthing spaces into medical wards of various capabilities. Level III hospitals provide comprehensive resuscitative surgery and medical care. Medical providers include general surgeons, and both surgical and medical sub-specialists, with comprehensive anesthesia and nursing support. Patients who are unlikely to return to duty are evacuated as soon as possible after stabilization.

Level IV has been traditionally represented by comprehensive theater hospitals variously designated as General, Field, Theater Area, or Station Hospitals. These large and poorly mobile facilities provided definitive medical and surgical care and were equipped

with a broad array of support services. Since today's operational requirements call for a more flexible and mobile medical facility, it is unlikely that a true Level IV Hospital capability will exist in future warfighting theaters of operation. Instead, enhanced Combat Support Hospitals in the theater, plus direct evacuation of "stabilized" patients to the United States, will meet this Level IV requirement. Two key exceptions to this continue to exist: the Navy's two 1,000-bed hospital ships (*USNS Mercy* and *USNS Comfort*), and any host nation hospitals with which the services may have developed official relationships. Both of these Level IV capabilities were in use and in theater during Operation Desert Storm.

Level V represents fixed hospitals located outside the theater of operations, and in the continental United States. These are primarily military medical facilities, augmented within the United States by Veteran's Administration, and civilian hospitals as part of the National Defense Medical System. Definitive and rehabilitative care of all types may be found in Level V facilities.

The numeric sequence of these Levels may appear to imply a rigid stepwise movement of patients from Level I to Level II, and so on. This may have been true in its earliest conception, but is too inflexible for the dynamic operational environment of modern warfare. A strict hierarchy of units and levels is unlikely to exist on the modern battlefield. Another major change in military medical doctrine is the increased forward availability of medical expertise and technology. "Forward Surgical Teams," whose expertise was previously available only at Level III facilities, are now located in traditional Level II units.

Transportation

The goal of combat medical evacuation (medevac) is the safe and effective movement of the casualties. Transportation modes might include manual carries, ground vehicles, aircraft, watercraft, or any combination of these.

In many military operations, the manual carry is the primary means of moving casualties from the point of injury or illness to a point of safety where the medical evacuation can begin. Despite tremendous advances in many other areas of evacuation, manual carries remain almost unchanged over the centuries. Manual carries can be exhausting work, and necessarily have a range limited to a few hundred or thousand meters.

Litter transportation offers modest improvements over manual carries. Some support and comfort is afforded the patient, and spinal immobilization, fracture splinting, oxygen therapy, and other static treatments can be often maintained during movement. Airway management, ventilation, and other dynamic care remain difficult to perform. Litter carries have the additional advantage that the work of transporting a patient can be shared by two to four persons. The shipboard environment poses constraints of difficult extraction and hazardous operating conditions. These are overcome by training, drills, a pervasive emphasis on safety, and innovations such as specialized stretchers and backpack transport of medical supplies to incident locations.

Ground vehicles are the most common platform used to move casualties over relatively long distances on the battlefield. Current U.S. military doctrine places dedicated ambulances in the warfighting maneuver units. In most scenarios, battlefield casualties will be carried or dragged several hundred meters to a casualty collection point where ground ambulances can pick them up. As a result, ground ambulances can be expected to get fairly close to the scene of injury.

The helicopter ambulance has been a valuable component of the medevac system since its introduction for this role during the Korean War. By the end of the Vietnam War, medevac helicopters offered speed and versatility unmatched by ground platforms.[16] They are largely unaffected by terrain and can reach remote areas inaccessible to ground vehicles. Disadvantages include their cost and vulnerability to small-arms fire. This latter factor accounts for the doctrine of keeping helicopter pickup points a safe distance from direct hostile fire. Helicopter evacuation is also very weather-dependent. Most casualties will still need to be carried to a point of safety by a combination of manual or litter carry and ground vehicle transportation.[17] The Army provides all dedicated helicopter medevac services for military units, and Army helicopter squadrons are designated as transportation assets for the Navy hospital ships.

Medevac shares two significant limitations: availability and limited patient-care en route. Battlefields and disasters are fluid and dynamic situations, making it challenging to anticipate where ambulances will most be needed. Field medical providers must be capable of improvising transportation when ambulances are not available. Using non-medical vehicles and personnel for casualty evacuation including trucks, buses, and non-medical helicopters, is a well recognized part of military contingency planning.[18]

The second limitation of tactical medevac is the difficulty in providing en route or ongoing care. Ground and air platforms are cramped, noisy, poorly illuminated, and prone to vibration, jarring, and sway. Patient access, assessment, monitoring, and interventions are difficult at best. Only in the most modern platforms are there provisions for onboard oxygen and suction. Airway, breathing, and monitoring equipment are not built-in, and thus must be brought separately. An attempt to compensate for this deficiency may be seen with the development of the Life Saving Treatment and Transport module (LSTAT). The LSTAT is a state-of-the-art patient stretcher that allows more sophisticated patient monitoring and treatment than has been possible in the past.

Equipment

Forward medical equipment is often limited by weight and space restrictions, but includes airway, breathing, circulatory, hemorrhage control, and splinting devices. Intravenous circulatory support and basic invasive procedures including needle and tube thoracostomies may be performed at the aid station. Simple lifesaving surgery may be performed at the forward support surgical team collocated with the medical company (clearing station, Level II), but definitive procedures are reserved for the hospitals further in the evacuation chain. Rear-area evacuation hospitals are capable of modern, sophisticated services. Military research commands continue to experiment with sophisticated technology aimed at improving survival and decreasing mortality. Such innovations as electronic "dog tags" that include important medical information, physiological monitoring vests, and collagen impregnated battle dressings, are but a few.

Communications

Much of the medical oversight, and many clinical or logistics decisions affecting patient-care and movement, take place from afar during combat operations. Medical communications networks are vital to these requirements. The direct radio supervision of field providers through radio communications in the tactical setting must be minimized for security reasons.[19] Because of communications bandwidth limitations, dedicated, sole-use medical communications systems have been rare in combat. However, continued research and development in audio, video, and data transmission technology ("telemedicine") show promise to link far-forward enlisted care providers with physicians farther in the rear. Pilot programs aboard ships and in remote outposts have demonstrated this potential. Because of weight, bulk, reliability, and cost concerns, the foreseeable future, however, will likely see only modest deployment of advanced communications equipment in the far-forward field environment.

Control

Control of tactical prehospital personnel and other medical resources is generally under the direct supervision of the unit commander, who is usually not a medical officer. This situation is analogous to the incident command system (ICS) where the medical sector is under the control of the Incident Commander, often a non-medical fire officer.[20] The reasons are again parallel to the civilian ICS example: the medical mission is often subordinate to the overall tactical mission. In this regard, the military command-and-control format is not unfamiliar and in fact underscores another aspect of modern EMS that draws its origins from the military. Although overall control of military medical units rests with the unit commander, day-to-day medical oversight and operational control are directed by the medical officers and noncommissioned officers (sergeants and petty officers) within the medical section or element. Owing to the dispersed nature of combat units, intervening independent-duty medics or physician assistants are often called upon as delegated representatives of the physician.

Military EMS during Peacetime

Each military installation is generally responsible for its own medical care under the direction and support of a centralized military medical command. The medical services of each installation are linked to the overall military medical care system. At smaller or more isolated locations, patients are referred to military hospitals at other locations for secondary care. These in turn are linked to a series of more sophisticated tertiary-care medical centers, each with special capabilities, consultants, and equipment. However, referral is not restricted to military systems. A patient may be referred to the closest appropriate hospital, whether military or civilian. Occasionally, civilian patients may be referred to a military facility when appropriate resources are not otherwise available.

Prehospital care at military installations has historically been the function of the supporting medical treatment facility, whether an outpatient clinic or a full-service military hospital, and the majority of installations are provided EMS services by these facilities. This model is becoming rarer in the civilian sector, where less than 5% of EMS agencies are operated by or from hospitals.

Installation needs and overall medical requirements drive levels of care and system design at military installations. The combined total population requiring EMS services at these sites approaches 3.5 million (more than each of the U.S. territories and 26 of the states). However, with over 800 worldwide military installations, the majority of military locations have populations, including resident dependents and civil servants, of less than 20,000. With its younger, healthier population, superficial inspection would suggest the incidence of significant medical problems requiring EMS would be low. This does not seem to be the case—one study revealed BLS and ALS level requirements similar to civilian communities, and this was borne out in a service-wide survey conducted in the Navy in 1998.[21,22]

Most states provide general exemptions from statutes and administrative codes for federal EMS services. Each of the three services has regulations governing installation EMS operations. In general, wide latitude is provided to medical treatment facility commanders in the provision of these services, but commanders are directed to meet community standards of care. Additionally, although not binding, the Government Services Chapter of the American College of Emergency Physicians, comprised primarily of active duty, reserve, and retired military medical officers, has recommended that installation EMS services meet or exceed community standards.[23] Difficulties arise in that no two communities are identical, standards of care may be insufficient or nonexistent at overseas locations, and none of the services has specifically identified the various standards with which to comply (e.g., response times, equipment, levels of providers, etc.). At a time of shrinking budgets and manpower, the services are struggling to ensure the optimal quality of this service for all beneficiaries without escalating costs at the expense of other medical services.

In general, access to services is through an installation-specific number, usually not through the national emergency number "9-1-1." The area of responsibility is normally restricted to federally owned land, although, at many overseas locations, beneficiaries reside in the local community, often without community EMS. At these locations, the catchment area may be extended. Dispatch may occur from a centralized location, or through the installation Fire Department or medical treatment facility. At most locations, Fire Department personnel (who are trained at either the First Responder or EMT-Basic level) perform nontransport first response functions. Installation of primary EMS response services is usually at the EMT-Basic level, although an increasing number of installations have upgraded to the EMT-Intermediate or EMT-Paramedic level. Ambulance service providers include supporting military hospitals or federal Fire Departments, contracted ambulances agencies, or community municipal agencies. Patients are delivered to the installation medical treatment facility, or, if the patient's condition exceeds the capabilities of that facility, they are directly transported to area hospitals.

Interaction with the Civilian Community

Military-civilian interactions may be considered in two parts: those occurring in the course of daily, routine operations, and those that may occur in response to disasters or other emergency exigencies.

At overseas locations, cooperative sharing of resources occurs under the auspices of written agreements between the United States and the host nation governments, referred to as Status of Forces Agreements (SOFA). SOFAs allow for utilization of each of the parties' capabilities to the mutual benefit of both. In the United States, this cooperative sharing arrangement occurs less frequently, due to issues of competition between local vendors and the federal government. There are notable exceptions, however.

Military hospitals occasionally provide the only resources, or augment scarce resources, in the civilian community. Many serve as specialty care centers for large geographic areas. Madigan Army Medical Center in Tacoma, Washington; Brooke Army Medical Center in San Antonio, Texas; William Beaumont Army Medical Center in El Paso, Texas; and Wilford Hall Air Force Hospital in San Antonio, Texas all serve as trauma centers in their communities. Madigan is an important provider of paramedic ambulance services for an otherwise underserved portion of Washington state; it also serves as an EMS direct medical control facility. Darnall Army Community Hospital in Killeen, Texas is the only hospital providing sophisticated emergency services in a large area of central Texas. Brooke Army Medical Center is an important international resource for burn victims.

The Military Assistance to Safety and Traffic (MAST) program exemplifies the use of military resources for community services.[24] Since 1969 the MAST program has provided military aeromedical evacuation capabilities to civilian communities. They have flown thousands of missions and transported tens of thousands of patients. This service has been accomplished safely and without expense to the patients; the military has benefited by maintaining aeromedical evacuation skills. Such services were the forerunners to the now prevalent civilian air medical programs. In developing civilian programs, much was learned from military air medical evacuation experience. Since the development of civilian helicopter systems throughout the United States, the number of MAST missions has declined dramatically, primarily because of the non-compete requirement placed on the military. Where civilian aeromedical systems exist, they must be accessed first and decline a mission before MAST may participate.[25]

In the event of a large-scale emergency or disaster situation, military response, including medical and EMS, is governed under a concept referred to as Military Support to Civil Authorities (MSCA). There are two levels of response. Under the MSCA doctrine, commanders, including medical commanders, may utilize existing military resources to assist local communities to preserve life or to mitigate or prevent major property loss. This may be done without higher-level authority, and is known as the "Immediate Response" clause of MSCA. In the case of a disaster of the magnitude that a larger force or more prolonged assistance would be necessary, all military actions are governed by the Stafford Act. Under the Stafford Act, each of the various federal agencies is assigned Lead Federal Agency responsibilities to assist the states and local communities in disaster response. The military is assigned a supporting role only, but has this role in all emergency support functions of disaster relief as described by the Federal Response Plan. For most disasters, ultimate coordination of the federal response is assigned to the Federal Emergency Management Agency. Medical support is assigned to the Department of Health and Human Services. In the event of specific terrorist acts involving weapons of mass destruction, the Federal Bureau of Investigation has overall Federal Lead Agency responsibilities for investigation of the crime scene only (known as "Crisis Management").

For overseas disasters or other humanitarian assistance missions, appropriate arrangements and details of provided support and services are developed by the Department of State and the supported nation.

The Military and the National Disaster Medical System

The Department of Defense is a prime initiator, planner, and current participant in the National Disaster Medical System (NDMS). Military resources are the transportation backbone for many NDMS missions. Military personnel and facilities assist in the coordination of participating hospital networks. Department of Defense leadership, medical personnel, and logistic groups may assist in relief efforts.[26,27,28]

The NDMS concept has been tested, primarily in the prehospital setting, and military medical providers have assisted other federal agencies in hurricane relief or other humanitarian assistance missions within the continental United States. For domestic disaster medical support, the Office of Emergency Preparedness has cognizance over the NDMS. This agency unfortunately possesses few facilities, and even fewer personnel, in comparison to the Department of Defense and the Veteran's Administration. Military personnel, physical resources, and facilities are crucial to the overall success of the NDMS.

Summary

The military pioneered systematic emergency care. Both the military and civilian sectors have come a long way in adapting wartime lessons to peacetime EMS. The sharing of resources and responsibilities by civilian and military communities can improve these services even more. Because much can be learned from each other, open professional exchanges and planning to meet the needs of the ill and injured must take priority over issues of jurisdiction, sources of payment, and patient eligibility. Working from these premises, the mission and goals of both sectors may be accomplished.

Reference

1. Boyd D, Edlilch R, Micik S, eds. *Systems approach to emergency medical care*. Norwalk, CT: Appleton-Century-Crofts; 1983.
2. Richardson GR. *Larrey: Surgeon to Napoleon's Imperial Guard*. London: John Murray; 1974.
3. Adams GW. *Doctors in Blue*. New York: Collier Books: 1961.
4. Stewart MJ. *Moving the Wounded: Litters, Cacolets and Ambulance Wagons, US Army 1776–1876*. Fort Collins, CO: The Old Army Press; 1979.
5. Summers MB, Bryan DN, De Lorenzo RA. *The US Army Medical Specialist*. In On-line supplement to American Academy of Orthopedic Surgeons. *Emergency Care and Transportation of the Sick and Injured*. 7th ed. Sudbury, MA: Jones and Bartlett; 1999.
6. Bellamy R. The causes of death in conventional land warfare: implications for combat casualty care research. *Military Medicine*. 1984;1495:55–62.
7. De Lorenzo RA. Improving combat casualty care and field medicine: focus on the military medic. *Military Medicine*. 1997;162(4):268–272.
8. De Lorenzo RA. Military and civilian emergency aeromedical services: achieving common goals with different approaches. *Aviation, Space and Environmental Medicine*. 1997;68(1):56–60
9. Department of the Army. *Field Manual 8-10: Health Service Support in a Theater of Operations*. Washington, DC; 1991.
10. De Lorenzo RA. 91W: Force XXI combat medic. *AMEDD Journal*. 1999;Oct–Dec:2–6.
11. De Lorenzo RA. Making the leap to 91W: a transition guide for leaders. *AMEDD Journal*. 2000;Jan–Mar:37–41.
12. De Lorenzo RA. Military medic: the original expanded-scope EMS provider. *JEMS*. 1996;21(4):50–54.

13. De Lorenzo RA. Special Training for Special Missions. Sidebar to accompany Military Medic: The Original Expanded-Scope EMS Provider. *JEMS*. 1996;21(4):52.

14. Department of the Army. *Field Manual 8-10-5. Brigade and Division Surgeon's Handbook*. Washington, DC; 1991.

15. Duggan B. Organization of military medical units. In Burkle F, ed. *Disaster medicine*. New York: Medical Examination Co.; 1984.

16. Baxt W.G., Moody P. The impact of rotorcraft aeromedical emergency care services on mortality. *JAMA*. 1983; 249:3047–3051.

17. Dorland P. *Dust Off: Army Aeromedical Evacuation in Vietnam*. Washington, DC, 1982: Center of Military History, United States Army; 1982.

18. Department of the Army. *Field Manual 8-10-6. Medical Evacuation in a Theater of Operations*. Washington, DC; 2000.

19. Bowen TE, Bellamy RF, eds. *Emergency War Surgery*, 2nd ed. US Department of Defense, Washington, DC; 1988.

20. De Lorenzo RA, Porter RS. *Tactical Emergency Care*. Upper Saddle River, NJ: Brady (Prentice Hall); 1999: 384.

21. Leonard F. Ambulance use in a military population: epidemiology and implications. *Mil Med*. 1992, May;157 (5):239–243.

22. Author (J. Mothershead) personal correspondence.

23. De Lorenzo RA, Mothershead JL, Rivera-Rivera E, Biggers W. Military emergency medical services systems (policy statement). *Ann Emerg Med*. 1997;30(4):561.

24. Army Regulation No. 500-4, Air Force Regulation 64-1, Military Assistance to Safety and Traffic (MAST). Washington, DC; 1987.

25. Interagency Executive Group. *Program manual for MAST programs*, Jan 1978.

26. Dolicker GJ. Preparing for the worst: the challenge facing NDMS. *JEMS*. 16(8):94–100.

27. Heaton LD. Army medical service activities in Vietnam. *Mil Med*. 1966;131:646.

28. National Disaster Medical Systems. *Concept of Operations*. Rockville, MD; 1998. (Draft), National Disaster Medical System.

International

Eelco H. Dykstra, MD
Jeffrey L. Arnold, MD

Introduction

E MS has developed rapidly throughout the world in the past two decades as evidenced by reports from numerous countries.[1-34] Multiple factors have promoted the recent global development of EMS, including rapid urbanization, ageing populations, economic growth, and social upheaval in a number of countries. The emergence of emergency medicine as a unique medical specialty throughout the world has supplied specialists in emergency medicine, who have been key proponents of EMS development in their countries.[6,35]

One of the most significant factors in the international development of EMS has been the increased mobility and migration throughout the world in recent years. This process of globalization has led to a sharp rise in expectations about the quality and performance of local EMS systems, irrespective of where they are in the world. As a consequence, the number of international efforts to meet these expectations is steadily growing. Among the better-known examples of establishing minimum international standards are the recommendations for resuscitation promulgated by the American Heart Association Emergency Cardiac Care Division (AHA/ECC) in cooperation with the International Liaison Committee on Resuscitation (ILCOR).

International EMS Systems

The international diversity of EMS systems is astounding. Worldwide, there are more approaches to the delivery of EMS than there are countries.[1-34] When one begins to appreciate that virtually every EMS system is unique, the problem of understanding and categorizing all of these diverse systems becomes nearly impossible. Only by analyzing the various system components that comprise EMS systems in other countries can we begin to unravel operations as complex and multidisciplinary as those belonging to EMS.

In this context it has been said that "a systems approach towards EMS is not a luxury, but a necessity."[39] An analysis of EMS systems worldwide reveals that all EMS systems share a number of essential components (table 9.1). All EMS systems have a mission or purpose. All EMS systems have various stakeholders (including both individuals and groups) whose interests are affected in some way by the functioning of EMS. All EMS systems have various operational, logistical, administrative, planning, and financial subsystems, which enable each overall system to carry out its defined mission. As one example, the several operational subsystems central to EMS systems worldwide include EMS access, regulation (emergency call screening and triage), dispatch, response, and medical oversight.

Major International EMS Models

Certain combinations of EMS systems components appear clustered together so often that they have come to be recognized as useful international EMS models. Although these models represent broad generalizations, they have found international acceptance as convenient "handles," which facilitate further discussion and analysis. The reader familiar with international EMS will recognize that exceptions to the rule occur, even within the same country. The major international EMS model types presented here are the Anglo-American, Franco-German, Netherlands, Sarajevo, and Japanese models.[35]

Anglo-American Model

The most salient component of the Anglo-American model of EMS is the provision of prehospital care by

TABLE 9.1
The Essential International Components of EMS Systems
EMS COMPONENTS
Mission

Stakeholders
  Public
  EMS personnel
  Other agencies
  Policy-makers
  Financiers

Operations
  Access
  Regulation
  Dispatch
  Response
  Medical control

Logistics
  Communication
  Transportation
  Equipment
  EMS facilities
  Definitive care facilities

Planning   Training

Administration
  Organization
  Information transfer
  Quality assurance
  Policy and law

Finance

Franco-German Model

The Franco-German model is based on the provision of prehospital care by physicians. Here, physician participation tends to be operational, with physicians typically serving as members of the EMS crew. Although in some cases paramedics can perform advanced interventions, it is only with the supervision of a physician at the scene. In Germany, the backgrounds, qualifications, and experience levels of these EMS physicians vary significantly, particularly in the more rural areas where physicians are hard to come by.

Another operational component in some countries, such as France, Spain, and many Latin American countries, is "medical regulation," which describes the placement of a physician at the dispatch step to field calls to EMS. This physician regulator then triages the call and matches it with available resources, dispatching the appropriate level of response. In some cases, the regulator may provide definitive medical advice, obviating the need to send any resources at all.

Advocates of the Franco-German approach speak about their "emergency physicians," but these are generally not comparable with their counterparts from the Anglo-American model. The major distinction is that clinical and academic recognition for EMS and emergency medicine is largely absent in the Franco-German model. Why is this important? First, without clinical recognition, it is impossible to offer a career perspective to young physicians with a lifetime commitment to EMS, emergency medicine, or both. Board certification is only possible in other specialties, such as anaesthesia, surgery, or internal medicine. Second, without academic recognition, it is nearly impossible to mobilize or maintain the volume and quality of the resources required for research in EMS or emergency medicine. The Franco-German model is found in many European and Latin American countries.

The Netherlands Model

The Netherlands model is based on the provision of advanced prehospital care by nurses. These ambulance nurses can best be compared with "nurse practitioners" in the United States. They are licensed to independently perform the full range of interventions in an EMS setting, independent of direct medical oversight. In general, the Netherlands model follows the Franco-German model in the sense that there is

non-physicians. Other characteristic components include regulation and dispatch of EMS resources by non-physician personnel, and the provision of prehospital life-support care by emergency medical technicians and paramedics.

Because non-physicians provide prehospital care in the Anglo-American model, the important operational component of medical oversight has evolved, through which emergency physicians provide direct or indirect supervision of non-physician emergency care providers. Here emergency physicians assume a strategic or directive role, serving as directors, educators, and arbiters of quality management. Accordingly, clinical and academic recognition exists for these emergency physicians. Proponents of the Anglo-American approach to EMS include the countries of Australia, Canada, Costa Rica, Hong Kong, New Zealand, Singapore, Taiwan, the United Kingdom, and the United States.

no clinical or academic recognition for EMS or emergency medicine. This model is not only found in the Netherlands, but also parts of Thailand.

The Sarajevo Model

The Sarajevo model utilizes community-based, free-standing EMS facilities or "emergency centers" to provide EMS and EMS-related services. Emergency centers not only provide traditional EMS functions, such as ambulance base stations, but may also contain central dispatch centers and clinical facilities, ranging from walk-in type clinics to full-scale emergency departments without any attachment to a particular hospital. Emergency centers may also incorporate auxiliary functions like EMS training, or interventions from the public or occupational health domains. This model can be found in parts of Eastern Europe and Asia.

The Japanese Model

The Japanese model of EMS is also based on "emergency centers," but in this case, the emergency centers are more akin to free-standing intensive care units than emergency departments. In this model, only the most critically ill or injured patients are brought by ambulance directly to an emergency care center, which usually consists of a 20- to 30-bed critical care unit surrounded by specialized facilities, including an operating room, intensive care unit, and often a cardiac catheterization unit. These emergency centers may stand independently or be physically attached to a larger hospital. One of the key components in this system is the presence of triage protocols that clearly define which patients should be delivered to emergency centers. While the Anglo-American model has been described as taking the patient to the hospital and the Franco-German model takes the hospital to the patient, the Japanese model brings the patient to the ICU. Approximately 150 of these emergency centers are spread throughout Japan. This model has also developed in Russia and has been exported to China.

Resources for the International Development of EMS

Several organizations and institutions throughout the world have played important roles in the development of international EMS systems in recent years.

Governmental organizations, such as the U.S. Department of Transportation, have made standards and training protocols for EMS personnel available to other countries. Nongovernmental organizations, such as the American Heart Association, have led an international movement to create universal standards for resuscitation from out-of-hospital cardiac arrest. In addition, the International Medical Corps and other organizations have initiated EMS development projects around the world.

An increasing number of international conferences has promoted the exchange of information about EMS in the world today. In the United States, the National Association of EMS Physicians (NAEMSP) has added an international section to its annual conference. In Europe, the Pan-European Center for Emergency Medical Management Systems (PECEMMS) has sponsored international conferences on EMS and emergency medicine throughout Europe since 1992. In Asia, the Asian Society for Emergency Medicine has organized a biennial conference on EMS and emergency medicine. Other organizations sponsoring international conferences include the International Federation of Emergency Medicine (Australia, Canada, Hong Kong, United States, and United Kingdom), European Society of Emergency Medicine, and various local and national societies of emergency medicine throughout the world.

Publications have been an important source of information exchange about EMS in other countries. Selected international journals of EMS and emergency medicine are listed in table 9.2. A number of web sites have also fostered the international exchange of information about EMS. Sponsored by a variety of organizations and institutions throughout the world, a selection of useful international EMS sites is listed in table 9.3.

Summary

The basic information contained in this chapter can be used as a frame of reference and a starting point when coming into contact with any aspect of international EMS. Virtually every EMS professional will encounter patients or colleagues from other systems and countries. Since the majority of the world has not yet decided which models to adopt, there are ample opportunities to become actively involved.

In order to facilitate involvement, a number of recommendations are listed in the form of "major lessons," which represent years of personal and institu-

TABLE 9.2	
Selected International Journals of EMS and Emergency Medicine	
COUNTRY/REGION	**JOURNAL**
Australia	*Emergency Medicine*
Brazil	*Brazilian Journal for Trauma and Emergency Medicine*
Canada	*Canadian Journal of Emergency Medicine*
China	*The Chinese Journal of Emergency Medicine*
Czech Republic	*The Journal of Emergency Medical Care*
Europe	*European Journal of Emergency Medicine*
France	*Reanimation Urgences*
Germany	*Der Notarzt*
Hong Kong (SAR)	*Hong Kong Journal of Emergency Medicine*
Italy	*Pronto Soccorso Nuovo*
Japan	*Journal of the Japanese Association for Acute Medicine*
New Zealand	*Emergency Medicine*
Philippines	*Lifeline/Philippine Journal of Emergency Medicine*
South Africa	*Trauma and Emergency Medicine*
South Korea	*Journal of the Korean Society of Emergency Medicine*
Spain	*Emergencias, Urgencias*
Sweden	*Journal of Traffic Medicine*
Taiwan	*Journal of Critical Care and Emergency Medicine*
Turkey	*Acil Tip Dergisi*
United Kingdom	*Emergency Medicine Journal (formerly Journal of Accident and Emergency Medicine), Pre-hospital Immediate Care*
United States	*Academic Emergency Medicine, American Journal of Emergency Medicine, Annals of Emergency Medicine, Journal of Emergency Medicine, Journal of Emergency Medical Services, Prehospital and Disaster Medicine, Prehospital Emergency Care*

tional experience.[36–38] These lessons describe the pitfalls that occur when attempting to compare EMS systems internationally and the problems encountered when helping to develop EMS systems. Either way, these recommendations are intended to help avoid the traps and errors that others have fallen into. They are perhaps the most important lessons to remember when considering any form of involvement in the field of international EMS.

1. Bear in mind that there is no standard nomenclature to describe EMS systems or components. Terms like "paramedic," "emergency physician," and even "EMS" are subject to many different interpretations in different parts of the world. The global confusion in comparing EMS systems is not in the least caused by a lack of internationally accepted definitions.

2. When comparing different EMS systems, remove words like "good," "bad," "better," and "worse." Keep in mind that the efficacy of *any* system of EMS has not yet been demonstrated. Instead, think always in terms of "different" ways of doing things.

3. Understand the limitations of direct comparisons between countries. Often overlooked, but very important for being able to accurately compare, is the geographic reality that the United States is more akin to a continent than a country. This means that most other coun-

	TABLE 9.3	
Selected International EMS and Emergency Medicine Web Sites		
WEB SITE	**COUNTRY/ REGION**	**INTERNET ADDRESS**
Australasian College for Emergency Medicine	Australia	www.acem.org.au
Royal Flying Doctor Service	Australia	www.rfds.org.au
Zavod Za Hitnu Medicinsku Pomoc Sarajevo	Bosnia	www.zhmpsarajevo.com
Canadian Association of Emergency Medicine	Canada	www.caep.org
Urgencias	Chile	www.interactiva.cl
Emergency Medicine in China	China	www.homestead.com/emchina/
Rallye Rejviz	Czech Republic	www.rallye-rejviz.cz
Adren@line	France	www.adrenaline112.org
Reanimation	France	www.reanimation.com
Hong Kong College of Emergency Medicine	Hong Kong	www.hkam.org.hk/colleges/em.htm
Italian Journal of EMS and Ambulance Staff	Italy	www.zen.it/nannini/
Japan Association for Acute Medicine	Japan	apollo.m.ehime-u.ac.jp/~jaam
Society for Emergency Medicine in Singapore	Singapore	www.sems.org.sg
Sociedad Espanola de Medicina de Urgencias y Emergencias	Spain	www.vigo.nu/sems
Ambulansforum	Sweden	www.ambulansforum.se
Society for Emergency Medicine, Taiwan	Taiwan, ROC	www.sem.org.tw
Emergency Medicine Association of Turkey	Turkey	www.deu.edu.tr/sempozyum/acil/ eindex.html
British Association of EMTs	UK	www.baemt.org.uk
American Academy of Emergency Medicine	USA	www.aaem.org
American College of Emergency Medicine	USA	www.acep.org
MERGiNET	USA	www.merginet.com
National Association of EMS Physicians	USA	www.naemsp.org
National Highway Transportation Safety Board EMS Division	USA	www.nhtsa.dot.gov/people/injury/ems/
National Society of EMS Educators	USA	www.naemse.org
Society for Academic Emergency Medicine	USA	www.saem.org

tries, including those in Europe, are, at most, comparable to the individual states in the United States. These and other factors, such as the lack of an internationally accepted EMS system model, make comparative EMS studies within and between countries difficult, although not impossible.

4. Be cautious with conclusions when insufficient information is available to describe overall EMS system design and system characteristics. Collecting clinical data from different EMS systems is one thing, but the interpretation of these data quite another. A myriad of medical, cultural, social, historical, and legal factors may

condemn a statistically significant study to functional and practical irrelevance.

5. Remember some of the lessons of system management. International EMS activities which over-emphasize one element generally lead to weaker performance of the system as a whole. An example is upgrading equipment and technology without considering elements such as medical direction and training.

6. Avoid becoming involved in the business of exporting EMS systems. There have been, and still are, many examples of entire EMS systems being exported in the "lock, stock, and barrel" mode from, for example, the U.S. to the Middle East. These ventures, often referred to as "turn-key" projects, generally fail miserably unless accompanied by early involvement, participation, and co-ownership of the local community.

7. Keep in mind that local sponsors of EMS development always understand local needs best. Local proponents of EMS understand the underlying agenda for establishing or developing EMS in their area, what the mission of EMS is, who the stakeholders are, and the range of political, economic, and cultural factors that impact development.

8. Remember that regional centers of excellence in EMS already exist in Asia, Europe, the Middle East, Africa, South America, and Central America. As EMS systems develop in different areas of the world, these local EMS systems have emerged as valuable regional models and their personnel may serve as regional experts for EMS development in neighbouring countries. For example, the local participants in recent EMS development in Hong Kong may offer more relevant insight and experience for EMS development in China than could experts in North American EMS.

References

1. Abbadi S, Abdallah AK, Holliman CJ. Emergency medicine in Jordan. *Ann Emerg Med*. 1997;30:319–321.
2. Adnet F, Jouriles NJ, Le Toumelin P, et al. Survey of out-of-hospital emergency intubations in the French prehospital medical system: a multicenter study. *Ann Emerg Med*. 1998;32:454–460.
3. Aghababian RV, Levy K, Moyer P, et al. Integration of United States emergency medicine concepts into emergency services in the New Independent States. *Ann Emerg Med*. 1995;26:368–375.
4. Algappan K, Cherukuri K, Narang V, et al. Early development of emergency medicine in Chennai (Madras) India. *Ann Emerg Med*. 1998;32:604–605.
5. Arnold JL, Song HS, Chung JM. The recent development of emergency medicine in South Korea. *Ann Emerg Med*. 1998;32:730–735.
6. Arnold JL. International emergency medicine and the recent development of emergency medicine worldwide. *Ann Emerg Med*. 1999;33:97–103.
7. Beveridge RC. Emergency medicine: a Canadian perspective. *Ann Emerg Med*. 1995;26:505–507.
8. Bresnahan KA, Fowler J. Emergency medicine in Turkey: current status and future directions. *Ann Emerg Med*. 1995;26:357–360.
9. Bossaert LL. The complexity of comparing different EMS systems—a survey of EMS systems in Europe. *Ann Emerg Med*. 1993;99–102.
10. Brismar B, Totten V, Persson BM. Emergency, disaster, and defense medicine: the Swedish model. *Ann Emerg Med*. 1996;27:250–253.
11. Bullard MJ, Liaw SJ, Chen JC. Emergency medicine development in Taiwan. *Ann Emerg Med*. 1996;28:542–548.
12. Burke FM, Zhang X, Patrick W, Kalinowski E, Li Z. Emergency medical services systems in the United States and China: a developmental comparison. *Prehosp Disas Med*. 1994;9:244–251.
13. Cameron PA, Bradt DA, Ashby R. Emergency medicine in Australia. *Ann Emerg Med*. 1996;28:342–346.
14. Church AL, Plitponkarnpim A. Emergency medicine in Thailand. *Ann Emerg Med*. 1998;32:93–97.
15. Clarke ME. Emergency medicine in the new South Africa. *Ann Emerg Med*. 1998;32:367–372.
16. Doezma D, Sklar DP, Roth PB. Development of emergency medical services in Costa Rica. *JAMA*. 1991;265:188–190.
17. Hu SC, Tsai J, Lu YL, Lan CF. EMS characteristics of an Asian metropolis. *Am J Emerg Med*. 1996;14:82–85.
18. Lasseter JA, Pyles JR, Galijasevic S. Emergency medicine in Bosnia and Herzegovina. *Ann Emerg Med*. 1997;30:527–530.
19. McHugh DF, Driscoll PA. Accident and emergency medicine in the United Kingdom. *Ann Emerg Med*. 1999;33:702–709.
20. Meskin S, Huyler F, Gupta SK. Delivery of emergency medical services in Kathmandu, Nepal. *Ann Emerg Med*. 1997;29:409–414.
21. Moecke H. Emergency medicine in Germany. *Ann Emerg Med*. 1998;31:111–115.
22. Musharafieh R, Bu-Haka R: Development of emergency medicine in Lebanon. *Ann Emerg Med*. 1996;28:82–86.
23. Nikkanen HE, Pouges C, Jacobs LM. Emergency medicine in France. *Ann Emerg Med*. 1998;31:116–120.
24. Osterwalder JJ. Emergency medicine in Switzerland. *Ann Emerg Med*. 1998;32:243–247.
25. Peralta PG, Sinon JB. Emergency medicine in the Philippines. *Ann Emerg Med*. 1995;26:743–745.
26. PoSaw L, Aggarwal P, Bernstein SL. Emergency medicine in the New Delhi Area, India. *Ann Emerg Med*. 1998;32:609–615.

27. Repetto C, Casagranda I, Overton D, Gai V. Emergency medicine: the Italian experience. *Ann Emerg Med.* 1998; 32:248–252.

28. Richards J. Emergency medicine in Vietnam. *Ann Emerg Med.* 1997;29:543–545.

29. Shimauchi A, Toki Y, Ito T. Characteristics of prehospital cardiac arrest patients in Japan and determinant factors for survival. *Am J Emerg Med.* 1998;16:209–213.

30. Tintinalli J, Lisse E, Begley A, Campbell C. Emergency care in Namibia. *Ann Emerg Med.* 1998;32:373–377.

31. Townes DA, Lee TE, Gulo S, VanRooyen MJ. Emergency medicine in Russia. *Ann Emerg Med.* 1998;32:239–242.

32. Tsai MC, Arnold J, Chuang CC, et al. A preliminary survey of emergency medicine in 12 Asian countries. *J Emerg Crit Care Med.* 1999;10:144–156.

33. Waisman Y, Amir LA, Or J. Emergency medicine in Israel: state of the art. *Ann Emerg Med.* 1995;26:640–642.

34. Wong TW. The development of emergency medicine in Hong Kong. *HKJEM.* 1994;1:79–84.

35. Dykstra EH. International models for the practice of emergency care [editorial]. *Am J Emerg Med.* 1997;15:209–219.

36. Kuehl AE. Perspectives on international EMS development. *Emerg Med Serv.* 1989;18:37–39.

37. Mitchell C. International EMS: lessons learned in Costa Rica. *Am J Emerg Med.* 1991;9:375–378.

38. Hauswald M, Yeoh E. Designing a prehospital system for a developing country: estimated cost and benefits. *Am J Emerg Med.* 1997;15:600–603.

39. Dykstra EH. 2nd Pan-European Conference on Emergency Medical Services, Abanao Terme, Italy, August 28–September 1, 1994.

Section Two

Sandra M. Schneider, MD

E L E M E N T S

In order for an EMS system to function, attention must be paid to each step or component of the process. Diverse systems must integrate flawlessly to provide effective care. A single flawed component may dismantle an otherwise excellent system.

A systems approach is essential both in and out of the hospital. It becomes more critical when the individual components must respond to unpredictable stresses. EMS faces unique issues of weather, geography, hazardous materials, and bystander activity. This section describes the choices available when designing a system. There is no ideal system. Each component of a system should be analyzed and optimized, given the challenges and resources unique to the system.

The role of the medical director is similar to that of the conductor of a symphony. Each component should be appropriately balanced and in step with the others. No single component can override the others. No weak component can be left unassisted.

In this section we analyze the components of an EMS system. The reader may note some duplication of material from one chapter to another. This is intentional. It is difficult to completely isolate our component from the others. Decisions in one area will affect the function of another.

Response Phases

Michael R. Gunderson, EMT-P

Introduction

Complex sequences of steps take place in several phases when an emergency response is initiated in a state-of-the-art EMS system. This chapter provides an overview of these phases to show their interrelationships and provide a context for subsequent chapters of this book. In the analysis of these phases, scenarios and processes are described that generally reflect those of a reasonably sophisticated urban EMS system in North America; there is a wide range of system and process designs in urban systems. The variations and differences in processes can be even more significant among major metropolitan areas, smaller cities and suburban areas, rural areas, and wilderness areas.

The phases of an EMS response will be examined in the following sequence:

1. Public Education and Prevention
2. Enrollment
3. Access
4. Triage
5. Response Configuration
6. Response Deployment
7. Pre-Arrival Instructions
8. On-Scene Care
9. Direct Medical Control
10. Disposition Options
11. Destination Selection
12. Transport
13. Transfer of Care
14. Data Collection
15. Recovery and Return to Service

Public Education and Prevention

Public education efforts by EMS systems are helpful in educating the community about the system itself and specific community health and safety issues. Public education efforts about the system are primarily directed towards assuring that the community knows what EMS is, what it is for, how to appropriately access its services, and what to do in the event of an emergency or urgency before crews arrive.

By using the large quantities of data available from responses made throughout their communities, EMS systems can identify many types of public health and safety risks. This identification allows systems to develop targeted public education and prevention programs, while continuing to monitor the impact of these interventions.

Some of the more successful EMS public education, prevention, and early intervention initiatives have been showcased in the annual Community Service Awards sponsored by the American Ambulance Association.[1] These programs have addressed:

- CPR and healthy heart living
- AED deployment
- Pediatric drownings
- Childhood immunizations
- Bicycle safety
- Helmet utilization
- Seat belt/child safety seat utilization
- Gun safety

A much broader scope of efforts may benefit from EMS involvement, particularly when conducted in collaboration with other healthcare providers, payors, and stakeholders.

Enrollment

There is strong interest in the integration of EMS information systems with the information systems of larger general healthcare providers, managed care organizations, and payors. This is particularly evident in nurse-staffed medical call centers that are being integrated with 9-1-1 emergency medical dispatch centers. Enrolling people into such systems before an EMS service request takes place provides field crews with information on their medical history, allergies, medications, attending physician, and hospital preferences before the crews even arrive on-scene. A similar pre-incident enrollment and clinical data collection process can occur in systems that operate ambulance/EMS service membership or subscription programs.

Access

There are many different reasons, circumstances, methods of access, and points of access for people seeking services from an EMS system. Each combination of these factors may have a different process by which the service request is routed, triaged, and managed (table 10.1).

The challenge for managers and medical directors is making sure that every case that results in contact with the EMS system gets the right care, at the right time, in the right place, from the right level of provider—regardless of the combination of reasons, circumstances, method of access, or point of access.

For example, there may be dramatic differences in how a call is handled among the following scenarios:

- An injured person calls 9-1-1 from his home telephone.
- A bystander contacts 9-1-1 via his cellular telephone to report an automobile crash with apparently serious injuries.
- A bystander drives up to a nearby EMS station and reports an automobile crash to the crew.

Triage

When someone dials 9-1-1, the call is routed to a 9-1-1 public safety answering point (PSAP), which is where an initial level of triage is made to determine the types of services required—police, fire, EMS, or any combination thereof. Since the overwhelming majority of 9-1-1 calls are for police services, most PSAPs are in police dispatch centers.

An important role of the system medical director is to assure that the processes used to make the initial triage decisions are clinically sound and consistently applied. To this end, PSAP protocols are typically employed. When the PSAP is managed by an agency other than the EMS system (i.e., police department), it can be a major political challenge for the EMS medical director to modify protocols.

TABLE 10.1			
Factors Influencing Access and Deployment of EMS Resources			
ACCESS POINT	**REASONS FOR CONTACT**	**CIRCUMSTANCES**	**METHOD OF CONTACT**
<ul><li>9-1-1 emergency call center</li><li>Emergency medical dispatch center</li><li>Nonemergency ambulance dispatch center or operator</li><li>EMS or fire/rescue station</li><li>EMS or fire/rescue unit while on the road</li><li>EMS or fire/rescue supervisor/manager/ administration unit on the road</li><li>Nurse-triage medical call center</li><li>Physician office, clinic or hospital</li></ul>	<ul><li>True emergency</li><li>Urgency</li><li>Minor problem</li><li>Chronic care needs</li><li>Medically related transportation need</li><li>Medical questions</li><li>Non-medical related needs</li></ul>	<ul><li>Location<ul><li>Home</li><li>Car</li><li>Public transportation</li><li>Remote location</li></ul></li><li>Ability to communicate</li></ul>	<ul><li>Standard telephone</li><li>Cellular telephone</li><li>TTD telephone</li><li>Third-party caller</li><li>Physical presence at EMS, fire, or healthcare facility</li><li>CB or HAM radio</li><li>E-mail</li><li>Fax</li></ul>

Most communication centers have call-takers and dispatchers. Call-takers primarily answer telephones and interact with callers. Dispatchers primarily talk on radios and interact with field personnel. This strategy provides a higher capacity for handling simultaneous emergency calls. Many systems subdivide the tasks even further by using separate dispatchers for police, fire, and EMS. In larger systems, dispatchers may not be in the same building as the call-takers. Once the call-taker has determined which public safety service is needed, the call itself (and any data collected on that call) is electronically transferred to the workstation of the appropriate agency's dispatcher for further handling.

If the primary need is for EMS, the PSAP call-taker transfers the call to an emergency medical dispatcher serving in a call-taker role. The dispatcher asks the caller specific sets of questions that allow efficient and reproducable information-gathering and clinical decision-making. The most basic issues for the dispatcher include the determination of the number of patients, their age, level of consciousness, breathing status, location, and the verification of the call-back number.

Response Configuration and Mode

If EMS resources will be sent to the scene, the levels of units (i.e., ALS and/or BLS units) and types of units (i.e., transport units, non-transport units) must be determined. This is called a response configuration. The mode of response for each of these units must also be determined:

- Emergency ("HOT")—with emergency lights and sirens
- Immediate ("COLD")—without lights or sirens
- Delayed—no immediate response required

Once the call-taker determines the response configuration and modes of response, that information can be passed on to a dispatcher. With medical call center integration, the case of a delayed response might be transferred to the nurse-triage medical call center for a broader range of services and potential dispositions that may or may not include further involvement from EMS.

Response Deployment and Notification

After the call-takers have obtained the information needed to deploy resources, the information is transferred to the workstation of a dispatcher, who will choose which units to send, and will notify the crews.

To understand the process of choosing which units to send, it is important to have a basic understanding of the two general models that are most commonly used for emergency vehicle deployment—static and dynamic.

Static deployment models use stations located throughout the service area. Vehicle locations remain the same between calls, excluding times when units are traveling to and from calls or other tasks. This is the method traditionally used by most fire departments and public EMS agency systems.

The most common dynamic model is called system status management (SSM).[2] It considers patterns in the location of calls for the particular time of day, day of week, and time of year. Vehicles are then placed at locations most likely to optimize the response to those anticipated call patterns. This approach is most commonly used by private ambulance companies.

The choice between these two models has a dramatic impact on the work environment of the crews. Although it is more comfortable for crews to respond from stations, response time intervals can be measurably improved when crews remain in their vehicles, located at key intersections based on the call pattern analysis. Thus, there are advantages and disadvantages to each strategy.

Multi-tierred systems often use a hybrid approach. Non-transport fire units often provide first-response services. They are operated with a dynamic SSM strategy. A hybrid approach can also be used in an ambulance-only system, with some units deployed under SSM and other units deployed at fixed stations.

To improve the selection and utilization of units, automated vehicle locator (AVL) technology is often used, which allows the real-time location of units to be displayed on an electronic map in the computer-aided dispatch (CAD) system. Global positioning satellite (GPS) technology is typically used in the vehicles to provide the real-time location data, which is updated on a minute-to-minute basis by direct radio link to the CAD. Once the response units are selected, they can be notified by any number of methods. If the units are in their station, an alarm system in the building is often used. In addition, the pagers worn by crew members assigned to a particular unit are activated, and a verbal message for the units is given on their assigned stand-by radio channel.

Pre-Arrival Instructions

After the call-taker passes the response configuration data to the dispatcher, he remains on the telephone with the caller to provide pre-arrival instructions (PAIs). The call-taker continues to interrogate in an effort to identify specific problems that may benefit from advice and coaching to the caller; the caller may provide interventions that can help the situation before the responding crews arrive. PAIs might include clinical instructions (i.e., airway and bleeding control), safety precautions, and preparations for the incoming crews (i.e., unlocking doors, putting dogs behind closed doors).

The call-taker activities, from the determination of a response configuration to PAIs, are usually directed by paper or computerized protocol systems. While there are several types and commercial versions of such protocols, the use of a structured protocol is advocated to avoid the problems associated with call-takers having to "invent" the process each time they handle a case.

On-Scene Care

First-response agencies are called simultaneously with ambulances when the response configuration protocols indicate their need. The first-response units are often fire trucks, but may include police units in some communities. The first-response crews may be formally certified as first responders or as EMTs. They typically provide basic care and automated external defibrillation. In some systems, the first-response crews provide advanced care with paramedics.

When the ambulance arrives, the transport crew is given an oral and written report on the situation by the first-response crew. In most instances, the transport crew is capable of providing advanced level care and will take the patient to the receiving facility without assistance from the first-response crew. The first-response crew can then notify its dispatcher that it is available for another call. In more serious cases, the transport crew may request someone from the first-response crew to travel with them to provide additional assistance while enroute to the receiving hospital.

The crews generally operate under two levels of medical protocol. The first level is for standing orders, which can be performed prior to making contact with direct medical oversight. The second level consists of interventions that can only be carried out under specific verbal authorization by direct medical oversight for a particular case.

Disposition Options

The care for a given patient has a variety of possible dispositions with regard to treatment and transport. A person may deny any illness or injury and refuse offers for assessment, treatment, or transport—or any combination thereof. Within the realm of transport, the dispositions can include paramedic transport, basic transport, and aeromedical transport. EMS systems generally limit the options presented to patients as one of two choices—transport to a hospital emergency department (ED) or refusal of transport.

Often system protocols are vague about how these various dispositions are reached, and how to handle refusals of assessment, treatment, or transport. Protocols and policies in most systems are also vague regarding the criteria to use in determining if a person is competent to make an informed refusal of assessment, treatment, or transport. There is very high potential liability for the system if these cases are handled inappropriately. EMS medical directors and managers should closely examine system processes and actual practices in this area.

Destination Selection

The process for deciding which hospital to take a patient to is becoming more complicated. The general policy in most systems is to take the patient to the hospital of choice. In other systems, the policy is to take the patient to the closest ED. Sometimes it is not such a simple issue. Patients may have restrictions in their healthcare insurance that dictate where they should be taken and under what circumstances. At other times, patients may insist on a particular hospital independent of insurance restrictions, hospital capabilities, or bed availability. There is also a growing trend of specialization for emergency-care designations at hospitals. There may be trauma centers, burn centers, chest pain centers, and stroke centers at different hospitals in the same community—which therefore complicates the destination selection process. During times of high patient census at hospitals and EDs, some hospitals may go on an official or unofficial "divert" status.

The EMS system may have considerations, related to the number of units available in the overall system or in a particular area, that can influence how far a transport might be allowed to go beyond the closest hospital. Protocols and policies in most systems are vague about how these considerations are balanced to reach a given decision. This is where direct medical oversight can be potentially helpful—if the people who provide direct medical oversight are properly trained and given adequate information about the status of the overall system to make good decisions.

Some communities utilize internet-based or wide-area network-based hospital bed status systems.[3] Participating hospitals log on to a specified website and update their status and the number of beds they have available. The EMS dispatch center and direct medical oversight can see the status of all hospitals and direct units accordingly. This system is particularly helpful when multiple hospitals are dealing with ED overcrowding issues or in times of disaster and multicasualty incidents.

Direct Medical Oversight

The main purpose of direct medical oversight during patient care is to provide a real-time quality assurance mechanism. The field provider presents a verbal report that includes the history, physical examination, field impression, interventions performed and planned, destination, rationale for the destination, and estimated time of arrival for the destination. Direct medical oversight determines if the plan and destination are appropriate, and provides feedback and consultation as needed. The direct medical oversight may be provided by receiving hospitals, designated hospitals, or designated staff equipped with radios or cellular phones. The personnel providing direct medical oversight are usually physicians, but may also include senior paramedics in a clinical manager role, or specially trained and qualified nurses or physician assistants.

The impact of direct medical oversight on patient outcome has not been clearly established. As a result, some systems allow field providers to operate almost entirely on standing orders. Even in such situations, there is usually a mechanism in place, at the discretion of the field providers, for obtaining a consultation with direct medical oversight. Other systems may require direct medical oversight contact in all high-severity cases.

Transport

Once a destination decision is made, the transport phase begins. There are three main steps in this phase. The first step involves transporting the patient from his current location to the vehicle; this can be anywhere from just a few steps from a fall on a public sidewalk to a very hazardous and extended transport from the upper floor of a tall building without an elevator (or with an elevator too small for the ambulance stretcher). It is important to recognize the significant limitations in assessment and treatment that are inherent to this step of the transport phase. The conscious patient may also experience very heightened anxiety and catecholamine release while being carried down stairs, over rough terrain, or under a tarp in extreme weather. It can be very difficult to manually maintain an airway, provide bag-valve-mask ventilation, do chest compressions and observe for cardiac rhythm anomalies, and so on, during this time. EMS medical directors and clinical managers should consider such issues when designing protocols and processes of care during transport from the scene to the unit.

The second step in the transport phase is from the location of the ambulance at the scene to the ambulance ramp of the receiving hospital. The clinical situation inside the ambulance is easier to address than that on a rolling stretcher enroute to the vehicle; however, there are limitations imposed by the ambulance compartment itself. Access to the patient is restricted by the space around the secured stretcher. Motion and noise in the patient compartment can also interfere with assessment and treatment.

From the scene or during transport, the ambulance crew may establish contact with the receiving ED if it is not the same facility that provided direct medical oversight, or if direct medical oversight contact was not made at all. The purpose of this contact with the receiving facility is to allow the ED to prepare for patient arrival, particularly if the patient will need immediate intervention. The policy requiring contact with the receiving ED prior to arrival varies considerably from community to community.

The third step involves the transport from the back of the ambulance onto the ED bed. Like the first step, the patient is being rolled along, hopefully with easier terrain and a shorter distance, but with the same limitations in assessment and treatment.

Transfer of Care

When the patient is brought into the ED, the crew provides a verbal report to the staff, which is in most cases an ED nurse. This verbal report is the primary information that will impact the initial phases of ED interventions. In most situations with an unstable patient, the written report is not yet completed upon arrival at the ED. With less extreme cases, the crew may have time to complete their written report during transport.

In many cases, the crews will finish up their written reports at a crew area in the ED, where they will be able to call their dispatch centers to obtain the interval times for the call. This information can be included on the report given to the ED. Crews often use these times from the dispatch center to interpolate times for their interventions in critical cases where charting was deferred in order to focus on priorities in patient care.

In some systems, EMS crews may submit their reports as long as 24 hours after they have transferred their patient to the ED. This is more common in systems where crews are under strong pressure to return to service as soon as possible due to other emergency calls. Delays in submitting completed reports should be discouraged and make the verbal reports all the more important.

Data Collection/Documentation

Data collection in the field is a difficult challenge for crews when they try to log their actions and observations concurrent with patient care. As a result, information is charted after the fact from imperfect recollections of events and times. Technology is slowly addressing this need with integration of data collection tools into various medical electronic monitoring devices such as defibrillator/monitors, pulse oximeters, and capnographs; however, the scope of data collection and documentation needs goes far beyond the physiological data gathered by these particular devices.

Narrative description of the event, circumstances, and relevant history is the most common format for conveying information from one caregiver to the next. If the narrative is handwritten, legibility is often difficult—especially when the next caregiver is looking at a second or third (or worse) generation copy of the report from one of the commonly used pressure sensitive multi-part paper forms.

Pen-based computers and other types of small portable computers have been steadily improving the field documentation process, but often require more time to complete the medical record, especially when the field crew member is not a competent touch typist. Field computer technology that allows crews to provide care while simultaneously gathering data remains an elusive goal. Voice recognition technology, combined with hands-free software packages, holds strong promise for the future of computerized field data collection.

At present, much of the documentation is done in handwritten formats with a combination of narrative, checkboxes, codes, and fill-in-the-blank types of fields on the prehospital care report forms. Some systems will have crews or data entry clerks type some of the information from their paper forms into a computer system after the call. Most commonly, this abstracting is limited to basic demographic and billing-related data.

Recovery and Return to Service

After the crew has transferred the patient to the ED bed and given its verbal and written reports to the receiving ED staff, it shifts to recovery activities: clean-up, and restocking the ambulance and carry-in equipment bags/boxes. This process can be relatively brief or very time-consuming, depending on the nature of the call just completed.

There may be a significant period of time before the crew and ambulance return to their normal service area if they are in a static vehicle deployment system and the receiving facility is a significant distance from their station. During the time while a unit is out of service or out of its service area, longer response times will occur, as units from outside the area try to cover more than their core area.

Summary

There are many phases in the response of an EMS system to a request for service. Each phase includes many simultaneous and complex processes. It is essential that EMS managers and medical directors understand how these phases and processes work in order to properly manage and improve them.

References

1. Contact the AAA for information regarding the recipients of their annual Community Services Awards—American Ambulance Association, 1255 Twenty-Third Street, NW, Suite 200, Washington, DC 20037-1174; (202) 452-8888; http://www.the-aaa.org.

2. Stout J: Ambulance system designs. *JEMS*. 1986; 11(1): 85–89.

3. For one example of an Internet-based hospital/bed status system, see EMSystem at http://www.emsystem. com.

CHAPTER 11

Levels of Providers

James E. Pointer, MD
Thomas J. McGuire, EMT-P

North America encompasses a wide spectrum of EMS systems including a diversity of prehospital providers. The following four levels of prehospital providers are common in North America: first responder (FR), emergency medical technician-basic (EMT-B), emergency medical technician-intermediate (EMT-I), and emergency medical technician-paramedic (EMT-P). Although national standards exist for these four levels of providers, various states have adopted more than 40 different sub-categories.[1]

The U.S. Department of Transportation (DOT) publishes the National Standard Curricula (NSC) as minimum standards for the four levels with suggested ranges of required training hours. The FR NSC were last revised in 1992, the EMT-B in 1994, the EMT-I in 1999, and EMT-P in 1998. The DOT only sets standards; it does not train or test. The National Registry of Emergency Medical Technicians (NREMT) is an independent, non-governmental agency established in 1970 that tests and registers FRs, EMT-Bs, EMT-Is, and EMT-Ps. The NREMT requires successful completion of an approved DOT training program. Approximately 39 states require NREMT registration for EMTs. Others perform testing through a state or local agency. Table 11.1 lists training hours ranges for the four prehospital provider levels based on DOT recommendations or field testing. Actual course hours will vary. Competence of the graduate is always the best criterion for judging program quality. A comprehensive guide to each state's and province's training and licensure/certification requirements (and scopes of practice) may be found at http://www.emergencymedicalservices.com.

Despite a paucity of scientific evidence, many urban areas have established complex and sophisticated paramedic systems.[2] The term *advanced life support* (ALS) is hopelessly vague; in some localities, it refers only to the paramedic level, and in others it traditionally refers to any intervention other than first aid and CPR. Iowa recently applied the term "paramedic" to EMT-Is, further confusing the correlation between the level of provider and the associated scope of practice.[3] The paramedic scope of practice varies considerably. Paramedics administer a variety of medications, use advanced procedures, and manage the cardiac arrest patient aggressively. Nearly all paramedic systems employ direct and indirect medical control. On the other hand, *basic life support* (BLS) classically has meant the provision of first aid, cardiopulmonary resuscitation (CPR), splinting techniques, and oxygen administration. BLS systems are characterized by little if any medical oversight, a superficial approach to patient assessment and treatment, and even less validating research than ALS sys-

TABLE 11.1				
Training Hours for Prehospital Providers				
LEVEL	**DIDACTIC**	**CLINICAL**	**INTERNSHIP**	**TOTAL**
FR	40	Optional	Optional	40
EMT-B	99–104	10	Optional	109–114
EMT-I	175–225	50–75	75–100	300–400
EMT-P (1994)	212–350	232–250	256–500	700–1100
EMT-P (1998) (including practical lab hours 185–666)	198–719	174–597	108–1160	654–3142

tems. To confuse the issue further, some states have an intermediate level between EMT-B and paramedic. These EMT-Is are essentially upgraded EMTs or downgraded EMT-Ps.

The final prehospital provider level is the FR. These municipal or volunteer personnel deliver basic first aid and CPR, and apply automatic external defibrillators (AEDs) until more highly trained EMTs or paramedics arrive. First responders are usually employed by police and fire agencies. In many urban areas, EMT-Bs and/or paramedics are the "first responders."

Table 11.2 gives sample scopes of practice for the four provider levels based on the DOT NSCs. The EMT-I drug list describes the national standard; local agencies can augment it as appropriate under local and state laws. The EMT-P NSC differ from the basic and intermediate NSC by not specifically pre-scribing what medications should be part of the paramedic's scope of practice. Instead, the curriculum follows a more traditional medical training model by introducing a wide range of drugs that a paramedic should be familiar with, but not necessarily deliver.

A number of factors are changing the classification of prehospital provider levels. First, the urban paramedic scope of practice has greatly expanded. Even in conservative states such as California, standing orders within the treatment protocols are prevalent, and in some states local jurisdictions can enact almost any addition to the paramedic armamentarium. Second, the EMT-B scope of practice has also grown ("technology creep"), blurring the distinction between EMT-Is and EMT-Bs. Third, fire service EMS has proliferated. Citizens have asked for and funded fire EMS personnel. These new services have forged new

TABLE 11.2
NSC Skills and Medications for Prehospital Providers

First Responder
CPR
First aid
Basic airway management
Patient assessment
Basic wound care
Deliveries
Safe patient movement
Assisted ventilation
Elective: AED

EMT-B
Scope of First Responders and:
Vital signs assessment
Oxygen administration
AED
Assist patient with nitroglycerine, inhalation meds
Activated charcoal, epi auto injector, oral glucose
On-scene triage
Splinting, spinal immobilization, helmet removal
Extrication and transport
Pneumatic Antishock Garment application
Elective: nasogastric tube, intubation of adults, infants, and children

EMT-I
Scope of EMT-B and some or all of the following:
Medical communications
Basic EKG
Multi-lumen, Combitube, adult and pediatric orotracheal intubation, oximetry, end-tidal CO_2
Naso- and oro-gastric tube
Basic determination of death
Manual defibrillation and pacing
Plural decompression
Meconium aspiration

Drug administration via IO, IV, rectal, inhalation, oral routes including:
Aspirin
Atropine
Adenosine
Bronchodilators
Diazepam
Epinephrine
Lasix
Lidocaine
Morphine sulfate
Narcan
Nitroglycerin
D50

EMT-P
Scope of EMT-I and some or all of the following:
Termination of resuscitation/grief support
Needle/surgical cricothyrotomy
Digital, transillumination intubation
Naso-tracheal intubation
PEFR testing
12-lead EKG
RSI and neuromuscular blockade

The current paramedic NSC does not make specific recommendations for an EMT-P pharmacopoeia (see text).
Reference:
http://www.dot.gov/people/injury/ems/nsc.htm

relationships and resulted in creative EMS configurations. Last and perhaps most important, "evidence-based" medicine has, hopefully, taken hold in EMS. Research and quality control, previously alien concepts to EMS, are beginning to test the hypotheses of out-of-hospital efficacy. The result of such scrutiny may be to limit future unproven components to scopes of practice at all levels.

This chapter describes the levels of prehospital providers in the context of changing needs, cost considerations, and evidence-based research.

First Responders

First responders (FR) are literally the first persons (citizens, public safety personnel, or prehospital professionals) to arrive at the scene of an emergency. In modern EMS systems the term FR usually refers to public safety personnel, usually firefighters or police. The DOT has developed standardized training curricula. These materials provide approximately 40 hours of training in educationally straightforward formats. The FR NSC were reviewed in the late 1970s and updated in 1995. The National EMS Education and Practice Blueprint describes the FR as using ". . . a limited amount of equipment to perform initial assessment and intervention and is trained to assist other EMS providers."[4] In the 1970s, fire departments began responding to medical calls. Now, many jurisdictions have trained firefighters to either the EMT-B or paramedic level, and FRs, in this context, are a dying breed.

Well trained FRs can deliver crucial care; they perform basic patient assessment including basic assessment of circulation and respiration. This information is not only important for initial treatment but it also provides a baseline for future therapy. Patients with a number of life-threatening conditions including airway obstruction, external hemorrhage, and fractures and dislocations can benefit from the skills of the FR. These personnel can assist ventilation, administer CPR, and (optionally) use AEDs. The AED and CPR are the two most important components of the scope of practice of the FR. These are arguably the most critical procedures in out-of-hospital care; in fact, they are the only treatment modalities that clearly improve patient survival. FRs also provide assistance in controlling often hectic scenes, and in calming bystanders and family members.

The AED is an elective skill in the DOT FR curriculum, and many jurisdictions have trained police and other public safety personnel to the FR level, largely to provide AED to citizens.[5] The AED component requires about four hours of additional training. Lay AED programs are now widespread. For some years, AED has been a standard of care in EMS systems.

Because of the AED component, FRs are now more often included in training and quality improvement programs than in the past. This is largely due to regulatory requirements and the recognition that, although the AED is very easy to operate, AED users require a knowledge of cardiopulmonary resuscitation *in addition to* the judgment and mechanics involved in operating the device itself.

Basic EMTs

The latest EMT-B NSC were field tested and rolled out in early 1994. The DOT has significantly upgraded the EMT-B scope of practice without a significant increase in required teaching hours. Additions to the scope of practice include AED, auto-injection of epinephrine, placement of the pneumatic antishock garment, administration of oral glucose and activated charcoal, and assisting the patient with nitroglycerin and inhaled respiratory medications (see table 11.2). The most controversial aspects of the EMT-Basic curriculum are the elective components, endotracheal and nasogastric intubation. Endotracheal intubation is the preferred advanced airway method, but this does not mean that every EMT-B should learn to intubate; endotracheal intubation is a high-risk skill. Due to training, confidence, or the frequent attendance of higher trained personnel, EMT-Bs are less frequently successful at intubating the trachea than are higher trained out-of-hospital providers.[6]

Perhaps the EMT-B, if practicing in an environment without a paramedic, should utilize the tracheopharyngeal lumen airway (Combitube), a device that is successfully placed blindly in about 90% of attempts.[7] Effective use of bag-valve-mask ventilation is also an essential skill, particularly in the pediatric population.[8]

In North America, training for EMT-B ranges from a minimum of 110 hours to over 300 hours.[9] The large majority of states and provinces use the DOT scope as a foundation, but many states add components. For example, California allows three optional components for EMT-Bs: endotracheal intubation, Combitube, and manual defibrillation.[10]

System planners must exercise extreme care in developing or selecting components to add to the EMT-B curriculum. It may be more rational to utilize a "modular" approach by making additions to the EMT-I scope rather than that of the EMT-B. In this way, the provider receives a higher level of basic training prior to performing skills or procedures that may require considerable judgment. With the increasing popularity of "one plus one" (a first responding paramedic is joined by a transport paramedic) and "one and one" (an EMT and a paramedic transport team respond together) systems, perhaps the most important duty of an EMT-B is to assist the accompanying paramedic. Even though intravenous cannulation is not a component of the Basic scope, it is a relatively safe skill that can be a very time-effective maneuver.

EMT-Bs are also extremely important in the provision of interfacility transports. They provide assistance in setting up intravenous lines, applying automated or semi-automated defibrillation, readying medications, and assisting with scene management. In some systems, EMT-Bs make triage decisions, initiate patient refusals, and dispatch and cancel aircraft. Perhaps this work component is the most promising for Basics, both medically and financially.

EMT-Bs are rarely included in quality improvement or medical oversight programs.[1] In fact, there has been very little research and literature that studies BLS personnel. In a recent analysis of a literature, only 7% of EMS-related peer-reviewed works included or described emergency medical technicians (EMT-Bs).[11] Again, we plead for the inclusion of BLS personnel into these programs. Direct medical oversight, a standard for paramedics, is usually not available for EMT-Bs, even those who perform the high-end optional scope. Basics do not have the training to make the necessary judgments prior to these procedures.

Intermediate EMTs

The EMT-I's scope of practice lies between that of EMT-Bs and paramedics. The scope of practice of the EMT-I ranges from that of an EMT-B with one additional skill to near the level of a paramedic. This intermediate level varies the most from state to state in scope of practice. The DOT NSC add additional patient assessment skills, administration of IV fluids, the Combitube, many medications, and medical communications to the EMT-B curriculum. Originally EMT-Is were implemented in rural or isolated areas

where paramedics were impractical due to fiscal or labor resources.

In most states, one usually becomes an EMT-I either by upgrading EMT-B skills through training and testing in appropriate add-on modules, or by training and testing at an established intermediate level. For example, California has an intermediate designation with a scope of practice containing about half of the paramedic elements but greatly augmented over that of an EMT-B. North Carolina uses the following four levels of EMS training: EMT-B, EMT-I, EMT-Advanced Intermediate, and EMT-P. Virginia has no intermediate category, but accomplishes the same goal through EMT modular upgrades.[9] For local EMS planners, it may be better to create the EMT-I through the addition of modules than through established state regulation. The DOT NSC, state regulations, and state statutes have created scopes of practice often too limited to fit local needs. The modular approach permits local medical directors to choose the skills needed for their jurisdictions. Whatever the mechanisms, the usual justification for EMT-Is is to provide some advanced skills in geographic areas that do not need or cannot afford paramedics. Indeed, the justification for advanced skills for rural EMS-Is and EMT-Bs is quite different from that for those same skills in urban areas where paramedics are readily available. It is crucial that the reaffirmed national levels of FR, EMT-B, EMT-I, and EMT-P be viewed locally as minimum levels rather than as ceilings. Too often in recent years state ceilings prevented innovative medical directors from adopting clinically proven advances such as AED.

EMS administrators must provide EMT-Is with medical oversight and inclusion in the quality improvement plan. Considering the lack of scientific evidence demonstrating the efficacy of the additional skills and drug administration used by paramedics, the most cost-effective prehospital system might be one that starts with the FR and adds interventions in a modular form as needed.[12]

Paramedics

Paramedics provide the most sophisticated prehospital care. Depending on law and local need, these providers administer an array of medications and initiate a large number of procedures. In some states, paramedics enjoy an exceptionally broad scope of practice. Paramedics have been the subject of extensive regulation and scrutiny during their short existence. The group has been required to test more frequently, complete more continuing education, and accept more direct supervision than any other healthcare professionals. Paramedics have often been subject to regulatory review without due process. Initially, physicians and nurses over-regulated paramedics to protect their own professions, expressing concern that paramedics might replace them in certain positions.

In the early days, EMS planners believed that strict control and supervision would compensate for the lack of experience with this new, advanced provider. Over the years the situation changed. Paramedics established a niche in the healthcare systems and are considered true professionals. Many paramedics are not just technicians; their ability and responsibility to provide complete patient assessment and technical skills often may separate them from other prehospital providers. Paramedics may in fact diagnose, not simply assess, a patient's condition.[13] Their scope of practice may expand to that of physician extender in the near future, thereby providing a crucial additional step on the career ladder.

The 1998 EMT-P NSC revised the 1985 standards and describe the minimum required information to be presented in training.[14] During development, the EMT-P NSC attracted considerable attention and controversy. Many warned that it created a new breed of practitioner, the need for which had not been determined. The NAEMSP and ACEP "formally opposed" early drafts as did individual authors.[15,16] These controversies about the paramedic scope of practice are, of course, not at all new. It is absolutely fascinating and timely to watch the 1972 premier episode of the television show "Emergency," which centers around these same issues and is in fact subtitled "The Wedworth-Townsend Act," for the embattled legislation that enabled newly trained California "paramedics" to practice.[17]

The final DOT document, certainly because of objections raised, is somewhat slimmer than earlier drafts. Still, the details of implementing the considerably enhanced curriculum remain complex. Individual states must identify necessary changes in statutes or regulations, update teaching staffs, and devise ways to bridge currently licensed personnel to the new levels.[18]

The matter of necessary course hours for paramedic training is always perplexing (see table 11.1). Cannon and his colleagues compared didactic training hours (1995 NSC) with NREMT-P examination results. Didactic course hours ranged from 62 to 1,594 (mean 377), yet had no correlation with successful completion of the exam.[19] After initial field testing of the 1998 NSC, a similar wide range of course hours occurred (see table 11.2). As the new NSC are rolled out across the nation, we will be better able to determine the requirements for delivering the new standards. Students certainly will feel the extra burden. One widely used paramedic text is 136% larger than its prior edition.[20]

These developments and the ongoing experience of EMS systems have produced inevitable and exciting areas of controversy such as the expanding scope of practice, competency of the new/inexperienced paramedic to practice alone, and cost-effectiveness. The evolution of these EMS system concerns will define future prehospital care. Tomorrow's systems will only vaguely resemble those of today.

Scope of Practice

In most systems the scopes of practice have been expanding. Not only has the number of paramedic drugs and procedures increased, but the circumstances and conditions under which a paramedic practices have also been augmented.

This broadened scope of practice is due to more affordable technology, more devices tailored to field use, and a willingness to move these devices and medications toward the front end of medical care. For example, pulse oximeters, cardiac pacers, and end-tidal CO_2 detectors are now conveniently available, (if not inexpensive) accessories to field cardiac monitors. In 1992 a local physician was actually criticized for *discussing* paralytic assisted intubation at a paramedic continuing education session. Today, this technique is part of the NSC.

The push to evidence-based medicine has caused medical directors to scrutinize more carefully additions to the paramedic scope of practice. Several rational models for expansion of the EMS armamentarium have been proposed.[21] The American Heart Association and others have attempted to use scientific studies and evidence in formulating clinical guidelines for all levels of practitioners.[22]

Such is the case with amiodarone, which has been rapidly added to paramedics' scope of practice for refractory ventricular fibrillation/pulseless ventricular tachycardia, possibly because of the paucity of evidence supporting the use of other medications (lidocaine, beryllium) used for this condition.

Amiodarone has been the subject of controversy because of its cost (about $150 per 300 milligram dose) and due to the results of the ARREST trial. The ARREST trial showed an increment in survival with amiodarone as compared with placebo for patients in refractory ventricular fibrillation. This improvement in survival was significant only to admission to the hospital. The study was not sufficiently powered to demonstrate survival to hospital discharge.[23] Some have pointed out that this situation is similar to the one a few years ago for high dose epinephrine.[24]

Because of shrinking healthcare resources, paramedics will function in a wide variety of clinical arenas. In the inner city or rural areas, prehospital services complement existing, under-funded community-health programs. Although not the original intent, paramedics sometimes work as technicians in emergency departments and hospital wards, partly because they are well suited to the task and the environment, but mostly because they are paid less than nurses and other medical professionals. Nursing associations, especially, have politicized these changes.

Cost

As the healthcare community becomes increasingly comfortable with the use of prehospital providers, it is also searching for improvements in system cost-effectiveness. These efforts have generally focused on the deployment of EMS resources, rather than issues of practice scope.[25]

For example, a two-tiered system using defibrillator-capable and advanced airway-trained first responders and EMT-Is may be more cost-effective and efficient than a one-tiered paramedic system.[26] Does a community of a thousand persons with a small but adequate hospital need *any* out-of-hospital care other than EMT basic-trained volunteer firefighters with automatic defibrillation capability?[22]

Prehospital providers may soon be educated to perform clinical tasks formerly reserved for physicians or physician's assistants. Urban EMS systems may not be able to respond to every call, in spite of the legal ramifications. It is not cost-effective to send two paramedics in an ambulance to assess a patient with a sprained ankle; however, one paramedic responding in a van with limited equipment and appropriate social service and medical referral back-up may accomplish more for less money. Some patients may be advised by telephone to seek medical help on an elective basis. Protocol-driven field triage may assist paramedics in pro-

viding certain patients appropriate alternatives to an ambulance ride to the emergency department.[27]

It is pointless and expensive for paramedics to consult direct medical oversight for every component of the scope of their practice or to rigidly perform a detailed patient history and physical exam without medical need. Better care is provided when direct medical oversight is required only in problem cases, and when standing orders are used for the majority of conditions.

The "value equation," a concept from industry, may find a foothold in EMS.[28] In this scheme, value equals function/cost or quality/cost. For example, the paramedic's cognitive training and armamentarium expand considerably, accompanied by the perceived need to place these personnel in first-response field settings. The value of this very expensive configuration is difficult to determine, but the cost is not. Its value certainly will be questioned.

Competence and the New Medic

Immediately following completion of training, a paramedic may be unprepared to practice alone or with an inexperienced partner. Invariably, paramedic competence is assessed by training institutions prior to licensure or certification. However, training can encompass as few as 900 hours.[9] Also, some EMS systems *do* require (mostly unstandardized) field internships or proctoring *after* licensure. However, in many jurisdictions nationally, and in virtually all of California, no system-wide standards exist for assessing, precepting, or proctoring paramedics *after* licensure and *before* solo practice. For example, it is possible for a California paramedic to be deemed competent to practice alone without ever having performed a live intubation.[29] The in-hospital literature shows a positive correlation between experience and outcome in a number of medical entities: myocardial infarction, pancreatic duodenectomy, carotid endarterectomy, percutaneous transluminal coronary angioplasty, and many other conditions.[30,31,32] Recently, Grubbs, in a critique of paramedic clinical education, said that therapeutic judgment required the knowledge of when not to, when to, when to modify, when to stop, how often to try, when to declare success, and when to recognize failure. The broad goal of clinical education is the development of therapeutic judgment. Most, if not all, of the components of therapeutic judgment require not only a classroom or an internship but a great deal of experience.[33]

One method to document a new medic's required experience is through benchmarking. Minimum benchmarks for a number of paramedic skills and activities, including patient contact, team leading/report writing, performance of endotracheal intubation, defibrillation, intravenous starts, and medication administration, can be required by the provider/EMS agency prior to practicing alone.[34]

Other methods for ensuring competency include prescription of a fixed number of ALS calls. An assessment using scenario-based techniques can also be employed. The importance of experience on outcome is only now just beginning to be appreciated. One must apply the many lessons from the hospital experience to the EMS arena, and further evaluate and refine these ideas to ensure that new/inexperienced paramedics demonstrate competence prior to "day one" on the job.[35]

Summary

The technologic advances of the 1990s, especially easy-to-use defibrillators, have clarified the role of prehospital care. However, much work remains in clearly proving that EMS benefits patients. Attempts to tailor services to local resources and needs continue to blur the distinction among the various levels of providers and between ALS and BLS. To continue advancing, EMS planners must be even more creative and flexible in system design, and in developing the curricula of the providers who drive those systems. In the optimal system, there may be no defined levels but rather a gradual continuum from FR to the ultimate prehospital provider accomplished through modules. Prehospital providers armed with physician extender education and standing orders might decompress and integrate our healthcare systems by assessing and treating a range of conditions in both the prehospital and the hospital environments.

References

1. *Emergency Medical Services—Agenda for the Future*, Washington, DC: National Highway Traffic Safety Administration; 1996.
2. National Academy of Sciences, National Research Council. *Accidental Death and Disability: The Neglected Disease of Modern Society*. Washington, DC: National Academy Press; 1966.
3. Garza M. State to call EMT-Is paramedics. *J Emerg Serv.* 2000;25:5,20.
4. *National EMS Education and Practice Blueprint.* Columbus: National Registry of Emergency Medical Technicians; 1993.
5. Davis E, Mosesso V. Performance of police first responders in utilizing automated external defibrillation on victims of sudden cardiac arrest. *Prehosp Emerg Care*, 1998; 2:101–107.
6. Spaite D. Intubation by basic EMTs: lifesaving advance or catastrophic complication? *Ann Emerg Med.* 1998;31: 276–277.
7. Ochs M, et al. Successful prehospital airway management by EMT-Ds using the Combitube. *Prehosp Emerg Care.* 2000;4:333.
8. Gausche M et al. Effect of out-of-hospital pediatric endotracheal intubation on survival and neurologic outcome. *JAMA.* 2000;283(6):783–790.
9. State and province survey. *Emerg Med Serv.* 1999;28: 217–249.
10. *California Code of Regulations*, Title 22, Social Security, Division 9: Prehospital Emergency Medical Services, Chapter 2, Article 2, ¶ 100064.
11. Brice J, Garrison H, Evans A. Study design and outcomes in out-of-hospital emergency medicine research: A ten-year analysis. *Prehosp Emerg Care.* 2000;4:144–150.
12. Callaham M. Quantifying the scanty science of prehospital emergency care. *Ann Emerg Med.* 1997;30:785.
13. Pons P, Cason D. *Paramedic Field Care: A Complaint Based Approach*. St. Louis: Mosby-Year Book, Inc.; 1997, xiii.
14. National Highway Traffic Safety Administration: http://www.nhtsa.dot.gov/people/injury/ems/nsc.htm. 2000.
15. Barney R. National EMS curriculum: guidelines or policies for practice. *Prehosp Disaster Med.* 1999;14:9.
16. Benson N, Henry G. ACEP/NAEMSP opposition [letter]. EMS-EDU-List, April 22, 1996.
17. Cinader RA, prod. *Emergency! World premiere episode.* Los Angeles, Emergency Productions; 1972. Available through: http://www.jems.com
18. National State EMS Training Coordinators, Inc. *State implementation guide, NHTSA.* 1999.
19. Gannon GM, Menegazi JJ, Margolis GS. A comparison of paramedic didactic training hours and NREMT-P examination results. *Prehosp Emerg Care.* 1998;2:141–144.
20. Bledsoe BE, Porter RS, Cherry RA. Paramedic Care: Principles and Practice. Upper Saddle River, NJ: Prentice Hall Health; 2000.
21. Spaite D, et al. Developing a foundation for the evaluation of expanded-scope EMS: a window of opportunity that cannot be ignored. *Ann Emerg Med.* 1997;30:791.
22. Guidelines 2000 for cardiopulmonary resuscitation and emergency cardiovascular care. *Circulation.* 2000;102 (suppl I):I-1.
23. Kudenchuk P, et al. Amiodarone for resuscitation after out-of-hospital cardiac arrest due to ventricular fibrillation. *NEJM.* 1999;341:871.
24. Callaham M, et al. A randomized clinical trial of high-dose epinephrine and norepinephrine vs. standard dose epinephrine in prehospital cardiac arrest. *JAMA.* 1992; 268:2667.

25. Stout J, Pepe PE, Mosesso VN Jr. Advanced life support vs. tiered-response ambulance system. *Prehosp Emerg Care.* 2000;4(1):1–6.

26. Ornato J, et al. Cost effectiveness of defibrillation by emergency medical technicians. *Am J Emerg Med.* 1998; 6:108.

27. Schmidt T, et al. Evaluation of protocols allowing emergency medical technicians to determine need for treatment and transport. *Acad Emerg Med.* 2000;7:663.

28. Lawrence D. Miles Value Foundation. Website: http://www.valuefoundation.org., 2000.

29. California Code of Regulations, Title 22, Social Security, Division 9: Prehospital Emergency Medical Services, Chapter 4, Article 3, ¶ 100159.

30. Birkmeyer JD, Finlayson SR, Tosteson AN. Effect of hospital volume on in-hospital mortality with pancreaticoduodenectomy. *Surgery.* 1999;125(3):250–256.

31. Hannan EL, Popp AJ, Tranmer B, et al. Relationship between provider volume and mortality for carotid endarterectomies in New York State. *Stroke.* 1998;29(11): 2292.

32. Kimmel SE, Berlin JA, Laskey WK, et al. The relationship between coronary angioplasty procedure volume and major complications. *JAMA.* 1995;274:1137.

33. Grubbs K. Current status of clinical education in paramedic programs: a descriptive research project. *Prehosp Disaster Med.* 1997;12(4):250–257.

34. Pirrallo R. Establishing biennial paramedic experience benchmarks. *Prehosp Emerg Care.* 1998;2:335–337.

35. Johnson J. Prehospital care: the future of emergency medical services. *Ann Emerg Med.* 1991;20:426.

CHAPTER 12

System Design

Jerry Overton, MPA
Jack Stout, BA

The acts of accessing emergency medical assistance, dispatching the appropriate resources, responding quickly, and rendering quality care in the prehospital setting seem simplistic and may be taken for granted by the patient, layperson, and even governmental officials. These acts, however, are only four components of the many that comprise today's cutting edge Emergency Medical Services (EMS) system. In the current environment, it is necessary not only to understand that each component is, in fact, complex, but also that each component is an integral part of the overall design of the EMS system. It is that design which will provide the patient, and the community, with the best chance of receiving quality care within economic reason. The most powerful force influencing an EMS system's ability to convert available financial resources into superior clinical performance and response-time reliability is system design.

Introduction

No forethought was given to the development of the EMS system prior to the late 1960s and early 1970s. The ambulance was viewed only as a means of transportation, and treatment in the prehospital setting by trained personnel was nonexistent. However, two sentinel events changed that perspective. First was the publication in 1966 of *Accidental death and disability: the neglected disease of modern society*.[1] The document identified many problems in emergency care, but its focus on the inadequacies in prehospital care was unique and began a shift of emphasis to an arena of care that previously had not been considered seriously.

The second event occurred late in 1973. Congress passed, and the President signed, the Emergency Medical Services System Act, and the word "system" was permanently added to the vocabulary.[2] The law, and its subsequent funding, addressed planning, "systems" development, research, and training. Propelled by more than $300 million in federal grants, the fed-

eral government's 15 components of EMS system design sent the nation in a conceptual direction from which it is still recovering. The 15 components were manpower, training, communication, transportation, facilities, critical care units, public safety agencies, consumer participation, access to care, transfer of patients, record keeping, public information and education, evaluation, disaster planning, and mutual aid.

Lacking fundamental elements such as medical oversight, financial structure, legal structure, a method of allocating market rights and responsibilities, or even a framework for describing performance expectations, the 15 components fell short of furnishing a conceptual basis for rational EMS system development. After brief national recognition, the conceptual direction and funds of the 1970s faded. Almost without exception, the high-performance systems of today were not recipients of federal EMS grants.

The 15 components failed in four ways to provide a foundation on which a nationwide network of quality prehospital care systems could be built. First, the 15 components were not developed from the patient's, or the consumer's, point of view. Second, as a systems approach, the 15-component framework violated key principles of systems engineering. Third, the 15 components failed to identify and organize essential elements of an effective EMS system into a useful framework. Fourth, the 15 components assumed a hopelessly oversimplified view of a complex function.

The American Heart Association introduced a clinical approach to EMS system design in 1991 with its "Chain of Survival."[3] The concept was important from two perspectives. First, it permanently introduced other components, or "links," into the EMS system (early access, early CPR, early defibrillation, and early advanced care). The calling party (Early Access) and the layperson bystander (Early CPR) were recognized as integral parts of the system. More important was the recognition of the interdependence of all the components and the analogy that a chain, or system, was only as strong as its weakest link or component. To be effective, all had to play their vital roles.

By 1991, however, most EMS systems had developed without clinical care as the primary driver. As history has demonstrated, prehospital system designs are not the product of policy decisions that deliberately select certain features and reject others with a full understanding of each option's demonstrated advantages and disadvantages. Rather, most system designs simply have evolved through a process of short-term, issue-driven policy decisions, or were loosely patterned after a television series.

This chapter presents the major elements of EMS system design that contribute to or detract from the system's ability to convert available financial resources into quality prehospital care. To understand those elements, an understanding must be gained as to why there is a need for EMS system design prior to arriving at a working definition of an EMS system.

The Need for EMS System Design

Before local and state governments were forced into tighter economic situations, EMS advocates could and would ask, "What is a life worth?" That has changed. Public needs of equal or perhaps even greater importance (for example, bioterrorism, prenatal care, infant nutrition, drug abuse prevention, law enforcement, and education) compete vigorously for the limited dollars available. Now, EMS administrators are facing that far more challenging question, "Is this the best we can do with the money we have?"

This question has created a dilemma for EMS administrators and medical directors. Priorities have been firmly established. Clinical sophistication, response-time reliability, performance accountability, and economic efficiency are no longer terms of art, but are requirements for those involved in administering, regulating, and funding EMS.

Expectations have increased as well. The patient and the physician expect a positive outcome. The patient and the local government official expect excellent response times at a reasonable, or reduced, cost. And the public expects its EMS system to be credible.

Often, priorities compete with each other, and expectations can be unreasonable. The situation will continue to worsen as the population grows older and as demand increases. It is estimated that the population of those more than 65 years of age will grow from 11.3% in 1980 to 13.1% in 2010, and EMS utilization will increase at an even faster rate.[4,5] It is estimated that the elderly are 4.4 times more likely to use EMS than the non-elderly, and that 48% of all intensive-care admissions fall within the geriatric age range.[6]

The conventional wisdom of EMS system design (for example, tiered response, specialized production strategy, 24-hour shifts in urban settings, use of fixed-post locations, and disorganized dispatch methods) has made status quo a higher priority than that of meeting the needs of patients. There exists a resistance to change. For the convenience of the system, patient care can be compromised.

Some EMS systems designed and managed for their own convenience have attempted to offset their ineffectiveness and inefficiencies by increasing local tax subsidization. Developing a tolerance for large amounts of subsidization, low-performance systems have become dependent on local tax support, with an unexpected result. Today, an imperfect but unmistakable inverse correlation exists between the level of local tax support (per capita per year subsidy) and the quality of patient care.[7]

Facing the political liability of a poorly performing EMS system design, elected officials too often fail to diagnose the system itself as the cause of the problem and, instead, treat the symptoms. Although too much money hardly is to blame when quality of prehospital care deteriorates, chronic symptoms of faulty system design are often misdiagnosed as a financial problem and, as a stopgap, are treated with more money.

The question is not whether an EMS system design is capable of consuming large sums of money; any design can. The question is whether, at any given level of financial support, one design generates more service of higher quality than another. Public officials in the 21st century will not take seriously EMS advocates who are unwilling or unable to grapple with the realities of economic efficiency, performance productivity, and the need to generate higher-quality service with limited financial resources.

Definition

The definition of an EMS system has changed as EMS has changed and developed. Definitions have ranged from being component-based, as evidenced by the EMS System Act of 1973, to clinical-based, inclusive only of the relationship of the clinical components.[8]

These and other definitions of EMS systems have developed from the viewpoint of the system itself. For example, systems based on the specialized production strategy define non-emergency patients, and the financial and other resources involved, as being outside the system. Thus, they avoid comparison with systems based on the flexible production strategy. The specialized production strategy employs two, three, or even four types of ambulances, each specializing in specific types of calls. The flexible production strategy employs a single ambulance staffed and equipped to respond to any type of call. Either strategy can incorporate the use of one or more types of First Responder units.

Similarly, other EMS system definitions assume that callers triage themselves reliably into emergency and non-emergency categories, dialing 9-1-1 for an emergency and a 7-digit telephone number for a non-emergency. The underlying assumption is that callers who do not dial 9-1-1 are not a responsibility of the EMS system because they failed to follow the access rules. As with systems based on specialized production strategies, these systems escape accountability for a segment of the patient population, including related costs and outcomes.

The term "EMS" reflects the original assumption that emergency patients can be distinguished from non-emergency patients, and that specialized production dedicated to each type of work will provide better service at a lower cost. This once-conventional wisdom failed to account for patterns of demand for prehospital care, and has proved false.[9,10]

If an EMS system is to serve patients, there must be a clear understanding of who the patients are. The following are the facts regarding consumer requests for medical assistance and transportation where a universal 9-1-1 number has existed for an extended period of time:

1. Slightly more than 70% of all medical requests enter the system through 9-1-1, with 30% entering the system through a 7-digit telephone number.
2. Approximately 20% to 30% of 9-1-1 medical requests are found to require Advanced Life Support (ALS) skills.
3. Approximately 12% of 7-digit number ambulance requests require ALS skills.
4. Many properly triaged emergency calls do not require ALS, whereas other properly triaged non-emergency calls require ALS en route (for

example, scheduled interfacility transport of a patient requiring advanced en route support—an increasingly common type of transport as hospitals and hospital cardiac care units consolidate).

Every EMS system has in common two inputs: patients and money. The system's most important input is the patient, yet money is also essential. Any organization that is required to provide a timely and medically appropriate response to each patient's request for service requires funds for its operation. The EMS system is a mechanism for converting financial resources into service.

Every EMS system also has common outputs, including patient assessment, treatment, and medical transportation. By linking input and output, the system converts dollars into service. Depending on efficiency, some EMS systems generate small volumes of low-quality service from a large dollar input, while others generate large volumes of high-quality service from a small dollar input (fig. 12.1).

An EMS system is comprised of organizations, individuals, and equipment, with some type of communications network and facility to house functions such as fleet maintenance, training, control center operations, billing and collection activity, and other support services. In addition, every EMS system has some type of information system, a mechanism for financing its operations, and a formal and informal legal structure defining organizational roles and responsibilities. Finally, almost every EMS system is required to have, or purports to have, some type of medical oversight structure.

Impact on patient outcome, the most important result of all this activity, is a function of two related but separate factors. First is efficacy of the system's protocols, including priority dispatch, and medical and ambulance deployment protocols. Second, and equally important, is system compliance with those protocols. These two factors must be dealt with separately, since a defect in one factor cannot be corrected by acting on the other. These two factors affect every aspect of the clinical, operational, and economic performance of the EMS system.

Understanding the dynamics of the inputs and outputs, and the importance of the functions of the related factors, provide a foundation for an all-encompassing definition of an EMS system defined from the patient's perspective. Therefore, for the purposes of this chapter, *an EMS system is defined as con-*

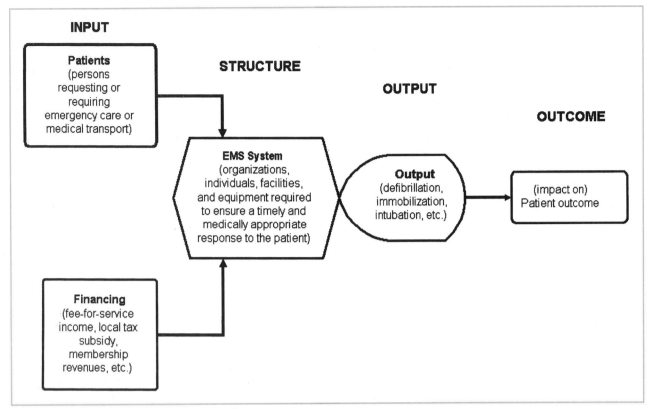

INPUT

STRUCTURE

OUTPUT

OUTCOME

Patients
(persons
requesting or
requiring
emergency care or
medical transport)

EMS System
(organizations,
individuals, facilities,
and equipment required
to ensure a timely and
medically appropriate
response to the patient)

Output
(defibrillation,
immobilization,
intubation, etc.)

(impact on)
Patient outcome

Financing
(fee-for-service
income, local tax
subsidy,
membership
revenues, etc.)

FIGURE 12.1. *Relationship of the "system" to its environment.*

sisting of those organizations, individuals, facilities and equipment whose participation is required to ensure timely and medically appropriate responses to each request for prehospital care and medical transportation.

In defining the system from the patient's point of view, all patients are included, regardless of how they access the system, whether system managers accept or reject responsibility for their care, and whether such patients ultimately require heroic intervention or just simple kindness and safe medical transport. In the end, the patient must always be the focal point of the EMS system.

Fundamentals

System design refers to the EMS system's underlying framework of legal, organizational, clinical, business, and financial structures, and the interrelationship and coordination among those structures. System design is critically important but not all-powerful. The following are its limitations:

1. Talented and motivated people can produce good results in a bad system design, but not for extended periods of time.

2. Incompetence can produce poor results in even the best system design.
3. Talented people tend to be attracted to system designs that will potentially nurture and showcase individual talents.
4. Talented people have options because they are talented. In general, the industry's most talented managers choose to avoid employment in EMS systems that hinder their abilities.
5. Good system design makes excellence possible and superior performance probable, but guarantees neither.
6. Bad system design makes excellence impossible and inferior service probable.
7. Sound system design cannot guarantee clinically appropriate and economically efficient performance. Poor system design can make consistent lifesaving performance extremely unlikely, if not impossible.

The term "system design" is uncomfortably vague. The first step in defining the concept is to identify the direct effects of an EMS system's design. Any EMS system design establishes eight major structural attributes:

1. *Geographic Scope.* The geographic scope of the system's primary service area (9-1-1 medical response area) affects economies of scale and can determine how less economically desirable areas are served.

2. *Standards setting and enforcement.* The process whereby performance standards are established (if established), monitored, and enforced is, in the long run, the most important aspect of an EMS system design. In general, if well designed, this process will eventually expose and correct defective aspects of the system's design.

3. *Division of functions.* Division of functional responsibilities among participating organizations (for example, first response, multiple ambulance providers, and medical oversight) impacts funding requirements and revenue options, affects distribution of liability, and can enhance or dilute organizational accountability of performance results.

4. *Production strategies.* The type of production strategies employed (for example, specialized production strategy vs. flexible production strategy, First Response for life-threatening emergencies vs. law enforcement First Response with AED) establish the system's productivity limit, thus more directly impacting production costs and funding requirements than any other single factor, including wages.

5. *Market allocation.* Selection of organizations to participate within the system (for example, bid competition, accident of history, political influence, default) sets the stage for all that follows. Only a few EMS systems deliberately award EMS market rights and responsibilities to the best-qualified organizations willing to commit to performance standards.

6. *Consequences of chronic failure to perform.* If and how a poorly performing organization can be replaced by one that is more qualified is a key element of EMS system design. Not surprisingly, this feature is least likely to be applied, as it is equally difficult to replace a governmental agency performing poorly as it is to terminate an agreement with a politically influential, long-standing private contractor.

7. *Business structure.* The sources, amounts, routes, and contingencies of dollar-flow into and within the system determine which organizational behaviors will be financially supported and which will not. In many lower-performance systems, these contingencies of financial rein-

forcement are either irrelevant to the system's reason for being, or downright contrary (for example, budget increases justified by deficient performance). Market-test comparisons with other systems that are serving similar markets and are known for their efficiency can be a powerful stimulant. In short, the system's business structure provides or fails to provide the critical link between the public interest and organizational motivation.

8 *Management level required.* Not all EMS system designs require the same level of management to extract the system's maximum potential. In general, policymakers must choose between low-performance designs capable of approaching their full but modest potential versus high-performance designs that are capable of achieving superior results but require leadership talents well above the norm.

Because of the number of factors impacting EMS performance and funding, an EMS system with high-performance potential demands a higher level of management. The chief advantage of low-performance EMS system designs is that the maximum performance, modest though it may be, can often be achieved by managers of limited interest or ability. For example, it is much easier to manage a system using the same level of staffing coverage with 24-hour shifts and fixed-response locations than to devise a deployment strategy that incorporates peak-load staffing and variable staffing schedules. As a result, the maximum performance of inferior designs falls far below that achieved by systems of superior design, even where substantial subsidies are available.

Impacts of an Inferior System Design

Regardless of the well-meaning intent of the governmental official, the commitment of the EMS administrator, or the tenacity of the medical director, the system design must be sound if the expected level of performance is to be possible. Aside from its obvious impact on patient outcome, an inferior system design can affect the delivery of care operationally and financially. The following negative impacts result from inferior system design:[11]

1. *Unequal socio-economic service base.* System designs that have no performance accountability and that are driven by economics can focus on

those neighborhoods or areas that result in a higher level of reimbursement, reducing service to poorer neighborhoods.

2. *Unequal response-time performance.* System designs that do not measure response-time reliability and performance accountability can ignore geographically challenging areas while deploying more resources in easier-to-serve, high response-volume areas. This is typical of systems that measure response times by averages.

3. *No incentive to grow.* Inferior system designs that use the static resource deployment method discourage efficiencies that may lead to volume growth and associated revenues.

4. *Inability to match the right patient with the right resources.* A system design that employs call screening, rather than call triage, and is not patient-focused, can easily send the wrong resource, that is, a non-emergency ambulance rather than an ALS ambulance, or even no ambulance, to the person accessing medical assistance. Not only is this detrimental to patient care, but this duplication of services for the same patient leads to inefficiencies, and is ultimately more expensive to the taxpayer, the patient, or both.

5. *Leaving the choice to the consumer.* The person experiencing a medical emergency or, if not the calling party, the person accessing help, is in no position to compare ambulance services, nor is he or she a medical expert able to determine the best and closest resource that will minimize the threat of death or disability. In effective system design, informed officials make this choice or decision prior to system implementation.

Comparing EMS System Designs

Communities across the United States and the world provide EMS to their citizens using a variety of different system designs. Presently, there are more than 30 different designs for providing this essential service. Design of the EMS system can range from service by local government agencies, such as municipal EMS and fire departments, to open-market competition among private ambulance companies.

The wide variation in system design has been problematic for those attempting to compare systems using any traditional methodology. Usually a comparison focuses on one specific aspect of the system,

such as staffing and resource patterns.[12] Other attempts have identified specific system designs and attempted to survey one component, such as cost.[7] Finally, the need to measure clinical outcomes has led researchers to examine variables both within systems and between systems, in an attempt to maximize both researcher knowledge of EMS system design attributes and patient outcome.[13]

The creation of a conceptual framework for comparing EMS systems of diverse design, one biased in favor of the patient, must track the system's response to every patient, including those who are not accessing the 9-1-1 emergency number and who are therefore excluded as not being part of its traditional function. Any conceptual framework that subordinates the patient to the system fails to provide a basis for fair comparison of the different system types. Since the patient's needs are not securely a part of the system's purpose, these conceptual frameworks are not stable platforms for comparing the advantages and disadvantages of system designs. If the decision to organizationally and operationally separate emergency service production from non-emergency transport production is clinically and financially sound, only a comparison of total system performance, clinical and financial, can test the proposition conclusively.

After nearly two decades testing more than 30 basic prehospital system designs, design features can be isolated that are more common and sometimes universal among better-performing systems, and less common or nonexistent among systems performing at low levels of efficiency. A growing number of today's better-performing EMS systems are products of an informed selection of structural features that deliver the best possible chance of survival without disability, using limited financial resources. Because of their ability to attain and sustain peak performance over long periods of time, these systems have been termed High Performance EMS (HPEMS) systems, and their track records are defining the future of EMS.

Performance

For purposes of examination, EMS systems can be divided into the following four categories:

- High quality with above average cost
- Low quality with below average cost (most common)
- Low quality with above average cost

- High Performance—above average service with below average cost (Syracuse; Tulsa/Oklahoma City; Charlotte, N.C.; Reno; Fort Wayne; Little Rock; Fort Worth; Kansas City; Richmond; Pinellas County; Clark County; Acadian System serving rural Louisiana; and East Texas EMS System serving rural eastern Texas).

The EMS systems in the high-performance category share key features of system design rarely associated with less cost-effective systems. All HPEMS systems share the understanding that economic efficiency, response-time reliability, and clinical performance are directly interdependent. Certain other system design characteristics also can influence and define efficiency potential.

It is necessary to understand that two broad objectives, when combined, furnish the basis for predicting and explaining the operational consequences of policy decisions affecting system design:

- The development of a basic working knowledge of the three measures essential to judging and comparing system performance
- The identification of EMS system design factors that contribute to or detract from the system's ability to convert financial resources into service.

Essential Measures

Just as nothing impacts a system's ability to turn financial resources into service more powerfully than system design, nothing impacts patient care more powerfully than the system's ability to convert financial resources into service. Clinical performance, response-time reliability, and economic efficiency are more than related; they are absolutely interdependent.

By shortening one or two sides of the triangle in figure 12.2, even a poorly structured, badly managed system can perform reasonably well on one or two measures, creating an appearance of competence when viewed from a favorable angle. The consequences of such distortion harm the patient, the taxpayer, or frequently both. For example, an unskilled manager can limit spending by allowing clinical quality and response-time reliability to deteriorate. Similarly, given enough money, even the most unskilled management team can generate something of value.

The challenge is to simultaneously generate clinical excellence, response-time reliability, and economic efficiency. Meeting that challenge qualifies any system and its personnel as high performance.

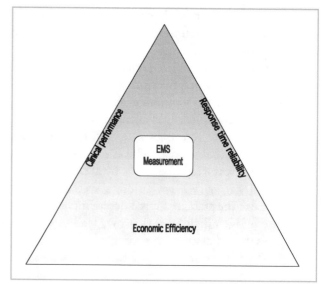

FIGURE 12.2. *The interdependence of EMS System Design.*

Comparing Clinical Performance

The EMS System Matrix (fig. 12.3) that follows provides a two-dimensional framework for documenting and comparing any system's clinical structure and performance with that of any other, regardless of design. The most important task of every EMS system is to generate a planned, coordinated, and medically appropriate response to every patient in need of its services. Thus, the matrix is deliberately driven from its left vertical axis, that is, a comprehensive, sequential list of system-response phases, from prevention through medical oversight of the response.

Documenting the clinical performance of an EMS system using the matrix is a formidable task, regardless of the system's design, and therein is its value. Using the matrix, any EMS system can be documented in detail and compared fairly with any other, regardless of differences.

A few comments should be made regarding the use of the matrix. Medical oversight is the only element appearing on both the vertical and horizontal axes. As an output, medical oversight requires the full range of structural components (such as a responsible organization, a legal basis, and funding) for which provision is made horizontally.

The three most important duties of medical oversight are formulating system performance specifications (that is, standards and protocols governing output performance), monitoring compliance with specifications, and initiating action for compliance as needed. Although most high-performance systems

OUTPUTS (Services)	STRUCTURE							SYSTEM STANDARDS AND PROTOCOLS
	A. Responsible Organization	B. Legal basis	C. Personnel	D. Equipment/ facilities	E. Info-Systems	F. Medical oversight	G. Finance (Sources, amounts)	
1. Prevention and early recognition								
2. Bystander action and system access								
3. 9-1-1 Call taking								
4. First Response dispatch/services								
5. EMS telephone inquiry and pre-arrival care								
6. Ambulance services								
7. Receiving facility interface								
8. Medical oversight								

FIGURE 12.3. *EMS System Matrix.*

employ independent medical oversight that is responsible for all components of the EMS system, others do not. Thus, provision is made vertically for listing a separate medical oversight entity, or specifying "none" for each output category.

To document and compare clinical capability, it is necessary to examine written protocols, personnel certification requirements, equipment standards, monitoring and quality improvement practices, patient-outcome measures, and other aspects of the following system outputs on the left axis of the EMS matrix:

1. Prevention and early recognition (for example, seat belt awareness, feet first, first-time water safety, early recognition of cardiac symptoms, anti-violence programs)
2. Bystander action and system access
   A. CPR instruction
   B. System Access
      1) Emergency (9-1-1)
      2) Non-emergency (7-digit number)
3. 9-1-1 call-taking function
4. First response dispatch/services
   A. Technical Rescue and Extrication
   B. Initial medical support and assistance
5. EMS telephone inquiry and pre-arrival instructions

6. Ambulance services
   A. Emergency responses (presumptively classified)
   B. Non-emergency transports (presumptively classified)
   C. Interfacility critical care transfers
   D. Helicopter transport (scene flights)
7. Receiving-facility interface
   A. Patient exchange procedures
   B. Participation in quality assurance
   C. Equipment exchange arrangement
   D. Information exchange arrangement
   E. Selection of hospital destination
   F. Facility Diversions
8. Medical Oversight
   A. Internal or external
   B. Advisory or authoritative
   C. Qualifications of physicians
   D. Level of funding and staff support

Comparing Response-time Reliability

It is estimated that an American will suffer a coronary event approximately every 29 seconds, and that someone will die from one approximately every minute. Those statistics, combined with the fact that at least

250,000 people a year die within one hour of the onset of the event, usually from ventricular fibrillation, define the need for EMS.[14]

Many systems today have built their response time around achieving "8-minute response-time reliability" but are unaware of the origins of that standard. Studies have shown that with the arrival of Basic Life Support and defibrillation, the third link in the "Chain of Survival," within four minutes and ALS, the fourth link, within eight minutes, patients in ventricular fibrillation have a significantly better chance of surviving out-of-hospital cardiac arrest.[15,16,17]

Just as an EMS system creates reliable or unreliable clinical performance, it creates reliable or unreliable response-time performance. Figure 12.4 demonstrates response-time distributions for two different EMS systems claiming "8-minute response-time reliability." Given what has been learned about the physiology of cardiac arrest, it is clear that System A's 8-minute *average response time* delivers poor and potentially life-threatening service to most patients.

In contrast, System B's 8-minute *fractile response time* (at the 90% level of reliability) delivers a real chance of survival more than 90% of the time. Because cardiac arrest is the most time-critical of all calls, response-time standards for both First Response

and ambulance service must be aimed at meeting the needs of patients experiencing a life-threatening event.

Average response time is not only a totally misleading indicator of response-time reliability, but it is also a clinically inappropriate goal. Deployment practices producing the most impressive-sounding average statistics are quite different from those generating 8-minute, 90% fractile reliability or a less stringent rural equivalent. It is impossible to pursue the lowest possible average response time and the highest percentage fractile reliability. A choice must be made.

The type of report shown in table 12.1 typifies performance by the ambulance component of the Richmond, Virginia, EMS system, and is widely used by high-performance systems to track response-time reliability. The report clearly shows the number of responses for each minute and the cumulative percentage. Clearly, the 50th percentile is achieved far before the 8-minute fractile requirement is achieved.

Response Time From the Patient Perspective

Response time typically is discussed as though what it is and how it is measured are understood. In real-

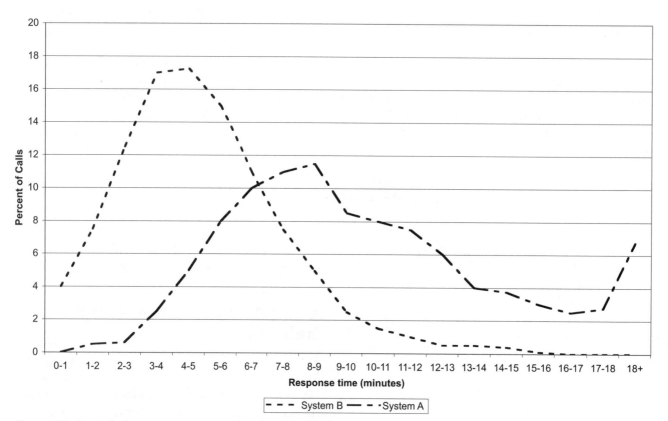

FIGURE 12.4. *Ambulance response time distributions for two systems.*

TABLE 12.1			
Fractile Response Time Distribution			
RESPONSE TIME (MIN.)	**RUNS (NO.)**	**TOTAL (%)**	**CUMULATIVE (%)**
<1	31	1.55	1.55
1–<2	57	2.85	4.40
2–<3	140	7.01	11.41
3–<4	221	11.06	22.47
4–<5	301	15.07	37.54
5–<6	339	16.97	54.50
6–<7	299	14.96	69.47
7–<8	253	12.66	82.13
8–<9	172	8.61	90.74
9–<10	58	2.90	93.64
10–<11	41	2.05	95.70
11–<12	28	1.40	97.10
12–<13	13	0.65	97.75
13–<14	14	0.70	98.45
14–<15	8	0.40	98.85
15+	23	1.15	100.00

poor performance. The solution is institutional, and includes enforcement of a standard which requires that there be no chronic pattern of response-time discrimination against any neighborhood, district, or zone as defined by local ordinance. Richmond, Virginia, and Kansas City, Missouri, as examples, have high expectations of response-time equity among neighborhoods, and local officials have divided each city into six zones to ensure this equity takes place. While it is recognized that this further requirement increases production costs for an already efficient provider of services, local officials made the policy decision to approach response times from the patient perspective, and absorb the additional costs. If the area-wide standard is already stringent, however, requiring a standard within each zone or district can raise the system-wide standard to an unattainable level.

Response Intervals

To begin the process of examining response times, it is advantageous to divide the response times into response intervals. An excellent template to start is one that also has the potential of determining clinical outcomes.[18] Response intervals allow a closer, quicker analysis, and often, changes made in a single response interval will greatly improve overall response-time performance. Specifically, the intervals of "call received to time of dispatch" and "time of dispatch to ambulance en route" are often too long. In HPEMS systems, both of these times are measured with the expectation that they will be achieved in 30 seconds or less, 90% of the time. It is much easier to impact these times than it is to impact travel time, because distance is constant, and pressure placed on field crews only adds stress to an already stressful situation, the result of which could be an at-fault accident.

Wherever response-time reliability is deficient, managers have developed persuasive arguments to account for this deficiency. It is true that call-density-per-square-mile, road systems, shape of the service area, caliber of mutual aid, traffic congestion, placement of hospitals, weather conditions, population fluctuations, and other factors define the limits of response-time reliability achievable from any given operating budget. These factors do, in fact, determine the maximum productivity level at any given level of response-time reliability. However, experience has shown that the most important factors in determining maximum, realistic response-time reliability at any given funding level are:

ity it is measured in many different ways by many different systems. Optimally, the response time would start the second the event occurs, and end with ALS at the patient's side. However, this is unrealistic. Patients cannot be expected to record an accurate time when suffering a medical or traumatic emergency. Similarly, external variables prevent response-time accountability between the second the vehicle arrives at the scene and the time the medic gains access to the patient.

The ALS clock starts the second the first request for help is received and can be recorded. It does not start when an extended telephone interrogation has been completed, the responding unit is alerted, the crew acknowledges the dispatch, or the unit starts en route. The ALS clock stops the second a fully staffed, equipped, and transport-capable ALS unit arrives on the scene.

It can be important to record the time of arrival at the patient side. To time-stamp this second, a "patient contact" button may be programmed on a portable radio with automatic number identification capability and interfaced to the Computer Aided Dispatch (CAD). The ALS clock does not stop when the First Response arrives on the scene, a supervisor arrives at the scene, or BLS mutual aid arrives on the scene.

Although a fractile response-time standard equalizes response-time reliability in a city or among various zones, districts, or neighborhoods of the service area, it still can leave geographic pockets of chronic

- understanding the response volume by time of day and day of week,
- knowing the geographic location of the responses, and
- using an algorithm to strategically locate the resources based on these predictors and the number of resources available to the system at any point in time.

Comparing Economic Efficiency

Having established a foundation for comparing the structures of clinical performance and response-time reliability, attention must be given to comparisons of economic efficiency. Diagnosing and correcting causes of poor economic efficiency requires a working knowledge of marginal cost analysis, amortized capital costs, the Unit Hour Utilization (UH/U) ratio, effective unit-hour production, average versus marginal unit-hour costs, and economies of scale. Nearly as complex are the revenue considerations and sources. The following fundamentals regarding costs and pricing must be understood prior to discussing some of these key concepts:

1. Price does not equal cost. In EMS, price, or the rates charged to transport the patient, rarely equals the total cost of providing service. Since subsidies distort pricing structures, some of the most efficient EMS systems charge the highest rates or user fees. The minimal charges of less efficient systems, which receive greater subsidy, therefore create the illusion of a bargain. Comparison of bottom-line efficiency must account for the combined effect of subsidies and user fees in different proportions among different EMS systems.

2. Component cost does not equal system cost. The cost of operating a system component (for example, 9-1-1 ambulance service or ALS First Response) is not the cost of operating the entire EMS system, even if the managers of that component have declared it to be the entire EMS system. For example, in cities where a subsidized government third-service handles 9-1-1 emergency requests and private firms provide non-emergency and interfacility transport, the total cost of the ambulance service component includes both the user fees paid to private firms, and the user fees and subsidy payments supporting the government-run third-service. That total often does not include the costs of public education, First Response, or medical oversight. All components and costs must be identified to fully compare the total system costs.

3. More subsidy does not equal better ambulance service. Subsidizing the ambulance service component of an EMS system reduces the rates (or user fees) to below cost. For example, assume a system's total annual subsidy divided by its total annual patient transports is $400. Further assume that this system also charges an average user fee (base rate plus mileage) of $250 per patient transport and currently experiences a 50% collection rate. A mathematical calculation reveals that, should the subsidy stop, this system theoretically would survive by increasing its average user-fee to $1,050. In today's reimbursement environment, this rate would not be acceptable, as no third-party payer, Medicare, or commercial insurance carrier would consider payment of this rate. Such an inefficient system would not survive economically and could not survive politically. The "zero-subsidy" user-fee level of many systems burdened with inefficient designs exceeds $1,000 per patient transport. Thus the only effect of the ambulance subsidy is to reduce price below cost, merely delaying the inevitability for a poorly designed system.

The Subsidy-Price Trade-Off Chart

Figure 12.5 shows a subsidy-price trade-off chart from seven EMS systems. This chart will assist other EMS systems when making similar comparisons and developing their own subsidy-price trade-off charts.

To plot the subsidy-price trade-off line for the ambulance component of a system, obtain or estimate total payments for all emergency and non-emergency ambulance services (including all providers in the market: public and private, emergency and non-emergency) from all sources (local tax support, patient payments, private third-party and HMO contract payments, Medicare, Medicaid, donated funds, subscription membership fees). Divide that total by the population of the primary service area and plot the result (that is, the total system cost per capita regardless of how financed) along the horizontal axis at the bottom of the chart. This point defines the amount of annual subsidy per capita that would sustain the system without revenue from any other source, one of two points along the system's subsidy-price trade-off line.

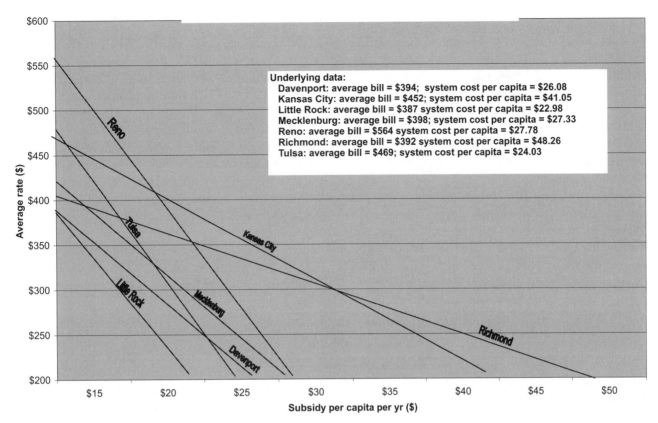

FIGURE 12.5. *Subsidy Price Trade-Off.*

Data shown in figure:

Underlying data:
Davenport: average bill = $394; system cost per capita = $26.08
Kansas City: average bill = $452; system cost per capita = $41.05
Little Rock: average bill = $387 system cost per capita = $22.98
Mecklenburg: average bill = $398; system cost per capita = $27.33
Reno: average bill = $564 system cost per capita = $27.78
Richmond: average bill = $392 system cost per capita = $48.26
Tulsa: average bill = $469; system cost per capita = $24.03

Next, estimate the current total average bill for ambulance service in the service area. Note that number, but do not plot it on the chart yet. Estimate the current per capita per year local tax subsidy of the system's ambulance service component. Using these two numbers (the current total average bill and the current per capita per year subsidy), locate where the current total average bill intersects the current per capita subsidy and plot the spot. This point defines the system's current actual position on its subsidy-price line, the second of the two points required to draw the system's current subsidy-price trade-off line. Connect the two marks, extending the left end beyond the plotted point to intersect the vertical axis. The result is the subsidy-price trade-off line.

Understanding Economic Efficiency

The basic measurement of efficiency in EMS is the Unit Hour Utilization (UH/U) ratio. This measurement has become the standard for determining effective deployment strategies, response patterns, unit and system productivity, and even scheduling practices.[19] To understand the importance of UH/U requires a basic understanding of the concept of a unit hour.

A unit hour is defined as a "fully equipped and staffed ambulance on a response or waiting for a response for one hour." Direct labor costs comprise more than 65% of the total costs of the average unit hour. The other 35% consists of the system infrastructure, including dispatch, administration, vehicles, equipment, and overhead. As a result, the cost of a marginal unit hour, or adding a unit to the existing schedule, is approximately 40% to 50% of the total unit hour costs.

Unit hour costs are affected powerfully by economies of scale. For that reason, they are a poor predictor of clinical quality and cost per transport. Only when the unit hour is productive does the cost to the system begin to decrease. That productivity is termed "utilization" and is defined as, "how frequently the unit hour is used."

Unit hour utilization is the measurement that results from dividing the utilization by the number of unit hours produced in a given time period. The equation for UH/U is as follows:

$$\frac{U\ (\text{Utilization})}{UH\ (\text{Unit Hours})} = \text{Unit Hour Utilization}$$

High-performance EMS managers use this ratio to measure the productivity of different actions with the system. While the most common is transports, the productivity of responses, patient contacts, post-to-post moves and workload also can be calculated by this equation. The UH/U is higher in urban areas because more patients are served in a smaller geographic area. As figure 12.6 shows, there is a direct correlation between UH/U and transports per 10,000 populations.

After calculating the UH/U for transports, the cost per transport can be determined. By using the following equation and dividing the cost per unit hour by the UH/U, the true cost of transporting the patient, not the revenue received per transport, is yielded:

$$\frac{\text{Cost per Unit Hour}}{\text{U/UH}} = \text{Cost per Patient Transport}$$

Such calculations are crucial in revealing the powerful impact of economic efficiency in EMS system design. For example, if the full cost of placing a fully equipped ambulance in service is $100 an hour (cost per unit hour) and a patient is transported once every three hours (U/UH), the cost per transport is approximately $300 ($100/0.33). If a patient is transported once every four hours, the cost climbs to $400 ($100/0.25). While it may be unrealistic to assume that productivity in any EMS system can increase from one patient every four hours to one patient every three hours, it is not unrealistic to assume that productivity can increase by eight minutes. If a patient were transported every three hours and 52 minutes, the cost per transport would decrease to $370 ($100/0.27). Although the $30 savings per transport might seem insignificant, the savings accumulate when multiplied over a large number of patients. For example, an EMS system would save $360,000 each year based on 12,000 patients transported annually.

High-performance EMS managers not only understand the importance of these calculations and the power of results, but study comparisons with similar HPEMS systems to ensure that they are achieving at least equal or better service at lower cost as those systems. Table 12.2 provides such a comparison of the highest performing systems in EMS.[20]

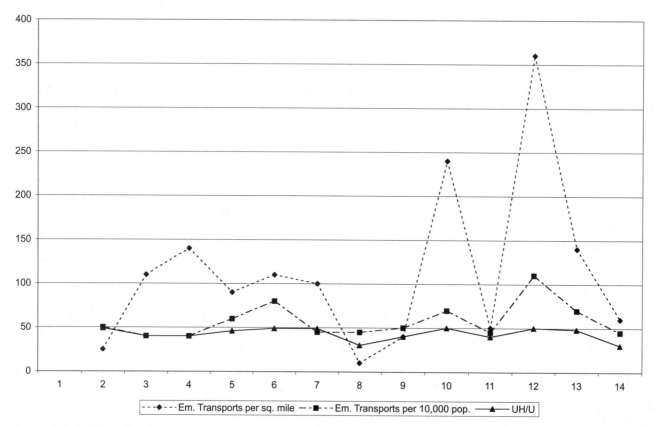

FIGURE 12.6. *UH/U Results.*

TABLE 12.2			
Economic Efficiency			
System	**Cost per Unit Hour**	**Unit Hour Utilization**	**Cost per Transport**
Davenport	$ 88.76	0.41	$216.49
Ft. Wayne	$116.96	0.38	$307.78
Ft. Worth	$ 75.78	0.29	$261.31
Kansas City	$105.84	0.34	$311.29
Lincoln	$118.77	0.28	$424.18
Little Rock	$ 62.19	0.20	$310.95
Mecklenburg	$ 85.97	0.26	$330.65
Monterey County	$ 91.18	0.17	$536.35
Nova Scotia	$ 26.24	0.10	$262.40
Oklahoma City	$113.88	0.26	$438.00
Pinellas County	$110.05	0.50	$220.10
Reno	$134.00	0.38	$352.63
Richmond	$114.38	0.39	$293.28
Tulsa	$ 91.86	0.31	$296.32
Mean	**$ 95.42**	**0.31**	**$325.84**
Median	**$ 98.85**	**0.30**	**$309.37**

Design Factors

Although an HPEMS system is the product of many different factors along with a commitment to ensure that those factors are consistently applied and maintained, four key elements impact the system's ability to convert financial resources into service. Those key elements, and the most significant design characteristics of each, are described in the following sections.

Service Area Definition

With the changing healthcare environment and the increasing sophistication of EMS, it is increasingly difficult to operate a small ambulance service at high clinical quality without high costs. The minimum requirement for high-performance operation is a service area population of approximately 100,000 people exclusively served (emergency and non-emergency) by a single ambulance service provider.

Where local populations are insufficient to generate optimum economies of scale, multi-jurisdictional systems are often the answer. For example, Emergency Medical Services Authority (EMSA), the first public utility model, serves both Tulsa and Oklahoma City, providing care to approximately 68% of all patients transported in the state of Oklahoma, including a large rural area with minimal tax support. In rural areas, the multi-jurisdictional approach is the only answer if any semblance of an HPEMS system is to be designed. Both Acadian Ambulance, based in Lafayette, Louisiana, and East Texas EMS, in Tyler, have been successful in bringing together smaller communities with the counties to form systems that can use the tools of high performance.

Population is not a guarantee of efficiency, as a large urban service area can be made to function as poorly economically as if it were a sparsely populated rural area. By allowing multiple firms to share the same geographic market, each firm's service area remains equally large, but call-density per square mile resembles that of a rural area, and efficiencies are lost.

Medical Oversight

High-performance EMS systems are driven by externally imposed and enforced clinical and response-time standards. To ensure adherence to protocols and system accountability, medical directors in these systems are actively involved in providing leadership and oversight. The characteristics of effective medical oversight are as follows:

External. The medical director is neither hired nor compensated by any organization whose work is the subject of medical oversight. The medical director's authority is independent of and superior to the organizations participating in the EMS system. Otherwise, it would be difficult or impossible for the medical director to settle disputes among participating organizations or people within those organizations.

Authoritative. On matters affecting the quality of patient care, the medical director directs; he or she does not advise. The system design assumes that the delivery of prehospital care is the medical director's practice of prehospital emergency medicine.

Scope of Authority. A single medical director oversees all organizations and individuals participating in the EMS system. The scope of authority is system-wide and extends to all output components of the EMS matrix and all organizations in the system. In multi-jurisdictional systems, this authority is legally recognized by all jurisdictions served.

Funding. Effective medical oversight requires a sustained commitment and continuing level of funding. This includes providing the tools to oversee the position and staff assistance, when needed.

First Response

Delivered by existing fire department personnel with fire apparatus or police departments with automatic external defibrillators, first response is without question the local government's best public service value. Studies have shown that the marginal cost per response at the EMT-D level, including training, fuel, medical supplies, accelerated vehicle maintenance and depreciation, and amortized costs of medical equipment, ranges from as high as $27 to as low as $8.[21] The characteristics of first response in high-performance systems include the following:

Utilization. Priority dispatch on all presumptively classified life-threatening calls usually equals 40% to 45% of the community's 9-1-1 medical requests. Proper utilization of first response resources means response only to these requests, unless specifically requested to the scene as a result of a special circumstance.

Service area. Unlike ambulance services that must respond and transport across geopolitical boundaries in conformance with medical-trade patterns, the most cost-effective form of first response is mono-jurisdictional. Thus, in multi-jurisdictional EMS systems, each participating first responder is responsible for serving its own jurisdiction, and the ambulance service component operates regionally to provide for best economies of scale.

Unit selection. In advanced multi-jurisdictional EMS systems, first response near geopolitical borders is dispatched on a "nearest-unit" basis, not on the basis of political affiliation. The Pinellas County, Florida, EMS system, with 17 participating fire departments and a single regional ambulance service provider, exemplifies this feature.

No discussion of first response would be complete without raising two questions:

1. How often are your first responders first?
2. Is early defibrillation early?

Even though fire department resources outnumber ambulance service resources in most, if not all communities, first responders arrive before ambulance crews achieving an externally monitored 8-minute, 90% standard of reliability, on or about 50% of responses. Proper use of first response, and the interaction with dispatch, are important for the preservation of resources in high-volume, densely populated areas.

Perhaps more important is the need to examine the second question. Even in HPEMS systems where first response is used appropriately and response-time reliability is strictly defined and attained, the percentages of cardiac arrest patients in ventricular fibrillation is still unacceptably low. This points to an access problem. All systems have 9-1-1, but the bystander is not placing the call, for multiple reasons. System design planners must be aware of this fact and must work actively to improve this situation (e.g., through community education) by ensuring the Early Access link of the Chain of Survival is incorporated into their definition of an EMS system.

Ambulance Service

Of all EMS system elements, ambulance service is the most costly, the most complex, and the most politically sensitive. The situation is exacerbated because the proven principles of high-performance ambulance operation conflict with conventional thinking. But the proof is in the results. Every ambulance service documenting externally monitored ALS response-time performance at the 8-minute, 90% level of reliability while maintaining minimal subsidization, exhibits the following characteristics.

Sole provider. Exclusive market rights to furnish emergency and non-emergency ambulance service are granted to a sole, and often competitively selected, provider. Local ordinance or state law bans "cream skimming" or "cherry picking" of non-emergency patients or facilities with contracts that have guaranteed payment mechanisms. Elected officials designing an EMS system face a difficult but inevitable policy choice. Two of the following three policies are possible, but not all three:

- High-quality ambulance service with clinically sound response-time reliability,
- Retail competition and consumer choice within the market, and
- Little or no local tax subsidy.

At predetermined intervals, an examination of the market place is conducted to ensure that the local government is receiving the best service for its cost-subsidy tradeoff. If it is not, it should conduct a competitive bid process for the exclusive right to serve the community, or negotiate an extension at its option.

Control center operations. The ambulance provider has control of the dispatch center, allowing the deployment and redeployment of resources based on soundly developed algorithms. In HPEMS systems, patient care begins when the telephone rings. The dispatchers are Emergency Medical Dispatch certified, perform priority dispatch interrogation, deliver Dispatch Life Support using pre-arrival instructions, and have field experience. All calls are triaged, and screening is prohibited.

Accountability. High-performance EMS systems have performance requirements that are either founded in local government ordinances, contracts, or both. Failure to perform will result in financial penalties or even replacement.

Revenue maximization. With finite sources of revenues, HPEMS systems incorporate a business function into their operations. Understanding fee-for-service billings and maximizing revenues from Medicare, Medicaid, and other third-party payers are not normally a function of local government, but it is a requirement of the EMS system if local tax subsidies are to be minimized.

Flexible production strategy. Rather than operating specialized ambulance fleets, HPEMS systems employ a single fleet of ALS units capable of handling any type of service request. Using advanced deployment practices, the all-ALS (single-tier) system guarantees that every patient, regardless of the presumptively coded dispatch, will receive the highest level of care, and the system will benefit from productivity levels significantly higher than those relying on the specialized (two-tier) production strategy.

The value of the flexible production strategy was shown in a recent study involving the 13 EMS systems in table 12.3. The purpose of the study was to determine the cost savings, if any, of the flexible production strategy when compared to specialized production. Savings were documented in all systems with a range of 4.9% to 19.82%, with a median of 12.9%. It was concluded that a substantial savings could be realized from implementing the flexible production strategy, with the percentage of savings determined by operational, demographic, and local regulatory factors.[22]

System Status Management. Since buildings are stationary and fires are rare, fixed-post locations make sense when deploying fire suppression. In contrast, temporal and geographic patterns of demand for

TABLE 12.3
ALS/BLS Systems Study Participants

SYSTEM	
Albuquerque	Oklahoma City
Arlington	Pinellas County
Fort Wayne	Reno
Fort Worth	Richmond
Kansas City	Syracuse
Las Vegas	Tulsa
Little Rock	

EMS vary widely, based on the movements of people and their changing patterns of activity. To meet that demand, high-performance systems have developed a technique that allows for the movement of ambulances in anticipation of where that ambulance will be needed next. The technique is System Status Management (SSM).

System Status Management is defined as "the art and science of matching the production capacity of an EMS system to the changing patterns of demand placed on that system."

Like all elements of the HPEMS system, SSM is protocol-driven. The rationale behind SSM is twofold. First, SSM must ensure the timely transport of both emergency and non-emergency patients. Second, SSM must *manage* the deployment and redeployment of resources to provide the coverage that meets emergency response-time performance requirements and non-emergency response-time expectations.

The foundation of SSM is the development and application of a System Status Plan (SSP). The SSP is an algorithm, or on-line protocol, for the deployment and redeployment of the system's unit hours. The SSP is developed from a report called a demand analysis, which is a statistical chart showing the historical call volume for each hour of the day and day of the week. To be effective and take into account unusual fluctuations, the demand analysis incorporates as many weeks as possible, but the minimum needed to ensure accuracy is 20 weeks.

The SSP must also consider the geography of the area and any specific geographical barriers. Rivers can be a specific problem, as can large city parks or other uninhabited regions of the primary service area. Time of day can also create a geographical problem, as population shifts away from a downtown area and toward the suburbs at night and back again in the morning. For this reason, those involved with SSM look on the SSP as being built on a continuum, balancing the temporal demand with the geographic demand of the EMS system.

Patterns of demand for EMS more closely resemble those for law enforcement than fire suppression. As a result, for the same reason urban police departments do not use 24-hour shifts, high-performance ambulance services in urban areas use few if any 24-hour shifts. Rather, HPEMS systems use peak-load staffing, comprised of shift schedules and staffing plans that match production with demand. Shifts can be 8, 10, 12, and even 16 hours in length. However, the needs of the crews must always be considered, and work loads distributed equally. The alternative to System Status Management is System Status Mismanagement, and the result will be detrimental to the system. To ensure the success of SSM, the following must be balanced:

- Concern for adequate coverage of high volume areas and peak-load periods
- Concern for adequate coverage of low volume areas and off-peak periods
- Concern for employee health, safety, skill, and job satisfaction
- Concern for economic efficiency and financial stability.

Summary

EMS has evolved into an integral part of the healthcare continuum in a relatively short period of time. As a result, the priorities and expectations of the patient, the public, local government officials, and the medical community are diverse, complex, and often, competing. Effective EMS system design provides those involved with the EMS system the essential measures and tools to be effective in this rapidly changing environment. High-performance EMS systems have the ability and flexibility to provide high levels of care and simultaneously be economically efficient. They are EMS systems designed from the patient's perspective.

The most complex element in EMS system design is the ambulance service. In choosing an ambulance service provider, a jurisdiction can select from one or two local government agencies and local and national private firms throughout the United States, several with excellent track records serving their own or other communities. The rational choice is the best-qualified organization willing to take the risk and take on the task. If that organization's credentials and track record clearly demonstrate an ability to generate the required clinical and response-time performance from the financial resources available, then whether that organization is a government agency or a private firm is not important. It is the commitment to perform and to be accountable that is tantamount because, in the end, that commitment is to service—service to the patient and to the community.

References

1. Committee on Trauma and Committee on Shock: *Accidental death and disability: the neglected disease of modern society*, Sep 1966, Washington DC, Fifth printing by the Commission on Emergency Medical Services, Jan 1970, American Medical Association.
2. *EMS System Act of 1973*, Public Law 93-154, Washington DC, 1973.
3. Cummins, RO, Ornato, JO, Theis, WH, Pepe, PE. Improving survival from sudden cardiac arrest: the "chain of survival" concept. *Circulation*. 1991;83:1832–1847.
4. Sanders, AB. Care of the elderly in emergency departments: where do we stand? *Ann Emerg Med*. 1992;21:792–795.
5. Meador, SA. Age-related utilization of advanced life support services. *Prehospital and Disaster Med*. 1991;6:9–14.
6. Strange, GR, Chen, EH, Sanders, AB. Use of emergency departments by elderly patients: projections from a multicenter data base. *Ann Emerg Med*. 1992;21:819–824.
7. Heyman, FW. *Sirens Are a Warning Sound*, Fort Wayne, IN: Three Rivers Ambulance Authority; 1985.
8. *EMS Agenda for the Future*. Washington DC: Department of Transportation, National Highway Traffic Safety Administration; 1996.
9. Wilson, B, Gratton, MC, Overton, J, Watson, WA. Unexpected ALS procedures on non-emergency calls: the value of a single-tier system. *Prehospital and Disaster Med*. 1992;7:380–392.
10. Ornato, JP, Racht, EM, Fitch, JJ, Berry, JF. The need for ALS in urban and suburban EMS systems. *Ann Emerg Med*. 1990;19:1469–1470.
11. *Contracting Guide for Ambulance Services*. Sacramento, CA: American Ambulance Association; 1994.
12. Braun, O, McCallion, R, Fazackerley, J. Characteristics of midsized urban EMS systems. *Ann Emerg Med*. 1990;19:536–546.
13. Eisenberg, MS, Horwood, BT, Cummins, RO, Reynolds-Haertle, R, Hearne, T. Cardiac arrest and resuscitation: a tale of 29 cities. *Ann Emerg Med*. 1990;19:179–186.
14. American Heart Association. *1998 Heart and Stroke Statistical Update*. Dallas, TX: American Heart Association; 1997.
15. Eisenberg, MS, Copass, MK, Hallstrom, A, Cobb, LA, Bergner, L. Management of out-of-hospital cardiac arrest: failure of basic emergency medical technician services. *JAMA*. 1980;243:1049–1051.

16. Eisenberg, MS, Bergner, L, Hallstrom, A. Out-of-hospital cardiac arrest: improved survival with paramedic services. *Lancet*. 1980;812–815.

17. Eisenberg, MS, Hallstrom, A, Copass, MK, Bergner, L, Short, F, Pierce, J. Treatment of ventricular fibrillation. *JAMA*. 1984;251:1723–1726.

18. Cummins, RO, Chamberlain DA, Abramson, NS, et al. Recommended guidelines for uniform reporting of data from out-of-hospital cardiac arrest: the Utstein style. *Ann Emerg Med*. 1991;20:861–874.

19. Stout, JL. System status management. *JEMS*. 1983;8:22–32.

20. Overton, J. *Market Study 2000*. Richmond, VA: National Association of Public Utility Models; 2000.

21. City Auditor. *Audit Report of First Responder Program (Audit Report Number 99-02)*. Richmond, VA: City of Richmond; 1998.

22. Overton, J. *ALS and BLS: A Cost Effectiveness Study*. Presentation to the National Association of EMS Physicians, Fort Myers, Florida, January 2000.

Funding

Robert A. Swor, DO

Introduction

Most citizens, politicians, and physicians would agree that the provision of out-of-hospital emergency care is, like police and fire protection, a basic service that must be provided to their communities. Very few, however, would agree on how this service should be provided, and even fewer would agree as to how it should be funded. In this section we will review the methods used to fund EMS systems in the past, and catalog some of the current funding methods. Development of adequate ongoing funding for EMS systems will be a crucial issue to all EMS systems in the future.

Initial EMS Funding

Prior to the development of organized EMS systems, the delivery of out-of-hospital care was fragmented. Perhaps the single largest providers of emergency care were funeral home operators, who owned vehicles that could transport a patient on a gurney. With the publication of "Accidental Death and Disability: The Neglected Disease of Modern Society," federal funding for emergency care in the streets started to become a priority.[1] Initial funds through the Department of Transportation were provided by Public Law 89-564, The Highway Safety Act of 1966, which funded EMS services through matching grant provisions to states. Funding was made available for EMS components such as ambulances, communications, personnel, and others (Section 402), and for special demonstration projects and studies (section 403). This program served as a catalyst for initiating EMS systems and developing public support. It did not, except for a few cases, stimulate development of organized EMS systems. These funds continue to flow to states for the provision of EMS training.

As interest in emergency care increased, it became apparent that medical, pediatric, and other sub-specialty patients would also benefit from a regionalized approach to emergency care. To that end, Congress approved federal funds in 1972 for so called "EMS demonstration projects" in five regions. The objective of this funding was to show that comprehensive EMS services could be supplied throughout a region.[2] The Robert Wood Johnson Foundation also became active in funding EMS demonstration projects. It funded projects on EMS response systems through a well publicized emergency medical telephone number, distributing grant monies to 33 regions from the period 1972–1977. A myriad of other federal projects also existed at this time, supplying monies for training, disaster preparedness, communications, and the like.

Emergency Medical Service Systems Act of 1973

The Emergency Medical Service Systems (EMSS) Act of 1973 became the first comprehensive federal approach to supporting regional development of EMS systems. This act enumerated 15 mandatory components needed in an EMS system and served as a template for program planners. The act was designed to promote development of systems that were able "to meet the individual characteristics of each community."[2] Funding was for a total of $185 million over three years and was granted to regional "lead agencies" which would direct disbursement of funds. Each region would have an average population of 700,000. Some 303 regions were initially created, although not all received funding each year. Funding was disbursed in two-year increments for:

Section 1202 Feasibility Studies and Planning
Section 1203 Initial Operations
Section 1204 Expansion and Improvement
Section 1205 Research

The level of funding expected to be needed by each lead agency for development of a successful and viable program was $1.5 to 1.75 million (1974 dollars). Funding was apportioned so that 25% of all monies went to rural areas. On a per-capita basis, regions received $1 for urban areas, $3.50 for rural areas, and $10 for wilderness areas to address the unique complexities of EMS care provision in less densely populated regions. The act was amended in 1976 and again in 1979, to take the program from its inception in 1974 until its termination in 1981. Emphasis was placed on securing other sources of funding so that services would continue when federal funding ceased.

This act also made available, for the first time, monies for emergency medicine residencies. Although in the history of the act no residency ever actually received funds for resident education, the carrot was sufficient to stimulate the development of emergency medicine resident training programs. The provision of funding for system development stimulated the parallel development of emergency physician, nursing, and trauma services, and resulted to a large degree in the EMS systems as we know them today.

The chief failure of the act was its inability to adequately stimulate local initiatives to fund EMS. When the "feds" went out of the EMS business, the sophisticated infrastructure that a number of EMS systems had, also died.

Preventative Health Block Grants

Federal funding for EMS systems was cut back dramatically with the introduction of Federal Block Grant programs (Omnibus Budget Reconciliation Act of 1981) by the Reagan administration.[2] This legislation folded Health and Human Service funds into seven blocks, with EMS funding folded into preventive health (PHHS) block grants. Programs now included with EMS funding were Hypertension Control, Rodent Control, Rape Prevention and Crisis Services, Fluoridation, Home Health Service, and Health Education. How these funds are dispersed was left to the discretion of state authorities. Funds were not to be used for costs of operation and purchase of equipment.[2]

The purpose of this legislation was to shift responsibility of funding EMS services to the states, while still funding lead agencies to direct EMS services.

The result of this policy shift was a significant decrease in total funding to EMS during the period 1981–1983 as documented by a General Accounting Office survey.[3] In the same survey of six states (California, Florida, Iowa, Massachusetts, Pennsylvania, and Texas), funding decreased 34% from 1981 to 1983, but was increased 28% during the following three-year period (1983–1985) by the states. It appeared that the concept of shifting funding to the states was successful (see below).[3] The result of this funding shift, however, was that EMS communities had to compete with the other constituencies served by the above programs for funding. In an area where EMS was not felt to be a priority, or the EMS community was not active in garnering support, funding suffered significantly. Since the inception of this block grant program there have been no new federal funds earmarked specifically for EMS funding.

Revenue Sources for EMS

Federal

Although federal funding of EMS systems has declined since the expiration of the EMSS Act, most states still receive significant federal funding. In one survey 35 states receive PHHS funds which are utilized for the provision of different aspects of emergency medical services. Another 25 receive funding through Department of Transportation Highway Safety Funds.[4] Most commonly, these funds are provided through Section 402 of the Highway Safety Act, and flow to the State Office of Highway Safety Planning.[4] In keeping with the intent of the PHHS act, funds are disbursed to the office of highway safety planning, which may use these funds for statewide administration of EMS or distribute them to local agencies for their use.

A wide variety of federal agencies are involved in EMS and disaster programs (discussed more fully elsewhere), which support state and local program operations and development. The most visible is that of the EMS division of the National Highway Traffic Safety Administration (NHTSA), a section of the Department of Transportation. NHTSA involvement in EMS stems from its role in assuring highway safety for citizens. Its predominant role is one of developing educational curricula for different levels of EMS providers, yet it also has served an important function in supporting EMS system evaluation (through its technical assessment program) and through funding of visionary projects such as the EMS Agenda For the

Future.[5] No EMS division funds flow to state or local EMS offices.

Periodically, state and local EMS programs are able to receive federal funds for specific programs. The most common of these are Emergency Medical Services for Children (EMS-C) funds, which are administered through the Maternal Child Health Bureau of the Health Resources and Services Administration (HRSA) of the Department of Health and Human Services. EMS-C was founded in 1984 with a mission to reduce child and youth disability and death due to severe illness or injury. Its goals are to ensure that state-of-the-art emergency medical care is available for all ill or injured children and adolescents; that pediatric services are well integrated into an emergency medical services (EMS) system; and that the entire spectrum of emergency services, including primary prevention of illness and injury, acute care, and rehabilitation, are provided to children and adolescents.[6] By EMS standards, EMS-C is a well funded program, with $15 million allocated for FY 1999 alone. EMS-C funds a myriad of EMS programs annually, with a philosophy that those programs that benefit all of EMS tend to benefit children as well. For that reason the EMS-C program has been an important source of support for EMS development.

Federal support for EMS system development was also provided by the Trauma System Planning and Development Act, which created a trauma program under HRSA from 1994 to 1998. While the amount of funding for this program was relatively small ($4 million annually), it did serve to stimulate trauma system assessment and development in a number of states.[7] The trauma system model supported by HRSA identified that trauma systems were an important component of comprehensive EMS systems. There has been no sustained federal funding for trauma system development, although an appropriation was made for a trauma office through HRSA in FY 2001.

A number of other federal agencies, such as the Federal Emergency Management Agency, the U.S. Fire Administration, branches of the armed services, and others, support vital EMS and disaster functions throughout the country. They do not, however, provide funds for direct support of EMS systems.

State

State support of EMS funding has become crucial for the continued viability of EMS systems. States sur-

veyed by the General Accounting Office in 1985 showed a 50% increase in EMS expenditures from the period 1981–85.[3] Methods of funding vary substantially from state to state. The most common is state general funds, with an annual allocation to support the state EMS office. In an annual survey of state EMS directors, a number of different categories of funding mechanisms were identified: ad valorem tax districts; fees for vehicle registration/driver's licenses, traffic violations, EMS service/vehicles, and civil penalties; excise taxes; tobacco taxes; and others (see table 13.1). The most common of these, ad valorem tax districts, provides legislation that allows local communities to tax themselves to organize EMS services. The fees typically range from 1 to 3 mills.[8] These funds may be used at the state level or redistributed to local regulatory or provider agencies. Utilization of funds is similarly variable, with funding disbursed for training, equipment, communications, operations, or administration. Virginia returns 25% of funds collected to the county in which a vehicle is registered. Some states also allocate special funds for unique EMS needs; California allocates $754,000 to high tourist impact areas, for instance. Level of funding by states is extremely variable, with states spend-

TABLE 13.1
State Methods of EMS Funding

Revenue From Vehicle or Driver Licensing
Virginia, New Mexico, Idaho, Colorado, Florida

Revenue from Motor Vehicle Violations
Florida—$5 per violation, $25 for Driving While Intoxicated
Arizona—$2.3 million from Driving while Intoxicated fines and other moving violations
Rhode Island—$1 surcharge per violation
Utah—$3 fee on fines or bail forfeiture
Mississippi—$5 fee per violation, $5 for bail forfeiture
Minnesota—$10 for failure to wear seatbelt
Indiana—Drunk Drivers pay uncollectable EMS fees for Motor vehicle accidents in which they're involved

EMS Service/Vehicle License Fees
Florida, Maine, Massachusetts, New Mexico, Oklahoma

Tax Districts
Alaska, Florida, Iowa, Kentucky, Mississippi, Missouri, New York, North Carolina, North Dakota, Oklahoma, South Dakota, Texas, Utah, Wyoming

*Adapted from Kleinholz[8]

ing per capita as much as $1.20 (Alaska) or as little as 3 cents (California).[4]

The state of Maryland is a unique example for its support of EMS and the creation of an integrated statewide EMS system. Initiated in 1973 by executive order of its governor, this system provided for: training of EMS personnel, nurses and physicians; development of a statewide helicopter emergency transport system; tertiary care centers for specialized medical conditions, most notably trauma care; and research facilities. A statewide 9-1-1 system has been developed as part of this system The system enjoys an enviable amount of support from the state general fund.[9]

Local

To this point, the chapter has discussed how State and Federal EMS systems' administrative elements have been put into place and are sustained. Far more relevant to patients, however, is how local EMS systems are financed so that they may be available for provision of emergency care. Local EMS funding sources are as varied as the number of EMS systems. System models are discussed elsewhere in this text, but fall into the general categories of private, public, volunteer, or some combination of these. Large urban areas are generally serviced by municipal EMS services, based in either the fire department or an autonomous division within the municipal government (third service). Suburban systems, because they are comprised of multiple smaller municipalities, may either be public or private or a blend of both. Rural systems, because of small run volumes and high fixed cost associated with EMS service implementation, are most commonly volunteer or paid on-call systems. Sources of revenue include tax subsidies, patient revenues, service charges, or subscriptions. Municipal systems tend to be supported by tax-generated revenue out of general funds of the municipality, with funds augmented through billings for service. Many communities have special assessments for EMS services. Some communities wish to minimize out-of-pocket expense for EMS services, and either have contracts or agreements (with or without a local subsidy) to provide for EMS service for their citizens. The vast majority of these continue to provide (and pay for) fire department-based first responders, which provide emergency care as a public service.

In addition to traditional sources of EMS revenue, fund-raising activities by communities play an important role in EMS system funding. Volunteer services, in particular, receive fund-raising support by local service organizations (Kiwanis, Lions Club, and many more). These organizations will frequently raise funds for specific capital equipment needs or desires (e.g., new ambulances, defibrillators, 12-lead EKG machines, etc). In addition to providing financial support for programs, fund raisers are an invaluable means of creating community awareness and support for the EMS system.

It should be noted that some systems are supported by operating revenues of hospitals and are managed as a separate division of the hospital corporation.

Public Utility Models

In an effort to develop cost-effective EMS services that are accountable to the public, a number of systems (Pinellas County, FL, Tulsa, OK, Oklahoma City, OK, Fort Wayne, IN) have evolved under a so-called "Public Utility Model" (PUM) or "High Performance System," a quasi-governmental system that utilizes a governmental oversight body and a private contractor to supply EMS services area-wide. A governmental ambulance authority is established that procures equipment, manages administrative expenses, handles all billings, and contracts for provision of services with a single ambulance provider. The ambulance provider manages all aspects of the delivery of EMS services in accordance with standards established by the medical control board. Unique features of this model include the provision of all ALS care and single-provider provision of all emergency and non-emergency transportation (which defrays the cost of emergency care). Another unique provision of this system is a franchise fee (typically $2–$5 per transport) charged to fund oversight of medical issues by the medical control boards.[10]

Although PUM models and variations on this model have been implemented in a number of communities as cost-effective systems, they have come under attack by municipal providers, predominately in the fire service, who advocate that the marginal cost of upgrading an existing fire service to provide all EMS care is a far more economically efficient method of service provision.[11] They also argue that the third-party reimbursement is an attractive means by which cities may leverage the costs of their fire services. The economics of this analysis are daunting and without a clear resolution. Decisions made regarding this issue ultimately are not based on economics.

Reimbursement

A fundamental philosophical question that impacts EMS system funding, and will impact it even more in the future, is whether EMS service provision is a public safety service, emergency medical care, or both. This issue begs the question as to whether third-party payers should be responsible for EMS service payment or whether it should be supported by local governmental funding, or both. In reality this issue depends less on philosophy and more on the affluence of the community. In many large poor urban communities the issue is moot. In one survey, reimbursement for ambulance services varied from 19% (Baltimore, MD) to 80% (Provo, UT).[11] At this lower end, the level of reimbursement generated may not even recover the cost of billing. Whether third-party reimbursement is able to cover the cost of service varies tremendously, based on the service demands on, and operating efficiency of, the service provider.

Third-Party Reimbursement

Regardless of whether EMS service is provided by public or private provider, reimbursement of services by insurers is crucial for the ongoing viability of the EMS system. Traditionally these services have only been reimbursed for transport of a patient to a hospital facility. A wide variety of insurers pay for ambulance services, and the list mirrors those of insurers for other types of healthcare coverage (one author quotes a list of 1,200 providers).[12] Payment may be for advanced or basic life support, and varies based on the service provided, not the level of responder that provides care. A major determinant of whether reimbursement is paid for transport is medical necessity. Definition of this medical necessity is extremely variable and a source of great frustration to EMS service providers.

Generally, ambulance services may charge for a variety of expenses including those related to: dispatch services, level of response (BLS or ALS and emergency or non-emergency), equipment utilized, medication and fluid administration, and distances traveled. Bills for service may include a single charge to reflect all services or may be itemized for each service provided. As ambulance transport disproportionately is supplied to the elderly, Medicare (Part B) pay-

ments are the largest single source of revenue for emergency providers. Other common sources of payment are state Medicaid programs, Blue Cross/Blue Shield, auto insurance plans for motor vehicle accidents, and an increasing number of Health Maintenance Organizations (HMOs) or Preferred Provider Organizations (PPOs). Historically, levels of reimbursement also vary based on the geographic region, as a result of the differences in costs to provide service. Some EMS experts have identified up to a fivefold difference in rate of payment for similar services across the country.[13]

During the late 1990s, billings for ambulance services to the Health Care Financing Administration (HCFA) which administered the Medicare program and is now called Center for Medicare and Medicaid Services (CMS), were identified as being one of the sectors of health care that had the greatest rate of increase. The reasons for this dramatic increase may have been been related to a number of factors, including the initiation of billing by volunteer services, the increasing number of EMS providers by expansion of the Fire Service, the aging of the population, and some alleged increasing ambulance billing fraud. Whatever the reasons, HCFA was given a mandate by the Balanced Budget Act of 1997 to revise ambulance reimbursement without increasing total Medicare costs.[13] As of this writing, the CMS has developed, through a complex negotiated rulemaking process, new regulations for ambulance reimbursement. These revisions will result in substantial changes in reimbursement to EMS organizations. Some agencies will suffer substantial decreases in payment compared to historical levels, which may impact the provision of emergency services to their communities. Other agencies, because of regional changes in CMS billing, may profit from these changes. At this time it is unclear exactly what impact the fee schedule will have on EMS services nationally. It does appear clear that funding for Medicare will not increase in the future at a level necessary to keep pace with the aging of the population and the corresponding increased need for EMS services. One possible scenario is that a greater portion of the cost of EMS services will be shifted to local communities. Depending on whether EMS services are provided by private services, some communities may be faced with the loss of their present services. The EMS community will need to be politically aggressive to garner legislative and financial support for EMS reimbursement if these trends are to be addressed.

Subscription Services

A common means of funding for many systems is to have so-called subscription services. The populace is offered the option of subscribing for EMS care, and pays an annual fee. Those who elected to subscribe receive EMS services without charge for that year. Others are charged on a fee-for-service basis. Results of fundraising on a local level can be quite variable. Use of professional fundraisers can increase the yield, but upfront costs can be very high.

Cost Effectiveness

Since their inception EMS systems and their costs have been under scrutiny, with the essential question being whether the costs of EMS services are justified.[14,15,16] While the answer to this question seems self-evident to all emergency care professionals, every aspect of medical care is being subjected to economic scrutiny. Answers to this question are complex and have been addressed in a number of venues. EMS outcomes are a subject of a major NHTSA-funded project, with a focus on defining potential measures of EMS effectiveness. These measures have been defined by Maio and others, and include measures of: death, disability, discomfort, destitution, and dissatisfaction. Under this model, cost savings and pain control, as well as decreasing morbidity and mortality, may be appropriate measures of EMS benefits.[17] Some work has been focused on cost-effectiveness of EMS services using cardiac arrest survival as a measure. Valenzuela calculated the cost/life saved and cost/year of life saved when implementing advanced life support services in Tucson, Arizona. He identified a cost/year of life saved as approximately $8,800 (1988 dollars), which compared favorably to treatment for other medical conditions such as heart or liver transplant, or chemotherapy for acute leukemia.[18] In another elegant work, Nichol estimated the cost per year of life saved for enhancements to an EMS system. He estimated the cost per quality adjusted life year (QALY) as $40,000 by adding additional AED-equipped vehicles to an existing EMS service.[19] In a subsequent work he estimated the cost/life saved of implementing a first response with AED-equipped police as $27,000/QALY.[20] These costs compare favorably with the costs of a variety of medical and non-medical interventions.[21]

Though cardiac arrest represents a small part of the value of EMS services, analyses and data such as these can be useful tools in a discussion of the value of EMS services.

Medical Oversight Funding

This issue is of vital importance to medical directors. Medical oversight requires a substantial degree of time, energy, expertise and organizational support. To perform the medical director's duties with the appropriate administrative structure requires adequate financial support. Many EMS medical directors receive a stipend for their time. Large communities either contract directly with the EMS medical director (EMSMD) or contract with the employer for time spent. Many big-city EMSMDs in the United States are university-based, but this is also variable. A few communities employ full-time EMS medical directors. Costs of medical oversight of systems are typically borne by governmental agencies in large areas (greater than 500,000 population) and by hospitals in less populated regions.[22] A survey in one relatively rural state (Colorado) identified that almost 75% of the medical directors served this function in a voluntary capacity.[23]

Public-utility model systems allocate a per-transport charge to provide for medical oversight. Third-party reimbursement occurs for on-line medical direction (Medicare has a billing code for on-line medical direction), but payment for it varies by the various CMA regions in the United States.

Summary

Funding of EMS systems is in peril. Changes in the mechanism for reimbursement at the federal level will have impacts on each system that are difficult to discern. However, it is clear that reimbursement for services provided will probably not cover the cost of EMS care provision for communities. This cost shifting will require local community subsidies to maintain the viability of the system. The EMS community will need to be more politically active to advocate for adequate levels for EMS reimbursement.

Resources available to support emergency medical systems will doubtlessly continue to change, and medical directors need to be cognizant of the issues. Reimbursement issues clearly impact EMS patient care; federal and state EMS funding often support program oversight, technical assistance, regulatory activities, and new approaches to EMS care, but will not fund local EMS provision.

References

1. *Accidental Death and Disability: The Neglected Disease of Modern Society.* Washington, DC: Division of Medical Sciences, National Academy of Sciences-National Research Council; Sept 1966.
2. Boyd DR. The History of Emergency Medical Services Systems in the United States of America. In: Boyd DR, Edlich RF, Micik S. *Systems Approach to Emergency Medical Care.* Norwalk, VA: Appleton-Century-Croft; 1983.
3. Report Assesses Leadership of States in Providing EMS Using Federal Grants. *EMS Communicator* 1986;13 (6):1–4.
4. State Survey, *Emergency Medical Services;* 2000. http://www.emsmagazine.com, 2001.
5. Snyder JA, Baren JM, Ryan SD, Chew JL, Seidel JS. Emergency medical service system development: results of the statewide emergency medical service Technical Assessment Program. *Ann Emerg Med.* 1995;25(6):768–775.
6. *Emergency Medical Services for Children—Program Information.* http://www.ems-c.org, 2001.
7. Bass RR, Gainer PS, Carlini AR. Update on trauma system development in the United States. *J Trauma.* 1999; 47(3 Suppl):S15–21.
8. Kleinholz SB, Doeksen GA. *State Legislation for Funding of Rural Emergency Medical Services.* Southern Rural Development Health Task Force; March 1991.
9. *Annual Report.* Maryland Institute for Emergency Medical Services Systems; 1986–1987.
10. Stout JL. System financing. In: Rousch WR, ed. *Principles of EMS Systems: A Comprehensive Text For Physicians.* Dallas: American College of Emergency Physicians; 1989.
11. *Revenue Recovery: Emergency Medical Services* [monograph]. Washington: IAFF; 1997.
12. Third party reimbursements—medicare, medicaid and other players. In: Fitch JJ, Keller R, Raynor D, Zalar C. *Beyond the Street.* Solana Beach, CA: Jems Publishing; 1988.
13. Overton J. Reimbursement in EMS. Presented at the Turtle Creek Conference, Dallas, 2001.
14. Urban N, Bergner L, Eisengerg MS. The costs of a suburban paramedic program in reducing deaths due to cardiac arrest. *Medical Care.* 1981;19(4):379–392.
15. Cretin S. Cost-benefit analysis of treatment and prevention of myocardial infarction. *Health Serv Res.* 1977;12 (3):174–189.
16. Hallstrom A, Eisenberg MS, Bergner L. Modeling the effectiveness and cost-effectiveness of an emergency service system. *Soc Sci Med.* 1981;15C:13–17.
17. Maio RF, Garrison HG, Spaite DW, et al. Emergency medical services outcomes project I (EMSOP I): prioritizing conditions for outcomes research. *Ann Emerg Med.* 1999;33(4):423–432.
18. Valenzuela TD, Criss EA, Spaite D, et al. Cost effectiveness of paramedic emergency medical services in the treatment of prehospital cardiopulmonary arrest. *Ann Emerg Med.* 1990;19(12):1407–1411.
19. Nichol G, Hallstrom AP, Ornato JP, et al. Potential cost-effectiveness of public access defibrillation in the United States. *Circulation.* 1998;97:1315–20.
20. Nichol G, Hallstrom AP, Ornato JP, Riegel B, Stiell IG, Valenzuela T, Wells GA. Potential cost-effectiveness of public access defibrillation in the United States. *Circulation.* 1998;97(13):1315–17.
21. Tengs TO, Adams ME, Pliskin JS, Safran DG, Siegel JE, Weinstein MC, Graham JD. Five-hundred life-saving interventions and their cost-effectiveness. *Risk Analysis.* 1995;(15)3,369–390.
22. Swor RA, Krome RL. Administrative support for EMS medical directors: a profile. *Prehosp Disaster Med.* 1990; 5(1):25–30.
23. Hall WL. Medical direction of prehospital personnel in Colorado. *Prehosp Emerg Care.* 2001;5(1):122.

CHAPTER 14

Reimbursement Trends

Jerry Overton, MPA

Introduction

The evolving Medicare fee schedule for medically necessary ambulance transportation has have a profound impact on emergency medical services (EMS) systems throughout the country. As the new Medicare rules are implemented, reimbursement for Medicare patients will be based largely on national relative value units that vary depending on the level of service provided, from basic life support to advanced life support emergency. Under the new fee schedule, nearly all EMS systems will lose money when compared with the actual cost of providing the service, particularly advanced life support services (ALS), rural services, efficient systems, and those that bill for services. The nonspecific term "ALS" in the federal rules on reimbursement prolongs the confusion caused when that term is used as a descriptor. To adapt to these impending changes, EMS administrators and medical directors must work together to diversify and solidify their revenue sources and to seek out ways to make their systems even more efficient, while maintaining a high quality of clinical care.

When patients are injured or sick and require the services of emergency medical personnel, they give little thought as to how the providers will be compensated for their care. However, reimbursement is a topic of considerable importance to EMS administrators and medical directors, who must cope with a complex and seemingly constantly changing reimbursement environment while ensuring that patient clinical needs are met.

Emergency medical services systems receive revenue from tax subsidization, third-party reimbursement, patient payment, or a combination. The sources of reimbursement for EMS are finite and include Medicaid, Medicare, private-paying patients, commercial insurance, and (in some systems), contracts with managed care or other payers. In systems responsible for responding to 9-1-1 emergencies, patient demographics create an environment in which Medicaid and Medicare typically make up the bulk of reimbursement. Medicaid is a federally authorized program that provides healthcare coverage for indigent and special-case patients. Although authorized by the federal government, Medicaid is administered by the individual states, and the states determine specific eligibility and reimbursement rates. Medicare is a federally authorized, regulated, and funded program that provides healthcare coverage for persons aged 65 and older. The program is administered by Medicare carriers, with individual carriers setting the reimbursement rates based on historical charges. Because there is no nationwide Medicare reimbursement rate, the rates vary from state to state and even within the same state.

Poised to have the greatest impact on EMS reimbursement is the proposed Medicare fee schedule for EMS transports, which is examined in detail here. This new fee schedule is, in part, the result of the rapid increase in Medicare expenditures for basic and advanced life support that has occurred over the past fifteen years or so. Another catalyst for changing Medicare fees was a series of Government Accounting Office reports on the potential for fraud and abuse in EMS and private ambulance systems, focusing on the use of ambulance transportation for nonmedically necessary, non-emergency cases. A third reason for changing the Medicare fee schedule is the lack of uniformity among Medicare carriers in program administration and reimbursement rates. Finally, for many years, ambulance transportation was the only service not on a Medicare fee schedule; it was being reimbursed at fee-for-service rates, which varied widely across the country. To get rising EMS Medicare costs under control, the federal government saw a need for changes in the system.

The Evolving Medicare Fee Schedule

The evolving Medicare fee schedule being implemented can be traced back to proposed federal regulations issued in 1996. These regulations proposed basing reimbursement for EMS on the patient's condition at the hospital. No consideration would be given to the patient's actual condition at the scene; the Medicare rules would predetermine whether the patient would be classified as basic life support or advanced life support. An appendix to these rules listed specific patient conditions, and assigned a level of service. The regulations also required physician certification statements for non-emergency transports. Needless to say, EMS providers actively fought these regulations, which would have had a devastating effect on EMS systems, and implementation was postponed.

A year later, as a part of the Balanced Budget Act of 1997, Congress succeeded in placing ambulance transportation services on a fee schedule. Legislators also mandated assignment for EMS, meaning that EMS systems must accept whatever the Medicare carrier pays for the services provided as their full payment. Also, with one exception, EMS systems would not be paid for their services unless they transported the patient. The only exception would be for services rendered to patients pronounced dead on scene after the arrival of EMS. The scheduled implementation date for these new rules was initially January 1, 2000, but was later extended to January 1, 2002.

In response to the publication of the new rules, the Center for Medicare and Medicaid Services (CMS), formerly the Health Care Financing Administration, which oversees the Medicare program, received the largest number of adverse comments in its history for any proposed rule. If the legislation had been implemented as written, a considerable number of both public and private EMS systems would have collapsed almost immediately. Given this outcry, the proposed Medicare fee schedule has still not been implemented.

In the new Medicare fee schedule, reimbursement rates are based on national relative value units (RVUs), which vary depending on the level of service provided, from basic life support (RVU = 1.00) to advanced life support level 2 (RVU = 2.75). Emergency medical services reimbursement is based on the RVU plus a regional cost index plus a national conversion factor plus mileage. The regional cost index is 70% of the base rate and the national conversion factor is currently proposed at $157, adjusted annually for inflation. As of December 2001 the actual reimbursement for ambulance transport under the Medicare fee schedule is shown in table 14.1. With mandatory assignment as part of the rule, EMS systems have no choice but to accept the proposed fees.

Additional aspects of the new Medicare fee schedule, which will be phased in over four years, include mileage reimbursement set as a national rate, with an added fee adjustment for rural services. Another section of the rule determines payment based on the patient condition at the scene, but the proposal does not address how the patient condition is to be coded. Reimbursement will be prorated for multiple patient transports. Missing from the proposal is any phase-in for ALS systems from their current payment for responding to all requests for service with an ALS vehicle, regardless of the patient condition.

As implemented, likely there will be more losers than winners under the Medicare fee schedule. The more heavily subsidized systems are likely to be winners, while those that depend largely on fee-for-service are likely to be losers. Emergency medical services systems in Tennessee, North Carolina, and Rhode Island will be more highly reimbursed than they are now. The greatest negative impact will be on any systems that bill for services, ALS systems, rural systems, and highly efficient unsubsidized systems.

The large number of losers is primarily due to the high percentage of Medicare patients served by EMS. In a typical system, 40% of billings are for Medicare patients, 20% for Medicaid, 25% for private pay, and 15% for commercial insurance or managed care. However, EMS providers, like other healthcare providers, have been cost shifting to make up for patients who cannot or do not pay. Thus, in a typical system, 55% of revenues comes from Medicare patients, 15% from Medicaid, 5% from private pay, and 25% from commercial insurance or managed care. The dependence on reimbursement from Medicare is likely only to grow. In 1990, persons aged 65 or older com-

TABLE 14.1	
Reimbursement Rates for Ambulance Transport Under the Proposed Medicare Fee Schedule, Adjusted for Inflation	
BLS	$163.51
BLS (emergency)	$262.61
ALS-1	$196.21
ALS-1 (emergency)	$310.66
ALS-2	$449.65

prised 12% of the population in the United States, and accounted for 36% of ambulance transports and 43% of emergency department admissions. Older persons also are 4.4 times more likely than the general population to use EMS. The elderly are currently the fastest growing segment of the population, which means systems can anticipate a greatly increasing demand for their services.

The financial impact of the new Medicare fee schedule has not been fully examined. To compare the new Medicare reimbursement with the actual cost of providing the transport, costs can be calculated by dividing utilization (U) by unit hours (UH) (the number of patients transported during a period divided by the unit hours produced during the same period). This calculation yields the productivity of the system. Further, dividing the cost per UH by productivity then yields the cost per transport, as shown in the following equation:

$$\text{Cost per UH} \div \text{Productivity (U/UH)}$$
$$= \text{Cost per Patient Transport}$$

This calculation provides the true cost of transporting the patient, not the revenue received per transport. For example, if the cost of placing a fully equipped ambulance on the street is $100 (cost per UH) and a patient is transported once every three hours (U/UH), the cost per transport is approximately $300 ($100 ÷ .33). If a patient is transported once every four hours, the cost per transport is $400 ($100 ÷ .25). Such calculations are crucial in revealing how few transports will be fully covered under the proposed Medicare fee schedule (table 14.1). Even the most efficient systems will find that Medicare reimbursement will not cover the actual cost of transporting a patient. When analyzed using this approach, the so-called winners under the new rules may also find that they are not fully reimbursed for their transport costs.

In Richmond, Virginia, first-year losses in the system under the Medicare fee schedule are estimated at $350,000 and will increase to a staggering $700,000 after four years. The difference between the actual costs of transport and Medicare reimbursement cannot be offset by reimbursement from other payers, including health maintenance organizations or commercial insurers. As an example, several third-party commercial payers have already notified ambulance services that they will be implementing the same payer codes and payment mechanisms.

Adapting to the New Rules

There are several options for systems as the Medicare fee schedule is implemented. One option that is **not** available is raising rates. With mandated assignment, rate increases will be meaningless, because systems will be required to accept whatever Medicare pays.

Additional Subsidization

For some systems, additional subsidization is an option. The Richmond Ambulance Authority predicts that, under the Medicare fee schedule, they will need a subsidy of about 29% of total revenues. This represents a 6% increase from the current level of 23%.

Service Alternatives

To stay afloat under the new Medicare rules, systems may need to explore various service alternatives. With personnel costs accounting for about 75% of the total unit hour in a system, administrators will be looking at ways to cut these costs, perhaps by staffing the ambulance with one paramedic and one emergency medical technician, rather than with two paramedics. Integrated transportation models that shift non-emergency patients to less costly modes of transportation or allow treatment of a patient at home are an option, but might not be feasible if providers are paid only if the patient is transported. Administrators are likely to focus on decreasing the number of non-emergency transports while increasing emergency response times; to save money, the increase in response time is likely to be considerable. However, deviating from a nationally recognized standard may be detrimental to patient care, jeopardizing the possibility of a positive outcome for a cardiac arrest patient. Deferring capital purchases is another cost-saving mechanism, but one that would force providers to work with older and less sophisticated equipment.

Improved Efficiencies

Changes in the systems, with an emphasis on functioning more economically, are also likely. Another option of systems under the proposed Medicare fee schedule is to improve efficiency, a goal that should be a joint effort of both administrators and medical directors. As described earlier, if the cost of placing an ambulance on the street is estimated at $100 and a patient is transported every four hours, the cost per transport is $400 ($100 ÷ .25). If a patient were transported every three hours and 52 minutes, the cost per transport would decrease to $370 ($100 ÷ .27). Although the $30 savings per transport might seem insignificant, when multiplied over a large number of patients, the savings accumulate. For example, based on 8000 patients transported per year, a system would save $240,000 annually.

Summary

When the new Medicare fee schedule will be totally implemented remains uncertain. In the meantime, organizations such as the American Ambulance Association and others continue their efforts to have CMS increase Medicare reimbursement rates. Efforts are also being made to obtain regulatory relief through the involvement of the Secretary of Health and Human Services and members of Congress.

Implementation of the proposed Medicare fee schedule has been delayed as many questions are resolved. Changes in Medicare rules can confuse EMS providers and Medicare carriers alike. One small Medicare change, applying to the inclusion of Zip codes, that went into effect in early 2001 ultimately resulted in nonpayment to EMS systems in at least ten states for more than six weeks while Medicare carriers made the appropriate electronic formatting change. Given this experience, a considerable concern is that carriers will be unable to effectively implement the new fee schedule.

Some of the recent initiatives taken by Congress indicate that the concerns of EMS systems are being heard. Members of Congress are beginning to recognize that at the proposed reimbursement rates, EMS systems will be unable to continue to afford to operate and provide quality care to patients, much less introduce any new technologies.

Over the coming months and years, EMS systems will be forced to change, as they adapt to a new Medicare fee schedule. As fee-for-service and subsidization become less assured sources of revenue, administrators will need to look for ways of diversifying and solidifying their revenue sources. Simultaneously, they must seek ways to increase efficiencies in their system. To survive in a changing environment, EMS systems need to take a proactive stance, rather that merely reacting to changes under way.

Medical Interventions

Kristi L. Koenig, MD
Angelo A. Salvucci, Jr., MD

Introduction

One of the fundamental issues all EMS systems must address is the development of medically appropriate patient-care protocols. The specific medical interventions utilized by EMS personnel are arguably the most important oversight role for the system medical director. Protocol development and oversight require a thorough understanding of local system design, resources, personnel, and medical convention as well as a knowledge of the medical literature.

Out-of-hospital advanced medical care was first provided by physicians in the 1960s in mobile cardiac care units. Paramedics, acting as physician extenders and operating under protocols, began to replace these physicians soon after, and the scope of advanced life support was expanded to include other than cardiac care. With the introduction of EMT-Bs, the distinction between basic and advanced providers has blurred. All types of responders require indirect medical oversight. The need for direct medical oversight varies among levels of providers and types of systems.

Progress in medical interventions and protocols has attempted to follow advances in medical knowledge. Yet the decision to add or eliminate a procedure has often been initiated by an anecdotal case and approved by cursory local review. As the body of knowledge in the specialty of EMS increases, decisions regarding interventions will be based more on a rigorous scientific process. External forces (healthcare financing reform, evidence-based medicine) and internal forces (increased physician oversight, outcome-oriented research) are driving the reexamination of EMS system design as well as specific medical interventions and protocols.

Protocols

Protocols are the laws by which the system runs. They specify the actions the system providers are to take, and normally encompass most aspects of both direct and indirect medical oversight. Protocols may also include rules for both administrative and clinical operations. Ideally, protocols will be developed to govern every situation that the provider might encounter, including clinical care given by direct medical oversight.

In defining protocols, whether establishing a new system or building on an existing one, one must first decide what, and then how, to treat. The medical director should consider the specific environment of the community and customize the protocols accordingly. For example, the average length and range of transport times would influence the type and extent of scene treatment. Furthermore, protocols must be tailored to the type of responders that exist in the system and to whether there is a tiered response. The level of responder who transports patients will also influence protocol structure. Finally, the medical director must be certain that the protocols do not require a level of care that exceeds the training or equipment capabilities of the providers or otherwise set standards that cannot reasonably be met.

Establishing a Treatment Philosophy

There are a number of basic philosophical issues that the medical director must resolve prior to choosing treatment modalities and designing specific protocols for their use. Many factors enter into the decision-making process, and include operational, financial, political, ethical, and legal concerns as well as the medical issues. The system must be tailored to meet local needs, and in doing so may differ from nationally accepted guidelines. The medical director must keep the overall system and the community of interest in mind.

Evidence-Based Decision Making

Implementing a decision-making process in system design has historically been quite difficult. Medical directors often assume oversight responsibilities of an existing system that has established practices in place. The perspectives of administrators, line personnel, fire chiefs, legislators, physicians, and hospitals can all be quite different, and because there has been no uniformity in the process, decisions have often been viewed as just "one doc's opinion."

Evidence-based medicine is an attempt to establish the critical review of clinical care research as a foundation on which to build clinical policy.[1] It has been defined as "the conscientious and judicious use of current best evidence from clinical care research in the management of individual patients."[2] As applied to EMS system design, there are three steps in the process. First, ascertain the current best evidence from existing literature. From this evidence, on a regional, state, or larger area basis, develop evidence-based clinical guidelines. Finally, use these guidelines to form specific local protocols.[3]

The medical director must consider the unique features of the local system, and even subsets of the system, in protocol development. For example, adding EMT automated defibrillation (EMT-D) capabilities to an EMS system will be effective only if: (1) all (or nearly all) first responders are trained as EMT-Ds; (2) EMT-D response times are short; and (3) the time interval between EMT-D arrival and paramedic arrival is relatively long.[4] Absent any of these, little survival benefit will be gained.[5] EMS systems that include both rural and urban areas, or areas with differing response times, will benefit from a detailed subsystem analysis before starting an EMT-D program.

EMS as a medical specialty has an advantage in this transition to evidence-based medicine because the majority of the practice is already protocol-driven. However, EMS is at a disadvantage in that the body of medical evidence, particularly the highest priority evidence, randomized controlled trials (RCTs), is very limited and not increasing very rapidly. In a review of publications referenced on MEDLINE between 1985 and 1995, there were 35 RCTs that examined out-of-hospital care.[6] Of those, virtually all found that new or standard interventions were no more effective than placebo, controls, or no intervention. Only one of these RCTs found that an intervention was effective or better than control (hypertonic saline was more effective than normal saline in

trauma).[7] A greater effort to publish this type of work is needed so that medical directors have sufficient material on which to base their decisions.

Standing Orders

Standing orders are those procedures that may be performed by out-of-hospital providers independent of direct medical oversight. Some systems operate entirely under standing orders with no requirement for provider contact with the direct medical oversight; others use no standing orders. The majority of systems have introduced some standing orders, after which voice communication may be established with the direct medical oversight.

Standing orders have the potential to improve the efficiency and quality of out-of-hospital care, although outcome studies have not yet been published. There is some evidence that standing orders result in closer adherence to the protocols.[8] A reduction in trauma scene times has not been shown.[9] Medical directors should consider using standing orders in those conditions which: (1) are time critical; (2) have little likelihood of clinically useful direct medical oversight orders; and/or (3) have been shown to be appropriately managed by field providers. Further research will better define the balance between direct medical control and standing orders.[10] If standing orders exist in a system, they should be included within the protocols, and their use closely monitored.

The medical director must be certain that all physicians providing direct medical oversight in the system know and understand the protocols. This director must determine if and how direct medical oversight is required, and under what circumstances the direct medical oversight should be allowed to override or exceed the existing protocols.[11,12] The permissiveness of the protocols is based upon the sophistication of the direct medical oversight as well as the philosophy of the system medical director. There are certainly some situations in which deviation from the protocols might provide for better patient outcomes. However, it is clearly undesirable and patently risky to allow the direct medical oversight to deviate routinely from the protocols. This practice would likely lead to inconsistent treatment and ultimately increased clinical errors. Rather than allowing the direct medical oversight to deviate independently from existing protocols, many medical directors have included optional sections in the protocols. In this way, uniformity can be maintained in educating the providers, while still allowing for individual physician clinical judgment. The system medical director has the ultimate responsibility for all aspects of both indirect and direct medical oversight.

Educational Requirements

Another basic consideration is the level of education that can be supported for the providers in the local system. If the medical director chooses to implement additional or more complex clinical protocols, will any additional education and cost be required? Furthermore, are there resources available to implement and continue this new training? For example, if after studying the clinical needs, allowable scope of practice, and the best medical evidence, the medical director wishes to add the skill of pediatric intraosseous infusion, a number of questions must be asked (table 15.1).

Personnel Safety

The safety of out-of-hospital personnel must remain paramount when designing protocols. Provider injury and illness prevention are necessary components of the system.[13] It may not be appropriate to ask the providers to perform certain procedures in unsafe areas or under difficult conditions. The decision of whether to send vehicles to and from the scene (HOT) or (COLD) (which is discussed later) is another example of taking provider safety into consideration.

Protection from violence is paramount. When the patients are victims of violent crimes, protocols in many urban settings specify waiting for police to secure the scene before initiating treatment. This protocol may increase response times and scene times, and may limit the performance of certain clinical procedures in the field, all of which must be understood in advance and carefully monitored. Restraints, both physical and chemical, are appropriate in many circumstances, for both provider and patient safety.[14] The indications and methods must be described in detail.

The use of naloxone is another example. The traditional administration of a 2-mg bolus to all patients with a suspected opioid overdose may precipitate violent behavior in some patients.[15] A slower titration to the clinical endpoint of an adequate respiratory rate may be more appropriate.

Exposure to infectious diseases is an increasing worry for all healthcare professionals. Considerable emphasis has been placed on the use of universal precautions. Although providers are generally aware of the importance of avoiding contact with blood and body fluids, compliance remains inconsistent.[16,17] Procedures that involve avoidable blood or body fluid exposure should be reexamined. For example, naloxone may be administered IM, or possibly submentally, rather than intralingually.[18,19] IV lines should be inserted only when necessary, preferably with self-capping catheters.[20] Protocols must also address other areas of job-related infections. For example, protection against airborne infections (e.g., tuberculosis, respiratory syncytial virus, rubella) must be included in protocols for airway management, bag-valve-mask ventilation, and endotracheal intubation. Fecal-oral (hepatitis A, salmonellosis) and direct contact (scabies, cutaneous herpes) precautions are important during patient evaluation and transportation.[21,22]

Specialty Receiving Centers

The medical director needs to determine which types of specialty receiving centers (SRCs) exist in the community. Specific SRCs may be designated for such clinical areas as: trauma, burn, hyperbaric medicine, replantation, toxic envenomation, spinal cord injury, neonatal, eye, behavioral, pediatric burn, pediatric trauma, poison, and chest pain. Protocols pertaining to transport to SRCs must be clear so that patients

---

TABLE 15.1

Questions to be addressed before adding a new skill:

1) Would this be implemented system-wide or in targeted areas? (Here, a small retirement community might be of lower priority than a populous area with many swimming pools and a school.)

2) What level providers exist in the system, and what would be the training requirements for each?

3) Are there available training institutions or other options to teach the providers this skill? (Options include performing the procedure on chicken bones or manikins.)

4) What is the mechanism to implement the protocol changes?

5) How will these changes affect the system?

6) Will there be sufficient field experience for the providers to maintain their skills, especially in the overall management of the critically ill or injured child? If not, can this be mitigated with other forms of training, perhaps even virtual reality?

7) Is there a quality management system in place, and can effective monitoring be done?

---

can be correctly triaged to the appropriate facilities. The goal is not necessarily to transport all patients to SRCs, a practice that would not be clinically or economically justified. Rather, the triage criteria and protocols must be based on a consideration of expected clinical outcome differences and community resources, and made with all parties involved, including managed care plans and other payers.[23,24] Issues to consider include sensitivity and specificity of triage criteria, SRC equipment and staffing standards, reporting requirements, and regional coordination. Furthermore, unstable patients may not be candidates for transport to SRCs. For example, a burn patient with an unstable airway might be appropriately intubated in the nearest ED and secondarily transferred to a burn center.

Treatment and Transport Dilemmas

Under what circumstances can a patient refuse treatment or transport, and what should be the approach to that patient? Management of these cases in the out-of-hospital setting can be particularly difficult. The patient's competence, legal rights, and medical condition all enter into the decision. EMS personnel have limited information, and these patients can be at risk for poor medical outcomes.[25] This is an excellent example of the importance of developing comprehensive protocols that have the specificity to direct the provider, along with the flexibility to allow adaptation to specific scene circumstances. The protocols should state at what point the direct medical oversight should be involved in transport and treatment decisions, and when a patient may be transported against his will.[26,27]

Field providers will frequently encounter situations where the use of patient restraint is appropriate. Some patients may be restrained by law enforcement personnel to facilitate transportation. Others will be either refusing care, or agitated to the extent that they are a danger to themselves or others. Physical restraints can cause sudden death, believed to be secondary to positional asphyxia.[28] Chemical restraints, such as benzodiazepines or droperidol, can be safe and effective.[14] It is important the protocols specify both when and how restraints are applied, as well as emphasize continuous patient monitoring.

There are several other philosophical questions regarding patient rights. For example, suppose a patient wishes to be transported to the hospital where his private physician practices, thereby bypassing other appropriate facilities. Since the hospital of choice is not the closest, how will this event affect the resources of the entire system? Will the ambulance be unnecessarily out of service for a long time? What if the patient is having chest pain, or becomes unstable enroute? In order to limit liability and provide the best system-wide care, methods for addressing these questions must be clearly delineated in the protocols.

When is it appropriate for the provider not to transport the patient? Consider a case in which the provider arrives on scene and feels that the patient does not have an emergency. In some systems, police are allowed to cancel further EMS response, either because they feel the patient does not have an emergency condition, or because the patient is dead and does not require resuscitation. There is a potential danger in allowing personnel with limited medical training to make such determinations.

While many systems have sufficient resources so that all patients who request it may be transported, in some the limited resources would be quickly overwhelmed. A decision must be made as to whether and under what circumstances a provider can refuse to transport a patient. A specific procedure must be developed and used to prevent individual variance that could lead to adverse patient outcomes.

The question of whether certain ambulance transports are "medically necessary" is receiving increasing emphasis in the current health care environment.[29] The medical director must keep in mind that this is a multifactorial issue involving healthcare access, costs, and patient education.[30] One system has addressed this issue by introducing a coordinated multiple-option response. Access to non-emergency transportation, advice centers, poison control, social services, and the patient's private physician are all potentially available to the patient who does not require immediate ambulance transportation.[31] The role of paramedics is being expanded further in some systems to include immunizations and other primary care, identification of at-risk elderly or domestic violence patients, and injury prevention.[32–34]

Withholding Treatment

The discussion of when it is appropriate to withhold or discontinue treatment of out-of-hospital patients has become increasingly relevant. With growing attention to medical appropriateness and cost-effectiveness, systems have implemented treatment protocols which provide for the discontinuance of care in cases in which it is considered futile.[35] For example, in San Francisco, patients in asystole secondary to a non-witnessed cardiac arrest or any traumatic etiology are determined to be dead by paramedics in the field. Studies suggest continued resuscitation efforts for victims of cardiopulmonary arrest in whom out-of-hospital resuscitation has failed are futile, except perhaps in patients with primary cardiac arrest and persistent ventricular fibrillation or patients with severe hypothermia or certain drug overdoses.[36] Potential problems such as body removal delays and access to grief support counseling must be anticipated, but this practice is accepted by family members.[37,38] Furthermore, in coroner's cases the providers must not be asked to declare a patient dead before the body is moved to a safe location (e.g., out of the traffic lane on a busy freeway). As with any protocol, the medical director should seek medical, legal, and ethical advice.

To help with transport decisions concerning patients in full arrest, it may be useful to categorize patients into "medical," "blunt-trauma," or "penetrating-trauma." Medical arrest patients can be further subdivided according to their initial cardiac rhythms. For example, a patient with a long down-time and a presenting rhythm of asystole probably should not be transported. In the past, patients with rhythms other than asystole were generally not considered to be appropriate for field determination of death. However, if providers have access to end-tidal carbon dioxide measurements, selected patients with pulseless electrical activity (PEA) may be declared dead on-scene. One study of patients in PEA reported no survivors in 150 patients in cardiac arrest who had an end-tidal carbon dioxide of 10 mm Hg or less after 20 minutes of resuscitation measures.[39] In the case of penetrating trauma, it may be most beneficial to transport the victim who presents in asystole to the nearest trauma center, especially if pericardial tamponade is suspected and down-time is short. The blunt-trauma victim in full arrest on arrival of personnel might best be determined to be dead. Both the providers and the direct medical oversight must have written guidance and understanding of the transport of "dead" patients.

There are situations in the out-of-hospital arena in which further medical care is futile, but social circumstances prohibit the determination of death. For example, if a large crowd of people has gathered and is observing the providers, it may be necessary to remove the patient from the scene prior to terminating resuscitative efforts. All circumstances under which resuscitation may be abandoned or withheld must be clearly defined. This will require the medical director to address the issue of do-not-resuscitate (DNR).[38,40–43] In some systems, DNR patients are given standardized documentation and/or medallions.

Level of Provider

A system-specific decision must be made concerning the level of provider to send to each call. Some systems work only with paramedics, some use EMT-B, and others send first responders to the scene. Law enforcement agencies are expanding their roles as well.[44] Some systems mix the levels of response, either within units or with separated tiers.[45] While it is simplest to send paramedics to all calls, this may be financially prohibitive. Conversely, if there were unlimited resources and a paramedic could be placed on every corner, there would not then be sufficient critical patients for the providers to maintain their psychomotor and assessment skills.

With the introduction of automated defibrillator capable EMTs, the distinction between ALS and BLS lost clinical relevance. The advanced skills of paramedics may no longer translate into improved patient survival.[46,46A] Today, EMT-B personnel may be capable of performing all of the medical interventions, which improve patient outcomes. If the originators of paramedicine had an AED in 1968, would they have bothered to teach firemen how to read a cardiac monitor?

Types of Vehicles

In a tiered system, matching provider level with vehicle type can be complicated, and systems have adapted in many ways. Should paramedics use motorcycles or other non-transport vehicles so that they can respond only when needed and be released quickly when not? If so, what if a paramedic is the first on the scene and finds a critical patient in need of immediate transport? The protocol must indicate, at least in broad brush, when such paramedics should transport in the "fly car." Should first responders be capable of transporting critical patients before arrival of the ambulance? Studies have suggested that for critical trauma patients, rapid transportation to the hospital, whether by medical personnel, police, or even private vehicle, may be most appropriate.[47,48] What should happen if a stable patient is being transported and a call comes in describing a critical patient who is located enroute to the hospital? Should the ambulance personnel be forbidden, permitted, or required to stop and assess the critical patient? This decision will involve direct medical oversight.

Hot versus Cold

Another operational issue to be addressed when writing a protocol is whether response vehicles should travel to and from the scene with lights and siren (HOT) or normally (COLD). Lights-and-siren (L&S) response and transportation on all calls were derived from the practice of other public safety agencies, and have been the historical standard. With the recognition that driving HOT contributes to accidents and injuries to both out-of-hospital providers and the general public, and is unnecessary in many cases, this practice has been reexamined.[49,50]

There is evidence that L&S response decreases response times, and one might expect that patient outcomes would be improved in certain time-critical cases (e.g., ventricular fibrillation).[51] Dispatch protocols can reliably determine which calls require a rapid response and which can safely be responded to more slowly.[52] Responding COLD to the lower priority calls may decrease the complications of EMS response without affecting patient care.

After on-scene evaluation and treatment by EMS personnel, the number of patients who require L&S transportation to the hospital will be relatively few, perhaps less than 10%.[53] Many systems have not addressed this, however, and L&S transportation is frequently overused.[54] One study showed an average decrease in transport time from the scene to the hospital of 3 minutes, 50 seconds, a time that was felt to be clinically significant in only 4 of 75 patients.[53a] The best way to decrease out-of-hospital time may be to carefully organize the response itself, rather than by driving quickly. The medical director must specify in each protocol whether the providers should respond and transport patients either HOT or COLD.

Use of National Guidelines

One general approach in designing protocols is to conform to the guidelines published by national groups. Examples of these are: Advanced Cardiac Life Support (ACLS), Advanced Trauma Life Support (ATLS), Neonatal Resuscitation, Pediatric Advanced Life Support (PALS), Resources for the Optimal Care of the Injured Patient, and Guidelines for the Man-

agement of Patients With Acute Myocardial Infarction.[55,56] However, so long as the medical director has the agreement of the local medical community, both EMS and others, it is not imperative to adhere to nationally endorsed guidelines. For example, indications for the pneumatic antishock garment (PASG) have been markedly limited or even eliminated in some systems long before being addressed in ATLS protocols. Obviously, the medical evidence must be supportive of such decisions.

National guidelines are developed through a committee process, and must necessarily involve a compromise position among all participants. This means the recommendations may conflict with practice in some systems. National guidelines also undergo a lengthy review process, which can delay publication for years; however, this may be an advantage, as it allows time for additional studies to be published. For example, several years ago many medical directors decided that the medical evidence favored the use of high-dose epinephrine in the treatment of cardiac arrest, and introduced it into their systems despite it not being endorsed by the American Heart Association. Only after further research demonstrated that there was no survival benefit was it removed.

Telemetry

The question of whether to require rhythm strip transmission must be addressed by the medical director.[57,58] The decision depends upon the level of out-of-hospital provider training, sophistication of clinical protocols, length of transport times, non-transport of patients in selected systems, and the type of patients who are likely to be encountered. Many systems require telemetry equipment be available, but utilize it only for complex cardiac rhythms in critical patients. Telemetry is required by law in some states.

Historically, telemetry has been limited to radio transmission of single-lead EKG data. However, with the emphasis on the rapid identification and treatment of patients suffering from acute myocardial infarction, some systems have added the capability to transmit a complete twelve-lead EKG.[59] Although the benefit is unclear, potential uses of this information are to (1) initiate out-of-hospital thrombolysis, (2) decrease time to ED administration of thrombolytics, (3) give advance notice for preparation for primary coronary angioplasty, and (4) triage of patients to regional cardiac centers.

MEDICAL INTERVENTIONS

Scene Time

An issue that should be considered when designing protocols is that of scene time. The key question to consider is whether there is anything that can be provided in the hospital, but not in the field. For example, a trauma patient with uncontrolled internal hemorrhage needs to get to an operating room as quickly as possible, whereas a patient in cardiac arrest from medical causes can receive most indicated interventions on-scene. The medical director must decide for which patients the providers should "load and go" and for which further scene treatment may be appropriate. Certainly, in the case of major trauma, scene time should be kept to a minimum. The optimal solution may not be to "scoop and run," but rather to "scoop and treat," that is, to start fluid resuscitation (when appropriate) and other treatments enroute. The protocols must, once again, be based on expected patient outcome.[60]

In non-traumatic medical emergencies, the issue of optimal scene time can be more complex. In a cardiac arrest, there is often little more treatment that can be provided in the hospital than in the field, and early transport of the patient may simply delay appropriate interventions. Obviously, certain procedures, such as defibrillation, should be performed immediately in the field. In cases of anaphylaxis, immediate administration of epinephrine is appropriate, but prolonged scene time for fluid boluses is not. The general goal of the out-of-hospital provider should be to perform those procedures that are time-critical to improve patient outcome. When necessary, these should be done on-scene, and if not, during transport. The protocols must delineate detailed steps for each medical condition.

The out-of-hospital providers may not be able to "scoop and treat" in all seemingly appropriate situations. In a case in which the providers are forced to remain on the scene due to a lack of destination or accepting facility, lack of a transport vehicle, or because of a prolonged extrication, the medical director must decide whether ad hoc deviations in the protocols are allowed. A case in point is the rare necessity for a field amputation, a procedure outside of the paramedic scope of practice in most systems.[61–63] While some might argue that a degree of vagueness could be useful, experience indicates that it is best to incorporate all reasonable possibilities into the protocols so that there is consistency and accountability in the handling of each situation.

Specialty Populations

The protocols must recognize the special needs of certain unique groups of patients. These include infants and children, the elderly, those with medical devices (e.g., tracheostomies, implantable defibrillators, infusion pumps), and dialysis patients. The EMS for Children program has as one of its objectives to "increase the number of EMS agencies that use pediatric protocols."[64] Patterns of use and medical conditions differ for the elderly as well.[65] The medical director must decide whether to design special protocols for each group, as is commonly done for children, or insert specific caveats in the general protocols where needed.

Summary of Treatment Philosophy

All protocols must be customized and endorsed according to local community standards. National guidelines should not be adopted into a system without review, modification, and local approval. Once all these philosophical and operational issues are considered, the system medical director develops the specific language for the system. Finally, the protocols require constant oversight and timely revision to remain medically and operationally appropriate.

Establishing Specific Treatments

This section does not attempt to cover every out-of-hospital clinical protocol. It will discuss some of the areas of controversy that the medical director will encounter when developing treatment protocols.

Airway Management

Many different devices and techniques exist for the management of the out-of-hospital patient's airway. Options include oral endotracheal (ET) tubes, nasotracheal (NT) tubes, esophageal obturator airways (EOA), esophageal gastric tube airways (EGTA), percutaneous transtracheal ventilation devices (PTV), surgical cricothyrotomy, laryngeal mask airway (LMA), pharyngeo-tracheal lumen airway (PTL), and the esophageal tracheal Combitube (ETC). In addition, the variability in patient types (premature newborns through bull-necked adults), clinical settings (e.g., cardiac arrest, multiple trauma, CHF), scene conditions (noise, lighting, temperature, space), provider training (First Responder, EMT, paramedic), and frequency of skill use (urban vs. rural) all serve to complicate the medical director's decision.

Bag-valve-mask (BVM) ventilation is often adequate and most appropriate. It has been shown to provide adequate oxygenation for pediatric patients when used by paramedics with the "squeeze, release, release" method.[66] In adults it is more difficult to maintain adequate volumes.[67] BVM should be considered in situations where short-term ventilation is needed (e.g., respiratory failure with a short transport time, opiate overdose) and/or when the provider is not trained in advanced airway skills. BVM does not prevent vomiting and aspiration, however, and would not be a good choice for patients at risk for these if alternative airway techniques were available. The protocols should specifically state when BVM is indicated and when advanced airways should be attempted.

Endotracheal intubation is the definitive airway of choice in the emergency department. Its role in the field has yet to be proven or defined, although it is generally accepted to be an appropriate technique if performed by well trained personnel. Properly performed, ET intubation provides a secure airway and limits aspiration. Options for ET tube insertion include direct laryngoscopy, digital guidance, and the lighted stylet.[68]

Issues to address when considering ET intubation include initial and ongoing training costs, frequency of use, and methods of monitoring. Its use in lower call-volume systems may be particularly problematic, as infrequent skill performance has been associated with an increase in unsuccessful intubation and other complications.[69] Its use in children is also controversial, where lower success and higher complication rates and a lack of survival benefit have been reported.[70] A large prospective randomized multi-center trial in Los Angeles, California is currently addressing this issue.[70a]

Confirmation of the correct placement of the ET tube has been the subject of considerable recent discussion. Unrecognized esophageal intubation is a usually lethal event, and occurs in a small but not insignificant percentage of cases. This has been well demonstrated in both hospital and out-of-hospital settings.[71,72] With the exception of the intubator definitively visualizing the tube passing through the vocal cords, clinical assessment (ET tube fogging, breath and epigastric sounds) does not have the necessary reliability to prevent this tragic outcome.[73] In one study, chest auscultation was shown to be inac-

curate in 15% of patients, even under ideal operating room conditions.[74] Considering the suboptimal auscultation conditions in an ambulance, intubations must be confirmed by other means.[75]

Two techniques have become generally accepted for use in out-of-hospital ET tube placement confirmation: expired carbon dioxide detection, and air aspiration. Pulse oximetry is less valuable because of the delay in hemoglobin desaturation.[76] Colorimetric CO_2 detectors are very specific, but can be insensitive in cardiac arrest, the condition for which patients are intubated most frequently in EMS systems.[77] When functional, they are useful to detect movement of the ET tube out of the trachea during patient treatment and transportation.

Air aspiration devices utilize either a syringe or self-inflating bulb which is connected to the ET tube. Air is readily aspirated from the cartilage-supported trachea but not from the collapsible fibromuscular esophagus. Data suggest the device is reliable, even in cardiac arrest, but can be insensitive in bronchospasm, pulmonary edema, and in the morbidly obese.[78–80] However, one report of its field use found that only 5 of 10 esophageal intubations were detected.[81] Accuracy in infants has not been well established, and it is not FDA-approved for use in patients less than 5 years of age.[82]

The National Association of State EMS Directors supports the universal use of endotracheal tube placement confirmation devices.[83] The exact clinical role of each device in the out-of-hospital setting has not yet been established, but training needs to emphasize that they must be used as adjuncts and not replacements for clinical judgment. Medical directors should consider the use of one or both for all intubations.

The use of neuromuscular-blocking agents to facilitate out-of-hospital ET intubation has been reported and is in use in some systems. It increases the frequency of successful intubations in both adults and children.[84,85] Outcome improvement has not been demonstrated, and some believe that the complication rate (e.g., unsecured airway in the paralyzed patient, aspiration) may argue against the technique.[86] Further investigation is needed.

The ETC, PTL, and LMA have been introduced as alternative or backup devices to ET intubation.[87,88] They do not require laryngoscopy, and training costs are less.[89] The ETC has become increasingly popular. Its position can be verified by the use of either an air aspiration device or CO_2 detector.[90,91]

In patients in whom other airway techniques are

unsuccessful, direct access to the trachea can be obtained through the cricothyroid membrane. This can be with a simple large-gauge catheter over a needle, a tube introduced via the Seldinger technique, or a surgical cricothyroidotomy.[92–94]

Respiratory Emergencies

The incidence, severity, and mortality of asthma in the United States is increasing, and EMS systems must be prepared to manage cases of acute and refractory exacerbations.[95] An inhaled beta-adrenergic agent is the most appropriate first-line medication.[96] Albuterol and metaproterenol are most commonly used, and their clinical profiles are not significantly different in this setting. Administration may be by nebulizer or metered dose inhaler, which are equally effective in mild or moderate severity cases.[97] In severe attacks, a nebulizer may be more appropriate.[96] Continuous nebulization is safe and at least as effective as intermittent doses, and should be considered for severe cases, including intubated patients, where it may offer additional benefit.[98,99] Investigations to date have not identified a maximum dose of inhaled albuterol in adults or children.

Inhaled anticholinergic agents (atropine, glycopyrrolate, ipratropium) are another treatment option. Their onset of action is slower than the beta agonists. Ipratropium may or may not have an additive effect when used with beta agonists; atropine and glycopyrrolate do not.[100–103] Subcutaneous terbutaline and epinephrine are no more effective than the inhaled beta agonists, their effects are not additive to the beta agonists, they are more uncomfortable for the patient, and they are potentially more toxic.[104,105] However, subcutaneous epinephrine is frequently used in patients in extremis who are "not moving any air," on the theory that aerosols would simply be deposited in the mouth and not reach the target organ.

Although not immediately effective, steroids are another mainstay of asthma therapy, and the medical director should consider a protocol for their oral administration, especially in systems with long ETAs.[105a] IV aminophylline has not been shown to provide additional benefit.[106–108] In fact, no intravenous agent, including IV fluids, has been shown to be beneficial, and protocols should address whether an IV should be inserted.[109] Additional hospital treatments, such as ketamine, intravenous epinephrine, or isoproterenol, and helium-oxygen have not been studied in the out-of-hospital setting.

Many patients continue to deteriorate despite aggressive treatment, and ultimately require assisted ventilation or ET intubation. Indications for intubation include altered mental status, severe fatigue, and profound hypoxemia. Intubation is associated with a high frequency of complications, such as pneumothorax and cardiac arrest.[110] The medical director must balance the clinical necessity of intubation with the risk of complications and specify the exact indications and types of airway management for these patients.

Inhaled beta agonists are also the preferred primary treatment for acute exacerbations of chronic obstructive pulmonary disease (COPD). The additional use of anticholinergic agents is better established.[100] Aminophylline is probably not effective.[111] Almost all patients with an exacerbation of COPD require supplemental oxygen, although its use in this setting is sometimes controversial. High-flow oxygen is not necessary for mild COPD exacerbations, but it is indicated for those who are severely dyspneic. The often cited "loss of hypercarbic respiratory drive" has never been shown to exist, and the hypercarbia associated with oxygen administration is probably due to changes in physiologic dead space rather than a reduced respiratory effort.[112,113] Since the risks of profound hypoxemia and subsequent cardiac ischemia in these usually elderly and chronically ill patients are great, oxygen should not be withheld.

In designing the treatment protocols for patients with respiratory emergencies, the medical director must be cautious in interpreting the assessment of the field providers. Paramedics may have difficulty accurately interpreting lung sounds under field conditions.[114] Auscultation in a moving ambulance is difficult.[75] Since the treatment for one respiratory condition may be ineffective or even harmful for another (e.g., epinephrine for acute pulmonary edema, or furosemide for a dehydrated patient with pneumonia), care must be taken in both developing and monitoring compliance with protocols.[115] In mildly ill patients with complex medical problems, it may be best to monitor and transport with minimal treatment aside from supplemental oxygen, particularly in short ETA systems. This is another situation in which the medical director may consider requiring direct medical oversight.[11]

Cardiac and Circulatory Emergencies

The treatment of patients with cardiac emergencies was the impetus for the development of advanced out-of-hospital medical care.[116] The knowledge of effective and ineffective treatments is progressing rapidly. For example, after a brief period of interest, high-dose epinephrine and active compression-decompression CPR have been shown not to have outcome benefit, and their use is not recommended.[117-120] In other areas, however, significant controversies remain.

The rapid delivery of an electrical countershock to a patient in ventricular fibrillation is the well established cornerstone of cardiac resuscitation, and survival rates increase with decreasing time to defibrillation. Initially, defibrillation was performed by physicians, and then paramedics.[116] With the introduction of automated defibrillators, EMTs and first responders have been utilized.[121,122] Defibrillation was available in 60% of EMS systems in 1993.[123] Continued improvements in the reliability, size, and ease of use of automated defibrillators have made them feasible for almost all systems.

The role of other resuscitation measures is less well established. The rapid provision of advanced life support measures, including ET intubation, cardiotonic medications, and cardiac pacing, has not been shown to improve patient outcome.[124,125] Systems that use BLS measures with defibrillation have reported survival rates consistent with paramedic systems.[46a,46b,124,126,127] Although ACLS guidelines for drug administration are not based on evidence obtained from RCTs, they have become standard in EMS systems and training programs, and should generally be followed.[128,129] Clearly, additional investigation is needed.

In the treatment of patients with acute myocardial infarction (AMI), the most important role of the EMS system in the reduction of mortality is to emphasize early recognition and treatment.[130] Education efforts are primary, and should include symptom recognition and use of 9-1-1.[130] Use of the EMS system can reduce treatment delay, but a tightly structured patient evaluation and treatment approach must be included in the protocols to prevent unnecessarily prolonging out-of-hospital time.[131,132] The benefit of advanced life-support care has not been well demonstrated, particularly in urban areas with short transport times.[133] A coordinated out-of-hospital and hospital system minimizes the time to treatment.[130]

Myocardial reperfusion, whether by thrombolytic agents or angioplasty, improves outcome in patients with AMI.[130] The role of the EMS system is being reexamined in a comprehensive effort to reduce the delay to myocardial reperfusion, the majority of which occurs in the time interval between the onset of symptoms and seeking of medical attention.[134] Since the benefit of thrombolytics decreases with time, one might expect field administration to be useful.[135] Paramedic thrombolytic initiation is feasible, and does reduce time to drug administration; however, mortality reduction has not been well demonstrated.[136,137] The American Heart Association and American College of Cardiology (AHA/ACC) recommend that out-of-hospital thrombolytic administration only be considered when transport times exceed 90 minutes.[130]

A second option is the out-of-hospital 12-lead ECG. Paramedics apply leads and transmit information via cellular telephone to the direct medical control. Training requires about 4 hours and increases on-scene time by less than five minutes.[138] This technique reduces door-to-needle time, or time to primary angioplasty.[139] Initially, the time reduction to thrombolysis was reported as 30 minutes or more, but it has more recently been shown to save only 10 minutes.[139,140] By itself, an emphasis on rapid ED evaluation and treatment can reduce the total door-to-needle time to less than 20 minutes.[141] Thus, it is unlikely that an out-of-hospital EKG would decrease this interval sufficiently to provide an improved clinical outcome. The National Heart Attack Working Group believes the clinical impact of the out-of-hospital EKG to be small.[142] However, one additional potential benefit is to provide the ability to triage patients to hospitals best equipped to manage acute MI, which might include those with angioplasty capabilities.[139]

The use of aspirin has been advocated in the out-of-hospital treatment of both unstable angina and acute MI.[143] Inhibition of platelet aggregation begins to occur within one hour, and the chewable form is more rapidly absorbed.[130,143] The Second International Study of Infarct Survival reported that aspirin was more beneficial when administered within five hours of symptom onset.[144] The ACC/AHA guidelines concluded that there is little evidence for a time-dependent effect on early mortality, but that aspirin reduces late mortality, and recommend that 160 to 325 mg of aspirin be administered promptly.[130] There is no evidence that shortening the time to administration by a few minutes in a short transport time system will improve outcome.

The treatment of CHF with acute pulmonary edema (APE) is complex. There has been a trend away from furosemide as a first-line treatment and toward a more liberal use of nitrates. One out-of-hospital study that examined the treatment of patients with presumed APE compared four regimens: nitroglycerin (NTG) plus furosemide, MS plus furosemide, all three, and NTG plus MS. The authors found that NTG is beneficial in the out-of-hospital management of APE, while MS and furosemide may not add anything and may be potentially deleterious.[145]

The out-of-hospital management of paroxysmal supraventricular tachycardia (PSVT) has evolved. Verapamil was the first reliable pharmacologic therapy to be utilized.[146] Thereafter, adenosine came into favor.[147] The two drugs are equally successful at converting PSVT, and adenosine is more costly than verapamil.[148] However, adenosine has numerous advantages over verapamil, including fewer contraindications (e.g., age, hemodynamic instability, pregnancy, wide-complex tachycardia, and preexcitation SVT), less-serious adverse effects, and short time of pharmacologic effect (10–60 seconds).[148] Its safer clinical profile is particularly important in the out-of-hospital setting, where studies consistently report a 21 to 39% rate of misdiagnosis of PSVT, and many of these incorrect diagnoses involve contraindications (e.g., ventricular tachycardia) to the use of verapamil.[148]

Out-of-hospital transcutaneous pacing has been reported by several authors. There is general agreement that pacing is unlikely to be useful in the treatment of asystole or PEA.[149,150] One small study did report a possible improvement in outcome of patients with hemodynamically significant bradycardia, but this needs confirmation with better controls and a larger sample size before it can be recommended.[150]

Trauma

After securing an unstable airway, the most important intervention in the care of the seriously injured patient is to expedite transportation to the site of definitive care. The operational issue of "scoop and run" versus on-scene treatment has already been addressed in this chapter. As opposed to many medical conditions (e.g., hypoglycemia, status epilepticus, opiate overdose, airway obstruction), the out-of-hospital care of most trauma patients is not to initiate definitive care, but to temporize and transport. Protocols and quality monitoring processes should focus on minimizing the on-scene time while providing necessary care.

The role of advanced levels of intervention in treating major trauma patients has been questioned. Two recent studies have reported that patients, mostly victims of penetrating trauma, transported to the hospital by non-medical police personnel or private vehicle have a greater likelihood of survival than similarly injured patients transported by paramedic ambulance.[47,48] Others have shown a decreased mortality with the implementation of paramedic programs.[151,152] Care must be taken in interpreting these reports. Optimal treatment of patients with differing injuries (e.g., blunt vs. penetrating), or in different settings (e.g., urban vs. rural) will not be identical. Trauma is not a single disease. Protocols must delineate treatments based on specific injuries and indicate the timing and amount of IV fluids that should be administered.

Another issue in the out-of-hospital treatment of trauma patients concerns the use of PASG. Unfortunately, the PASG became part of the treatment armamentarium without studies to test its efficacy. In a position paper by the National Association of EMS Physicians, the PASG was considered acceptable for use in pelvic fractures with or without hypotension, uncontrolled lower-extremity hemorrhage, severe traumatic hypotension, and spinal shock.[153] However, these recommendations were not based on controlled outcome-based studies.[154] The four prospective randomized trials in the out-of-hospital setting published to date have concluded that outcome is unaffected by the use of the PASG.[155–158] No definitive evidence to support the use of the PASG exists at this time.[159]

The efficacy of intravenous fluid administration in injured patients has also been questioned. Traditional training has emphasized aggressive fluid resuscitation of hypotensive trauma patients. However, studies have not shown a survival benefit in either adults or children.[160–162] In a study of hypotensive patients with penetrating torso injuries without concomitant head injury, outcomes were improved when intravenous fluids were delayed until surgery.[163] Worse outcomes with aggressive fluid resuscitation may be due to accelerated hemorrhage, either from disruption of a thrombus, dilution of clotting factors, or lowering of blood viscosity.[163] However, in another report, IV hypertonic saline increased both the blood pressure and likelihood of survival in head-injured patients.[7]

The role of secondary brain injury in the ultimate outcome of head-injured patients is being increasingly recognized.[164] The two most important determinants of secondary brain injury are hypoxia and hypotension. A single systolic blood pressure measurement less than 90 was associated with worse outcome in one study.[165] Hyperventilation can reduce intracranial hypertension, but if too aggressive can result in cerebral ischemia.[166] Protocols must address the avoidance of hypotension and hypoxia in these patients with aggressive fluid resuscitation and oxygenation. A retrospective study concluded that out-of-hospital intubation of severely head-injured patients improved outcome.[167] A group in San Diego is currently investing the possible role of rapid sequence intubation in the field.[167a]

Indications and methods of spinal immobilization have been modified both in the emergency department and in the field. Traditional teaching has been for field providers to immobilize any patient with an even remote clinical suspicion of spinal injury onto a rigid backboard. The rigid boards cause significant discomfort, even to healthy volunteers.[168] Vacuum splints can be more comfortable and are equally effective.[169] Emergency department-based studies have demonstrated that use of clinical criteria can reduce the number of cervical spine radiographs, and a large multi-center study is underway to further define this.[170] Clinical criteria associated with cervical spinal injury have been reported: altered mental status, neurological deficit, intoxication, spinal pain, and suspected extremity fracture.[171] Protocols must balance patient comfort and ease of transport with the clinical suspicion of a spinal injury.

Finally, one of the most important things the field providers can do to alleviate patient suffering is to provide analgesia. In the setting of trauma, this practice is generally discouraged. Although not well studied, administration of opioid analgesia in the presence of intra-abdominal hemorrhage and head trauma is thought to deleteriously affect vital signs, mental status, and accuracy of further evaluation. The medical director must decide whether any type of analgesia will be allowed in the setting of trauma. For example, if a patient has an isolated long-bone fracture, should providers be permitted to administer intravenous morphine? Although there is concern about abuse potential and maintaining an appropriate scavenger system, nitrous oxide is successfully used for analgesia in some systems.[172,173]

Management of Neurologic Emergencies

Management of the patient who presents with an altered level of consciousness (ALOC) is a common out-of-hospital problem. In addition to basic measures, including oxygen, protocols must address additional drugs to administer. Historically all of these patients received IV dextrose. There is some evidence, however, that the indiscriminate use of intravenous dextrose can worsen outcome in patients suffering from myocardial infarction, stroke, or other conditions that place them at risk for cerebral ischemia.[174,175] Others have concluded that the hyperglycemia seen in sicker stroke patients is a stress response, and that treatments aimed at lowering glucose are not beneficial.[176] Rapid reagent tests for blood glucose can be used, but may be inaccurate in 6 to 8% of cases, particularly if reagent strips are exposed to heat or light, and clinical presentation must also be considered in the decision to administer glucose.[177] If a rapid reagent test is unavailable, all patients with suspected hypoglycemia should receive dextrose.[178] In patients with suspected or confirmed hypoglycemia, but no intravenous access, intramuscular glucagon may be included as a protocol option.[179]

Some concern has been raised about whether to administer thiamine prior to, or concomitant with, dextrose to prevent precipitating an acute Wernicke's encephalopathy.[180] Symptom onset was hours to days following dextrose administration in the one report that addressed this question.[181] Since cellular thiamine uptake is slower than glucose, there is no clinical or pharmacologic justification to withhold dextrose until thiamine is administered.[178] Patients who are not transported to the ED for further care will be at greater risk, however.

Another commonly used medication for patients with ALOC is naloxone. Naloxone is safe and effective, and the adverse reactions are generally inconsequential.[182] Patients with concomitant sympathomimetic effect (e.g., cocaine) can have more severe reactions, although these are rare.[183] Some authors recommend administering a low dose (0.1–0.2 mg IV) to reduce the likelihood of violent behavior and adverse reactions, although adverse reactions have been reported with doses of 0.1 mg as well.[15,178,184] Clinical assessment can be used to determine which patients with ALOC require naloxone.[185] Naloxone may be administered IV, IO, or IM, and the IM route is used customarily in some systems in patients with a measurable blood pressure.[18,184] There is no evidence that other routes (submental, intralingual, endobronchial) are more rapid or effective.[19]

Flumazenil, a specific benzodiazepine antagonist, is an additional medication to consider. It has a potential to cause refractory seizures, especially in patients who are benzodiazepine addicted, have an underlying seizure disorder, or have taken an overdose of drugs such as tricyclic antidepressants, which have anticholinergic effects. Because of this risk and the relatively benign course of patients with benzodiazepine overdose, it cannot be recommended for out-of-hospital use at this time.[178,186]

A second out-of-hospital neurologic emergency is status epilepticus. Most systems use diazepam, either IV or rectally for treatment of this entity.[187] A more recent option, in use in Australia, is the use of IM midazolam. One in-hospital study in children found it to be as effective, and more rapid in onset compared to IV diazepam, largely because of the inherent delay in obtaining IV access in a seizing child.[188] Propofol has also been effectively used in the out-of-hospital setting in patients who fail diazepam treatment.[189] A study underway in San Francisco is comparing outcomes of status epilepticus patients given diazepam, lorazepam, or placebo. The investigators hope to determine whether it is beneficial to treat this condition, or whether the risk of creating an unstable airway and respiratory depression may worsen outcomes in a short ETA system.

Management of Childbirth

Management of out-of-hospital childbirth is part of the EMT curriculum and therefore is not always addressed in the paramedic protocols. Since many systems are developing protocols for all levels of providers, a childbirth protocol is appropriate and should specify under what circumstances delivery should be prepared for and performed in the field as opposed to initiating transport of the patient to the hospital. Certainly, it is generally better to bring the patient to the hospital, yet a precipitous delivery in a moving ambulance can be even more chaotic and dangerous than one prepared for in the field. Protocols must also address the management of complications.[190]

Management of Other Medical Emergencies

A controversial area is the prehospital management of poisonings or overdoses. While it used to be common to give ipecac in the field, this technique has fallen out of favor in most systems. Especially in suicidal adults, the nature of the ingestion cannot always be reliably determined. Therefore, it may be dangerous to give ipecac since the patient may develop a de-creased level of consciousness enroute (as in the case of a tricyclic antidepressant overdose). This could lead to vomiting in a patient without a controlled airway. In fact, gastric emptying has not been shown to be beneficial.[191] Some systems use activated charcoal in the field.[192] Further studies are needed to determine whether this is beneficial.

Anaphylaxis is one of the few medical emergencies that, in the absence of treatment, can proceed rapidly to death. Therefore, BLS personnel can be taught to use epinephrine preparations specifically for this purpose.[193,194] In addition, the medical director may adopt a protocol that allows BLS providers to administer the patient's own epinephrine. These issues need to be carefully examined if such protocols are used at the BLS level, since state laws may not be permissive, BLS providers do not traditionally make contact with the direct medical oversight, and the treatment is not without complications.[195]

Summary

The medical director considers basic philosophical issues, tailors them to the local system, devises specific interventions, and formally writes the protocols, presumably with the general support of the medical community. There must be a system in place to monitor the protocols and to revise them as necessary. As medical evidence supports new treatments, they must also be considered for introduction into the local system, with timely modifications of protocols as appropriate. There is a delicate balance between being the first and the last to introduce an intervention.

References

1. Evidence-Based Medicine Working Group. Evidence-based medicine. *JAMA.* 1992;268(17):2420–2445.
2. Sackett DL, Rosenberg WMC, Gray JA, Haynes RB, Richardson WS. Evidence-based medicine: what it is and what it isn't. *BMJ.* 1996;312:71–72.
3. Haynes RB, Sackett DL, Gray JM, et al. Transferring evidence from research into practice: developing evidence-based clinical policy. *ACP Journal Club.* 1997;126(2):A14–A16.
4. Kellermann AL, et al. Impact of first-responder defibrillation in an urban emergency medical services system. *JAMA.* 1993;270:1708–1713.
5. Watts DD. Defibrillation by basic emergency medical technicians: effect on survival. *Ann Emerg Med.* 1995;26(5):635–639.
6. Callaham M. Quantifying the scanty science of prehospital emergency care. *Ann Emerg Med.* 1997;30(6):785–790.

7. Vassar MJ, Fisher RP, O'Brien PE, et al. A multicenter trial for resuscitation of injured patients with 7.5% sodium chloride: the effect of added dextran 70. The Multicenter Group for the Study of Hypertonic Saline in Trauma Patients. *Arch Surg.* 1993;128:1003–1011.

8. Holliman CJ, Wuerz RC, Meador SA. Decrease in medical command errors with use of a standing-orders protocol system. *Am J Emerg Med.* 1994;12:279–283.

9. Gratton MC, et al. Effect of standing orders on paramedic scene time for trauma patients. *Ann Emerg Med.* 1991;20(12):1306–1309.

10. Holliman CJ, Wuertz RC, Vasquez-de Miguel G, Meador SA. Comparison of interventions in prehospital care by standing orders versus interventions by direct (on-line) medical command. *Prehosp Disaster Med.* 1994;9(4):202–209.

11. Hoffman JR, et al. Does paramedic-base hospital contact result in beneficial deviations from standard prehospital protocols? *West J Med.* 1990;153:283–287.

12. Salerno SM, Wrenn KD, Slovis CM. Monitoring EMS protocol deviations: a useful quality assurance tool. *Ann Emerg Med.* 1991;20:1319–1324.

13. Gershon RRM, Vlahov D, Kelen G, et al. Review of accidents/injuries among emergency medical services workers in Baltimore, Maryland. *Prehosp Disaster Med.* 1995;10(1):14–18.

14. Rosen CL, Ratliff AF, Wolfe RE, et al. The efficacy of intravenous droperidol in the prehospital setting. *J Emerg Med.* 1997;15(1):13–17.

15. Gaddis GM et al. Naloxone-associated patient violence: An overlooked toxicity? *Ann Pharmaco.* 1992; 26(2):196.

16. Marcus R, Srivastava PU, Bell DM, et al. Occupational blood contact among prehospital providers. *Ann Emerg Med.* 1995;25(6):776–779

17. Eustis TC, Wright SW, Wrenn KD, et al. Compliance with recommendations for universal precautions among prehospital providers. *Ann Emerg Med.* 1995; 25(4):512–515.

18. Sporer KA, Firestone JF, Isaacs SM. Out-of-hospital opioid overdoses in an urban setting. *Acad Emerg Med.* 1996;3(7):660–667.

19. Salvucci AA, Iscovich AL, Eckstein M. Submental injection of naloxone. *Ann of Emerg Med.* 1995;25(5): 719.

20. O Conner RE, Krall SP, Megargel RE, et al. Reducing the rate of paramedic needlesticks in emergency medical services: the role of self-capping intravenous catheters. *Acad Emerg Med.* 1996;3:668–674.

21. Sepkowitz KA. Occupationally acquired infections in health care workers. Part I. *Ann Int Med.* 1996;125: 826–834.

22. Sepkowitz KA. Occupationally acquired infections in health care workers. Part II. *Ann Int Med.* 1996;125: 917–928.

23. Koenig KL, Salvucci A, Zachariah B. EMS systems and managed care integration. *Prehosp Emerg Care.* 1998; 2(1):67–69.

24. Slack DS, Koenig KL, Bouley D. Paramedic accuracy in estimated time of arrival: significance in the managed care environment. *Acad Emerg Med.* 1995;2(10): 943–944.

25. Burstein JL, Henry MC, Alicandro J, et al. Outcome of patients who refused out-of-hospital medical assistance. *Am J Emerg Med.* 1996;14(1):23–26.

26. Alicandro J, Hollander JE, Henry MC, et al. Impact of interventions for patients refusing emergency medical services transport. *Acad Emerg Med.* 1995;2:480–485.

27. Adams JA, Verdile V, Arnold R, et al. Patient refusal in the out-of-hospital setting. *Acad Emerg Med.* 1996; 3:948–951.

28. Stratton SJ, Rogers C, Green K. Sudden death in individuals in hobble restraints during paramedic transport. *Ann Emerg Med.* 1995;25:710–712.

29. Billittier AJ, Moscati R, Janicke D, et al. A multisite survey of factors contributing to medically unnecessary ambulance transports. *Acad Emerg Med.* 1996;3(11): 1046–1052.

30. Rucker DW, Edwards RA, Burstin HR, et al. Patient-specific predictors of ambulance use. *Ann Emerg Med.* 1997;29:484–491.

31. Koenig KL. Unscheduled access to health care: reengineering the 9-1-1 system. *Acad Emerg Med.* 1996; 3(11):989–991.

32. Garza MA. Paramedics—the next generation. *JEMS.* 1993;8:89–96.

33. Kinnane JM, Garrison HG, Coben JH, Alonso-Serra HM. Injury prevention: is there a role for out-of-hospital emergency medical services? *Acad Emerg Med.* 1997;4(4):306–312.

34. Landis JM, Sorenson SB. Victims of violence: the role and training of EMS personnel. *Ann Emerg Med.* 1997;30:204–206.

35. Kellermann AL, Hackman BB, Somes G. Predicting the outcome of unsuccessful prehospital advanced cardiac life support. *JAMA.* 1993;270:1433–1436.

36. Bonnin MJ, Pepe PE, Kimball KT, Clark PS. Distinct criteria for termination of resuscitation in the out-of-hospital setting. *JAMA.* 1993;270:1457–1462.

37. Delbridge TR, Fosnocht DE, Garrison HG, Auble TE. Field termination of unsuccessful out-of-hospital cardiac arrest resuscitation: acceptance by family members. *Ann Emerg Med.* 1996;27(5):649–654.

38. Koenig KL, Tamkin G, Salness KA. Do-not-resuscitate orders: where are they in the prehospital setting? *Prehosp Disaster Med.* 1993;8(1):22–26.

39. Levine RL, Wayne MA, Miller CC. End-tidal carbon dioxide and outcome of out-of-hospital cardiac arrest. *N Engl J Med.* 1997;337(5):301–306.

40. Iverson KV. A simplified prehospital advance directive law: Arizona's approach. *Ann Emerg Med.* 1993;22: 1703–1710.

41. Fitzgerald DJ, Milzman DP, Sulmasy DP. Creating a dignified option: ethical considerations in the formulation of a prehospital DNR protocol. *Am J Emerg Med.* 1995;13(2):223–227.

42. Hall SA. An analysis of dilemmas posed by prehospital DNR orders. *J Emerg Med*. 1997;15(1):109–111.

43. Koenig KL, Salvucci AA. Out-of-hospital do-not-attempt-resuscitation in the suicidal patient: a special case. *Acad Emerg Med*. 1997;4(9):926.

44. Alonso-Serra HM, Delbridge TR, Auble TE, et al. Law enforcement agencies and out-of-hospital emergency care. *Ann Emerg Med*. 1997;29(4):497–503.

45. Braun O, McCallion R, Fazackerley J. Characteristics of midsized urban EMS systems. *Ann Emerg Med*. 1990;19:536–546.

46. Mitchell RG, et al. Can the full range of paramedic skills improve survival from out of hospital cardiac arrests? *J Accid Emerg Med*. 1997;14:274–277.

46A. Ranier TH, et al. Paramedics, technicians, and survival from out of hospital cardiac arrest. *J Accid Emerg Med*. 1997;14:278–282.

47. Branas CC, Sing RF, Davidson SJ. Urban trauma transport of assaulted patients using non-medical personnel. *Acad Emerg Med*. 1995;2(6):486–493.

48. Demetriades D, Chan L, Cornwell E, et al. Paramedic vs private transportation of trauma patients: effect on outcome. *Arch Surg*. 1996;131:133–138.

49. Saunders CE, Heye CJ. Ambulance collisions in an urban environment. *Prehosp Disaster Med*. 1994;9(2):118–124.

50. National Association of Emergency Medical Services Physicians (NAEMSP) and the National Association of State EMS Directors (NASEMSD). Use of warning lights and siren in emergency medical vehicle response and patient transport. *Prehosp Disaster Med*. 1994;9:133–136.

51. Billittier A IV, Ciotoli M, Patel V, Lerner EB. Ambulance response time with and without lights and siren in urban and suburban/rural settings. 1996 *ACEP Research Forum Abstracts*. 1996;131.

52. Kallsen G, Nabors MD. The use of priority medical dispatch to distinguish between high- and low-risk patients. *Ann Emerg Med*. 1990;19:458–459.

53. Kupas DF, Dula DD, Pino BJ. Patient outcome using medical protocol to limit "lights and siren" transport. *Prehosp Disaster Med*. 1994;9(4):226–229.

53A. O'Brien DJ, Price TG, Adams P. The effectiveness of lights and siren use during ambulance transport by paramedics. *Prehosp Emerg Care*. 1999;3(2):127–130.

54. Lacher ME, Bausher JC. Lights and siren in pediatric 9-1-1 ambulance transports: are they being misused? *Ann Emerg Med*. 1997;29:223–227.

55. Committee on Trauma, American College of Surgeons. *Resources for Optimal Care of the Injured Patient*. Chicago, American College of Surgeons, 1993.

56. Ryan TJ, Anderson JL, Antman EM, et al. ACC/AHA Guidelines for the management of patients with acute myocardial infarction: a report of the American College of Cardiology/American Heart Association Task Force on Practice Guidelines (Committee on Management of Acute Myocardial Infarction). *J Am Coll Cardiol*. 1996;28:1328–1428.

57. Cayten CG, et al. The effect of telemetry on urban prehospital cardiac care. *Ann Emerg Med*. 1985;14:976–981.

58. Erder MH, Davidson SJ. Telemetry in prehospital care [letter]. *Ann Emerg Med*. 1987;16:923.

59. Aufderheide TP, Kereiakes DJ, Weaver WD, et al. Planning, implementation, and process monitoring for prehospital 12-lead diagnostic programs. *Prehosp Disaster Med*. 1996;11:162–171.

60. Koenig KL. Quo vadis: scoop and run, stay and treat, or treat and street? *Acad Emerg Med*. 1995;2(6):477–479.

61. Koenig KL, Schultz CH, Bade R. In-field extremity amputations. *Prehosp Disaster Med*. 1993;8:205.

62. Krommer, et al. In-field, extremity amputations: prevalence and procedure in emergency services. *Prehosp Disaster Med*. 1992;7(Suppl. 1):33s.

63. Koenig KL, Schultz CH, DiLorenzo R. The crush injury cadaver lab: a new method of training physicians to perform fasciotomies and amputations on survivors of a catastrophic earthquake [abstract]. *Ann Emerg Med*. 1992;21:613.

64. US Department of Health and Human Services, Health Resources and Services Administration, Maternal and Child Health Bureau. *5-year plan: Emergency Medical Services for Children, 1995–2000*. Washington, DC: Emergency Medical Services for Children National Resource Center; 1995.

65. Dickinson ET, Verdile VP, Kostyun CT, Salluzzo RF. Geriatric use of emergency medical services. *Ann Emerg Med*. 1996;27(2):199–203.

66. Gausche M, Stratton SJ, Henderson FP, et al. Bag-valve-mask ventilation for children in the out-of-hospital setting. *Acad Emerg Med*. 1996;3(5):404.

67. Cummins RO, Austin D, Graves JR, et al. Ventilation skills of emergency medical technicians: a teaching challenge for emergency medicine. *Ann Emerg Med*. 1986;15:1187–1192.

68. Margolis GS, Menegazzi J, Abdlehak M, Delbridge TR. The efficacy of a standard training program for transillumination-guided endotracheal intubation. *Acad Emerg Med*. 1996;3:371–377.

69. Johnson JC. Prehospital care: the future of emergency medical services. *Ann Emerg Med*. 1991;20:426–432.

70. Nakayama DK, Gardner MJ, Rowe MI. Emergency endotracheal intubation in pediatric trauma. *Ann Surg*. 1990;211:218–223.

70A. Gausche M, Lewis RJ, Stratton SJ, et al. Effect of out-of-hospital pediatric endotracheal intubation on survival and neurological outcome: a controlled clinical trial. *JAMA*. 2000;283(6):783–790.

71. Schwartz DE, Matthay MA, Cohen NH. Death and other complications of emergency airway management in critically ill adults. *Anesthesiology*. 1995;82:367–376.

72. Jenkins WA, Verdile, VP, Paris PM. The syringe aspiration technique to verify endotracheal tube position. *Am J Emerg Med*. 1994;12:413–416.

73. White SJ, Slovis CM. Inadvertent esophageal intubation in the field: reliance on a fool's gold standard. *Acad Emerg Med*. 1997;4(2):89–91.

74. Andersen KH, Schultz-Lebahn T. Oesophageal intubation can be undetected by auscultation of the chest. *Acta Anaesthesiol Scand*. 1994;38(6):580–582.

75. Brown LH, Gough JE, Bryan-Berg DM, Hunt RC. Assessment of breath sounds during ambulance transport. *Ann Emerg Med.* 1997;29(2):228–231.

76. Guggenberger H, Lenz G, Federle R. Early detection of inadvertent oesophageal intubation: pulse oximetry vs. capnography. *Acta Anaesthesiol Scand.* 1989;33:2.

77. Ornato JP, Shipley JB, Racht EM, et al. Multicenter study of a portable, hand-size, colorimetric end-tidal carbon dioxide detection device. *Ann Emerg Med.* 1992;21:518–523.

78. Baraka A. The esophageal detector device in the asthmatic patient. *Anaesthesia.* 1993;48:275.

79. Wee MKY. Comments on the oesophageal detector device [letter]. *Anaesthesia.* 1989;44:930–931.

80. Baraka A, Choueiry P, Salem R. The esophageal detector device in the morbidly obese. *Anesth Analg.* 1993; 77:400.

81. Pelucio M, Halligan L, Dhindsa H. Out-of-hospital experience with the syringe esophageal detector device. *Acad Emerg Med.* 1997;4:563–568.

82. Burnnett YL, Brennan MP, Salem MR. Efficacy of the self-inflating bulb in verifying tracheal tube placement in children. *Anesth Analg.* 1995;80:S63.

83. Resolutions of the National Association of State EMS Directors: 1995. *Prehospital Disaster Medicine.* 1996; 11:240–242.

84. Hedges JR, Dronen SC, Feero S, et al. Succinylcholine-assisted intubation in prehospital care. *Ann Emerg Med.* 1988;17:469–472.

85. Sing RF, Reilly PM, Rotondo MF, et al. Out-of-hospital rapid-sequence induction for intubation of the pediatric patient. *Acad Emerg Med.* 1996;3:41–45.

86. Hadzic A, Vloka JD, Sanborn K. Rapid-sequence induction for pediatric intubation [letter]. *Acad Emerg Med.* 1997;4:80–81.

87. Atherton GL, Johnson JC. Ability of paramedics to use the Combitube in prehospital cardiac arrest. *Ann Emerg Med.* 1993;22(8):1263–1268.

88. Pepe PE, Zachariah BS, Chandra NC. Invasive airway techniques in resuscitation. *Ann Emerg Med.* 1993; 22:393–403.

89. Rumball CJ, MacDonald D. The PTL, Combitube, laryngeal mask, and oral airway: a randomized prehospital comparative study of ventilatory device effectiveness and cost-effectiveness in 470 cases of cardiorespiratory arrest. *Prehosp Emerg Care.* 1997;1(1):1–10.

90. Butler BD, Little T, Drtil S. Combined use of the esophageal-tracheal Combitube with a colorimetric carbon dioxide detector for emergency intubation/ventilation. *J Clin Monit.* 1995;11:311–316.

91. Waifai Y, Salem MR, Baraka A, et al. Effectiveness of the self-inflating bulb for verification of proper placement of the esophageal tracheal Combitube. *Anesth Analg.* 1995;80(1):122–126.

92. Spaite DW, et al. Prehospital cricothyrotomy: an investigation of indications, technique, complications, and patient outcome. *Ann Emerg Med.* 1990;19:279.

93. Johnson DR, et al. Cricothyroidotomy performed by prehospital personnel: a comparison of two techniques in a human cadaver model. *Am J Emerg Med.* 1993; 11:207.

94. Jacobson LE, Gomez GA, Sobieray BA, et al. Surgical cricothyroidotomy in trauma patients: analysis of its use by paramedics in the field. *J Trauma.* 1996;41: 15–20.

95. Centers for Disease Control: Asthma—United States 1982–1992. *JAMA.* 1995;273:451–452.

96. Jagoda A, Shepard SM, Spevitz A, Joseph MM. Refractory asthma, part 1: epidemiology, pathophysiology, pharmacologic interventions. *Ann Emerg Med.* 1997;29:262–274.

97. Colacone A, et al. A comparison of albuterol administered by metered dose inhaler (and holding chamber) or wet nebulizer in acute asthma. *Chest.* 1993;104(3): 835.

98. Shresta M, Bidadi K, Gourlay S, et al. Continuous vs intermittent albuterol, at high and low doses, in the treatment of severe acute asthma in adults. *Chest.* 1996;110:42–47.

99. Rudnitsky G, Eberlein R, Schoffstall J, et al. Comparison of intermittent and continuously nebulized albuterol for treatment of asthma in an urban emergency department. *Ann Emerg Med.* 1993;22:1842–1846.

100. Patrick D, Dales R, Stark R, et al. Severe exacerbations of COPD and asthma: incremental benefit of adding ipratropium to usual therapy. *Chest.* 1990;98:295–297.

101. Karpel JP, Schacter EN, Fanta C, et al. A comparison of ipratropium and albuterol vs. albuterol alone for the treatment of acute asthma. *Chest.* 1996;110:611–616.

102. Diaz JE, Dubin R, Gaeta TJ, et al. Efficacy of atropine sulfate in combination with albuterol in the treatment for acute asthma. *Acad Emerg Med.* 1997;4(2):107–113.

103. Cydulka R, Emerman C. Effects of combined treatment with glycopyrrolate and albuterol in acute exacerbation of asthma. *Ann Emerg Med.* 1994;23:270–274.

104. Zehner WJ, Scott JM, Iannolo PM, et al. Terbutaline vs albuterol for out-of-hospital respiratory distress: randomized, double-blind trial. *Ann Emerg Med.* 1995;26:686–691.

105. Quadrel M, Lavery RF, Jaker M, et al. Prospective, randomized trial of epinephrine, metaproterenol, and both in the prehospital treatment of asthma in the adult patient. *Ann Emerg Med.* 1995;26:469–473.

105A. Creese AT, Christy DE, Levitt MA. Is there a substantial delay in steroid administration to patients with acute asthma exacerbations? *Ann Emerg Med.* 1997; 30(3):426.

106. Littenberg B. Aminophylline treatment in severe, acute asthma. *JAMA.* 1981;259:1678–1684.

107. Coleridge J, et al. Intravenous aminophylline confers no benefit in acute asthma treated with intravenous steroids and inhaled bronchodilators. *Aust N Z J Med.* 1993;23(4):348.

108. Goodman DC, et al. Theophylline in acute childhood asthma: a meta-analysis of its efficacy. *Ped Pulm.* 1996;21(3):211.

109. Potter PC, Klein M, Weinberg EG. Hydration in severe acute asthma. *Arch Dis Chil.* 1991;66:216–219.

110. Leatherman J. Life-threatening asthma. *Clin Chest Med.* 1994;15:453–479.

111. Murata GH, et al. Aminophylline in the outpatient management of decompensated chronic obstructive pulmonary disease. *Chest.* 1990;98(6):1346.

112. Hanson CW, Marshall BE, Frasch HF, Marshall C. Causes of hypercarbia with chronic obstructive pulmonary disease. *Crit Care Med.* 1996;24:23–28.

113. Dick CR, Liu Z, Sassoon CS, et al. O2-induced change in ventilation and ventilatory drive in COPD. *Am J Respir Crit Care Med.* 1997;155(2):609–614.

114. Wigder HN, Johnson DR, Cohan S, et al. Assessment of lung auscultation by paramedics. *Ann Emerg Med.* 1996;28:309–312.

115. Wuerz RC, Meador SA. Effects of prehospital medications on mortality and length of stay in congestive heart failure. *Ann Emerg Med.* 1992;21:669–674.

116. Eisenberg MS, Pantridge JF, Cobb LA, Geddes JS. The revolution and evolution of prehospital cardiac care. *Arch Int Med.* 1996;156:1611–1619.

117. Barton C, Callaham M. High-dose epinephrine improves the return of spontaneous circulation rates in human victims of cardiac arrest. *Ann Emerg Med.* 1991;20:722–725.

118. Callaham M, Madsen CD, Barton CW, et al. A randomized clinical trial of high dose epinephrine and norepinephrine vs standard-dose epinephrine in prehospital cardiac arrest. *JAMA.* 1992;268:2667–2672.

119. Schwab TM, Callaham ML, Madsen CD, Utecht TA. A randomized clinical trial of active compression-decompression CPR vs standard CPR in out-of-hospital cardiac arrest in two cities. *JAMA.* 1995;273:1261–1268.

120. Stiell IG, Paul HC, Wells GA, et al. The Ontario trial of active compression-decompression cardiopulmonary resuscitation for in-hospital and prehospital cardiac arrest. *JAMA.* 1996;275:1417–1423.

121. Eisenberg MS, Cummins RO. Defibrillation performed by the emergency medical technician. *Circulation.* 1986;74(suppl):IV9–IV12.

122. White RD, Asplin BR, Bugliosi TF, Hankins DG. High release survival from out-of-hospital ventricular fibrillation with rapid defibrillation by both police and paramedics. *Acad Emerg Med.* 1996;3:422.

123. Keller RA. 1993 EMS salary survey. *JEMS.* 1993;18:76–91.

124. Callaham M, Madsen CD. Relationship of timeliness of paramedic advanced life support interventions to outcome on out-of-hospital cardiac arrest treated by first responders with defibrillators. *Ann Emerg Med.* 1996;27:638–648.

125. Guly UM, Mitchell RG, Cok R, et al. Paramedics and technicians are equally successful at managing cardiac arrest outside hospital. *BMJ.* 1995;310:1091–1094.

126. Sedgewick ML, Dalziel K, Watson J, et al. Performance of an established system of first responder out-of-hospital defibrillation: the results of the second year of the Heartstart Scotland Project in the Utstein Style. *Resuscitation.* 1993;26:75–88.

127. Eisenberg MS, Horwood BT, Cummins RO, et al. Cardiac arrest and resuscitation: a tale of 29 cities. *Ann Emerg Med.* 1990;19:179–186.

128. Stiell IG, Wells GA, Hebert PC, et al. Association of drug therapy with survival in cardiac arrest: limited role of advanced cardiac life support drugs. *Acad Emerg Med.* 1995;2:264–273.

129. Kloeck W, Cummins RO, Chamberlain D, et al. The universal advanced life support algorithm: an advisory statement from the Advanced Life Support Working Group of the International Liaison Committee on Resuscitation. *Circulation.* 1997;95:2180–2182.

130. Ryan TJ, Anderson JL, Antman EM, et al. ACC/AHA guidelines for the management of patients with acute myocardial infarction: a report of the American College of Cardiology/American Heart Association Task Force on Practice Guidelines (Committee on Management of Acute Myocardial Infarction). *J Am Coll Cardiol.* 1996;28:1328–1428.

131. National Heart, Lung, and Blood Institute. *9-1-1: Rapid Identification and Treatment of Acute Myocardial Infarction.* Bethesda, Maryland: US Department of Health and Human Services, Public Health Service, National Institutes of Health; May 1994. NIH Publication 94-3302.

132. Kereikes DJ, Weaver WD, Anderson JL, et al. Time delays in the diagnosis and treatment of acute myocardial infarction: a tale of eight cities. Report from the Pre-hospital Study Group and the Cincinnati Heart Project. *Am Heart J.* 1990;120:773–780.

133. Shuster M., et al. Effects of prehospital care on outcome in patients with cardiac illness. *Ann Emerg Med.* 1995;26(2):138–144.

134. Gurwitz JH, McLaughlin TJ, Willison DJ, et al. Delayed hospital presentation in patients who have had acute myocardial infarction. *Ann Int Med.* 1997;126(8):593–599.

135. Fibrinolytic Therapy Trialists (FIT) Collaborative Group. Indications for fibrinolytic therapy in suspected acute myocardial infarction: collaborative overview of early mortality and major morbidity results from all randomised trials of more than 1000 patients. *Lancet.* 1994;343:311–322.

136. Weaver WD, Cerqueira M, Hallstrom AP, et al. Prehospital-initiated vs hospital-initiated thrombolytic therapy: the Myocardial Infarction Triage and Intervention Trial. *JAMA.* 1993;270:1211–1216.

137. European Myocardial Infarction Project Group (EMIP). Prehospital thrombolytic therapy in patients with suspected acute myocardial infarction. *NEJM.* 1993;329:383–389.

138. Aufderheide TP, Keeland MH, Hendley GE, et al. The Milwaukee Prehospital Chest Pain Project: phase I. Feasibility and accuracy of prehospital thrombolytic candidate selection. *Am J Cardiol.* 1992;69:991–996.

139. Kereikes DJ, Gibler WB, Martin LH, et al. Cincinnati Heart Project Group. Relative importance of emergency medical system transport and the prehospital electrocardiogram on reducing hospital time delay to therapy for acute myocardial infarction: a preliminary report from the Cincinnati Heart Project. *Am Heart J.* 1992;123:835–840.

140. Canto JG, Rogers WJ, Bowlby LJ, et al. The prehospital electrocardiogram in acute myocardial infarction: is its full potential being realized? *J Am Coll Cardiol.* 1997;29:498–505.

141. Haynes BE, Orange County, California EMS Director: personal communication; 1997.

142. Selker HP, Zalenski RJ, Antman EM, et al. An evaluation of technologies for identifying acute cardiac ischemia in the emergency department: a report from a National Heart Attack Alert Program Working Group. *Ann Emerg Med.* 1997;29:13–87.

143. Eisenberg MJ, Topal EJ. Prehospital administration of aspirin in patients with unstable angina and acute myocardial infarction. *Arch Int Med.* 1996;256(14):1506–1510.

144. ISIS-2 (Second International Study of Infarct Survival) Collaborative Group. Randomized trial of streptokinase, oral aspirin, both, or neither among 17,187 cases of suspected acute myocardial infarction: ISIS-2. *J Am Coll Cardiol.* 1988;12(6 Suppl A):3A–13A.

145. Hoffman JR, Reynolds S. Comparison of nitroglycerin, morphine and furosemide in treatment of presumed pre-hospital pulmonary edema. *Chest.* 1987;92:586–593.

146. Shaw LC, Eitel DR, Walton SL, Pollack M. Prehospital use of intravenous verapamil. *Am J Emerg Med.* 1986;5:207–210.

147. Gausche M, Persse DE, Sugarman T, et al. Adenosine for the prehospital treatment of paroxysmal supraventricular tachycardia. *Ann Emerg Med.* 1994;24(2):183–189.

148. Brady WJ, DeBehnke DJ, Wickman LL, Lindbeck G. Treatment of out-of-hospital supraventricular tachycardia: adenosine versus verapamil. *Acad Emerg Med.* 1996;3(6):574–585.

149. Cummins RO, Graves JR, Larsen MP, et al. Out-of-hospital transcutaneous pacing by emergency medical technicians in patients with asystolic cardiac arrest. *NEJM.* 1993;328(19):1377–1382.

150. Barthell E, Troiano P, Olson D, et al. Prehospital external cardiac pacing: a prospective, controlled clinical trial. *Ann Emerg Med.* 1988;17:1221–1226.

151. Jacobs LM, Sinclair A, Beiser A, D Agostino R. Prehospital life support: benefits in trauma. *J Trauma.* 1984;24(1):8–13.

152. Messick WJ, Rutledge R, Meyer AA. The association of advanced life support training and decreased per capital trauma death rates: an analysis of 12,417 trauma deaths. *J Trauma.* 1992;33:850–855.

153. Domeier RM, O'Conner RE, Delbridge TR, Hunt RC. Use of the pneumatic anti-shock garment (PASG). *Prehosp Emerg Care.* 1997;1(1):32–35.

154. O'Conner RE, Domeier RM. An evaluation of the pneumatic anti-shock garment (PASG) in various clinical settings. *Prehosp Emerg Care.* 1997;1(1):36–44.

155. Mattox KL, Bickell WH, Pepe PE, et al. Prospective randomized evaluation of anti-shock MAST in post-traumatic hypotension. *J Trauma.* 1986;26:779–786.

156. Bickell WH, Pepe PE, Bailey ML, et al. Randomized trial of pneumatic anti-shock garments in the prehospital management of penetrating abdominal injuries. *Ann Emerg Med.* 1987;16:653–658.

157. Mattox KL, Bickell W, Pepe PE, et al. Prospective MAST study in 911 patients. *J Trauma.* 1989;29:1104–1112.

158. Chang FC, Harrison PB, Beech RR, Helmer SD. PASG: does it help in the management of traumatic shock? *J Trauma.* 1995;39:453–456.

159. Salvucci AA, Koenig KL, Stratton S. The pneumatic anti-shock garment (PASG): can we really recommend it? *Prehosp Emerg Care.* 1998;2(1):86–87.

160. Kaweski SM, Sise MJ, Virgilio RW. The effects of prehospital fluids on survival in trauma patients. *J Trauma.* 1990;30(10):1215.

161. Dalton AM. Prehospital intravenous fluid replacement in trauma: an outmoded concept? *J R Soc Med.* 1995;88(4):213P–216P.

162. Teach SJ, Antosia RE, Lund DP, Fleischer GR. Prehospital fluid therapy in pediatric trauma patients. *Ped Emerg Care.* 1995;11(1):5–8.

163. Bickell WH, Wall MJ, Pepe PE, et al. Immediate versus delayed fluid resuscitation for hypotensive patients with penetrating torso injuries. *NEJM.* 1994;331(17):1105–1109.

164. Chestnut RM, Marshall LF, Klauber MR, et al. The role of secondary brain injury in determining outcome from severe brain injury. *J Trauma.* 1993;34(2):216–222.

165. Fearnside MR, Cook RJ, McDougall P, et al. The Westmead Head Injury Project outcome in severe head injury: a comparative analysis of pre-hospital, clinical, and CT variables. *Br J Neurosurg.* 1993;7:267–279.

166. Obrist WD, Langfit TW, Jaggi JL, et al. Cerebral blood flow and metabolism in comatose patients with acute head injury. *J Neurosurg.* 1984;61:241–253.

167. Winchell RW, Hoyt DB. Endotracheal intubation in the field improves survival in patients with severe head injury. *Arch Surg.* 1997;132:592–597.

167A. Ochs, M. The use of neuromuscular blocking agents and advanced sedation by field EMT-Paramedics for more effective airway management in adult trauma patients with Glasgow Coma Score of 8 or less. Trial study interim report to the California Commission on Emergency Medical Services, Sacramento, CA. June 28, 2000.

168. Chan D, Goldberg R, Tascone A, et al. The effect of spinal immobilization on healthy volunteers. *Ann Emerg Med.* 1989;18:918–924.

169. Johnson DR, Hauswald M, Stockoff MS. Comparison of a vacuum splint device to a rigid backboard for spinal immobilization. *Am J Emerg Med.* 1996;14:369–372.

170. Hoffman JR, Schriger DL, Mower W, et al. Low-risk criteria for cervical-spine radiography in blunt trauma: a prospective study. *Ann Emerg Med.* 1992;21:1454–1460.

171. Domeier RM, Evans RW, Swor RA, et al. Prehospital clinical findings associated with spinal injury. *Prehosp Emerg Care.* 1997;1(1):11–15.

172. Pons PT. Nitrous oxide analgesia. *Emerg Med Clinics N America.* 1988;6:777–782.

173. Johnson JC, Atherton GL. Effectiveness of nitrous oxide in a rural EMS system. *J Emerg Med.* 1991;9:44–53.

174. Browning RG, et al. 50% Dextrose: antidote or toxin? *Ann Emerg Med.* 1990;19:683–687.

175. Nielsen MM, Barsan WG, Dimlich RVW. Effect of IV glucose on survival and neurologic outcome after cardiac arrest [abstract]. *Ann Emerg Med.* 1991;20:454.

176. Tracey F, Crawford VLS, Lawson JT, et al. Hyperglycemia and mortality from acute stroke. *Quart J Med.* 1993;86:439–446.

177. Jones JL, Ray VG, Gough JE, et al. Determination of prehospital blood glucose: a prospective controlled study. *J Emerg Med.* 1992;10:679–682.

178. Hoffman RS, Goldfrank LR. The poisoned patient with altered consciousness: controversies in the use of a coma cocktail. *JAMA.* 1995;274(7):562–569.

179. Vukmir RB, Paris PM, Yealy DM. Glucagon: Prehospital therapy for hypoglycemia. *Ann Emerg Med.* 1991;20:375–379.

180. Reuler JB, Girard DE, Cooney TG. Wernicke's encephalopathy. *NEJM.* 1985;312:1035–1039.

181. Watson AJS, Walker JF, Tomkin GH, et al. Acute Wernicke's encephalopathy precipitated by glucose loading. *Ir J Med Sci.* 1981;150:301–303.

182. Yealy DM, Paris PM, Kaplan RM, et al. The safety of prehospital naloxone administration by paramedics. *Ann Emerg Med.* 1990;19:902–905.

183. Merigian KS. Cocaine-induced ventricular arrhythmias and rapid atrial fibrillation temporally related to naloxone administration. *Am J Emerg Med.* 1993;11:96–97.

184. Osterwalder JJ. Naloxone for intoxications with intravenous heroin and heroin mixtures: harmless or hazardous? A prospective clinical study. *Clin Tox.* 1996; 34(4):409.

185. Hoffman JR, Schriger DL, Luo JS. The empiric use of naloxone in patients with altered mental status: a reappraisal. *Ann Emerg Med.* 1991;20(3):246–252.

186. Gueye PN, Hoffman JR, Taboulet P, et al. Empiric use of flumazenil in comatose patients: limited applicability of criteria to define low risk. *Ann Emerg Med.* 1996;27:730–735.

187. Seigler RS. The administration of rectal diazepam for acute management of seizures. *J Emerg Med.* 1990;8: 155–159. *Ped Emerg Care.* 1997;13(2):92–94.

188. Chamberlain JM, Altieri MA, Futterman C, Young GM, Ochsenschlager DW, Waisman Y. A prospective randomized study comparing intramuscular midazolam with intravenous diazepam for the treatment of seizures in children. *Ped Emerg Care.* 1997;13(2):89–91.

189. Kuisma M, Roine RO. Propofol in prehospital treatment of convulsive status epilepticus. *Epilepsia* 1995; 36(12):1241–1243.

190. Verdile VP, Tutsock G, Paris PM, Kennedy RA. Out-of-hospital deliveries: a five-year experience. *Prehosp Disaster Med.* 1995;10(1):10–13.

191. Pond SM, Lewis-Driver DJ, Williams GM, et al. Gastric emptying in acute overdose: a prospective randomized controlled trial. *Med J Austr.* 1995;163:345–349.

192. Crockett R, Krishel SJ, Manoguerra A, et al. Prehospital use of activated charcoal: a pilot study. *J Emerg Med.* 1996;14(3):335–338.

193. Lindbeck GH, Burns DM, Rockwell DD. Out-of-hospital provider use of epinephrine for allergic reactions: pilot program. *Acad Emerg Med.* 1995;2:592–596.

194. Fortenberry JE, Laine J, Shalit M. Use of epinephrine for anaphylaxis by emergency medical technicians in a wilderness setting. *Ann Emerg Med.* 1995;25(6):785–787.

195. Horowitz BZ, Jadallah S, Derlet RW. Fatal intracranial bleeding associated with prehospital use of epinephrine. *Ann Emerg Med.* 1996;28:725–727.

CHAPTER 16

Communications

James J. Augustine, MD

Introduction

How much information is needed by the emergency physician and the Emergency Medical Technician (EMT) to improve the clinical care of a patient in the prehospital setting? When, and in what form, should that information be presented to the emergency physician? How can data be collated to efficiently perform quality improvement activities for medical and administrative operations of EMS organizations? And how can the uncounted new technologies be implemented in time and cost-effective ways to improve all facets of system operations?

These are areas for medical directors' input to EMS systems upon entry to the new millennium. Communications technology has progressed so rapidly that multimedia presentation of patient information may overwhelm those providing medical oversight. This chapter will review the many components of communications that must be addressed by EMS leaders.

Prehospital medical care systems interact with numerous public groups in the provision of services. Ideally, the communications system integrates the various delivery components into the smooth, seamless operation desired and expected by the public. Therefore, emergency medical services must have an efficient and coordinated system for communication with:

- Persons requesting assistance (systems access and dispatch)
- Fire, law enforcement, and other EMS units
- Medical oversight
- The community (public education)
- Community service agencies
- Hospital personnel (medical records)
- EMS administration (administrative records)
- Disaster service providers

Each system must consider the unique nature of its resources, geography, and funding to provide a functional and cost-efficient system. Rapid changes in the communication needs of the EMS community and the available equipment require continual monitoring by the medical directors. The system medical director must provide oversight for all elements that affect emergency medical care.

Objectives of a Communications System

The EMS communications system integrates the components, service providers, and administrators to provide quality emergency medical care. It establishes the protocols for day-to-day operations, with flexibility and redundancy necessary for disasters and other special needs. The efficiency of the system must be measured locally, as each EMS provider has unique geography, medical service providers, and public expectations to consider in system design. Common components of a comprehensive system are described in this and subsequent chapters on dispatch, data collection, and medical control.

Communication system priorities differ somewhat between rural and urban systems. Rural providers usually service large geographic areas, have relatively long prehospital response and transport times, and operate with a variety of response providers. Communication technology appropriate for the service's terrain and distance is necessary. Rural systems generally have lower service volumes and a greater prevalence of volunteer providers, factors that increase the importance of skilled and available direct medical oversight. A 1988 survey of state EMS programs by the National Association of State EMS Directors (NASEMSD) revealed that 31 states and territories had inadequate EMS radio system coverage in some rural areas. There is no indication that all deficiencies have been addressed. Radio frequency congestion or interference was reported in 32 states, primarily in urban areas.[1]

Urban systems generally will have higher call volumes and propensity for radio congestion. These factors will differentiate the radio frequencies most useful for the services and the modes for integrating dispatch and medical control. The relative importance of trained emergency medical dispatching may also be greater in rural settings, to allow for use of pre-arrival instructions, and provide a timely and appropriate response of personnel and equipment.

The Medical Directors' Responsibility

Medical directors oversee the provision of quality emergency medical care, and prioritize those aspects of the communications system that promote optimal care. This oversight begins with a public education program that encourages appropriate and timely use of EMS. Single-number access (such as 9-1-1) provides timely activation and is easily accepted and taught. Scene medical care is facilitated by support from dispatch, communications protocols, and inter-agency linkages with fire, law enforcement, and other EMS units. Medical conversations with medical oversight physicians should be easily available, but evaluation and treatment protocols will promote timely standardized care. Medical records document that care, and provide input for quality improvement and research activities.

Administrative information systems, though not directly patient-care related, maintain the service available for patient care. Administrative information on nuts-and-bolts issues of vehicle maintenance, equipment and supplies, personnel licensure and education, and facility upkeep are necessary. Human-resource issues of due process, health surveillance, and employee recognition are other components of the management information system supporting direct medical care.

Components of an EMS Communications System

Access

Researchers and providers have identified a clear deficit in public recognition of emergency medical situations and activation of the EMS system.[2,3] The advancement in timely emergency care options for acute heart disease, strokes, and trauma have driven many public education activities about activation of 9-1-1. Activation is accomplished in a six-step process: (1) a need is detected; (2) a location is determined; (3) an appropriate method of transport and facility to provide that care is decided upon; (4) a provider of that service is identified; (5) a communications device and/or telephone number is located to access; and (6) contact is made directly or indirectly with the emergency service.[1]

The system must facilitate each of these steps, and educate members of the general public about the proper process.[4] In its simplest form, the system must provide a mechanism by which any citizen with an urgent medical need can easily and reliably access emergency providers. The most common access system remains the landline telephone, but the popularity of the cellular phone is challenging many EMS systems to locate emergency call sites. A combination access and location system is available through the Global Positioning System tied to cellular phones. Mainly vehicle-based, this system is activated by a single button in the vehicle, which connects the caller to an operator who automatically is able to locate the position of the emergency site. The operator can then connect the caller to the closest indicated Public Safety Answering Point (PSAP).

In certain geographic areas, the phone systems are supplemented with emergency call boxes, citizen and marine band radios, and direct intercom systems. In the United States, emergency number 9-1-1 for access to all emergency providers is being implemented with federal, state, and local government support. Seven-digit numbers are difficult to remember and may cause a time delay in requesting emergency assistance. The enhanced 9-1-1 (or E9-1-1) system, activated from a landline, permits automatic caller locations and phone number identification to be displayed at the dispatching site. This feature identifies the caller address to eliminate telephone queries about emergency location in many situations. This modification, although slightly more expensive, can reduce false alarm requests and offer assistance to those callers unable to communicate due to age or nature of injury. This identification can be automatically tied to a system status computer, which will then immediately display the closest available emergency responders.

There is now recognized that 9-1-1 systems increase public safety demands.[5] Some members of the public now view 9-1-1 as the access to non-emergency services, which has resulted in some "gridlock" conditions and rollover of calls to answering systems. System demands also increase as emergency units must respond to "hang-up" calls. These calls are made by curious citizens or youth, testing the system to see how it works, but have also originated from portable phones that dial random numbers as their batteries fade.

In those areas without 9-1-1, access to the emergency system should be made as easy as possible with a single telephone number, publicized as widely as possible. In some areas dialing 9-1-1 gets an operator who will manually relay the call to the appropriate emergency agency. However, in some areas this operator is hundreds of miles from the emergency and may have difficulty in contacting local emergency providers.

Cellular phones do not have automatic caller identification, and often these calls are forwarded to a central PSAP, which may be the state police or other regional law enforcement organization. The caller must then identify the location of the call, which may be a challenge. There is an opportunity to apply newer technology to define the location of the cellular phone, and the federal government is attempting to implement this technology as a national standard.

Dispatch

The responsibility and function of the EMS dispatcher have evolved as demand for EMS services has grown and public expectations for a higher level of care have evolved. Just as the television show "Emergency" raised public awareness of highly trained and equipped prehospital care providers, the show "Rescue 9-1-1" has emphasized the role of the individual receiving the emergency call.

The emergency medical dispatcher now has the role of call receiving, interrogation, determining response configuration and mode, and delivering any appropriate pre-arrival instructions to the caller.[6] Following the initial response, the dispatcher supports field operations with additional information regarding scene location, a complete description of the medical complaints, road conditions, potential hazards, special approaches, and simultaneous fire and police response. The dispatcher may designate which channel and hospital to use for medical control, and may also assist in linking field and hospital personnel. In some configurations, dispatch assists in research data collection, time logging, and prompting for re-

peat drugs, procedures, or scene times. Dispatchers should be knowledgeable of the entire emergency response system, and be able to access all necessary support resources. Any medical protocols used should be reviewed by medical oversight. Properly administered, emergency medical dispatch (EMD) in metropolitan areas will shorten average response times for urgent patients, decrease unnecessary use of backup resources, improve public perception of emergency services, and help minimize the inappropriate use of emergency resources.[6] EMD may also encourage the system to reduce use of "lights and siren" response, decreasing the likelihood of vehicle accidents.

Many systems provide prearrival instructions to the caller until emergency medical personnel arrive. Cardiopulmonary resuscitation and other first-aid skills are taught or guided by this telephone link. In some localities, the dispatcher operating under medical standing orders will provide these instructions. In other areas, the radio dispatcher is separate from the person performing the interrogation and providing telephone instructions.

Ideally, one dispatch center should operate in an EMS system with trained emergency medical dispatchers. Central dispatch will usually save money, manpower, and equipment when compared to individual dispatch centers for each community. It will also minimize time delays in coordinating scene responses, particularly near jurisdictional borders. The dispatch center will coordinate activities among responding vehicles, including special rescue units, support services, police, fire, utilities, and tow vehicles. Without timely coordination and communication, the full life-saving potential of the system may not be realized.

Medical Oversight Communications

One of the hallmarks of early EMS development was the initiation of medical communications between trained field technicians and direct medical oversight. This development allowed the delegation of complex medical tasks and equipment from a licensed physician to the out-of-hospital scene. Direct medical oversight is best provided by experienced physicians who are immediately available for medical guidance of field personnel. This availability has resulted in a continuous improvement process in the hardware designed for field to hospital medical communications. Early EMS systems utilized radio communications from the field to the system medical director. If there are a large number of receiving hospitals, this arrangement may not be practical in terms of available radio frequencies or equipment/personnel expenses. Under these circumstances, direct medical oversight is provided by a single resource hospital "base station." When the EMS system uses a non-receiving base station for direct medical oversight, it may become the responsibility of the base station to notify the receiving facility of the emergency situation, the patient's condition, the treatment, and the expected time of arrival. It is the responsibility of the regional EMS authority to determine system needs considering the number of receiving hospitals and field units requiring communication channels. When voice communication is not used for direct medical oversight, the receiving hospital should be notified, through the dispatcher, of the patient's condition, expected time of arrival, and other pertinent medical data that will make the receiving facility better able to respond at the time of the patient's arrival.

The next generation of medical communication devices added another radio linkage that allowed further assessment of patient condition by medical control. This system was glorified in the series Emergency, with Johnnie and Roy transmitting biotelemetry information to the Rampart base station. These communication devices came to be implemented in many EMS systems, transmitting EKG rhythm strips (biotelemetry) from field to hospital. Multiple studies have suggested that in systems with paramedics well trained in rhythm interpretation, telemetry does not improve patient care.[7,8] A later derivation, however, using twelve-lead EKG transmission has evolved as a useful tool for minimizing the time to administration of thrombolytic therapy.

The next advances in documentation came with the use of cellular phones, broadening the options and reliability of the system. Direct medical oversight communications between physician and provider may be by telephone (fixed or cellular), radio, or combinations of the two. Selection of equipment for hospital-to-ambulance communications must take into consideration transmission interference and distances, as previously outlined.

Many systems have purchased instant developing cameras for photo documentation of the emergency scene; ED personnel found great value in this photographic addition to the prehospital care report (PCR).[9] Use of video documentation has led to videocamera use, digital cameras, and even the use of media film footage to add critical information to a verbal report Media coverage of major incidents in the community, with ground and helicopter-based cameras, can be an incredibly valuable method of communicating scene information to medical direction, hospitals, and other public safety decision-makers. This electronic media presence at major incident scenes, and the media's ability to disseminate messages very rapidly to a wide audience, allow safety planners to consider the electronic media as the "fourth public safety agency."

The next generation of direct medical oversight communications devices is in early implementation phases, particularly in the U.S. military.[10] These devices will allow multimedia exchange between field personnel and physicians, with immediate and simultaneous audio, video, and biodata exchange. Such systems were field tested in Atlanta during the 1996 Olympic games, when concerns about terrorist activity prompted the use of videolinking technology from the scene directly to the Pentagon.

Another electronic interface useful for timely documentation are devices for computerizing the care records. A variety of hardware devices from hand held devices to laptop computers have been designed with software for prehospital use. The software can be designed for instantaneous transmission to the receiving hospital, integrated quality assurance, data collection, and linkage to digital cameras. ED providers value typed PCRs because they are legible and formatted consistently. There are designs that now package standing protocols, dosage calculators, medical references, and guides to other hazards. They can also be married to global positioning devices and cellular phones for further utility.

Direct Medical Oversight and Communication Options

Protocols for evaluation and treatment have complemented training objectives, and improved the standard for patient care.[11] Requirements for voice contact have been shown to increase scene times, and may actually increase the inappropriate use of drugs and intravenous lines.[12,13] Physician contact rarely resulted in significant changes in therapy, and those patients who would benefit were easily identified through evaluation protocols.[14] Protocol errors were uncommon in another study, and about half the errors were by the base hospital.[15] For the multiple trauma patient, direct medical oversight may increase the accuracy of triage to a trauma facility.[16] In all systems, standing orders must be available to provide a backup system for patient care in the event of communications failure.

When EMT-to-hospital communication is advantageous for patient care, the conversation will be direct and standardized.[17] The prehospital provider identifies himself and gives an estimated time to arrival. The patient's age, chief complaint, pertinent history, and physical exam should be conveyed. Vital signs should be identified as stable; if not stable, only then, the values given. Standing orders already performed (airway, IV, drugs given) should be reported, and further orders requested as necessary. Any orders given by direct medical oversight should be repeated to insure accurate conveyance of medical information. Detailed reports should wait until hospital arrival.[18]

Hardware

System hardware requirements will be specific to the area's geography, budget, and communication goals. In all systems, there should be redundancy and flexibility engineered and available. Fixed bases are established in the communications centers, medical facilities, and EMS vehicle stations. For large service areas, repeaters are necessary. These may be ground-based or satellite units. The mobile radio (in vehicles) and portable radio components are integrated. In most areas of the country, cellular phone systems may be linked as another communication alternative. Air ambulance units, if part of the system, must also be integrated into the communications system. Advantages and disadvantages of various communication system configurations are described below.

VHF Radio Systems

Many rural and suburban EMS systems utilize VHF (Very High Frequency) high band radios that, without repeaters, have approximately a 15-mile range on flat terrain. VHF radio systems are simplex, which means messages can be sent only one way at a time.

Under the current Federal Communications Commission (FCC) rules, EMS frequencies are licensed in the Special Emergency Radio Service (SERS), which does not allow repeaters in the VHF band. This regulation results in some range limitations in rural areas. Other factors affecting range include antenna height and power output.

UHF Radio Systems

Generally, more heavily populated areas rely upon UHF (Ultra High Frequency) EMS radio systems. UHF systems usually are duplex systems, which means that messages can be sent and received simultaneously. The FCC has designated 10 UHF medical channels within the UHF spectrum in the SERS. Licensees are authorized to use all 10 channels and, although these frequencies usually do not have the range of VHF frequencies, they can penetrate buildings better; mobile relays or repeaters may be added to extend range.

In both VHF and UHF radio systems, many EMS agencies have installed some type of coded squelch system to prevent monitoring or interference of medical communications by unrelated agencies. Coded squelch systems can prevent other agencies from hearing radio transmissions, but they do not prevent other transmissions on the same frequencies from interfering with or blocking messages. Some areas, especially in the western United States, interface EMS radios with mountaintop microwave base stations. Depending upon the height of the mountains, this system can extend EMS radio system coverage to large geographic areas.[19]

Radio Telephone Switching Systems

A few areas have installed radio telephone switching systems (RTSS) to enable ambulance crews to talk to hospital staffs or dispatch centers beyond the normal ranges of VHF or UHF radio systems. These systems enable mobile radios, usually UHF, to interface with telephone lines and extend radio system coverage to rural areas. The RTSS enables full duplex systems and, with appropriate equipment, accommodates EKG telemetry with physician-provider interrupt capabilities.

Microwave Relays

EMS radio systems also can be interfaced with microwave relays extending along major highways, extending the ranges of the radio system up to hundreds of miles by converting radio frequencies into telephone/microwave frequencies and back to radio frequencies on the receiving end. Microwave systems can accommodate a wide variety of radio systems for state and local emergency services, and for non-emergency services such as highway maintenance crews.

800 MHz Public Safety Trunking Systems

The FCC has designated 800 MHz public safety radio frequencies (821–824 MHz and 866–869 MHz) to be used in public safety trunking radio systems. EMS agencies have participated in the planning process with the local chapter of the Associated Public Safety Communications Officers (APCO). Trunked systems, which usually are computerized, allow more efficient use of frequencies because the computer automatically searches for an open frequency when a call is made. Thus the caller is not required to select a frequency manually each time, helping to prevent radio frequency congestion and interference. Trunking is currently permitted by the FCC in the 800 MHz frequency band, including the UHF bands.

A major difficulty has evolved in 800 trunked systems with frequency compatibility. The FCC allowed different manufacturers to use different protocols or "architectures" for equipment design, so one system may not match another. This mismatch causes problems with communication between adjacent service areas if two different systems are used. Another challenge is posed by 800 MHz systems in that vehicle repeaters are not allowed, so EMS responders who need communications while caring for patients inside homes or other settings away from the ambulance may not be able to access the closest tower.

In some areas with 800 MHz trunked systems, EMS agencies have opted to stay on UHF frequencies, while other public safety agencies have switched over to the 800 MHz frequencies. Even in these situations, it is important for EMS entities to be involved in the planning process, and to have some mechanisms to communicate with other public safety responders. A major drawback to 800 MHz radio systems for rural areas is the limited range of these frequencies. Many more repeaters are usually needed to cover a given geographic area than would be required with lower band frequencies, which can significantly increase the cost of providing 800 MHz radio systems in rural areas.

Cellular Telephone

Cellular telephone systems are becoming common in urban areas and are beginning to spread to rural areas as well. Advantages of cellular telephones for EMS communications include: they provide an alternate means of communicating in some radio dead spot areas; they are easy to use; they provide easy access to the telephone systems; and they provide du-plex voice capabilities. They can also provide mobile 9-1-1 emergency access. Disadvantages of cellular systems include: dedicated lines usually are not available or are costly; they may become overloaded during disaster situations; and, in multi-unit or multi-agency responses, it can be operationally difficult to coordinate multiple cellular users in the field (because different users cannot monitor each other's transmissions). Taking into account these limitations, cellular telephone can provide a good supplement to EMS radio systems, but they should not be relied upon exclusively.

Land Mobile Satellite Communications

In sparsely populated, remote rural areas, providing EMS radio system coverage can be very expensive. Land mobile satellite communications may provide a cost-effective alternative to terrestrial radio systems in rural areas. Several companies are now developing this technology. Some plan to use satellites in "fixed" geostationary orbits, while others plan to use multiple low-orbit satellites. These systems will use omni-directional antennas, more compact than the traditional satellite dishes that must be pointed at a satellite in a fixed point in the sky.

Digital Technology

New digital technologies have been developed that will enable radios to utilize narrower frequency bands, thereby significantly increasing the number of frequencies available within each band. However, converting to this new technology requires costly replacement of existing radio systems.

Integrating Fire, Law Enforcement, and EMS Response

There are three common organizational structures for EMS communications centers: (1) A single center houses all staff communication equipment for dispatch and coordination of police, fire, and EMS; (2) The communication center is located in and operated by a police or fire department, with EMS dispatch responsibility; (3) Each public service division, police, fire, and EMS has a separate communication center. While recognizing local priorities, the configuration of the center is not as important as the mechanism to ensure that vital functions of EMS are coordinated. It is desirable for EMS, police, and fire personnel to have the capability of communicating directly with each other regarding needs for additional personnel or equipment, traffic or geographic problems, and to better coordinate activity in multiple response situations. Coordinated communications are essential in special circumstances such as hazardous materials incidents, multiple casualty incidents and disasters.

A state EMS communications plan is available in most states to assist local areas in emergency interfaces. Radio frequency coordination is a common problem locally and nationally. The FCC regulates public safety services, as with all radio frequency users. Presently EMS radio users are licensed under the SERS, competing with veterinarians, hospitals, school buses, rescue, and relief organizations for available frequencies. In some locations, severe radio congestion has occurred. The FCC has been petitioned to designate a separate Emergency Medical Radio Service, to be included within the public-safety radio service and overseen by groups more familiar with the special needs of EMS. This change would help alleviate congestion on current and future radio frequency bands. Detailed reference on radio frequency spectrum usage is available.[20]

EMS Communications Planning

A comprehensive state EMS communications plan is available in most states to assist local areas in emergency communications systems development. As technologies and frequency regulating requirements change, state EMS communications plans should be periodically updated. To help address this need, the NASEMSD contracted for development of a two-volume planning guide, "Planning Emergency Medical Communications." One guide deals with planning at the state level and the other deals with planning at the local level.

Major Incident Communications

Emergency service communications is *the* critical component of any major incident or disaster plan. Communication procedures to be used during a major incident should be easily identified so resources can be coordinated under stress. Procedures should resemble the day-to-day communication patterns as much as possible. The ability must exist to override components of the communications system and block

out nonessential communications. Backup procedures and equipment should be available in the event of component failure. Certain community-wide disasters often render the public telephone system temporarily inoperable, so emergency radios should be available and alternate radio frequencies designated if usual channels become overloaded. To overcome the problem of incompatible radio frequencies among emergency response agencies working together in a disaster situation, some systems have installed inexpensive radio scanners in response vehicles and dispatch centers. These scanners allow the responders to listen in on each other, to improve the communications net despite otherwise incompatible radios.[21]

Hospital Communication Systems

Hospitals providing direct medical oversight ideally should establish a communications network with other hospitals in the system regarding the availability of beds and other resources. This network becomes especially important during multiple-casualty incidents when triage and transportation of many victims must occur in a timely manner. Hospital-to-hospital communication usually involves VHF high-band or dedicated landlines, although microwave is another consideration. Ideally, hospital communications systems should use more confidential modes of transmission, since they include more sensitive medical information. Hospital networks also include dedicated air and ground ambulance units that supplement the system.

Emergency Medical Care Records

Communications with other medical personnel and legal documentation of the patient interaction is provided by the medical report. Copies of this document should be kept in the patient's permanent hospital medical record, filed with the EMS service, and available for many reporting and auditing purposes. The components of the interaction record should represent a total picture of the EMS service provided. A minimum data set has been proposed, but the perfect incident report system remains to be designed.[22,23] Since the prehospital care report (PCR) is often the only documentation of the field situation and care, medical directors should stress the importance of historical points and observations at the scene, includ-

COMMUNICATIONS

ing environmental and situational factors.[24] Education should stress the importance of a PCR that is accurate, precise, comprehensive, legible, objective, and time-sequenced.[25] Proper documentation may prevent some lawsuits and dramatically improve the defense in others.[26] Documentation is particularly important for calls that do not result in patient transport, because of questions of informed consent and abandonment.

Several documentation formats have been proposed to structure the PCR.[27] The provider must select a memory cue that is appropriate and can be consistently applied, with an audit and review system that reinforces documentation priorities. Medical director overview is a requirement. The key document components are:

- Patient demographics
- Incident times
- Dispatch information and nature of call
- Vital signs recorded and timed
- Objective observations, of patient, environment, and situation
- Assessments, treatments, and reassessment
- Direct medical oversight received
- Pertinent oral statements made by the patient or bystanders
- Unusual circumstances arising during the incident

The medical documentation process is completed by the medical review and audit process, with quality management (QM) feedback to the provider.[28]

Administrative Records

Administrative records are necessary for the efficient operation of an EMS service and the provision of quality care. Certification and continuing education of personnel should be logged to ensure appropriate provider qualification. For services using controlled drugs, state licensure is required. Vehicle, equipment, and supply purchase and maintenance are recorded. Documentation of equipment problems and their resolution are particularly critical, especially patient-care equipment. Public relations and service commitments are an increasing responsibility of EMS agencies. Service complaints from the public served by the system should be recognized as opportunities for ser-

vice improvement, and respected as well for liability potential.

Communicating with Public and Media Relations

The EMS system continually interacts with the general public, the same public that ultimately funds the system. System administrators and providers should respect this relationship and acknowledge their responsibility. Informal and inexpensive public interaction programs, like school displays and blood pressure checks, may be as effective as more formal and expensive demonstrations. The least expensive and most effective communication program is the everyday interaction with patients, bystanders, and family. Each run has the potential for extensive public interaction, with serious and large incidents drawing media coverage. Media involvement should be positive and productive, as tremendous damage can be inflicted to those systems that ignore or antagonize these communications experts.[29] Many systems design programs that combine public and media interaction; drunk-driving demonstrations, open houses, and extrication or disaster drills can foster good relationships among these important groups, and facilitate an ongoing productive partnership with the service community.

Setting up the Communication Network

A critical planning item is the need for information sharing between the various public safety agencies, and within the component elements of the EMS system. Integrating information systems within the EMS agency will facilitate:

- Crew scheduling
- Vehicle maintenance
- Medical properties inventory
- Service billing
- Regulatory compliance
- Equipment maintenance
- Management reporting
- Quality management
- Risk management
- Customer service efforts

Outside the EMS agency, efforts to integrate information systems may include

- Fire service dual reporting
- Integration with hospital information systems
- The regional disaster service agency
- Media reports
- Regulatory agency reporting

The communication system sets the stage for high-quality patient care. A needs assessment should be performed, and objectives outlined for the various communication components. Respecting geographic, environmental, and operational factors, hardware and appropriate licenses are obtained.

New configurations of system access, dispatch, and medical communications are becoming available. Smart radio systems integrate medical and administrative roles.[30] System status management and vehicle locator systems are other efficiency tools to facilitate medical care and allow administrative oversight.[31]

Medical and administrative protocols further improve operational efficiency. Medical standing orders, based on patient complaint (e.g., short of breath) or problem (e.g., through the chest), guide the EMT through evaluation and care delivery. With regular QM and medical review, protocols also guide the educational process, personnel evaluation, and recognition programs.[32]

Administrative protocols should guide system personnel in such diverse areas as management of bodily substance exposures, restocking of care supplies, handling of controlled substances, nontransports situations, "Do Not Resuscitate" requests, complaint response, and vehicle maintenance.

Integrating with Other EMS Priorities

The wide variety of communication needs in 21st century EMS will be well served by the World Wide Web. The extension of internet-based communication systems will influence each component of the EMS system, from provider education, to on-line medical direction, to regulatory compliance. A vast library of linkages can serve the needs of individual providers and EMS system leaders.[33] The communication system will facilitate the delivery of high-quality emergency medical care. It can enable productive relationships with the general public and other emergency responders. It can bring the guidance of the direct medical oversight physician to each patient interaction. It is the foundation for appropriate and timely response to multiple casualty and disaster incidents. It provides the input material for data collection, system evaluation, and quality improvement programs.

With these ideals, communications is relegated a high priority in EMS system design and operation. The medical director should approve those communication components affecting medical care. As communication hardware improves the linkage between EMS provider and direct medical oversight, the system medical director should oversee the application to avoid data overload. Care enhancement will occur through skillful application.

References

1. Johnson M. The States of EMS Communications, unpublished. *National Assoc of State EMS Directors.* Carlsbad, CA, 1988.
2. Mayron R, et al. The 9-1-1 Emergency Telephone Number. *Amer J Emerg Med.* 1985;2:491–493.
3. Knolle LL, et al. Knowledge of Access to and Use of the EMS System in a Rural Illinois County. *Amer J Preventive Med.* 1989;5:164–169.
4. Edwards K. Emergency—When to call the squad. *Ohio Med.* 1990;Sept:12–13.
5. Doyle I. Communications—The Critical Link. *Rescue Emerg Med Ser.* 1992;2(1):26–27.
6. Slovis CM, et al. A Priority Dispatch System for EMS. *Ann Emerg Med.* 1985;14:1055–1060.
7. Pozen MW, et al. Cost and Utility Considerations in Implementing Ambulance Telemetry. *Heart & Lung.* 1980;9:866–872.
8. Cayten CG, et al. The Effect of Telemetry on Urban Prehospital Cardiac Care. *Ann Emerg Med.* 1985;14:976–981.
9. Hunt RC. Comparison of Motor Vehicle Damage Documentation in EMS Run Reports Compared with Photographic Documentation. *Ann Emerg Med.* 1993;22:651–656.
10. Nordberg M. Taking it to the Streets: Telemedicine Update. *EMS Magazine.* 1999;28(8):37–39.
11. Hunt RC, et al. Standing Orders vs. Voice Control *JEMS.* 1982;7(11):26–31.
12. Pointer JE, et al. Effect of standing orders on field times. *Ann Emerg Med.* 1989;18:1119.
13. Pointer JE, et al. The impact of standing orders on meds & skill selection: paramedic assessment, and hospital outcome. *Prehosp Disaster Med.* 1991;6:303.
14. Hoffman JR, et al. Does PM-base hospital contact result in beneficial deviations from standard prehospital protocols? *West J Med.* 1990;153:282.
15. Wasserberger J, et al. Base station prehospital care. *Ann Emerg Med.* 1987;16:867.

16. Champion H. Effect of Medical Direction of Trauma Triage. *J Trauma*. 28:235–239.

17. Augustine J. Medical Direction and EMS. *EMS Magazine*. 2001;30(5):65–69.

18. Shanaberger C. If It Isn't Written Down . . . *JEMS*. 1990;15(6):79–80.

19. Holliman CJ. Maximizing prehospital radio communications. *JEMS*. 1990;15(5):5–9.

20. Johnson MS, et al. Is EMS communicating with the FCC? *JEMS*. 1989;14(6):51–56.

21. Garshnek V. Telecommunications Systems in Support of Disaster Medicine: Applications of Basic Information Pathways. *Ann Emerg Med*. 1999;34:213–218.

22. Shanaberger C. The Unrefined Art of Documentation. *JEMS*. 1992;(17)1:155–157.

23. Hedges JR, et al. Minimum Data Set for EMS Report Form: Historical Development and Future Implications. *Prehospital & Disaster Med*. 1990;5(10):383–384.

24. Brown-Nixon C. Field Documentation Myths. *Emerg Med Ser*. 1990;19:8,18–21.

25. Strange J. Does Your Documentation Reflect Your Care? *Emerg Med Ser*. 1990;19:8.

26. Lazar RA, et al. Presumed Insufficient. *JEMS*. 1990; 15(8);23–29.

27. Ball R. Documentation—The Overlooked Aspect of Emergency Care. *JEMS*. 1990;15(5):31–32.

28. Pointer JE. The ALS base hospital audit for medical control in an EMS system. *Ann Emerg Med*. 1987;16:557.

29. Stephens K. Effective news media handling critical at accident sites. *Emergency Medicine & Ambulatory Care News*. June 1989;5.

30. Adler S. Smart Radio Systems. *Emergency Medical Services*. 1988;17:37–38.

31. Stout J. System status management. *JEMS*. 1989;14(4): 65–71.

32. Stewart C. Communications with EMS providers. *EMCNA*. 1990;8:103.

33. Reeder Lee. Best EMS Web Sites. *JEMS*. 1996;21(8):56–57.

Emergency Medical Dispatch

Jeff J. Clawson, MD

Introduction

Surviving a life-threatening medical emergency is predicated by a series of actions that optimally occur within precisely defined periods of time. If all necessary actions occur within the prescribed time periods and are performed according to defined standards, the patient has a significantly increased chance of survival. The series of actions that must take place for one to survive a medical emergency has been called the "chain of survival." Survival is not the only issue. If the prescribed actions are performed late or inappropriately, the patient may survive, but impaired brain function or paralysis may result.

Occupying the first link in the chain of survival, the pre-response link, is the emergency medical dispatcher (EMD). Following recognition of an emergency, the caller must know whom to call and how to call them, and be willing to perform basic lifesaving measures immediately if necessary. The caller must also avoid certain actions that may make the situation worse.

It is important to inform and educate the public in recognizing medical emergencies, notifying the emergency care system, instituting basic lifesaving measures, and refraining from doing further harm. The failure of the public to perform any one of these four tasks reduces the chance for survival, results in postincident impairment, or actually worsens the situation. Inappropriate action by the public can also render subsequent medical actions ineffective.

During the last 20 years it has become apparent that the public will access 9-1-1 for a range of medical problems, from minor ailments to genuine life-threats.[1] Properly trained 9-1-1 communications center staff can perform specific functions that enhance the efficiency and effectiveness of prehospital care. The dispatcher can rapidly elicit reasonably accurate symptom pictures from frightened callers, allowing more accurate medical categorization of victims. In addition, the dispatcher can activate the configuration of responders optimally suited to deal with the specific emergency. It is not enough to mindlessly send paramedics on all cases; it is necessary to accurately determine the need for these highly trained individuals.[2] If this is not done for all calls, the number of available providers will be reduced because of their inappropriate use.[3] A paramedic team located too far from the next patient may be ineffective solely due to excessive response distance.

In the 1970s, this dilemma stimulated the development of emergency medical priority dispatching and its training process.[4] The goals are sending the right thing, to the right person, at the right time, in the right way, and doing the right things until help arrives. Because the dispatcher is often the least medically trained provider in the chain of survival, these goals are accomplished through the careful use of a comprehensive protocol, including the items in table 17.1.

Unrestricted use of scarce medical resources gambles with the possibility of a concurrent need for those resources. Availability of paramedics is a relative issue. Even in the best-covered system, if a defibrillation-capable unit is used unnecessarily, precious minutes may be added to the arrival at the next call. In most systems those extra minutes are lethal. The value of dispatch prioritization in such situations, not

---

TABLE 17.1

Items in the Emergency Medical Dispatch Protocol

- Systematized, scripted formal caller interrogation process
- Systematized, scripted post-dispatch and pre-arrival instructions (dispatch life support)
- Clinical/situational problem descriptors and associated codes that match the dispatcher's evaluation of the injury or illness type and severity with vehicle response mode and configuration
- Support and definitional reference information

to mention pre-arrival telephone interventions, is obvious. Even if the family and the media never know that the closest appropriate unit did not respond, the medical director still must endeavor to establish a system that balances all factors affecting appropriate medical dispatch.

The development and rapid growth of EMS have redefined the individual roles of prehospital providers and EMS physicians. Even the citizen has been identified as a potential key player in the evolving roster of the prehospital care team. However, the last in a long line of individuals identified as vital to the optimal functioning of the EMS system was the EMD. This key role for the dispatcher was accurately defined in 1978 when Salt Lake City Fire/EMS identified the medical dispatcher as the "weak link" in the chain of survival.[5] Until then the average medical dispatcher had less than one hour of formal medical training.

The emergence of structured EMD protocols and training as vital elements of appropriately functioning EMS systems was a phenomenon of the 1980s. A number of factors contributed to the delay in recognition. Early medical directors rarely observed the dispatch function because for most emergency physicians a prehospital case begins when the telemetry radio announces a call. The dispatcher's function regarding the mechanics of dispatch and the decision-making process was unknown to the medical community. Whether the closest appropriate unit was sent, a paramedic unit was unavailable because of previous assignment to a "cat bite" call, or the first assigned vehicle never arrived because it was involved in an unnecessary lights-and-siren accident remained hidden from most traditional EMS physicians.[6]

Myths of Medical Dispatch

There are seven commonly held and virtually universal myths regarding medical dispatch that delay the development of sound programs; these are malignant myths rather than innocent misconceptions (see table 17.2).[7] One by one these myths were proven false, as the practice of emergency medical dispatching was more carefully studied and better understood. They often are believed not only by police chiefs, fire chiefs, EMS administrators, politicians, and field personnel, but also by medical directors and dispatchers themselves.

One of the more common myths is that most callers are hysterical. In 1986, Eisenberg compared the emotional levels of 640 callers reporting cardiac ar-

TABLE 17.2

The Eight Myths of Medical Dispatch

1. The caller is too upset to respond accurately.
2. The caller does not know the required information.
3. The medical expertise of the dispatcher is not important.
4. The dispatcher is too busy to waste time asking questions, giving instructions, or flipping through card files.
5. Phone information from dispatchers cannot help victims and may even be dangerous.
6. More personnel and more units at the scene are always better.
7. It is dangerous not to maximally respond or not respond to lights-and-siren.
8. All you need is protocol and training to do EMD.

rest with other complaints.[8] A standard emotional scale from 1 to 5 was used; 1 represents "normal conversational speech" and a 5 represents an individual "so emotionally distraught that information (for example, the address) could be obtained only with great difficulty." Of the 146 callers in non-cardiac arrest cases, the mean emotional score was 1.4. Contrary to popular belief, the mean emotional quotient of the 494 callers reporting cardiac arrest was only 2.1. In 1990 a study of 160 random callers in Los Angeles revealed an average Emotional Content/Cooperation Score (ECCS modified) of 1.2.[9] No callers were rated at 5. More recent studies revealed an ECCS of 1.05 in 3,019 cases reviewed in British Columbia and 1.21 in 3,430 cases in Monroe County (Rochester, NY).[10]

A second myth is that the callers do not know the required information. In dispatch, the common classifications for standard callers are first-, second-, third-, and fourth-party. A first-party caller is the patient. A second-party caller is someone with the patient or intimately familiar with the patient's current condition. A third-party caller is someone who is neither with the patient nor knows the patient (for example, "I just saw a car accident out the window and it looks really bad!"). Fourth-party callers are related agency personnel who transfer field requests for EMS response (i.e., police dispatchers, airport authority, security companies). Sixty percent of callers can be classified as first- or second-parties; 40% are third-parties.[11] The high incidence of third-party callers is often the reason dispatchers fail to obtain complete information.

In reality this is the result of the dispatcher not asking the right questions rather than lack of knowledge on the part of the caller. This can be demonstrated by comparing interrogation sequences using formal protocols with those not using such protocols (fig. 17.1). Dispatchers left on their own usually invent questions to ask the caller, who routinely responds, "Look, I don't know." Rarely will an ad-libbing dispatcher ask the following structured series of questions:

1. Is s/he **awake**?
2. Did you ever hear her/him **talk** (cry)?
3. What was s/he **doing**—standing, sitting, or lying down?
   a. (Sitting or lying) Is s/he **moving at all**?
4. Where **exactly** is s/he?

None of the questions in this series are medical in nature; rather, they are situational. A caller may never have gotten any closer than 50 yards from the patient, yet could easily answer the majority of the questions. A talking, moving, sitting patient is not in cardiac arrest and that is the major dispatch concern when dealing with "unknown problem" or "man down" situations.

The myths regarding the medical training of dispatchers and their use of protocols are disproved as EMS systems establish programs for EMD training and use medically approved protocols.[12] Hundreds of dispatch systems provide pre-arrival instructions, with almost universal positive results medically, politically, and legally.[13] The National Association of EMS Physicians (NAEMSP) stated in its consensus document on EMD that "standard telephone instructions by trained EMDs are safe to give and in many instances are a morally necessity" (see appendix I).

The myths that EMDs are "too busy" are usually coupled with the need to increase dispatcher coverage when implementing a medical priority dispatching system. No dispatch center has ever been forced to increase the number of dispatchers as a result of

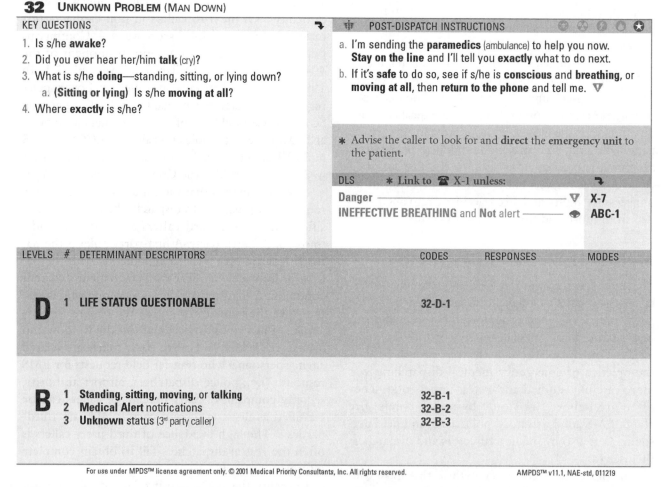

FIGURE 17.1. *Unknown Problem (Man Down) Protocol (from MPDS v11, ©2001 NAEMD, used with permission).*

using a priority dispatch system. Once a complete priority dispatch system is phased into dispatch operations, the provision of patient-directed interrogations does not become another time burden for the dispatchers. During the implementation phase of formal EMD in Los Angeles, interrogation time actually decreased. The time to dispatch on critical cases (cardiac arrest and choking) shortens because the protocol identifies the most important items and addresses them first. An appropriate response is dispatched, followed by more questions or telephone treatment. Adding the EMD to the high-call-volume Los Angeles center did not affect the call waiting time before being answered by the dispatcher; it averaged 7 seconds both before and after implementation.[14]

Of the seven misconceptions, the last two are the result of the illogical extrapolation of lights-and-siren use by other public safety responders to EMS.[14] More attention is being focused on using lights-and-siren for all EMS responses. Currently, there are neither data nor studies supporting the routine use of lights-and-siren. No published data establish the amount of time saved by lights-and-siren or by maximal response. The NAEMSP position paper, "Use of Lights-and-Siren in Emergency Medical Vehicle Response and Patient Transport," strongly supports the preplanned, medically overseen, deliberate use of lights-and-siren only when indicated from a patient-care standpoint.[14] The following three positions from that document relate to the impact of medical dispatching protocols on the use of lights-and-siren:[15]

NAEMSP Lights & Siren Position Paper

The use of lights-and-siren during both response and transport must be based on sound patient-problem assessment or on objective situational protocol. Written prospective protocol for the use of lights-and-siren during transport must be in place and approved by the medical director. In the absence of such protocol the paramedic or EMT on the scene should make contact with the base station hospital to clarify the vehicle Response Mode for transport of a given patient.

Dispatch prioritization is an essential element in any EMS system for it establishes the appropriate level of care initially required including vehicle response configuration and mode of urgency. All medical dispatch centers must institute and monitor adherence to dispatch prioritization protocols that clearly delineate appropriate lights-and-siren use from those that do not.

All jurisdictions allowing the use of lights-and-siren by emergency medical vehicles must require training and professional EMD certification of their dispatchers and mandate the use of priority medical dispatch protocols approved by the local medical director that clearly delineate lights-and-siren use.

Emergency Medical Dispatcher

The role of the EMD in a modern EMS system is extensive, and requires a detailed base of knowledge.[5] The typical role is multifaceted, with at least six subroles. These include (1) interrogator; (2) radio dispatcher; (3) triager; (4) logistics coordinator; (5) resource provider; and (6) pre-arrival aid instructor. Specific training in each of these facets is essential. However, they represent only a portion of the skills requisite to the functioning of a public safety dispatcher.

A sound basis in generic telecommunication techniques is the first prerequisite for optimal emergency medical dispatching.[16] Many high-volume systems use computer-aided dispatch (CAD) to divide responsibilities between the calltakers (input and evaluation) and the dispatchers (output and allocation). The following discussion applies to both groups of EMDs.

The EMD requires specific training in what is commonly referred to as the dispatch priorities. It is an oblique cross-section of prehospital medicine unique to dispatch-appropriate interrogation, vehicle allocation, pre-arrival instructions (PAIs) given to the caller, and concise information regarding the clinical situation and scene conditions given to the responding provider en route. The properly trained EMD must be a sophisticated healthcare professional because the fund of knowledge from which the dispatch priorities are gleaned is the same as that of the emergency physician, nurse, or paramedic; however, the types of treatments performed over the telephone are generally more elemental. The basic components of EMD are chief complaint identification, key question interrogation, dispatch life support instructions, and prehospital medical care dispatch coding and response configuration setup. They are covered in more detail in subsequent sections of this and the next chapter.

Medical Oversight

The inclusion of the dispatch process in medical oversight lagged behind that of prehospital field care. For years, medical oversight was blissfully unaware of the pre-arrival phase of EMS. One reason for this was that fire services commonly were step-parents of EMS in the 1970s; for example, before 1990, no EMS physician had stepped inside the fire-EMS dispatch center for the District of Columbia (now NAEMD-accredited). Resistance to medical oversight has been encountered when the medical community first examines the practices of the medical dispatch center. It is the medical director's responsibility to work with the EMS agency administration to establish appropriate, medically sound practices and quality management programs for EMD (see appendix I).[17]

The concept of EMD obviously encompasses more than training. In fact, a practice standard has evolved that not only defines the role of the EMD but also the supervision, quality management, and risk management that must accompany it.[17,18] Medical oversight at dispatch is essential and is a key element of quality management for medical directors. The implementation process begins with training and certification. The standard instruction period for an EMD course is 24 hours.[17] Training is a critical basis for the rapid, precise decisions required. NAEMSP described some of the difficulties in designing EMD:

> In order to prioritize calls properly, the EMD must be well-versed in the medical conditions and incident types that constitute their daily routine Training in these priorities must be detailed and dispatch-specific; not just EMT or paramedic training per se. Since, much of the knowledge and many of the skills required by the EMD are dispatch-specific. A curriculum for their training differs substantially from those used in the preparation of EMTs or paramedics. Training as an EMT or paramedic does not adequately prepare a person for the role of an EMD. Much of the required EMD curriculum cannot be found in standard EMS training curricula. It consists of content and emphasis which differ significantly from that used for the training of all other health professionals and public safety dispatchers (see appendix I).

Quality Management

A quality management (QM) program is essential to the successful implementation and maintenance of an EMD program. To assure quality in practice there must be an understanding of how quality is defined. Inherent in the notion of EMD is the development of objective measurements of the performance of EMD activities. These measurement tools have four goals:

1. To assure that dispatchers understand policy, practice, and protocol;
2. To assure that dispatchers comply with policy, practice, and protocol;
3. To assure that policy, practice, and protocol are correct and effective; and
4. To correct or improve any deficiencies in EMD policy, practice, and protocol.

QM Components

The 11 components of a comprehensive QM program for EMD are listed below:[19]

1. Selection
2. Orientation
3. Initial training
4. Certification
5. Continuing dispatch education
6. Medical oversight
7. Data generation
8. Performance evaluation or case review and feedback
9. Recertification
10. Risk management
11. Decertification, suspension, and/or termination

SELECTION. If dispatchers are to be involved in the emergency medical care of patients, the selection of new dispatchers must take that into account. Abilities to read written scripts, follow instructions, carry out multiple tasks, and exercise good judgment and self-control in stressful situations must be assessed. There are a number of attributes and predictors of success that should be incorporated into selection criteria.

ORIENTATION. EMDs must be inculcated from the start with the paradigm that EMS exists to help people, not just to save lives. Because the majority of callers do not have a time-critical or life-threatening medical emergency, unless EMDs are help-oriented they will view these callers as either undeserving of their assistance or a waste of time. Through proper orientation, EMDs learn that although they cannot save the life of every caller, they can help everyone who calls. This orientation leads to enhanced self-esteem, higher morale, reduced frustration, and optimal customer relations.

INITIAL TRAINING. The training of EMDs must revolve around the use of medically appropriate and approved dispatch protocols. The difference between guidelines and protocols is profound; guidelines are permissive, protocols are not. EMDs use protocols to carry out their unique role in the chain of patient care. In the absence of medical dispatch protocols, dispatch quality management is simply not possible.

As the types of EMD training programs burgeoned over the years, two distinctly different methodologies have emerged. In one type the EMDs are trained without a significant or knowledgeable review of a specific protocol; in the other the protocol sets the practice standard, because it defines the actions of the dispatcher throughout the call. A crucial element of any EMD curriculum is review by the teacher of each medical dispatch protocol; without review the EMD is left only with generalities. Understanding and practice of the protocols are essential to effective EMD training.

CERTIFICATION. No informed patient prefers the care of a non-certified provider to that of a certified one. Formal certification of EMDs, whether by state or national standard-setting organizations, is an essential component.[12,17] Certification attests that the EMD has been exposed to a defined body of medical dispatch knowledge and obligates the EMD to conform to a standard of care. There is a clear and growing trend toward professional certification; and medical directors must be involved. Minimum certification standards should include all of the items in table 17.3.

The mission statement preceding the regulation rules for EMD in Utah states, "The purpose of these rules is to provide for the establishment of minimum standards to be met by those providing medical dispatch services in Utah so as to promote the health and safety of the people of this State."[20] In the 1990s there is no question of the dispatcher's ability to achieve these goals.

CONTINUING DISPATCH EDUCATION. The half-life of medical knowledge is about five years. Much of what the EMD learns in initial training becomes obsolete as medicine moves forward. It is now technologically possible to defibrillate over the telephone and even view the person on the other end of the line. The physicians responsible for medical oversight must take an active role in the quality management process and in providing sound continuing dispatch education (CDE). Such developments will have profound implications for the future practice of EMD. CDE keeps EMDs abreast of the changes and progress in medical dispatching. A formal continuing education program allows the EMD to share experiences with colleagues. Identified patterns in the medical dispatch practices of a given agency can be illuminated and discussed in an academic and non-threatening forum. Positive behavior is reinforced, and negative behavior is discouraged.

CDE is essential to reinforce initial concepts and build on the science of dispatch priorities.[19] As the operational experience of new EMDs expands, CDE becomes their link with the changing aspects of medicine. Regular exposure to appropriate medical concepts as they relate to dispatch increases understanding and fosters application of medical principles at the point EMS actually begins—the dispatch center. Medical directors must take an active role in the quality management process by providing appropriate CDE for dispatchers. The fact that EMD is an emerging and changing field mandates an active CDE program to keep the dispatchers current.

Traditionally the major educational, occupational, and supervisory influences of dispatchers are related to public safety rather than medicine. A closer-to-equal balance of emphasis needs to emerge in combined dispatch centers; an active CDE program is required to keep EMDs current with medical standards and the ideas specific to their daily routine. A minimal CDE investment of one hour of education per month is now the national standard.[21] As more experience is gained in the application of CDE, the exact amount and type of training will be redefined.

PHYSICIAN OVERSIGHT. All medical activities demand physician involvement and guidance. There should be physician involvement in the planning, or-

TABLE 17.3
EMD Certification Standards
■ The use of a medical dispatch protocol system should be required and generically defined.
■ A comprehensive quality management program should include significant performance evaluation through an ongoing medical case review process.
■ A state or regionally approved training and certification program should include provision of medical oversight and a process for approval of individual agencies' written medical dispatch protocols.

ganization, and clinical oversight of EMD activities. In reality, EMDs and other prehospital providers are physician extenders. Ultimately the medical director is responsible and accountable for the performance, the personnel, and the adequacy of medical dispatch policy, practice, and protocol.

NAEMSP states, "Medical oversight for the EMD and the dispatch center is a part of the EMS physician's responsibilities" (see appendix I). This responsibility includes initial training, CDE, medical dispatch case review, protocol review, and approval. The formal reviews should be performed on both the response assignments and the need for lights-and-siren responses. Although these activities are time-consuming, they deserve adequate recognition. Once involved with dispatch the physician often becomes fascinated, because medical dispatch lies at the core of EMS philosophy. Analogously, the dispatch response protocols are the "messenger RNA" of the EMS system, putting planned desires of medical oversight into play for the desired "replication" of the response system each time a call is processed. Thus, sound medical input at dispatch influences the makeup and deployment of the system. The establishment of dispatch priorities often requires an unprecedented review of why the system does what it does.

To most medical directors the dispatch center is somewhat of an unknown, because traditional direct medical oversight begins when the telemetry radio signals. Medical dispatch activities, because they occur before this event, are often excluded from the activities of the average medical director. Dispatch case review is the equivalent to prehospital care report (PCR) review. This review is accomplished through a medical management oversight committee process.

It is essential that the medical director attend an EMD training course taught by an credentialed instructor with significant EMD training experience. There is a one-day, leadership-level training program for dispatch managers and medical oversight physicians taught by several national standard-setting orga-

nizations. Once physicians understand both the knowledge base required for such training and the medical basis for dispatch priorities, they can provide adequate medical oversight for their dispatchers.

DATA GENERATION. EMD managers and administrators must define what data are needed to evaluate objectively the effectiveness of an EMD program and the performance of the EMDs (see fig. 17.2).[14]

Raw data must be analyzed and converted into useful information. A random sampling of roughly 3% to 5% of all cases should be generated for EMD protocol compliance. Special dispatch life support (DLS) pre-arrival instruction cases should also be reviewed for protocol compliance. Field responders' feedback, obtained through the use of a formal reporting mechanism, is another means by which the efficacy of dispatch can be measured.[22] Other data that may be affected by EMD program performance are vehicle fuel consumption, maintenance requirements, and accidents. More commonly, communications centers utilize automated priority dispatch protocols dynamically linked to CAD systems to generate meaningful statistical and EMD performance data or system improvement. Central to data reporting are the totals and frequencies of all call types, by both chief complaints and determinant levels (see appendix II). Determinant levels are assigned to prioritize responses and use as levels, OMEGA, ALPHA, BRAVO, CHARLIE, DELTA, and ECHO. (See chapter 18.)

PERFORMANCE EVALUATION/CASE REVIEW. The fundamental issue in the evaluation of EMD performance is protocol compliance.[23] Protocol was either followed or it was not. The goal of case review is to assist EMDs in improving performance and protocol compliance. While, case reviewers can listen to a case repeatedly; the EMD has only one chance.

The review of a case should begin with listening to the entire call to get an overall sense of the case. The call should then be reevaluated successively for compliance to case entry (primary survey) and key ques-

Case Entry (%)	Key Questions (%)	CLEVELAND August 1992 (%)	MONTREAL September 1992 (%)	LOS ANGELES 1989 (%)
100	100	88	92	93
<100	100	83	86	82
100	<100	54	50	75
<100	<100	53	72	37

FIGURE 17.2. *Does protocol compliance during evaluation affect Determinant Code correctness (and response)?*

EMERGENCY MEDICAL DISPATCH

tion (secondary survey) protocol, selection of correct dispatch code for appropriate unit response and mode, and adequacy of pre-arrival instructions.

Random review of cases assures that each dispatcher's actual state of practice (specifically compliance to protocol) is studied. In addition, review of smaller numbers of both exemplary and problem cases is useful. These cases are often identified by external sources. The involvement of field personnel in reporting incidents that represent dispatch-related problems is beneficial to the performance and policy evaluation process.[22]

Careful review leads to the identification of the elements of success or the specific problems of compliance, understanding, policy, or protocol. Without adequate case review, dispatcher compliance to protocol generally falls below 50% to 80% (depending on the scoring category examined) even when mandatory compliance is a formal policy requirement (fig. 17.3). The level of compliance of every dispatcher should be collected and cumulatively compared with established levels of acceptable practice. Studies have shown that case reviews, and the feedback of compliance levels directly to each EMD, improves compliance dramatically.

RECERTIFICATION. EMD recertification is the logical result of CDE education. Without the condition that EMDs maintain certification, there is little incentive to stay current. More important, unless maintenance of certification is mandatory for EMDs, there is little incentive to participate in ongoing CDE. Recertification is being required by more states, provinces, and shires.

RISK MANAGEMENT. Risk management is the legal equivalent of preventive medicine. All the elements of EMD quality management contribute to a healthy EMD risk management environment and significantly reduce the chance of a dispatch disaster and subsequent litigation.[19]

DECERTIFICATION, SUSPENSION, AND/OR TERMINATION. Disciplinary actions involving EMDs should be progressive. Formal documentation of deficiencies and corrective actions are basic ingredients for successful remediation of individual EMD problems.[21] The unnecessary loss of an employee, who was recruited, selected, trained, and developed, is costly. Therefore, care must be taken to ensure that the employee has every reasonable opportunity to achieve acceptable levels of performance.

These 11 components of dispatcher QM are essential to maintain the type of employment environment that assures that safe, effective patient evaluation and care initiate every EMS call.

Supervision at Dispatch

It is essential that effective and supportive operational supervision is available for these "air traffic controllers of the ground." Supervision should be delivered by individuals who have extensive training in EMD. To identify problems prospectively, the professional supervisor must have both EMS and EMD knowledge and be responsible for all quality and risk management processes. All managers who supervise EMDs must be EMD-trained themselves.

It is essential that well planned, active medical oversight exist to integrate all the components of a comprehensive QM program. This medical management process usually follows a path separate from the regular chain of command; it consists of a linked set of QM oversight committees.[14] The medical dispatch review committee (MDRC) functions at the middle management level, initially reviewing and directing the activities of the QM process. The second functional oversight group is the dispatch steering committee, whose membership is upper management and includes representatives of the chief administrative officer, the medical director, the dispatch supervisor, and the QM unit leader. Based on QM case review and other issues, the MDRC makes recommendations to the steering committee, which generally approves, disapproves, or sends suggestions back for further development. Dispatch and field personnel should both sit on these committees.

Pre-Arrival Instructions

Trained EMDs are the "first" first responders. They provide the initial professional intervention, reducing the response time almost to zero for specific problems. There is no better justification for the provision of PAIs than landmark legal opinion delivered by James Page to the Aurora, Colorado, Fire Department in 1981:

> "After years of arriving 'too late' at the scenes of hundreds of life-threatening emergencies, it is difficult for me to offer a detached and unemotional opinion. Throughout the United States, we have spent billions of dollars constructing systems to respond to medical emergencies and we have done

In the first month that EMDs were provided with performance feedback, there was an average increase of over 12 percent in the six components of the protocol—and four of the six components showed further increases in the following month. In fact, with continued feedback to the EMDs regarding their recent performance, four years after this study the center reported over 99 percent total compliance to the protocol. A properly designed and uniformly applied quality management process results in improved compliance to nearly all components of an emergency medical dispatch protocol.

Compliance to Protocol

The Impact of a Comprehensive Quality Management Process on Compliance to Protocol

Protocol Component	Before Feedback	After Feedback	P Value
CE	92.3	98.6	p = .002
CC	89.9	91.6	p = .271
KQ	65.8	96.2	p < .0001
Level	79.6	93.3	p < .0001
PDIs	40.8	95.8	p < .0001
PAIs	92.9	100.0	p = .005

	Sept.	Oct.	Feedback begins	Nov.	Dec.
CE	92.3	87.4		**97.2**	**98.6**
CC	89.8	87.3		**94.9**	91.6
KQ	65.8	73.4		89.3	96.2
PDI	40.8	75.4		**93.8**	95.8
PAI	92.9	**95.2**		**99.0**	**100.0**
Level	79.6	81.8		**99.0**	93.3
Total	79.1	80.4		**93.3**	**97.4**

__Bold__ indicates compliance at Accreditation standards.

Legend for Table

CE = Case Entry (primary survey)
CC = Chief Complaint
KQ = Key Questions (secondary survey)
PDI = Post-Dispatch Instructions
PAI = Pre-Arrival Instructions
Level = Response Determinant Coding

Improving the Accuracy of Determinant Levels

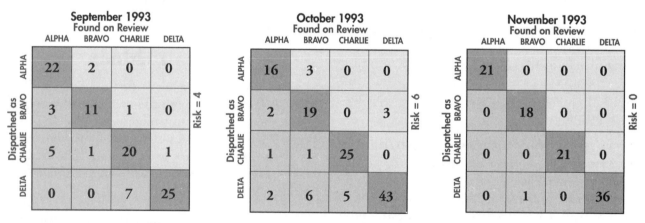

FIGURE 17.3. *Impact of Case Review and Feedback on Compliance to Protocol and Determinant Code Selection Accuracy* [20]

little to cure the deadly 4-minute gap at the front of the system. While we race through city traffic to get to the scene, a brain dies from lack of CPR (oxygen). Frankly, I don't understand how any public safety or health care worker can accept these recurring tragedies without actively seeking a solution to the 'response time' problem, which proves fatal in so many cases."[24]

There are many recurring and predictable situations that must be uniquely addressed and corrected before terminating a call at dispatch. To the field provider, a cardiac arrest victim is a pulseless, motionless, non-breathing patient; however, the same patient initially presents to the dispatcher in the following fashion:

"Is he conscious?"   "No!"

"Is he breathing?"   "Uh, I'm not sure. He's making funny noises."

In this case the funny noises, a common telephone description of the agonal respirations, must be correctly interpreted.[4] To the trained EMD, until proven otherwise, this situation represents an unconscious victim with an uncontrolled airway that must be cleared, or worse, a patient in the agonal throes of death. Just as the provider at the scene would immediately establish airway control rather than defer it to someone else later, the EMD must act appropriately and immediately.

Because the responsibility to provide initial care applies to EMDs, they must be trained to give PAIs. Some PAIs are simple commands such as "Don't move the patient," "Call back if the patient's condition worsens," "Gather the patient's medications and write down the name of your doctor," and "Turn on the outside lights." Other PAIs are more detailed, for example, mouth-to-mouth breathing, the Heimlich maneuver, direct pressure hemorrhage control, childbirth assistance, and CPR. The more sophisticated or

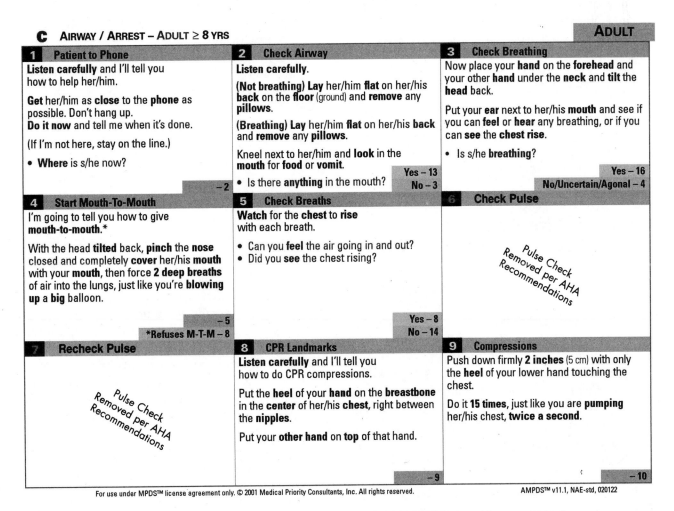

C   AIRWAY / ARREST – ADULT ≥ 8 YRS   **ADULT**

1 Patient to Phone	**2 Check Airway**	**3 Check Breathing**
Listen carefully and I'll tell you how to help her/him. **Get** her/him as **close** to the **phone** as possible. Don't hang up. **Do it now** and tell me when it's done. (If I'm not here, stay on the line.) • **Where** is s/he now? – 2	**Listen carefully.** **(Not breathing) Lay** her/him **flat** on her/his **back** on the **floor** (ground) and **remove** any **pillows.** **(Breathing) Lay** her/him **flat** on her/his **back** and **remove** any **pillows.** Kneel next to her/him and **look** in the **mouth** for **food** or **vomit.** • Is there **anything** in the mouth? Yes – 13 / No – 3	Now place your **hand** on the **forehead** and your other **hand** under the **neck** and **tilt** the **head** back. Put your **ear** next to her/his **mouth** and see if you can **feel** or **hear** any breathing, or if you can **see** the **chest** rise. • Is s/he **breathing**? Yes – 16 / No/Uncertain/Agonal – 4
4 Start Mouth-To-Mouth	**5 Check Breaths**	**6 Check Pulse**
I'm going to tell you how to give **mouth-to-mouth.*** With the head **tilted** back, **pinch** the **nose** closed and completely **cover** her/his **mouth** with your **mouth**, then force **2 deep breaths** of air into the lungs, just like you're **blowing up a big** balloon. – 5 *Refuses M-T-M – 8	**Watch** for the **chest** to **rise** with each breath. • Can you **feel** the air going in and out? • Did you **see** the chest rising? Yes – 8 / No – 14	*Pulse Check Removed per AHA Recommendations*
7 Recheck Pulse	**8 CPR Landmarks**	**9 Compressions**
Pulse Check Removed per AHA Recommendations	**Listen carefully** and I'll tell you how to do CPR compressions. Put the **heel** of your **hand** on the **breastbone** in the **center** of her/his **chest**, right between the **nipples.** Put your **other hand** on **top** of that hand. – 9	Push down firmly **2 inches** (5 cm) with only the **heel** of your lower hand touching the chest. Do it **15 times**, just like you are **pumping** her/his chest, **twice a second.** – 10

    AMPDS™ v11.1, NAE-std, 020122

FIGURE 17.4. *Dispatch Life Support protocols (from MPDS v11, ©2001 NAEMD, used by permission).*

intricate PAIs are given through the use of DLS protocols (fig. 17.4). These protocols are algorithmic scripts using binary (and trinary; yes/no/unknown) logic branching that the EMD reads to the caller. Dispatcher-imposed variation is reduced to a minimum. The protocol scripts encourage dispatcher intervention through the reduction of fear and anxiety as well as through the development of learned phrasing by repetitive use.

Pre-arrival instructions are not only an essential dispatcher practice but are a clear public expectation.[25] The failure to provide appropriate PAIs is described as negligent by a growing number of plaintiff attorneys. Although the notion that dispatch agencies will be successfully sued for providing PAIs has been a roadblock to their use, there has been only one dispatcher negligence lawsuit filed following the provision of PAIs since that practice took form in 1975. On the contrary, an increasing number of recent lawsuits, completed or in progress, cite the omission of PAIs (or dispatcher abandonment, as legal terminology now describes it) as either the primary or the associated allegation.

The American Heart Association (AHA) states that:[26]

> EMDs have been identified as a vital but often neglected part of the EMS system. All communities should provide formal training in emergency medical dispatch and require the use of medical dispatch protocols, including pre-arrival instructions for airway control, foreign body airway obstruction, and CPR by telephone.

Dispatch Life Support

The concept of DLS provides the basis for establishing the actual content and application method of the special treatment protocols used by medical dispatchers.[27] In 1989, NAEMSP defined DLS as "the knowledge, procedures, and skills used by trained EMDs in providing care through pre-arrival instructions to callers. It consists of those life support principles that are appropriate to application by medical dispatchers" (see appendix I). Because of the "blind" nature of the provision of PAIs and the need to rapidly teach the caller relatively intricate procedures in real-time (without practice tries or visual verifications), the protocols must be written succinctly and followed strictly.

The AHA life support procedures are based on the trainer's ability to teach in person the application of a physical procedure to a willing student, often over a significant period of time. Unfortunately, the EMD does not have such luxuries. The dispatcher (the instructor) must teach the caller (the unwilling student) a physical procedure (the PAIs) in real-time (seconds) without any visual aids or practice. There is verification neither of correct application nor of any follow-through by those at the other end of the line.

For example, although the chin lift is not a difficult psychomotor skill to teach in person, over the phone it becomes difficult and time-consuming. However, the head-tilt method of airway control can be easily taught to the caller as follows: "Put one hand on his forehead and your other under his neck. Lift up on the hand under his neck and push down on the hand on his forehead. This will open his airway." EMDs are instructed to be aware of hazards in neck manipulation if the patient has also incurred a significant mechanism of injury; this is rarely present in the routine PAI situations. DLS more realistically incorporates the fact that, although many treatments dispatchers provide are similar to basic life support, they simply must be different in content, process, and real-time instruction.

Unfortunately, a common problem for medical oversight during the initial review and adoption of DLS treatment sequence protocols is erroneous deviation from other current treatment standards such as those of the AHA.[27] In reality the dilemma is understanding the special limitations of the dispatch situation, not the dispatch protocol itself. As NAEMSP stated: "Training and recertification in basic life support, as is *appropriate to application by medical dispatchers*, is necessary to maintain and improve this unique, and at times, lifesaving, nonvisual skill" (see appendix I).

Dispatch life support was formally defined to clearly establish the necessary functional differences between the dispatcher process and field care as legitimate. EMD training contains many dispatch-specific methods of description and caller application found in neither field provider training nor protocol.

Medical directors and others involved in the creation of CPR and ACLS standards continue to broaden their perspectives on how these standards should apply to PAIs. As the science of EMD evolves, medical dispatch experts and professional medical dispatcher organizations are being more involved in the development of new standards that affect EMDs and their remote patients. Currently there is an improving dialogue between the AHA and NAEMD in solving these apparent dilemmas.

Compliance to Protocol

Inherent in DLS is the necessity for medical dispatchers to adhere to written protocols for the provision of telephone treatment in a standard, reproducible way.[9] Although there is growing interest and effort among public safety agencies to provide telephone instruction to callers, only about 5% to 10% of centers provide correct, non-arbitrary, medically approved PAIs read directly from detailed protocol scripts.

It is essential for the medical director to understand the difference between PAIs and telephone aid; the two very different methods of patient care initiated by dispatchers are:[28]

PREARRIVAL INSTRUCTIONS are telephone-rendered, medically approved, written instructions given by trained EMDs to callers to aid the victim and control the situation before prehospital personnel arrive. The protocols for PAIs are used word for word as is feasible.

TELEPHONE AID is ad lib advice provided by dispatchers based on their own experience and training in a procedure or treatment, but not following a written PAI protocol. This method exists in a system either because no protocols are used or because protocol adherence is not required.

There is a dramatic difference between the DLS process of PAIs and that of telephone aid. Telephone aid simply assures that the dispatcher has attempted to provide some sort of care to the patient through the caller, but does not assure that the care is necessary, correct, standard, or medically effective. Often, the use of telephone aid is sporadic and arbitrary.

Telephone aid provides the illusion of PAIs without consistently delivering high-quality and accurate advice. The following are common errors seen during medical dispatch case reviews in agencies providing telephone aid:

1. Failure to correctly identify conditions requiring telephone interventions, and therefore prearrival instructions, in the first place. For example, "saving" an infant having a febrile seizure who was incorrectly identified as needing CPR because of the failure to follow protocols designed to verify the absence of breathing before the initiation of potentially dangerous dispatcher invasive treatment such as chest compressions.

2. Failure to accurately identify the presence or lack of interim signs and symptoms during the provision of telephone intervention. For example, dispatchers who ad lib CPR sequences often fail to ask important non-visual verifiers such as "Did you see the chest rise?" or "Did you feel the air go in?"

3. Failure to perform, describe, or teach multiple step procedures such as CPR care in a consistent and reproducible fashion. For example, quality management reviews often reveal that dispatchers in the same center (or even the same dispatcher) perform care differently on each occasion if they do not follow the scripted PAI protocols exactly.

4. Lack of medically approved protocols for use as a template for evaluating dispatcher performance during the case review and quality management processes. Non-mandatory guidelines cannot be quality assured.

The requirement of medical appropriateness within the dispatch center through effective medical oversight is an essential element for assuring the correct, safe, and efficient application of dispatcher telephone intervention.

Psychological Components

Although it may seem to the casual observer that the emotional or hysterical behavior of callers is random or unpredictable, there are predictable, generic components present in most caller interrogation processes and PAI situations.[14] The following are the most common:

THE HYSTERIA THRESHOLD. All distraught callers have a threshold of hysteria control that can be reached through repetitive persistence. Bringing callers below the threshold is usually quite easy if the appropriate techniques are utilized by properly trained EMDs. Once below the hysteria threshold, callers are often in complete emotional control and can repeat instructions word perfect.[29]

THE REPETITIVE PERSISTENCE METHODOLOGY. The most successful method of crossing the hysteria threshold is repetitive persistence, which is performed by the EMD repeating in the same exact wording a request to calm down or perform any other desired act.[29] For example, "You're going to have to calm down, ma'am, if we're going to help your baby," should be repeated firmly to gain initial control of the caller. Usually this approach works after only two or three repetitions. Alterations in wording are perceived by callers as signs of indecision or lack of control on the part of the EMD.

THE "BRING THE PATIENT TO THE PHONE" PROBLEM. It is striking how many times PAIs are begun only to be interrupted by the caller yelling, "Bring him in here to the phone!"[30] Obviously this wastes time and interrupts the EMD's train of thought and provision of instructions. At the beginning of the telephone treatment sequence the EMD should always ask, "Where is the patient?"

THE "REFREAK" EVENT. There are three points at which callers may be reminded of the distressing state of the victim, "refreak," and cause the EMD to lose critical control.[29,30] "The first is when the victim is brought to the phone, and the caller is immediately reminded of how bad the victim appears. The second is when the EMD asks for verification of the absence of vital signs (breathing or pulse). The third is when the caller fails to revive the patient through the performance of CPR or the Heimlich maneuver, becomes frustrated, and may stop trying.

THE "NOTHING'S WORKING" PHENOMENON. Average callers harbor the misconception that because they are following the EMD's instructions the victim will respond or immediately be revived. This belief results in a specific type of frustration refreak that can interrupt the treatment sequence. In despair, callers will commonly state "nothing's working." The EMD can easily overcome this with appropriate encouragement and repetitive persistence, and by mentioning that they are "keeping the victim going until the paramedics get there."[30]

THE PARAMEDICS "AREN'T COMING" NOTION. During PAIs callers may often wonder fearfully if help is truly on the way and often repetitively ask, "Are they coming?"[30] This may relate to the average citizen's skepticism regarding "the check's in the mail." The dispatcher need only confirm that the paramedics have left the station and are on their way. It is important that this be relayed in "lay terms" for easy comprehension because the distraught caller may not understand professional terms such as "en route."

THE "RELIEF" REACTION. A less common but relevant situation may occur when a patient's condition improves. The "relief" reaction is caused when feeling of relief, guilt, remorse, or fear of what might have been strike the caller. When the patient apparently no longer needs the immediate assistance of the caller, the caller has the opportunity to vent built-up emotion and may begin crying. Tasking the caller with important monitoring assignments or reaffirming the patient's status are effective ways to deal with this event.[14]

The realization that these events will occur as predicted allows the EMD to prepare for them and then react appropriately. This "cause and effect" understanding is as valuable to the dispatcher as a road map would be to a traveler on an unknown journey.

Further identification of the psychological aspects of PAIs and the interrogation of people in crisis will add significantly to the effectiveness of medical dispatching. Understanding the predictable actions and reactions of callers and those at the scene of a critical event increases the effectiveness and confidence of the EMD when dealing with these stressful and difficult situations.

Medical Dispatch Priorities

The development of dispatch priorities was a pivotal event in the evolution of EMD.[5] These priorities lie at the heart of optimal medical dispatch functioning; they are the sum basis of the knowledge, decisions, and treatment of the dispatcher. Dispatch priorities are not a new concept to the emergency physician. In fact they are the subset of medical urgency science on which emergency department triage decisions are usually based (see appendix II).

Because the EMD is often the least trained professional in the EMS chain of survival, the protocols should be fully understood and carefully adhered to. An EMD protocol consists of the following three components: key questions (KQs), PAIs, and dispatch priorities including determinants and response (see figs. 17.1 and 17.5). An additional information dispatch card section should always be "in sight" and therefore "in mind," continually familiarizing the EMD with important medical information and axioms (fig. 17.5).

Every key question asked on a dispatch priority card is included for one or more of the following reasons:

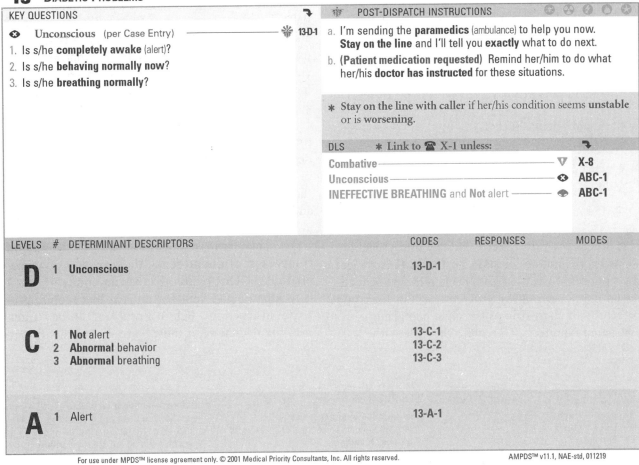

KEY QUESTIONS

✪ Unconscious (per Case Entry) ——————— ✿ 13-D-1

1. Is s/he **completely awake** (alert)?
2. Is s/he **behaving normally now**?
3. Is s/he **breathing normally**?

POST-DISPATCH INSTRUCTIONS

a. I'm sending the **paramedics** (ambulance) to help you now. **Stay on the line** and I'll tell you **exactly** what to do next.

b. **(Patient medication requested)** Remind her/him to do what her/his **doctor has instructed** for these situations.

* Stay on the line with caller if her/his condition seems **unstable** or is **worsening**.

DLS * Link to ☎ X-1 unless:

Combative ——————————————————— ▽	X-8
Unconscious ——————————————————— ✪	ABC-1
INEFFECTIVE BREATHING and Not alert ——— ◉	ABC-1

LEVELS	#	DETERMINANT DESCRIPTORS	CODES	RESPONSES	MODES
D	1	**Unconscious**	13-D-1		
C	1	**Not** alert	13-C-1		
	2	**Abnormal** behavior	13-C-2		
	3	**Abnormal** breathing	13-C-3		
A	1	Alert	13-A-1		

AMPDS™ v11.1, NAE-std, 011219

FIGURE 17.5. *Protocol consists of key questions, pre-arrival (post-dispatch) instructions, and dispatch priorities (determinants and responses) based on the dispatch priorities (Diabetic Problems protocol, from MPDS v11, ©2001 NAEMD used by permission).*

- It gleans information that is necessary to determine the appropriate response assignment.
- It identifies and verifies conditions that require pre-arrival instructions.
- It obtains information required by response personnel to pre-plan and address the scene and patient (fig. 17.6).
- It provides for scene safety in minimizing the hazards and risks to patients, laypersons, and professional responders (fig. 17.7).

A key question group that leaves any of these necessary indications uncovered is defective, and will result in an unsound interrogation. Often a system adopting a priority dispatch system is tempted to make pre-implementation modification to existing key question sets, PAIs, and dispatch determinants.

This common error is the equivalent of buying a new ambulance then changing the timing, wiring, and other sundry parts without road-testing it first.

To a large extent the prime reason for the structure of the key questions is the identification of the most appropriate mobile response (that is, the dispatch priority) that reflects predetermined distinctions in response urgency. For example, the EMD's determination of the level of consciousness in a diabetic problem case results in one of three basic determinants: "conscious and alert" or "conscious but not alert" or "unconscious but breathing" (fig. 17.5). The clear division among these determinants makes dispatch response assignments relatively simple for this particular chief complaint. The response section of the dispatch protocol matches each of these determinants with the most appropriate mobile response available in the system.

In the past, many medical dispatchers were given lists of medical conditions considered in need of great urgency or a higher level of response. These lists were diagnoses, not the dispatch "priorities," and might have included the following:

- Appendicitis
- Anaphylactic shock
- Heart attack
- Heat stroke
- Pneumothorax
- Pulmonary embolus

Unfortunately, the effectiveness of using such lists was severely limited, because for the EMD to select the right response, the right problem had to be diagnosed first.[5] Each of the problems on this list could present with chest pain as the chief complaint or an associated symptom. To require the caller—the least medically trained person in the EMS system—to initially diagnose the problem (before interrogation or a scene evaluation) is flawed logic. Priority dispatch uses chief complaint indices that are symptom- or incident-based rather than diagnosis-based. Because medical problems such as cardiac difficulties are usually reported by either the patient or a second-party caller, actual symptoms are more readily obtained than in traumatic situations. In those latter cases the determination of the type of incident or mechanism of injury is the basis of the initial response, because the calls are usually made by a third or fourth party, and access to individual patient symptoms may be less available.

The answers to key questions lead to the second component of the protocol, the provision of appropriate PAIs. One reason that key questions are asked is to identify and verify conditions that require pre-arrival instructions. Before a problem can be treated over the telephone, it must be reasonably confirmed

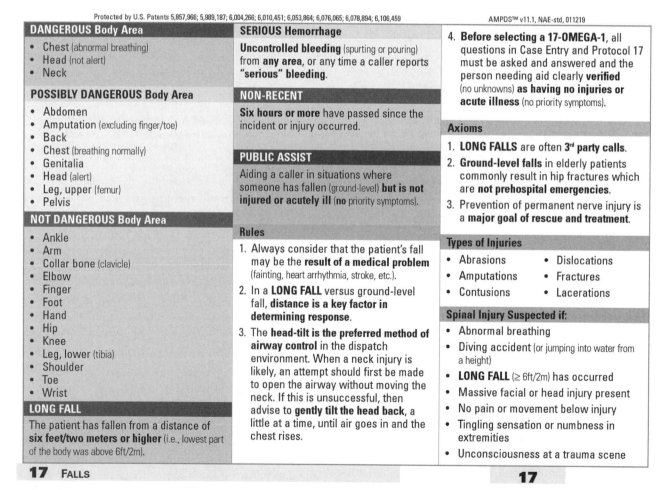

AMPDS™ v11.1, NAE-std, 011219

DANGEROUS Body Area
- Chest (abnormal breathing)
- Head (not alert)
- Neck

POSSIBLY DANGEROUS Body Area
- Abdomen
- Amputation (excluding finger/toe)
- Back
- Chest (breathing normally)
- Genitalia
- Head (alert)
- Leg, upper (femur)
- Pelvis

NOT DANGEROUS Body Area
- Ankle
- Arm
- Collar bone (clavicle)
- Elbow
- Finger
- Foot
- Hand
- Hip
- Knee
- Leg, lower (tibia)
- Shoulder
- Toe
- Wrist

LONG FALL
The patient has fallen from a distance of **six feet/two meters or higher** (i.e., lowest part of the body was above 6ft/2m).

SERIOUS Hemorrhage
Uncontrolled bleeding (spurting or pouring) from **any area**, or any time a caller reports "serious" bleeding.

NON-RECENT
Six hours or more have passed since the incident or injury occurred.

PUBLIC ASSIST
Aiding a caller in situations where someone has fallen (ground-level) **but is not injured or acutely ill** (no priority symptoms).

Rules
1. Always consider that the patient's fall may be the **result of a medical problem** (fainting, heart arrhythmia, stroke, etc.).
2. In a **LONG FALL** versus ground-level fall, **distance is a key factor in determining response.**
3. The **head-tilt is the preferred method of airway control** in the dispatch environment. When a neck injury is likely, an attempt should first be made to open the airway without moving the neck. If this is unsuccessful, then advise to **gently tilt the head back**, a little at a time, until air goes in and the chest rises.

4. **Before selecting a 17-OMEGA-1**, all questions in Case Entry and Protocol 17 must be asked and answered and the person needing aid clearly **verified** (no unknowns) **as having no injuries or acute illness** (no priority symptoms).

Axioms
1. **LONG FALLS** are often 3rd **party calls**.
2. **Ground-level falls** in elderly patients commonly result in hip fractures which are **not prehospital emergencies**.
3. Prevention of permanent nerve injury is a **major goal of rescue and treatment**.

Types of Injuries
- Abrasions
- Amputations
- Contusions
- Dislocations
- Fractures
- Lacerations

Spinal Injury Suspected if:
- Abnormal breathing
- Diving accident (or jumping into water from a height)
- **LONG FALL** (≥ 6ft/2m) has occurred
- Massive facial or head injury present
- No pain or movement below injury
- Tingling sensation or numbness in extremities
- Unconsciousness at a trauma scene

17 FALLS   **17**

FIGURE 17.6. *Additional information dispatch card (Falls Protocol from MPDS v11, ©2001 NAEMD, used by permission).*

that it exists. Pre-arrival instructions cannot stand alone.[28] They must follow as the result of proven interrogation scripts that identify those who need treatment and those who do not. Therefore, PAIs are only one component, albeit an essential one, of a competent medical dispatch system. Systems that provide telephone instructions without proper medically approved interrogation and evaluation of the patient's situation first are at significant medical and legal risk. This should never be done.

In medicine, planning and knowledge aforethought are crucial to the effective functioning of medical providers. Emergency nurses, trauma surgeons, and aeromedical personnel clearly have a medical advantage if they have some idea of the emergency they are about to encounter; prehospital providers are no different. Information that is succinct, yet contains scene situation essentials, is crucial to responders. Until someone actually arrives, no one knows more about the scene than the EMD, who is "scene commander" until someone else visually evaluates the scene. The EMD must determine the "big picture" and paint a verbal image for adequate en route preparation of the field providers.

Hazardous materials, the mentally disturbed, patients on drugs, and the "just plain mean and nasty armed to the teeth" pose significant risks to responders, the caller, bystanders, and the patient. Obtaining and transmitting, as a priority, information forewarning those who could benefit from such knowledge is within the role of the EMD (fig. 17.7). Failure to uncover essential information during an interrogation has cost the lives of responders.

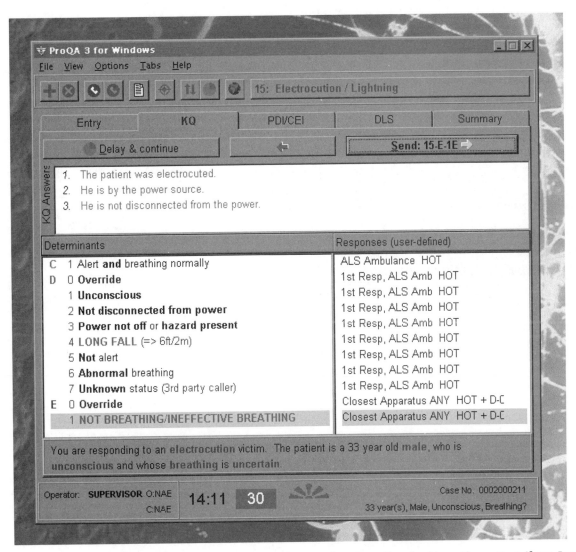

FIGURE 17.7. *Information required by response personnel to preplan the call and address the patient (from ProQA Software v3.3, © 2001 Medical Priority, Inc., Salt Lake City, UT., used with permission).*

Dispatcher Configurations

In dispatch centers where several dispatchers are on duty, medical dispatching is best performed by dividing individual responsibilities between call interrogation and dispatch functions.[14] This team approach is called "horizontal" dispatching. The interrogating calltaker follows the entry-level and key question protocols while the radio dispatcher processes the response elements of the call (fig. 17.8). This binary approach frees the interrogator to progress into PAIs without deciding which of the two functions, unit dispatching or PAIs, is more important. In some smaller centers where this approach is used, the dispatcher may have listened to the calltaker's interrogation and therefore can give the prehospital responders accurate information regarding the situation. In large and busy horizontal dispatching systems, dispatchers and interrogators may operate at physically separate but interactive computer terminals without the dispatcher ever monitoring the conversation between interrogator and caller.

"Vertical" dispatching holds each calltaker/dispatcher responsible for a given geographic area and requires that one individual handle all functions for each call. This is the default condition of dispatcher functioning in small centers only having one person on duty. The vertical dispatch configuration is less effective for EMDs using priority dispatch protocols, because important choices are often made simultaneously, but it works well with a careful understanding of and adherence to protocols. Obviously, single-dispatcher centers have no alternative other than to vertically dispatch.

Medicolegal Issues

The fascination with legal aspects of EMS has also played a major role in retarding the development of EMD by perpetuating a myriad of inappropriate fears and supposed pitfalls awaiting this relatively new field. Specifically, there has been considerable concern about the potential liability that dispatchers might incur when giving telephone instructions or prioritizing calls. With the exception of a 1984 dispatch incident in Dallas (related to a noncompliant call screener), there are no public records of any lawsuits (successful or unsuccessful) addressing either area,

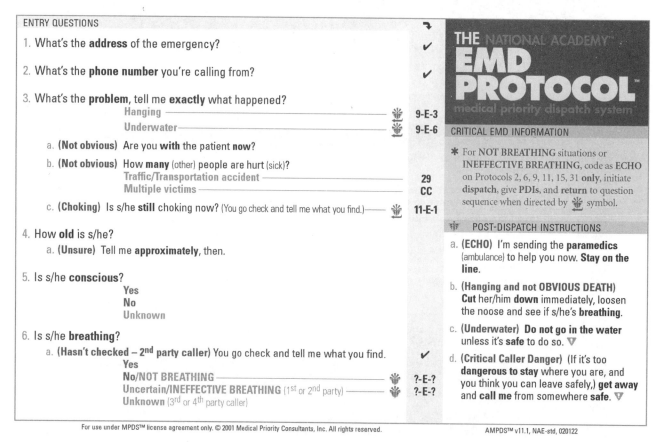

FIGURE 17.8. *Case Entry Protocol (from MPDS v11, © 2001 NAEMD, used by permission)*

even though thousands of communities now perform both functions routinely.

The legal climate is getting warmer in all areas of medicine, and EMS is no exception. As the legal community has learned more about the workings of the prehospital care system, it has discovered the dispatch center as well; however, at this time *failure* to provide PAIs and "screening out" stand out as the major areas of risk. Legal cases involving dispatch misadventures have become common enough that plaintiff's attorneys have coined a term for it—dispatcher abandonment.

The medical director must understand the four essential components of negligence in a court of law. These are: (1) duty, (2) breach of duty, (3) damages, and (4) causation. Most malpractice cases are won or lost in the area of causation by success or failure to show that acts of omission by the defendant were the "proximate cause" of the untoward result (damages). However, the concept of duty may play a more prominent role as medical dispatching evolves. Prosser states in regard to duty, "Changing social conditions lead constantly to the recognition of new duties. No better general statement can be made than that the courts will find a duty where in general reasonable men would recognize it and agree that it exists."[31]

In 1981, Page wrote:

> I personally feel that the highly successful 'medical self-help' program introduced by the Phoenix Fire Department, may have started a process which will redefine a municipality's duty to its citizens. Similarly, the Emergency Medical Dispatch Priority Card System, created by Clawson in association with the Salt Lake City Fire Department, may have further advanced the municipality's duty. In other words, I can foresee a day when a citizen might allege that the municipality (which maintains a full-time public safety dispatching service) was negligent for failing to implement and operate such a service. In view of the fact that implementation of this new level of service does not constitute a major expenditure to the municipality—and thus is basically an organizational/management/training issue, rather than a funding/taxation issue—I feel the case for a legal obligation (duty) to provide it becomes stronger.[24]

In 1993 the *Journal of Emergency Medical Services* reported that, on the basis of their annual 200-city survey, 94% of communication centers operated by EMS agencies were offering some sort of pre-arrival instructions to callers. However, only 70% of fire departments and 68% of police-operated centers offered pre-arrival instructions.[32] The courts must decide whether or when such a duty, therefore a standard of care, is actually created. This issue is moot in many states, as statutes and regulations required them. Legitimate concerns have been raised concerning pre-arrival instructions. The common expression is, "Doctors don't even give advice over the phone. Why should dispatchers?" However, in thousands of cases, trained EMDs have given excellent instructions via the telephone. Because the alternative is literally nothing, more intelligent concerns should focus on the questions listed in the table 17.4:

TABLE 17.4
Pre-Arrival Instruction Concerns
1. Is there **adequate identification** of the problems requiring dispatcher "invasive" treatment?
2. Are dispatchers **uniformly trained**?
3. Do dispatchers use sound, **medically approved algorithms** that give more detailed instructions such as CPR?
4. Is there **adequate quality management and medical oversight** at dispatch **including call review**?

The answers to each of these questions play an important role in the risk management aspect of EMD. Because dispatchers are not any less accountable, just less accessible, than other EMS practitioners, the answers to these questions should obviously be in the affirmative. In 1981 George stated in the *EMT Legal Bulletin*:[33]

> An 'upfront' clearly articulated written policy in support of telephone screening of emergency calls coupled with sound guidelines and protocols for use by dispatchers would provide a ray of legal light in an otherwise murky area of heavy potential liability. A reasonable system of call screening can provide a good legal defense for both the EMS dispatcher and his employer should a charge of negligent handling of emergency calls be raised by a plaintiff.

The less structure that is built into the interrogation, the more questions are asked and the longer the interrogation lasts. Without structure, key elements are often omitted, and unnecessary and anecdotal queries are interjected; the unfortunate result is that the four objectives of key questioning are not adequately or consistently covered. When a paramedic is shot because the dispatcher failed to ascertain the potential for violence at the scene, it becomes painfully apparent that "a hole" could exist in more than just the system.

The absence of standard protocols makes it difficult to reproduce the same sequence of interrogation or the same answers in relation to a given chief complaint. As George further warned:[33]

> EMS dispatchers must always avoid the appearance of responding to or categorizing emergency calls in a haphazard or arbitrary manner. A unified procedure will provide an excellent method of safeguarding against arbitrary decision-making. Without a unified system, one dispatcher may decide that a crucial situation exists primarily on the level of emotion he detects in the caller's voice, while another may depend on his own "gut" reaction, without being able to articulate a clear reason for his decision.

Some places provide various forms of legal immunity to public safety personnel. Governmental immunity may not always protect an individual or their employer from liability damage recovery, as in the *Kazmerowski v. Chicago*, Supreme Court of Illinois decision.[34] Immunity should never be provided to dispatchers without being clearly linked to appropriate training and certification, use of medically approved protocols, compliance with protocol, quality management mechanisms, random case review and feedback, continuing dispatch education, and recertification. If all these are not assured, then public safety dispatchers and their employers should be responsible for negligent actions.

Summary

At times, application of common sense seems impossible in a world of self-protectionism, political correctness, and "what if" mentality. Had EMS and EMD appeared in the 1930s, legal discussions would have been largely unnecessary. In those earlier times, actions themselves were considered more important than the imagined consequences. Today, however, this professional concern precludes more constructive activities by dispatchers in many systems. Optimal dispatching requires the courage to practice medicine at dispatch the same way it is done in the field. Many of the key decisions and diagnoses in medical practice are based on statistical predictability or the likelihood of finding a specific problem using standard evaluations and tests. Medical priority dispatching concepts were born of this "physician-based" process.

The EMD's role differs in major ways from that of the field provider. Street practitioners act as advocates for individual patients assumed to be dying until it is proven otherwise. EMDs are the advocate for the well-being of the entire system and they must constantly juggle the concepts of "allocate versus conserve" and "hurry versus wait." This requires a philosophy of training and protocol quite different from that of field personnel. The EMD's multiple roles of interrogator, prioritizer, and pre-arrival intervenor are analogous to the physician's tasks of history taking, evaluation, categorization, and treatment. It is no wonder that the modern medical director feels comfortable with the philosophy of EMD, and in providing medical oversight.

The advocacy of the system versus the individual patient is the dilemma faced in providing safe and efficient dispatch priorities. EMS physicians responsible for medical dispatch programs are repeatedly forced to deal with that dilemma.

Today, many EMS systems lack the money and human resources to respond maximally to every medical request. The improvements in patient care and survival, and the appropriate tiering of response through structured call prioritization, provide one answer to the spectre of political or financial self-destruction in EMS.[33,35,36]

Focusing on the EMS system, not paying appropriate attention to dispatch, is analogous to picking up a deadly snake by the tail instead of just behind the head. The unexpected "bite" of medical dispatch has injured a number of unwary medical directors. Excellence at dispatch encourages excellence down the line. Nursing QM expert Smith-Marker stated it well regarding telephone-based medical triage:[37]

> Telephone triage can function according to defined purposeful expectations or by intuition. A medical dispatching system can operate in a designated manner or haphazardly. Patient care by phone can be delivered by design or by impulse and habit. Standards either exist or they do not. If they exist, they must be detailed, consistent, and comprehensive or they will be shallow, irrelevant, and worthless.

In conclusion, the core of emergency medical dispatching, as in most aspects of medical practice, is the provision of the correct medical interactions at the right time by appropriately trained practitioners. The critical functions of EMDs in prehospital medicine are unique and crucial parts of the responsibility of medical oversight.

References

1. Roberts B. EMS dispatching: its use and misuse. Dallas Fire Department internal report, 1978.

2. Bailey E, et al. The use of emergency medical dispatch protocols to reduce the number of inappropriate scene responses made by advanced life support personnel. *Prehosp Emerg Care.* 2000;4:2.

3. Curka P, Pepe P, Ginger V. Emergency medical services priority dispatch. *Ann Emerg Med.* 1995;22:1668.

4. Zachariah B, Pepe P. The development of emergency medical dispatch in the USA: a historical perspective. *European Journal of Emergency Medicine.* 1995;2:109–112.

5. Clawson J. Dispatch priority training: strengthening the weak link. *JEMS.* 1981;6:2.

6. Clawson J. Medical priority dispatch: it works! *JEMS.* 1993;8:2.

7. Clawson J. Priority dispatching after Dallas: another viewpoint. *Journal of Emergency Medical Services.* 1984;9:36–37.

8. Eisenberg M, et al. Identification of cardiac arrest by emergency dispatchers. *Am J Emerg Med.* 1986;4:4.

9. Clawson J. The value of protocol compliance. *Journal of the National Academy of EMD.* 1990;1:3.

10. Clawson J, Sinclair R. The emotional content and cooperation score in emergency medical dispatching. *Prehosp Emerg Care.* 2001;5:1.

11. Keene K. Promises, promises: does EMD really work? *Emerg Med Services.* 1990;19:9.

12. Clawson J. Regulations and standards for emergency medical dispatchers: a model for state or region. *Emerg Med Services.* 1984;13:4.

13. Keller R. EMD in the fire service. *Fire Chief.* 1992;36(5):46.

14. Clawson J, Dernocoeur K. *Principles of Emergency Medical Dispatch. 3rd ed.* Salt Lake City, UT: Priority Press; 2000.

15. Clawson J. The maximal response disease-red lights and siren syndrome. *JEMS.* 1987;12:1.

16. National Academies of Emergency Dispatch. *Emergency Telecommunicator Course Manual.* Sudbury, MA: Jones & Bartlett Publishing; 2001.

17. American Society for Testing and Materials. *Standard Practice for Emergency Medical Dispatch Management.* Pub No F1560-94, Philadelphia, PA, 1994.

18. American Society for Testing and Materials. *Standard Practice for Emergency Medical Dispatch.* Pub No F1258-95, Philadelphia, PA, 1995.

19. Clawson J. Quality assurance: A priority for medical dispatch. *Emerg Med Services.* 1989;18:7.

20. Emergency Medical Dispatcher Rules of the Utah Emergency Medical Services System and Standards Act, Title 26, Chapter 8.

21. Quality Improvement Case Review and Remediation Actions Policy, Salt Lake City Fire Department, 1998. In: *Principles of Emergency Medical Dispatch. 3rd ed.* Salt Lake City, UT: Priority Press; 2001.

22. Clawson J. Medical dispatch review: "run" review for the EMD. *JEMS.* 1986;11:10.

23. Clawson J, Cady G, Martin R, Sinclair R. Effect of a comprehensive quality management process on compliance with protocol in an emergency medical dispatch center. *Ann Emerg Med.* 1998;32:578–584.

24. Page JO. *EMT's Legal Primer.* Solana Beach, CA: Jems Publishing Co; 1985.

25. Billettier A, et al. The lay public's expectations of pre-arrival instructions when dialing 9-1-1. *Prehosp Emerg Care.* 2000;4:3.

26. Guidelines for cardiopulmonary resuscitation and emergency cardiac care. *JAMA.* 1992;268:2172.

27. Clawson J, Hauert S. Dispatch life support: establishing standards that work. *JEMS.* 1990;15:8.

28. National Institutes of Health. *Emergency Medical Dispatching: Rapid Identification and Treatment of Acute Myocardial Infarction.* NIH Publications, No 94, 1994.

29. Clawson J. The hysteria threshold: gaining control of the emergency caller. *JEMS.* 1986;11:8.

30. Clawson J. Psychological components of pre-arrival instructing. In: *Emergency Medical Dispatcher Training Program Manual.* Salt Lake City: Medical Priority Consultants; 1986.

31. Keeton P, ed. *The Law of Torts,* 5th ed. St. Paul, MN: West Publishing Co; 1984.

32. Cady G. EMS in the United States: a survey of providers in the 200 most populous cities. *JEMS.* 1993;18(1):71.

33. George J. EMS triage. *Emergency Medical Technician Legal Bulletin* 1981;5:4.

34. American National Bank & Trust Co., *Special Adm'r for the Estate of Renee Kazmierowski, Deceased Appellant, v. City of Chicago, et al.,* Appellee; Illinois Supreme Court Decision docket #86215, Nov. 1999.

35. Stratton S. Triage by emergency medical dispatchers. *Prehosp Disast Med.* 1992;7:263.

36. Valenzuela T, et al. Estimated cost-effectiveness of dispatcher CPR instruction via telephone to bystanders during out-of-hospital ventricular fibrillation. *Prehosp Disast Med.* 1992;7:379.

37. Wheeler S. *Telephone Triage: Theory, Practice and Protocol Development.* Albany, NY: Delmar Publishers; 1993.

Appendix I

Emergency Medical Dispatching*

The following document expresses the positions developed by the membership of the National Association of EMS Physicians (NAEMSP). This position is based on the Consensus Document for Emergency Medical Dispatching.

Introduction

Medical Dispatching has been the last major area in the prehospital emergency medical services chain of care to be identified and developed. The "health" of many EMS systems can be gauged by the appropriateness of training, protocols, and medical control and direction of dispatchers. The involvement of prehospital EMS physicians in the world of dispatch is relatively new but unquestionably essential. For this reason, the National Association of EMS Physicians has taken the following position relative to Emergency Medical Dispatching.

Position

The trained Emergency Medical Dispatcher (EMD) is an essential part of a prehospital EMS system. Medical direction and control for the EMD and the dispatch center also constitutes part of the prescribed responsibilities of the Medical Director of the EMS system. The functions of emergency medical dispatching must include the use of predetermined questions, pre-arrival telephone instructions, and pre-assigned response levels and modes. The EMD must understand the philosophy and psychology of interrogation and telephone interventions, basic emergency medical priorities and interventions, and be expert in dispatch life support. Minimum training levels must be established, standardized, and all EMDs must be certified by governmental authority.

Position Statements

1. The medical aspects of emergency medical dispatching and communications are an integral part of the responsibilities of the Medical Director of an EMS system.
2. Proven knowledge and skills in the area known as basic telecommunications are requisite for all public safety telecommunicators.
3. Understanding the philosophy of medical interrogation and the psychology of providing Pre-Arrival Instructions is integral to the training and functioning of EMDs.
4. Pre-arrival instructions are a mandatory function of each EMD in a medical dispatch center.
5. Dispatch prioritization is an essential element in any EMS system for it establishes the appropriate level of care including the urgency and type of response. Standard medically approved telephone instructions by trained EMDs are safe to give and in many instances are a moral necessity.
6. Training as EMDs is required for all dispatchers functioning in medical dispatch agencies and requires unprecedented cooperation between the diverse disciplines of telecommunications and emergency medicine necessary to provide this unique teaching forum. This training includes content and results in competence which differ substantially from that standardly provided for EMTs and paramedics. It must be taught by specially-trained instructors.
7. Quality Assurance, Risk Management, and Medical Control and Direction are essential elements to the management of medical dispatch operations within the EMS system.
8. Certification and authorization by government agencies in accordance with standards promulgated by NAEMSP in conjunction with other organizations must be required.

Definitions

Emergency Medical Dispatching: the reception and management of requests for emergency medical assistance in an EMS system.

Emergency Medical Dispatcher (EMD): a specially trained public safety telecommunicator with the specific emergency medical knowledge essential for the appropriate and efficient functioning of emergency medical dispatching.

Medical Dispatch Center: any agency that routinely accepts calls for EMD assistance from the public and/or that dispatches prehospital emergency medical personnel pursuant to such requests.

Public Safely Telecommunicator: an individual trained to communicate by electronic means with persons seeking emergency assistance and with agencies and individuals providing such assistance.

Basic Telecommunications Skills: the generic body of knowledge and skills necessary to function as a

Public Safety Telecommunicator whether performing specifically in the role of medical, fire, law enforcement, aeromedical, park service dispatcher, or in any combination of these roles.

Medical Director*: the management and accountability for the medical care aspects of an EMD program including: (1) the direction and oversight of the training of the EMD, (2) development and monitoring of both the operational and the emergency medical priority dispatch protocol systems, (3) participation in EMD system evaluation, and (4) directing the medical care rendered by the EMDs.

Medical Oversight Control*: the EMS physician(s) responsible for the provision of education, training, protocols, critiques, leadership, testing, certification, decertification, standards, advice, and quality control through an official authoritative position within the prehospital EMS system.

Medical Priority Dispatch System: a medically approved system used by a medical dispatch center to dispatch appropriate aid to medical emergencies, which include: (1) systematized caller interrogation, (2) systematized Pre-Arrival Instructions, and (3) protocols which match the dispatcher's evaluation of the injury or illness type and severity with vehicle response mode and configuration.

Pre-Arrival Instructions: telephone-rendered, medically approved, written instructions given by trained EMDs through callers which help to provide aid to the victim and control of the situation prior to arrival of prehospital personnel.

Dispatch Life Support: the knowledge, procedures, and skills used by trained EMDs in providing care through Pre-Arrival Instructions to callers. It consists of those BLS and ALS principles that are appropriate to application by medical dispatchers.

Quality Management Assurance: the comprehensive program of setting standards and monitoring the performance of the clinical, operational, and personnel components of the medical dispatch center in relation to these accepted standards.

Risk Management: a sub-component of the Quality Assurance program designed to identify problematic situations and to assist EMS Medical Directors, dispatch supervisors, and EMDs in modifying practice behaviors found to be deficient by quality assessment procedures; to protect the public against incompetent practitioners; and to modify structural, resource, and protocol deficiencies

*Relates specifically to Emergency Medical Dispatch

that may exist in the emergency medical dispatch system.

Vehicle Response Configuration: the specific set of vehicle(s) in terms of types, capabilities, and numbers responding as the direct result of actions taken by the emergency medical dispatch system.

Vehicle Response Mode: the manner of response used by the personnel and vehicles dispatched which reflects the level of urgency of a particular required treatment or transport (e.g., use of emergency driving techniques such as red-lights-and-siren vs. routine driving).

Discussion

The Emergency Medical Dispatcher (EMD) is the principal link between the public in need of emergency medical assistance and the EMS system. As such, the EMD plays a key role in the ability of the EMS system to respond to a perceived medical emergency. Most often, all of the information obtained is through telephone communications with a caller who often is distressed and out of control. The EMD must have skills which allow him/her to match the personnel and equipment dispatched to the perceived emergency. Thus, the EMD must be able to discern the nature and the urgency of the illness(es) and/or injury(ies) in a manner which allows selection of the most appropriate response configuration and mode.

Therefore, the EMD must possess special knowledge and a set of medical and technological skills which are unique for the EMS system. They need to know sufficient medical knowledge in lay terminology to acquire an appropriate medical history and be cognizant of all of the characteristics inherent within the EMS system in which they function. Furthermore, recent studies indicate that EMDs may play a very important role in the provision of instructions by which a caller may initiate appropriate treatment and life support prior to the arrival of any of the EMS responding vehicles and personnel. The capable EMD provides "first responder" care through the surrogate caller. Such skills have been shown to help preserve lives, prevent further injuries, and even assist with the delivery of babies.

Without these specially trained, talented, dedicated, and skilled professionals, an EMS system cannot function optimally. Unfortunately, in most situations, persons performing the dispatch functions have had little more training than the average layperson. Inadequate personnel and equipment may be dispatched for major problems while too comprehensive a portion of the system may be mobilized for minor problems. This latter circumstance may result in depriving others in need of the committed services to be deprived of them. Any break in these important functions result in failure of the entire EMS system. An EMS system only can be as good as its EMDs.

Since emergency medical dispatching is key to the successful operation of any prehospital EMS system, the policies and procedures utilized by trained EMDs must conform to national standards and local capabilities. The history obtained by telephone and both the medical care dictated by the EMD and the responses initiated are functions of the type and level of medical care possible from the specific EMS system. The quality of all of the medical care delivered by a system is the responsibility of the medical director of that prehospital system. Therefore, all of the policies and procedures used by the Medical Dispatch Center in terms of medical care rendered are part of the responsibilities of the Medical Director and hence, must be approved by the Medical Director of the system. Key to the Medical Director's role in the management of medical dispatch centers is his or her detailed understanding of the concepts of EMD and its physical operation, involvement in all aspects of quality assurance of medical dispatch, and medical direction and accountability for the protocols, policies, and procedures relevant to the medical dispatch activities of the EMD. In summary, the medical aspects of emergency medical dispatching and communications are an integral part of the responsibilities of the Medical Director of each EMS system.

Certain skills are common to all public safety communicators. These include the theory and operation of complex communication equipment, troubleshooting the same, and basic radio and telephone communication skills. Serious liability for dispatch centers commonly results due to the lack of these essential skills. The training and certification of the EMD is built upon this baseline of knowledge and skills, which is generic for performing in the role of medical, fire, law enforcement, aeromedical, park service dispatcher, or any combination of these services.

The ability to interact with anxious, uncooperative, and, at times, hysterical callers rests on the ability of the EMD to anticipate the actions of the undirected caller, assist the caller in regaining control, and then, convert the caller into a calmer, first responder is a special one. Each is an essential step in the performance of the prescribed duties and contributes to the substantial responsibilities delegated to the EMD by the Medical Director and the Medical Dispatch Center. Each of these steps requires special training and the development of different skills. This knowledge and special set of skills are not part of the standardized EMT or paramedic curricula. Each is specific to medical dispatch training.

Since the value of EMDs providing Pre-Arrival Instructions to callers in attendance with victims of cardiopulmonary arrest was first demonstrated 14 years ago, Pre-Arrival Instructions have become a mandatory function of the EMD. In essence, the EMD is the first "first-responder" and through immediate action effectively can eliminate the often deadly gaps which may occur between receipt of the call and the beginning of treatment which is delayed until after the arrival of the responding vehicles and personnel. First response consists of telephone instructions provided by trained EMDs functioning from standard, medically approved protocols. Such instructions are safe and, in many instances, are a moral necessity. The telephone instructions are given through the caller to help another person or the caller protect the victim(s) from further harm or injury, to initiate life-impacting treatments, and to transform an undirected caller into a calmer scene rescuer who no longer needs to be helpless. Training, certification, and recertification in Dispatch Life Support (DLS), which includes that portion of BLS appropriate to application by medical dispatchers is necessary to maintain and continually upgrade this unique, and, at times, life-saving, nonvisual skill. Hence, it is essential that EMDs understand the philosophy of medical interrogation and the psychology associated with the provision of Pre-Arrival Instructions. This knowledge and the associated skills must be integral parts of the training, direction, and management of EMDs and any Medical Dispatch Center.

Dispatch Prioritization is an essential element in EMS and requires careful attention by both the EMD, his or her supervisor, and the EMS physician responsible for medical control. These priorities must reflect the level of appropriate response including types of personnel (ALS vs. BLS vs. first responder), response configuration (numbers and types of vehicles responding), and mode of response (red-lights-and-siren vs. routine). Haphazard or arbitrary dispatch decisions have been shown to place victims of serious illness or injury at unnecessary risk, and have resulted in significant liability to systems lacking these essential protocols, procedures, and policies.

With the use of unified, standard protocols, the emergency medical dispatcher's conduct will be less vulnerable to charges of careless or reckless judgment. For example, without a unified system of standard protocols, one dispatcher may decide that a crucial situation exists primarily on the basis of the level of emotion he/she detects in the caller's voice, while another may depend on his or her own "gut" reaction without being able to articulate a clear reason for a decision. A unified procedure provides an excellent method of safeguarding against arbitrary decision-making. Similarly, EMS employers can point to such guidelines as a system of risk management in an area in which human error and its dire consequences clearly are foreseeable. The appropriate prioritization of the type, number, and manner of responses is essential to effect an appropriate reduction of responding vehicles traveling red-lights-and-siren, and therefore unnecessary vehicle accidents. This will assure that emergency crews will not be committed inappropriately to non-emergency cases, and that the right care will be sent in the right way to the right patient at the right time.

The necessity to prioritize responses is evident in the majority of EMS systems today. In order to prioritize calls properly, the EMD must be well versed in the medical conditions and incident types that constitute their daily routine. Training in these priorities must be detailed and dispatch-specific (not EMT or paramedic training per se). The development of dispatch priorities for an agency or locality must be carefully thought out and ultimately approved by those physicians responsible for medical control.

Since much of the knowledge and many of the skills required by the EMD are dispatch-specific, a curriculum for their training differs substantially from those used in the preparation of EMTs or paramedics. Training as an EMT or paramedic does not adequately prepare a person for the role of an EMD. Much of the required EMD curriculum cannot be found in standard EMS training curricula. It consists of content and emphasis which differ significantly from that used for the training of all other health professionals and public safety dispatchers. The unique teaching forum necessary to provide this essential training requires unprecedented cooperation between the diverse disciplines of telecommunications and prehospital and emergency medicine. Instructor requirements should include line dispatch experience as a trained EMD for the Primary Dispatch Instructor and a minimum of advanced life support training and experience for the Medical Dispatch Instructor who is responsible for teaching the core course materials, specifically the medical dispatch priorities. All instructors should have successfully completed a credible EMD course prior to assuming a teaching role. Essentially, training of EMDs is required for all dispatchers functioning in medical dispatch agencies, and contains significant content and competence which differs substantially from that standardly provided to EMTs and paramedics.

Quality management assurance, risk management, and medical direction and control are essential elements for the ongoing well-being of any EMS system. Routine medical reviews of the activities of EMDs and medical dispatch centers in general is vital to the health of all EMS systems. Dispatch review committees constitute one method of providing quality assurance for EMD activities and the medical aspects of the operation of a medical dispatch center. Such committees should be composed of prehospital EMS physicians and those responsible for the provision of medical control, dispatch supervision and management personnel, EMTs and/or paramedics, and EMDs. Each must be familiar with all aspects of EMS communications, specifically the medical dispatch process, and must be involved in an ongoing way with its function relative to medical issues, operations, and patient care.

Recognition of the important role of emergency medical dispatchers in the delivery of prehospital emergency medical services by responsible governmental agencies, and by the public in general, is important for the public health and protection. Without such recognition and action, it is unlikely that the training of these important professionals will be mandated. An ever-increasing number of states, regions, counties, and municipalities certify or at least require standard training of EMDs. This constitutes an essential prerequisite to the practice by EMDs. Minimum standards must be developed and promulgated for the training, certification, and or licensure of all public safety telecommunicators, specifically Emergency Medical Dispatchers.

Conclusion

In order to assure the professionalism of this key aspect of prehospital emergency medical care, EMS physicians should participate actively in the development, training, quality assurance, medical control and direction oversight of EMDs and medical dispatch centers. Oversight physicians should be intimately involved in the any decision-making regarding all aspects of medical response. The Emergency Medical Dispatcher provides an all-important professional link in the overall EMS chain of care and survival.

Appendix II

Analysis of Call Types by Determinant Level

Cleveland Emergency Medical Services Master Dispatch Analysis, 1995

Determinant Level	Incidents	% of all Calls
DELTA	32,534	37.3%
CHARLIE	16,136	18.5%
BRAVO	24,814	28.5%
ALPHA	13,719	15.7%
Total	**87,203**	**100.0%**

Analysis of Call Types by Chief Complaint

1 ABDOMINAL PAIN/PROBLEMS — 2,847 incidents — 3% of all complaints

DETERMINANT LEVEL	INCIDENTS/ LEVEL	PERCENT/ CHIEF COMPLAINT	DETERMINANT CODES	INCIDENTS/ CODE	PERCENT/ CODE
CHARLIE	**1,186**	**41.7%**			
			1-C-0	9	0.32%
			1-C-1	563	19.78%
			1-C-2	483	16.97%
			1-C-3	60	2.11%
			1-C-4	71	2.49%
ALPHA	**1,661**	**58.3%**			
			1-A-1	1,661	58.34%

2 ALLERGIES/HIVES/MED REACTIONS/STINGS — 672 incidents — 1% of all complaints

DETERMINANT LEVEL	INCIDENTS/ LEVEL	PERCENT/ CHIEF COMPLAINT	DETERMINANT CODES	INCIDENTS/ CODE	PERCENT/ CODE
DELTA	**62**	**9.2%**			
			2-D-1	25	3.72%
			2-D-2	34	5.06%
			2-D-3	3	0.45%
CHARLIE	**254**	**37.8%**			
			2-C-1	254	37.80%
BRAVO	**267**	**39.7%**			
			2-B-1	267	39.73%
ALPHA	**89**	**13.2%**			
			2-A-1	89	13.24%

3 ANIMAL BITES/ATTACKS   230 incidents   < 1% of all complaints

DETERMINANT LEVEL	INCIDENTS/ LEVEL	PERCENT/ CHIEF COMPLAINT	DETERMINANT CODES	INCIDENTS/ CODE	PERCENT/ CODE
DELTA	43	18.7%			
			3-D-1	34	14.78%
			3-D-4	2	0.87%
			3-D-5	2	0.87%
			3-D-6	5	2.17%
BRAVO	93	40.4%			
			3-B-0	2	0.87%
			3-B-1	82	35.65%
			3-B-2	9	3.91%
ALPHA	94	40.9%			
			3-A-1	80	34.78%
			3-A-2	14	6.09%

4 ASSAULT/RAPE   7,228 incidents   8% of all complaints

DETERMINANT LEVEL	INCIDENTS/ LEVEL	PERCENT/ CHIEF COMPLAINT	DETERMINANT CODES	INCIDENTS/ CODE	PERCENT/ CODE
DELTA	1,232	17.0%			
			4-D-1	196	2.71%
			4-D-2	218	3.02%
			4-D-3	350	4.84%
			4-D-4	468	6.47%
BRAVO	5,559	76.9%			
			4-B-1	3,207	44.37%
			4-B-2	167	2.31%
			4-B-3	2,185	30.23%
ALPHA	437	6.0%			
			4-A-1	316	4.37%
			4-A-2	121	1.67%

5 BACK PAIN (NON-TRAUMATIC)   671 incidents   1% of all complaints

DETERMINANT LEVEL	INCIDENTS/ LEVEL	PERCENT/ CHIEF COMPLAINT	DETERMINANT CODES	INCIDENTS/ CODE	PERCENT/ CODE
DELTA	9	1.3%			
			5-D-1	9	1.34%
CHARLIE	35	5.2%			
			5-C-0	8	1.19%
			5-C-1	27	4.02%
ALPHA	627	93.4%			
			5-A-1	572	85.25%
			5-A-2	55	8.20%

6 BREATHING PROBLEMS — 12,116 incidents — 14% of all complaints

DETERMINANT LEVEL	INCIDENTS/ LEVEL	PERCENT/ CHIEF COMPLAINT	DETERMINANT CODES	INCIDENTS/ CODE	PERCENT/ CODE
DELTA	8,032	66.3%			
			6-D-0	9	0.07%
			6-D-1	2,894	23.89%
			6-D-2	996	8.22%
			6-D-3	4,133	34.11%
CHARLIE	4,084	33.7%			
			6-C-1	2,576	21.26%
			6-C-2	1,275	10.52%
			6-C-3	233	1.92%

7 BURNS/EXPLOSIONS — 376 incidents — < 1% of all complaints

DETERMINANT LEVEL	INCIDENTS/ LEVEL	PERCENT/ CHIEF COMPLAINT	DETERMINANT CODES	INCIDENTS/ CODE	PERCENT/ CODE
DELTA	45	12.0%			
			7-D-0	1	0.27%
			7-D-1	12	3.19%
			7-D-3	3	0.80%
			7-D-4	29	7.71%
CHARLIE	129	34.3%			
			7-C-0	1	0.27%
			7-C-1	16	4.26%
			7-C-2	112	29.79%
BRAVO	40	10.6%			
			7-B-0	1	0.27%
			7-B-1	39	10.37%
ALPHA	162	43.1%			
			7-A-1	154	40.96%
			7-A-2	8	2.13%

8 CARBON MONOXIDE/INHALATION/HAZMAT — 107 incidents — < 1% of all complaints

DETERMINANT LEVEL	INCIDENTS/ LEVEL	PERCENT/ CHIEF COMPLAINT	DETERMINANT CODES	INCIDENTS/ CODE	PERCENT/ CODE
DELTA	40	37.4%			
			8-D-1	20	18.69%
			8-D-2	8	7.48%
			8-D-3	10	9.35%
			8-D-4	2	1.87%
CHARLIE	32	29.9%			
			8-C-1	32	29.91%
BRAVO	35	32.7%			
			8-B-1	35	32.71%

9 CARDIAC/RESPIRATORY ARREST — 2,054 incidents — 2% of all complaints

DETERMINANT LEVEL	INCIDENTS/ LEVEL	PERCENT/ CHIEF COMPLAINT	DETERMINANT CODES	INCIDENTS/ CODE	PERCENT/ CODE
DELTA	1,717	83.6%			
			9-D-1	1,704	82.96%
			9-D-2	13	0.63%
BRAVO	337	16.4%			
			9-B-1	337	16.41%

10 CHEST PAIN — 7,480 incidents — 9% of all complaints

DETERMINANT LEVEL	INCIDENTS/ LEVEL	PERCENT/ CHIEF COMPLAINT	DETERMINANT CODES	INCIDENTS/ CODE	PERCENT/ CODE
DELTA	4,531	60.6%			
			10-D-0	1	0.01%
			10-D-1	140	1.87%
			10-D-2	297	3.97%
			10-D-3	4,093	54.72%
CHARLIE	2,447	32.7%			
			10-C-1	1,064	14.22%
			10-C-2	1,110	14.84%
			10-C-3	16	0.21%
			10-C-4	257	3.44%
ALPHA	502	6.7%			
			10-A-1	502	6.71%

11 CHOKING — 555 incidents — 1% of all complaints

DETERMINANT LEVEL	INCIDENTS/ LEVEL	PERCENT/ CHIEF COMPLAINT	DETERMINANT CODES	INCIDENTS/ CODE	PERCENT/ CODE
DELTA	418	75.3%			
			11-D-1	196	35.32%
			11-D-2	208	37.48%
			11-D-3	14	2.52%
ALPHA	137	24.7%			
			11-A-1	137	24.68%

DETERMINANT LEVEL	INCIDENTS/ LEVEL	PERCENT/ CHIEF COMPLAINT	DETERMINANT CODES	INCIDENTS/ CODE	PERCENT/ CODE
DELTA	2,305	58.1%			
			12-D-1	1,964	49.51%
			12-D-2	329	8.29%
			12-D-3	12	0.30%
CHARLIE	365	9.2%			
			12-C-0	20	0.50%
			12-C-1	46	1.16%
			12-C-2	105	2.65%
			12-C-3	83	2.09%
			12-C-4	111	2.80%
BRAVO	201	5.1%			
			12-B-0	12	0.30%
			12-B-1	189	4.76%
ALPHA	1,096	27.6%			
			12-A-1	1,096	27.63%

DETERMINANT LEVEL	INCIDENTS/ LEVEL	PERCENT/ CHIEF COMPLAINT	DETERMINANT CODES	INCIDENTS/ CODE	PERCENT/ CODE
DELTA	323	23.0%			
			13-D-0	3	0.21%
			13-D-1	320	· 22.82%
CHARLIE	764	54.5%			
			13-C-1	585	41.73%
			13-C-2	179	12.77%
ALPHA	315	22.5%			
			13-A-1	315	22.47%

DETERMINANT LEVEL	INCIDENTS/ LEVEL	PERCENT/ CHIEF COMPLAINT	DETERMINANT CODES	INCIDENTS/ CODE	PERCENT/ CODE
DELTA	30	81.1%			
			14-D-1	20	54.05%
			14-D-2	2	5.41%
			14-D-3	3	8.11%
			14-D-4	4	10.81%
			14-D-5	1	2.70%
BRAVO	6	16.2%			
			14-B-1	6	16.22%
ALPHA	1	2.7%			
			14-A-1	1	2.70%

15 ELECTROCUTION 51 incidents < 1% of all complaints

DETERMINANT LEVEL	INCIDENTS/ LEVEL	PERCENT/ CHIEF COMPLAINT	DETERMINANT CODES	INCIDENTS/ CODE	PERCENT/ CODE
DELTA	26	51.0%			
			15-D-1	5	9.80%
			15-D-2	7	13.73%
			15-D-3	4	7.84%
			15-D-4	2	3.92%
			15-D-5	5	9.80%
			15-D-6	1	1.96%
			15-D-7	2	3.92%
CHARLIE	25	49.0%			
			15-C-1	25	49.02%

16 EYE PROBLEMS/INJURIES 283 incidents < 1% of all complaints

DETERMINANT LEVEL	INCIDENTS/ LEVEL	PERCENT/ CHIEF COMPLAINT	DETERMINANT CODES	INCIDENTS/ CODE	PERCENT/ CODE
DELTA	6	2.1%			
			16-D-1	6	2.12%
BRAVO	91	32.2%			
			16-B-0	1	0.35%
			16-B-1	90	31.80%
ALPHA	186	65.7%			
			16-A-1	90	31.80%
			16-A-2	96	33.92%

17 FALLS/BACK INJURIES (TRAUMATIC) 4,384 incidents 5% of all complaints

DETERMINANT LEVEL	INCIDENTS/ LEVEL	PERCENT/ CHIEF COMPLAINT	DETERMINANT CODES	INCIDENTS/ CODE	PERCENT/ CODE
DELTA	1,423	32.5%			
			17-D-0	2	0.05%
			17-D-1	175	3.99%
			17-D-2	639	14.58%
			17-D-3	326	7.44%
			17-D-4	281	6.41%
BRAVO	1,517	34.6%			
			17-B-0	11	0.25%
			17-B-1	117	2.67%
			17-B-2	114	2.60%
			17-B-3	1,275	29.08%
ALPHA	1,444	32.9%			
			17-A-1	1,096	25.00%
			17-A-2	348	7.94%

18 HEADACHE — 729 incidents — 1% of all complaints

DETERMINANT LEVEL	INCIDENTS/ LEVEL	PERCENT/ CHIEF COMPLAINT	DETERMINANT CODES	INCIDENTS/ CODE	PERCENT/ CODE
CHARLIE	519	71.2%			
			18-C-0	1	0.14%
			18-C-1	42	5.76%
			18-C-2	92	12.62%
			18-C-3	199	27.30%
			18-C-4	179	24.55%
			18-C-5	6	0.82%
ALPHA	210	28.8%			
			18-A-1	210	28.81%

19 HEART PROBLEMS — 177 incidents — < 1% of all complaints

DETERMINANT LEVEL	INCIDENTS/ LEVEL	PERCENT/ CHIEF COMPLAINT	DETERMINANT CODES	INCIDENTS/ CODE	PERCENT/ CODE
CHARLIE	117	66.1%			
			19-C-0	1	0.56%
			19-C-1	17	9.60%
			19-C-2	91	51.41%
			19-C-3	8	4.52%
BRAVO	14	7.9%			
			19-B-1	14	7.91%
ALPHA	46	26.0%			
			19-A-1	46	25.99%

20 HEAT/COLD EXPOSURE — 119 incidents — < 1% of all complaints

DETERMINANT LEVEL	INCIDENTS/ LEVEL	PERCENT/ CHIEF COMPLAINT	DETERMINANT CODES	INCIDENTS/ CODE	PERCENT/ CODE
DELTA	32	26.9%			
			20-D-1	32	26.89%
CHARLIE	6	5.0%			
			20-C-1	6	5.04%
BRAVO	64	53.8%			
			20-B-1	31	26.05%
			20-B-2	33	27.73%
ALPHA	17	14.3%			
			20-A-1	17	14.29%

21 HEMORRHAGE/LACERATIONS   3,421 incidents   4% of all complaints

DETERMINANT LEVEL	INCIDENTS/ LEVEL	PERCENT/ CHIEF COMPLAINT	DETERMINANT CODES	INCIDENTS/ CODE	PERCENT/ CODE
DELTA	1,109	32.4%			
			21-D-0	1	0.03%
			21-D-1	1,051	30.72%
			21-D-2	55	1.61%
			21-D-3	2	0.06%
BRAVO	1,813	53.0%			
			21-B-0	1	0.03%
			21-B-1	1,812	52.97%
ALPHA	499	14.6%			
			21-A-1	499	14.59%

22 INDUSTRIAL/MACHINERY ACCIDENTS   43 incidents   < 1% of all complaints

DETERMINANT LEVEL	INCIDENTS/ LEVEL	PERCENT/ CHIEF COMPLAINT	DETERMINANT CODES	INCIDENTS/ CODE	PERCENT/ CODE
DELTA	18	41.9%			
			22-D-0	1	2.33%
			22-D-1	6	13.95%
			22-D-2	11	25.58%
BRAVO	25	58.1%			
			22-B-1	25	58.14%

23 OVERDOSE/INGESTION/POISONING   2,220 incidents   3% of all complaints

DETERMINANT LEVEL	INCIDENTS/ LEVEL	PERCENT/ CHIEF COMPLAINT	DETERMINANT CODES	INCIDENTS/ CODE	PERCENT/ CODE
DELTA	256	11.5%			
			23-D-0	1	0.05%
			23-D-1	242	10.90%
			23-D-2	13	0.59%
CHARLIE	777	35.0%			
			23-C-0	1	0.05%
			23-C-1	360	16.22%
			23-C-2	189	8.51%
			23-C-3	69	3.11%
			23-C-4	79	3.56%
			23-C-5	15	0.68%
			23-C-6	64	2.88%
BRAVO	1,187	53.5%			
			23-B-0	14	0.63%
			23-B-1	1,173	52.84%

DETERMINANT LEVEL	INCIDENTS/ LEVEL	PERCENT/ CHIEF COMPLAINT	DETERMINANT CODES	INCIDENTS/ CODE	PERCENT/ CODE
DELTA	**1,142**	**35.8%**			
			24-D-0	3	0.09%
			24-D-1	72	2.26%
			24-D-2	38	1.19%
			24-D-3	713	22.36%
			24-D-4	310	9.72%
			24-D-5	6	0.19%
CHARLIE	**1,395**	**43.7%**			
			24-C-0	12	0.38%
			24-C-1	1,383	43.37%
BRAVO	**234**	**7.3%**			
			24-B-0	1	0.03%
			24-B-1	225	7.06%
			24-B-2	8	0.25%
ALPHA	**418**	**13.1%**			
			24-A-1	171	5.36%
			24-A-2	247	7.75%

25 PSYCHIATRIC/SUICIDE ATTEMPT   **1,346 incidents**   **2% of all complaints**

DETERMINANT LEVEL	INCIDENTS/ LEVEL	PERCENT/ CHIEF COMPLAINT	DETERMINANT CODES	INCIDENTS/ CODE	PERCENT/ CODE
DELTA	**39**	**2.9%**			
			25-D-0	2	0.15%
			25-D-1	37	2.75%
CHARLIE	**871**	**64.7%**			
			25-C-1	54	4.01%
			25-C-2	676	50.22%
			25-C-3	141	10.48%
BRAVO	**133**	**9.9%**			
			25-B-0	1	0.07%
			25-B-1	132	9.81%
ALPHA	**303**	**22.5%**			
			25-A-1	303	22.51%

DETERMINANT LEVEL	INCIDENTS/ LEVEL	PERCENT/ CHIEF COMPLAINT	DETERMINANT CODES	INCIDENTS/ CODE	PERCENT/ CODE
CHARLIE	**1,556**	**25.3%**			
			26-C-0	19	0.31%
			26-C-1	721	11.73%
			26-C-2	816	13.28%
BRAVO	**705**	**11.5%**			
			26-B-0	7	0.11%
			26-B-1	698	11.36%
ALPHA	**3,885**	**63.2%**			
			26-A-1	3,083	50.16%
			26-A-2	802	13.05%

DETERMINANT LEVEL	INCIDENTS/ LEVEL	PERCENT/ CHIEF COMPLAINT	DETERMINANT CODES	INCIDENTS/ CODE	PERCENT/ CODE
DELTA	**1,635**	**86.0%**			
			27-D-0	1	0.05%
			27-D-1	1,486	78.17%
			27-D-2	43	2.26%
			27-D-3	61	3.21%
			27-D-4	44	2.31%
BRAVO	**263**	**13.8%**			
			27-B-1	188	9.89%
			27-B-2	1	0.05%
			27-B-3	74	3.89%
ALPHA	**3**	**0.2%**			
			27-A-1	3	0.16%

DETERMINANT LEVEL	INCIDENTS/ LEVEL	PERCENT/ CHIEF COMPLAINT	DETERMINANT CODES	INCIDENTS/ CODE	PERCENT/ CODE
CHARLIE	**672**	**62.4%**			
			28-C-0	7	0.65%
			28-C-1	523	48.56%
			28-C-2	142	13.18%
BRAVO	**180**	**16.7%**			
			28-B-0	5	0.46%
			28-B-1	175	16.25%
ALPHA	**225**	**20.9%**			
			28-A-1	225	20.89%

29 TRAFFIC ACCIDENTS		10,054 incidents		12% of all complaints	
DETERMINANT LEVEL	INCIDENTS/ LEVEL	PERCENT/ CHIEF COMPLAINT	DETERMINANT CODES	INCIDENTS/ CODE	PERCENT/ CODE
DELTA	**4,331**	**43.1%**			
			29-D-0	6	0.06%
			29-D-1	1,682	16.73%
			29-D-2	1,468	14.60%
			29-D-3	258	2.57%
			29-D-4	466	4.64%
			29-D-5	246	2.45%
			29-D-6	195	1.94%
			29-D-7	10	0.10%
BRAVO	**5,707**	**56.8%**			
			29-B-1	3,579	35.60%
			29-B-2	2,128	21.17%
ALPHA	**15**	**0.1%**			
			29-A-1	15	0.15%

30 TRAUMATIC INJURIES, SPECIFIC		2,737 incidents		3% of all complaints	
DETERMINANT LEVEL	INCIDENTS/ LEVEL	PERCENT/ CHIEF COMPLAINT	DETERMINANT CODES	INCIDENTS/ CODE	PERCENT/ CODE
DELTA	**273**	**10.0%**			
			30-D-0	3	0.11%
			30-D-1	185	6.76%
			30-D-2	7	0.26%
			30-D-3	78	2.85%
BRAVO	**1,322**	**48.3%**			
			30-B-0	8	0.29%
			30-B-1	1,152	42.09%
			30-B-2	162	5.92%
ALPHA	**1,142**	**41.7%**			
			30-A-1	856	31.28%
			30-A-2	286	10.45%

DETERMINANT LEVEL	INCIDENTS/ LEVEL	PERCENT/ CHIEF COMPLAINT	DETERMINANT CODES	INCIDENTS/ CODE	PERCENT/ CODE
DELTA	**3,093**	**73.6%**			
			31-D-0	1	0.02%
			31-D-1	2,412	57.43%
			31-D-2	99	2.36%
			31-D-3	581	13.83%
CHARLIE	**902**	**21.5%**			
			31-C-0	5	0.12%
			31-C-1	485	11.55%
			31-C-2	149	3.55%
			31-C-3	35	0.83%
			31-C-4	205	4.88%
			31-C-5	23	0.55%
ALPHA	**205**	**4.9%**			
			31-A-1	205	4.88%

DETERMINANT LEVEL	INCIDENTS/ LEVEL	PERCENT/ CHIEF COMPLAINT	DETERMINANT CODES	INCIDENTS/ CODE	PERCENT/ CODE
DELTA	**364**	**6.8%**			
			32-D-0	12	0.22%
			32-D-1	352	6.54%
BRAVO	**5,021**	**93.2%**			
			32-B-1	2,383	44.25%
			32-B-2	562	10.44%
			32-B-3	2,076	38.55%

CHAPTER 18

Priority Dispatch Response

Jeff J. Clawson, MD

Introduction

EMS resources are limited.[1] This is increasingly evident as pressures to contain the costs of medical care rise and elected officials agonize at the addition of even a single EMS unit to an already over-taxed fleet. It is impractical for a community to have ambulances on each block; even if enough personnel could be trained, they would never get enough call volume to adequately retain their skills. Thus the use of the EMS system must be judicious and balanced. Prioritizing calls is one way to effectively and safely accomplish this.[2-4] Prioritization provides a logical method to deal with what appears at times to be apparent chaos of response choices.[5] Instead of having the system whirl in a version of EMS roulette, paramedic units are sent to appropriate calls rather than those that come in first.[6-9] The EMD must adhere to clearly established, medically approved protocols to safely and effectively accomplish this essential task.[10-11] It has been reasonably demonstrated that the science of medical dispatching requires non-arbitrary adherence to these protocols for response decisions made in the time-based environment of dispatch to be medically reliable.[12-14]

The core purpose underlying the creation of the EMD's protocol was the need to control more rationally the process of EMS response.[15] During the beginnings of modern EMS (circa 1970) the standard method of vehicle and crew deployment was what is now referred to as "maximal response."[16] Thirty years later, the need to regulate response has taken on greater implications. The issues include:

- Response configuration (numbers and types of crews and vehicles)
- Response mode (routine driving vs. lights-and-siren use)
- Referral to alternate care and evaluation methodologies (nurse advice, specialty center triage, non-EMS transport)
- Economics of response
- Politics of response
- Personnel satisfaction and crew burnout
- Responder and public safety secondary to emergency response modes
- Prioritization risk management and legal concerns

The central issue from a patient-care standpoint is getting "the right thing to the right place at the right time in the right way." The central issue from a systems standpoint is not running out of response teams by balancing need with resource dynamically.

The Maximal Response Dilemma

Millions of EMS responses occur every year. Before priority dispatch and call screening, virtually every response was run with lights-and-siren, not only to the scene, but often back to the hospital as well. This is an example of "maximal response" and is a combination of always responding with lights-and-siren or always sending multiple vehicles.[13,16,17]

Maximal response takes root in three traditional myths. First, "It's an emergency; we've got to hurry!" Years ago when hurrying was all that was done for the victim, speed had some value because it got the victim to the hospital for treatment. Second, many systems have confused EMS response logic with that of fire response. A fire gets worse by the second, but a single cardiac arrest does not spread geometrically in the manner of fire. Although medical problems do progress, the vast majority involve a single patient, usually in a less-than-life-threatening crisis. Third and least acceptable, running lights-and-siren is fun and seems important. After the fire department management in Salt Lake City discussed sending first-response engines without lights-and-siren (Cold), a paramedic captain remarked, "What are you guys going to do, take away the last thing on this job that's fun?"

Maximal response often has been touted as the method ensuring that those in dire straits rapidly get help. But without medically appropriate prioritization plan for the dispatcher to follow, everyone will get help—some too much and some too little, too late. In the recent past, maximum EMS response was sent always to "avoid errors in judgment." Today, however, medical oversight may be unable to medically or legally defend a significant delay in arrival at a critical emergency because a paramedic team was sent to a minor "cat-bite" call.[18] Systems capable of tiered response or all-paramedic configurations that still send a "one of each" shotgun response, rather than use their first responder personnel or EMT-B ambulance crews efficiently, are not functioning at an appropriate level of medical responsibility.[19] Fortunately, maximal response is a dinosaur in progressive systems; medical priority dispatching is the route of its extinction.[2,20]

Fire and EMS dispatching are more similar to each other than either is to police dispatching. The majority of both fire and EMS calls are initially considered escalating emergencies, but that is true for only a small portion of police requests. However, there remains a subtle and less understood difference between fire and EMS dispatching that contributes to maximal response thinking. Because combined fire and EMS dispatch is common, medical directors must have a clear understanding of the difference between the two. The changing dispatch role during an incident can be thought of graphically as the variable width of a wedge (see fig. 18.1).[18]

A report of a fire begins at the point of the wedge. The initial role of dispatchers is straightforward; they must get the location, discern what is burning, determine the safety of the caller, and then send the right resources based on those factors. Once the first arriving crew sees the active fire scene, the process escalates and the wedge expands as on-scene command relays the specifics of the fire and requests additional responses. The dispatcher also gets busier with information relay as multiple command sectors are established and additional units stage. Move-ups and mutual aid are often necessary, and other agencies such as police and EMS are notified if needed. The small point at the beginning of the fire dispatch wedge represents the need to get suppression units on the road quickly without extensive questioning of the caller. Since the extent of the fire can rarely be determined initially, it is assumed that it is getting worse each second. In fire surpression, seconds count.

But this pattern of response should not be extrapolated to EMS cases. The greatest responsibility of the EMD occurs at the beginning of each call. The wedge is therefore reversed in EMS calls. The interrogation process should be the fulcrum on which the correct and efficient nature of the response rests.

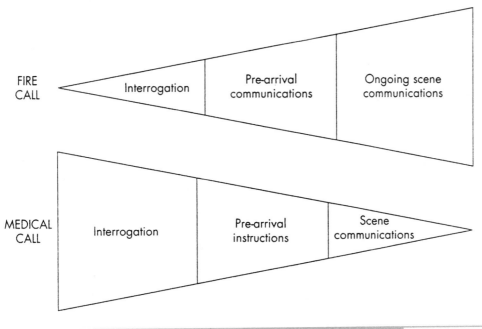

FIGURE 18.1. *Wedge of Fire vs. EMS call comparison. (From PSMO 2nd Edition. Page 142.)*

Medical priority dispatching is an effective and safe method to determine the nature of the emergency at the time the call is received, eliminating the need for the classical maximal response in most cases.[6,7,9,15,19–21]

Moreover, the maximal response philosophy does not eliminate dispatch errors. It just replaces them with less apparent errors such as paramedic units tied up on medically simple but administratively complex calls, first responders used unnecessarily, and emergency vehicle accidents. As evaluation of systems becomes more sophisticated, the inefficiencies and dangers of routine maximal response are more evident and incur a much greater liability than the occasional less-than-optimal result of a measured response. In 1991 the effectiveness of using priority dispatch methods to select calls for "only EMT-B initial responses" was studied.[7] In 14,100 cases dispatched over a 90-day period, a reasonable process was successfully used to determine response requirement, making paramedic units available more often. The negative effect on patient outcome as a result of paramedic delay was negligible. In EMS the maximal response should be reserved for only the highest level of actual or potential crisis (see appendix I).

Emergency Medical Vehicle Collisions

Thousands of emergency medical vehicle crashes occur every year in North America as a result of lights-and-siren and multiple unit responses.[17,22–25] According to U.S. Department of Transportation statistics, 40% of all reportable accidents involve an injury and 0.7% involve a fatality. In addition, hot (lights-and-siren) responses cause many more crashes that involve other vehicles when the EMS unit slips safely by.[26] There are significant questions regarding the effectiveness and safety of light-and-siren use.[27–29]

Obviously, efforts made to appropriately limit hot responses and extraneous responding vehicles reduce the number of accidents.[15,30,31] The original premise of medicine, "First to do no harm," still applies.[32] The EMS philosopher Page asks:[33]

> "What is the likelihood you'll get sued? Let's start by putting things in proper perspective. By far the greatest legal hazards facing EMTs arise from ambulance vehicle accidents. For some reason or other, we don't like to talk about ambulance vehicle accidents. Even though most of them are preventable. Instead. we are fascinated—in a morbid kind of way—with the whole subject of 'medical malpractice'."

More recently, EMS literature has become replete with articles addressing emergency medical vehicle accident problems and various solutions to prevent and avoid them.[27,29] Unfortunately, few of them suggest significantly reducing the use of lights-and-sirens.[34,35] However, in 1992 the NAEMSP published its position paper, "Lights-and-Siren Use in Emergency Medical Vehicle Response and Patient Transport" (appendix I). Among its 14 wide-ranging positions, the following are key:

1. Quality management (QM), loss control, safety risk management, and medical control and direction are essential elements in the management of emergency medical vehicle (EMV) response within the EMS system. The medical aspects of EMV operation and patient transport rationale are integral responsibilities of the medical director of an EMS system and lights-and-siren response and transport protocol must be ultimately approved by the medical director. Discretionary variation by EMS field personnel must be limited.
2. The use of lights-and-siren during both response and transport must be based on sound patient-problem assessment or on objective situational protocol. Written prospective protocol for the use of lights-and-siren during transport must be in place and approved by the medical director. In the absence of such protocol the paramedic or EMT on the scene should make contact with the base station hospital to clarify the vehicle response mode for transport of a given patient.
3. The use of lights-and-siren must be restricted to only those situations of dire circumstance in which response time reduction has been proven to improve patient survival.
4. Other than in critical cases or multiple patient incidents the lights-and-siren response of more than one EMV is unnecessary and should be limited by medical dispatch center policy.

There exist no data that prove the use of lights-and-siren saves lives, although that premise can be clinically but narrowly inferred only in true time-life situations.[36]

Tiered Response

Before discussing the steps in assigning dispatch priorities, it is crucial to understand the concept of tiered response. A tiered response is one of the most common methods of response deployment. The availability of more than one type of either response vehicle or level of personnel is required. Usually, tiered responses are found in larger municipal systems, particularly those that are fire department-based. The various types of response components may include first response non-transporting units (fire engines or squads staffed with first-responder firefighters), vehicles that do not transport (paramedic squads or paramedic fire engines), and transporting ambulances.

Tiered response systems make maximum use of dispatch priorities when the goal is to send "the right thing in the right mode to the right patient at the right time." The following (fig. 18.2) is a generic example of possible dispatch response choices in a tiered system using Emergency Medical Technician-Basic (EMT-B) fire engines, EMT-B ambulances, and paramedic ambulances. Hot indicates lights-and-siren response; cold indicates routine travel.

A popular response configuration alternative to tiered response is the "all-paramedic ambulance" system in which all transporting vehicles are paramedic ambulances, sometimes referred to as the "high performance" or Stout model.[37] Unfortunately, few all-paramedic systems, even with the benefit of excellent system status management, can provide initial response times of under five minutes without integration of more ubiquitously located units such as fire engines. These all-paramedic systems often use priority response determinations through the addition of "first responders" when necessary and the determination of whether the initial ambulance response requires a hot mode. When properly used through application of dispatch priority codes and medical oversight, the sometimes overlooked resource of public safety first responders or EMT-B units can markedly reduce response times for specific life-and-time-priority cases.

Justification

Whereas the applicability of the key question and pre-arrival instruction components of the dispatch protocol varies little by system, choosing the appropriate local response assignments is greatly dependent on the specific model of the local system and the types of personnel and vehicles available. The development of local response configurations often requires an unprecedented and threatening review of why the system does things the way it does. There are a few basic questions each system must legitimately attempt to answer before formulating dispatch priorities (see General Rules of the Response Planning Process in this chapter).[36]

Reviewing the generic response levels available best begins the process of formulating response assignments based on the dispatch priorities. This will guide local development along well established, tested paths that can be modified by formal interaction between the EMS administration and medical oversight. When multiple agencies are dispatched by a single central dispatch entity, it is important to adopt a single dispatch protocol agreed upon through joint development and consensus. If different protocols are required for each jurisdiction and dispatching is done centrally, often no protocol is followed. The frustrated dispatchers resort to using their own personal variation of available protocols in a "collage" format. This creates an extremely dangerous risk management situation.

Dispatch call prioritization had its early roots in the evolution of multiple levels of response vehicles and the system abuse that initially surfaced in larger municipalities.[1] In addition, burgeoning numbers of

Baseline Response Example
All actual response assignments are decided by local Medical Control and EMS Administration

Level	Response	Mode
ECHO	Closest Apparatus—Any (includes Truck Companies, HAZMAT, or on-air staff)	**HOT**
DELTA	Closest BLS Engine Paramedic Ambulance	**HOT** **HOT**
CHARLIE	Paramedic Ambulance	**COLD**
BRAVO	Closest BLS Engine BLS Ambulance (alone HOT if closest)	**HOT** **COLD**
ALPHA	BLS Ambulance	**COLD**
OMEGA	Referral or Alternate Care	

FIGURE 18.2. *An Example of Baseline Response Choices to the Determinant by Level (from* Principles of EMD, *3rd Edition, ©2001 NAEMD, used with permission).*

response vehicles arriving at single-patient scenes drew the attention of insightful system administrators, risk managers, and fiscal directors.[19]

There are two common misconceptions regarding dispatch prioritization. The first is a misunderstanding of the six-level determinant system (OMEGA, ALPHA, BRAVO, CHARLIE, DELTA, and ECHO). These levels are not related in an ascending linear order or urgency; the relationship is two-dimensional (see fig. 18.3). The horizontal axis shows variations in the type of scene personnel required, and the vertical axis separates cases requiring immediate first response from those needing only prompt but solitary secondary response by the appropriate vehicle and crew. Regardless of the type of system used in a given jurisdiction, the correct prioritization of determinants assists in determining the optimal use of those resources.

The second misunderstanding lies in the false belief that one must have a tiered system to use priority dispatch protocols. The name "priority" was chosen because this methodology was first employed to prioritize the actions of the dispatcher, not just the response.[18] The selection of response assignment and mode is always at the discretion of the local agency. However, medical oversight ultimately should approve the process.

The benefits of medically approved dispatch response prioritization are many. By bringing more accurate information into the dispatch office through a more precise interrogation process, EMDs are better able to recognize and understand the true medical condition. Therefore, such protocols allow for planned, safer responses (fewer units responding in the dangerous lights-and-siren mode), fuel and energy savings, reduced personnel burnout, and conservation of scarce paramedic teams for appropriate emergencies.[2]

Prioritization versus Screening

Unfortunately, there is a lack of distinction between call prioritization and call screening; these terms are often incorrectly used interchangeably. The distinction is the inclusion of the "no-send" option as a dispatch choice in call screening; that is, some calls are actually "screened out."[3]

Callers have long been denied an EMS response (or non-mobile referral evaluation) and care by some large systems both with and without protocol; however, correct use of standard dispatch priority protocols does not include this option. Dispatch prioritization allows only for the decision of *what* to send, not *whether* to send. Screening out significantly increases the legal and media exposure of a system.[18,38] A "low-send," as opposed to a "no-send," approach is legally, medically, and politically safer.

Recently, attention has been given to the concept of alternative care rather than a traditional EMS response. For example, this has been done for many years with ingestions in children under age 12 without clinical symptoms. Such an OMEGA response is accomplished by electronically transferring the caller to a regional Poison Control Center (this is not advised for ED-based systems) for further evaluation and possible home care. EMS is promptly called back for a "send" if any unanticipated problems are encountered by the experts at Poison Control.

The area of alternate care warrants considerable discussion and review. Until significant progress is made regarding the modification of protocolized dispatch priorities to include routine alternative care tiers, as opposed to the "no-send" choice, significant risks remain. Certainly, documentation of very high compliance to protocol is a necessary prerequisite to implementation of an alternative care option.[14] The complete OMEGA process (affecting 21 of the 33 chief complaints) is currently only used by communication centers with National Academy of Emergency Medical Dispatch (NAEMD) accreditation

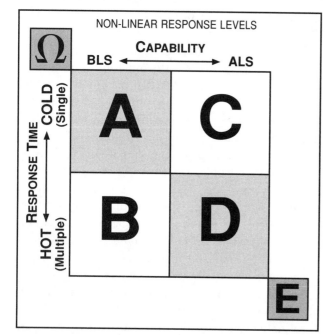

FIGURE 18.3. *Determinant Matrix (from MPDS v11, ©2001 NAEMD, used with permission).*

TABLE 18.1

Chief Complaints

CHIEF COMPLAINTS BY PROTOCOL TYPE

Medical Incident Protocols
1. Abdominal Pain/Problems
2. Allergies (Reactions)/Envenomations (Stings, Bites)
5. Back Pain (Non-Traumatic or Non-Recent Trauma)
10. Chest Pain
12. Convulsions/Seizures
13. Diabetic Problems
18. Headache
19. Heart Problems/A.I.C.D.
20. Heat/Cold Exposure
23. Overdose/Poisoning (Ingestion)
25. Psychiatric/Abnormal Behavior/Suicide Attempt
26. Sick Person (Specific Diagnosis)
28. Stroke (CVA)
33. Interfacility/Palliative Care

Traumatic Incident Protocols
3. Animal Bites/Attacks
4. Assualt/Sexual Assault

7. Burns/Explosion
16. Eye Problems/Injuries
17. Falls
21. Hemorrhage/Lacerations
22. Industrial/Machinery Accidents
27. Stab/Gunshot/Penetrating Trauma
29. Traffic/Transportation Accidents
30. Traumatic Injuries (Specific)

Time-Life Incident Protocols
6. Breathing Problems
8. Carbon Monoxide/Inhalation/HAZMAT
9. Cardiac or Respiratory Arrest/Death
11. Choking
14. Drowning (Near)/Diving/Scuba Accident
15. Electrocution/Lightning
24. Pregnancy/Childbirth/Miscarriage
31. Unconscious/Fainting (Near)
32. Unknown Problem (Man Down)

and compliance scores above 95%. Alternate care and referral require not only extremely high compliance to protocol but dedicated and continuous quality management.

DISPATCH DETERMINANT THEORY. The science emergency medical dispatch relies on a reproducible and internally consistent problem coding system. In 1995, a de facto standard list was federally identified, listing 32 chief complaint protocol divisions (table 18.1).

Each chief complaint protocol contains one or more determinant levels which define various theoretical groups of response assignments based on responder capability (first-responder vs. BLS vs. ALS) and rapidity of response mode (hot vs. cold). Once the EMD determines the severity of concern, using the answers to key questions and the additional information definitions and problem lists, the proper dispatch determinant can be selected. There are six dispatch determinant levels in the reference system:

E = ECHO-level
D = DELTA-level
C = CHARLIE-level
B = BRAVO-level
A = ALPHA-level
Ω = OMEGA-level

A vital principle is that the names of the dispatch determinants listed above do not change. EMS systems implementing priority dispatch must understand that the responder agency can prospectively assign preferred responses to each determinant as best fits their needs (see Response Theory and Local Development in this chapter). Each system must decide which resources each level best requires. For example, ALPHA-level may mean basic life support cold, and DELTA-level mean advanced life support hot.

Such determinants are vital for meaningful data collection and QM evaluation.[6] For example, priority dispatch systems maintained by national standard-setting organizations have the ability to gather meaningful statistical data with a standard coding system allowing performance comparisons among cities, regions, and even countries. In this sense, priority dispatch systems are the first EMS data collection systems with more than a local meaning. Such unified systems have an international scope. The capacity to participate in a broad-spectrum priority dispatch database is useful in an era where procedures, outcomes, and (more recently) payments for emergency services are increasingly scrutinized.

Use of the statistics generated through use of the determinants can demonstrate accurately what types and severity of calls a system has spent its resources handling. For example, there is a perception within EMS that 5% to 10% of calls are of a life-threatening nature, but no one really knows if this is accurate. Standardized priority dispatch coding allows for evaluation and verification that the system is being used appropriately and effectively.[6-9]

Dispatch determinants do not merely indicate the severity of a situation. That is, the determinant levels (E-D-C-B-A-Ω) are not related in a linear sense of becoming progressively worse. Rather, they define how many responders will go, and, when there are various tiers of capability, which levels of expertise are needed, and how rapidly they should arrive. This can be depicted in a two-dimensional, non-linear matrix (see fig. 18.3).

The vertical axis on the grid relates to response time. Could responders travel cold, or are they needed hot? The horizontal axis relates to rescuer ability. Could basic life support providers handle this or are advanced life support providers needed?[6-9] The matrix has nothing to do with what is actually available response-wise within any particular EMS system; it forms a grid for understanding the general clinical "value" of individual determinant codes within any given system.

Priority dispatch has replaced the traditional "more is better" concept. When a responder's training and manpower are matched to a particular situation, it can more efficiently be handled. For example, basic-level EMTs are experts at splinting, bandaging, and other basic skills. There is no reason they cannot be trusted to handle basic-level situations, freeing ALS providers (who are usually fewer in number) for appropriate situations.[7] In a 1992 study of the Long Beach, California system, Stratton, concluded:

"Emergency Medical Dispatchers, medically controlled and trained in a nationally recognized dispatcher triage system, were able to provide medical triage to incoming emergency medical 9-1-1 calls with minimal error for under-triage of ALS runs and high selectivity for non-emergency situations."[9]

Understanding Determinant Terminology

Implementers of priority dispatch are sometimes confused by the terminology, especially since the terms such as "determinant," "determinant code," "determinant level," "response code," and "response mode" sound so similar.[39] The following discussion should take the mystery out of the determinant response section of the protocol (see fig. 18.4).

Determinant Coding Components

First, consider the E,D,C,B,A (and in some instances Ω) determinant classification. Within each of these levels there can be a number of determinant descriptors, listed roughly in order of decreasing significance. The determinant descriptors within a level have a medical relationship to each other, which suggests a similarity of response. Put the two together (level plus description) with the number of the protocol (e.g., 12)—and the determinant code is the result. For example, after interrogating the caller on protocol 12, (Convulsions/Seizures) the EMD determines that the most appropriate classification is the "continuous or multiple seizures" descriptor under the delta level. This results in a "12-D-2" determinant code (see fig. 18.5).

Response Assignment Components

The response assignment process, which is where the dispatching agency determines how resources should be assigned, and their mode of travel to the scene is developed prospectively for all determinant codes. Each agency, through medical oversight and administration, establishes which response assignment prospectively best fits each determinant code—given the agency's available resources, geography, and political mandates *prior* to using a priority dispatch system on-line.

The response assignment included the response level and response mode. The response level defines the type of responders—specifically, their training or

LEVELS	#	DETERMINANT DESCRIPTORS	CODES	RESPONSES
D	1	**Not** breathing (**after** Key Questioning)	**12-D-1**	
	2	**CONTINUOUS** or **MULTIPLE** seizures	**12-D-2**	
	3	**Irregular** breathing	**12-D-3**	
	4	Breathing regularly **not** verified ≥ **35**	**12-D-4**	

FIGURE **18.4.** *Convulsions/Seizures Protocol (from the MPDS v11.1, ©2001 NAEMD, used with permission).*

PRIORITY DISPATCH RESPONSE

Determinant Coding Components				
Protocol Number	**Determinant Level**	**Determinant Number**	**Determinant Descriptor**	**Determinant Code**
12	D	2	**CONTINUOUS** or **MULTIPLE** seizures =	12-D-2

FIGURE 18.5. *Components of the Response Determinant Code (from* Principles of EMD, *3rd Edition, ©2001 NAEMD, used with permission).*

certification level—most commonly, advanced life support versus basic life support personnel.

Finally comes the response mode, which is what the dispatching agency determines the urgency of response travel to the scene to be. This is done by designating a hot (lights-and-siren) or cold (routine) response. The evaluating EMD always has the option to override the recommended response assignment and send a higher level of response if circumstances warrant it. Obviously, this should be the exception rather than the rule (less than 0.5 percent in systems using automated priority dispatch protocols). Sending a lower response is not allowed unless subsequently patient symptoms or situations are determined to have improved.

Defining response assignments is the responsibility of each agency's medical oversight physician, Medical Dispatch Review Committee, and Steering Committee. Using the 12-D-1 determinant code as an example, Medical Dispatch Oversight Committees may decide that an ALS unit responding with lights-and-siren with an ambulance is the most appropriate response assignment, thus generating the response assignment of "ALS Amb hot" (see fig. 18.6).

Priority dispatch has two very important coding systems. The first, the determinant codes, are developed and maintained by national standard-setting organizations, according to current medical practices, user feedback, and ongoing evaluation. The second,

the response assignment, is determined and maintained by each agency according to its available resources, user feedback and ongoing evaluation. In a properly established priority dispatch environment, the determinant code and response areas of the system work together to ensure that EMDs choose the most appropriate clinical determinant and assign the most appropriate responses. Figure 18.2 is an example of a hypothetical system's local baseline response assignments to each determinant level, but not necessarily to each chief complaint. This would be their starting point for developing responses to match each individual determinant descriptor and code.

Avoiding Response Code Confusion

It is important to clarify how to set response assignments, or more specifically, how to properly assign system resources to the determinants codes. Typically, an agency new to priority dispatch requests to make changes in the determinant section of the protocols in an effort to match them to existing local field responses. Frustration results when EMDs or their managers confuse the determinant codes with unit response assignments. Each determinant code is just that—a code. These "clinical" codes have no response value as such. In essence, these codes are the

Response Assignment Components		
Response Level	**Mode**	**Response Assignment**
Advanced Life Support (Amb)	HOT =	ALS Amb

FIGURE 18.6. *Components of the Response Assignment (from* Principles of EMD, *3rd Edition, ©2001 NAEMD, used with permission).*

dispatch equivalent to a type of medical coding system called diagnosis-related groups (DRGs) or ICD-9 codes used by most hospitals and clinics to bill patients. While these groups are universal (like priority dispatch codes of national standard-setting organizations), the specific amount billed for each code by one hospital may differ from that billed by another (just like different agencies may respond differently to the same determinant code). It is unnecessary to change or move the determinant code in either case, as they only represent the clinical classification determined by the system, and not the response assignment to it per se. Changing determinant code numbers or positions is not routinely allowed by national standard-setting organizations; changing local response assignments is.

In the case of priority dispatch, response assignments are always selected by the responder agency, approved by the medical director, and then listed in local terminology in the Responses-Modes section. On printed protocols, responses and modes are usually located to the right of the determinant code (numerals). It is not necessary to assign the same response (or approved referral for OMEGA) to all determinant codes within a specific determinant level. By virtue of their medical relationship to one another, determinants are grouped into one of the six levels. On a local response basis, however, it is not necessary to adhere to this grouping concept by assigning the same response to all determinants within a given level. For example, if an agency wishes to assign a response group to the "exotic animal" determinant code (3-D-5) that is different from the baseline response group assigned to the five remaining DELTA determinant codes, they should not attempt to move the determinant descriptor text into another determinant level; rather, they should designate the desired response assignment to code 3-D-5 "where it lies" (see fig. 18.7).

An agency should begin by initially assigning a baseline response to each different major determinant level—ECHO through OMEGA. ECHO responses, as discussed earlier, may involve different resources on different protocols (refer to fig. 18.3). These baseline response assignments are, in essence, the most commonly used response modes for each level, not the only ones possible. They represent the six basic responses (one for each determinant level) and are initially agreed to independent of any particular chief complaint. This forms a common starting point from which to specifically examine if each chief complaint's various determinant codes can be appropriately handled by the agency's baseline response types or not.

With these initial baseline responses in mind, each protocol should then be carefully reviewed by local medical oversight groups, with special attention given to any determinant code whose optimal response assignment (from the agency's and medical director's perspective) doesn't exactly fit the baseline response for that determinant level clinically. Such special response assignments are therefore "exceptions" to the baseline. From a legal standpoint, it is essential to document the rationale for why each exception to the

LEVELS	#	DETERMINANT DESCRIPTORS	CODES	RESPONSES	MODES
D	1	**Unconscious** or **Arrest**	**3-D-1**	Priority 1	
	2	**Not** alert	**3-D-2**	Priority 1	
	3	**DANGEROUS** body area	**3-D-3**	Priority 1	
	4	**Large** animal	**3-D-4**	Priority 1	
	5	**EXOTIC** animal	**3-D-5**	Priority 2 ←	
	6	**ATTACK** or **multiple** animals	**3-D-6**	Priority 1	
B	1	**POSSIBLY DANGEROUS** body area	**3-B-1**	Priority 2	
	2	**SERIOUS** hemorrhage	**3-B-2**	Priority 2	
	3	**Unknown** status (3rd party caller)	**3-B-3**	Priority 2	
A	1	**NOT DANGEROUS** body area	**3-A-1**	Priority 3	
	2	**NON-RECENT** injuries (≥ 6hrs)	**3-A-2**	Priority 3	
	3	**SUPERFICIAL** bites	**3-A-3**	Priority 3	

FIGURE 18.7. *Example of an intra-level locally chosen response or Protocol 3 (from* Principles of EMD, *3rd Edition, ©2001 NAEMD, used with permission).*

PRIORITY DISPATCH RESPONSE

LEVELS	#	DETERMINANT DESCRIPTORS	CODES	RESPONSES	MODES
E	1	**INEFFECTIVE BREATHING** *(to be selected from **Case Entry** only)*	6-E-1	Closest Staff (any) HOT Paramedic HOT	
D	1	**SEVERE RESPIRATORY DISTRESS**	6-D-1	Closest BLS/Paramedic HOT	
	2	**Not** alert	6-D-2	Closest BLS HOT/Paramedic COLD	
	3	**Clammy**	6-D-3	Closest BLS/Paramedic HOT	
C	1	**Abnormal** breathing	6-C-1	Closest BLS/Paramedic HOT	
	2	**Cardiac** history	6-C-2	Paramedic COLD	

Add suffix "A" to Determinant Code for Asthma

FIGURE 18.8. *Sample of Response Assignments (from* Principles of EMD, *3rd Edition, ©2001 NAEMD, used with permission).*

baseline response was preferred. This documentation then becomes the agency's self-defined standard of practice for response.

Each agency, therefore, may define specific response assignments for any one of several hundred separate determinant codes that are found within priority dispatch systems. Theoretically, it is conceivable that an agency could have dozens of different response assignments in a single protocol set, although the average agency appears to only use approximately three main types. For example, the CHARLIE-level determinants on the Chest Pain protocol could appear as shown (see fig. 18.8).

Additional confusion may occur if an EMS agency uses the same names or letters for their response groups that are used within the protocol for its codes—for example, ALPHA, BRAVO, CHARLIE, DELTA, or ECHO. When this is the case, baseline exceptions to response assignments can be extremely confusing (i.e., "send a BRAVO response for an AL-PHA determinant code"). It is highly recommended that agencies choose response group terms such as numerals, proper names, or unused letters of the phonetic alphabet such as X-RAY, YANKEE, and ZULU to avoid this inevitable "alphabet soup" confusion (see fig. 18.9).

In accordance with NAEMD, individual users are not to make changes to, or deletions from, the approved protocols. Such revisions are properly implemented only through the NAEMD Council of Standards, and may be requested by a user submitting a formal "Proposal for Change" form (see Appendix II) with appropriate rationale, case studies, data, or research.

Certain protocols also have special determinant code suffixes. These suffixes are used to aid in the computerized relay of specific subtypes within a chief complaint to CAD systems which need to identify these differences for add-on responses such as scene security by police in violent situations. For example,

LEVELS	#	DETERMINANT DESCRIPTORS	CODES	Correct RESPONSES	Incorrect MODES
D	1	**Not** alert	1-D-1	Zulu HOT	~~Delta HOT~~
C	1	**Fainting** or **near fainting** ≥ 50	1-C-1	Yankee COLD	~~Charlie COLD~~
	2	**Females** with **fainting** or **near fainting** 12–50	1-C-2	Yankee COLD	~~Charlie COLD~~
	3	**Males** with **pain above navel** ≥ 35	1-C-3	Zulu HOT	~~Delta HOT~~
	4	**Females** with **pain above navel** ≥ 45	1-C-4	Yankee COLD	~~Charlie HOT~~
A	1	Abdominal pain	1-A-1	X-ray COLD	~~Alpha COLD~~

FIGURE 18.9. *Sample of "correct" vs. "confusing" response assignment localizations (from* Principles of EMD, *3rd Edition, ©2001 NAEMD, used with permission).*

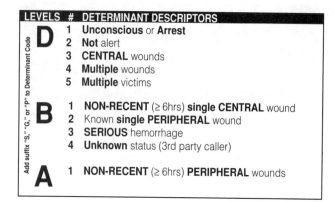

LEVELS	#	DETERMINANT DESCRIPTORS
D	1	**Unconscious** or **Arrest**
	2	**Not** alert
	3	**CENTRAL** wounds
	4	**Multiple** wounds
	5	**Multiple** victims
B	1	**NON-RECENT** (≥ 6hrs) **single CENTRAL** wound
	2	Known **single PERIPHERAL** wound
	3	**SERIOUS** hemorrhage
	4	**Unknown** status (3rd party caller)
A	1	**NON-RECENT** (≥ 6hrs) **PERIPHERAL** wounds

(left margin: Add suffix "S," "G," or "P" to Determinant Code)

FIGURE 18.10. *Stab/Gunshot/Penetrating Wounds protocol (from MPDS v11, ©2001 NAEMD, used with permission).*

it is important to differentiate a stabbing situation from a shooting for responder safety reasons. You can shoot a gun a lot farther than you can throw a knife. In the Stab/Gunshot/Penetrating Trauma, a 27-D-3s (stab) versus a 27-D-3g (gunshot) versus a 27-D-3p (other penetrating wound) makes it possible to relay this distinction electronically (see fig. 18.10).

Well delineated determinants allow for even more accurate information. For example, note that the CHARLIE-level determinants for Convulsions/Seizures, are numbered one through three (see fig. 18.11).

There are various benefits to knowing which of the underlying conditions (pregnancy, diabetes, or cardiac history) were associated with a convulsion or seizure. For example, a 12-C-3 determinant code means the caller reported a person with a cardiac history who was having a seizure. Field crews receive more accurate information, and the patient theoretically receives the benefit of helpers carrying the cor-

rect equipment. The data collected are more useful, and the quality improvement manager has better information.

Response Theory and Local Development

At a certain point during initial priority dispatch implementation, a committee including medical oversight physicians, field personnel, managers, and administrators faces the task of designating the response assignments to each chief complaint/incident type protocol. The goal of local response setting is to match local EMS capability with the various dispatch determinant descriptors and codes found on each protocol. It does not change the protocol; rather, it allows for each community to choose what resources to send for each of the determinant codes.

The political element of establishing localized responses for the dispatch determinants is probably the biggest hurdle an EMS system faces when implementing priority dispatch systems. Different EMS services within a region (each possibly a bit protective of its territory), different hospital base stations, and different medical directors, may initially complain to priority dispatch advocates that "this concept may work elsewhere, but won't work here."

The more relevant point is to look at what these somewhat diverse entities have in common: a desire to serve the public, and a commitment to emergency patients and the safety of responding crews. They must eventually sit together and objectively assess the purpose and structure of priority dispatch and resultant rational control of system response. Implementation may be an initial challenge, but it is has been accomplished successfully in the full range of EMS system designs and community sizes around the world.

Not every EMS system is like the example shown. Currently the diversity of response capability (not to mention response desires) from system to system is amazing. But each EMS system, with its unique characteristics, can maximize the efficiency of its response with correct use of a priority dispatch process.

Not usually understood, nearly every volunteer service can benefit from priority dispatch because it is no longer necessary for every available volunteer to respond on every call. Volunteer time and talent can thus be used more appropriately. Busy volunteer systems might configure their baseline responses as shown here:

LEVELS	#	DETERMINANT DESCRIPTORS
D	1	**Not** breathing (**after** Key Questioning)
	2	**CONTINUOUS** or **MULTIPLE** seizure
	3	**Irregular** breathing
	4	Breathing regularly **not** verified ≥ 35
C	1	**Pregnancy**
	2	**Diabetic**
	3	**Cardiac** history
B	1	Breathing regularly **not** verified < 35
A	1	Not seizing now **and** breathing regularly (verified)

FIGURE 18.11. *Convulsions/Seizures protocol Determinant Descriptors (from MPDS v11.1, ©2001 NAEMD, used with permission).*

ECHO: Police hot; on-call EMTs hot; Backup crew hot

DELTA: On-call EMTs hot; Backup crew hot

CHARLIE: On-call EMTs hot; Backup crew cold (for extra manpower if needed)

BRAVO: On-call EMTs hot; Backup crew stand-by at home

ALPHA: On-call EMTs cold

Priority dispatch responses can also be configured for rural BLS services. In some cases, there are so few calls per year that everyone is more than willing to drop everything to respond. The main issue is whether they should drive hot or cold.

For this example, let us also say this group has distant ALS backup, such as a helicopter:

ECHO: Police hot, on-call hot; Backup crew hot

DELTA: Everyone hot; Helicopter dispatched

CHARLIE: EMTs hot in EMS unit; EMT cold with personal vehicle; Helicopter on stand by

BRAVO: EMTs hot in EMS unit; EMT cold with personal vehicle

ALPHA: EMTs cold in EMS unit

Knowing that priority dispatch is being used to determine a critical rapid transport need (i.e., ECHO or DELTA-level situation) would increase the flight service's comfort level with an "early" dispatch command to launch.

General Rules of the Response Planning Process

There are five rules for system planners to remember when assigning field responses to the dispatch determinant codes.[36]

1. **Will time make a difference in the final outcome?**

   In other words, is the patient's problem one of the few true time/life priorities requiring the fastest possible response time, with a goal of less than five minutes? Most systems identify the most time-critical calls as cardiac or respiratory arrest, airway problems (including choking), unconsciousness, severe trauma or hypo-

volemia, and true obstetrical emergencies.[40] The early identification of these chief complaints means a maximum response is sent. For the majority of other problems, planners need to carefully consider using a less than all-out response. For example, situations that tend to generate a misdirected sense of urgency (in both the EMD and in field personnel) are those involving "dispatcher hysteria." One classic case is abdominal pain. Unexplained abdominal pain is frightening, yet true abdominal pain, except in rare instances, is not a *prehospital* medical emergency. This is not to say it is not a *surgical* emergency, however. The great majority of patients with abdominal pain face a lengthy workup in the emergency department. Through careful use of the key questions, the EMD can determine whether a person is within the parameters of those rare situations that might be time-critical. To have an ambulance crew, or worse yet, a full-tiered response, running hot to any but those rare cases is unnecessary and hazardous.

2. **How much time leeway is there for this problem?**

   That is, what range of time is appropriate for the problem? In medicine, this ranges from seconds to minutes to hours to days. The trained EMD knows that time can make a difference in life-threatening situations, so there is little time leeway; emergency crews must arrive at the scene as quickly as possible. However, the majority of calls lie in a range from those warranting prompt (but not breakneck) responses to those where there is significant time leeway for minor and clearly non-escalating problems.

3. **How much time can be saved by responding hot?**

   Accurate information about hot vs. cold response times is uncommon but increasing.[35,35] Response times from time of call to patient contact (vs. pulling up at the address) have not been well reported. Typical local traffic patterns, time of day, how fast local ambulances actually roll, typical roadway conditions such as stoplights, roads that demand frequent deceleration or acceleration, and local speed limit laws for emergency units should be some of the oversight committee's concerns. If an EMS unit has to respond a mile or two, are the very few seconds saved running hot worth the disruption to traffic and pedestrians, not to mention the safety of the motoring public and prehospital crew?

New studies published regarding whether time is actually saved running hot reflect clinically minimal time differences between responding hot and cold—yet the relative safety of a cold response is well demonstrated and also medically appropriate.[18,25,34]

The collective perception of lights-and-siren is that their use indicates a real emergency situation. The principles of priority dispatch have resulted in a redefining of what an emergency really is. Reducing the use of lights-and-siren is, in itself, a concept that can save lives.[17,25] When a person's life clearly depends on quick action and rapid motion, lights-and-siren is an important tool. However, there are many times when a situation that appears urgent in the field will not be helped by the use of lights-and-siren. The time saved using them (either going to the patient or to the hospital) is long gone before the patient benefits from definitive care. An ever-increasing number of public safety agencies are adopting the more responsible approach of limiting lights-and-siren use to potentially critical emergencies.

4. **What time constraints are present in the system?**

Each system design has limitations. In some areas, the crews are all-volunteer, and it routinely takes 10 minutes or more to get to the ambulance shed. There is a greater inherent time constraint there than a setup in which prehospital personnel await calls from inside an ambulance stationed on a street corner when the posting selection is done through use of a well designed system status plan fluidly redeploying available units based on call-frequency predictive analysis.[37] Their departure is immediate and their arrival significantly shortened overall.

5. **When the patient gets to the hospital, will the time saved using lights-and-siren be significant compared to the time spent awaiting care?**

This is the most ignored rule. When the critical needs of the patient do warrant the fastest possible response time to the hospital, proper advance notification of the emergency department staff results in immediate, continuing definitive care after arrival.

However, except for the most critical cases, patients do a great deal of waiting. Each usually first sees the ward clerk (who has to generate paperwork), and the health aide (who dresses the patient in proper emergency department attire). Only then might a nurse or a doctor enter the room. Non-critically ill or injured people in an emergency department wait for their turn with the doctor, then for transport for X-rays, for the person who will take blood for lab tests, for test results, for the doctor's decision, and for finalization either of admission to the hospital or subsequent release. This process can take several hours and requires much endurance. Did the hot ride in really help? In essence, was it medically (or publicly) ethical?[36]

Take, for example, a not-so-mythical EMS system where a private ambulance company provides basic life support-level transport services for a fire department-based EMS system. Each fire station has EMT-level first responders. Advanced life support is provided by firefighter/paramedics at a few of the strategically placed fire stations. Since the ambulance always responds, there are five tiers available to the system and six response-group options. With this sort of configuration, the response section next to the determinants truly demonstrates the user-defined flexibility of priority dispatch (see fig. 18.12).

Summary

While the paper development of a dispatch response plan is a medical/system process, assigning response configurations to all determinant codes is also a very political process. It is essential that the medical oversight physician be involved and is heard. Having a reasonable understanding of the concepts described in this chapter will give the average physician wading through the entire EMS process, a dry leg up.

Response development is a process, not an event. The more data are harvested from the dispatch coding system, the more refined, effective, and safe it will be for patients, the responders, and the EMS system in general. No one can expect to sit at a meeting table and hammer out every possible contingency. Something normally handled cold may—due to weather, traffic, or other unusual circumstances—someday at some particular time warrant a hot or maximal re-

ECHO-LEVEL

Closest apparatus of any kind hot, ALS responders hot.

Local rationale: The correct use of ECHO now allows this system to implement reasonable use of non-standard EMS responders such as truck companies, the hazmat unit, and other approved on-air staff to immediately aid patients who are literally dying right now. ECHO-initiated crews must be at minimum basic life support trained and understand scene safety entry procedures. For 9-E-1 patients, several police units that now carry AEDs are dispatched as "first in."

DELTA-LEVEL

Maximal response (both basic and advanced life support providers).

Local rationale: While advanced life support providers would always go hot, the basic life support transport unit may respond hot to cases of critical trauma where rapid transport is essential, or they may respond cold when a medical cardiac arrest patient will be worked for 20 to 30 minutes at the scene. There will always be situations that warrant having every appropriate responder travel hot to the scene.

CHARLIE-LEVEL

Closest advanced life support unit cold (occasionally hot), basic life support transport cold.

Local rationale: Facets of the caller's interview have identified a need for the expertise, judgment, and skills of advanced life support providers. Also, the need for patient transport is likely, so basic life support transport is dispatched cold, since advanced life support crews will take a few minutes to evaluate and treat the patient at the scene.

BRAVO-LEVEL

Closest basic life support unit hot (occasionally cold).

Local rationale: Something about the situation merits a rapid response, but the entire system does not need to be mobilized. Since there are inevitably more basic life support providers than advanced life support, they are usually not only closer, but also more available. Depending what the "first-in" crew finds, BRAVO-level calls may

result in occasionally discovering a patient who needs advanced life support evaluation or care, and they can request such a response while providing on-scene basic life support.

ALPHA-LEVEL

Closest basic life support transport unit cold.

Local rationale: Basic EMTs are educated to handle anything that appears in this category. Since the transport company has EMTs driving their ambulances, the fire department does not need to respond at all, leaving that resource available in case of other emergencies. The Salt Lake City Fire Department decreased the need for its EMS fire apparatus at 33 percent of its calls in the first year of full prioritization. The private ambulance company handling basic life support (fortunately under the same medical control as the fire department) was able to handle the majority of ALPHA-level calls without any compromise to patients.

OMEGA-LEVEL

Special referral and special response as approved.

Local rationale: This system's high compliance to protocol assures that patient situations identified as OMEGA can be safely and more effectively handled by non-traditional response means. An appropriate joint policy with the regional Poison Control Center allows caller transfer for in-depth evaluation and handling of certain types of asymptomatic poisoning and ingestion cases. Carefully evaluated expected deaths are more correctly and tactfully handled without EMS responders. Customer service to callers in need of physical help for people who are uninjured but have fallen or need aid returning to their usual resting place can be aided by various crews sent non-urgently under their new public assist assignment program. This system is seeking its national standard-setting organization's accreditation designation (which is based on very high protocol compliance parameters) so that it can safely implement all 21 OMEGA protocol determinant levels in the near future, many efficiently and effectively handled in conjunction with an established nurse advice line service and other professional referral specialty centers.

FIGURE 18.12. *An example of one EMS system's response configuration thinking.*

sponse. The EMD can be provided with the flexibility to choose other options as clearly defined in locally written dispatch policies. Sound, reasonable judgment should be the hallmark of well trained, protocol-equipped EMDs. The process should obviously be backed up by strong, attentive medical oversight.

References

1. Roberts B. EMS dispatching: its use and misuse. Dallas Fire Department internal report, 1978.
2. Clawson J. Dispatch priority training: strengthening the weak link. *JEMS*. 1981;6:2.
3. Robinson V. Call screening targets false emergencies. *International Fire Chief*. 1980;47:16.
4. Zachariah B, Pepe P. The development of emergency medical dispatch in the USA: a historical perspective. *European Journal of Emergency Medicine* 1995;2:109–112.
5. Murphy R. Priority dispatch system effectiveness proven. *APCO Bulletin*. 1985;59.
6. Bailey E, et al. The use of emergency medical dispatch protocols to reduce the number of inappropriate scene responses made by advanced life support personnel. *Prehosp Emerg Care*. 2000;4:2.
7. Curka P, Pepe P, Ginger V. Emergency medical services priority dispatch. *Ann Emerg Med*. 1995;22:1668.
8. Kallsen G, Nabors M. The use of priority medical dispatch to distinguish between high- and low-risk patients. *Ann Emerg Med*. 1990;19:458–459.
9. Stratton S. Triage by emergency medical dispatchers. *Prehosp Disast Med*. 1992;7:263.
10. American Society for Testing and Materials. *Standard Practice for Emergency Medical Dispatch*, Pub No F1258-95 revised, Philadelphia, PA, 1995.
11. National Institutes of Health. *Emergency Medical Dispatching: Rapid Identification and Treatment of Acute Myocardial Infarction*. NIH Publications, No 94, 1994.
12. American Society for Testing and Materials. *Standard Practice for Emergency Medical Dispatch Management*. Pub No F1560-94, Philadelphia, PA, 1994.
13. Clawson J. The value of protocol compliance. *Journal of the National Academy of EMD*. 1990;1:3.
14. Clawson J, Cady G, Martin R, Sinclair R. Effect of a comprehensive quality management process on compliance with protocol in an emergency medical dispatch center. *Ann Emerg Med*. 1998;32:578–584.
15. Clawson J. Medical priority dispatch: it works! *JEMS*. 1983;8:2.
16. Clawson J. The maximal response disease: red lights and siren syndrome in priority dispatching. *JEMS*. 1987;12:1.
17. Clawson J. Running 'Hot' and the case of Sharron Rose. *JEMS*. 1991;16:11–13.
18. Clawson J, Dernocoeur K. *Principles of Emergency Medical Dispatch*. *3rd ed*. Salt Lake City, UT: Priority Press; 2000.
19. St. John D, Shephard R Jr. EMS dispatch and response. *Fire Chief*. 1983;26:142–144.
20. Clawson J, Sinclair R. "Medical Miranda"—Improved emergency medical dispatch information from police officers. *Prehosp Disast Med*. 1999;7:263.
21. Slovis C, et al. A priority dispatch system for EMS. *Ann Emerg Med*. 1985;14:1055–1060.
22. Auerbach P, Morris J, Phillips J Jr, et al. An analysis of ambulance accidents in Tennessee. *JAMA*. 1987;258:1487–1490.
23. Clawson J. Ambulance accidents. *JEMS*. 1989;13:23.
24. Caldwell LH. Hard lessons. *Fire Command* 1990;57:20–21.
25. Leonard W. What a waste when the system fails. *Ambulance Industry Journal*. 1991;22:6–7.
26. Clawson J, Martin R, Cady G, Maio R. The wake effect—Emergency vehicle-related collisions. *Prehosp Disast Med*. 1997;12:274–277.
27. DeLorenzo R, Eiler M. Lights and siren: A review of emergency vehicle warning systems. *Ann Emerg Med*. 1991;20:1331–1334.
28. Skeiber S, Mason R, Potter R. Effectiveness of Audible Devices on Emergency Vehicles. Washington, DC: U.S. Department of Transportation, National Highway Traffic Safety Administration, Pub No DOT-TSC-OST-77-38, 1977.
29. Solomon S. Ambulance accident avoidance. *Emergency*. 1985;17:34–35, 44.
30. Clawson J. Hit or myth. *JEMS*. 1989;14:8.
31. Elling R. Dispelling myths on ambulance accidents. *JEMS*. 1989;14:60–64.
32. George J, Quattrone M. Above all—Do no harm. *Emerg Med Tech Legal Bull*. 1991;15:4.
33. Page J. *The EMT's Legal Primer*. Solana Beach, CA: Jems Publishing Co.; 1985.
34. Hunt R, et al. Is ambulance transport time with lights and siren faster than that without? *Ann Emerg Med*. 1995;25:507–511.
35. Kupas D, et al. Patient outcome using medical protocol limit "lights and siren" transport. *Prehosp Disast Med*. 1994;9:226.
36. Clawson J. The red-light-and-siren response. *JEMS*. 1981;6:2.
37. Stout J. System status management: the strategy of ambulance placement. *JEMS*. 1983;8:22–32.
38. George J. EMS triage. *Emergency Medical Technician Legal Bulletin*. 1981;5:4.
39. Clawson J. Avoiding response code confusion. *Journal of the National Academy of EMD*. 1997;8:1.
40. Dernocoeur J. The ten-minute goal. *JEMS*. 1982;7:51–52.

Appendix I Lights-and-Siren Position Paper

Use of warning lights and siren, emergency medical vehicle collisions, effectiveness of lights and siren, position statements, protocols and guidelines, inappropriate use of lights and siren, wake effect, risk of emergency response, emergency medical vehicle operator, collision reporting systems, ambulance accidents, dispatch protocols, patient transport, emergency medical vehicle response, warning lights and siren protocols, Prehospital and Disaster Medicine, 1994, Emergency Medical Response Task Force, position paper, National Association of Emergency Medical Services Physicians (NAEMSP)

Prehospital and Disaster Medicine, April–June 1994, Vol. 9, No. 2

This paper was developed for NAEMSP by the Emergency Medical Response Task Force: Jeff J. Clawson, MD, Chair; Robert Forbuss; Scott A. Hauert; Fred Hurtado; Alexander E. Kuehl, MD; W.H. "Bill" Leonard; Peter A. Maningas, MD; Joseph L. Ryan, MD; and Donald R. Sharpe.

Use of Warning Lights and Siren in Emergency Medical Vehicle Response and Patient Transport

Introduction

The use of warning lights and siren (L&S) by prehospital emergency medical services (EMS) vehicles is a basic component of emergency response and patient transport. This public-safety practice predates modern EMS by 50 years. Despite the long-term reliance on L&S, it is not a risk-free practice. There are many reports of emergency medical vehicle (EMV) collisions during L&S response and transports. These collisions often result in tragic consequences for the EMV occupants and those in other vehicles, and may cause significant delays to medical care for the patient the EMV was responding to or transporting. While there is no systematic collection of EMV collision data, some authors have suggested that the available information underestimates the extent of the problem. In addition, to date there have been few published analyses regarding the effectiveness of L&S as a modality that improves response times or, more important, patient outcome.

Despite the lack of data, it generally is accepted that the use of L&S is a privilege granted to emergency medical responders that should be reserved for those situations in which patient welfare is at stake. To provide guidance to the states' EMS medical directors and system managers, the National Association of EMS Physicians (NAEMSP) and the National Association of State EMS Directors (NAEMSD) endorse the following positions regarding the use of warning L&S in EMV response and patient transport.

Position Statements

1. *Emergency medical services (EMS) medical directors should participate directly in the development of policies governing EMV response, patient transport, and the use of warning lights and siren.*

Emergency medical vehicle response policy decisions involve many medical care and medical direction issues including patient outcome, quality improvement, patient and emergency medical provider safety, and risk management. Therefore, EMV response and patient transport decisions should be guided, reviewed, and approved by the EMS medical director.

2. *The use of warning lights and siren during an emergency response to the scene and during patient transport should be based on standardized protocols that take into account situational and patient problem assessments.*

Written protocols and guidelines should delineate when to use L&S during scene response and patient transport. These protocols should be based on a reasonable identification of situations for which a reduction in response and transport times might improve patient outcome. The protocols should be developed in conjunction with local emergency response practices and statutes and should receive approval from the EMS director. Final protocols should be distributed to all dispatch and EMS entities. Warning lights and siren protocols should be enforced, and inappropriate use of L&S by EMS personnel will be limited.

3. *EMS dispatch agencies should utilize an emergency medical dispatch priority reference system that has been developed in conjunction with and approved by the EMS medical director to determine which request for prehospital medical care require the use of warning lights and siren.*

Sound dispatch prioritization systems establish a patient's level of severity, which then allows the determination of the type of vehicle (s) that should respond and the urgency of that response. Emergency medical dispatch centers should institute the protocols and monitor adherence to them.

4. *Except for suspected life-threatening, time-critical cases or cases involving multiple patients, L&S response by more than one EMV usually is unnecessary.*

Guidelines for the multi-EMV L&S response should be outlined in emergency medical response policies and dispatch procedures.

5. *The utilization of emergency warning L&S should be limited to emergency response and emergency transport situations only.*

Alternative practices, such as returning to a station or quarters using L&S or using L&S for "staging" or moving to designated areas to stand-by for a response, should be discontinued. Exceptions to such a policy would include extraordinary circumstances such as a disaster, or situations in which patient outcome could be affected.

6. *All agencies that operate EMVs or are responsible for emergency medical responders should institute and maintain emergency vehicle operation education programs for the EMV operators.*

Initial and continuing education of EMS personnel should include instruction in safe and appropriate EMV driving techniques and should take place prior to initial EMV operation. Knowledge and demonstrated skill in EMV operation are prerequisites for all public-safety vehicle operators.

7. *Emergency medical vehicle-related collisions occurring during an emergency response or transport should be evaluated by EMS system managers and medical directors.*

Such evaluations should include an assessment of the dispatch process, as well as initial (at the beginning of the transport) and final patient conditions.

8. *A national reporting system for EMV collisions should be established.*

Data are needed regarding the prevalence, circumstances, and causes of EMV collisions, including related injuries and deaths, and "wake effect" collisions. Collection of the information should start at the state and local levels; the information collected should include uniform data elements for tabulation and nationwide comparison.

9. *Scientific studies evaluating the effectiveness of warning L&S under specific situations should be conducted and validated.*

These important research efforts should be supported by both public and private resources.

10. *Laws and statutes should take into account prudent safety practices by both EMS providers and the monitoring public.*

The major emphasis and focus should remain on the exercise of prudent judgment and due regard by EMV operators. Laws and statutes also should emphasize the motoring public's responsibility to clear a lane or access way for EMVs.

11. *National standards for safe EMV operation should be developed.*

Such standards should mandate that EMV operators should approach intersections safely and have a clear view of all lanes of traffic before proceeding through. Standard also should set appropriate speed limits for emergency responses and transports in urban and rural settings, and for responses that occur under adverse road, traffic, and weather conditions.

Discussion

The Risk of Emergency Response

Response to and transport of emergency patients are integral components of the EMS chain of care. Since the beginning of modern EMS, the usual response mode has involved the use of L&S. Since this type of response was consistent with the practices of other public-safety agencies that use emergency vehicles (i.e., law enforcement and fire service), the practice was implemented initially without question. As an understanding of EMS call histories and patient outcomes had evolved, it has become evident that the use of L&S by EMS vehicles is not necessary for every response or patient transport.

There is risk associated with the use of warning L&S: emergency medical vehicles running "hot" (with L&S) have been involved in many collisions that have resulted in injuries and death in a high number of cases. The monetary loss derived from EMV collisions, including property damage, increases insurance premiums, and any other negligence-related EMS problem. This situation exists at a time when published data demonstrating the use of L&S in response or patient transport is effective in improving patient outcome are lacking. In fact, the U.S. Department of Transportation has reported that sirens may never become an effective warning device. Even if warning L&S eventually are shown to be useful in certain time-critical situations (e.g., cardiac arrest or penetrating chest injuries), it is unlikely that L&S will be proven beneficial for each and every EMS response and transport.

Concern about patient welfare, combined with inadequate information on a patient's actual condition, often pressures emergency medical technicians and paramedics to rush to and from scenes in order to "save lives". As Auerbach states, ". . . loose interpretation of what constitutes an emergency has essentially given [EMV operators permission] to operate their vehicles as they see fit while carrying victims who are essentially stable by anyone's definition."

Medical Director Involvement

Since EMS response and patient transport are prehospital medical "tools," accountable EMS medical directors should be involved in the development of emergency response and transport policies.

Additionally, EMS medical directors should evaluate EMV collisions for the medical correctness of the dispatch process, the patient's condition on arrival at the scene and when the transport began, and the patient's eventual outcome. For those medical directors who may need assistance with this aspect of prehospital care, advice is available from colleagues in NAEMSP, NASEMSD, and other EMS organizations.

Standardized Dispatch, Response, and Transport

Sound emergency medical dispatch protocols should be established and used as the basis for determining those situations that would benefit from the appropriate use of warning L&S. Research is emerging that supports the concept that medically sound protocols safely delineate which patients do and do not require emergency advanced life support. Such protocols, as well as proper emergency medical dispatch system. The American Society for Testing Materials state in their Standard Practice for Emergency Medical Dispatch document that "this practice may assist in overcoming some of the misconceptions . . . that red lights, siren, and maximal response are always necessary." Ideally, the use of L&S should be reserved for those situations or circumstances in which response and transport times have been shown to improve a patient's chances for survival or quality of life. Examples of such situations included cardiac or respiratory arrest, airway obstructions, extreme dyspnea, critical trauma, childbirth, and problems with pregnancy, drowning, and electrocution. In some of these cases, a rapid response is important (e.g., cardiac arrest), whereas in others rapid transport is necessary (e.g., breech birth).

Nevertheless, a large number of calls to 9-1-1 are for non-emergency problems that require neither rapid response nor rapid patient transport. Systems utilizing non-L&S response modes for such low priority calls have experienced few problems. This issue, however, requires more in-depth study in order to determine the specific positive and negative effects of L&S utilization on patient outcome in the various types of high- and low-priority cases.

In the typical EMS model, once a patient is evaluated and provided appropriate emergency treatment, transport by an EMV is initiated to move the patient to a definitive care facility. Many patients to whom EMS respond do not require L&S for patient transport. However, many EMS systems do not have protocols governing L&S use during patient transport, and few endorse contact with an on-line medical control base-station for advice or consent on the use of L&S transport.

Response of Multiple Emergency Medical Vehicles

The use of warning L&S by all EMVs responding to a single incident has been scrutinized in many systems and many of those systems have adopted a modified approach. From a medical point of view, the response of more that one unit utilizing L&S is necessary only on those situations involving suspected life-threatening, time-critical cases, or multiple patients. Likewise, the practice of returning to a station or quarters using L&S so as to "be in position" for the next call has no support in most responsible public-safety communities.

The Emergency Medical Vehicle Operator

While prevention of EMV collisions will depend on the application of sound dispatch protocols, dispatcher training, and direct involvement of the EMS medical director in developing dispatch and transport policies, attention also should be direct at the EMV operator. Before a driver of an emergency vehicle takes the wheel, their driving records should be carefully screened, and each should be trained in the proper use of EMVs. Rigorous education and control of EMV drivers should reduce EMV collisions, create a more standard approach and practice to EMV operation, and improve EMV longevity. Fortunately, there are detailed instruction guides for proper EMV operation. Emergency medical services provider education should include instruction in "low force" driving techniques. In addition, all personnel operating EMS vehicles should be involved in agency quality improvement programs including continuing education courses on EMV operation.

Some state laws requires that EMV operators exercise what is called "due regard." New Jersey law (N.J.S.A. 39:4–91) states it ". . . shall not relieve the driver of any authorized emergency vehicle from the duty to drive with due regard for the safety of all persons, nor shall it protect the driver from the consequences of his reckless disregard for the safety of others." Using laws of this nature, a number of prosecutors recently have charged and convicted ambulance operators of involuntary manslaughter. Most state laws, however, fail to place clear responsibility for the use of L&S on the EMS operators themselves. While much talk has ensued regarding the public's responsibility to "watch out" or "get out of the way," EMS should not blame the public for the problem of EMV collisions.

The EMS Profession

Responsibility rests with the EMS profession and local governments to establish minimum standards for the safe operations of EMS vehicles and to monitor the use of such standards. An example of such a standard would be a formal policy stating that EMVs should not exceed the locally posted speed limit by more than 10 miles per hour in rural areas, and that EMVs should not travel at any speed that is unsafe for current road, traffic, or weather conditions.

Nationally, EMS-related organizations should work together in helping to create standards that detail the positions in this document. Organizations that should be involved in an effort to set standards for emergency medical response and transport included the American Ambulance Association, the American College of Emergency Medical Physicians, the Association of Public Safety Officers, the International Association of Fire Chiefs, the International Association of Fire Fighters, the National Association of Emergency Medical Technicians, the National Association of EMS Physicians, the National Association of State EMS Directors, the National Association of State EMS Training Coordinators, the National EMS Alliance, and the National Fire Protection Agency.

Reimbursement

The reimbursement profiles of many EMS agencies contain an extra charge for the use of warning L&S. This occurs because the federal Health Care Financing Administration reimbursement policies recognize L&S use as a special circumstance. Insurance reimbursement for "emergencies" also may be predicated on L&S use, further perpetuating this problem. Unless these types of policies and profiles are modified by the government, insurance companies, and the EMS profession itself, adjustments in L&S use (as recommended in this document) may be viewed as adversely affecting EMS reimbursement. Therefore, without reimbursement policy modifications, the L&S reform process may be slowed.

Emergency Medical Vehicle Collision Reporting

The amount of data available on EMV collisions in general is fragmented and has not been obtained using any systematized or scientific format. The Fatal Accident Reporting System (FARS) may underestimate EMV collision occurrence and outcome. In 1990–1991, a national press clipping service documented 303 EMV collisions in one year resulting in 711 injuries and 78 deaths. (Clawson, unpublished data). The number of fatalities discovered in this newspaper review eclipses those reported by FARS involving EMVs for the same time period.

An acknowledged, but little-studied result of L&S use is the "wake effect," in which use of L&S results in collisions that involve only civilian vehicles and not the EMV itself. The ratio of wake effect collisions to those actually involving an EMV may be as high as five to one. However, this only can be adequately assessed with a comprehensive EMV collision reporting system.

There are models for EMV collision reporting systems. The National Fire Protection Agency has had in place a uniform process for reporting and quantifying fire fighting-related collisions and injuries for many years. Utah and Tennessee have "ambulance accident" reporting systems. As Auerbach has reported about Tennessee's system: "Before the requirement for accident reporting was imposed, [EMV collisions] analysis would have been impossible. Prehospital [EMV collision] data collection is essential if emergency medical services physicians are to exert reasonable control and make knowledgeable recommendations involving clinical care and professional regulations." Ideally, the federal government will initiate a national reporting system for EMV collisions. Any reporting system should be uniformly structured, track the multiple different types of responding agencies and vehicles including both volunteer and fire-based first responders (not just "ambulances"), and also provide a mechanism for the identification and reporting of wake effect collisions.

Research

Regrettably, there currently are few published investigations of dispatch protocols for L&S use. Also, there are no published studies attempting to evaluate the effectiveness of L&S use in terms of patient outcome. Worse still, there are no studies in either refereed or public safety trade journals that demonstrate that the use of L&S saves significant time over routine driving methods. In 1987, Auerbach demonstrated that the mean delay to hospital care after an EMV collision in Tennessee approached 10 minutes.

The use of warning L&S in EMS rests primarily on the unsupported tradition that has evolved from police and fire-response practices. In some cases, these practices may adversely affect EMS patients and providers. Therefore, a series of objective, well-structured, scientific studies aimed at identifying both the positive and negative effects of L&S use should be pursued.

Conclusion

In order to ensure that we "first do no harm," sound rationale and corresponding protocols and policies for the use of warning L&S in EMV response and patient transport should be developed and instituted in all EMS systems. All EMV operators should be trained adequately and regulated. The judicious use of warning L&S in the initial response and subsequent transport of patients likely will result in a more balanced system of appropriate care with minimization of iatrogenic injury and death.

Appendix II Proposal for Change form

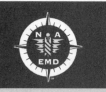

NA◆EMD
National Academy of Emergency Medical Dispatch

Medical Priority Dispatch System™-Ver. 11.0
PROPOSAL FOR CHANGE

LOG#: _____

Protocol Number(s) & Section(s) affected: _____

Protocol Version#: _____ **Language(s):** _____ **Type(s):** _____

DESCRIPTION OF PROPOSED CHANGE

To the Academy: Please accept for your review, the attached Proposal for Change to the MPDS protocol section and version noted above, SUMMARIZED as follows:

_____

_____

_____

I have included the following supportive material:

☐ Graphic or written description of proposed change
☐ Explanation of problem with current version
☐ Explanation of desired effect of proposed change
☐ References or copies of cited studies, articles, case transcripts, tapes, etc. (if applicable)

The number of attached pages is: _____ (indicate date and organization/agency on all papers)

I rate the necessity (URGENCY) for this change at: _____ (rate **1-10**, 1 = minimal, 10 = urgent)

RECOMMENDING CONTACT PERSON

_____   _____
Signature   DATE Submitted

_____   _____
Full Name (please print)   Primary PHONE Number

_____   _____
Title(s) or Academic Credentials   FAX and/or ALTERNATE PHONE Number

_____
Organization/Agency Representing

_____
Address for Correspondence

_____
City   ST/Prov.   Zip/Postal Code   Country

OVERSIGHT APPROVAL

The Academy takes all proposals for change very seriously and enters them into a formally defined process for review. To expedite official approval, please recommend potential *solutions* whenever possible and attach approval signatures from your local Dispatch Review or Steering Committee(s) as appropriate.

_____   _____
Dispatch Review Committee Signature   Steering Committee Signature

_____   _____
Full Name (please print)   Full Name (please print)

RLM:COF/MedicalChangeForm - © 5/5/2000, NAEMD

SETTING THE COURSE FOR EMD WORLDWIDE

Response Choices

David E. Persse, MD

Introduction

The entity of emergency medical services (EMS) has enjoyed a popular reputation for "saving lives." However, this public notion has recently come under scrutiny and the value of certain prehospital critical care services has been debated. In contrast, the evolving science of resuscitation medicine has provided greater opportunity for EMS systems to restore the lives of victims of out-of-hospital cardiac arrest—provided the system elements allow the greatest opportunity for success.

One of the most important elements to be considered in this endeavor is the resource deployment strategy (i.e., what resources go to which calls). There are nearly as many resource deployment strategies as there are systems in existence. There is no "perfect" resource deployment scheme. It is similarly held that each community must carefully design its deployment strategy to best meet the community's needs and resources (particularly financial resources). While this may sound good and well, the key phrase in the previous sentence is "carefully design." The art and science of system design are only recently beginning to develop, using patient outcome measures as production goals. Traditionally, response times and utilization rates have dominated the reason and rationale behind deployment strategies used in many EMS systems across America. An enlightened public has come to expect medical expertise to be among the characteristics of its emergency responders. Therefore, the goal of modern system designers is to achieve maximal medical success combined with prompt service and prudent financial practices. The purpose of this chapter is to explore evolving trends in deployment schemes, and to compare and contrast their advantages and disadvantages.

Reports of survival from out-of-hospital cardiac arrest were the seed from which modern EMS systems have grown. Response times then became an obvious and easy-to-understand yardstick of operational and medical success during the 1970s and 1980s when multiple scientific journal articles reported that improved cardiac arrest survival was inversely proportional to EMS response intervals. Since ambulance and other EMS vehicle response intervals were already tracked and relatively easy to collect as compared to actual survival rates, they became the mainstay of defining and determining quality in EMS. The majority of the prehospital cardiac resuscitation rates published during this time period boasted remarkable survival rates of as much as 43%, and predicted potential survival rates of 80% if appropriate community emergency care systems featuring short response intervals were put into place. Fittingly, civic leaders began seeking ways to implement EMS systems into their communities.

The federal government supported these efforts with several funding programs, including the EMS Act of 1973. Tragically, while the EMS Act of 1973 defined 15 "essential components" of EMS, it neglected to include medical oversight or clinically oriented outcome measures as essential components.

The economics of modern EMS began to change. Abundant federal support to survival through efficient use of resources balanced against fee-for-service generated revenues or taxpayer subsidies. Utilization rates became an increasingly important parameter for system directors. System designs often were directed toward remaining fiscally solvent, while at the same time boasting short average response intervals.

More recently, experts in EMS have been critical of actual survival rates measured in many metropolitan centers across America, citing disappointingly low numbers of survivors in spite of the expenditure of millions of taxpayer dollars. While some communities have demonstrated impressive survival statistics for out-of-hospital cardiac arrest, other communities have published survival rates so low that some have questioned the value of having paramedics in these urban settings. One major metropolitan system documented a reduction in survival rates for ventricular fibrillation from 30% to 0% between 1975 and 1995, in spite of significant investment into the system by the community.

Similarly, beginning in the mid-1980s and throughout the 1990s trauma surgeons debated the value of "scoop and run" versus "stay and play" strategies for caring for victims of severe trauma. As a result of outcomes measured in several well performed studies, most EMS systems today provide severely injured trauma patients potentially life-saving interventions while enroute to the closest trauma center. The new goal of prehospital trauma care is to provide the minimal amount of care on-scene, and not delay transport. Similar scrutiny of prehospital care led to many questioning the value of a variety of interventions provided by prehospital personnel. Consequently, the 2000 International Guidelines on Cardiopulmonary Resuscitation have been established on evidence-based criteria as opposed to expert opinion. Critical evaluation of patient outcomes has provided EMS leaders with a new and arguably more valuable system performance indicator to guide development.

Financial Efficiency vs. Medical Efficacy

Today EMS system design is often directed either toward financial efficiency or medical efficacy, suggesting there is little or no overlap and that these are two mutually exclusive and competing goals. A recent gathering of internationally recognized EMS experts tried to address this issue. The expert discussion compared the all-paramedic system design against the multi-tiered system design. The experts discussed convincing evidence of the operational-financial efficiency of the all-paramedic deployment scheme even though they also discussed the operational efficiency of fire-based tiered systems. Financial efficiency is argued to be best achieved through a community-wide ambulance system serving all stretcher transport needs using a single-tiered deployment of one paramedic/one EMT ambulance, with variable staffing matching anticipated call density for the 24-hour, seven-day coverage period. Such design minimizes or eliminates certain overhead inherent in priority dispatching: maintenance, staffing, and supply of multiple unit types, as well as differential response configurations. This type of deployment has been said to require the lowest cost

per participant and is characterized as "High Performance"—fewest input dollars per patient transported. The paradmedic deployment was, however, noted to have significant clinical disadvantages as compared to the tiered deployment, which has demonstrated improved clinical skill performance as well as response intervals to critical events.

Tiered systems have been criticized for poor financial efficiency due to the upkeep and overhead costs required for both basic ambulances and separate paramedic ambulances, particularly when responding only to emergency calls. Proponents of tiered systems generally concede some degree of financial inefficiency, especially in systems with provider agencies that will not deviate from static staffing schedules. The clinical superiority of tiered systems is commonly cited as the justification for any financial inefficiencies present. While the two deployment schemes were compared and contrasted, the experts did agree that the least effective and least efficient deployment scheme is an all paramedic system that is not involved in non-emergency and interfacility transports.

An important distinction which begins to come to light in these discussions is that financial efficiency is a function of overall system design, while medical efficacy may be a function of resource deployment strategy.

Between the two extremes of "all-paramedic, for all transports" and "tiered, emergency response only" is a spectrum of deployment schemes. System response should be tailored to the particular characteristics of the community. Communities differ from one another in a variety of ways. These differences will impact the resource deployment schema utilized. One characteristic of a community is the absolute geographic coverage in terms of square miles. This characteristic is compounded by mountain ranges, large bodies of water, freeway systems, hospital locations, and extremes of climate, including blizzards or floods. Another characteristic to be considered is population densities or, more appropriately, call densities. The economic makeup of the residents within the community will have an impact on the call density, contrasting with the actual population densities. The International Association of Fire Fighters indicates that call volumes can be predicted based on economic characteristics of a neighborhood. White-collar community residents can be expected to call for EMS assistance once every 24 hours for each 10,000 residents. Urban dwellers may call 1.5 to 2 times per 10,000 residents during each 24-hour period, while residents in "high violence" areas will call 4.2 to 5 times for each 10,000 residents in a 24-hour period.

Another closely related aspect of a community is the payor mix. For example, a 1997 Market Survey for the National Association of Public Utility Models found that Medicaid patients comprise 19% of the ambulance patient population in Richmond, but only 6% in Tulsa and only 1% in Reno. Conversely, Medicare patients represent 44% of the Tulsa transports and 46% of the Little Rock transports, but only 28% of the Reno transports. Private paying patients comprise only 2.2% of the Pinellas County payor mix, but 30.6% of those patients transported in Kansas City. Another important difference among systems which must be considered is the type of provider agency: municipal third service, public utility model, private ambulance company, volunteer, or fire-based. Is there a single provider for all ambulance needs or multiple providers, and do they all provide emergency service?

Clearly, the financial support of any EMS system is of vital importance to its success and survival. A growing amount of expertise in financial support of systems in an ever more complicated medical economic environment will benefit the EMS providers of the future.

Coupled closely with the economic viability of a system is its patient-care success. For decades it has been assumed that intense training of providers will result in quality care. Investigations into cardiac arrest survival have shed doubt on the assumption that ample training and quick response will provide good outcomes. Therefore, more critical approaches to EMS delivery strategies are being developed to enhance clinical success. The right combination of financial strategy and deployment strategy to achieve fiscal buoyancy and clinical success should be the goal of each system designer. A method to characterize EMS systems according to their cardiac arrest survival rates has been proposed.

Type A: A system that has been proven to positively impact cardiac arrest survival.

Type B: A system where it is not clear whether it impacts cardiac arrest survival.

Type C: A system that has evaluated cardiac arrest outcomes and shown to be extremely poor.

Type C1: A system with financial, logistical, or operational barriers such that it will never be able to demonstrate a benefit to the community by producing cardiac arrest survivors.

Type C2: A system with geographical/population density barriers such that it will never be able to demonstrate a benefit to the community by producing cardiac arrest survivors (wilderness).

This classification of EMS systems is based on clinical success of cardiac arrest resuscitation. Cardiac arrest resuscitation is one marker for the clinical quality of a system, as it represents the greatest medical triumph a system can produce and infers clinical expertise in the care of other critically ill or injured patients. More indepth quality monitoring of all injury and illness patients and their outcomes would allow medical oversight a better assessment of actual proficiency of care delivery. The ability to closely monitor most if not all care delivery also should be a marker of high-quality system design. Monitoring of actual quality-of-care delivery is important, as the products delivered by EMS systems are *quality care, and saved lives.*

The consumer defines overall quality of service, generally retrospectively. Unfortunately, most consumers still consider rapid response to be the ultimate quality marker. It is not until after they are informed of significant differences in survival potential that they reconsider their position. Most Type A systems utilize some form of dispatch prioritization. An inherent risk of any prioritization scheme is that a true life-threatening emergency might be under-triaged and have inadequate resources deployed on initial dispatch, resulting in a life lost. When considering the entire system, the designers can easily be lulled into a sense of security against under-triage tragedies by deploying a maximum response to all calls. Unfortunately, current research suggests this approach may actually result in a greater loss of life when the entire system is considered. For example, if a medium-sized city had a witnessed ventricular fibrillation cardiac arrest survival rate of 10% resulting in 15 long-term survivors, with no cases of undertriage due to an all-paramedic response scheme, most members of the community would feel comfortable with the system performance. However, if it were known that a nearly identical community utilizing an aggressive tiered deployment scheme had a witnessed ventricular fibrillation survival rate of 20% resulting in 30 long-term survivors, but also had one case of potentially life-threatening under-triage per year, observers may wonder if 14 or 15 lives were unnecessarily lost due to the operational, financial, and emotional advantages of the single-tiered system.

The incentive to employ aggressive deployment schemes stems from decreasing revenue sources supporting systems coupled with increasing expectations of clinical performance. For decades the public was satisfied to know that if they called the local emergency number someone would respond to quickly manage the emergency. It is a standard expectation in urban, suburban, and even some rural areas of America that emergency services are available to quickly respond. Community standards, including standards of care, are ultimately determined by juries in courts of law. They "evolve" in part according to public expectations as those expectations are honed by the professions in their literature and forums, and reported in the press and media.

As EMS has matured, the expectations of the public have grown. Television portrayed tremendous clinical success of EMS systems. More recently, medically oriented television dramas have shown patients dying in spite of the heroic efforts of the medical personnel portrayed. Nonetheless, many members of the public still believes that most people who have CPR performed on them survive. In reality, some systems have consistently achieved survival rates of 25 to 30%, while many others remain less than 10%. Therefore, it should be considered reasonable for the public to expect that the local EMS system will focus its efforts on maximizing cardiac arrest survival, at least to the same degree as response time and the fiscal health of the organization.

When considering what resources should be sent to any given emergency request there is generally unrecognized potential for improved financial efficiency as well as medical efficacy. When configured correctly, rapid response times will also be a feature of sophisticated resource deployment schemes. However, in order to be optimally successful the system administrators must invest personnel and resources to the monitoring, interpretation, and modifications of resource deployment to emergency requests.

Probably the simplest deployment scheme in the United States, yet most common when considering square mile coverage, is an All EMT-B staffed ambulance system that handles all patient transports within a community. Many wilderness, rural, and some suburban communities rely on EMT-B personnel, many on a volunteer basis, to provide the ambulance service, both emergency and non-emergency. Low call volumes and limited financial support are generally the motivating factors leading communities to have such a system. The low call volume generally prohib-

its financial support for paramedic training, or maintaining clinical expertise through experience. Resource utilization issues are fairly simple in this setting, as the same resource is sent on all requests. Any single-level response system is operationally simpler and is without the costs involved in differential response configuration. The addition of another level of response defines any system as "tiered." An example would be a EMT-B ambulance system that responds to all calls, but also sends local fire- or police-based first responders to emergency calls. Once a system becomes "tiered" or there is any prioritization of resources sent based on caller information, the system administration and medical oversight are obligated to closely monitor clinical and operational trends and seek to achieve optimal clinical performance based on the patient outcome data generated.

One of the greatest advances of the information and technology age to benefit EMS has been the progress made in the discipline of emergency dispatch. Sound scientific research has shown that sophisticated emergency medical dispatch centers can reliably identify less-emergent 9-1-1 requests for service. Such accuracy allows system designers to confidently consider more aggressive deployment schemes. Further incentive comes from recent investigations demonstrating a survival benefit for cardiac arrest patients in aggressively deployed systems. Requests for emergency service fill the spectrum from falsely triggered automatic medical alerts to an unconscious person, not-breathing. Modern dispatch prioritization systems give the system operators the ability to reliably categorize calls by their severity. Even for the conservative system operator there is great confidence in the prioritization system's ability to reliably identify less-emergent requests for service.

A remarkable percentage of calls to 9-1-1 can accurately be identified as either requiring no prehospital care and transportation or requiring BLS service only. Investigations have also shown an under-triage rate of less than one in 1400 calls. Undertriage is identified as an initial BLS resource dispatch, later requiring any degree of ALS level care. In Houston only 1.6% of all initial BLS dispatches later required the services of a paramedic; of those 0.3% received drugs and less than 0.04% had a true potential for advantage in outcome if a paramedic had been initially dispatched. At the same time, priority dispatch spared paramedics from over 40% of initial dispatch, keeping them available for the next call. By keeping the paramedics available, and in their "first-in" territory, the priority dispatch system *reduced* response times for paramedics to critical level calls.

The single largest line item of any budget is personnel. It is now common in many communities across America for firefighters and police officers to be utilized in the capacity of first responders. Using existing personnel and equipment offers tremendous financial and clinical advantage to a system. Through a medical dispatch prioritization scheme, first responders can quickly respond to an emergency scene, and more accurately determine their needs. This approach allows an opportunity to even more effectively respond the right resources to the right call. By sparing these resources from unnecessary calls, they are more available, and result in shorter response times to patients requiring critical interventions beyond those which can be provided by the first responders.

During the implementation, and after several subsequent audits of the Houston first responder program, it has been determined that the entire program costs (medical supplies, fuel, vehicle maintenance) were less than the overall operating and personnel costs for one additional ambulance per year. Pursuing aggressive deployment schemes, resulted in improved financial efficiency as well as improved clinical performance. Such schemes maximize the benefit of the financial support for the system and deliver the highest life-saving potential to the community. In the most sophisticated and aggressive EMS systems, calls of the lowest medical priority would be identified by dispatch and have the minimal resources deployed to confirm low medical need and to provide the necessary care.

It may not even be necessary to deploy an ambulance to some of the lowest priority calls. Automatic medical alert, 9-1-1 hang-ups, and reports of motor vehicle collisions where the caller can provide no detailed information generally did not require ambulances. Ninety percent of the automated medical alerts were false alarms where the device was unknowingly activated or malfunctioned. Of the remaining ten percent of automated calls, 90% of the patients were stable, with medical problems that were not time-critical and in fact required no medical intervention from EMS personnel. In 1% of the automated reports to 9-1-1 the patients received no care other than transport from the EMS personnel. In fact, in only 0.1% of these cases did paramedic-level treatment play a role in the patient's care. Hang-ups prior to any information being gathered by the call taker (other than the address obtained through the enhanced 9-1-1 systems) had similarly low necessity for rapid medical care. In cases of callers to 9-1-1 reporting a motor vehicle collision, but unable to answer any of the standard prioritization questions, it was found in over 60% of the cases there was either no patient or no acute care necessary and no transportation provided. In almost all of the remaining cases non-time dependent BLS care was sufficient to meet the patient's needs. In 2.4% of the calls patients required some degree of ALS care. Critical ALS care was required for 0.17% of all calls in this category. Interestingly, the need for either basic or advanced care was statistically greater if the caller could answer even one of the standard priority questions.

Adding more information into a prediction index other than the standard medical priority questions resulted in an even greater potential for sparing precious EMS resources. Investigators in the Detroit system considered determination of the geographic location and time of day, as well as the caller's description of the medical problem. Consideration of all these factors resulted in a further reduction of workload on the EMS system by accurately identifying probable false runs. Another study demonstrated that dispatching non-transport capable first responders to 9-1-1 calls, where the caller provided no information beyond the address, saved a large urban system over $500,000 in operating expenses and effectively added one ambulance to the system. Investigations looking into the ability of priority dispatch systems to correctly isolate those requests necessitating ALS care were also successful. It has been determined that in a system serving a community of over 200,000 priority dispatching spared ALS resources from approximately 25% of all initial dispatches.

Establishment and maintenance of clinical expertise are fundamental doctrines of modern medicine. The commonly spoken axiom of "the more you do something, the better you are at it!" applies to EMS personnel the same as it would to any medical professional. Some of the most important skills possessed by providers have little to do with eye-hand coordination and more to do with critical thinking. History taking and performance of a good physical exam are intellectual skills which must be performed to the best of an individual's ability on each patient encounter. Critical thinking skills specific for seriously ill and injured patients are even more important due to the nature of the patient's problems. The need for excellence when performing eye-hand coordination skills combined with critical decision-making settings prompts many medical directors to mandate frequent retraining and/or evidence of continuing expertise for such interventions as cricothyroidotomy and pharmacologically assisted intubation. Recent studies have strongly suggested the need for such tight control of more common interventions such as "routine intubation" among paramedics who rarely perform these skills.

The need for expertise in performing critical skills is not controversial. What is controversial is whether training alone can provide the necessary level of expertise. One recent investigation compared witnessed ventricular fibrillation cardiac arrest survival within one large system where all paramedics were trained at the same institution, exposed to the same continuing education, operated off the same protocols, and differed only in resource deployment strategy. In this community a targeted deployment strategy (tiered) was used in the higher call volume region of the city while a uniform deployment strategy (all-paramedic) was used in low call volume areas. The two critical intervention skills tracked (intubation and IV success) were statistically significantly different between the two deployment strategies. The patients in the targeted deployment region successfully intubated 99% of patients, compared to 92% in the uniform deployment region. It is interesting to note that most all paramedic systems reporting intubation success in the literature report approximately 92% success. Intravenous success was similarly improved in the tiered targeted deployment region, with 98% success compared to 83% for the uniform deployment region. More importantly, return of spontaneous circulation, survival to admission, and survival to hospital discharge were all statistically significantly improved in the targeted deployment region (see table 19.1).

Summary

Since the birth of modern EMS in the early 1970s, quality of out-of-hospital emergency care and success of system operations have been tightly linked to response times. Current research has strongly suggested that this dogma remains true for capable AED first responders, but may not apply to the significantly more complicated and experience-dependent interventions offered by paramedics.

This having been said, communities are then left to decide which type of EMS system they wish to have. It would seem that those communities seeking

TABLE 19.1		
Outcomes of Deployment Strategy		
	ALL PARAMEDIC	**TIERED**
Male	83%	73%
Mean age (years)	63.3	61.5
Response time (min.)	9.0	7.7
Bystander CPR	63%	43%
Intubation success	92%	99%
IV success	83%	98%
Return of spontaneous circulation	33%	56%
Admitted	29%	51%
Discharged alive	4%	24%

to have Type A systems must invest the resources necessary to custom design the resource deployment strategy to provide AED-capable first responders within 5 minutes.

Bibliography

Anderson BD, Manoguerra AS, Haynes BE. Diversion of 9-1-1 poisoning calls to a poison center. *Prehosp Emerg Care*. 1998;2(3):176–179.

Bachman JW. Cardiac arrest in the community: how to improve survival rates. *Postgrad Med*. 1984;1;76(3):85–90, 92–95.

Baer NA. Cardiopulmonary resuscitation on television: exaggerations and accusations. *N Engl J Med*. 1996;335(21): 1604–1605.

Bailey ED, O'Connor RE, Ross RW. The use of an emergency medical dispatch system to reduce the number of inappropriate scene responses made by advanced life support personnel. *Acad Emerg Med*. 1997;4(5):15.

Bailey ED, O'Connor RE, Ross RW. The use of emergency medical dispatch protocols to reduce the number of inappropriate scene responses made by advanced life support personnel. *Prehosp Emerg Care*. 2000;4(2):186–189.

Becker LB, Ostrander MP, Barrett J, et al. Outcome of CPR in a large metropolitan area—where are the survivors? *Ann Emerg Med*. 1991;20:355–361.

Border JR, Lewis FR, Aprahmian C, et al. Prehospital trauma care—stabilization or scoop and run. *J Trauma*. 1983; 23:708–711.

Bourn S. Give me proof—is EMS really worth it? *J Emerg Med Services*. 1992;17:83–85.

Cady G, Linberg C. 200 City Survey. *JEMS*. 2001;26(2):36–41.

Curka PA, Pepe PE, Ginger VF, et al. Emergency medical services priority dispatch. *Ann Emerg Med*. 1993;22(11): 1688–1695.

Curka PA, Pepe PE, Ginger VF, Sherrard RC, Ivy MV, Zachariah BS. Emergency medical services priority dispatch. *Ann Emerg Med*. 1993;22(11):1688–1695.

Eisenberg MS, Bergner L, Hallstrom A. Cardiac resuscitation in the community: importance of rapid provision and implications for program planning. *JAMA*. 1979; 4; 241 (18):1905–1907.

Eisenberg MS, Bergner L, Hallstrom A. Paramedic programs and out-of-hospital cardiac arrest: I. Factors associated with successful resuscitation. *Am J Public Health*. 1979; 69(1):30–38.

Ginsburg W. Prepare to be shocked: the evolving standard of care in treating sudden cardiac death. *Ann J Emerg Med*. 1998;16(3):315–319.

Huang RR, McGraw S, Zalenski R, et al. The emergency medical service transportation index (EMSTI): a mathematical index for improving the effectiveness of EMS dispatch response. *Acad Emerg Med*. 1997;4(5):415–416.

International Association of Fire Fighters. *Emergency Medical Services—A Guide Book for Fire-Based Systems*. 1995, 11.

International Guidelines on Cardiopulmonary Resuscitation. *Circulation*. 2000;102:1–1.

Key CD, Persse DE, Pepe PE, et al. Automated alarms for urban 9-1-1 EMS response: evaluating the feasibility of sending first responders without ambulances. *Acad Emerg Med*. 1997;4:414.

Key CD, Persse DE, Pepe PE, et al. Safety of first-responder only utilization for motor vehicle incidents when the 9-1-1 caller is unable to answer standard medical priority dispatch questions. *Acad Emerg Med*. 1997;4:414.

Key CD, Persse DE, Pepe PE, et al. Urban emergency medical services response to automated 9-1-1 alarms: a prospective evaluation of the safety and operational advantages of dispatching rapidly-responding first responder crews without ambulances. *Acad Emerg Med*. 1998; 5(5):441.

Kostoulakos NM, Bradley DR. Overestimation of the effectiveness of cardiopulmonary resuscitation. *Percept Mot Skills*. 1997;84(3 pt.2):1409–1410.

Lombardi G, Gallagher J, Gennis P. Outcome of out-of-hospital cardiac arrest in New York City: the pre-hospital arrest survival evaluation (PHASE) study. *JAMA*. 1994; 271:678–683.

Marsden AK. Getting the right ambulance to the right patient at the right time. *Accid Emerg Nurs*. 1995;3(4):177–183.

Neely KW, Eldurkar JA, Drake M. Do Emergency Medical Services dispatch nature and severity codes agree with Paramedic Field Findings? *Acad Emerg Med*. 2000;174–180.

Palazzo FF, Warner OJ, Harron M, Sadana A. Misuse of the London ambulance service: how much and why? *J Accid Emerg Med*. 1998;15(6):368–370.

Palumbo L, Kubincanek J, Emerman C, Jouriles N, Cydulka R, Shade B. Performance of a system to determine EMS dispatch priorities. *Am J Emerg Med*. 1996;14(4):388–390.

Pepe PE, Monnin MJ, Mattox KL. Regulating the scope of EMS services. *Prehosp Dis Med*. 1990;5:59–63.

Persse DE, Key CB, Bradley RB, et al. Impact of a paramedic deployment strategy on cardiac arrest survival in a large urban EMS system. *Acad Emerg Med*. 2000;7:746.

Persse DE, Key CB, Pepe PE. Effect on work force of utilizing non-transport first responders instead of ambulances to respond to EMS requests with no information. *Prehosp Emerg Care*. 1997;1(3):171.

Ritter G, Wolfe RA, Goldstein S, et al. The effect of bystander CPR on survival of out-of-hospital cardiac arrest victims. *Am Heart J*. 1985;110(5):932–937.

Smith JP, Bodai BI, Hill AS, et al. Prehospital stabilization of critically injured patients: a failed concept. *J Trauma*. 1985;25:65–70.

Spaite D. Expanded Scope EMS: a word of caution. National Meeting National Association of EMS Physicians, Naples, Florida, 1991.

Stout J, Pepe P, Mosesso V. All-advanced life support vs. tiered-response ambulance systems. *Prehosp Emerg Care*. 2000;4:1–6.

Stratton S, Niemann JT. Effects of adding links to "The Chain of Survival" for pre-hospital cardiac arrest: a contrast in outcome in 1975 and 1995 at a single institution. *Ann Emerg Med*. 1998;31:471-477.

Zachariah BS, Pepe PE, Curka PA. How to monitor the effectiveness of an emergency medical dispatch system: the Houston model. *Eur J Emerg Med*. 1995;2(3):123–127.

First Responders

Alan A. Katz, MD
Michael Cassara, DO
Christine M. Houser, MD

Introduction

First responders constitute the initial line of defense against potentially life- or limb-threatening medical events. First responder deployment for the management of real and potential emergencies has increased dramatically in recent years.

A first responder is generally defined as any person arriving first at the scene of a medical emergency in the prehospital environment, regardless of the individual's type of credential.[1] The term was used interchangeably with the term *Certified First Responder*, and signified completion of the objectives and requirements outlined by the curriculum developed by the National Highway Traffic Safety Administration (NHTSA) and individual states. Heightened awareness of the need for rapid assessment and intervention during critical out-of-hospital medical emergencies, such as cardiac arrest, coupled with recognition of the delay inherent with more advanced provider response, has led many to broaden the first responder definition. Many consider a first responder as simply an individual attempting to aid another in trouble.

More EMS system protocols have expanded the role of first responder to include those persons with a duty to respond to medical emergencies, including members of the police and fire departments, park rangers, airline attendants, security personnel, and occupational and mass gathering safety officers. Many have proposed that, with the ability to universally distribute new technologies such as, the automated external defibrillator (AED), the first responder should include the lay public as well. The use of lay public first responders provides both another level of provider and complexity to current emergency medical response systems. In some circles, there is still debate and uneasy acceptance of untrained laypersons in first responder roles and over the scope of their practice. Future use of laypersons in the role of first responder requires a more thorough understanding of what in-fluences the likelihood of helping behavior in response to medical emergencies, and how the effectiveness of that helping behavior may be improved.

In this chapter, these issues surrounding the first responder will be discussed. To better understand these issues, the history and development of first responder programs will be presented, including the requirements necessary for achieving formal certification as a Certified First Responder (CFR). The current roles and responsibilities of generic first responders will be described. Helping behavior will be reviewed from the social psychology perspective. Innovations in first responder use will be presented, and the chapter will conclude with comment on the future roles of first responders, both in the community and in the work place.

History and Development

Formal education of non-physician emergency medical personnel in the United States dates back to the 1950s, with the creation of training programs for ambulance attendants by both the American College of Surgeons and the American Academy of Orthopedic Surgeons. Training of prehospital personnel did not move toward a unified standardized protocol until 1971, when the EMT-Ambulance standard curriculum was created by a third-party contractor for NHTSA. The success of the EMT-Ambulance curriculum led to the development of other curricula providing varying levels of prehospital certification, including NHTSA's 40-hour *Crash Injury Management for the Law Enforcement Officer* training program. This curriculum, designed to address the perceived lack of prehospital care training of law enforcement personnel, is considered the foundation on which the first responder curriculum is based. The first national standard curriculum for first responders was written in 1979. Despite many changes in content, nomenclature, and teaching methods in the other curricula created for the EMT-Intermediate and Paramedic, the first responder curriculum had remained essentially unchanged until 1990, when NHTSA sponsored its Consensus Workshop on Emergency Medical Services Training Programs. At this meeting, the groundwork to revise the first responder training course curriculum was begun. The revised first responder curriculum, utilizing the revised *EMT-Basic: National Standard Curriculum* and the *National EMS Education and Practice Blueprint* as a basis, was accepted in 1995. It remains today as the national standard for CFR education and practice.

The peaked interest in the first responders as an important component of an EMS system is linked by many to the innovations in prehospital defibrillation. For most of the past 40 years, laypersons and basic-level prehospital care providers were limited in the number and quality of interventions that they could perform at the scene of a cardiac emergency. Airway maneuvers, methods of rescue breathing, and cardiopulmonary resuscitation represented the extent of the interventions that both trained and layperson first responders could perform. The reasons why these basic level providers were limited in their ability to deliver more in the emergency cardiac care setting are many. Defibrillation was an advanced cardiac life support intervention requiring a level of training greater than that of the basic level provider. Use of the manual defibrillator demanded a significant time commitment to achieve the medical sophistication necessary to interpret arrhythmias. Initial prehospital defibrillation protocols, therefore, held defibrillation as an advanced life support skill. In addition, use of manual defibrillators by *any* prehospital care personnel was also limited because of criticism from some physicians who felt defibrillator use by non-physicians was akin to practicing medicine without a license. Resistance to non-physician defibrillation was based also on the perception that risks to the patients and prehospital providers were too great.

The successful use of defibrillators by paramedics put an end to all controversy. Defibrillation by non-physicians received widespread support after repeated observations revealed that better patient outcomes were achieved with rapid defibrillation, particularly in cases of cardiac arrest secondary to ventricular fibrillation in the setting of myocardial infarction.[2,3] Much support was generated for universal defibrillator use in all systems. The use of defibrillators, however, remained limited because of the extensive training required to operate the manual machines.

The advent of the AED brought with it the hope of increasing public access to defibrillation. The AED is a defibrillator equipped with programming for cardiac rhythm analysis and with programming to prompt intervention. Briefly, when the monitoring pads of an AED are applied to a patient in cardiac arrest, the patient's rhythm is interpreted by the AED processor as one of two possible entities: a rhythm requiring defibrillation (i.e., ventricular fibrillation) or a rhythm not requiring defibrillation (i.e., asystole). When the AED detects a rhythm requiring defibrillation, it initiates a charging sequence. AEDs are now manufactured to a variety of specifications, and newer models incorporate the latest advances in defibrillation technology, including biphasic waveforms.

With the development of the AED, individuals with no medical training could perform defibrillation; *any* first responder could use the same technology in the cardiac arrest situation as a physician. In addition, AEDs could be incorporated into existing systems easier and faster than standard units.[4,5] Recent studies indicate that they function as well as traditional machines requiring rhythm interpretation by experienced practitioners, and produce a faster time to initial shock than their manual counterparts.[3–10] They seem to be easier to use, easier to learn, and easier to integrate into existing EMS systems. The success of the AED program has directly led to the heightened interest and attention that first responders now enjoy.

Current First Responder Curriculum and Training

The *First Responder: National Standard Curriculum* defines, outlines, and nationally standardizes the roles and responsibilities of CFRs. This curriculum defines the first responder as the first individual who arrives at the scene of a medical emergency, regardless of the type of credential.[11] *The National EMS Education and Practice Blueprint* expands this definition by stating that the first responder "uses a limited amount of equipment to perform initial assessment and intervention."[11] The curriculum supports the first responder as an important first level of response; however, the curriculum is clear in noting that first responders are not sufficiently prepared or certified to work independently on ambulances.

The pedagogical philosophy of the first responder curriculum places an emphasis on "need-to-know" information, while trying to avoid more advanced, but potentially confusing, "nice-to-know" subject material.[1] This philosophy also emphasizes the development of assessment-based problem-solving skills, rather than the development of problem-solving skills based on a specific diagnosis. The curriculum is designed to provide a standard foundation of knowledge regardless of the geographic location and the provider's previous experience. The curriculum contains 40 hours of coursework divided into seven modular components: a preparatory module (6.5 hours); airway (7 hours); patient assessment (6 hours); circulation (6 hours); illness and injury (6.5 hours); childbirth and children (5 hours); and EMS operations (3 hours). Each of these modules contains several prepared outlined lesson plans detailing specific objectives. Candidates must demonstrate knowledge of the objectives by passing both a written and a practical skills examination to achieve certification. Advanced provider skills (i.e., automated defibrillation, vital signs, supplemental oxygen) may be incorporated into the first responder curriculum. NHTSA recommends that the inclusion of more advanced content (i.e., AED instruction and training) should receive approval by each state EMS provider certification board and should remain within the framework of *The National EMS Education and Practice Blueprint*. In addition, candidates seeking to receive certification from the American Heart Association (AHA) for cardiopulmonary resuscitation (CPR) coursework must complete additional requirements and show competence in accordance with AHA standards.

The Role of First Responders

First responders are an important part of any emergency medical service, and perform a number of essential functions during the first few minutes of an emergency. As the initial healthcare provider to arrive at the scene, first responders have a responsibility to survey the scene to insure safe access to the injured. Once the scene is deemed safe, first responders assess the number of injured people and the nature of each person's injuries. After insuring that the EMS system has been activated, the first responder should initiate care up to the level of their training. First responders should continue in their patient-care assessment and treatment responsibilities until more advanced prehospital care providers arrive. First responders should then assist these advanced prehospital care providers in patient-care activities and transportation.

First responders, traditionally, are most recognized for their role in prehospital cardiac emergencies. Prior to the introduction of the AED, first responders were at best able to provide only CPR upon arrival at the scene of a cardiac arrest. Although early CPR has been shown to be important in improving outcomes in the setting of cardiac arrest, it is generally accepted that if defibrillation capability arrives 6 or more minutes after the onset of cardiac arrest, resuscitation will be less successful.[2,6,10,12–15] With the advent of the AED, the first responder has been given access to a proven intervention that can improve outcomes without the need for extensive training, and in a cost-effective manner.[16–18]

Many investigators have studied the use of the AED by different levels of prehospital providers. The results of their research have supported the use of the AED in prehospital cardiac emergencies. In a controlled clinical trial by Cummins comparing EMT use of the AED with the use of standard defibrillators, use of the AED was demonstrated to produce a faster initial shock.[5] Although AED use in this study did not demonstrate a significant difference in patient outcome compared with standard defibrillators, AED use appeared to hold advantages over standard defibrillators with regard to training, skill retention, and ease and speed of operation. Cobbe described a 12.5% survival to hospital discharge rate among patients defibrillated by ambulance crews equipped with AEDs as part of the first year of the Heartstart Scotland Project.[4] They also comment that AEDs were "introduced rapidly, with limited training implications and costs." Sedgwick reported a similar level of success with AED use by ambulance crews in the project's second year.[19] In addition, this study demonstrated that AED use has an acceptable sensitivity and high specificity for detecting appropriate rhythms to shock, and for initiating defibrillation.[9]

With the strength of the data, investigators began to study the use of the AED by personnel assuming the specific role of first responder. Hoekstra compared the effect of first responder AED use on specific time intervals to critical therapeutic interventions (i.e., initial shock, IV access, endotracheal intubation, adrenergic drug therapy).[7] Kellerman and Hackman studied first responder defibrillation in an urban environment.[20] Callaham studied first responders with defibrillators, paramedics with advanced life support capabilities, and patient outcomes.[6] These studies describe shorter times to initial countershock. Callaham noted that early defibrillation by first responders was associated with a nine-fold improvement in survival.[6] In addition, Hoeckstra reported by delegating initial countershock to first responders, significantly shorter times from paramedic arrival to IV access, endotracheal intubation, and initial drug therapy interventions resulted.[7] In summary, these studies showed that AED use by first responders produces favorable, comparable results while making access to early defibrillation more widespread.

Others sought to study AED use by first responders with a duty to respond. In most of these studies, the personnel were trained members of local fire and police departments. In many respects, the results mirrored the previously mentioned studies of first responders. White reported a high rate of survival among patients in ventricular fibrillation after AED use by police officers in Rochester, Minnesota.[21] Mosesso also demonstrated decreased time to defibrillation with police use of the AED.[22] Police first responder defibrillation was also noted as an independent predictor of survival.[22] Weaver demonstrated improved survival with AED use by firefighter first responders.[3]

With the inception of the AED, many have questioned whether the device could be placed in the hands of laypersons. Layperson use of the AED has been mentioned in the literature since the mid-1980s. In 1986 and in 1987, Moore studied the homes and families of patients who suffered cardiac arrest as a result of ventricular fibrillation and survived.[8,23] Moore found that approximately half of the homes and families studied could potentially use the AED, and that laypersons could learn to use the AED safely and correctly.[8,23] In addition, his group commented that the laypersons taught to use the AED were able to deliver shocks an average of eight minutes faster than typical response times of EMTs.[8] Chadda described the use of the AED by laypersons who witnessed cardiac arrest before the arrival of prehospital care providers.[24] Sixteen percent of the patients in this small series survived to hospital discharge. In 1988, Cummins noted that a high percentage of deaths associated with commercial air travel were of cardiac origin, and commented that perhaps some of these deaths could be avoided if laypersons or airline personnel had access to the AED.[25,26] Over the past decade, many have started to study the effect of laypersons in the workplace trained to use the AED as a first responder during cardiac emergencies. Despite these studies, there is still insufficient research on layperson defibrillation, and much more is required if the dream of universal defibrillation is to become a reality.[17,18,27-30]

Although much of the interest in first responders has focused on their role in cardiac emergencies, they can also function efficiently and effectively in other prehospital emergency settings as well. Although literature on the subject is sparse, the use of first responders has been increasingly described in the initial response plans for imagined and real mass casualty incidents, including acts of biological or chemical terrorism or war.[31-34] Each of these selected examples from the literature bring up interesting questions and comments on the role of first responders in response to acts of war, acts of terrorism, or multiple casualty incidents.

Sharp describe the use of a variety of multidisciplinary personnel types (fire department personnel, police department members, emergency department staff members, prehospital response staff) as first responders for the 1996 Atlanta Olympic Games.[34] In particular, first responders were deployed to help counter the threat posed by the use of a biological or chemical agent by terrorist groups. First responders were given the responsibility for recognizing a biological or chemical agent should multiple patients present with a known "toxidrome." They were trained to identify the major chemical and biological agents, the associated clinical syndromes for each, the methods of decontamination necessary, and the therapeutic interventions necessary. Keim and Kaufmann noted the important role of first responders in the initial response to acts of bioterrorism.[32] They make an important observation that first responder training in biological terrorism recognition and response tactics is not standardized, nor is it universally distributed.

Hogan in his discussion of the Oklahoma City terrorist bombing, described the initial EMS response team interventions.[31] He noted that the majority of prehospital interventions included spinal immobilization, wound management, and IV fluid administration. This account of the bombing suggested that first responders, trained in basic first-aid skills, could have provided a majority of the required patient-care skills.

Rivkind, in his study of the medical preparedness and response in Israel during the Gulf War, stated that "many of the people who sought ED care for burns, lacerations, and cuts could have been treated with the use of simple first-aid skills outside the hospital."[33]

In sum these studies suggests that:

- There are limited resources in the setting of any multiple casualty incident.

- In many disaster plans, first responders will be relied upon to provide initial situational information (i.e., presence of a real or suspected chemical or biological weapons or weapons of mass destruction).

- In many multiple casualty incidents, most of the medical problems encountered can be initially handled by first responders adequately trained in basic first-aid techniques.

- First responders require additional, standardized training concerning their roles in multiple-casualty incidents in order to be utilized correctly.

Helping Behavior

Students and theoreticians of human behavior have analyzed helping behavior in an effort to understand why such behavior developed in human societies at all, and what determines when such behavior occurs in modern situations. Helping behavior amongst humans is initially thought to have developed in early human society, somewhere between one-half and two million years ago.[35] Although it may seem that helping behavior must have always been a part of human existence, from an evolutionary perspective helping another, even if it costs the helper, is thought to have developed as a way to increase the probability of one's genes being passed on. For example, when a parent helps a child to survive even if the parent's survival is risked, the probability of a percentage of the parent's genes continuing in the gene pool will be enhanced. More typical types of helping behavior initially consisted of cooperative divisions of labor or cooperative behaviors for the defense of a related group of individuals from outside threats (such as fighting together against intruders or hunting together to obtain large prey). Sociobiologists and social psychologists have attempted to clarify those circumstances which lead to a first helping response being made. An understanding of these factors should alter our training and system design to improve the probability of first response and to understand how these mechanisms sometimes break down.

Both the sociobiology field (which tends to focus on animal behavior research) and the social psychology field (which examines human social interactions) have concluded that help is most likely to be offered when one individual is in close proximity to the one requiring assistance, when the physical characteristics of the two are similar, when the individual requiring assistance is familiar to the other individual, and when the two perceive each other as belonging to the same group.[35] Individuals in need of assistance are also more likely to be helped if the problem does not appear to be one they created for themselves.[36]

Among individuals, the more rewards and generally positive experiences a particular person has had with helping behaviors, the more likely the individual is to engage in that behavior in the future.[37] Observing others behaving in the same helping manner has also been demonstrated to increase the tendency to do the same when placed in a similar situation.[38] A clear need for assistance or direct request for assistance is a major factor determining the likelihood of help being offered. Even in cases of quite severe need for assistance, if the bystander is uncertain that help is needed or desired, it is unlikely to be offered.[39-41]

The role the outside environment plays has also been examined. The higher the load of sensory stimulation, the less likely individuals are to help. For example, someone walking along a busy street with a high noise level is less likely to aid another individual than someone walking down a calmer, quieter, street.[42] This difference in likelihood of helping is maintained even if neither of the two individuals is particularly busy themselves. The pioneering, but disturbing, work of Milgram indicated the importance of authority figures in directing behavior. Milgram's initial research was conducted shortly after World War II in response to atrocities that had occurred. It was designed to test the effects of authority figures on the behavior of average U.S. citizens. Milgram found that by introducing an authority figure (even as mild as someone in a white coat) the majority of individuals continued to "perform as directed" by delivering electric shocks to fellow subjects even when he believed the subject's life was at risk (and despite hearing someone screaming in response to the simulated shocks delivered). This dramatic demonstration of the power of authority indicates that persons in a perceived position of authority can work either for or against helping behavior, depending what the person who is perceived to have authority directs other individuals to do. In cases of incident command structures, this can contribute to a general chain of command pattern of behavior which enhances effective delivery of assistance. In cases in which authority is improperly taken by an individual or incorrectly assumed by another, it can work to the detriment of helping behavior.

It has also been noted that an individual must feel that it is appropriate for them to help before they will engage in this behavior. For example, individuals who are in charge in a situation are more likely to offer help or direct others to do so.[35] This highlights a very important aspect of helping behavior. One critical component of the likelihood to help is the presence of bystanders and their actions or verbalizations. If one bystander takes action or states that action should be taken, others are likely to do so. Similarly, it has been found in numerous studies that increasing numbers of bystanders decrease the likelihood of a helping intervention being made. Large numbers of bystanders not taking any action to provide assistance makes it increasingly unlikely that the individual in need will receive assistance. This is thought to be due to a number of factors. One is the negative modeling provided by the various bystanders to each other in which each sees the other not taking action. Another factor is that individuals may doubt the appropriateness of taking action given that no one else seems to be assessing the situation in the same way. Finally, responsibility for action-taking is thought to diminish in the setting of multiple bystanders as each hopes or thinks that another may take action ("diffusion of responsibility"). Research on this phenomenon burst to the forefront of social science after the infamous murder of Kitty Genovese in Queens, New York, in 1964. Thirty-eight individuals were documented to have witnessed the incident, which occurred over a lengthy period of time, yet no one intervened when she was attacked.

Individuals closest to the event have the best chance of being motivated to respond. Individuals who perceive themselves as belonging to the same group as the affected individual and who may be familiar with that person, are more likely to respond. In order to fully take advantage of these factors, the largest possible number of people must be trained within a community. This training optimizes the chances of someone close to the individual requiring help being familiar with that victim or at least perceiving the victim as part of their community group.

Training serves other purposes. A trained individual can serve as an authority figure for those around them until more technically qualified assistance is available, as well as providing a model of bystander intervention which others are likely to follow, either during that incident or in later events. Training increases the likelihood of an individual feeling that their intervention is appropriate. Those left "in charge" have been noted to be more likely to take helping actions. When helping behavior has been accomplished or attempted, every effort should be made to reward the behavior and publicize it so as to demonstrate the model of helping behavior to as many individuals as possible.

Finally, individuals can be instructed through public education efforts to remove some of the effects of diffusion of responsibility and bystander inaction. They can be taught to request help and direct a particular person to take action. This direction can "break the spell" that prevents otherwise well-intentioned individuals from providing assistance.

Individuals who are trained to respond and who see it as their duty to respond, such as physicians in a hospital or paramedics on a call, do render appropriate assistance. The challenge is to create this same tendency to respond among non-medical first responders and to expand the types of assistance first responders render by increasing the perception of what is appropriate helping behavior for them in a new variety of settings. The *EMS Agenda for the Future*, emphasized the same potential for enhanced community health and welfare through increased roles for first responders and EMS systems.

The Future

The roles first responders perform in the EMS system of the future have the potential to be dramatically varied in the years ahead. The *EMS Agenda for the Future* offers a vision of what first responders could do if the training, technology and infrastructure necessary were dedicated to EMS systems.[43] First responders could be recognized as an important component of the prehospital care provider network. They could include the lay public and those with a duty to respond, as well as the CFR, and other members of the EMS response team. Their training would be expanded to serve as a foundation for a career in prehospital care. Training standards would be universal, and additional testing for multiple state certifications would be unnecessary. College-level credit and an even more-recognized licensure would be bestowed upon first responders. Financial assistance for advanced training and continuing medical education coursework would be provided. First responders would have at their disposal newer and more accessible diagnostic and therapeutic modalities resulting from technological advances. In addition, the roles of first responders would be greatly expanded to more than just that of a healthcare provider. First responders would be community activists for accident and injury prevention. They would have the capability to provide follow-up care and general community health monitoring. They would possess the capability to assist in the development and implementation of policies concerning the delivery of prehospital emergency health care. Finally, EMS systems would receive adequate funding to maintain, train, and support the efforts of first responders.

The preceding is a summary of the vision presented in the *EMS Agenda for the Future*. Unfortunately, that vision of the first responder has not yet been realized; first responders are still limited in numbers. To effect improvement in the current level of functioning of EMS, there must be a critical mass of enthusiastic first responders trained and ready to respond, however, although volunteers serve more than 25% of the nation's population, the number of EMS volunteer organizations is decreasing.[44-46] EMS systems should expand the definition of those who may function as first responders, including the lay public. Fire and police department personnel have already demonstrated the effectiveness of serving as first responders during cardiac emergencies.[3,19,21,22] Despite these studies, the universal use of these workers as first responders during cardiac emergencies is lacking. Alonso-Serra surveyed 800 police organizations nationwide.[19] Of those surveyed, 80% already respond to one or more types of emergencies, 50% provide some level of patient care, and 60% state they should be involved and that their officers are willing to undertake extra medical training. Less than 5%, however, distribute AEDs to their officers. There is already existing formal support for the training of lay persons as first responders, especially in response to cardiac emergencies.[8,23,27,47-49] Despite this support, a nationally coordinated, multidisciplinary-supported effort to mobilize laypersons as first responders in cardiac emergencies has yet to be realized. Perhaps the residual effects of earlier articles in the literature concerning AED use by first responder providers are still to blame.[50-54]

Changes must also be made in how first responders are trained. The development of multiple curricula for prehospital care providers over the past 40 years has resulted in the proliferation of providers with similar titles, but with greatly divergent capabilities.[44] The *National EMS Education and Practice Blueprint* and the corresponding national standard curricula clearly define the four levels of prehospital care provider (CFR, EMT-basic, EMT-intermediate, EMT-paramedic) and their responsibilities. However, universal implementation of these guidelines is still lacking; a CFR in rural New York has not necessarily

received the same training nor has the same responsibilities as a CFR in urban Los Angeles. Improvements and standardization in training methods and curricula content would be better achieved if training were moved to university-affiliated training centers. Instructor quality could be improved, standardization of course content would be easier to regulate, and, successful course graduates could receive college credit. These changes have been suggested by many; however, the implementation of these changes is still moving slowly.

Finally, the services first responders provide must be expanded. First responders must do more than just respond to cardiac emergencies. First responders should be more active in the setting of traumatic emergencies and multiple casualty incidents. Many accounts of these events suggest that first responders are overlooked, underutilized, and insufficiently trained to assist in the care of patients when these events occur. Yet, the authors of these accounts also state that the majority of the medical problems seen at the scene of these events require only basic medical skills as part of their initial management.[31,33] First responders should be thought of as an integral component of any disaster plan, and those personnel who will serve as first responders as part of that plan should be adequately trained. First responders should be engaged in more preventative, as opposed to reactive, patient interventions. Garrison supported the inclusion of primary injury prevention as part of the services provided. EMS providers are a natural choice for involvement in primary injury prevention activities because "they are widely distributed among the population, reflect the composition of the community, and enjoy high credibility. EMS policy makers should prioritize their resources and align their economic incentives towards prevention."[55] Such participation by first responders and other prehospital care providers in injury prevention initiatives is sporadic and highly variable, and "EMS is not optimally engaged in providing education that improves community health through prevention, early identification of medical problems, and treatment."[44]

Summary

Despite the shortcomings discussed, the first responder, as a recognized prehospital care provider, has made much progress over the past 40 years. With astute planning, thought, and action on the part of EMS policy makers, curricula writers, and those who serve as first responders in the workplace and in the community, first responders will continue to evolve and provide the highest level of service.

References

1. *National Standard Curriculum: First Responder.* Washington, DC: National Highway Traffic Safety Administration; 1995

2. American Heart Association Medical/Scientific Statement: Improving survival from sudden cardiac arrest: the "chain of survival" concept. *Circulation.* 1991;83:1832–1847.

3. Weaver WD, et al. Use of the automatic external defibrillator in the management of out-of-hospital cardiac arrest. *N Engl J Med.* 1988;319(11):661–666.

4. Cobbe SM, et al. "Heartstart Scotland"—initial experience of a national scheme for out of hospital defibrillation. *BMJ.* 1991;302:1517–1520.

5. Cummins RO, et al. Automated external defibrillators used by emergency medical technicians: a controlled clinical trial. *JAMA.* 1987;257:1605–1610.

6. Callaham M, et al. Relationship of timeliness of paramedic advanced life support intervention and outcome in out-of-hospital cardiac arrest treated by first responders with defibrillators. *Ann Emerg Med.* 1996;27:638–648.

7. Hoekstra JW, et al. Effect of first-responder automated defibrillation on time to therapeutic interventions during out-of-hospital cardiac arrest: the Multicenter High Dose Epinephrine Study Group. *Ann Emerg Med.* 1993;22(8):1247–1253.

8. Moore JE, et al. Layperson use of automatic external defibrillation. *Ann Emerg Med.* 1987;16(6):669–672.

9. Sedgwick ML, et al. Efficacy of out-of-hospital defibrillation by ambulance technicians using automated external defibrillators: the Heartstart Scotland Project. *Resuscitation.* 1992;24:73–87.

10. Truong JH, Rosen P. Current concepts in electrical defibrillation. *J Emerg Med.* 1997;15(3):331–338.

11. *National Emergency Medical Services Education and Practice Blueprint.* Columbus: National Registry of Emergency Medical Technicians; 1993.

12. Cummins RO. Emergency medical services and sudden cardiac arrest: the "chain of survival" concept. *Ann Rev Public Health.* 1993;14:313–333.

13. Eisenberg MS, et al. Cardiac arrest and resuscitation: a tale of 29 cities. *Ann Emerg Med.* 1990;19(2):179–186.

14. Nichol G, et al. Effectiveness of emergency medical services for victims of out-of-hospital cardiac arrest. *Ann Emerg Med.* 1996;27:700–710.

15. Vukov LF, et al. New perspectives on rural EMT defibrillation. *Ann Emerg Med.* 1988;17(4):318–321.

16. Killien SY, et al. Out-of-hospital cardiac arrest in a rural area: a 16-year experience with lessons learned and national comparisons. *Ann Emerg Med.* 1996;28:294–300.

17. Nichol G, et al. Cost-effectiveness analysis of potential improvements to emergency medical services for victims of out-of-hospital cardiac arrest. *Ann Emerg Med.* 1996;27:711–720.

18. Ornato JP, et al. Cost-effectiveness of defibrillation by emergency medical technicians. *Am J Emerg Med.* 1988;6(2):108–112.

19. Alonso-Serra HM, et al. Law enforcement agencies and out-of-hospital emergency care. *Ann Emerg Med.* 1997;29:497–503.

20. Kellerman AL, Hackman BB, et al. Impact of first-responder defibrillation in an urban emergency medical services system. *JAMA.* 1993;270:1708–1713.

21. White RD, Asplin BR, et al. High discharge survival rate after out-of-hospital ventricular fibrillation with rapid defibrillation by police and paramedics. *Ann Emerg Med.* 1996;28:480–485.

22. Mosesso VN, Davis EA, et al. Use of automated external defibrillators by police officers for treatment of out-of-hospital cardiac arrest. *Ann Emerg Med.* 1998;32:200–207.

23. Moore JE, et al. Home placement of automatic external defibrillators among survivors of ventricular fibrillation. *Ann Emerg Med.* 1986;15(7):811–812.

24. Chadda KD, et al. Successful defibrillation in the industrial, recreational, and corporate settings by laypersons (abstract). *Circulation.* 1987;76(suppl IV):IV–12.

25. Cummins RO, et al. Frequency and types of medical emergencies among commercial air travelers. *JAMA.* 1989;261:1295–1299.

26. Cummins RO, et al. In-flight deaths during commercial air travel: how big is the problem? *JAMA.* 1988;259:1983–1988.

27. American College of Emergency Physicians: Early defibrillation programs. *Ann Emerg Med.* 1999;33:371.

28. Cummins RO. From concept to standard-of-care? Review of the clinical experience with automated external defibrillators. *Ann Emerg Med.* 1989;18:1269–1275.

29. Eisenberg MS. Defibrillation and public expectation. *Acad Emerg Med.* 1997;4:535–536.

30. Eisenberg MS. The shocking state of external defibrillation. *Acad Emerg Med.* 1995;2:761–762.

31. Hogan DE, Waeckerle JF, et al. Emergency department impact of the Oklahoma City terrorist bombing. *Ann Emerg Med.* 1999;34:160–167.

32. Keim M, Kaufmann AF. Principles of emergency response to bioterrorism. *Ann Emerg Med.* 1999;34:177–182.

33. Rivkind A, Barach P, et al. Emergency preparedness and response in Israel during the Gulf War. *Ann Emerg Med.* 1998;32:224–233.

34. Sharp TW, Brennan RJ, et al. Medical preparedness for a terrorist incident involving chemical or biological agents during the 1996 Atlanta Olympic Games. *Ann Emerg Med.* 1998;32:214–223.

35. Horowitz IA. Effect of choice and locus of dependence on helping behavior. *Journal of Personality & Social Psychology.* 1968;8:373–376.

36. Rushton JP, Teachman G. The effects of positive reinforcement, attributions, and punishment on model induced altruism in children. *Personality & Social Psychology Bulletin.* 1978;4:322–325.

37. Rushton P. Altruism & society: a social learning perspective. *Ethics.* 1982;92(3):425–446.

38. Yakimovich D, Saltz E. Helping behavior: the cry for help. *Psych Sci.* 1971;23:427–428.
39. Clark RD III, Word LE. Why don't bystanders help? because of ambiguity. *Journal of Personality & Social Psychology.* 1972;24:392–400.
40. Korte C, Ypma I, Toppen A. Helpfulness in Dutch society as a function of urbanization and environmental input level. *Journal of Personality & Social Psychology.* 1975;32:996–1003.
41. Solomon LZ, Solomon H, Store R. Helping as a function of number of bystanders and ambiguity of emergency. *Pers Soc Psychol Bull.* 1978;4:318–321.
42. Milgram S. *Obedience to authority.* New York: Harper; 1974.
43. *EMS Agenda for the Future.* National Highway Traffic Safety Administration. 1996.
44. Delbridge TR, Bailey B, et al. EMS agenda for the future: where we are . . . where we want to be. *Ann Emerg Med.* 1998;21:251–263.
45. Fitch JJ. Volunteers. In Kuehl AE, ed. *Prehospital Systems and Medical Oversight.* 2nd ed. St. Louis: Mosby-Year Book: 1994;339–344.
46. McNally VP. A history of the volunteers. *Fire House.* 1986;11:49–53.
47. Bachman JW. The good neighbor rescue program: utilizing volunteers to perform cardiopulmonary resuscitation in a rural community. *J Fam Pract.* 1983;16:561–566.

48. Cummins RO, et al. Training laypersons to use automatic external defibrillators: success of initial training and one-year retention of skills. *Am J Emerg Med.* 1989;7:143–149.
49. Haynes KA. Red Cross plans lifesaving courses on using defibrillators. *Los Angeles Times.* March 26, 1999.
50. Food and Drug Administration Defibrillator Working Group. Defibrillator failures: causes of problems and recommendations for improvement. *JAMA.* 1990;264:1019–1025.
51. Ornato JP, et al. Inappropriate electrical countershocks by an automated external defibrillator. *Ann Emerg Med.* 1992;21(10):1278–1282.
52. Ornato JP, et al. Limitation on effectiveness of rapid defibrillation by emergency medical technicians in a rural setting. *Ann Emerg Med.* 1984;13:1096–1099.
53. Richless LK, et al. Early defibrillation program: problems encountered in a rural/suburban EMS system. *J Emerg Med.* 1993;11:127–134.
54. Sweeney TA, Runge JW, et al. EMT defibrillation does not increase survival from sudden cardiac death in a two-tiered urban-suburban EMS system. *Ann Emerg Med.* 1998;31:234–240.
55. Garrison HG, Foltin GL, et al. The role of emergency medical services in primary injury prevention. *Ann Emerg Med.* 1997;30:84–91.

Bibliography

Hunt RC, et al. Influence of emergency medical services and prehospital defibrillation on survival of sudden cardiac death victims. *Am J Emerg Med.* 1989;7:68–82.

Krebs DL, Miller DT. Altruism and aggression. In: Lindzey G, Aronson E, ed.: *Handbook of Social Psychology.* New York: Random House; 1985.

Ornato JP, et al. Impact of improved emergency medical services and emergency trauma care on the reduction in mortality from trauma. *J Trauma.* 1985;25(7):575–579.

Sedgwick ML, et al. Performance of an established system of first responder out-of-hospital defibrillation: the results of the second year of the Heartstart Scotland Project in the "Utstein Style." *Resuscitation.* 1993;26:75–88.

Stratton S, Niemann JT. Effects of adding links to the "chain of survival" for prehospital cardiac arrest: a contrast in outcomes in 1975 and 1995 at a single institution. *Ann Emerg Med.* 1998;31:471–477.

Resuscitation Issues

Paul E. Pepe, MD, MPH

Introduction

Most resuscitation efforts are initiated at a moment's notice, usually unexpectedly, and most often, in the out-of-hospital setting, with little knowledge of the patient.[1] The very nature of the typical resuscitative situation seldom lends itself to a calm, rational, or informed decision-making process. Recognizing that any delay in resuscitation uniformly increases the chance of developing irreversible damage to the brain and other key organs, most patients are resuscitated without discrimination—but not always without question.[2–7]

With the discovery that most out-of-hospital cardiac arrests are due to sudden ventricular fibrillation (VF) and that with immediate defibrillatory countershock these cases are highly reversible, out-of–hospital rescuers have now devoted themselves to rapid response and aggressive resuscitative efforts.[8–11] Unfortunately, VF is not a static process, and the possibility of successful resuscitation declines with each minute that passes, even when bystanders immediately perform cardiopulmonary resuscitation (CPR).[8–10,12–14] With the clear recognition that the chance of full recovery deteriorates temporally, the provision of rapid response has become a paramount focus of such rescuers, and even the lay public at large.[1,8,15] In fact, today a rapid response from emergency medical services (EMS) crews has become a *de facto* societal imperative.[16]

Moreover, this rapid response imperative extends across all populations of cardiac arrests patients, even though many patients have had an unwitnessed arrest and are discovered after lengthy periods of extended ischemia.[16–21] Although such cases usually are beyond reversibility using currently available techniques, rare and unexpected survivors from these circumstances have encouraged the philosophy to provide urgent and universal resuscitative efforts for all persons found apneic and pulseless.[16,20,21] Today, with the exception of persons found to have *rigor mortis*, dependent lividity, or *advanced* directives, the accepted standard is to provide a trial of interventions.[10,16]

Therefore, the true difficulties are the psychological, ethical, and philosophical concerns that come with the societal and medical obligation to act in situations in which all efforts appear to be (and are most likely will be) futile.[17] EMS practitioners routinely initiate and conduct certain resuscitations with reluctance. Their emotions tell them that resuscitation of an asystolic jaundiced 90-year-old man reported to have metastatic cancer is a fruitless endeavor. Furthermore, it can be rationalized that allowing that person to die from a sudden cardiac arrest is more humane than attempting to prolong a life that may only be a painful, bedridden existence. Beyond this consideration is the philosophical notion that any intervention at all interferes with a natural process, and that the waiving of resuscitative efforts is not an active act of negligence but rather a realistic acceptance of the human condition. In essence, this line of thinking would constitute a general recognition of "the right to die with dignity."

On the other hand, there are arguments that any attempts to discriminate between those who should and should not be aggressively resuscitated is the first step on the road to genocide.[17] Who should decide, how old is "too old to resuscitate?" How long is "too long to resuscitate?" Where does one draw the line? In this line of thinking, failure to attempt resuscitation defies the Hippocratic Oath because it neglects an individual's "ultimate right"—the right to live.

Even when accepting the concept that universal attempts at resuscitation must be performed, the decision to terminate resuscitation efforts is also difficult and often wrought with emotion and controversy.[22–24] To give up on a young child or a relatively young man in front of his wife and children is a scenario that can evoke strong emotions and guilt feelings among family and rescuers. How does one help the family bridge the chasm of loss, and the rescuer get beyond the sense of inadequacy, when a bitterly tearful ten-year-old boy stares at a lifeless father and says, "Wake up, daddy, please wake up!"? How can "futility" be explained to this child?

No matter what rationalizations and arguments are used, be they internalized or openly expressed, heartfelt or rhetorical, they are not always clear-cut. Decisions concerning who should be resuscitated and for how long, involve issues ranging from religious, moral, ethical, legal, humanistic, and medical to considerations of patient rights, the effects on family, and even the availability of medical and financial resources.[16]

Also, beyond these issues is the consideration that the worst place for self-fulfilling prophecy is in the arena of resuscitation medicine. In the past, decisions to initiate resuscitative efforts, often have been based on probabilities of success.[2,25–27] Today, there is objective data based on current techniques;[5,16,28–32] however, in the future, with the development of improved resuscitative techniques, the standards may need to be modified.[16,33] The ultimate decisions must be based on sound medical data and the interpersonal skills of experienced practitioners.

As an example, a decision to discontinue resuscitation efforts at the scene of a cardiac arrest and pronounce a patient as "dead" is first based on medical knowledge of established outcome statistics, and then on principles of compassion in the interaction with the family and other bystanders. Take the case of a patient who has presented to paramedics with asystole and who is flaccid and without neurologic response. Bystanders report that they found him "not breathing" and called for help. In addition, there was a known response interval for the medical rescuers of 10 minutes, and no basic CPR was performed during that period. This was followed by a failure to develop any electrical complex on the electrocardiogram (EKG), or any other clinical response, after the provision of CPR, endotracheal intubation, proper ventilatory techniques with 100% oxygen, "three rounds" of standard intravenous (IV) drug therapy, and even an attempt at transcutaneous pacing.

In such a scenario, most providers would feel comfortable with stopping subsequent efforts, since there is now an enormous collective experience that provides us with a well-established general knowledge base that under these circumstances no one has been known to survive.[12,16] But clearly, the next step is more difficult. Whenever EMS personnel first arrive at the scene and the family's body language and tone

appear already to be accepting the occurrence of death by stating calmly "I think he's dead," there is less anxiety about decisions to terminate resuscitation efforts. However, whenever they arrive and there is a young mother at the doorway, grasping a child, pointing in a state of terror to the bedroom screaming, "Oh please, please . . . he's in there!!" then our compassion and "care-giving" come to the forefront. Decisions to pronounce the patient as dead must be tendered with what is now the best "care" for the surviving family. The cardiac arrest victim may be beyond our help, but these loved ones are now our patients. They are now in the greatest of pain and they need us to "care" for them as well. This is where our compassion and interpersonal skills must come to the forefront.

This chapter examines the various arguments for and against universal resuscitation attempts, and also examines the validity and caveats of the medical and scientific data influencing these positions. Also, since most lifeless patients will at least receive an initial resuscitation attempt at resuscitative efforts, it will also examine more closely the decisions to discontinue such efforts. The following discussion will also closely examine certain caveats and special circumstances surrounding resuscitations, and also offer some technical advice on how to handle termination of resuscitations in the out-of-hospital setting.

Even after consensual discussions with family, the accountable provider will effectively be the human being responsible to waive resuscitation attempts or, once initiated, to discontinue any further resuscitation efforts. Such decisions, as complex as they are, should be based on a sound understanding of the concepts and data supporting them. The chapter will attempt to describe to the latest information and rationales influencing these decisions, and address some of the medical, ethical, legal, and social aspects.[34] It must be recognized, however, that as new data and new medical advances become available, these comments may become outdated. Still, the basic concepts of humane caring and the key principles of compassionate oversight of medical resuscitations, as interwoven throughout this discussion, will persist.

Initial Resuscitation Decisions

There are three major decision issues that providers must face in resuscitations:

1. Should resuscitation attempts be *initiated*?

2. If initiated, *when* should resuscitation attempts be terminated?
3. If they are to be terminated, *where* should the resuscitation efforts be ended?

The first part of the following discussion will discuss the rationales for and against universal resuscitation attempts. Subsequent sections will then deal with considerations regarding the termination of initiated efforts.

Against Universal Resuscitation Attempts

There are four traditional concerns with unconditional resuscitation attempts:

1. Some patients have an obvious irreversible condition, the treatment for which is beyond the current capabilities of any available medical resources. These are generally obvious and well accepted reasons for not initiating resuscitation efforts;

2. The patient involved expressly did not wish to have any "heroic measures" implemented because he had a documented, terminal, irreversible process and even documented this wish in a written, legal advanced directive.[35–39] This has been accepted by most state legislatures and constitutes acceptable practice;

3. The brain is permanently damaged sooner than the cardiovascular systems. Therefore, there is a risk of creating a population of neurologic cripples if the number of cardiovascular resuscitations regularly exceed the number of salvaged nervous systems. Also, resuscitations without neurological recovery create unnecessary healthcare expenditures, even if the patient is pronounced "brain dead" several days after the event.[4,25,40]

4. It is unrealistic, extraordinarily expensive, and even potentially dangerous for the rescuers, "innocent" uninvolved bystanders, or others in traffic, to have EMS respond to and treat all victims of cardiopulmonary arrest, particularly since the situation will often be irreversible without certain unique conditions being present. For example, it is unlikely that anyone will survive.[2,27,29] One could argue that it would be unnecessary to race the rescue vehicle on a dark, rain-slicked highway to a probable futile situation.

The first and second are good rationales for waiving resuscitation efforts. Today, by most standards, conditions such as decapitation, incineration, *rigor mortis*, and dependent lividity are accepted as *absolute conditions of irreversibility*. Likewise, the possession of legally binding advanced directives and "do not attempt resuscitation" (DNAR) orders are routinely accepted, as reasons not to attempt resuscitations. Nevertheless, in both of these cases, there are still certain caveats that must be considered.

The final and fourth may be considered rationalizations more than rationale. The risk of restoring life, but with permanent neurological injury, is emotionally compelling. However, there are certain reasons that argue against this concern. The most controversial consideration for not attempting resuscitations rests with the fourth concern stated above. The concept that an extremely low probability of success suggests not attempting out-of-hospital resuscitation is debatable. The key issue lies is the concept of irreversibility; therefore, it is worthwhile to consider the concept of what constitutes death and irreversibility.

Defining Death

Although religious definitions vary, most scientists would define death as a progressive and ongoing process that involves a continuum of events usually beginning with oxygen deprivation to certain critical tissues, followed by a cascade of ischemic events and by depletion of adenosine triphosphate (ATP) in certain organs, manifested by clinical signs such as *rigor mortis*, and, finally, the decay process. In other words, a finite point in time at which death is present is an oversimplified view.

Since no one has yet to demonstrate a device that provides the capability of seeing a "soul" leaving the body, providers are left with somehow identifying that point in time beyond which certain key elements of this process are irreversible. In the following discussion, various anatomic, temporal, and physiological concepts are reviewed to see if irreversibility can be determined reliably.

Anatomic Considerations

Notwithstanding the perfunctory caveats about hypothermia and perhaps certain drug overdoses, it is generally accepted that a person with non-traumatic circulatory arrest is in an *absolutely* irreversible condition when found to be cold, stiff with *rigor mortis*, and/or marked with dependent lividity. The same acceptance of irreversibility applies to those persons with complete incineration or decomposition. Traumatic conditions such as transected torsos, decapitation, anatomical decerebration, and massive, explosive penetration across the midline of the brain are currently considered to be beyond salvage.

However, in many situations, there are no clear-cut clinical signs that tell the would-be rescuer if that critical point of a "biological death" has occurred. Inexperienced rescuers may also mistake certain discolorations for lividity, and lividity may be unidentifiable in dark-skinned persons. Thus there are caveats to consider when using such signs for "irreversibility."

Certain types of injuries to the heart or great vessels, not easily apparent from external inspection, are often beyond repair. Nevertheless, as technology and medical discoveries evolve, these injuries, that we often called "lethal" injuries, may eventually be treatable. Therefore, with the clear signs stated above, anatomical indicators are not always easy to recognize, and they may be a moving target in terms of future therapies.

Certain traditional descriptions of death signs also may be inaccurate. Pupils may fixate in dilation within 90 seconds of anoxia or because of some ophthalmological or pharmacological reason. Therefore, a lack of initial pupillary response is not a definitive indicator of potential outcome. In addition, individual patients have different responses and tolerances to those processes which cause irreversible states.

Age of the Patient

In many hospital situations, resuscitation attempts for the elderly often are limited.[40] However, in the out-of-hospital setting, age does not appear to be a criterion for resuscitation efforts.[5,6,28,41,42] Results from multiple studies in the United States and Belgium support the recommendation for aggressive efforts for the elderly in the out-of-hospital setting, particularly those with ventricular dysrhythmia.[5,6,28,41,42] In a prospective study that examined survival by age group in out-of-hospital cardiac arrests, 15% of patients aged 70 or older presenting with ventricular fibrillation or ventricular tachycardia survived to hospital discharge, and almost all were neurologically intact.[28] Other studies, however, have shown no survival potential for patients older than age 90.[16,41,42] Therefore, although survival may be lower for the elderly because of co-morbidities, the evidence indicates that resuscitation efforts are still worthwhile, at least for those younger than age 90.[16]

One other consideration is to recognize that these studies concerning age actually dealt with non-traumatic arrest. In trauma-associated cardiac arrest, specific data regarding age are lacking. It is generally well accepted that the older the patient is, the worse the outcome will be; co-morbidity is the main factor and the older the patient, the more likely the co-morbidity. Nevertheless, chronological age is still not an absolute predictor of outcome. The current criteria for waiving resuscitation, as discussed below, are also determined more by factors other than age in trauma patients.[16]

Elapsed Interval of Arrest

While age and previous state of health both correlate with outcome, they are only modest correlations in comparison to the elapsed time interval between arrest and the initiation of advanced life support. This concept has been particularly well studied in non-traumatic arrest.[8–10,12–14] For example, survival rates from sudden ventricular fibrillation (VF) fall about 10% per minute, but this figure combines two populations of arrest victims, those who receive immediate CPR by witnesses and those who do not receive immediate bystander CPR.[10,13] Survival chances may exceed 40% even at 12 minutes after the onset of the arrest when the collapse is witnessed and bystanders perform CPR.[9] The 12 minutes typically includes about 2 to 3 minutes for recognition, the call for help and time for dispatch, 8 minutes to respond to the location, and 1 to 2 minutes to reach the patient's side and shock. In contrast, without bystander CPR, survival chances may be less than 5% within five minutes after the collapse.[8,9] These probabilities of survival reflect the individual quality of bystander CPR, and other factors.

While accepting that in general, the elapsed response interval, usually measured as the time of the first telephone ring at the public safety answering point (PSAP) until arrival at the street location, has been shown to be one of the strongest predictors of survival rates following cardiac arrest, the reported time intervals: "collapse to call" and "scene arrival to intervention," are neither always accurate, nor are they totally reliable indicators of outcome in individual cases.[8,14]

Permanent, significant brain injury can occur within 3 minutes after sudden complete cessation of either breathing or heartbeat, but some patients can tolerate twice that time. It is possible that new technologies may change this paradigm.[43,44] And what about those who do not have sudden and complete cessation of cardiopulmonary function? Some patients have ill-defined intervals of arrest, such as those who started out with a gradual depression of cardiovascular function. They may have permanent or severe damage of critical organs even before complete clinical cessation of cardiopulmonary function.

Reports of elapsed time from both witnesses and rescuers following a sudden arrest are inaccurate pieces of information. Minutes may have "seemed like hours" to those distraught relatives in the home who are anxiously awaiting help. Likewise, rescuers' perception of elapsed time usually underestimate the actual time. Meanwhile, even when response times are documented by rescuers to be quite long (a dispatch-to-patient-contact interval of greater than 10 minutes), patients occasionally are resuscitated successfully and even achieve long-term survival, particularly with early bystander CPR. Furthermore, although witnesses report that the patient suddenly went unconscious right at the time of the initial call for her help, on closer questioning, it may be revealed that the patient "was still breathing a little" just up to the time of arrival of the rescuers. This might represent agonal breaths, but it might also represent some limited spontaneous circulation that may have been present, as occurs in some cases of ventricular tachycardias. In summary, estimated arrest intervals are a very general predictor of outcomes.

It is also important to recognize that time elements are even less precise and less predictable in non-VF cases. Patients may have a degree of hypoperfusion or hypoxia prior to signs of arrest; the hypoxia led to the arrest. Likewise, trauma patients usually do not arrest until some other severe circulatory insult (i.e., severe hemorrhage, pericardial tamponade, tension pneumothorax) precipitates the arrest.[16] Such patients may have even less capacity for salvage, but still the variability in the timing and degree of systemic insult make the time factor even more inaccurate.

Quantifying the Signal in Ventricular Fibrillation

The presenting EKG rhythm, though somewhat indicative, is not always accurate in predicting outcomes in non-traumatic arrest. While "coarse" VF may predict a better outcome than "fine" VF, neither is an absolute guarantee of the patient's eventual outcome.[45] In addition, technological (gain/display/lead), physiological (myocardial/biochemical status), and anatomical (body habitus/lung disease) variations may alter the EKG interpretation of heart activities.

Certainly those patients who receive defibrillation, but have no residual rhythm despite several minutes of good oxygenation, CPR, and adrenalin administration, have been without adequate coronary artery circulation for a significant period of time (figure 21.1). Occasionally, some patients respond well to initial therapeutic interventions, but their general hemodynamics eventually dwindle.[46]

Presumably, this might occur either because of a significant coronary artery occlusion that may have precipitated the event or because of a state of refractory peripheral vascular "paralysis" due to the ischemic sequelae to the vascular smooth muscle. On the other hand, a few patients who have a poor initial response may still do well after persistent efforts.

These exceptional cases, however, *are* the exception to the rule. While not absolute, the response to initial therapy is one of the more reliable indications of the prognosis, in the patient with VF.[47] Although an initial presenting rhythm of coarse VF is more apt than fine VF to be converted to an organized rhythm associated with spontaneous circulation, this observation is much less reliable than the actual response to initial therapeutic interventions.[12,48–50]

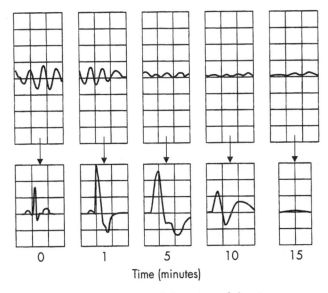

FIGURE 21.1. *An illustrated depiction of the time course of the ventricular fibrillation waveform* (top) *demonstrating a deterioration of coarse to fine fibrillation. The lower panel shows samples of the typical conversion rhythms one might expect as time elapses.*

Recently, the use of various technological measurements of the EKG signal in cases of VF may provide improved predictions of both response to initial therapy and outcome.[46,50-53] The use of quantitative analyses such as median frequency and scaling exponents have been demonstrated to correlate well with the initial response to therapy and even outcome.[46,50-53] Above certain median frequencies or below certain scaling exponent levels, VF is expected to immediately respond to defibrillatory countershocks. Below certain levels of median frequency or above certain scaling exponent levels, the patient will not convert successfully into a rhythm with associated pulse and blood pressure. Under such circumstances, certain other therapies should be attempted prior to countershocks, and these therapies may improve the receptivity to defibrillation attempts.[46,50-56] In fact, increased receptivity may be indicated by improvements in the EKG signal (i.e., coarser VF, higher median frequency, lower scaling exponents). Conversely, lack of improvements in the EKG signal may indicate persistent unresponsiveness and futility.

While these concepts in power spectrum analysis of VF are promising, absolute predictors of outcome have not been determined. With the advent of new technological advances, there may be patients who respond at higher scaling exponents or lower median frequencies than previously predicted with countershocks. For example, new countershock waveforms (biphasic, recti-linear) may be capable of successfully converting hearts in a more ischemic condition. Also, other new therapies (e.g., active compression-decompression devices or minimally-invasive direct cardiac massage) may shift the EKG signal to a more positive level through better coronary artery blood flow than is currently available.[43,44] This concept has not yet been addressed in terms of the other (non-VF) rhythms (figure 21.2).

Other Than Ventricular Fibrillation

Prospects for surviving are much worse for patients presenting with asystole or pulseless electrical activity (PEA).[2,16,20,21,57] However, while pulseless patients who present with agonal complexes, idioventricular rhythms, or even normal-looking EKG complexes have a much bleaker chance of surviving than those presenting with coarse VF, some still do survive neurologically intact.[16,20,21] Some clinicians have advocated that a presentation of less than 20 per minute

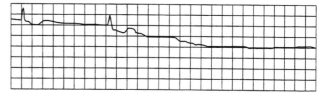

FIGURE 21.2. *The typical electrocardiograph tracing seen in the "dwindling heart" scenario as it deteriorates from pulseless idioventricular to asystole.*

with asystole or with agonal complexes is generally irreversible, and that resuscitation attempts should be waived in such cases. [2,58,59] However, current data show that the use of those EKG presentations is not an absolute criterion despite an initial picture of apparent cardiac standstill.[16,21,60]

The conclusions that resuscitation efforts should be attempted in all non-traumatic arrest patients has also withstood several other challenges. For example, the potential for better defining objective criteria for waiver of resuscitation by using EKG findings, combined with clinical circumstances, was initially investigated in a 1994 study involving two comprehensive cardiac arrest registries.[60] Investigators prospectively followed out-of-hospital cardiac arrests for two years in Seattle and Houston. They specifically analyzed the chance of survival when the following three parameters were present: (1) the initial on-scene EKG demonstrated asystole; (2) the initial event was unwitnessed; and (3) bystander CPR was not performed. Of 1,143 consecutive adults presenting with unmonitored asystole, 1.7% survived. However, 279 were unwitnessed and received no bystander CPR; *none* of these 279 patients survived, despite aggressive efforts.[8,9,20] These results strongly supported the recommendation for waiver of resuscitation efforts when the three combined criteria were present, although the authors argued that, based on the small numbers, further investigation was indicated. In fact, that additional investigation was accomplished several years later in a Milwaukee-based study.[21] In that retrospective study of 3,767 out-of-hospital asystole cases occurring over a 15-year period, 15 asystole survivors were found (and most of them neurologically intact) even when the initial event was unwitnessed and no bystander CPR had been performed. While the frequency of survival is extremely low for these patients, these results support the current recommendation to provide some period of attempted resuscitation to confirm that such efforts are futile.

The Medical Resolution

In all of these discussions of anatomical signs, elapsed intervals, presenting EKG, or waveform analyses, the word "probability" continually creeps in, and the word "absolute" is hard to find. Conceptually, with the certain exceptions stated previously aggressive initiation of resuscitation should be undertaken for most cardiac arrest cases to *test* irreversibility. This philosophy is shared by most medical and legal organizations.[61] The *Uniform Determination of Death Act*, which has been adopted by some states and which is endorsed by the American Bar Association and the American Medical Association, states that:

> An Individual who has sustained either: (1) irreversible cessation of circulatory and respiratory functions; or, (2) irreversible cessation of all functions of the entire brain, including the brain stem, is dead. A determination of death must be made in accordance with accepted medical standards.

This implies that resuscitative efforts should begin in almost all cases where there has been no advance directive. Without testing the responsiveness of the circulatory system through attempts at resuscitation, one cannot determine the true irreversibility of circulatory and respiratory function.[17] Likewise, one cannot state whether brain function is irreversible. Therefore, no matter where the resuscitation is conducted and no matter who is conducting it, it is critical that the trial of resuscitative measures is carefully detailed and chronologically recorded to validate the hopelessness of the case. By documenting the failure to respond to resuscitative efforts, the criterion of irreversibility of the cessation of circulatory and respiratory function can be established. This will help to end any speculation as to the recoverability of the brain. Simply stated, without re-establishing circulation, the brain will not survive.

Sociological Confounders

WAIVING RESUSCITATION BECAUSE OF HEARSAY

All of the previous considerations argue in favor of the current standard that, in the absence of *rigor mortis*, lividity, or decapitation, resuscitation efforts should be initiated in the prehospital setting.[16] The responders are compelled to initiate the resuscitation attempt despite protests from family, bystanders, or self-proclaimed authorities such as lawyers or even "doctors" on the phone. However, this becomes difficult when crews arrive and a family member says,

"Papa has cancer and this is his doctor on the phone and says not to do anything." Even with a living will or a durable powers of attorney in hand but without documented medical records, or without the unfamiliar physician on the phone being able to provide evidence that he is the patient's physician, the medical care provider still may be at medical-legal risk when waiving resuscitation.

Although recent expert medical consensus supports a more liberal attitude toward waiver of resuscitation efforts in reportedly terminal patients, the chance of making a "mistake" remains worrisome.[10] While a person with diagnosed acquired immunodeficiency syndrome (AIDS) or small-cell carcinoma of the lung may be dead within two years, it must be recognized that any given individual may return to a reasonable lifestyle for at least several months if resuscitated early in the course of the disease. Therefore, the statement that "the patient has lung cancer" should not be considered an absolute rationale, particularly when the condition is generically classified as "lung cancer" and reported as hearsay. In the absence of a documented DNAR status, the most reasonable rationale for stopping a resuscitation is the lack of response to initial resuscitative measures.

Living wills and advanced directives usually require physician interpretation and formulation into a treatment plan. They do not necessarily indicate "No CPR" by themselves. So for the most part, in the absence of decapitation, incineration, lividity, or *rigor mortis*, the prehospital providers take a degree of risk when waiving resuscitation without a bona fide physician directive. Ideally, the pronouncing physician should be known to the providers and a well defined, well clarified, well accepted prospective decision should have been reached. This may require initiation of resuscitation efforts until that physician directive can be obtained. Nevertheless, common sense and compassion should always take major roles in the decision process.

Better yet, if the family or legal guardians wished no resuscitation, they should not activate the EMS system. For example, in hospice programs, if it is the established and accepted will of the patient to die of his terminal illness, the caretakers or family should not call the EMS system to "pronounce" or evaluate patients. Nevertheless, distraught, uncomfortable families may call 9-1-1 for help or a medical examiner may contact the police, who inadvertently call EMS. Therefore, it would be better that such patients be registered with the medical examiner's office or other appropriate authorities and they be notified accordingly. To that end, programs have been established in several states so that persons with terminal disease can be registered with the EMS program as having a Do Not Resuscitate (DNR) disposition.[10] With official documents and identification mechanisms (photo identifications, wristbands) being part of the "system," such approaches can avoid difficult scenarios.

FAMILY PROTEST

Often EMS personnel are called but are told on arrival that "the family wants nothing done." It is common for personnel to be called to a residence where they find an elderly person in cardiopulmonary arrest. Despite family protests that the patient "has cancer" and should be left alone, the rescue personnel should usually initiate the resuscitation. Despite threats of legal action, the providers and their direct medical oversight physicians actually would be ill-advised to waive resuscitation without better documentation. Commonly, it is the stated wish of the family that no "heroic" or "extraordinary" measures be taken and that they do not want their loved one "kept alive" by artificial means. Often they are reflecting the patient's own statements from some previous occasion . . . or so they say.

While it is becoming more and more acceptable among lay persons to let their loved ones "die with dignity," it must be clear in the provider's mind that there is no hope of survival when "following the family's wishes." Unfortunately, selfish motivations can exist, especially when elderly sick patients create a financial and emotional burden for the family, or when inheritance is a concern. Therefore, without prior knowledge of circumstances and prospective decisions, the EMS personnel should generally provide aggressive resuscitation. On the other hand, they should also attempt to aggressively resolve the situation by acquiring pertinent confirmation of an irreversible condition if at all possible. Again, common sense and compassion are still two of the most important tools in such difficult circumstances.

NEUROLOGICALLY IMPAIRED PERSON

Resuscitation of a patient with severe neurological impairment is another difficult area, but is akin to the approach used in terminally ill patients with malignancies. Like the oncologist who can render a prognostic opinion concerning the type of malignancy with and without therapy, the neurologist or neurosurgeon may be able to provide similar documenta-

tion. But outcome is often more difficult to define with severe neurological impairment, and surprises are known to occur.

Even for previously healthy persons, the argument exists that there is a potential for creating a population of neurological cripples by overzealous resuscitation efforts. Perhaps two or three in a hundred of those patients who survive long-term may enter a limbo of severe neurological impairment following "successful" cardiac arrest resuscitation. Generally, patients either survive and eventually awaken neurologically intact, or they go on to have progressive neurological deterioration and even systemic deterioration with ensuing death. Collective experience suggests that the odds are overwhelmingly in surviving with a reasonably intact neurological state and not a state of vegetation. The major exceptions, perhaps, are the premature infant, the severe head-injured patient, or the cerebral vascular accident patient whose outlooks are much harder to predict at the time of initial resuscitation.

Summarizing the Concepts of Initial Resuscitation Decisions

Without a clear-cut DNAR status, resuscitation should probably be initiated in any victim of nontraumatic cardiopulmonary arrest who is not in a state of *rigor mortis* or who does not have dependent lividity, regardless of the presenting EKG. Even when it seems "hopeless," there are rare anecdotes that vindicate the philosophy of universal initiation of aggressive resuscitation efforts.

Beyond the medical futility issue is the usually unspoken issue that the more EMS providers perform their skills, the better they are able to handle the next case. Although it may appear a little irreverent, there is a social obligation to perform resuscitation skills as often as possible so that subsequent patients get better care. So even the elderly, asystolic patient with an unknown elapsed interval of arrest should receive aggressive resuscitative attempts, not only because of the occasional surprise survivor, but also because every resuscitation attempt improves the subsequent performance of practitioners in terms of both skills and experience. This philosophy can be viewed as one that is life saving in the long run. Rather than an invasion of an individual's right, it is more of a method to better guarantee the ultimate right of others to live—and occasionally that very individual's right to live.

Rationales for Stopping Resuscitation

Termination of Efforts

Since there are rare occasions when the initiation of resuscitations are waived, the real issues come after the resuscitation effort has begun. How far and how long to go? There are several arguments in favor of stopping a resuscitation effort. Documentation may become available that the patient has a terminal process with an imminent death. Another example would be a situation in which there is no response to initial therapy and the chances of hurting rescuers far outweigh the chances of patient survival.[10] This argument is often very reasonable, but it also deserves close scrutiny and understanding on the part of the accountable physician before it is accepted routinely.

Criteria for Termination

Recent data have provided fairly discrete criteria for terminating resuscitative efforts on-scene. Specifically, adult patients will not survive an out-of-hospital arrest if all of the following criteria are present: (1) unmonitored arrest (not associated with trauma, primary respiratory etiology, drug overdose or temperature aberration); (2) absence of spontaneous circulation within 25 minutes of the initiation of standard advanced cardiac life support (ACLS) techniques; (3) absence of persistently recurring/refractory VF; and (4) absence of any neurological signs.[12,16,62]

The corresponding time frame for monitored arrest is 30 minutes.[12] The only exceptions to these time frames are hypothermia and refractory or persistently recurring VF.[12,16] A 20–25-minute criterion also has been strongly supported in studies of end-tidal carbon dioxide ($ETCO_2$) measurements.[30,31] In patients with cardiac arrest, a persistent $ETCO_2$ level of 10 mm Hg or less, measured by digital capnography 20 minutes after the start of ACLS, uniformly predicts death and, in turn, can also be used as an objective determinant to halt CPR efforts.[30,31]

These criteria are applicable independently of the reported "downtime" or CPR interval. Although there are no guarantees for survival, those with persistently recurring VF or a transient return of pulses may occasionally survive despite more than 25 minutes of ACLS. Therefore, continued in-hospital efforts are appropriate. However, using today's standard approaches, there are no other apparent exceptions. If future therapeutic advances are to be tested,

these criteria should be modified. Resuscitation medicine is the last place for self-fulfilling prophecies. For example, recent preliminary experience with new devices such as the active-compression-decompression pump has demonstrated survivors with 30 minutes of pulselessness.[43]

On-Scene Pronouncements of Death

If efforts are to be terminated at the scene, it may be advisable for the patient to be pronounced dead by standing protocols or by the direct medical oversight.[10,16] This may obviate the dangers of racing through busy traffic with the unlikely-to-be-saved patient, a situation which may endanger the lives of both the rescuers and bystanders. In addition, it avoids the distraction of emergency department personnel and resources from other serious cases, and it circumvents emergency department expenses.[63]

While this practice seems logical, however, there are several caveats to be considered. First, the physician is not truly present to pronounce the patient as "dead" even though the intermediaries are legally considered "the eyes and ears of the physician." Second, many families are emotionally attached to the concept of taking the patient "to the hospital" as providing the ultimate in care. Alternatives to on-scene termination would then be hospital transport without lights and siren (cold) when further efforts appear futile, but this may also carry the perception of suboptimal effort. Local medical oversight, in conjunction with governmental authorities, should determine the best policy for each community.[16]

Initiating the Termination Process

On-scene pronouncements can be very acceptable as long as the responsible physician meticulously trains the personnel and has confidence in their abilities and judgment, both medically and interpersonally with families. As with other EMS medical care, the physician may delegate an act of medical practice to the EMS personnel, as long as the physician involved is willing to take responsibility for that decision.[34] It is therefore a good practice that pronouncements be confirmed after consultation with the direct medical oversight physician.[10] This practice also should be considered in EMS systems with EMT-A providers as well, particularly when lengthy transports are involved. Otherwise, state and local authorities should be encouraged to develop protocols for the initiation and discontinuation of CPR in areas where more advanced care is not available. Prospective training is a must. More importantly, the example of the physician role model who is compassionate and professional is a key element to the success of such a policy.[16]

A suggested approach to on-scene termination of efforts is for the responsible on-scene provider to establish early interpersonal contact and interaction with family members. This early contact can be made to convey information about the initial findings and actions, or to ask about past history and medications. Once it becomes apparent that resuscitation will be unlikely (i.e., no response to intubation and first round of drugs), it would be appropriate to begin the termination procedures by informing the family of the gravity of the situation in a strategic, compassionate manner. For example, by "apologizing" for being blunt, but wanting the family to be fully informed, the EMS personnel can establish better credibility and trust.

In this first approach about termination, common sense statements can help. One approach might include the following statement: "As you're probably already thinking, his heart has stopped and that is obviously very bad. Occasionally, with our treatments, we can revive some people. Unfortunately, everyone we revive would have responded by now. So we need to face the likely reality that he is beyond our ability to do anything for him."

Giving that first salvo some time to settle in, a follow-up would be: "But I'll tell you what—we will keep working on him for a while longer and check with our doctors for any other suggestions. Still, you need to know, we don't think he will make it."

This provides the rescuers a chance to gauge the family's reaction and to bridge them into the sudden reality that has just overtaken them. Medical oversight contact can be made at this time if there are no standing orders.

As this interaction probably takes place about ten minutes into the clinical interventions, the following ten minutes provides a reasonable interval for the initial conversations to settle in. At this point, the rescuers can resume the termination conversation with the family, stating that "We weren't able to get him back" and make an offer (if the protocol calls for it) to have them speak directly to the EMS doctor. Once the family understands the futility, actions to be taken (including non-transport, police, and medical examiner issues) should be explained. Then comes the question: "So, with your permission, we're going to stop." If the family is still concerned and wants more done, then transport may be warranted. They are now our primary patients and our treatment depends on their wishes. If on-scene termination is the consensus, then the grieving-assistance should begin.

Many services provide chaplaincies, social workers, or other grievance counselors. They may also provide EMS supervisors who can stand by, while releasing the providers back into service.

Special Circumstances
Post-Traumatic Circulatory Arrest

Although traditional criteria for initiation of CPR (i.e., lifeless appearance, pulselessness, and apnea or agonal breathing) may be present, the heart itself might still be viable but simply failing to create adequate circulation because of factors such as severe hypovolemia, cardiac tamponade, or tension pneumothorax.[16] Though true cardiac arrest usually ensues within minutes, there may still be opportunity for reversibility under certain circumstances. Such circumstances may be difficult to distinguish on initial clinical examination.

Based on the scientific literature, four primary questions must be answered before determining resuscitation pathways in post-traumatic circulatory arrest: (1) Is the injury primarily blunt or penetrating? (2) What is the initial EKG rhythm on-scene? (3) Is there an intact airway, preferably with endotracheal intubation? and (4) What is the duration of pulselessness?[16]

Blunt Trauma

For blunt trauma with a clearly associated lethal mechanism of injury, data indicate that there is no survival for adults and children with an absence of perceptible pulse and respiration at the scene and an EKG heart rate less than 40 per minute, regardless of endotracheal tube placement or duration of pulselessness. Therefore, medically speaking, any on-scene resuscitation could be waived or terminated under such circumstances.[16,64-66] However, caution should be taken to first ensure that the lack of respiration is not due to a simple obstructed airway, and that sudden VF as an associated event is not present.[16]

Exceptions might be considered, however, for the pediatric patient with obvious lethal injuries who has agonal breathing and no pulse. In these cases, initial life support efforts might be encouraged, if only for the potential of organ donation.[16,64] For example, consistent with the other studies of pediatric post-traumatic arrest, a study reported no functional survivors among 38 pediatric victims of blunt trauma who presented to the ED in a pulseless cardiac arrest or with severe hypotension.[30] Specifically, 11 of the 12 patients who were transferred to the pediatric intensive care unit eventually died, and the single survivor had profound neurologic impairment six years after hospitalization.[30] However, 6 of the 12 admitted patients were eligible organ donors, and this resulted in four multi-organ donors during the seven-year study.

Another potential exception to the termination criteria for the patient with blunt trauma, adult or child, is the circumstance in which there is a loss of perceptible pulse or respiration 2 to 3 minutes before arrival at a trauma facility, where expanded opportunity for salvage (i.e., immediate rescue thoracotomy) is almost immediately available.[67] Nevertheless, it is still recommended that on-scene apnea and pulselessness are still valid criteria for either waiving or terminating resuscitation efforts in patients with blunt injury who have a clearly associated (lethal) mechanism of injury, no ventricular fibrillation, and no airway obstruction.[16]

Penetrating Injuries

The outcomes of patients with penetrating trauma who are without pulse and respiration on-scene also are bleak. Although an initial transient pulse can be restored after thoracotomy in some cases, no long-term survival is seen in cases in which endotracheal intubation was not performed and pre-thoracotomy CPR efforts lasted more than 5 minutes.[16,68] Better outcomes have been reported with successful endotracheal intubation and thoracotomy within ten minutes.[67,68]

Despite the better potential for salvage in patients with penetrating injuries, once true cardiac arrest ensues, survival diminishes. Even when endotracheal intubation is accomplished and proper ventilatory strategies are used, survival will not occur once asystole has occurred. Patients with penetrating injuries who become asystolic on-scene or en route, or those who remain pulseless and apneic for 15 minutes despite endotracheal intubation, will not survive.[67,68] In cases of asystole or in cases with the longer transport periods, on-scene termination or termination during transport, are medically indicated. These are important considerations to make prior to activation of air medical rescue or before proceeding with rapid transport through traffic.

Ruling Out Other Mechanisms

Whatever policy is used, the presence of a potentially reversible underlying medical condition that led to the patient's fall or motor vehicle collision must be considered. For example, an occasional patient with ventricular tachycardia may be involved in an automobile crash and be found "dead" by EMS crews. It is possible that ventricular tachycardia was initially sustained with some minimal perfusion and then evolved into a VF just before the arrival of EMS personnel. Therefore, aggressive therapy for the medical condition is still warranted. Likewise, even an asystolic patient may be the victim of a sudden hypoxic event (seizure or choking) that is still potentially reversible. Placement of an endotracheal tube would help to clarify this issue; if severe injuries are apparent and airway/respiratory procedures do not improve the situation, the injury patient with asystole is a clear candidate for termination of efforts.

Regardless of the overall bleak results, however, patients with post-traumatic circulatory arrest who present with persisting electrical activity (EKG complexes) but no signs of life can pose difficult decisions for EMS personnel. Nevertheless, the clear conclusion is that blunt trauma victims who are pulseless and have asystole or bradycardiac electrical cardiac activity (heart rate <40 beats/min) can be pronounced dead.[16,65] It could be argued that those with audible heart beats or with heart rates >80 beats/min may be the exception and that, although chances for intact survival are negligible, considerations for initial attempts at resuscitation may be still given under those circumstances.[16,65]

Pediatric

In the case of children (aged 17 years or younger), the decisions of when to resuscitate, how long to continue, and when to terminate resuscitation are based on fewer data.[48] Nevertheless, the available data do indicate that, with the exception of post-traumatic arrest, EMS providers should attempt to resuscitate any patient who does not have clear signs of lividity or rigor. As with adult patients, there are no clear-cut prospective criteria for waiving resuscitation. In fact, in many cases that retrospectively involved lividity or *rigor mortis,* providers have attempted resuscitation.[48]

In terms of terminating efforts, the criterion of no pulse (absence of spontaneous circulation) within 20–25 minutes of resuscitation initiation (unless there is hypothermia or persistently recurring VF) also applies.[32] In a prospective study of 300 pediatric patients with cardiac arrest, none of the 267 children who did not achieve on-scene return of spontaneous circulation survived.[48]

However, termination of resuscitation or on-scene pronouncement for children has not been universally recommended, because of the psychosocial impact on the family and because of the psychological comfort of the EMS providers.[10,24] A blinded survey of EMS personnel regarding comfort levels with on-scene pronouncement was reported in 1997 using a rating scale of 1 (not comfortable) to 10 (very comfortable).[24] This study found that veteran paramedics (n=201) are very comfortable (average score, 10) with the pronouncement of an adult on-scene but not with pronouncement of a child (average score, 2). Therefore, with the greater availability of extensive in-hospital support services for the family of pediatric patients, and considering the EMS providers' potential concerns with on-scene pronouncement, termination of resuscitative efforts for children may be best performed in the hospital. Nevertheless, it has also been emphasized that once medical futility is determined, personnel should take care during transport not to create additional risks in traffic, and in-hospital personnel might adopt modified procedures that limit further resuscitation and resource utilization.

Pregnancy

If on-scene witnesses report that a pregnant woman lost respirations 10 minutes previously and that they had been doing CPR somewhat ineffectively *and* the witnesses appear reliable about their timing and CPR performance, it is unlikely that any intervention will be successful. While it is generally believed that there exists enough oxygen in the placental intervillous space to support *fetal* metabolism for eight minutes or more after sudden arrest in the mother, only five minutes of fetal distress will usually result in an Apgar score of 5. Under the best of circumstances, in a premature infant, the prognosis would be more dismal and, if the fetus is less than 32 to 33 weeks old, survival is less likely. In addition, in trauma cases, the circulatory compromise is progressive, indicating the probability of even more prolonged compromise. While one needs to try to obtain a history of when the baby is due, these data, while helpful, usually are not available nor completely reliable, and one must pragmatically approach the situation with a clinical guess at fetal age. A fundus that is round and the size of a large bowling ball is probably reflective of a 6-month-old fetus and survival is less likely, even in the hospital setting. On the other hand, a football-shaped fundus half way between the umbilicus and xlphoid process probably reflects a 32-week-old or older fetus and there is an outside chance of success in a witnessed arrest. If the mother decompensates in front of the EMS personnel, they should treat the mother as usual, which would most likely mean provision of airway and rapid transport to a definitive care-providing facility. If the time elements are still reasonable, delivery and resuscitation of the baby still may be appropriate.

Advanced Life Support Not Available

In certain rural communities or in wilderness conditions, advanced care providers may not be available. This situation raises a potential dilemma in terms of when to terminate resuscitative efforts. Most guidelines for terminating resuscitation were based on studies in which ALS procedures were used.[10,12,29–32,63] In fact, the established criteria for the appropriate timing of termination of efforts have been based on intervals of ALS procedures, irrespective of prior intervals of CPR or estimated periods of cardiac arrest duration.[12,29,32,62] In addition, some might argue that until ALS procedures are performed, the ability to resuscitate someone has not really been tested.

Nevertheless, current consensus is that when ALS is not going to be available for a half hour or more, it is likely that performing CPR for more than that period of time will be futile. The rationale here is that if a 20 to 25 minute trial of ALS without the return of pulses constitutes futility, then 20 to 25 minutes of CPR would not be any more advantageous. The American Heart Association has taken the position that a half hour trial of CPR or ALS is a reasonable interval following which to declare futility.[10]

The usual exceptions, of course, are persistent VF or hypothermia.[12] In the case of persistent VF, if an automated external defibrillator (AED) is available and shocks are still advised, then one might choose to prolong resuscitative efforts. If the AED does not indicate the need to shock, resuscitative efforts can be halted after a half hour or when the CPR provider becomes fatigued. Hypothermia is a difficult problem. Although unlikely, survival after prolonged cardiac arrest may be achieved in certain cases of clear hypothermia (e.g., submersion in extremely cold waters).[69] Under such circumstances, more prolonged CPR efforts can be considered. Logistics, rescuer fatigue, safety, and other factors must be considered and a personal judgment must be made, particularly if communication with direct medical oversight is not available.

Multiple Casualties

Triage decisions at the multiple casualty incident (MCI) are often difficult and probably only 80% accurate even when the most experienced medical personnel make the priority judgments. The standard approach is not to become preoccupied with pulseless patients if there are multiple patients with serious injuries. Of course, if there are 40 patients, 39 of whom are "walking wounded" and the other one is in a state of cardiopulmonary arrest, the resuscitation is quite appropriate. But in circumstances in which life-threatening but reparable injuries are present in several patients and available personnel resources are limited, waiving resuscitation for a pulseless, apneic patient is probably appropriate.

The best guideline is to do what will save most lives in the long term. For example, even if there are critically ill or injured patients, the "walking-wounded" or "normals" should be evacuated first if hazards still exist. They are more apt to survive long-term, unless they become injured by ongoing hazards. When hazards are not present, then the usual triage routine of "sickest first" applies. Among those whose state is immediately life-threatening, who should be the first resuscitated? Again, who is more apt to survive long-term? The severe head-injured patient (unconscious and barely responsive to anything but deep painful stimuli) who has a blood pressure of 85 mm Hg has a much poorer prognosis than the nearby "shocky appearing" patient with abdominal trauma, also with a blood pressure of 85 mm Hg but who is very lucid. Therefore the second patient should receive priority for evacuation, as the probability of long-term survival is greater despite a similar degree of hypotension.

The patient with a femur fracture, although it is a potentially life-threatening injury, is unlikely to die immediately, and evacuation/treatment can be delayed even though the patient has an even better chance of long-term survival than the abdominal trauma case. All things considered, both patients can be salvaged, especially if other assistance will be shortly available. Within the group of patients who are determined to be the most serious because of immediately life-threatening injuries, one should con-sider the resources available and then triage according to best chances of long-term survival.

Subtle Values of Resuscitation Efforts

Positive communications from families of cardiac arrest victims have not only come from the survivors, but more often from the families of those patients who died. Most of the time these families are grateful for their impressions that the EMS system and the receiving hospital (as applicable) did "everything possible" and that they were given the satisfaction that their loved one got "the best shot he could have had." In addition, they also mention the perspective that even the two or three days of transient "survival" gave the family members a better chance to adjust and come to terms with the loved one's demise.

In essence, the aggressive resuscitation efforts made the transition easier for them, and the hospital costs were not so much a major burden in their minds. Perhaps the insurance company actually relieves the burden, and this approach translates into higher medical costs for us all. For now, though, the sociological consensus appears to be that when there is any question or possibility of salvage, one should always provide initial aggressive care. In fact, asking families at the time of a failing resuscitation attempt whether or not they feel that the patient should receive further care is usually unfair and a difficult burden to place on them. This does not preclude informing them or discussing options, but in most cases, they will avoid having the overwhelming responsibility of "ending it all." Therefore, termination policies set in place by medical community consensus should be established to take this burden from the family. Again, termination policies should still be considered a tool, not a shackle, for direct medical oversight.

Summary

Universal attempts at resuscitation will probably continue to be questioned, particularly as medical resources become sparse. The great majority of patients who are victims of cardiac arrest will die, even under the most optimum circumstances. But the collective body of knowledge that we now have compels us to at least try an initial attempt at resuscitation in almost all cases in which there are no documented, prospective determinations of DNR status. The issue of when to stop these initial attempts has become less difficult to pinpoint. Recent data have provided better guidelines and criteria for termination of efforts. But such decisions usually depend on the ultimate decision of an accountable physician. It is that physician who must directly or through EMS personnel pronounce death and inform family and friends that their loved one is gone forever. The Golden Rule should apply. If it were a member of the physician's family, how would he decide? The decision is not one that should be mandated by some law or protocol, but rather by sound, informed medical judgment and, most importantly, a little wisdom.

"Wisdom" is most often defined as accumulated philosophic or scientific learning, meaning that research efforts and improved methods of identifying those who will or will not be salvaged must be continually sought. In addition, the search for better resuscitation techniques and technologies must continue, particularly those applied in the out-of-hospital setting. Furthermore, it means that this seeking must always be combined with humanity and compassion.

References

1. Eisenberg MS, Bergner L, Hallstrom AP. Cardiac resuscitation in the community—importance of rapid provision and implications for program planning. *JAMA*. 1979;241:1905–1907.

2. Kuisma M, Jaara K. Unwitnessed out-of-hospital cardiac arrest: is resuscitation worthwhile? *Ann Emerg Med*. 1997;30:69–75.

3. Charlson ME, et al. Resuscitation: how do we decide? *JAMA*. 1986;255:1316–1322.

4. Rosemurgy AS, Norris PA, Olson SM, Hurst JM, Albrink MH. Prehospital traumatic cardiac arrest: the cost of futility. *J Trauma*. 1993;35:468–473.

5. Longstreth WT. Does age affect outcomes of out-of-hospital cardiopulmonary resuscitation? *JAMA*. 1990;264:2109–2110.

6. Tresch DD, et al. Should the elderly be resuscitated following out-of-hospital cardiac arrest? *Am J Med*. 1989;86:145–150.

7. Iserson KV. Forgoing prehospital care: should ambulance staff *always* resuscitate? *J Med Ethics*. 1991;17:19–24.

8. Cummins RO, Ornato J, Thies WH, et al. State-of-the-art review—Improving survival from sudden cardiac arrest: the "chain of survival" concept: statement for Health Professionals from the Advanced Cardiac Life Support Subcommittee and the Emergency Cardiac Care Committee, American Heart Association. *Circulation*. 1991;83:1832–1847.

9. Eisenberg MS, Bergner L, Hallstrom A. Paramedic programs and out-of-hospital cardiac arrest. I: Factors associated with successful resuscitation. *Am J Public Health*. 1979;69:30–38.

10. American Heart Association Emergency Cardiovascular Care (ECC) Committee and Subcommittees. Ethical aspects of CPR and ECC. Part 2: Guidelines 2000 for cardiopulmonary resuscitation and emergency cardiovascular care. *Circulation*. 2000;102 (Suppl I): I–12 to I–21.

11. Becker LB, Pepe PE. Ensuring the effectiveness of community-wide emergency cardiac care. *Ann Emerg Med*. 1993;22:354–365.

12. Bonnin MJ, Pepe PE, Kimball KT, Clark PS. Distinct criteria for termination of resuscitation in the out-of-hospital setting. *JAMA*. 1993;270:1457–1462.

13. Weaver WD, Cobb LA, Hallstrom AP, et al. Considerations for improving survival from out-of-hospital cardiac arrest. *Ann Emerg Med*. 1986;15:1181–1186.

14. White RD, Hankins DG, Bugliosi TF. Seven years' experience with early defibrillation by police and paramedics in an emergency medical services system. *Resuscitation*. 1998;39:145–151.

15. Cobb LA, Hallstrom AP. Community-based cardiopulmonary resuscitation: what have we learned? *Ann New York Acad Sci*. 1982;382:330–342.

16. Pepe PE, Swor RA, Ornato JP, et al. Resuscitation in the out-of-hospital setting: medical futility criteria for on-scene pronouncement of death. *Prehosp Emerg Care*. 2001;5:79–87.

17. Bioethics Committee, American College of Emergency Physicians. Medical moral, legal and ethical aspects of resuscitation for the patient who will have minimal ability to ultimately survive. *Ann Emerg Med*. 1985;14:919–926.

18. McIntyre KM. Medicolegal considerations in cardiopulmonary resuscitation and emergency cardiac care. In: *Medical Control in Emergency Medical Services Systems*. Washington, DC: National Academy Press; 1981.

19. Nordeman LJ, Pepe PE. Alpha and omega: studying resuscitation at the beginning and end stages of life. *Prehosp Emerg Care*. 1997;1:120–122.

20. Pepe PE, Levine R, Fromm RE, et al. Cardiac arrest presenting with rhythms other than ventricular fibrillation: contribution of resuscitative efforts toward total survivorship. *Crit Care Med*. 1992;21:1838–1843.

21. Larabee TM, Tamblyn ER, DeBehnke, et al. Asystolic, unwitnessed out-of-hospital cardiac arrest and no bystander CPR as a criterion for waving resuscitation efforts (abstract). *Acad Emerg Med*. 1999;6:446.

22. Delbridge TR, Fosnocht DE, Garrison HG, Auble TE. Field termination of unsuccessful out-of-hospital cardiac arrest resuscitation: acceptance by family members. *Ann Emerg Med*. 1996;27:649–654.

23. Schmidt TA, Harrahill MA. Family response to out-of-hospital death. *Acad Emerg Med*. 1995;2:513–518.

24. Myers JH, Sirbaugh PE, McCurren RH, et al. Consideration of paramedics' perspective in determining policies for on-scene termination of resuscitation efforts (abstract). *Acad Emerg Med*. 1997;4:496.

25. Brain Resuscitation Clinical Trial I Study Group. Neurologic recovery after cardiac arrest: the effect of ischemia. *Crit Care Med*. 1985;13:930–931.

26. Eisenberg MS, Cummins RO. Termination of CPR in the prehospital arena. *Ann Emerg Med*. 1985;14:1106–1107.

27. Smith JP, Bodai SI. Guidelines for discontinuing prehospital CPR in the emergency department. *Ann Emerg Med.* 1985;14:1093–1098.

28. Bonnin MJ, Pepe PE, Clark PS. Survival in the elderly after out-of-hospital cardiac arrest. *Crit Care Med.* 1993;21:1645–1651.

29. Kellerman AL, Hackman BB, Somes G. Predicting the outcome of unsuccessful prehospital advanced cardiac life support. *JAMA.* 1993;270:1433–1436.

30. Wayne MA, Levine RL, Miller CC. Use of end-tidal carbon dioxide to predict outcome in prehospital cardiac arrest. *Ann Emerg Med.* 1995;25:762–767.

31. Levine RL, Wayne MA, Miller CC. End-tidal carbon dioxide and outcome of out-of-hospital cardiac arrest. *N Eng J Med.* 1997;337:301–306.

32. Pepe PE, Key CB, Sirbaugh PE, Shook JE, Kimball KT. Distinct criteria for the termination of resuscitation efforts for cardiopulmonary arrest in children (abstract). *Acad Emerg Med.* 1996;3:475.

33. Pepe PE. Out-of-hospital resuscitation research: rationale and strategies for controlled clinical trials. *Ann Emerg Med.* 1993;22:17–23.

34. Pepe PE, Bonnin MJ, Mattox KL. Regulating the scope of EMS. *Prehosp Disast Med.* 1990;5:59–63.

35. Rosner F. The living will. *Chest.* 1986;90:441–442.

36. Haber JG. The living will and the directive to provide maximum care—the scope of autonomy. *Chest.* 1986;90:442–444.

37. Raffin TA. Value of the living will. *Chest.* 1986;90:444–446.

38. McCarthy P. Do not resuscitate: administrative and ethical considerations in prehospital arrests. *J Emerg Med Services.* 1983;9:26–30.

39. Understanding the living will. *Senior Medical Review.* 1986;1:4–6.

40. Taffet GE, Teasedale TA, Luchi RJ. In-hospital cardiopulmonary resuscitation. *JAMA.* 1988;260:2069–2072.

41. Van Hoeyweghen RJ, Bossaert LL, Mullie A, et al. Survival after out-of-hospital cardiac arrest in elderly patients. *Ann Emerg Med.* 1992;21:1179–1184.

42. Swor RA, Jackson RE, Tintinalli JE, Pirrallo RG. Does advanced age matter in outcomes after out-of-hospital cardiac arrest in community-dwelling adults? *Acad Emerg Med.* 2000;7:762–768.

43. Plaisance P, Lurie KG, Vicaut E, et al. A comparison of standard cardiopulmonary resuscitation and active compression-decompression resuscitation for out-of-hospital cardiac arrest. *N Engl J Med.* 1999;341:569–575.

44. Buckman RF. Direct cardiac massage without major thoracotomy: feasibility and systemic blood flow. *Resuscitation.* 1997;34:247–253.

45. Weaver WD, et al. Amplitude of ventricular fibrillation wave-form and outcome after cardiac arrest. *Ann Intern Med.* 1985;102:53–55.

46. Angelos MG, Menegazzi JJ, Callaway CW. Bench to bedside: resuscitation from prolonged ventricular fibrillation. *Acad Emerg Med.* 2001;8:909–924.

47. Bonnin MJ, Pepe PE, Clark PS. Key role of prehospital resuscitation in survival from out-of-hospital cardiac arrest (abstract). *Ann Emerg Med.* 1990;19:466.

48. Sirbaugh PE, Pepe PE, Shook JE, et al. A prospective, population-based study of the demographics, epidemiology, management, and outcome of out-of-hospital pediatric cardiopulmonary arrest. *Ann Emerg Med.* 1999;33:174–184.

49. Brown CG, Martin DR, Pepe PE, et al. Standard versus high-dose epinephrine in out-of-hospital cardiac arrest: a controlled clinical trial. *N Eng J Med.* 1992;327:1051–1055.

50. Pepe PE, Abramson NS, Brown CG. ACLS—does it really work? *Ann Emerg Med.* 1994;23:1037–1041.

51. Brown CG, Dzwonezyk R. Signal analysis of the human electrocardiogram during ventricular fibrillation: frequency and amplitude parameters as predictors of successful countershock. *Ann Emerg Med.* 1996;27:184–188.

52. Cobb LA, Fahrenbruch CE, Walsh TR, et al. Influence of cardiopulmonary resuscitation prior to defibrillation in patients with out-of-hospital ventricular fibrillation. *JAMA.* 1999;281:1182–1188.

53. Noc M, Weil MH, Gazmuri RJ, Sun S, Biscara J, Tang W. Ventricular fibrillation voltage as a monitor of the effectiveness of cardiopulmonary resuscitation. *J Lab Clin Med.* 1994;124:421–426.

54. Yakaitis RW, Ewy GA, Otto CW, Taren DL, Moon TE. Influence of time and therapy on ventricular defibrillation in dogs. *Crit Care Med.* 1980;8(3):157–163.

55. Niemann JT, Cairns CB, Sharnia J, Lewis RJ. Treatment of prolonged ventricular fibrillation: immediate countershock versus high-dose epinephrine and CPR preceding countershock. *Circulation.* 1992;85:281–287.

56. Kern KB, Garewal HS, Sanders AB, et al. Depletion of myocardial adenosine triphosphate during prolonged untreated ventricular fibrillation: effect on defibrillation success. *Resuscitation.* 1990;20:221–229.

57. Wigginton JG, Pepe PE, Bedolla JP. Gender-related differences in the presentation and outcome of out-of-hospital cardiopulmonary arrest: a multi-year, prospective population-based study. *Crit Care Med.* 2002 (special supplement); in press.

58. Silfvast T. Initiation of resuscitation in patients with prehospital bradyasystolic cardiac arrest in Helsinki. *Resuscitation.* 1990;19:143–150.

59. Brown C. Limiting care: is CPR for everyone? *Clin Issues Crit Care Nurs.* 1990;1:161–168.

60. Pepe PE, Cobb LA, Persse DE, et al. Improved criteria for waiving resuscitation efforts for out-of-hospital primary cadiac arrest (abstract). *Ann Emerg Med.* 1994;23:619.

61. Emergency Cardiac Care Committee, American Heart Association. Standards and guidelines for cardiopulmonary resuscitation and emergency cardiac care. *JAMA.* 1986;255:2841–3044.

62. Pepe PE, Brown CG, Bonnin MJ, et al. Prospective validation criteria for on-scene termination of resuscitation after out-of-hospital cardiac arrest (abstract). *Acad Emerg Med.* 1994;1:315.

63. Kellermann AL, Staves DR, Hackman BB. In-hospital resuscitation following unsuccessful prehospital advanced cardiac life support: 'heroic efforts' or an exercise in futility? *Ann Emerg Med.* 1988;17:589–594.

64. Hazinski MF, Chahine AA, Holcomb GW, Morris JA. Outcome of cardiovascular collapse in pediatric blunt trauma. *Ann Emerg Med*. 1994;23(6):1229–1235.

65. Battistella FD, Nugent W, Owings JT, Anderson JT. Field triage of the pulseless trauma patient. *Arch Surg*. 1999;134(7):742–745, Discussion 745–746.

66. Rothenberg SS, Moore EE, Moore FA, Baxter BT, Moore JB, Cleveland HC. Emergency department thoracotomy in children—a critical analysis. *J Trauma*. 1989;29:1322–1325.

67. Copass MK, Oreskovich MR, Bladergroen MR, Carrico CJ. Prehospital cardiopulmonary resuscitation of the critically injured patient. *Am J Surg*. 1984;148:20–26.

68. Durham LA, Richardson RJ, Wall MJ Jr., Pepe PE, Mattox KL. Emergency center thoracotomy: impact of prehospital resuscitation. *J Trauma*. 1992;32:775–779.

69. Nemiroff MJ. Near-drowning. *Respir Care*. 1992;37:600–608.

Information Systems

Greg Mears, MD
Joseph Zalkin

Introduction

Emergency Medical Services (EMS) is the practice of medicine involving the evaluation and management of patients with acute traumatic and medical conditions in an environment outside the hospital (prehospital). EMS is the intersection of public health, public safety, and acute patient care. EMS requires working talents in business, logistics, disaster preparedness, telecommunications, and public relations. The ingredients for success lie in understanding the health and medical care of populations through systems.

Emergency Medical Services might be more functionally termed Emergency Medical Systems. As our world grows with respect to population, technology, public expectations, and medical care capabilities, EMS is forced in a role of rapid growth and change. Services must expand to meet these growths, either in numbers or in the quality or quantity of care that they can provide. It is these stress factors that place a critical importance on information systems.

EMS is no longer isolated as an expensive source of transportation. It is held accountable for its response times, the quality of its service, the medical care it provides, and its cost or value to the customer (citizen). It is held to the standards of other medical specialties to prove its effect on patient outcome as a justification for its existence. Finally, as part of the healthcare system, EMS is required to interact with the rest of the system at the local, regional, state, and federal levels through the exchange of information.

History and Overview

Any discussion of EMS information systems draws heavily from historic documents and events that have shaped the current EMS system structure. The following events are helpful in defining an EMS information system.

1973 EMS Enactment

In 1973, the Department of Health, Education and Welfare defined 15 components of an EMS system. Although an information system was not listed as one of the 15 components, each component was shaped or defined as a piece to a puzzle. The puzzle when completed required a significant amount of data to interact and monitor each of the pieces or components. Even more importantly, federal funding was provided to agencies that modeled their system after these components. This was the first legislation for EMS, which required data or documentation of services through a coordinated patient record, and a formal review and evaluation process.

1991 Utstein

In 1991, the American Heart Association published the "Recommended Guidelines for Uniform Reporting of Data From Out-of-Hospital Cardiac Arrest: The Utstein Style." This was the first major document to specifically address EMS systems and their performance with respect to patient outcome. Other documents had addressed patient outcome as an endpoint, but the Utstein Criteria were a standard data set with standard definitions for measuring cardiac arrest survival across systems. The Utstein Criteria required the exchange of information between the 9-1-1 dispatch center, the EMS system, and the hospital. Table 22.1 lists the recommended Utstein data set.

1993 Uniform Prehospital Dataset

In 1993, the National Highway Traffic Safety Administration (NHTSA) developed a consensus document, which defined 81 elements important to an EMS information system. Of the 81 elements, 49 were considered essential and 32 were considered desirable (table 22.2). These elements were created in an effort

TABLE 22.1	
Utstein Criteria Cardiac Arrest Core Dataset	
TEMPLATE DATA FOR SURVIVAL MEASUREMENT	**TIME EVENT DATA**
Population served	Time of collapse/Time of recognition
Confirmed cardiac arrests considered for resuscitation	Time of call receipt
Resuscitations not attempted	Time first emergency response vehicle is mobile
Resuscitations attempted	Time vehicle stops
Cardiac etiology	Time of arrival at patient's side
Non-cardiac etiology	Time of first CPR attempts
Arrest witnessed	Time of first defibrillatory shock
Arrest not witnessed	Time of return of spontaneous circulation
Arrests after arrival of emergency personnel	Time intubation achieved
Initial rhythm ventricular fibrillation	Time intravenous access achieved
Initial rhythm asystole	Time medications administered
Initial rhythm ventricular tachycardia	Time CPR abandoned/death
Other initial rhythm	Time departure from scene
Determine presence of bystander CPR	Time arrival at emergency department
Any return of spontaneous circulation	
Efforts ceased in field or emergency department	
Admission to intensive care unit	
Patient died in hospital and within 24 hours	
Discharged alive	
Death within 1 year of discharge	
Alive at 1 year	

to allow an EMS system to benchmark itself with respect to the service, patient care, personnel performance, patient outcome, and data linkage with other organizations or larger datasets. Perhaps even more important than the elements themselves, is the creation of a standard definition for each element, which is critical for any information system.

1996 EMS Agenda for the Future

In 1996, NHTSA published the EMS Agenda for the Future. This is the most important modern EMS document to date in that it addresses EMS as a community-based health management system, fully integrated with the overall healthcare system. Included in this document were recommendations on the development of 14 distinct attributes of EMS (table 22.3). The goal of the document was to improve the quality of community health, result in more appropriate use of acute healthcare resources, and yet allow EMS to remain as the public's emergency medical safety net. One of the 14 components addressed in the document was Information Systems.

Five recommendations for information systems were issued from the EMS Agenda for the Future:

1. EMS must adopt a uniform set of data elements and definitions to facilitate multi-system evaluations and collaborative research.

2. EMS must develop mechanisms to generate and transmit data that is valid, reliable, and accurate.

3. EMS must develop and refine information systems that describe the entire EMS event so that patient outcomes and cost-effective issues can be determined.

4. EMS should collaborate with other healthcare providers and community resources to develop integrated information systems.

5. Information system users must provide feedback to those who generate data in the form of research results, quality improvement programs, and evaluations.

1998 EMS Agenda Implementation Guide

Finally, NHTSA in 1998 produced a follow-up document to the EMS Agenda for the Future entitled "The EMS Agenda for the Future Implementation Guide." This document took the 14 components of the original agenda and outlined suggestions or approaches to their development. Directly or indirectly, this document reinforces the need for a standardized information system for every one of the essential EMS components identified. The information system, in fact, is the backbone for the development of these components. The future of EMS will be based on information systems.

TABLE 22.2	
1993 NHTSA Uniform EMS Dataset	
ESSENTIAL	**DESIRABLE**
Incident address	Complaint onset date
Incident city	Complaint onset time
Incident county	Date unit notified
Incident state	Time of arrival at patient
Location type	Patient care record number
Date incident reported	Crew member identification number (3)
Time incident reported	Crew member type/level (3)
Time dispatch notified	Patient street address
Time unit notified	City of residence
Time unit responding	County of residence
Time unit arrives at scene	State of residence
Time unit left scene	Telephone number
Time unit arrives at destination	Social security number
Time back in service	Age
Lights and sirens to scene	Chief complaint
Service type	Injury intent
Incident number	Factors affecting ems delivery of care
Response number	Time of first CPR
Agency/unit number	Provider of first CPR
Vehicle type	Time CPR discontinued
Crew member identification number (1)	Time of witnessed cardiac arrest
Crew member identification number (2)	Witness of cardiac arrest
Crew member type/level (1)	Time of first defibrillatory shock
Crew member type/level (2)	Return of spontaneous circulation
Patient name	Initial cardiac rhythm
Zip code of residence	Cardiac rhythm at destination
Date of birth	Respiratory effort
Gender	Skin perfusion
Race/ethnicity	Glasgow coma score (total)
Destination/transferred to	Revised trauma score
Destination determination	Procedure attempts
Lights and/or sirens used from scene	Treatment authorization
Incident/patient disposition	
Cause of injury	
Provider impression	
Pre-existing condition	
Signs and symptoms present	
Injury description	
Safety equipment	
Alcohol/drug use	
Pulse rate	
Respiratory rate	
Systolic blood pressure	
Diastolic blood pressure	
Glasgow eye opening component	
Glasgow verbal component	
Glasgow motor component	
Procedure or treatment name	
Medication name	

1997 DEEDS

In 1997, the National Center for Injury Prevention and Control published a document entitled Data Elements for Emergency Department Systems (DEEDS). This document was similar in concept to the EMS Data Set from NHTSA, except it was targeting the emergency department. This document extended the concept of an information system by providing standards for data collection and linkages back to EMS and forward to hospital discharge.

TABLE 22.3

EMS Agenda of the Future: Emergency Medical Services Attributes

Integration of health services
EMS research
Legislation and regulation
System finance
Human resources
Medical oversight
Education systems
Public education
Prevention
Public access
Communication systems
Clinical care
Information systems
Evaluation

Existing Registries and Healthcare Databases

Trauma Registries

At the state and/or national level, trauma registries have been implemented which have served as a valuable descriptive and quality management tool for trauma centers and trauma systems. These registries contain detailed information regarding the management of patients as they progress through the trauma system. Trauma registries capture some EMS data, but a link with EMS data is extremely important to complete the description of trauma care from event through hospital discharge or rehabilitation. Currently there are several commercial trauma registry software vendors who provide software to trauma centers and systems at the local or state level. Currently, there are two national trauma registries that group data centrally from participating trauma centers and states. The National Trauma Databank is maintained by the American College of Surgeons; Tufts University maintains the National Pediatric Trauma Registry.

Motor Vehicle Crash Database

At the state and national level, crash data are collected and maintained through either the Department of Transportation or through law enforcement. The Department of Motor Vehicles also maintains a database of information with respect to drivers and vehicles. Both of these data sources have potential interaction with an EMS information system.

NHTSA has a program known as CODES (Crash Outcomes Data Evaluation System), which uses probabilistic linkage to match state data from law enforcement, EMS, and the Emergency Department/hospital. CODES is a collaborative approach to generating medical and financial outcome information relating to motor vehicle crashes and using this outcome-based data as the basis for decisions related to highway traffic safety. Federal financial assistance is available to states that have the ability to capture data at the state level from these three venues. CODES has been in existence since 1992, and is currently working with 25 states.

Other Databases

Several other healthcare-related databases and information systems exist at the local, state, and national level. Most states have some form of a hospital insurance or admission/discharge database. These databases may or may not capture information on patients who are not admitted to the hospital, such as those seen in the emergency department and released.

Each state maintains a Medical Examiners Database, which records information on all deaths, including the cause of death. Most states have some form of Public Health and/or Injury Surveillance database. The amount of information and usefulness of these databases vary greatly from state to state.

EMS Information System Design

The raw material for information is data. Information systems collect and arrange data to serve particular purposes. Following the recommendations of the EMS Agenda for the Future, uniform data elements with uniform definitions, which can describe an entire EMS event, is the goal of an information system. An EMS event begins with layperson or patient recognition of a problem, which leads to activation of the system through the 9-1-1 or communications center. The end of an EMS event is the transfer of care of a patient to another healthcare provider outside the EMS system, release of the patient from EMS care by EMS, refusal of EMS care by the patient, or death. To measure and draw conclusions through research, patient outcomes, quality management, or evaluation, the end of an EMS event must include some information regarding emergency department care, hospital care, and final disposition.

Information systems must also provide a mechanism for storage and retrieval of EMS events in the form of historic medical records. The knowledge of previous medical care or EMS usage can be crucial in true acute care situations when little patient information can otherwise be obtained. This information should be available in a format that can be accessed prior to or during patient care.

An EMS information system must be able to include data from several sources. The communication center (9-1-1) can provide time-related data such as dispatch and arrival times, dispatch complaint information, vehicle response information, and Emergency Medical Dispatch (EMD) data. Emergency Medical Dispatch protocols identify general demographics of the patient, the chief complaint, the protocol used for the response, and pre-arrival instructions. A patient or event identifier should be established to link this data with the EMS patient care record.

The Utstein Criteria (table 22.1) and the NHTSA Uniform Data Set (table 22.2) combined give an important definition standard to prehospital data points. It is important to work within these recommendations to create an environment where information can be linked with other databases, systems, and registries. Through this uniform data, standardized evaluation, research, and outcome measures can be obtained. It is important to note that these two data sets are recommendations for a minimal data set. For complete documentation of an EMS event, other data elements must be created to include standards of medical care documentation such as current medications taken by the patient, drug allergies, medical and injury related risk factors, examination results, narrative interactions or treatment exceptions, and disposition details or instructions. As EMS moves outside of its traditional treatment and transport modalities, the need to create a medical document with the consideration of treatment and referral or treatment and release must be considered. This requires increased documentation of disposition instructions and patient education.

Much of the information collected during an EMS event can be improved through the use of medical devices. Information collected by a medical device, stored, and later downloaded into the information system is essential to the future of EMS information systems. Direct data collection from medical devices removes many of the inherent data entry errors, improves the completeness of the medical record, and frees personnel to provide patient care. Currently, prehospital medical devices do not have a universal capability to transfer all the numeric and waveform data to information systems outside their proprietary software. It is typical for a single EMS system to have multiple devices from multiple manufacturers that perform the same function. This duplication requires a system to have the proprietary software from each manufacturer to download and archive data. Because of the multiple proprietary systems, the ability to combine and functionally use the data is limited, especially if waveforms from monitor/defibrillators is included. This same problem makes it impossible to create an electronic medical record in a timely manner for use immediately after patient care, and makes the retrieval of previous EMS events for comparison extremely difficult. Manufacturers must create an open architecture where device data, numeric and waveform, can be moved from database to database within an information system in a time frame to allow electronic record retrieval or generation.

Information systems must be designed to interface with the other healthcare providers who will be participating. The DEEDS dataset published through the CDC is the recommended standard for an emergency department data set. It provides definitions for each recommended data point and includes coding and documentation that can provide information for patient outcome; emergency departments are only now beginning to follow its recommendations.

Communication with the hospitals is critical with respect to the identification of data points that will allow linkage between the two databases. There is a significant problem with respect to patient confidentiality and the ability to obtain hospital information with respect to patient care and outcome. States should work toward improving EMS law and regulations so that information can flow in both directions. The future of EMS is dependent on the ability to obtain outcome information in a timely manner.

Systems are now more than ever in the position of financial accountability; and are held accountable for the quality of their service, patient care, and finances. All EMS information systems should incorporate any information that is required for billing and reimbursement in a format that will allow interaction with billing software, and fulfill government regulations for Medicare reimbursement.

EMS event data must have the capability to be reliably linked at the regional or national level. Trauma Registries, state EMS databases, injury prevention databases, law enforcement databases, medical examiner databases, and the NHTSA Crash Outcomes Data Evaluations System (CODES) are some of the possibilities.

Finally, EMS data collection and use must be based on system design and workflow. Failure to consider these two issues will result in incomplete data, useless information, and failure of the information system. Many EMS data collection systems have failed for the lack of understanding and consideration of the end user and workflow.

EMS System Types

Systems by nature are extremely variable. Boundaries, jurisdictions, geography, politics, equipment, manpower, and training are never the same for two systems. System design is an art. There are some concepts that have universal implications, such as response times for cardiac arrest survival, or decreased scene times in multi-system trauma, but very few concepts have been proven through research. Stout has introduced several models of EMS delivery and management through the analysis of several urban-based EMS systems. Using methods of system status management it is postulated that the ideal size for efficiency is a population base of just over 1,000,000. These same operational and management concepts have not been proven in systems with a population base of less than 250,000. There are no current guidelines or literature that propose a standard EMS delivery plan for rural or wilderness populations.

EMS information systems mirror the lack of standards and the diversity. Urban systems have very different data and communication needs from rural. In an urban environment resources are often constrained, call volumes are high, and issues such as trauma center use and hospital diversions are important. In a rural environment, response times and resources are also affected, but for different reasons; it is more difficult to maintain education and skills with limited patient contact. Funding or resources may not be available for paramedic level care. Rural systems are often volunteer-based.

When implementing an information system it is critical to consider each and every attribute of the system. Urban systems require more data to be more efficient for day-to-day operations. Rural systems require data more for the ability to monitor and improve the system through patient outcome measures and quality management, and to maintain service in their community. The amount, method, and mechanism for data documentation, computer data entry, and data analysis are very different for each system. If any differences or similarities in patient outcomes or overall system successes or failures are gained by comparing data between urban and rural settings, information system design is critical.

There are several common variables in EMS systems, which can allow some grouping and generalization. Systems are typically defined as either volunteer (or not for profit), private service (for profit), or third service (governmental based). Each of these types has information needs that are very different and distinct. For instance, a private service will be more interested in capturing the required billing information on each encounter. A volunteer service may not be interested in billing at all. These issues must be considered in the development of any EMS information system.

EMS data must also be considered from a time perspective. Documentation of an EMS event should include information regarding the entire EMS event, from dispatch through either releasing or turning the patient over to another medical care facility. This involves information pre-event, the actual patient encounter, and the post-event disposition and documentation.

The data should be defined and analyzed based on sound business principles. These include documentation with the ability to analyze performance based on the service, the provider, and the patient.

EMS data must take into account the system workflow. Definitions of the data must be clear and understandable, collection must be as automated as possible, and it should have a positive effect on the systems performance by improving the technician's time with each patient, improving the treatment and care for individuals, and providing real-time (or near real-time) feedback to the system and technicians.

EMS Operations from a Data Perspective

An EMS event begins with the recognition by the victim or bystander of a medical or traumatic event in need of medical care. There is an established workflow from 9-1-1 call activation through hospital discharge. The sequences of call-taking and dispatch have critical system time stamps. These time stamps document when the call arrived in the dispatch center, when the responders were alerted to the call, when the unit rolled out of the station, arrived at the scene, arrived at the patient, departed the scene, arrived at the facility, and was again ready for service. These time stamps describe the "action" times of an EMS response. Much debate exists at this time with respect to what each of these intervals should appropriately be, but they are quality indicators that define the system, and are a necessity for quality improvement initiatives. Computer aided dispatch (CAD) entry in the current model is dependent on operator coding of events. Future models will incorporate "dual" time stamps—operator and automated—recorded into the CAD information for incident reporting. The busier the 9-1-1 centers gets, the more likely the radio-acknowledged time stamps will be inaccurate. By adding checks and balance with automated time stamps, the events have a fail-safe method of recording accurate times.

9-1-1 Call Center

Early in the chain of events the public is processed through a series of data management systems. Some of the earliest examples of information systems involve the emergency access number (7-digit or 9-1-1) to the communications center. From the landline-based telephone system an account number can be obtained (phone number) along with an Automated Number Identifier (ANI), also known as Caller ID. In addition to the number of the caller, additional information is provided by the computerized system. These data include the location of the caller via an Automated Location Identifier (ALI) screen, and the appropriate Police, Fire, and EMS agency for that district or location. These agencies are identified through an Emergency Service Number (ESN) that is cross-referenced with the caller data. ESNs are maintained by each county and coordinated with a regional emergency telecommunications agency. The local coordinator defines the responders in a given area. This is ultimately a perpetual process, with annexation and response lines changing almost daily. The ESN changes with a broad change in responders; that is, City Police, City Fire, City EMS would represent one triplet of responders and would receive a 3-digit identifier, whereas City Police, County Fire, City EMS would get a different identifier to reflect changes in the responders.

Once the ESN and/or Road Name, Block Number, and Direction are shared from the ALI information, the telecommunicator types the required information into the CAD System. In generic terms, CAD systems are configured to accept information and make unit assignments based on pre-configured response standards. In a large center, calls may be taken at one console in the same room as the radio dispatchers, or may go to a central answer point—a public safety answer point (PSAP) that may provide all caller inquiry and dispatch, or may route calls to EMS agencies secondary answer points for emergency medical dispatch processing.

Dispatch priority can be assigned to the EMS call. A high-priority call can involve multiple-agency response. Data sharing among responders may involve voice, alpha-pagers, mobile data printers, and mobile data terminals. Voice communication to responders provides a traditional medium to communicate information. However, few communities have well integrated emergency communication systems across all Public Safety agencies. Often services are in an electronic "Tower of Babel": VHF, UHF, 800Mhz, Cellular, PCS, and others during large scale or mutual aid events.

A key measure of system effectiveness is reasonable response times. EMS must navigate the shortest distance to a call and to a healthcare facility. Often, responders must avoid hazards to get to a scene. Rerouting requires knowledge of streets and landmarks, further complicated in mutual aid response to unfamiliar areas. Technology in the dispatch center and the response unit can assist in call assignment to closest unit, suggested route from current location, and key time stamps for event documentation. A modern CAD system with supplemental automated vehicle locator and in-vehicle navigation can determine closest unit by nature of the call and direct the responders via an electronic map with the shortest distance of travel. This will maximize efficiency and give a system control of its response times and performance.

Data typically captured by an Emergency Medical Dispatch (EMD) system is listed in table 22.4.

EMS System for 2010

Personnel 2010

EMS personnel equipped with handheld multifunctional devices capable of assessing and monitoring vital signs (non-invasive BP, pulse oximetry, pulse, respiratory rate, cardiac rhythm, 12-lead EKG, CO_2, and blood glucose) and providing needed external pacing, defibrillation, and cardioversion are now used to evaluate all patients. The device is quickly attached

TABLE 22.4
Emergency Medical Dispatch Datapoints
Time into 9-1-1 center
Time CAD incident started
Time of initial EMD entry questions started
Caller's location
Caller's location verified?
Caller"s phone number
Caller's phone number verified?
Chief complaint defined
Age of patient
Level of consciousness defined
Level of breathing defined
Caller's class: 1st party–4th party
Time of EMS dispatch/notification
Key questions asked?
Completely?
In order?
Post dispatch information given?
Appropriate?
Possible
EMD call class by call-taker
EMD call class by reviewer

patient. On arrival to the ED, the EMS personnel proofread the EMS patient-care report, collect all the necessary signatures via the touch screen, and finalize the report. Once the report is finalized, it prints out both at the hospital and the administrative EMS office, while all data are stored centrally on a database with a web browser/internet interface. Billing information is also transmitted directly to the billing office for generation of the necessary financial forms. Concerned about another call that has just been paged out, the EMS personnel quickly restock the ambulance based on the list of used supplies provided on the handheld data unit's tabulations, and the EMS crew activates the button on the handheld unit, signifying they are back in service. At the end of the day, the EMS provider generates a quality management report from this specific call which indicates all care was provided appropriately based on the complaint and protocol and the patient was admitted for a successful angioplasty and positive cardiac enzymes. The cardiologist was able to access the EMS 12-lead EKG over the EMS internet-based information system to document a ventricular dysrhythmia which provided the necessary documentation to qualify the patient for an internal defibrillator.

Ambulance 2010

A comprehensive vehicle-based data unit will incorporate currently available technologies and glean from other commercial transportation models. The ambulance/aid cars of the year 2010 will use Global Positioning System (GPS) to identify where the unit is in a common navigational language—latitude and longitude. Adding a radio beacon to the GPS equipment, we have an Automated Vehicle Locator (AVL) device that can be queried for the location, speed, and direction of the unit. Matched with CAD information on the caller's location, a quick match can be made in a matter of seconds. Priority calls will be assigned to units that AVL and CAD have defined as "near" to the caller. In addition, a data display in the unit will assist the driver to locate the call, even if there is a roadblock due to other events in the area. The Display will be compatible with either driver or attendant operation. New "heads-up" display will place critical information in 3D fashion in the driver's field of view, reducing eye-to-screen movement. Greater use of "smart" systems will mark events based on the status of the ambulance and crew. Field radios "mark event" buttons record arrival at patient side, and so on. There are currently experiments with

to the patient and automatically performs these functions while EMS personnel spend time interviewing the patient and performing the needed physical exam and treatment. Personnel enter data as they perform their assessment and provide treatment into a second handheld device that allows data to be entered in a combination of ways. Verbal information is entered by voice recognition. Treatment and procedures are entered by a combination of touch screen and barcode scanning. Scanning the barcode of the patient's driver's license or personal ID enters patient's demographic data. The handheld then communicates back with a central database through a wireless interface to determine if this patient has received EMS services in the past and, if so, provides the most recent past medical history, medication, and allergy list. It copies all other pertinent information already in the system to minimize data entry of the personnel. The advanced monitoring device communicates with the handheld data unit through a wireless or infrared interface to complete the patient record along with the 9-1-1 dispatch information that was retrieved over the same wireless network. EMS personnel choose from a list of destinations and this information is automatically relayed to the receiving hospital prior to the arrival of the EMS unit and

INFORMATION SYSTEMS

transmission of uplink video, bio-telemetry, and audio from the ambulance treatment area to a receiving station in the ED. Taking advantage of telemedicine concepts opens up the potential of future "mobile clinics" and care and release options.

Medical Devices

In the 1970s, 3-lead EKGs in the field were standard; the 1980s added pacing, and the 1990s extended 12- to 15-lead EKGs to patient side. External defibrillation has progressed from large bulky machines weighing over 20 pounds, to automated external defibrillators (AED) which weigh less than 8 pounds.

The medical devices in most hospitals currently have a means of connecting and communicating through a protocol for standard communications between devices, both in like-manufactured and unrelated equipment. A network exists within a hospital that provides the highway for this information exchange. Due to the disconnected and varying environments EMS must operate in, the protocol has not been implemented successfully in the prehospital environment. Prehospital medical devices have very limited data transmission, storage, retrieval, or analysis capabilities at this time outside of the proprietary software provided from each manufacturer.

EMS, like the rest of the healthcare field, has become more complex and sophisticated, with systems that can monitor waveform trends and provide computer-assisted diagnosis and decision support systems using artificial intelligence to monitor and shape a patient's course. An example is the automated external defibrillator: using waveform frequency and amplitude measures of EKG, a decision support system alerts rescuers that the patient is in a life-threatening cardiac rhythm. This data store becomes critical for EMS systems. The ability to capture, store, aggregate, and analyze this data is critical to the evaluation of the system's performance, finance, and resource management. Also, medical devices such as AEDs are moving into the lay public where the ability to obtain data from these devices is critical to maintaining the continuum of care through the healthcare system (Figure 22.1). Medicare reimbursement for the insertion of an internal defibrillator requires a rhythm strip documenting a ventricular dysrhythmia. Without this AED data, this would be impossible if a patient were resuscitated by a public-access AED.

In modern EMS systems, communications is the most expensive recurring fixed cost beyond the ambulance. To assist crews and management in decision support, appropriate data and voice communications require systems that provide broad coverage and simple operation. In jurisdictions with wide response areas, there may be separate radio systems in each community. This is also an issue where remote support to an EMS or disaster response can create a "tower of Babel" where multiple EMS personnel on the same scene cannot communicate due to disparate equipment.

Consumer communications using digital cell systems interfaced with orbiting satellites can provide voice and data support worldwide. Commercial communications networks, like Nextel, provide digital voice and group "radio" communications. Note of caution: non-public safety grade systems (commercial cellular, Nextel) are likely to be busy or out of service in a major event. The integration of alpha paging either by direct or commercial carriers adds another means of messaging to single crews or groups in a

---

**Typical Information
Captured by an AED**

Initial time on
Date
Battery self test
Battery status
Initial ekg waveform
Commit to treat
Shocks delivered count
EKG after treatment
Joules of shock
Ohms of resistance
Estimated delivered energy
Alert messages (push to shock,
    no shock indicated)

FIGURE 22.1

**Medical Devices with
Data Transfer Capabilities**

Automated external defibrillator (aed)
Standard monitor defibrillator/pacer
Pulse oxymetry
Capnograph (waveform co_2)
Non-invasive bp monitor
Ventilator/respirators

FIGURE 22.2

Non-Medical Devices

Global Positioning System (GPS)

Radio/Communications
VHF
UHF
800 MHz
900 MHz
2.4 GHz
Satellite

Cellular
Analog
Digital
PSC
Iden

Paging Systems
Alpha-Numeric
2-Way Paging
Event Loggers (tattlers)

FIGURE 22.3

timely manner in a relatively secure means. Two-way paging allows for messaging both to a pager and returned to the sender. Today's modern CAD system can coordinate status messages to supervisors on fleet readiness and inform medical directors of events in the district. The transportation industry has used devices to record the speed, braking use, turning force, and other parameters to monitor compliance with regulation and policy. Vehicle maintenance can be reduced by driver education and both policy and preventive maintenance procedures. Electronic monitors (black box, tattlers) help to define the actions of the driver during normal and emergent operation of the EMS unit.

Global positioning systems (GPS) once were limited to military usage until the late 1980s. Established to assist troop and missile guidance in wartime, the 24 GPS satellites establish in less than 3 minutes the location of the GPS equipment by latitude and longitude. New FCC requirements will make triangulation to determine the location of 9-1-1 cellular callers a mandate.

The easy access to internet connectivity by dial-up lines adds a portal to exchange information from far and wide. Cellular data packet devices (CDPD) and dedicated data channels in 800 and 900 MHz systems extend the connectivity options to web-like private networks at patient side. EMS managers must concern themselves with the adaptability of onboard data systems with safety equipment—air bags, chang-

ing light conditions, and ergonomics. Most mobile solutions are an outreach of law enforcement-based data projects that do not take the special nature of the EMS unit into account. Two distinct systems emerge—one for patient data collection and one for navigational assistance. Some pilot projects are using handheld computers to gather patient and treatment interventions and then dock and transfer the data to either a laptop computer in the mobile, or a desktop computer in the hospital or EMS base. Some early pilot systems exist that communicate back to a central database through a wireless network.

EMS Information System Components

Dataset

EMS Information Systems must begin with a well-structured and defined dataset. There are existing datasets that fulfill much of this requirement. The NHTSA prehospital dataset does define a standardized set of data elements with specific definitions. This dataset is currently only in version 1.0 and is only a start. Many other data elements are required to reconstruct a complete EMS event. As a system develops these datapoints, it is important to use as many national standards and definitions as possible.

Patient care data can be divided into four broad categories.

- **Patient Information:** Demographics, Billing Information, Medical History

Data Entry Devices

Personal Data Assistance
 Palm Pilot
 CE Devices-
 Palmtops

Pen Tablets
 Fujitsu
 Dauphin
 IBM ThinkPad 370
 Symbol
 Panasonic CF-25

Laptops

Desktops

FIGURE 22.4

- **Surveillance Data:** Injury Risk/Mechanism, Cardiac Arrest, Review of Systems
- **Current Diagnostic/Physiological Monitoring:** Vital Signs, Physical Exam
- **Interventional:** Procedures and Treatment (pharmacology), Disposition

Hardware

Modern computer technology has done much to remove barriers of collecting and using data across devices and various types of hardware. Most databases can either exist or move data back and forth through desktop computers, mainframe computers, handheld personal digital assistants, and other devices, with the exception of specialized medical devices. The design of any information system should develop specifications which provide for this data interchange ability.

Software

Computer software can be defined in many ways and comes in many varieties. Three common types of software are used by EMS systems for documentation and report generation. Database programs are the central component of an information system. These store, retrieve, and provide the ability to analyze data that is entered into the system. Front-end programs that are typically database forms, or some commercial package that allows for data entry, are used to add logic and provide a user interface for data entry. Good front-end programs provide a significant amount of error checking, and work to merge workflow with data entry from a user perspective. Back-end programs are typically report generators that provide the ability to ask a question and generate an answer from an existing database. Other programs exist that perform or make these tasks easier. These can include spreadsheet programs such as Excel, statistical analysis packages such as SAS, and support software such as mapping or communications software. Current technology uses network environments and leverages the internet. Web browser-based information systems, such as the North Carolina PreMIS system (**www.premis.net**) allows EMS systems to enter, analyze, and generate reports through an internet-based web server. Through a web browser, such as Internet Explorer or Communicator, EMS systems are provided with an EMS information system and no special software is required by the individual EMS system. Access to the system requires only a computer with a web browser and an internet connection.

Through this route data entry and retrieval are possible for any location that has internet access.

Many systems will continue to rely on paper documentation for some time. This may be in the form of a written document with little structure, or may be complex in nature. The use of computer technology, even when documents are written, is possible. Many EMS systems use documents generated by computer software that allows handwritten documentation, which is then faxed or scanned into a database. This technology has been used in the law-enforcement community for several years and can be implemented in EMS.

Maintenance

All computers and computer software require ongoing maintenance and support. This is even more true for EMS information systems. The nature of EMS, being in unpredictable and disparate locations and conditions, provides many opportunities for equipment and software failure, malfunction, or system overload. Although computer base data entry and retrieval should be the goal of every EMS system, paper backup systems will always be required.

With any EMS information system, a formal educational program, support, and maintenance structure must be planned, developed, and maintained. The quality and service provided in this one area will determine the success and failure of an EMS information system.

Security

Security of an EMS information system is critical and can be split into two areas: security of the patient's information and confidentiality, and the security of the EMS system's information and confidentiality.

EMS system security is important for many reasons. EMS is a political entity and is subject to public and private scrutiny. EMS is also a component of the healthcare system that comes with a significant amount of medical-legal risk. EMS is also many times in a competitive market where details of operational and system issues, if made available outside of the agency, could be detrimental. Finally, EMS, as part of the healthcare system, is responsible for quality management and benchmarking. This process provides a continuing analysis of patient care and system operations in an ongoing fashion for improved service delivery and care.

An EMS information system should be designed from the ground up to provide top-level security to the EMS system and its personnel. Policies and procedures should be developed that define access and use of the system, complete with appropriate disciplinary actions to assure their compliance.

Any information system that aggregates data from multiple EMS systems should have adequate policies and procedures in place to prevent the identity of EMS systems from being disclosed to any outside agencies, or the public, without the consent of that EMS agency.

Patient security is also critically important to an EMS information system. Policies and procedures should be developed and implemented to provide appropriate access to EMS personnel in need of patient data, but protect the patient from undue or unneeded exposure.

In 2000, the U.S. Department of Health and Human Services released regulations protecting patients and healthcare data that is transmitted electronically. This regulation has significant implications for all of health care, including EMS. The regulation is known as the Health Insurance Portability and Accountability Act (HIPAA). This act provides detailed requirements relating to healthcare information that is collected by any healthcare entity. Much of the document addresses electronic transactions with respect to reimbursement, but there are significant sections on patient confidentiality and security, including definitions of what data are defined as identifiable and when they may be released, what requires patient consent prior to release, and punishment that can occur when this act is not followed.

From an EMS information system perspective, HIPAA basically divides security and confidentiality into four major components:

- Patient Privacy and Confidentiality
- User Policy and Procedure
- Physical Security
- Software Security

At the time of this publication, the HIPAA document has just been released in its final form. For that reason, much of the interpretation has not been finalized.

Clear definitions are provided which define when a patient's record can be released from the healthcare provider. This includes detailed information with respect to what information that identifies a patient can be released, and how permission for the release of this information must be obtained.

Any healthcare data or information system must have detailed policy and procedure describing who, when, where, how, and why any personnel can access the system, including user rules and disciplinary policy.

Any healthcare data or information system must meet the physical security requirements of HIPAA, including issues such as locked, controlled access, and entry logs.

Finally, any healthcare information that is transmitted electronically, must meet the HIPAA requirements, including issues such as user authentication and data encryption.

Reimbursement

Modern EMS services are costly to operate. The reasonable costs for service and the amount of payment in a usual and customary manner are slim margins for EMS managers to address. In general, patients with insurance will provide the agency information to bill the insurance provider. If the claim is deemed valid (based on the core data elements and medical necessity) reimbursement from third party payors may result in 80 to 100% of the fee. Prehospital Care Reports (PCRs) are subject to audit to reduce fraud and verify medical need. In 2000, the Health Care Financing Agency (now called the Centers for Medicare and Medicaid Services) reviewed the fees for service and the applicability of data related to care. EMS agencies across the nation were forced to quantify and qualify the care given to establish a fee assign-

---

Essential Reimbursement Data Elements

Patient demographics (name, social security number, age, address)

Payor information (insurance account numbers, both primary and secondary)

Relationship of the insured (if a minor)

Work related?

Auto crash?

Medical condition (chief complaint)

Care provided (Transport, EKG, IV, Medication)

How patient was transferred (stretcher, assisted, wheelchair, etc.)

Loaded miles with patient

FIGURE 22.5

ment. New Medicare reimbursement schedules were defined by negotiated rule. Agencies will be allowed to bill for service in two broad categories—BLS and ALS—as defined by chief complaint; in addition, fees for loaded miles may be included in the total charges. As with most medical fee systems, the federal guidelines will be used by commercial insurance groups to justify claims.

Pitfalls of Information Systems

Now that devices, data elements, and collection methods have been discussed, it is important to understand the limits and potentials of the actual database architecture and structure. Database software is designed to allow data to be stored, manipulated, and retrieved with various levels of complexity and speed, based on a specific database format. Databases are typically either a flat file format or a relational format. Flat file format is a design where all information is entered into a single table, much like a spreadsheet. This is the most basic database design. It allows for data to be manipulated, but only allows a small number of variables to be considered at a time. A relational database allows multiple flat file tables to be connected or linked together by a data element that is common to each table. An example would be a table containing part numbers and part descriptions that could be linked with a table containing part numbers and part prices. A relational database has the structural capability to build a complex information system.

Databases are also described as stand-alone or client-server. A stand-alone database is a database that resides on a single computer designed to work with a single user at one time. A client-server database is designed to be placed on a network where many individuals can use the database simultaneously.

Relational client-server databases allow multiple tables or sources of data to be linked together into a true information system. From this system, documents can be created that pull information from each source of data and combine it into a single report. This report may be in the form of a EMS patient-care report, or it may generate specific reports to track skills, protocol compliance, system status measurement, personnel performance, vehicle maintenance, billing, risk management documents, or patient outcome reports, to name a few.

There are several qualities that can be identified in successful information systems. The design of an information system must start by defining what information is needed and can be collected. Each of these data points must be identified and defined through a consensus of the front-end data entry personnel as well as the back-end data maintenance and processing personnel. The methods of data entry must be considered based on the equipment, training, experience, and education of the EMS provider. A well designed system is often called "user friendly" to mean that the individual users' experience and the functionality of the equipment and software are integrated to maximize performance and satisfaction.

As datapoints are defined, classifications or schemes must be derived to allow information to be sorted into useful groups. This is a difficult process, in that no standard diagnostic or reimbursement coding system was designed with EMS as a primary user. EMS documents are based on chief complaint, rather than diagnosis; providers at all levels have difficulty in translating EMS records into usable ICD-9 or E-code parameters. The depth of these coding systems is much too complex for day-to-day operations. It is critical for the success of an EMS information system to have a standardized problem-based classification scheme, which can objectively and reliably cross over to other EMS and data systems. This will also be the foundation for true EMS billing and reimbursement based on services provided, rather than transportation of a patient from one location to another. Orange County, North Carolina has implemented a classification scheme based on an initial medical, or trauma classification, followed by a description of the problem or injury in a tree-based structure, beginning with the anatomic system and/or organ system and expanding to more detail. This has been shown to be an easy, effective classification for EMS providers, but has not been thoroughly tested against ICD-9, or E-code Standards. An EMS database should be well designed just as a PCR. It should be grouped and formatted in the order that the information is discovered or recorded by the EMS provider.

The introduction of new data systems requires that several issues be addressed. Both initial and continuing education will require time and funds. A successful project will have designated technical and operational staff. An implementation team made up of core individuals who can represent the end user can assist in identifying logistical impediments.

Around the clock support from vendors is a must if the system is to be accessible. Locally created systems will need similar support mechanisms.

If ambulance-based hardware is part of the project, care for safety (airbags clearance and locked mounts), security, lighting (visible in night and day) and power (most EMS units kill power in the station) must be addressed.

New wireless technologies are expanding connected devices in areas where traditional "wire-based" connections were costly or impossible.

Summary

EMS data are needed for system and resource management, quality improvement, injury or population surveillance, and reimbursement. At the same time, EMS is becoming more complex and stressed by quality and quantity issues. More time is needed for hands-on patient care, yet more information must be documented. Modern EMS systems must adopt information systems and documentation as a component of the EMS service. The institutionalization of information provides time, training, and resources to quality information to be recorded, stored, retrieved, and applied.

A system to collect, monitor, and report the activities of an EMS system in an efficient manner makes the medical director's job easier. Huge collections of unqualified data that have been collected for traditional reasons with little feedback will lead to failure of the data system and reduced cooperation among the agencies. Modern biomedical equipment, sophisticated 9-1-1 systems, and integration of hospital care and billing information are attainable in most communities. Medical directors should partner with EMS management and healthcare facilities to assure these sometime separate data stores can blend together. A modern EMS system relies on access to data to manage the health of the system and to make informed decisions.

Bibliography

Braun O. EMS system performance: the use of cardiac arrest timelines. *Ann Emerg Med.* 1993;22:52–61.

Cone DC, Jaslow DS, Brabson TA. Now that we have the Utstein style, are we using it? *Acad Emerg Med.* 1999;6(9):923–928.

Cummins R. The Utstein style for uniform reporting of data from out-of-hospital cardiac arrest. *Ann Emerg Med.* 1993;22:37–40.

Cummins R. Why are researchers and emergency medical services managers not using the Utstein guidelines? *Acad Emerg Med.* 1999;6(9):871–875.

Durch JS, Lohr KN, eds. *Emergency Medical Services for Children.* Washington, DC: National Academy Press; 1993.

Emergency Medical Services: Agenda for the Future. Washington, DC: National Highway Traffic Safety Administration; 1996.

Emergency Medical Services Systems Act of 1973: Public Law 93-154, Title XII of the Public Health Services Act. Washington, DC; 1973.

Emergency Medical Services: Agenda for the Future. Implementation Guide. Washington, D.C: National Highway Traffic Safety Administration; 1999.

EMS Outcomes Evaluation: Key Issues and Future Directions. Proceedings from the NHTSA Workshop on Methodologies for Measuring Morbidity Outcomes in EMS. Washington, DC: National Highway Traffic Safety Administration, April 11–12, 1994.

Garrison HG, Foltin G, Becker L, et al. *Consensus statement: The Role of Out-of-Hospital Emergency Medical Services in Primary Injury Prevention.* Consensus Workshop on the Role of EMS in Injury Prevention, Arlington, VA, August 25–26, 1995, Final Report.

Joyce SM, Brown DE. An optically scanned EMS reporting form and analysis system for statewide use: development and five year experience. *Ann Emerg Med.* 1991;20:1325–1330.

Meislin HW, Spaite DW, Conroy C, Detwiler M, Valenzuela TD. Development of an electronic emergency medical services patient care record. *Prehosp Emerg Care.* 1999;3:54–59.

Nagai M, Yamamoto M, Numata T. Current assessment and proposed improvement to emergency medical information systems in Japan. *Med Inform.* 1994;19:21–36.

National Academy of Sciences, National Research Council. *Accidental Death and Disability: The Neglected Disease of Modern Society.* Washington, DC: National Academy Press; 1966.

National Center for Injury Prevention and Control. *Data Elements for Emergency Department Systems:* Release 1.0. Atlanta, GA: Centers for Disease Control and Prevention; 1997.

North Carolina Prehospital Medical Information System, http://www.premis.net.

Peters J, Hall GB. Assessment of ambulance response performance using a geographic information system. *Social Science & Medicine.* 1999;49:1551–1566.

Shahein H, Zaky MM. ESMIS—A computer-based emergency medical services management information system. Part 1: Design procedure. *Int J Bio-Medical Computing.* 1983;14:451–462.

Shahein H, Zaky MM. ESMIS—A computer-based emergency medical services management information system. Part 2: Database design. *Int J Bio-Medical Computing.* 1984;15:9–22.

Siscovick DS. Challenges in cardiac arrest research: data collection to assess outcomes. *Ann Emerg Med.* 1993;22:92–98.

Spaite DW, Criss EA, Valenzuela TD, Guisto J. Emergency medical services systems research: problems of the past, challenges of the future. *Ann Emerg Med.* 1995;26:146–152.

INFORMATION SYSTEMS

Spaite DW, Valenzuela TD, Meislin HW. Barriers to EMS system evaluation—problems associated with field data collection. *Prehosp Disaster Med*. 1993;8:S35–S40.

Svenson JE, Spurlock CW, Calhoun R. The Kentucky Emergency Medical Services information system: current progress and future goals. *KMA Journal*. 1997;95:509–513.

Swor RA. Out-of-hospital cardiac arrest and the Utstein style: meeting the customer's needs? *Acad Emerg Med*. 1999;6: 875–877.

Uniform Pre-Hospital Emergency Medical Services (EMS) Data Conference. *Final Report*. Washington, DC: National Highway Traffic Safety Administration; 1994.

CHAPTER 23

Evaluation

C. Gene Cayten MD, MPH

Introduction

The evaluation of EMS systems is a difficult but critical task of the medical director. Yet in many EMS agencies, evaluation is a low priority; it should not be. Evaluation is necessary to ascertain whether the system is fulfilling its goals. Without evaluation, expenditures cannot be objectively prioritized. To make the most of limited resources it is critical that evaluation efforts be sharply focused. Evaluation must provide periodic data relating to EMS operations and quality of care and data for future planning. This chapter discusses an EMS systems model, an overall evaluation model, a strategic evaluation model, and methodologic issues.

EMS Systems Model

More than many other aspects of medical care, the handling of emergency cases depends on the harmonious coordination of community resources. Past neglect, however, has caused emergency care in many communities to rely on a fragmented assortment of transportation, communication, hospital, and physician services. Hospitals frequently have been concerned only with the operation of their own emergency departments. Ambulance organizations and police and fire departments have set up their own procedures for responding to requests for emergency assistance; little emphasis has been given to coordination among emergency transportation services and hospital emergency departments.[1]

There are multiple aspects to an EMS care continuum. The phases of care include prevention, prehospital, hospital, and rehabilitation. Evaluation of a system is only possible if the goals and objectives define the desired results. In defining the goals, the limits of the program are also defined. Program designers structuring the system must appropriately balance the resources available for each aspect of emergency health care. Furthermore, they must determine how resources should be organized and operated to coordinate the various system elements. This involves two key concepts: goal orientation and feedback loop. Goal orientation is a set of realistic, general goals for the system that must be agreed on and prioritized. The feedback loop ensures that as old goals are achieved new goals are set. As experience indicates needed modifications, goals and programs are changed appropriately.[2]

As illustrated in figure 23.1, the general planning process involves the following activities:[2]

1. Evaluating program progress with consequent modification of goals and alternative approaches
2. Setting general goals
3. Describing the status of the system under consideration
4. Developing specific objectives consistent with the general goals
5. Devising alternate strategies for achieving objectives
6. Selecting and structuring the alternative programs
7. Implementing the program

General goals for EMS systems often are set by political government agencies. The staff is then responsible for turning these broad objectives into specific programming actions. A detailed description of the system being planned is essential for the development of such actions. A description should include the current demand for services, the nature of services provided by the system, and the resources currently employed within the system (and any constraints on their use). A chronological listing of actions taken on behalf of a typical emergency patient is also a valuable part of the system description. Together these data indicate where improvements are

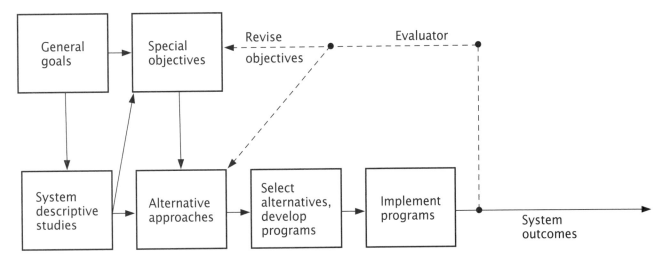

FIGURE 23.1. *The EMS planning process.*

Aspects of EMS Planning

Specific objectives are necessary for the planning and evaluation process to maintain continuity relative to indicators of system performance. Comparison of system structure and performance with available standards or EMS systems developed in other communities may aid in identifying inadequacies and further defining objectives. At this level, each objective should be stated in terms of the difference between the current value of the system performance measure and its desired value. Each objective should also include a target time for its achievement. For example, a specific one-year objective might be to decrease the proportion of ambulance responses taking longer than ten minutes to less than 5%. Associated with each objective should be several viable courses of action that could be taken to satisfy the objective. These alternatives may be devised by local system managers and planning experts, or they may be suggested from the experiences of other communities.

Having gathered data and set objectives, EMS personnel next select strategies and implement programs. Evaluation techniques for selecting among alternatives differ with the type of decision being made. In some cases a simple cost analysis might be used. In others, sophisticated statistical and operations research methods, such as queuing analysis, computer simulation, or optimization techniques, might be required. When the needed resources or expected outcomes are difficult to quantify, subjective assessments by local experts or trained consultants using a consensus technique may be the basis for decisions.

In selecting particular approaches for accomplishing objectives, managers should first specify the criteria alternatives which will be compared. Other considerations are the cost and the time period required before results will be observed. Potential problems that may be encountered when implementing a prospective approach should also be addressed.

To complete the process there must be ongoing evaluation. Such evaluation is a key aspect of system management and planning. Information on system performance helps answer questions asked by public officials, the general public, and other agencies, about EMS provided to the community. Evaluation also indicates where further changes in the system structure or medical procedures are most needed.

Thus, system evaluation is considered broadly as covering an assessment of the total system, and quality improvement is considered more narrowly as process evaluation focusing on the performance of personnel in the system. For example, if a community has a high percentage of cardiac patients who are not successfully resuscitated in the field, despite adequate numbers of well trained responders compared with other communities, the agency should compare response times. If response times are appropriate, the following planning options should be considered: (1) increase the number of responder units (2) develop an emergency medical technician-defibrillation (EMT-D) program (3) train fire department personnel as defibrillation-capable first responders and (4) develop a program of public cardiopulmonary resuscitation (CPR) training. Implementation time and special problems, such as dealing with unions or specific agencies, must be considered when deciding on an alternative or combination of alternatives. Once the new program is defined and implemented, it must be monitored and evaluated to determine whether the prehospital cardiac resuscitation rate has in fact improved. If not, the program may need to be modified or supplemented by others.

In summary, planning, management, and evaluation as described in the aforementioned steps are aspects of an ongoing process, not isolated or onetime activities. They are an integral part of system management and control, providing the objectives to be pursued by the system and feedback on the effectiveness of programs already undertaken.

Overall Evaluation Model

During the past 30 years many publications have been devoted to the development and implementation of evaluation models. In the field of medical care evaluation, Donabedian proposed a basic framework of structure, process, and outcome that has been effectively adapted to EMS system evaluations.[3]

Structure evaluation (or input evaluation) measures the credentials and level of personnel training, the adequacy of facilities and equipment, and the method of organizing resources in the EMS system. Gibson compiled an extensive list of structural criteria for EMS system evaluation.[4] Although system inputs may be measured easily and statistically, the validity of structural standards remains uncertain. Unfortunately, research has not demonstrated that fulfilling the input standards, that is, meeting all available standards for facilities, equipment, and personnel of a "model" EMS system, has any impact on patient health. In many cases input standards are considered "necessary but not sufficient" for achieving the optimal outcome.

Process evaluation assesses the performance elements of medical care. Process assessment techniques include analysis of the appropriateness of care, the patterns of care, case reviews using implicit or explicit criteria, and the data used for clinical decision making. Currently, most process evaluation methods consist of record audits to establish compliance with protocols. Validity and reliability problems have been noted when explicit process criteria are employed in medical record audits. For example, the degree to which prehospital care reports (PCR) reflect the care provided is frequently questioned. Although research has indicated somewhat stronger correlation between process indicators and patient outcome measures, process-outcome relationships are considered weak for most medical conditions.

Because outcome measures are the most important indicators of overall system success, they should be incorporated in all system evaluation efforts.[2] However, patient outcome measures reflecting mortality and morbidity are insensitive to the individual phases of emergency care; thus, other indicators must be employed as well. Also, ultimate-outcome measures are not sensitive measures of the early phases of emergency care. The further one moves toward measuring ultimate or long-term outcome, the less can be said regarding the quality of the initial emergency care.

To study the results of care, intermediate-outcome measures have a closer temporal relationship to the care being rendered, and are more relevant than long-term measures.[2] Figure 23.2 indicates where intermediate-outcome measures may be useful indicators of system status and effectiveness. For each phase of the EMS program, measures selected should reflect the specific objective pursued. For instance, to monitor the effectiveness of care provided at the scene, intermediate-outcome measures (outcome III) might include the number or proportion of patients suffering cardiac arrest who are successfully resuscitated in the field. Prehospital trauma care could be assessed by change in trauma score (TS) or revised trauma score (RTS) from initial field status to initial emergency department status.[5] Pozen et al used the intermediate-outcome measures of survival to ICU admission, 24-hour survival and morbidity measures, and survival to discharge.[6]

Strategic Evaluation Model

Because any attempt to evaluate an entire system on a day-to-day basis is a costly and time-consuming process, the medical director must focus evaluation efforts on several specific "tracer" medical conditions using structure, process, and outcome measures selectively. The following represents a possible approach:

1. Use intermediate-outcome measures, that is, choose a set of outcome measures that reflect care given at a selected phase along the EMS system continuum (see fig. 23.2).

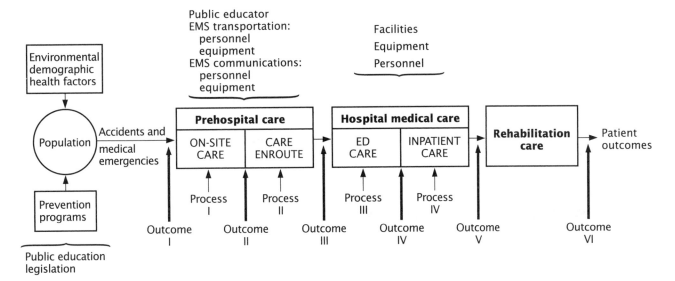

FIGURE 23.2. *Aspects of EMS evaluation.*

2. Use structural (or input) measures to supplement the intermediate-outcome measures.
3. Use process measures to supplement the intermediate-outcome measures.

As defined by Kessner and Kalk, a "tracer" condition should meet the following criteria: it should have a significant functional impact on those affected, be well defined and easy to diagnose in field and practice settings, be sufficiently prevalent to permit the collection of adequate data, have a natural history that varies with use and effectiveness of medical care, have a well defined medical management approach, and be well understood in terms of its socioeconomic effects.[7]

Although other medical conditions and outcome methods can be used, evaluation systems usually begin with cardiac and trauma tracers. Cardiac arrest and major trauma deaths often are used as tracers for medical care evaluation of a system outcome. For cardiac arrest, ventricular fibrillation survival to the hospital and survival until discharged are good measures of a system impact because there are good comparative data available. Attempts to study prehospital cardiac-care outcomes have been limited because of a lack of consistency in the type of sample studied. The literature identifies the following four sampling strategies for prehospital cardiac-care evaluation: (1) patients with out-of-hospital cardiac arrests (2) patients with a final diagnosis of myocardial infarction in hospital discharge records (3) patients with an emergency room diagnosis ruling out myocardial infarc-

tion and (4) those identified by prehospital providers as suspected myocardial infarction patients. Each of these samples has its own potential biases that must be considered when interpreting results. Hearne compiled a comprehensive analysis of cardiac-arrest outcome studies, including case definitions, methodologic characteristics, and summary outcome data.[8] Because of the great variation in definitions of outcome measures, Eisenburg proposed a uniform reporting system.[9] This was followed by the Utstein style for reporting cardiac arrest, which arose from an international conference in 1990.[10] The Utstein style utilizes templates with uniform definitions, resuscitative endpoints, and standard methodologies (fig. 23.3). This has enabled the meaningful comparison of resuscitation efforts in different countries as well as within countries. Prehospital cardiac arrest registries, as in Seattle, have also been developed.[9]

For major trauma, actual survival is often compared with the probability of survival using the injury severity score (ISS) alone or in combination with the TS or RTS (that is, the TRISS method).[11] The American College of Surgeons Committee on Trauma Major Trauma Outcome Study (MTOS) provides data for comparison purposes.[12]

To evaluate trauma care systematically, trauma patient data must be collected on a regional basis. One such example is the organized approach described by Shackford for San Diego County.[13] It is a multidisciplinary, concurrent audit of the quality of medical care in a trauma system. A committee of physicians, nurses, and health officials representing trauma

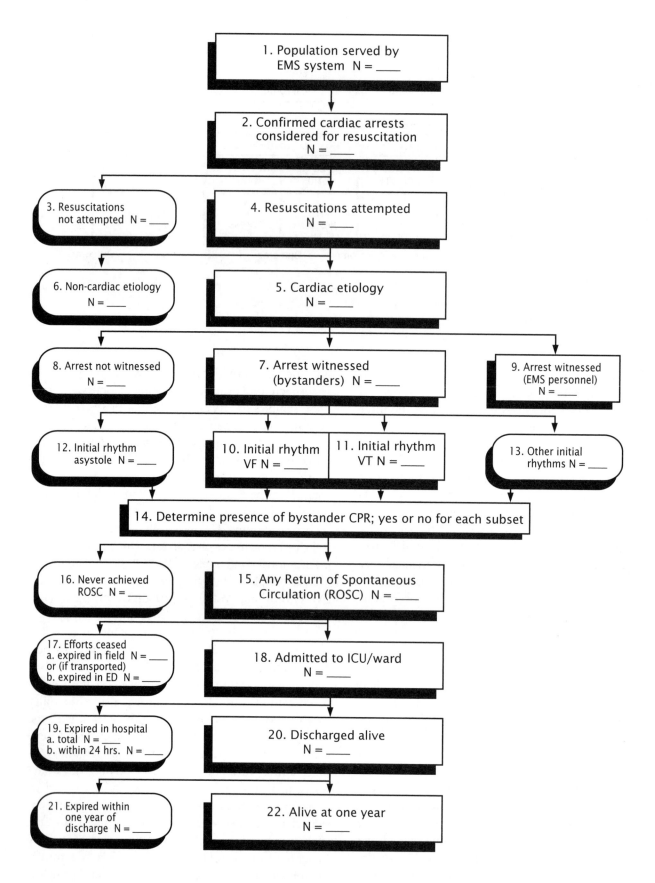

Modified from Annals 20:8:865, 1991.

FIGURE 23.3. *Utstein Style.*

centers, nontrauma hospitals, the public agency administering the trauma system, and a computerized trauma registry are the primary tools. Another approach to outcome assessment for trauma patients is a preventable death study, which can be done by an autopsy method using 500 consecutive deaths caused by motor vehicle accidents. Patients who died from central nervous system or prehospital cardiac arrest injuries are not included; they cannot be effectively studied by this method.[14,15] Each record is assessed by a group of surgeons and emergency physicians according to a set of criteria focused on whether death was preventable. Although this technique is relatively inexpensive, its reliability in different settings is questionable.[16] The clinical method requires only 250 consecutive deaths from motor vehicle accidents obtained by reviewing death certificates.[17] In such a study prehospital, hospital, and medical examiner reports are used. Even though the team used criteria-based worksheets, the degree of subjectivity inherent in these judgments precludes comparing results among geographic areas.

If the proportion of observed deaths is higher than predicted by data from other sources, the medical director should focus evaluation efforts on a basic structural evaluation. Structural evaluations are relatively easy and inexpensive. For example, if the ventricular fibrillation survival rate is low, the evaluator should determine variables such as how many advanced life-support units per 100,000 population the community provides relative to areas reporting better survival rates, the number of paramedics on each run, and the presence or absence of an accompanying basic life support (BLS) response.

Once readily available input standards have been used, attention should be turned to process evaluation. System process measures, such as response time for trauma and cardiac cases and time from injury to operating room in penetrating abdominal cases, are especially useful.[4,13] These simple measures should indicate the system's efficiency in dealing with critical patients. If any of these measures is grossly out of line with national standards or recommendations, action must be taken to improve it.

Assessing individual provider performance is an important part of the ongoing evaluation of prehospital care. Specific analysis formats should be designed for this purpose. Data coded for performance evaluation should also be used for system evaluation. Care must be taken to focus such ambulance run-report analysis to complement the outcome and structural (input) components of the system evaluation

approach. Wading through reams of PCR cross-table analyses is an extremely time-consuming and costly approach to evaluation. If carefully planned, review of PCRs can identify areas of strength and weakness in a system. Considerable experience and data processing sophistication should be used in designing an EMS report form and analysis scheme.

Methodological Issues

In EMS systems there are distinct methodologic issues that must be considered in any evaluation effort. These issues are EMS outcome severity indices, difficulties in developing process criteria, and the reliability and validity of the data.

EMS Outcomes

Recently research has focused on developing nonmortality outcome measures for determining the effectiveness of EMS. Maio, Garrison, and Spaite looked at the six "Ds": survival (death), impaired physiology (disease), limited function (disability), alleviate comfort (discomfort), satisfaction (dissatisfaction) and cost effectiveness (destitution).[18] They used frequency data of EMS services and expert opinion to rank order conditions for children and adults based on their potential value for the study of effectiveness of care. The group has done further work on the development of instruments to measure these various outcomes. A critical factor for this endeavor is to establish outcome measures proximate enough to interventions to reflect their effect.

Severity Indices

To perform acceptable medical outcome evaluation, it is essential that the status of the ill or injured patient be adequately quantified and controlled. Unless control patients for case mix are provided, the results of outcome studies are difficult to interpret and impossible to reproduce.

Although numerous indices quantify the status of injured patients, indices for medical patients remain largely untested. Injury status indices have been designed for a number of purposes including triage, epidemiologic studies, clinical studies, and system studies. An index should be selected with care, as many were not developed with the necessary methodologic rigor to ensure that valid interpretations can be made. Injury indices developed along two lines: anatomic and physiologic. Presently the abbreviated injury scores (AIS) and the injury severity score (ISS) that derived from it are the most widely used anatomic severity scores. The RTS is the most widely used physiologic severity score; the TRISS method, derived from the RTS, the ISS, and age, also has been accepted.

Abbreviated Injury Score

The AIS was first published in 1971 to scale injuries caused by motor vehicle accidents.[19] It grades each of six anatomic regions on a scale of 1 through 5, with 1 considered minor and 5 considered fatal.[20] The AIS was revised in 1976, 1980, 1985, and 1990. The revisions increased the specificity of the coding and assured that the AIS is useful in assessing patients with penetrating injuries. Studies show that the AIS can be reliably abstracted, particularly by physicians and nurses. The average time required per medical record is 10 to 30 minutes, depending on the complexity of the case and the clinical skills of the abstractor.

The values and limitations of the AIS must be taken into consideration. Because it was initially designed for motor vehicle injuries, recent versions attempted to improve it for scaling penetrating injuries. The AIS is not a linear progression; the difference between an AIS 1 and 2 may not be the same as the difference between an AIS 4 and 5.[21] Also, a 3 in a given body area may not be the same as a 3 in another area, although an effort was made to make them roughly comparable. The AIS contains injury codes, and does not code the results of injuries such as blindness. The AIS cannot be determined directly from codes.[22] According to McKenzie, only 67% of the International Classification of Disease (ICDA) codes can be translated directly into AIS codes. However, many of the noncompatible ICD-9 CM codes are infrequently used. McKenzie also found that intrarater abstracting reliability is higher for patients with blunt injuries than patients with penetrating injuries. An AIS cannot be reliably coded from emergency department records, as it requires the complete hospital record. This is particularly true for patients with penetrating injuries. Because hospital record face sheets and computerized hospital data sets do not provide a comprehensive list of all injuries, conversion tables based on current versions of the AIS and ICD-9 CM should be used only for statistical analyses of large data sets looking at trends as areas for further investigation.[23]

Injury Severity Score

The ISS was developed by Baker based on the AIS.[24] The ISS combines the patient's injuries in a single score representing the overall severity of injury. The score is the sum of the squares of the highest AIS value in each of the three most severely injured regions of the body. If there is a score of 6 in any one body system, the maximum overall score of 75, indicating a fatal injury, is given. Injury severity scores range from 1 to 75. Bull and Stoner studied the validity of the ISS and found that it is correlated with such outcomes as length of hospital stay, time of death, disability, necessity for surgery, and plasma cortisol concentrations, but correlated less firmly with mortality and morbidity rates.[25] By itself the ISS explains only 49% of the variance in mortality. Also, a small error in AIS scoring results in a large ISS difference because the AIS is squared.

Osler and Baker have suggested that the ISS be reconfigured to use the AIS values of each of the most severe injuries, regardless of body regions.[26] This modification is called the New Injury Severity Score (NISS). Thus, if a patient has a gunshot wound causing two severe injuries within the abdomen, both are used in calculating the score rather than just the most severe injury. Osler performed retrospective calculations of NISS and comparison of NISS with prospectively calculated ISS, and found NISS to outperform ISS in predicting mortality.[26]

ICISS

Rutledge developed an injury severity scoring system based on the actual survival ratios for each separate injury incurred by a patient.[27] It is called ICISS (International Classification of Disease, 9th Revision Injury Severity Score). Survival risk ratios are calculated for each relevant ICD-9 CM code from the Agency for Healthcare Policy and Research Health Care Utilization Project (HCUP) data base. For each ICD-9 CM code the SRR is calculated by dividing the number of patients in the HCUP having the code who died in the hospital by the number of patients with the code. The product on these ratios yields a predicted probability of survival. Rutledge found that ICISS outperformed both ISS and TRISS as predictors of patient survival, hospital charges, and hospital length of stay.[28] Also, since ICSS is derived directly from ICD coded discharge diagnosis, AIS severity coding is not necessary.

Hannan used New York State Trauma Registry data for patients with blunt injury to predict mortality using three statistical models: (1) the original TRISS based on the Major Trauma Outcome Study coefficients, (2) the new TRISS model, using coefficients derived from New York State data, and (3) ICISS, which predicted values obtained from HCUP.[29] They found that the ICISS model has a better C statistics and better Hosmer Lemeshow statistics while predicting mortality for all adults with blunt injuries. None of the three models predicted mortality accurately for victims of motor vehicle crashes or victims of low falls. The ICISS model had a statistically significantly higher C statistic for other blunt injuries and for motor vehicles crashes. Hannan also noted that both TRISS and ICISS models tested in their study could have been improved by using each of the elements of the Revised Trauma Score as separate independent variables, rather than choosing prior weights for the RTS.

Trauma Score

The TS is a physiologic index derived from the Champion and Sacco Triage Score, which was developed using logistic regression to determine the physiologic variables that best predict mortality.[21] It is not designed for use in small children. The TS is based on systolic blood pressure, respiratory rate, respiratory effort, capillary refill, and the Glasgow Coma Scale (GCS). The TS explains 73% of the variance in trauma mortality.[23]

The data to calculate TS are frequently not available from retrospective studies. Many field providers do not routinely collect GCS scores or capillary refill.[30] The TS has a sensitivity rate of approximately 80%.[23] Thus, 20% of patients with severe injuries will not be identifiable by the TS because they physiologically compensated, or because response time is so fast that decompensation did not take place. The specificity rate for the TS is approximately 75%; it overestimates severity of injury when physiologic changes are related to factors other than hypovolemia, cerebral edema, or hypoxia.[23]

The RTS has dropped capillary refill and respiratory expansion because they are unreliable when collected in the field. It includes only the GCS, systolic blood pressure, and respiratory rate.

TRISS and ASCOT

The TRISS method combines the anatomic ISS, the physiologic TS, and age.[12] Age was added because the MTOS found that a patient age greater than 55 years significantly increased mortality. When ISS is used alone, the score would be identical for a patient with a gunshot wound to the abdomen who was brought promptly to the operating room, and a patient who has spent many hours in the field bleeding into an irreversible shock state. On the other hand, patients with identical TS scores could have vastly different ISS scores, depending on the amount of time following the injury when the TS is measured and on the physiologic response of the patient. Using ISS, TS, age, and coefficient based on whether the injuries were blunt or penetrating, a probability of survival (PS) for a group of patients can be calculated and compared with a large data base such as the MTOS.[11,31,32] Such a comparison uses the Z statistic to relate the observed to the predicted survival rates in two populations. The M statistic assures that different ranges of trauma scores between the two populations do not distort the comparison. The M statistic comparison prevents the bias that results when a population with fewer injured patients and a high percentage of survival is compared with a population with more severely injured patients and a lower percentage of survival. The RTS replaced the TS in the TRISS method for developing outcome norms.

Sacco and Champion developed an Anatomic Profile based on AIS but giving more weight to severe head and chest injuries than to abdomen and extremity injuries. They use the Anatomic Profile together with the Revised Trauma Score and age as an index called ACSCOT (a severity characterization of trauma).[33] Though it is a somewhat better predictor of survival, it has been more complicated to calculate and less widely utilized than TRISS.[8] The Anatomic Profile has been further modified to demonstrate even greater discrimination and calibration.[34]

Both TRISS and ACSCOT use large data bases to develop coefficients to calculate the probability of survival for each patient. Separate coefficients are used for both blunt and penetrating injuries. Cayten found that hospital comparisons can be done more effectively where penetrating injuries use separate coefficients for gunshot wounds and stab wounds, and blunt injuries use separate coefficients for motor vehicle crashes, low falls, and other blunt injury categories.[35] This has been confirmed in further studies.[23]

Process Criteria

Explicit criteria are specific, written criteria used to evaluate care; *implicit* criteria are in the minds of evaluators when judging the quality of care. The use of explicit criteria is more objective and reliable. There are several different methods by which explicit process criteria can be developed. All methods attempt to achieve some degree of consensus either by reference to textbooks, expert panels, small group discussions, questionnaires to larger groups, or statistical summaries.[36]

It is often difficult to establish process criteria, particularly if they need to be detailed and specify the sequencing of treatments.[37] Once process criteria are established, they are usually employed in a checklist format to score prehospital, direct medical control, and emergency department forms. Generally, such criteria are used to screen for cases that should be reviewed in more depth. Few attempts have been made to weigh process criteria for EMS evaluation, although this has been attempted for other types of medical audit.

One of the most sophisticated approaches to the use of process criteria for EMS system evaluation has been developed by Wolfe.[38] The criteria are algorithms that are weighted and programmed allowing PCR data to be computer-scored. The computer compares recommended treatment with the treatment actually recorded, and the appropriateness of each step is scored. Cases in which the treatment provided varies significantly from that specified by the algorithm are screened out by the computer for in-depth medical review. Although the criteria require that certain actions are taken within specified periods of time, the scoring system does not take into account sequences of actions when multiple actions are required during the same period of time. An in-depth discussion on using process criteria is in the chapter on quality management.

Reliability, Validity and Abstraction

The satisfactory quality of data used for evaluation should not be taken for granted. Both the reliability and validity of the data should be considered. Reliability is the extent to which measurement results are free from experimental error and are therefore reproducible. Reliability depends on the consistency of the characteristic being measured from individual to individual (homogeneity across individuals) and its stability over time. A measurement can be reliable with-out being valid. Reliability, however, establishes the upper boundary of validity because an unreliable scale cannot be a valid one. Validity is the extent to which the data are unbiased and relevant to the characteristic being measured. In this sense, data measurement should be free of systematic error caused by the measuring instrument itself, the user of the instrument, the subject, or the environment in which the scaling procedure is administered.

In terms of the overall design of evaluation efforts, Sherman presented a case study describing his evaluation of mobile intensive care units; 18 threats to the validity of the evaluation and methods used to control these threats were discussed.[39] He concluded that the major threats to validity are the effects of history, maturation, instrumentation, regression, and the potential interaction of selection and experimental unit composition. A list of these potential parameters and the methods to control them might be a useful guide to EMS evaluators in the planning stage. Through identifying and documenting potential threats to validity, the overall quality and credibility of EMS evaluations should improve.

There are two additional concerns. The first is the validity with which the care providers make the observations or measurements, and the second is the reliability of the data abstracting and recording processes. Cayten conducted a study assessing the validity of EMS data.[22] Emergency department nurses and EMT-As took simultaneous vital sign measurements with nurses who were specially trained and standardized against measuring devices. Tolerance limits were developed for the quantitative variables. Table 23.1 shows that emergency care personnel did better assessing qualitative variables than quantitative. Among quantitative variables, diastolic blood pressure was the least accurately assessed. Certain participants had a tendency to "err" in the sense that they disagreed with the standard on several of the variables. This study indicates that users of basic clinical data must establish their level of validity before interpreting the results based on them. When it is essential that all the data are of high quality or that critical medical decisions will be based on the data, multiple measurements may be necessary, as well as an ongoing emphasis on carefully obtaining accurate data.

Hermann investigated the interobserver reliability in the collection of EMS data.[40] In this study, charts were selected from five hospitals to test the interobserver reliability of nurse abstractors. Different nurses reabstracted the charts. The results show that there is

		TABLE 23.1		
		Comparison of ED Nurses and EMT-As in Vital Sign Observations		
VARIABLE	**GROUP**	**OBSERVATIONS WITHIN LIMITS**	**TOTAL OBSERVATIONS**	**PROPORTION WITHIN TOLERANCE LIMITS**
Systolic BP	ED Nurses	66	80	.825
	EMT-As	91	115	.791
Pulse rate	ED Nurses	65	80	.813
	EMT-As	86	116	.741
Respiration rate	ED Nurses	56	80	.700
	EMT-As	84	116	.724
Diastolic BP	ED Nurses	51	80	.638
	EMT-As	61	114	.535

	EMT Observations in Agreement with Standard		
VARIABLE	**OBSERVATIONS WITH AGREEMENTS**	**TOTAL OBSERVATIONS**	**PROPORTION WITH AGREEMENT**
Age	116	116	1.00
Neck vein distention	114	116	.983
Pupil size equality	113	116	.974
Level of consciousness	112	116	.966
Pupil reactivity	112	116	.966
Pupil size	110	116	.948
Obesity	108	116	.931
Pulse character	104	116	.929
Respiration character	99	115	.861
Pulse regularity	98	116	.845

considerable variability in the accuracy with which the different variables were abstracted. Intraobserver abstracting reliability was consistently better than interobserver abstracting reliability. For the 26 variables studied, intraobserver values ranged from 0.62 to 0.99 with most falling above 0.80. This means vital signs had interobserver agreement of 0.95 or better; however, final diagnosis, emergency department diagnosis, condition on arrival, and elapsed time since onset had interobserver values of less than 0.60.

Linn similarly found that the accuracy with which data are abstracted from medical records leaves a great deal to be desired.[41] He found that when nurse clinicians abstracted medical record data using 33 data elements, there were discrepancies in 16% of the cases. In coding the major diagnosis, there was a 46% discrepancy. Therefore, when system evaluation requires abstraction of data from records, periodic review of both intraobserver and interobserver reliability testing must be performed.

Population-Based Evaluation

Population-based studies provide information on all patients in a given region, state, or country. This is particularly important for EMS systems, since many patients never get into the system. Population-based goals have been used extensively in the Centers for Disease Control goals for the United States: Health People 2000.[42] When prehospital cardiac case was in its infancy Crampton used population-based data to establish its value.[43] Mullins and Mann recently reviewed the population-based research assessing the effectiveness of trauma systems. He listed the types of databases used as follows: death certificates, hospital discharge claims data, and fatal accident reporting system (FARS).[44] Though limited in the clinical information available in these sources, population-based studies can be used to monitor the aggregated impact of multiple initiatives.[45]

Population-based evaluation also lends itself to data set linkages. The National Highway Safety Administration (NHTSA) has supported state data linkage projects (CODES) to assess the impact of various injury prevention initiatives such as the use of passenger restraint devices. Data linked included police crash reports, PCRs, hospital discharge abstracts, and death certificates. Where a common identifying number is not found on the data sources to be linked, computer-matching software programs have been used.

Summary

EMS system evaluation should be viewed as an ongoing process; the general goals of the system and each of its components provide a framework for planning, management, and evaluation. Initially the adequacy of the various components of the EMS system must be assessed. Objectives then give rise to alternative courses of action, and from these alternatives, specific programs are selected for implementation. Thereafter, system and subsystem performance are monitored continually to evaluate effectiveness of programs and determine whether objectives have been achieved.

Evaluation is a key aspect of the EMS planning process. Its purpose is to indicate whether EMS systems are effective in diminishing death and reducing disability; more important, they demonstrate where improvements are needed. Techniques for evaluating EMS systems include assessments of system structure, medical care process, and patient outcomes. System evaluation studies the results of system and subsystem function, regardless of specific programs designed for each area.

In EMS system evaluation the case mix must be precisely described and reliable. In addition, valid process criteria and outcome measures must be developed. In general, two techniques have been employed to define case mix: specifying tracer medical conditions by diagnostic codes, and using severity indices. It is also essential to develop explicit criteria for assessing the quality of care when process evaluation is used. The limitations of severity scales must be fully understood.

Care must be taken to assure that the data used for EMS evaluation are valid and reliably collected. Specialized data collections for evaluation and research purposes alone are expensive and often do not provide sufficient sample size for statistical significance. Because in many situations EMS system evaluators will be interested in using data that are collected on an ongoing basis, it is essential for EMS medical directors and researchers to develop quality controls in the data collection process.

References

1. Thomas W, Cayten CG. Emergency medical services planning and evaluation. In: Schwartz GR, ed. *Principles and Practice of Emergency Medicine*. Philadelphia: WB Saunders Co.; 1986.

2. Cayten CG, Evans WJ. EMS systems evaluation. In: Boyd D, Edlich R, Mycik S, eds. *Systems Approach to Emergency Medical Care*. Appleton-Century-Crofts; 1983.

3. Donabedian A. *A Guide to Medical Care Administration*. Vol. 2. Medical care appraisal—quality and utilization. New York: American Public Health Association; 1969.

4. Gibson G. Guidelines for research and evaluation of emergency medical services. *Health Serv Res.* 1974;89:99.

5. Jacobs LM, et al. Prehospital advanced life support: benefits in trauma. *J Trauma.* 1984;24:8–13.

6. Pozen M. *Confirmation Parameters for Assessing Prehospital Care.* Final Report. Hyattsville, MD: National Center for Health Services Research; 1980.

7. Kessner DM, Kalk CE, Siner J. Assessing health quality: the case for tracers. *N Engl J Med.* 1973;288:1891–1894.

8. Hearne T. The development of emergency medical services. In: Eisenberg MS, Bergner T, and Hallstrorn AP, eds. Sudden Cardiac Death in the Community. New York: Praeger Publishers; 1984.

9. Eisenberg MS, Bergner L, Hearne T. Out-of-hospital cardiac arrest: a review of major studies and a prospered uniform reporting system. *Am J Public Health.* 1980;236–240.

10. Cummins RO, Chamberlin DA, Abramson NS, et al. Recommended guidelines for uniform reporting of data from out-of-hospital cardiac arrest: The Utstein Style. Task Force of the American Heart Association, the European Resuscitation Council, the Heart and Stroke Foundation of Canada, and the Australian Resuscitation Council. *Ann Emerg Med.* 1991;20:861–874.

11. American College of Surgeons Committee on Trauma. Quality assessment and assurance in trauma care. *Bull Am Coll Surgeons.* 1986;71:4–23.

12. Boyd CR, Tolson MA, Copes WS. Evaluating trauma care: the TRISS method. *J Trauma.* 1987;27:370–378.

13. Shackford SR, et al. The effect of regionalization upon quality of trauma care as assessed by concurrent and it before and after institution of a trauma system: a preliminary report. *J Trauma.* 1986;26:812–820.

14. West JG. An autopsy method of evaluating trauma care. *J Trauma.* 1981;21:32–34.

15. West JG. Validation of autopsy method for evaluating trauma care. *Arch Surg.* 1982;117:1033–1035.

16. MacKenzie EJ, Steinwachs DM, Bone LR, et al. Inter-rater reliability of preventable death judgments. *J Trauma.* 1992;33:292–303.

17. Cales R. *Medical evaluation in trauma care systems.* Rockville, MD: Aspen Publications; 1986.

18. Maio RF, Garrison HG, Spaite DW, et al. Emergency medical services outcome project I (EMSOP I): prioritizing conditions for outcomes research. *Ann Emerg Med.* 1999;33:423–432.

19. Petrucelli E, States JD, Homes LN. The abbreviated injury scale: evaluation, usage and future adaptability. *Accid Anal Prev.* 1981;13:29–35.

20. American Association for Automotive Medicine. *The Abbreviated Injury Scale.* 1985 revision. Arlington Heights, IL: The Association; 1985.

21. Champion HR, Sacco WJ, Hung TK. Trauma severity scoring to predict mortality. *World J Surg*. 1983;7:4–11.
22. Cayten CG, et al. Assessing the validity of EMS data. *J Am Coll Emerg Physicians*. 1978;7:390–396.
23. MacKenzie EJ. Injury severity scales: overview and directions for future research. *Am J Emerg Med*. 1984;2:537–548.
24. Baker SP, et al. The injury severity score: a method for describing patients with multiple injuries and evaluating emergency care. *J Trauma*. 1974;14:187–196.
25. Bull JP. The injury severity score of road traffic casualties In relation to mortality, time of death, hospital treatment time and disability. *Accid Anal Prev*. 1978;7:249.
26. Osler T, Baker SP, Long W. A modification of the Injury Severity Score that both improves accuracy and simplified scoring. *J Trauma*. 1997;43:922–926.
27. Rutledge R, Fakhry S, Baker C, Oller D. Injury severity grading in trauma patients: a simplified technique based upon ICD-9 coding. *J Trauma*. 1993;435–497.
28. Rutledge R, Osler R, Emery S, et al. The end of the Injury Severity Score (ISS) and the Trauma and Injury Severity Score (TRISS): ICISS and international classification of diseases, ninth revision-based prediction tool, outperforms both the ISS and TRISS as predictors of trauma patient survival, hospital charges, and hospital length of stay. *J Trauma*. 1998;44:41–49.
29. Hannan EL, Farrell LS, Garthy CH, et al. Predictors of mortality in adult patients with blunt injuries in New York State: a comparison of TRISS and ICISS. *J Trauma*. 1999;47:8–14.
30. Moreau M, et al. Application of trauma score in the prehospital setting. *Ann Emerg Med*. 1985;14:1049–1054.
31. Champion HR. Major trauma outcome study. Bulletin to participants, Feb 1986.
32. Champion HR, Frey CF, Sacco WJ. Determination of national normative outcomes for trauma. *J Trauma*. 1984;24:651.
33. Champion HR, Copes WS, Sacco WJ, et al. Improved predictions from a severity characterization of trauma (ASCOT) over trauma and injury Score (TRISS): Results of an independent evaluation. *J Trauma*. 1996:40:42–49.
34. Sacco WJ, Mackenzie EJ, Champion HR, et al. Comparison of alternative methods for assessing injury based on anatomics descriptors. *J Trauma*. 1999;47:441–447.
35. Cayten CG, Stahl WM, Murphy JG. Limitations of the TRISS method for interhospital comparison: a multihospital study. *J Trauma*. 1991;31:471.
36. Romm FJ, Hulka BS. Developing criteria for quality of care assessment: effect of the delphi technique. *Health Serv Res*. 1979;14:309–312.
37. Cole L, et al. Prehospital cardiac care—illusion of consensus. *J Am Coll Emerg Physicians*. 1977;6:552–555.
38. Wolfe H. Computerized model for EMS performance. PHS 80–3271. Washington, DC: Department of Health and Human Services; 1980.
39. Sherman M, et al. Threats to the validity of emergencies services evaluation: a case study of mobile intensive care units. *Care*. 1979;17:127–138.
40. Hermann N, et al. Interobserver and intraobserver reliability in the collection of emergency medical services data. *Health Serv Res*. 1980;15:127–143.
41. Linn BS. Effort of Burn Education on Quality of Emergency Care. Washington, DC: National Center for Health Services Research Management Series; 1975–1978.
42. U.S. Department of Health and Human Services. *Healthy People 2000. National Health Promotion and Disease Prevention Objectives*. Washington, DC: Public Health Services; 1991.
43. Crampton RS, Aldrich RF, Gascho JA, et al. Reduction of prehospital, ambulance and community coronary death rates by the community-wide emergency cardiac care system. *Am J Medicine*. 1975;58:151–165.
44. Mullins RJ, Mann NC. Population-based research assessing the effectiveness of trauma systems. *J Trauma*. 1999; 47:441–447.
45. Cayten CG, Quervalu I, Agarwal N. Fatality analysis reporting system demonstrates association between trauma system initiative and decreasing death rates. *J Trauma*. 1998;46:751–756.

Research

Donald M. Yealy, MD

Introduction

Prehospital care administrators experienced a "honeymoon" from the early 1970s until recently. Therapeutic interventions and system configurations were employed based on limited scientific data. Treatments usually were extrapolated directly from the hospital setting, even though the prehospital environment is markedly different.[1,2] EMS must prove what is beneficial. EMS researchers have begun to respond to this need, conducting large trials on the value the role of each facet of the prehospital "chain of survival"—from bystander CPR to basic automatic defibrillation to system use of paramedics.[3,4,5] Additionally, academic prehospital-care physicians interested in professional advancement must show the same ability to expand the knowledge base of their chosen field as the more traditional medical academicians.

This chapter highlights the basic features, and identifies the potential benefits and pitfalls of prehospital research. This chapter is not a cookbook for EMS research, nor does it obviate the need for accessing other sources on research design. The following section helps medical directors start or better supervise research and avoid certain traps.

Benefits of Prehospital Research

The first benefit of prehospital research is that data obtained can help improve the care of those treated. This fact contrasts the perception that care is variable in a randomized research trial and some patients will have a worse outcome. Patients treated within a well designed protocol generally receive high-level, homogenous care. The knowledgeable investigator tries to control all outside influences and ancillary treatments to detect the effect of the study intervention. Data from inpatient research suggests that many patients in an experimental trial demonstrate greater

subjective and objective improvement than those with similar diseases treated outside a study protocol.[6,7] These benefits may occur even when subjects are randomized to an intervention that eventually proves less effective. This result is due to a well defined, consistent study treatment plan (including ancillary treatments) coupled with vigilant monitoring for benefit or harm. To reap these advantages the investigator must carefully plan the trial so the study intervention and ancillary care are practical, medically sound, clearly defined, and monitored.

When a trial is well designed, closely monitored, and successful in answering a question, many benefit. All involved gain insight in the pathophysiology of the problem studied. The authors and the system gain academic recognition. The field providers derive satisfaction from seeing "science in the field" impact care.[8] The people in the system learn that medical practice is dynamic, and gain better understanding about the natural evolution of care. Thus clinical skills, judgment, and *esprit de corps* are improved

Basic Research Design

Although cellular and animal experiments are common in biomedical research, EMS research largely focuses on the investigation of humans, including both patients and providers. The interventions that have been studied range from a drug to a method of managing resources.

Research trials can be performed using a variety of formats. The researcher and medical director must choose between less sophisticated but more "doable" designs and more detailed but difficult designs. The reader is referred to other works for a more "nuts-and-bolts" approach to research design and implementation.[6,9–12]

Research designs can be broadly divided into the following two categories: *observational* and *experimental* studies. In observational designs, events are monitored and analyzed without attempts to manipulate or alter the outcome. Traditional quality management (QM) often follows this format. For example, the administration of a specific drug by paramedics can be monitored and analyzed to discover the patterns that govern its use. Although this design is simple, it cannot define cause-and-effect relationships. *Qualitative* studies are a variant of observational designs in which events are analyzed without attempts to measure outcomes in traditional "unit" values, but rather measure more subjective features.

Experimental designs introduce an intervention (or exposure) and monitor its effect on outcome. Most experimental designs in human research are *quasi-experiments*. The latter term reflects the lack of absolute control over all events and characteristics (variables) needed to create a true experiment.[9,10] Although animal and human trials seek to control all interventions and treatments, in clinical practice this is impossible. Particularly in prehospital investigations, not every factor that can influence outcome may be recognized, and therefore not controlled (confounders). This lack of control can cloud or magnify any difference noted after treatment. True experiments occur only when all variables influencing outcome are identified and controlled. For convenience, the term "experiment" in this chapter is used to denote both true and quasi-experiments.

In general, observational studies are easier to perform than experimental studies; however, experimental studies afford the investigator an improved ability to define any cause-and-effect relationship. Prehospital research, especially disaster medicine, lends itself to observational studies because the events studied are sporadic, beyond control, and unpredictable. In these specific investigations, meticulous attention to obtaining data in a detailed and structured format produces information better able to define potential causality. Events that occur more frequently or more predictably are studied better using an experimental design once the problem is defined.

Another factor in choosing a specific research design hinges on the length of time subjects will be studied. *Cross-sectional* designs measure all variables at one time; the traditional survey is an example of a cross-sectional design. The trials are easy to perform, and provide data on the prevalence of an outcome or other measured variable in a population. However, cross-sectional designs cannot prove a cause-and-effect relationship among variables or events.

Longitudinal studies follow a group of subjects over time and can better determine a cause-and-effect relationship. This benefit is not without cost; longitudinal studies usually require more time and effort than cross-sectional designs. Longitudinal designs can be further categorized based on the timing of outcome measurement relative to patient identification and enrollment. *Case-control* studies identify a specific outcome and then find what past actions or characteristics could account for the outcome. *Cohort* designs identify potential enrollees without the desired outcome and follow them over time to detect differences in outcomes (sometimes after differing exposure to a treatment) or measured variables.

Prospective designs are those that follow subjects forward in time—that is, the investigators identify a question and create a tool to measure before any care, exposure, or observations occur. *Retrospective* designs look backward in time to answer a question, often using chart reviews or tools designed to measure outcomes for another purpose. For example, a retrospective case-control study of cardiac arrest could identify survivors and then compare their treatments and characteristics with those of non-survivors. A prospective cohort design could enroll patients in cardiac arrest, observe or manipulate therapies, and measure outcomes. Most case-control designs are retrospective, and most cohort designs are prospective, but exceptions exist. For example, a large cohort can be studied over time and a question asked after the observation interval is complete. Using a tool designed to extract information—a retrospective cohort design can be created. In EMS, cardiac arrest database studies offer this potential; the recent Ontario Prehospital Advanced Life Support (OPALS) trial was an experimental cohort design, but the rich data set created potential for future retrospective cohort and case-control designs.[3,7]

Although both types of longitudinal studies enhance the ability to define causal relationships compared with cross-sectional designs, well designed prospective cohort trials are less prone to biases and error than retrospective and case-control trials. The researcher can specify when and what interventions, measurements, and ancillary treatments are to be performed during a prospective trial. In retrospective and case-control designs the investigator is "at the mercy" of what was done and recorded. Again the benefits of a prospective trial usually require more time, effort, and money.

Because of these limitations, observational and cross-sectional designs are useful to generate and refine questions rather than solve problems. A retrospective study can further refine the question and provide preliminary data regarding the answer. When an event or outcome is rare (for example, survival from asystole), a retrospective case-control design may be the most practical method of evaluating a problem. Prospective experimental designs are best used for mature research questions (that is, those questions well refined by previous studies) pertaining to common or predictable events. Thus an investigator with a question in previously "uncharted waters" creates the basis for a series of works, beginning with cross-sectional and observational studies and culminating in a prospective experiment.

Randomization and Blinding

Two features can limit the biases that creep into prospective experimental designs: randomization and blinding. *Randomized* assignment of subjects is done to ensure that the characteristics of each group are similar at entry into a trial, and that any unknown influences throughout the trial are evenly distributed between groups. Randomization does not obliterate all inqualities between groups in a comparative trial, but it does lessen the potential. *True randomization* means that each subject has an equal chance of being assigned to any of the treatment groups. This is usually done with a text or computer-generated table of random numbers, although the time-honored "coin flip" is equally valid. Alternatives to true randomization including "every other" patterns (for example, every other patient, every other day or week) or assignment based on seemingly haphazard variables (for example, birthdate, social security number) ease the perceived logistic difficulties with in-field randomization. These alternatives should be used sparingly, because the benefits are slight and the protection from group inequalities is less than that provided by randomization.

Some investigators employ the *natural assignment* method, where exposures or treatments are allowed to occur in groups that appear otherwise matched. This includes "off/on" or "run in" trials, where an intervention is allowed to occur "on its own" or with some prompting, but not in a rigorous method. Natural assignment is useful when it is impossible to otherwise assign treatment—for example, in the OPALS design where the presence of paramedic care could not be added nor removed for experimental purposes.[7] This design may be the "best compromise," even with the known threats to validity.

Blinding refers to actions that prevent participants from knowing which specific intervention is being used during the trial. If only the study subject is unaware, the design is single-blinded. If the study subjects and data collectors are unaware, the design is double-blinded; triple-blinding means the subjects, data collector, and caring providers are all unaware. Blinding limits natural biases about the utility of any interventions. Some interventions cannot be blinded, especially device applications such as pneumatic anti-shock garments, immobilization devices, or airway products.

Even when blinding appears simple, the researcher must vigilantly ensure that it occurs. Curiosity can spur patients and care providers to devise ingenious methods to unblind a trial. For example, a prehospital trial comparing outcomes in patients with electro-mechanical disassociation treated with dexamethasone or a saline placebo fell prey to this ingenuity.[13] Some of the field providers tasted the study solution before administering it; a salty taste identified the placebo, thus unblinding the trial. The effect of this knowledge on the other events occurring during resuscitation is unclear; a potential bias existed that could not be resolved by data analysis.

Experimental designs often compare a new intervention to the current standard therapy; this is termed a *controlled* trial. A "no-treatment" control also helps identify the natural course of events in the trial. In the absence of a control group, the experimental effect may be overestimated. *Concurrent* controls are those observed at the same time interval as the experimental group, while *historical* controls are drawn from the past. As expected, concurrent control groups limit confounding effects and biases (especially changes in populations or care over time, called *secular* influences) compared to historical controls, though the latter design is easier.

Both the experimental (new) and control (standard or absent) treatments may be amenable to blinding, especially in drug trials. Although intended to be pharmacologically or physically inactive, *placebos* may produce a subjective or objective benefit, though aside from analgesic trials, the effect of this is unproven. This fact justifies their use in trials involving nonlife-threatening diseases. When a standard of care exists, irrespective of its absolute effectiveness, it should be used as the control agent in the experiment.[14,15]

A prospective, randomized controlled experiment, particularly when coupled with blinding procedures, is best able to provide data to define a cause-and-effect relationship. These trials are the "gold standard" in biomedical research, but are not the most common design in current published EMS literature.[16] This is because of the effort, practical barriers, and finances required to complete such trials.

Data Analysis

The basic goal of statistical analysis is to help organize and compare information from research trials. *Descriptive* statistics allow a large body of data to be summarized, thus painting a picture of what happened during the observational or experimental period in a compact and organized form. A measurement of the central tendency (the average) such as the mean, median, or mode, and a measurement of the variability of the individual scores (the standard deviation and range) are helpful.[12,17] When reporting on exclusive events (such as survived or died, male or female, improved, worsened or no change) frequency tables and cumulative totals organize the results. Some data are easier to interpret if grouped in more meaningful sets such as percentiles or quartiles.[11]

Analytic statistics compare groups by determining whether a difference truly exists or can be excluded. Since many trials intend to prove that a different outcome occurs after an intervention, the major goal of analytic evaluation is to provide a mathematic estimate of the probability that any observed difference could have been the result of chance alone. This estimate is communicated as the familiar p (for probability) value. The p value asks "How likely is it that my data are fooling me and chance alone could account for any differences?" When a chance event is erroneously thought to be due to a treatment effect, a Type I (or alpha) error is committed. One can never eliminate the possibility of a Type I error, but before data are collected and analyzed the acceptable probability of error should be set. By convention, if p is less than or equal to 1 in 20, results are considered significant.

If no mathematic difference is seen between two or more groups, analytic statistics can define the Type II (or beta) error. A Type II error occurs when a true treatment effect was not detected. This usually results from inadequate sample size or excessive variability among individual observations. Analogous to the p value is the power calculation, which estimates the likelihood that a difference could have been detected given the study population and variability. Thus it answers for us, "How hard did we look for a difference?" The power estimation is related to the Type II error and is equal to 1 – beta. The conventionally acceptable Type II error is 1 in 5 (0.20) or less. This value correlates to a power of 0.80 or higher.

A more popular way to analyze data comparatively is to use confidence intervals (CI).[12,18] These calculate the likely range of values that could exist if the experiment or observations were continued on infinitely. Either a 95% or a 99% CI can be calculated—saying that "if measured again and again in new subjects with the same design, 95% or 99% of the time the population mean effect would fall in this range." When CIs do not overlap between therapies or after different exposures, it suggests the effect difference is both present and unlikely due to chance (similar to p value calculation).

Contrary to popular belief, analytic testing does *not* evaluate the clinical importance of the observations. Low p values, big differences in CIs, and high power estimates do not mean more important observations, but merely estimate the mathematic likelihood of error. There are a multitude of analytic tests to compare data, and the choice is driven by the type of data collected and the specific comparison sought. Also, likelihood ratios, predictive probabilities for diseases or outcomes, and "number needed to treat" calculations can offer insight into differing therapies. The reader is referred to more exhaustive works for further details on these issues.[6,9–11,12] In practice, it is best to consult with a research design and analysis person early in the process of asking questions—they can help avoid analytic problems as the question and outcomes of interest are defined.

Pitfalls in EMS Research

Well designed prehospital research provides many benefits, but certain pitfalls must be avoided. Identifying these traps before and during a study creates research that improves patient care and reduces frustration.

Ask a Focused Question

The conclusions reached from a study depend on why the data were obtained. A common reason that a trial fails to get "off the ground" or is rejected for publication is the absence of a clear and important question. Without a question, an answer cannot follow. Information from an unfocused investigation will produce data that are difficult to interpret.

The question asked should be important to the researcher and to others in the field. Embarking on the project simply because it has "never been investigated" may waste resources. Many problems that arise during data collection, analysis, and publication can be corrected, but an unimportant question is irreparable. One should ask colleagues and other experts for advice before investing resources in an idea. Simply put, the question must pass the "So what?" test.

Although useful information may be gleaned from a trial intended to answer a question on an unrelated topic, this is the exception rather than the rule. Good research is focused; ask a specific question, then design a trial that answers that question. One helpful exercise is to write in one or two succinct sentences the questions that are important before starting any research endeavor. After generating a list, set priorities and focus the first trial on the most important questions. The question may be modified later, but starting with a clear focus improves the quality of both the design and the data collected. If a long list of questions is created, initially focus on the top two, the rest will serve as incentive for later trials.

Write a Clear Hypothesis

Not only must a question be asked, but it must be focused; a hypothesis is generated based on the question. The hypothesis is a declarative thought to be disproven or not disproven (it can never be definitively "proven"). The null hypothesis states that no difference will exist between two or more groups after treatment. The research (or alternated) hypothesis states that a difference or change will be seen between groups. The research hypothesis can be either directional (that is, states whether improvement or worsening in an outcome will be noted) or nondirectional (that is, does not indicate which therapy is better or worse). A study of adenosine use in the prehospital treatment of narrow complex tachycardia could test any one of the following hypotheses:

Null—Heart rate and blood pressure will be unaltered after treatment with adenosine.
Research (nondirectional)—Heart rate and blood pressure after adenosine therapy will differ from pretreatment values.
Research (directional)—Heart rate will be significantly lower and blood pressure higher after adenosine therapy compared with pretreatment values.

Each hypothesis differs slightly, although all are acceptable and overlap. Usually the null hypothesis is chosen in formal research design because comparative statistics either reject or fail to reject this statement.

The use of a null hypothesis is not mandatory; the key is choosing a clear, concise hypothesis.

Some observational designs simply intend to describe "what's happening," or generate background information on a disease, population, intervention, or system. A formal hypothesis is not appropriate; however, a clear, simple objective must be stated. For example, "We sought to describe the EMS providers' attitudes about cessation of field resuscitation in our system" is a clear objective, while "We followed the results of our field resuscitation termination protocol" is ambiguous.

First Search the Literature

After a specific research question is created, the literature must be reviewed in at least two computerized searches (using Medline or another search service), followed by a manual review of the cited references. Sometimes the question will be answered and validated by previously published works, obviating the need for a trial. More commonly, information about unanticipated problems or useful methods to measure outcomes is discovered; then the question can be refined or the design adjusted to avoid potential traps. The search may eliminate the need to "reinvent the wheel" during protocol development. When the search is complete, the investigator should be an expert on the topic.

Before a prospective trial is conducted, the available data should suggest that each treatment has an equal chance of benefitting the subjects. Although final analysis may demonstrate that one treatment is better than another, knowledge of this before the trial obviates the need for an investigation. Usually, the investigators *believe* one treatment will be more beneficial before designing a trial; however, this belief does not constitute scientific knowledge.

Decide What to Measure and Then Seek Bias

Once the hypothesis is generated and refined, the next step is deciding what measurements are needed. The characteristics and responses quantified are *variables*; these range from age, sex, weight, and height to blood pressure, survival rates, and neurologic function scores. Three types of variables are seen in research trials; often, events that are one type of variable in a particular design serve a different function in another design.

Dependent (or response) variables are measured to define the outcomes of a study and the effect portion (for example, blood pressure, peak flow rate, or survival after treatment) or any cause-and-effect relationship. *Independent* (or classification-treatment) variables defining the cause are factors brought into a study (for example, age, sex, weight) or imposed by the investigator (for example, dose of drug). Extraneous variables are also called noise or confounding variables; as the names suggest, these events or characteristics are beyond control or not recognized, yet still influence observations.

Bias is a distortion of any relationship between cause-and-effect; it occurs when extraneous variables alter results or when the dependent or independent variables are not properly controlled or measured. The investigator must anticipate all sources of bias and seek to reduce them. This is best done through careful thought and "bouncing" the idea around with colleagues.

Define the Population

Before enrolling subjects, the researcher must ask, "What is my target universe?" and "Do I have access to that or a similar group?" The target universe is all people who could be studied (for example, all patients with out-of-hospital arrest or all patients with severe pulmonary edema). Once they have defined the universe, investigators must determine if they have access to part of it; in practice, no one has access to the entire target universe. If a group that is similar to the target universe is accessible, a research trial is feasible. If only a dissimilar group or a very small number of subjects similar to the target universe are accessible, a study will not be meaningful.

Seek Help with Statistics

Before writing a protocol, an investigator who is unfamiliar with this area should seek the help of a statistician, especially in an experimental comparative trial. In addition to formulating a strategy for data tabulation and analysis, the statistician can determine the size of the study population needed. Sometimes, it is obvious that the question asked requires such large numbers of subjects that it cannot be done in a timely or economic fashion. This consultation prevents the investigator from performing a study that cannot provide the information desired, or worse, provides misleading information. It also prevents unnecessarily enrolling too many subjects.

Before approaching the statistician, the investigator decides what measurements are the most important and how much difference between groups is clinically important. These two factors guide the sample size determination; often, investigators decide on these after the trial is complete, based on the results of mathematic manipulations. The latter produces data with statistical significance but without clinical significance.

Create a Protocol

The key to protocol development is precise identification of the actions taken and information collected. It must be clear who is eligible for enrollment, what measurements are to be made by whom, and what interventions will occur. Measurements as simple as weight (estimated, in metric or English units) and blood pressure (palpated, auscultated, by whom, and with what technique) are a source of confusion and error if not specifically defined.

Unless similar trials have been completed previously, research protocols usually require multiple drafts to refine. These drafts are circulated among colleagues and local or national experts to improve the quality of data collected. At this point it is wise to involve those responsible for data collection and subject treatment. The actual providers are often ignored in this stage of research. Often a "street-smart" prehospital provider provides practical tips to streamline the protocol.[8]

Whenever economically feasible and practical, persons collecting data should not be responsible for providing clinical care. Having a research assistant with medical knowledge ride along to ensure protocol adherence improves the quality of the data collected. This approach, although costly, reduces the perception of "extra work" by the field providers. Often, students, off-duty medics, or others perform this task on a voluntary or stipend arrangement.

Regardless of who treats subjects and collects data, each action should be as simple as possible. It is tempting to collect mountains of data. Although data uncollected are lost forever, there is a diminishing return to recording more information in the field. Clinical experience suggests that the accuracy of data collection is inversely proportional to the complexity and number of data points. Use the specific hypothesis as a reference point—actions interfering with attaining an answer should be eliminated.

The ideal data form is simple, and focused, incorporating familiar, well defined terms; this may differ from the traditional prehospital care report (PCR), which serves more general purposes. Organizing the study form so information is recorded at the time of each intervention or measurement and using a "checklist" or electronic bar coding, improves the quality and consistency of the information. A cumbersome form that requires redundant information or lengthy prose produces inconsistent data that are often incomplete and hard to interpret.

When planning a trial, the researcher must outline other specific steps in the protocol. The handling of any experimental drug or device must be defined, and criteria to terminate treatment must be specified. If blinding procedures are used, the indications and methods for unblinding must be clear and practical. These steps ensure that the clinical care of each patient can be tailored if a problem arises. Finally the data accumulated are analyzed at defined intervals by individuals not directly involved with patient enrollment. This identifies any inappropriate enrollment of subjects or unexpected harm. If compelling, these preliminary data may require the trial to be modified or terminated.

Get IRB Approval and Devise a Consent Strategy

Institutional review boards (IRBs) evaluate research protocols to ensure that patient autonomy and safety are maintained. IRBs are based on federal guidelines that mandate inclusion of lay and professional members. Any institution can create an IRB by contacting the Department of Health and Human Services (DHHS) for guidance and approval. Most IRBs are university- or hospital-based, although pharmaceutical companies and other research-oriented organizations also develop IRBs.

Until recently, most published EMS research trials did not receive the same IRB evaluation required of in-hospital trials.[16,19] EMS research is not exempt from this process, but identifying the appropriate IRB can be problematic. Non-hospital affiliated providers or those affiliated with multiple hospitals often scramble to access established IRBs. Usually the institution most closely related to the EMS system or the principal investigator reviews the proposal. In certain circumstances a separate IRB is created to serve the needs of prehospital researchers unable to access more traditional, established boards. The latter approach is time-consuming, labor-intensive, and associated with certain administrative costs, and therefore is best reserved for organizations performing research frequently.

As a rule of thumb, *any trial involving humans needs IRB review*. Often, this is brief, called "expedited" or "exempt," where the latter means "exempt from full Board review" but *not* exempt from any review. EMS researchers should consult their local IRB and review the published DHHS guidelines for the exemption criteria. In general, the IRB guidelines, including those for consent, center on the risk to the participants, the need for the data, and the ability of those involved understanding and agreeing to participation.

After IRB submission, the investigator may encounter difficulties. Prehospital care is unfamiliar to many hospital-based physicians, nurses, or laypersons. Researchers should educate members about EMS. This may be done through the protocol, a cover letter, or personal contact if permitted. In the absence of this step, gaining approval is slow and difficult. The wise investigator approaches the IRB concerns as opportunities to improve the protocol or educate the members.

Time can be an ally in gaining IRB approval. The first proposals submitted to an IRB unfamiliar with EMS are often closely scrutinized. As more high-quality protocols are submitted, members of the IRB become familiar with and accepting of prehospital research. Another mechanism that aids the process is becoming involved. Physicians can volunteer to serve on the IRB and become an educator "from within"; over time this is the most useful way to ease the process.

Obtaining and documenting informed consent for prehospital research presents special challenges.[16] By definition, informed consent is voluntarily obtained from a competent patient who is aware of the alternatives, risks, and benefits. This process ensures that the patient maintains autonomy and control throughout the study. The tradition of reading and signing a document that outlines the trial design and patient rights is cumbersome in the field, and the physician investigator is rarely present at the time of enrollment. As a solution, consent can be gained by proxy through field providers or by distant contact such as over a radio or telephone. This consent is obtained after a brief oral description of the design, and it is documented by initialing a smaller document or recording radio or telephone communications. In certain groups of patients known to frequently access the EMS system (for example, those afflicted with asthma or sickle cell disease), consent is obtained before any acute exacerbations; this is termed *prospective consent*.

Most field research should be done with contemporaneous consent, using the strategies above. However, when studying patients with critical illnesses—especially resuscitation research—this cannot occur. Based on feedback from multiple disciplines, new guidelines for this specific circumstance were enacted by the federal government in 1996. The DHHS and FDA both oversee research; together, their provisions allow an IRB to waive the requirement for informed consent only if the following conditions are met:[20]

1. There is minimal risk to the subject (see below).
2. The subject is confronted by a life-threatening situation requiring the drug.
3. Informed consent cannot be obtained because of impaired communication or inability to obtain legally effective consent from a surrogate.
4. The research could not be carried out otherwise.
5. Time does not permit obtaining consent from the subject's legal representative.
6. There is no other reliable alternative therapy that provides an equal or greater likelihood of saving the patient's life.

In addition, the investigators must disclose the research design and goals to the public and seek community input and approval to invoke a waiver of consent. This last stipulation, newly introduced in 1996, often requires a series of media releases and/or community hearings to assure that knowledge and public approval exists.[20]

Deferred consent as an alternative to obtaining formal consent is no longer recognized as adequate. It allowed enrollment of subjects with little or no initial information. Later, full disclosure and options for withdrawal were presented to the subject or representative. Deferred consent was *de facto* "assumed consent" and was eliminated and replaced by clearer waiver guidelines

When faced with consent issues in prehospital research, the best plan is to contact the IRB and other local and national experts. No one rule solves all problems, and the EMS physician should expect some ambiguity and negotiating. The entire process involves balancing the needs of the individual with those of society, a task formidable even for seasoned ethicists.

Interact with the Providers

Before and during a field trial, all personnel should be educated about the goals.[8] Emphasis on the importance of each EMS provider's role and the practical and scientific benefits increases enthusiasm for the project. This is done through continuing education or mandatory conferences with the field teams. Although large meetings make the task easier for investigators, it is best to follow them with smaller group sessions to further educate the teams. The use of adult education techniques such as videotape and public service television broadcasts are beneficial.

Questions and potential problems should be solicited from the field teams. If the investigator does not seek these opinions, unanswered problems and concerns can undermine the field teams' confidence in the trial, negatively impacting enrollment and data collection, and fostering a feeling of distance from the investigator.[8]

For example, in a randomized controlled experiment the field providers must administer a specific treatment based on a factor outside their control (the randomization table or a coin flip). If blinded, the provider does not know which therapy is used at the time of treatment. Specific measurements must be taken at set intervals even if inconvenient. These actions are a source of confusion and concern for the provider accustomed to treating each patient individually. Also troublesome to field personnel is the possibility that one group of patients receives less optimal treatment. These conflicts are mitigated by close attention to proper design and implementation, and communication of the scientific benefits of the prospective, randomize, controlled, and blinded design.

Use Pilot Trials

Often a smaller group of subjects is studied initially to detect any problems with the protocol. This is particularly true when studying an area new to the investigator or the EMS system. These pilot trials may not produce "usable" data, especially if significant changes are required based on the initial evaluation. Thus the focus of the pilot phase differs from the actual trial; problem identification and resolution assume more important roles. If minimal or no changes are needed, pilot data are incorporated with those of the actual trial.

Keep the Ball Rolling

The major reason a field trial hits "operational obstacles" (such as missed enrollment or protocol non-adherence) is that the field teams lose faith or enthusiasm in the usefulness of the trial. As they did in the preparatory phases, investigators must continually seek input from field providers and answer any concerns raised during the trial. Scheduled frequent meetings with the supervisors and field providers identify concerns or problems before they mushroom.[8] Without this contact, research is often perceived as increased work with no benefit. A trial of nebulized albuterol for the field treatment of wheezing suffered from the problem.[21] The investigators planned to collect objective data concerning the severity of symptoms before and after treatment, using a miniature computerized pulmonary function testing device. The field teams were educated about the importance of these data before the trial started. When the trial was complete, compliance with the protocol was found to be poor. The field teams felt that the pulmonary testing did not influence decisions of the direct medical oversight physicians and the pulmonary function data were unimportant. As a result the study failed to answer the intended question.

The inclusion of one or more field providers in the design and implementation of a trial builds support from within the system. These colleagues aid the principal investigator in "keeping the ball rolling" after data collection begins, especially if any difficulties arise. Studies without this involvement may have problems with perceived or real shortcomings in the protocol identified by the field providers. The medical director and researcher should be sure that the field teams and the system are always recognized during professional and lay dissemination of the study intent or results. This again fosters a "team approach."

Pitfalls in Interpreting Data

Observational, cross-sectional, and retrospective designs uncover shortcomings in patient care and resource allocation, and identify areas for prospective research. These designs do not interfere with clinical care; thus, the diligence of the investigator is the major stumbling block in completing the trial. In addition to the cause-and-effect shortcoming outlined previously, these designs face challenges based on the validity of the data recorded and conclusions reached.

Internal validity refers to the truth within a study. Simply put, internal validity means investigators measured what they thought they were measuring. For example, if using a change in the Glasgow Coma Score (GCS) to assess the effect of a treatment in trauma care, it should be calculated by the same observer or by observers with similar training. Comparing GCS at the scene (estimated from the prehospital record or calculated by the field provider) with those judged by an attending emergency department physician is invalid; any change may be the result of a treatment effect, different observers, charting anomalies, or a combination. Problems with internal validity are best sought and addressed before data collection.

External validity refers to the ability to generalize results and conclusions from a study population to other systems or geographic areas. Some data are system-specific, and others reflect features shared by many systems. Quality management projects crafted into research trials after the fact are prone to problems of limited external validity. For example, poor outcome in out-of-hospital cardiac arrest may reflect problems within that system alone (such as faulty defibrillators, long response times, a skewed population). Although this information is a useful quality tool within the system, it has a limited external validity. There are no rules to determine the external validity of collected data and conclusions; the investigator merely asks before and after the trial, "What do my observations mean to others?"

Finally, data from all patients enrolled in a trial should be analyzed. This analysis is based on "an intention to treat," and it uncovers benefits or harm that might have been missed if only those who completed the protocol were examined. For example, a trial investigating the effect of inhaled nitrous oxide/oxygen for pain that analyzes only those who completed a minimum five minute course of treatment may overlook side effects experienced by those who refused further participation after one to two minutes.

What to Do with Research Data—Choosing an Outlet

Not all investigators deserve to be published, and the choice of where to publish or present is perplexing. If the data collected have limited external validity or utility, they should not be submitted just "to get something published." Editors and reviewers are knowledgeable; it is not often that this process results in publication. In these cases the information is used for individual system refinement.

Sometimes, data obtained from a quality management investigation is useful to others, and therefore submitted for publication.[5,18,22] These trials, along with well designed prehospital experiments or observational studies, should be matched to the right audience. Each journal and each meeting focuses on different audiences and themes; the author should ask, "What do I want to impact and how do I best access that group?" This guides the choice of venue, both written and oral. For example, dispatch-related studies are better suited to EMS administrators and medical directors; the audience reading a general medical journal may not include these key people. Conversely, a breakthrough intervention that dramatically affects a disease encountered by a broad group of providers (for example, cardiac arrest or trauma) is better presented in a meeting or journal that attracts a wide audience.

Research and Education

The interactions of emergency medicine residents and EMS fellows with faculty is described by the following documents focusing on the rescue requirement and on the contract.

Emergency Medicine Resident Research Requirement

An original research project of "presentable" quality is a requirement for graduation from this program. All graduating residents must present their project at the Annual EM Resident Research Day that is scheduled at the end of the academic year.

Quality research takes time. Each resident should identify a project and a faculty advisor by September 1 of the R2 year. It is very important to develop a time line for your project that incorporates enough time to submit the project to both the Emergency Department Research Review Committee (EDRRC) and to the Institutional Research Subject Review Committee (RSRB).

Residents are encouraged to submit their projects for consideration to regional and national meetings (such as the SAEM Annual Meeting and the ACEP Research Forum). Residents will receive financial support to present their research projects.

Emergency Medicine Resident/ Faculty Research Contract

Role of the Resident

It is the resident's responsibility to:

1. Choose a research advisor. (This person must be on faculty but does not have to be on the Emergency Medicine faculty.)
2. Make and keep appointments with the research advisor to develop and work on the project.
3. Develop a research hypothesis or study objective.
4. Perform an intensive literature search.
5. Read and be familiar with the literature relevant to the project.
6. Work closely with the faculty advisor to design a project that is feasible and that will "answer" the research question.
7. Consult with a statistician during the design phase of the project.
8. Prepare a proposal for the Departmental Research Committee and for submission to the RSRB.
9. Collect data (research enrollers may be used to gather data for some projects).
10. Analyze the importance of the results.
11. Understand the limitations of the study.
12. Prepare a 10-minute slide presentation.

Role of the Faculty Advisor

It is the faculty advisor's responsibility to:

1. Guide the project, being sure that the research proposal is feasible, well designed, and possible to complete as a resident.
2. Help the resident set a time-line for completion of the project, and hold the resident to deadlines.
3. Proofread and make sure the final version of the research proposal is complete prior to its submission to the Departmental Research Committee.
4. Attend the Departmental Research Committee meeting at which the project is discussed.
5. Read and sign off on the proposal before it is sent to the RSRB.

6. Review the end-of-year presentation and make a strong effort to attend.

I have read and agree to fulfill my obligations as outlined above:

Resident: _____ Date: _____

Faculty Advisor: _____ Date: _____

Summary

Prehospital research can be rewarding for investigators, field providers, systems, and patients. The choice of a specific design is based on the question asked and resources available. By investing time during the preparatory phases and preventing common pitfalls in design and implementation, data collection and analysis are eased. Finally, the people involved in the daily aspects of a field trial—the care providers and supervisors—must be included in the process.

References

1. Gibson G. Emergency medical services: the research gaps. *Health Serv Res.* 1974;9:6–21.
2. Delbridge TR, Bailey B, Chew JL Jr, et al. EMS agenda for the future: where we are . . . where we want to be. *Ann Emerg Med.* 1998;31:251–263.
3. DeMaio VJ, Stiell IG, Wells GA, et al. The relationship between out-of-hospital cardiac arrest survival and community bystander CPR rates. *Ann Emerg Med.* 2001. (In press).
4. Mosseso VN, Davis EA, Auble TE, Paris PM, Yealy DM. Use of automated external defibrillators by police officers for treatment of out-of-hospital cardiac arrest. *Ann Emerg Med.* 1998;32:200–207.
5. Spaite DW, Valenzuela TD, Meislin HW, et al. Prospective evaluation of a new model for evaluating emergency medical services systems by in-field observation of specific time intervals in prehospital care. *Ann Emerg Med.* 1993;22:638–645.
6. Iber FL, Riley WA, Murray PJ. *Conducting Clinical Trials.* New York: Plenum Publishing Corp.; 1987.
7. Stiell IG, Wells GA, Spaite DW, et al. The Ontario prehospital advanced life support study (OPALS): rationale and methodology for cardiac arrest patients. *Ann Emerg Med.* 1998;32:180–190.
8. Warnke WJ, Bonnin MJ. Direction and motivation of prehospital personnel to do research: how to do it better. *Prehosp Disast Med.* 1992;7:79–83.
9. Campbell DT, Stanley JC. *Experimental and Quasi-Experimental Designs for Research.* Boston: Houghton Mifflin Co.; 1963.
10. Cook TD, Campbell DT. *Quasi-Experimentation: Design and Analysis Issues for Field Setting.* Boston: Houghton Mifflin Co.; 1979.
11. Elston RC, Johnson WD. *Essentials of Biostatistics.* Philadelphia: FA Davis Co.; 1987.
12. Hulley SB, Cummings SR. *Designing Clinical Research.* Baltimore: Williams & Wilkins; 1988.
13. Paris PM, Stewart RD, Deggler F. Prehospital use of dexamethasone in pulseless indioventricular rhythm. *Ann Emerg Med.* 1984;13:1008–1010.
14. Hrobjartisson A, Gotzsche PC. Is the placebo powerless? an analysis of clinical trials comparing placebo with no treatment. *N Engl J Med.* 2001;344:1594–1602.
15. The Coronary Drug Project Research Group. Influence on adherence to treatment and response of cholesterol on mortality in the coronary drug project. *N Eng J Med.* 1980;303:1038–1041.
16. Yealy DM, Scruggs KS. Study design and pre-trial peer review in EMS research. *Prehosp and Disaster Med.* 1990;5:113–118.
17. Menegazzi JJ, Yealy DM. Method of data analysis in the emergency medicine literature. *Am J Emerg Med.* 1991;9:225–227.
18. Simon R. Confidence intervals for reporting results of clinical trials. *Ann Intern Med.* 1986;105:429–435.
19. Yealy DM, Scruggs KS, Weiss LD. Informed consent in prehospital research. *Am J Emerg Med.* 1989;5:560.
20. Biros MH, Fish SS, Lewis RJ. Implementing the Food and Drug Administration's final rule for waiver of informed consent in certain emergency research circumstances. *Acad Emerg Med.* 1996:1272–1282.
21. Heller MB, et al. Data collection by paramedics for prehospital research. *Ann Emerg Med.* 1988;17:414–415.
22. Holyrod B, Knopp R, Kallsen G. Medical control, quality assurance in prehospital care. *JAMA.* 1985;256:1027–1031.

Section Three

Robert Bass, MD

Section three addresses a number of core issues related to medical oversight. Beginning with an overview, the section defines more specifically the process of direct and indirect medical oversight and the role of the EMS physician. What seems evident is that, as EMS systems have matured, the process of medical oversight has evolved. Noticeably diminished, except in historical references, is the traditionally paternalistic and solo approach of medical control replaced by the more sophisticated and collegial concept of medical oversight. Similar to trends in industry in the past several decades, more emphasis is being placed on a systems approach to medical oversight, including evaluation of processes and outcomes. Rather than reducing the role of the EMS physician, these trends have placed even more emphasis on the importance of the EMS physician as an essential component of EMS systems; as EMS systems have become increasingly sophisticated, the demand for knowledgeable and skilled EMS physician has increased as well.

Section three discusses the role of the EMS physician in education, quality management, and risk management. In all three areas, the role of the EMS physician is changing but not diminishing. Medical directors of EMS education programs are essential to insure that EMS providers are receiving training that is clinically appropriate, and that students are competent to provide patient care at the completion of their education. This can be accomplished through a didactic process that recognizes the expertise and role of the educators, while enabling the EMS physician to provide appropriate medical oversight. In the area of quality management and risk management, EMS physicians must provide the leadership and serve as participants in processes to ensure that patients receive the highest quality care by bringing their skills, knowledge, and experience to support these essential components of an EMS system.

To provide quality medical oversight, the EMS physician must be appropriately empowered by the system. To survive, EMS physicians must be aware of the myriad of political, legal, and ethical challenges that can impact the EMS system and their role as medical directors. Empowerment and survival are the subject of the final part of section three, which attempts to define critical factors that can make or break an EMS medical director. Empowerment is easy to define, but much more challenging to obtain. It is essential that EMS physicians understand the importance of empowerment and the methods by which they may be authorized to provide effective medical oversight, but being empowered by the EMS system is not enough. All too frequently, medical directors succumb to forces that, if recognized early enough and addressed effectively, could have been overcome. The skills to succeed and survive as a medical director are likely as important as the clinical expertise and experience brought to the job by the EMS physician.

25

Medical Oversight

Alexander E. Kuehl, MD, MPM
Eileen F. Baker, MD

Introduction

Medical oversight is the activity of physicians and other healthcare professionals to ensure that EMS providers and EMS systems provide optimal medical care. While the authority of a physician providing medical oversight may vary from state to state, there remains a core set of principles related to the oversight of EMS systems by physicians.[1] First and most importantly, every EMS system should have an identifiable physician with the authority to provide medical oversight. In some EMS systems, medical oversight authority is alternately vested in a body of physicians. The physician or body of physicians with the authority for medical oversight usually delegates certain medical oversight activities to other qualified physicians or healthcare professionals. While these activities may be delegated, the ultimate responsibility for medical care remains that of the physician or body of physicians with medical oversight authority. It is therefore essential that medical oversight authorities provide appropriate supervision to those who are performing delegated activities.

Medical oversight activities may be broken down into two categories: direct and indirect. Direct medical oversight activities are those wherein a physician makes contemporaneous decisions about patient care. These decisions may be rendered in the form of a consultation or as medical orders to EMS providers. Indirect medical oversight activities are all other activities performed prospective, concurrent, and retrospective to the prehospital care of the patient.

Most prehospital medical emergencies occur in locations that are removed from a medical facility. In some countries a mobile response team brings a physician to the scene of the medical emergency to provide care. In the United States, however, the acutely ill or injured patient is usually transported to the physician. For most prehospital medical conditions, patient outcome is assumed to be beneficially influenced by early medical intervention, and contemporary prehospital care systems are a well defined practice of medicine in the United States.[2] The World Trade Center and Pentagon terrorist attacks in 2001 highlight the need for an organized and effective system of EMS medical care and transport.

One of the most important aspects of prehospital medicine is medical oversight. However, the evolution of EMS systems in general, and medical oversight in particular, is varied. This is caused by a variety of factors including state, public health, philosophical, geographical, economic, legal, and demographic variations.

Historically basic life support (BLS) providers did not require physician oversight, while advanced life support (ALS) providers did. Today medical oversight is generally required for all levels of prehospital care. The proliferation in the number of intermediate providers has blurred the lines that traditionally separated the two levels of care. Despite these changes, the terms BLS and ALS remain, especially with regard to ambulance reimbursement.

The medical oversight of prehospital and disaster medicine continues to evolve. In the 1970s, federal funds were allocated for EMS with the passage of the Emergency Services Act of 1973. Those states that complied with the design stipulated by the Act were awarded monies to start EMS services. State responses varied, resulting in EMS systems with a range of medical sophistication, systems design, and medical oversight. Each state designated a "lead agency," usually within the state health department, to oversee EMS system operation. EMS Advisory councils were also created, comprised of EMS providers, nurses, physicians, public safety representatives, and the public at large. EMS councils were to advise the lead agencies on policy, education, protocols (usually in a complaint-based format), and other relevant issues. A state EMS director was designated in each state to provide program supervision. Initially, training for paramedics was performed by the medical directors themselves. At that time, many physicians practicing in emergency departments were not trained in emergency medicine, and their experience in prehospital care was limited.

When federal funding was reduced in 1981, the EMS advisory councils that had been created suffered a variety of fates. In many regions, these councils were left in place. In others, they continued to exist in name alone, or established themselves as the regional EMS authorities. A general observation, not universally true, is that states that were slower to establish EMS systems were often able to learn from the experience of other states and were more likely to adopt statewide protocols and more uniform standards. Conversely, states that were first to develop EMS systems in the 1970s have tended to retain more diversity.

As experience in providing EMS was gained, many states in the 1980s attempted to define the roles and responsibilities of the physician medical director. Requirements usually included familiarity with the design and operation of EMS systems and experience in the care of patients. Medical directors were expected to participate in base-station medical oversight of EMS, train prehospital providers, and provide "audit review and critique" of care provided. While "routine active participation in emergency department management of the acutely ill or injured patient" was required in some states, others required that the physician providing medical oversight for a given service only be licensed to practice in that state, without regard to training or practice specialty.

Over the past ten years, similar to the practice of medicine as a whole, the role and process of medical oversight has undergone a significant metamorphosis. Until the early 1990s quality management (QM) was not a significant aspect of medical care. Evidence-based medicine had not begun to have impact upon the daily practice of medicine. There was no assessment-based approach for basic out-of-hospital care, and little discussion of expanded scope of practice. There was no *EMS Agenda* and no concept of community-based EMS, nor any interest in the role of EMS in public health. BLS providers generally did not have medical oversight. Also over the past 10 years, there has been a trend in many EMS systems to include more non-physician healthcare professionals, with appropriate supervision, in the process of medical oversight. We have seen the term "medical control" become "medical direction," and more recently "medical oversight." This evolution in terminology likely represents the continued professional maturation and sophistication of both EMS systems and EMS physicians. More than ever, EMS systems require the involvement of physicians trained and experienced in the provision of EMS to achieve the level of quality medical care that the public expects and more recently demands.

The EMS Provider as a Physician Extender

EMS care in the United States is generally effected, with medical oversight, through the use of non-physician providers who assess patients and deliver defined care based on medical protocols. Before 1970, emergent patient care was provided in separate, independent segments, and the care provided in the prehospital phase was often not coordinated with that provided in the hospital phase. The physician treated the patient only after arrival at the emergency facility, with little or no input in the prehospital management. As knowledge of the pathophysiology of acute illness and injury advanced, it became evident that good patient outcomes necessitated that care be coordinated through each phase of treatment including prehospital, emergency department, and inpatient. It is a physician responsibility to oversee the clinical management of patients provided by the prehospital system and providers. This responsibility, and requisite authority, is EMS medical oversight.

Initially, it was the application of sophisticated medical interventions, such as manual defibrillation, intravenous access, medication administration, and invasive airway management, that necessitated physician participation in the supervision of prehospital care by ALS providers. After 1974, most states, localities, or county medical societies required that a licensed physician be accountable for prehospital care provided at the paramedic level.[1] As physician involvement increased, it became clear that the provision of quality prehospital medical care required medical oversight not only for paramedics, but also for First Responders, EMTs, system operations, call reception, and dispatch.[2,3]

In many states an important legal principle for medical oversight is based on the American Law Institute's Restatement of the Law of Agency, which defines the doctrine of "borrowed servant" as follows: "A servant directed or permitted to perform services for another may become the servant of such other in performing the services. He may become the other's servant as to some acts and not as to others." In prehospital care this concept means that the medical oversight physician is the borrower of another's surrogate. The paramedic employee of the ambulance service is borrowed to perform certain acts sanctioned by the responsible physician. Furthermore the concept of *respondeat superior* states that the borrower of the servant is ultimately liable for the acts and omissions of the surrogate as long as the surrogate is under the borrower's supervision. In the prehospital arena, the physician with authority for medical oversight may bear legal responsibility for the medical acts of the providers. Despite these legal dictums, it has taken a number of years for physicians in many EMS systems to be granted the requisite authority to provide appropriate medical oversight of EMS personnel, systems, and educational programs.

Usually the authority for medical oversight is based in law. All states mandate medical oversight for paramedic systems, and most now mandate medical oversight for all EMS providers.[1] As physician involvement is further encouraged and required for the entire scope of prehospital care, the confusing differentiation between basic and advanced providers becomes relatively moot. In California, each local EMS agency must have a physician medical director "to provide medical control and ensure medical accountability throughout the planning, implementation, and evaluation of the EMS system."

In 1991, the Emergency Medical Services Act of Alabama provided for implementation of medical oversight for all aspects of prehospital care. Physicians are responsible for the management of patient care, including the issuance of physician orders and establishing transportation requirements. Each region was required to appoint "a medical director who shall be a physician with experience and knowledge of EMS."[4] While most other states have taken a similar tack, a few states still do not address medical oversight responsibility in state law.[1,5] Few states mandate training for EMS medical directors; fewer still specify training requirements.

Models of Medical Oversight

For an EMS system to function effectively, there must be a seamless combination and coordination of both direct and indirect medical oversight, functioning under the medical oversight authority. Together the two categories of medical oversight facilitate the delivery of clinical care in a unique fashion. By analyzing the available prehospital and hospital resources in a particular community, medical oversight should be structured to meet the needs of the prehospital providers, the emergency department physicians, the hospitals, and ultimately the public. As technology, hospital capabilities, and patient populations change, the relative balance between indirect and direct medical oversight may shift. For example, if a community originally required base-station approval for a procedure such as thoracic decompression, an enhanced educational program driven by the QM process may allow the procedure to be performed under standing orders without direct medical oversight. Ideally the medical oversight structure nurtures and directs the system's educational and QM components.

The physician responsible for medical oversight of an EMS agency seldom acts alone. Most commonly, this physician seeks the advice or approval of a group of physicians familiar with the management of acutely ill or injured patients. The formal relationships among the medical oversight physician (usually referred to as the medical director), the EMS agency, the providers, and the participating physician groups vary greatly from system to system. Those relationships are increasingly being defined by state or local law.

In its simplest form, medical oversight is the authority and responsibility of a single appointed physician medical director with the authority to make independent decisions regarding all the medical aspects of an EMS service. In theory, this medical director provides all indirect and direct medical oversight, and does not need formal approval from other physicians or organizations before taking action. Even with such an authoritarian model, it is advantageous for the chosen physician to lead by first developing consensus.

Alternatively, an EMS system or jurisdiction appoints a single physician medical director who functions at the pleasure of the appointing authority and a medical oversight committee. The physicians on the committee may, as a group, be granted medical oversight authority. As a committee, they form consensus regarding medical issues, and assist or direct the system medical director in decision making. A medical oversight committee model has the advantages of involving many physicians in the decision-making process and providing peer support for the medical director.

A medical director or medical oversight committee may be responsible for an individual service, a group of providers, an agency, a group of agencies, a geographic region, or an entire state. Logically a given agency or EMS provider should have only one oversight physician or committee; however, there remain many ambiguous situations. The medical oversight authority may delegate specific direct or indirect medical oversight tasks to other physicians, especially in large systems. Indeed, only the ultimate responsibility of medical oversight itself cannot be delegated.

Medical oversight models are as varied as the systems they serve. A particular model may function well in one locality yet not at all in another. Some well accepted and useful models may not be allowed under local or state law. If a system's medical oversight relationship does not serve the interests of its patients, the medical director should seek change.

In order to have a positive impact upon the provision of patient care in any prehospital system, a formal relationship must be established between the prehospital providers and the physician with medical oversight authority. Given the nature of prehospital illness and injury, medical oversight must provide consistent clinical guidance under a variety of circumstances. The terms used to describe EMS medical oversight both structurally and operationally are still evolving. Although one physician (or in some jurisdictions a group of physicians) should retain final responsibility and ultimate authority, in larger systems many aspects of medical oversight are delegated. Because of the diversity of possible approaches to medical oversight, it can be somewhat difficult to prepare potential medical directors for their roles. At least one model EMS curriculum has been published and EMS fellowships have grown exponentially since 1980.[6] Specialty or subspecialty certification seems unlikely for the foreseeable future, although prehospital activities were one of the unique activities originally used to justify the establishment of emergency medicine as a distinct specialty.

Direct Medical Oversight

Direct medical oversight has also been called "on-line," "base-station," or "immediate" medical control. Direct medical oversight is the contemporaneous physician direction of a field provider, usually by a physician. This concurrent oversight may be via radio, telephone, or on-scene physician. The advantage of direct medical oversight over the use of standing orders is the contemporaneous ability of the physician to order or withhold clinical interventions based on the assessment given by the on-scene provider.[7,8] This activity requires the establishment of effective communication between the EMS provider and the physician providing direct medical oversight. Although direct medical oversight epitomizes the concept of the field provider being the "eyes and ears" of the physician, there remains ongoing debate regarding the impact of direct medical oversight on comprehensive patient care.[2,7,9]

The organization and delivery of direct medical oversight in any given system should be determined by the specific characteristics of the system. When direct medical oversight is used, it may be accomplished via communications with the receiving facility base station or an EMS system physician. In some systems a physician or surrogate responds to the scene to provide direct medical oversight, occasionally even assuming hands-on patient care.

There are two divergent trends occurring. On the one hand, clinical protocols for all levels of providers are including more interventions under standing orders, thus avoiding the need for direct medical oversight. On the other hand, on-scene involvement by physicians appears to be growing in popularity as a treatment tool, a QM activity, and an education method. To be accurate, the latter two activities should be thought of as concurrent indirect medical oversight.

Indirect Medical Oversight

In the early 1970s an "off-line" or "project" medical director was defined by the federal government as a "physician directing the lead agency in the overall system design, implementation and evaluation; and (who) is responsible for the ultimate medical accountability and appropriateness of the entire regional (multi county) system," in other words, medical oversight.[5] Within the scope of medical oversight, everything that is not direct medical oversight is indirect. This includes, but is not limited to, medical protocol and policy development, quality assurance and improvement, education, communications, system design, operations, and disaster management. In the 1970s the "off-line" or "project" medical director had ultimate medical responsibility and accountability. However, today the medical oversight of field providers is usually an extension of the practice of physicians functionally located closer to the provider. Although a medical director may not be immediately available to provide direct medical oversight, protocols and standing orders, reviewed and approved by the medical director, are accepted tools to guide the EMS system and providers in the care that is delivered in the field. The medical director may delegate aspects of indirect medical oversight to other physicians or health professionals. The medical director remains ultimately responsible and must supervise those tasks if they are delegated to others.

The process to balance direct medical oversight with the use of standing orders in a given EMS system should develop from the bottom up.[10] First, a needs assessment should determine what clinical interventions are most beneficial in a given community. Then, weighing the skills and experience of the EMS providers against the clinical tasks at hand, medical oversight must identify the available provider levels, usually established by state law, that will be most effective in carrying out the required clinical interventions. Occasionally jurisdictions will have the ability to develop specifically tailored levels of providers for their area; this usually occurs only when the system is first established. In most cases, some existing state-defined provider level is chosen. Next, the frequently difficult decision must be made as to where to draw the line between standing orders and direct medical oversight. This decision should include a detailed analysis of the capability of the providers, the call volume, and the capability and availability of those who will be responsible for direct medical oversight. It is little wonder that the variation among systems is so great!

Of all the components of an EMS system, indirect medical oversight activities require the most physician effort and provide a foundation for clinical excellence. They also require that the physicians who participate in medical oversight are knowledgeable of operational, financial, and political issues that affect the ultimate delivery of clinical care. Historically, few physicians have formal training in these disciplines. The development of a system of medical oversight is a dynamic process that enables the EMS system to evolve and provide optimal patient care.

As systems become more sophisticated, the delivery of quality clinical care results not only from strong medical oversight, but also from collaborative efforts among physicians, operations managers, field providers, administrators, public officials, and community leaders. For example, medical directors often must either justify the cost-effectiveness of a specific field intervention or prioritize program development based on available resources. A solid understanding of the complex forces involved in such decision processes helps the medical director optimize overall patient care. The most astute, innovative EMS physician cannot have an impact upon prehospital patient care if the jurisdiction does not provide sufficient financial and political support.

Medical oversight authority may choose to delegate certain tasks related to indirect medical oversight to other physicians or healthcare professionals. Examples of delegated tasks include the medical oversight of dispatch, protocol development, education, or quality improvement. Since each of these components is intimately related to the other, it is essential that medical oversight authority supervise and coordinate these delegated tasks, lest the prehospital care system become fragmented and potentially ineffective.

System Design

Few physicians will ever have the opportunity to design an EMS system without restrictions; rather, most are charged with creating evolutionary change in response to the evolving environment. One of the most important aspects of system design is the choice of provider levels of care. This decision is based on the availability of resources, the geographic characteristics of the service area, the annual call volume, the amount of available physician support, and the public health needs and priorities of the community as determined by the medical director.

Because the pathophysiology of acute illness and injury begins at the time of the insult and not at provider arrival, medical oversight must assure that patient care begins at the time of public access to the EMS system. Call-takers and dispatch personnel must provide pre-arrival instructions in an effort to minimize morbidity while EMS is en route. The sequence and content of caller interrogation should allow dispatchers to reliably send the appropriate resources to the patient in a timely fashion. Similarly the EMS system should predetermine ambulance and personnel placement to minimize the interval from call receipt to arrival at the patient. Most acute clinical management is as dependent on a timely response as it is on adequately educated and equipped providers.

Protocol Development

Medical oversight develops protocols with input from EMS providers, physicians, and other healthcare professionals so that a consensus is established.[11] A clinical protocol is a pre-authorized course of care for use by prehospital providers in managing the medical problems of patients. Protocols may be in the form of clinical guidelines that must be approved by direct medical oversight before the EMS provider may initiate care, or standing orders that specify care that the EMS provider may initiate prior to contacting a physician. There are three important principles in protocol development. First, the protocol must be medically appropriate, which is a medical decision. Second, the protocol must be capable of being implemented in the field, which requires input from EMS providers. Third, the protocol must be cost-effective, which requires input from EMS administration. In addition to clinical protocols, medical oversight is responsible for developing appropriate triage protocols such as those used during a multiple victim incident (MVI) or for determining the level of response in a tiered system.[2,8] Medical oversight should assume a leading role in planning disaster response and in developing MVI drills and training. Transport protocols must also be developed to route patients to appropriate specialty centers based on clinical criteria. A thoughtful, objective, collaborative approach to patient destination protocols minimizes the financial and political pressures on and from the hospitals participating in the system. Medical oversight should be actively involved in the process of designating specialty referral centers such as trauma centers, burn centers, cardiac specialty centers, hazardous materials receiving facilities, stroke centers, and pediatric centers.

As in all of medicine, EMS physicians should rely on scientific literature to establish the foundation of all protocols. Individualizing protocols to fit a particular system is central to the art of prehospital medicine. Protocols, especially of a clinical nature, require a significant degree of local medical consensus.

Education

The National EMS Education and Practice Blueprint and the National Registry of EMTs both recognize four levels of providers: First Responder, EMT-Basic, EMT-Intermediate, and Paramedic.[12] The pivotal role of provider education in successfully implementing these levels is often overlooked by medical oversight. Medical oversight activity related to education is an investment in quality. Medical oversight of EMS educational program must provide the leadership in establishing standards for entry level and continuing medical education, course content, and educational performance. A comprehensive educational program provides the necessary assessment, diagnostic, and therapeutic skills to carry out clinical mandates adequately and meet the requirements of the state agency that certifies or licenses the EMS provider.

Quality Management

Webster's dictionary defines quality as "a degree of excellence."[13] QM in prehospital care provides continuous feedback to medical oversight about the effectiveness of the EMS system. It allows the medical director to modify the clinical objectives, to reshape the educational program, and to obtain data supporting change or reevaluation of the system. While the overall responsibility for QM rests with medical oversight, involving EMS providers and other healthcare professionals in the QM process will both enhance the identification of improvements in quality and, conversely, factors that impede improvement.[6]

The analysis of the outcome of prehospital care can be a difficult task. A key factor in that difficulty is that patients are frequently delivered to a multitude of institutions that may be reluctant to give access to patient medical records. It is often both legally and logistically difficult to collect outcome data for QM purposes.[14] Nevertheless such data is essential not only to monitor system performance, but to assess the impact of various treatment modalities on prehospital morbidity and mortality.

Summary

The physician or group of physicians responsible for medical oversight is the cornerstone of every EMS system. Through the use of direct and indirect medical oversight, the EMS system can be designed and can function to provide optimal prehospital patient outcomes. A successful and collaborative relationship between EMS physicians, community physicians, receiving facilities, field providers, administrators, and other personnel will improve patient care. An EMS physician must constantly learn from the collective experience of the system to build his or her expertise and, ultimately, the effectiveness of the system. Rapidly emerging scientific literature, newly developed technologies, and constantly changing political and financial climates mandate the constant evaluation and modification of the medical oversight of contemporary EMS systems.

References

1. Snyder JA, et al. Emergency medical service system development: results of state-wide EMS service technical assessment program. *Ann Emerg Med.* 1995;25:768–775.

2. Pointer SE, et al. The impact on standing orders on medication and skill selection, paramedic assessment, and hospital outcome: a follow-up report. *Prehospital and Disaster Medicine.* 1991;6(3):303–308.

3. *Emergency Medical Technician: Basic National Standard Curriculum.* Washington, DC: USDOT-NHTSHA, 1994.

4. Emergency Medical Services Act of Alabama, Section 132, 1991.

5. Boyd DR, et al. Medical control and accountability of emergency medical services (EMS) systems. *IEEE Transactions on Vehicular Technology.* 1979;T-28:249–262.

6. Swor RA, et al. Model curriculum in EMS for EM residencies. *Ann Emerg Med.* 1989;18:418–421.

7. Erder MH, Davidson SJ, Cheney RA. On-line medical command in theory and practice. *Ann Emerg Med.* 1989; 18:261–268.

8. Wuer RC, et al. Online medical direction: a prospective study. *Prehospital Disaster Med.* 1995;10:174–177.

9. Grefton MC, et al. Effect of standing orders on paramedic scene time for trauma patients. *Ann Emerg Med.* 1991;20:1306–1309.

10. Pointer, SE, Osur MA. Effects of standing orders on field times. *Ann Emerg Med.* 1989;18:1119–1121.

11. Bonnin MI, Swor RA. Outcomes in unsuccessful field resuscitation attempts. *Ann Emerg Med.* 1989;18:507–512.

12. *The Future of EMS Education: A National Perspective.* Washington, DC: Joint Review Committee on Educational Program for EMT-P; 1994.

13. *Webster's New Collegiate Dictionary.* Springfield, Mass: Merriam-Webster Inc.; 1975.

14. Stout JL. Organizing quality control in EMS. *JEMS.* 1988;13:67–74.

Indirect Medical Oversight

26

Edward M. Racht, MD

Introduction

Internationally, there are countless delivery models for the provision of emergency medical care outside of a hospital setting. In many countries, physicians routinely staff ambulances or rapid response vehicles that travel to the patient's side to render aid. In the United States, out-of-hospital emergency medical care is most commonly provided by non-physicians (first responders, emergency medical technicians, and paramedics) functioning under the direction and guidance of a designated physician or group of physicians. This very important concept of a delegated practice model led to the development and promulgation of contemporary Emergency Medical Services (EMS) throughout the United States. The basic premise of authorizing the provision of medical care and delegating the actual delivery of care to a non-physician is the clinical cornerstone of every U.S. EMS system.

While seemingly simplistic, this conceptually complex notion requires physicians to be an integrated component of all EMS systems. The reality is that physicians are not commonly present at the patient's side to supervise and participate in the delivery of all medical care (direct medical oversight). Even though the physician is not routinely present, the public expects to receive equivalent care by the EMS providers.

Medical oversight is the ultimate authority and responsibility for the medical aspects of the entire EMS system and its impact on patient care. Indirect medical oversight is the vehicle that provides for comprehensive physician involvement in all aspects of the EMS system. The easiest definition of indirect medical oversight is one of exception: *any physician involvement in an EMS system that is NOT Direct Medical Oversight.* Indirect medical oversight covers physician involvement "behind the scenes" and in "all the nooks and crannies." In essence, indirect medical oversight is the stamp of physician involvement in everything that has the potential to impact the clinical care delivered to patients. If done well, it is difficult to pick apart specific areas of physician involvement through indirect medical oversight.

Conceptually, it is helpful to think of an EMS system as a practice of medicine. Patients access the system with an expectation that they will be evaluated by competent practitioners, that appropriate examinations and testing will occur, and that some form of conclusion and plan of care will be initiated by a capable individual in the appropriate time frame with the right tools. The differences between an office- or facility-based practice of medicine and an EMS system are the methods used to effectuate the process. Although the overwhelming majority of calls in an EMS system are not true emergencies, EMS systems must be designed to deploy rapidly the right resources when the initial information regarding the nature of the illness or injury suggests a reasonable probability that a potentially serious condition exists. Thus, in addition to the need for a clinically sophisticated system, the response must also be structured to rapidly arrive at the patient's side wherever they may be. Indeed, in the initial phases of acute illness or injury, the most prevalent public expectation is that someone arrives soon after emergency care is requested.

Requirements

The requirements for physicians providing indirect medical oversight have been refined over the years as the profession continues to evolve. In 1986, Holroyd and his colleagues described the requirements of a medical director who provided "off-line medical control" (now referred to as indirect medical oversight) as:[1]

> "knowledge and demonstrated ability in planning and operation of prehospital EMS systems, experi-

ence in the prehospital provision of emergency care for acutely ill or injured patients, experience in the training and ongoing evaluation of all levels of participants in the prehospital care system, knowledge and experience in the application of medical control to an EMS system, and a knowledge of the administration and legislative processes affecting regional and/or state prehospital EMS systems."

The credentials and experience of physicians who provide indirect medical oversight are as varied as the communities and EMS systems they serve. Similarly, specific areas of involvement or job responsibilities are usually defined locally. In an effort to standardize the qualifications and requirements for Medical Oversight, the National Association of EMS Physicians (NAEMSP) developed a position paper for *Physician Medical Direction of EMS* in 1997.[2] In addition to defining required and desired training and continuing education elements, the Position Paper defines the following qualifications for EMS Medical Directors:

Essential qualifications

- Licensed to practice medicine or osteopathy
- Familiar with local/regional EMS activity

Desirable qualifications

- Board certification or board preparedness in emergency medicine (American Board of Emergency Medicine or American Board of Osteopathic Emergency Medicine)
- Active clinical practice of emergency medicine
- Completion of an EMS fellowship

Acceptable qualifications

- Board certification or board preparedness in a clinical specialty approved by the American Board of Medical Specialists or the American Osteopathic Association

This defined set of qualifications and educational guidelines provides a level of consistency to EMS medical oversight in an effort to enhance the physician's role in very diverse environments and systems.

Structure

The actual structure of indirect medical oversight is most commonly determined by the individual EMS agency, a governmental entity (such as a municipal-

ity, taxing authority, or hospital board), the local medical community (medical societies), or by local, regional or statewide regulation or legislation. Wydro and colleagues summarize the tremendous variation in regulatory requirements for physician participation in EMS activities at the advanced life support (ALS) level.[3] There is no "best way" or preferred structure that works best for any specific system. Medical oversight in its entirety is comprised of both direct and indirect components. In order for an EMS system to be clinically sophisticated and accountable, both components of medical oversight must be well integrated. The relationship among the components of medical oversight is in large part defined by the structure of the EMS system. It is important to note that many EMS systems have a long-established model of medical oversight that may not serve the interests of patients or the EMS system well. It is just as important for physicians to evaluate the medical oversight structure as it is to focus on the specifics involved in providing clinical care.

There are two basic principles that define the medical oversight structure. They are:

- Authority/reporting structure
- Scope and integration of oversight

The authority and reporting structure of medical oversight defines the physician's relationship in the EMS system. If the medical director provides only advice and is not integrated into the organizational decision-making processes, it is difficult to monitor clinical care in the system and facilitate change. As the individual charged with the ultimate responsibility for all patient care, the medical director must have defined authority and direct access to the "decision makers" within the system. In order to be an effective patient advocate, a physician must always have the ability to address patient care issues in the system openly and honestly and bring those issues to the appropriate policy makers for analysis and resolution.

Authority of the medical director is often a politically charged issue. Physician authority may be seen as a threat to administrators or other professionals. Many systems have developed a medical oversight advisory board to assist the medical director with his decision-making activities and approval processes.

Scope of oversight pertains to the various different components of an EMS system such as communications, public education, protocols, etc. It is important to always remember that clinically appropriate care must be delivered in an operationally appropriate manner. It becomes artificial to attempt to separate clinical care from operational delivery in most circumstances. Integration refers to how the various components of an EMS system come together to provide "seamless" care to the patient. Integration of medical oversight becomes very important when two or more physician medical directors have responsibility for agencies that may have simultaneous responsibility for a single incident, for example, mutual aid responders from two different localities, first responder agencies and transport agencies, or ground ambulance and aeromedical programs.

Every physician medical director must have a well defined scope of authority and responsibility. If ever there was a "square one" in medical oversight, this would be it.

Components

There are many components of an EMS system that may not be considered "clinical" that still have a profound impact on patient care. For example, an EMS system with a high ambulance breakdown rate may have significantly delayed response intervals that impact morbidity and mortality. Provider schedules may have an impact on clinical performance. Deployment strategies impact response intervals. Communication strategies regarding clinical errors have the potential to improve care throughout the system or to increase potential liability if done inappropriately.

It is obviously not appropriate, nor should it be the intent, for the physician medical director to "run" all aspects of an EMS system. It is, however, important to consider all the components of an EMS *system* that may impact patient care. To that end, indirect medical oversight is the physician's vehicle for providing appropriate clinical guidance and structure for the system. It is also important to note that indirect medical oversight may very well cross multiple agency or jurisdictional lines, and can be the one element that ties several independent agencies together under the unified mission of quality patient care. The medical director must have ultimate authority for clinical care delivered by an EMS system.

The NAEMSP *Position Paper on Physician Medical Direction in EMS* provides a useful template for physician involvement in several of the various components of the EMS system.[1]

Communications

Communications is often the initial contact the patient or caller has with the EMS system. Emergency medical communications includes three important responsibilities:

- correctly obtaining necessary information from the caller,

- rapid selection and dispatch of appropriate responding resources, and

- provision of appropriate instructions to the caller regarding what to do before help arrives.

Obtaining correct information from the caller requires a consistently applied approach to caller interrogation. Subsequent decisions regarding dispatch of resources and caller instructions are based on the ability to gather appropriate information. The communication questioning sequence may be part of a commercially available emergency medical dispatch (EMD) program or may be locally developed. Physician medical directors should evaluate carefully initial EMD program selection, development, implementation, and ongoing performance.

Because individual system design is variable, information gathered at the time of the initial call is essential to assign appropriate resources to the incident. For example, in a tiered system, initial call information will dictate whether an ALS or BLS resource is sent and whether the resources are sent "hot" (with lights and sirens) or "cold." Culley and her colleagues demonstrated an increased efficiency of a system by significantly reducing ALS responses to incidents not requiring ALS through the use of criteria-based dispatch.[4] Thus, a criteria-based dispatch system has the potential to reduce morbidity and mortality not only through timely response, but also by improving resource availability for subsequent requests for service. The physician medical director should evaluate not only the dispatch criteria, but the designated system responses as well.

As systems strive to match more efficiently EMS resources to patient needs and become more integrated into the local healthcare system, there is a real interest in being able to use information gathered at the time of the initial call as a potential predictor of either critical or non-urgent patient conditions. The physician medical director should be familiar with local system capabilities and what criteria are being evaluated. Neely reviewed audio recordings of dispatch conversations for three conditions (fall, sick, trauma) to identify whether dispatcher questions in one urban center could predict patients with important clinical field findings.[5] In their review of 430 recordings, caller answers to the questions asked did not appear to be useful when the goal was to identify patients without an important clinical finding. While the analysis focused on a small subset of patients, it demonstrates the importance of in-depth review of whether the "right" questions are asked.

Rapid deployment of the appropriate resources to any request for service is a public expectation as well as an important decision point in any time-dependent illness or injury. Medical oversight adds significant value by looking at "the big picture" of the medical response to the incident. For example, patients who are entrapped or difficult to access may benefit from additional or specialty resources early in the response that can provide specific medical evaluation or treatment during extrication.

Assignment of resources is based on the local medical practice standard as well as regional and national guidelines. A common example illustrates this issue. If a caller activates 9-1-1 for an "obviously dead" patient, does the EMS system send a single vehicle response without lights and sirens to process paperwork and provide family emotional support, or does it send the "cavalry" to potentially initiate resuscitative efforts? What constitutes "obviously dead" at dispatch? How accurate is the caller in identifying "obvious"? These are clearly medical questions that have a significant potential impact on patient outcome.

Pre-arrival instructions have become an important vehicle for delivering medical care via telephone by "coaching" callers through the appropriate steps of providing medical care until help arrives. Although a 1993 National Highway Traffic Safety Administration study found that 86% of states had not established dispatch standards, a recent study by Billittier of 524 respondents regarding their knowledge of 9-1-1 systems revealed that 76% expected pre-arrival instructions for specific medical emergencies.[6,7] In addition to accurate, consistent caller interrogation and appropriate, timely dispatch of resources, television has created public expectations about what should happen when they call 9-1-1.

Several studies have examined pre-arrival instructions for cardiac arrest, specifically the efficacy of telephone CPR instructions, the influence of pre-arrival instructions on improving bystander CPR, and the ability of dispatchers to accurately identify patients in cardiac arrest.[8-10] The National Heart Attack Alert Program and the American Heart Association (AHA) Operation Heartbeat programs both advocate aggressive implementation of pre-arrival CPR instructions.[11] The EMS Agenda for the Future and the American College of Emergency Physicians (ACEP) policy statement on emergency medical dispatch both advocate for appropriate emergency medical dispatch as part of an EMS system.[12,13] While some would still argue whether pre-arrival instructions have become a standard of care, it is clear that a strong organizational and public expectation exists supporting the concept.

Physicians should also be actively involved in establishing criteria for level of medical training of calltakers and dispatchers, continuing education requirement and content, processes for evaluating dispatch protocols, and quality management (QM) activities.

EMS call-taking, dispatch, and provision of pre-arrival instructions are a unique and challenging component of any system. Most physicians have little or no experience in a communications environment. As with all aspects of a system, the more time physicians spend in the environment learning and participating in the activities, the more opportunity the medical director will have to understand and improve the varied factors that influence patient care.

Protocols of Clinical Practice

Of all the components of an EMS system, most medical directors spend the largest amount of time on field clinical practice. And rightfully so; field clinical practice encompasses the very heart and soul of medicine: direct patient care. Support of field clinical practice is the bulk of traditional indirect medical oversight. Because the physician is not on the scene of every patient encounter, the delegated practice concept requires the development of protocols for providers to use when caring for patients. These documents or plans should reflect the expectations of the medical director, and provide specific guidance on the approach to managing particular situations.

Development of this aspect of an EMS system puts the physician's signature on the system, literally and figuratively. In most states, written protocols or standards are required by regulation or legislation, and empower providers to act in accord with the physician's orders. Individual systems have traditionally developed formats useful for their organization.

In addition to the content of the documents, the medical director must communicate his or her philosophy regarding *how* the protocols or standards are used. They may be an absolute requirement, a guideline or a recommendation. There is more variability in protocol design and application philosophy among EMS systems than the actual content itself.

It is important to note that the process used to develop protocols is just as important as the end product. Field medicine is a unique blend of operational and clinical decision trees. Any process used to develop guidelines, policies, standards, or protocols must address several key issues:

- Is there a need for a particular protocol?

- Is there evidence based on solid study design in the literature to support the protocol?

- Is there a financial or administrative impact associated with the protocol? If so, is it feasible and acceptable to those responsible for making those decisions? If not, what is the priority of the change? Should something else be moved "up or down" to accommodate a higher priority?

- Is there an educational or "roll out" requirement?

- What performance measures can be used to measure the impact of the protocol?

- Is there consensus among all conceivable stakeholders for development and implementation of the protocol?

At all stages of development, the protocol must be reviewed by stakeholders in the system for input. Done appropriately by the right people, this review process is crucial for a successful, contemporary, clinically sound document. Some communities have a formal review and approval process (often dependent on a physician review committee), while others seek out voluntary input from practitioners familiar with the out-of-hospital environment and practice. As with most medical projects of this magnitude, time invested up front is well worth the effort. Consensus of the medical community not only makes good clinical sense, but it provides the system and medical director with valuable liability protection.

There are several important topics that should be addressed in every system by protocol. In general, these "must haves" represent commonly encountered situations or difficult circumstances requiring specific

direction. They can be broken down into practice management issues and patient-care issues.

Given the complexity of most systems, it is wise for the medical director to address both practice management and patient-care issues through development of a written protocol:

Practice management issues

- Definition of a "patient" versus a non-patient (while this may seem obvious, the dramatic increase in cellular telephones has increased third-party callers who may not be aware of the need or lack of need for EMS)

- Definition of a minor (state statutes and local guidelines may conflict)

- Transport vs. non-transport criteria (including transport against a patient's will)

- Refusal of care process and requirements

- Criteria for initiation and termination of field resuscitation attempts

- Criteria for assessment of patient competency

- Criteria for direct medical oversight and on-scene physician authority

- Transport destination requirements (including trauma patient categorization and cardiac receiving centers)

- Hospital diversion criteria

- Credentialing and decredentialing requirements for all levels of provider (including specific authority to limit or restrict provision of medical activities of patient care for cause)

- Scene authority for patient care

- Use of and training for specific equipment used in patient care

- Patient record documentation requirements

- Mass casualty triage requirements and operational structure

Addressing practice management issues defines the "rules" for how specific situations are handled. Careful attention and appropriate legal guidance in areas of practice management can be of great value to the medical director in reducing potential liability.

One of the most important concepts addressed in practice management protocols is credentialing. Credentialing requirements should be established by the physician. In essence, credentialing is the process of evaluating the competency of an individual to provide the expected level of care in a specific system using specific protocols. When done well, credentialing critically evaluates the ability of a new provider to "cut the mustard" according to the medical director's expectations.

There is no clearly defined process for evaluation of the competency of new providers. In an excellent article that discusses experience and mentoring requirements for paramedics, Pointer suggests that systems and medical directors should establish benchmarks for specific events such as ALS assessment, endotracheal intubation, defibrillation, and other skills that are evaluated by experienced, training officers.[14] A professional development evaluation should follow the field mentoring and precede the physician "signing off" on the medic practicing alone. Pirrallo has suggested establishing specific measurable benchmarks in order to maintain clearance to practice.[15] The Milwaukee system ensures competence by requiring a minimum number of these specific skills. It is improbable and impractical to expect every medic to encounter specific types of patients during their credentialing process in order to demonstrate their abilities to a training officer. As such, using a benchmarking system, the medical director can define acceptable alternatives to actual patient encounter. These may include simulation, use of manikins, alternate training sites such as the operating room, or case review and discussion.

Patient-care issues

- Protocols that address specific elements of clinical practice pertinent in the communications component of the system
- Protocols that address specific elements of the clinical practice in the field
- Criteria for determination of death
- Specific criteria for performance of clinical procedures and interventions

Patient-care protocols should include details pertinent to evaluation and management of specific symptoms or diagnoses. In order to be useful, patient-care protocols should be easy to understand and retain, and should follow a logical flow. Medical directors who develop and promulgate complex, difficult-to-follow protocols may doom the provider, patient, and system to failure in a fast-paced, chaotic field environment. It is always prudent to allow field practitioners an opportunity to review and comment on any proposed, new, or changed protocol prior to widespread implementation.

As the medical director develops protocols, a philosophic decision (based in large part on system specifics and medical director comfort with perceived competence of providers) is how much of what the providers do clinically is contemporaneously medically directed and how much is covered by standing orders. While the value of direct medical oversight has been controversial, Rottman compared on-scene times, appropriateness of medical therapy, and accuracy of paramedic clinical assessments when prehospital care was provided by direct medical oversight (EMS certified base station nurses) versus paramedics using chief-complaint based protocols.[16] He concluded that use of the protocols resulted in small improvements of on-scene time without a change in agreement between the paramedics and physicians. Holliman reviewed the error rates of paramedics and direct medical oversight physicians before and after the implementation of a standing order system.[17] He describe a decrease in physician error rates (2.6% to 1.2%) from standing orders with no increase in scene time. McErlean describes no differences in scene time, time to nitroglycerin dose, oxygen use, IV access, EKG monitoring, or measurement of vital signs by paramedics using direct medical control or protocol for management of adult chest pain patients.[18] Indeed, the contemporary trend has been a migration toward more standing orders and less direct medical oversight for patient management.

An increase in proportion of indirect medical oversight does not negate the need for direct medical oversight. An appropriate balance must be developed based on the clinical sophistication of the system as well as the receiving hospital community. Wuerz and colleagues reviewed the frequency with which direct medical oversight resulted in orders, and the nature of the orders. They conclude that despite detailed standing orders, direct medical oversight resulted in orders for clinical interventions in 19% of the cases evaluated. Cone reports the impact of direct medical oversight on patient-initiated refusals in a hospital-based suburban EMS system.[19] Ambulance report documentation was better with direct medical oversight than without. Additionally, 13% of the patient initiated refusals were admitted to the hospital within a few days. This study suggests there may be a role for direct medical oversight in improving dispositions in patient-initiated refusals, an historically high medico-legal risk category.

With the development, promulgation, and availability of several nationally recognized curricula such as Advanced Cardiac Life Support (ACLS), Pre-Hospital Trauma Life Support (PHTLS), Basic Trauma Life Support (BTLS), and Pediatric Advanced Life Support (PALS), the medical director must define how concepts and specific recommendations of these programs integrate into the field practice of the system. If a medical director requires a specific course for providers, there should be clear guidance regarding what components of the course may be used in patient care in the EMS system. For example, some medical directors may allow all the principles and algorithms in PALS to be used by providers in the field even if not specifically defined in a local protocol. Others may restrict field practice to only those topics covered by local protocol. In order to make an informed decision, physicians should be familiar with the curricula of applicable programs.

Finally, as protocols are developed, an effort should be made to appropriately integrate voluntary guidelines. Voluntary guidelines are developed by many professional societies or governmental agencies addressing issues of interest to the EMS community. There has been much controversy, for example, regarding the AMA 2000 guidelines for management of cardiac arrest. In a landmark *Joint Position Statement on Voluntary Guidelines for Out-of-Hospital Practices* issued by the NAEMSP, the National Association of State EMS Directors, and ACEP, those organizations emphasized that voluntary guidelines should be used to supplement and enhance the overall local EMS structure and function, and are not required standard of care for EMS systems.[20] As medical directors develop or modify protocols, this position paper reinforces the importance of carefully evaluating all available data, including voluntary guidelines.

Education

Education provides the foundation for a clinically sophisticated EMS provider; unfortunately, initial education varies widely. A medical director-developed credentialing process as described earlier helps "level the playing field" and improves consistency in practice. A comprehensive orientation process helps new providers understand the clinical and operational expectations of the system.

The science and art of EMS practice changes rapidly, and a system must adapt. Provider education is important not only for change in practice but also to clarify questions regarding current clinical care. How education is delivered can be as important as the content itself. EMS providers live in a very practical world, and require common-sense approaches to delivering care in an unpredictable environment. Using actual case presentations dramatically increases the impact of an educational program. There are also innovative methods to deliver information that directly improves field care, such as computer-based manikins and automated patient care simulations.

Several states have adopted re-certification or re-licensure requirements that are based solely on obtaining appropriate continuing education over a defined period. Like many other health professions, education has become the focus of continuous professional development. More than ever, it is important that educational curricula be contemporary, scientifically sound, and relevant to the EMS environment.

In a 1997 NAEMSP/ACEP *Joint Policy Statement on the Role of EMS Physicians in EMS Education*, the role of the physician medical director was described as:[21]

■ To approve the medical and academic qualifications of the faculty, the accuracy of the medical content, and the accuracy and quality of medical instruction given by the faculty;

■ To routinely review student performance and progress and attest that the students have achieved the desired level of competence prior to graduation; and

■ To have a significant role in faculty selection and curriculum development, authority over presentation of medical content, and authority to assure that faculty teach established medical practices.

The medical director should have significant input to the entire educational program, including public education, dispatch, continuing medical education, and base station physicians. The curricula should reflect topics identified as important through the QM process or contemporary needs. For example, after the September 11th, 2001 tragedies, and with many EMS systems responding to concerns of bioterrorism or chemical weapons, systems were well served to develop educational programs targeting these new potential threats.

Finally, when developing an educational program, the medical director must never underestimate the power of training programs that bring several different levels of providers (dispatchers, paramedics, EMTs, nurses) together to address a specific topic. While course content obviously must be modified to target the audience appropriately, multi-level, multi-disciplinary training can have significant practical value and lead to better understanding and integration.

Evaluation

Measuring performance has become an important medical, political, and financial tool. Measurement of patient intermediate and long term outcomes is essential not only for individual systems, but also for individuals. Specific tools for system evaluation are covered in great depth elsewhere in this text. Likewise, the medical director must have significant involvement in every aspect of QM of an EMS system. After all, measuring performance is the ultimate indicator of effectiveness of the infrastructure created to care for patients. A healthy system thrives on QM data to fuel programs in other clinical areas. To be effective, the medical director should play a significant role in establishing measurable standards that accurately reflect the goals of the system, medical community, and consumers. Data collected must be as "clean" as possible; often in EMS we struggle with bad data. It is well worth the effort to establish a data collection system that captures the right information.

A medical director should actively seek input from the local physician community concerning system performance. Some systems have established committees, medical oversight boards, or medical societies that participate in the oversight of the system; others do not. Providing appropriate system performance information to the medical community establishes accountability and credibility. It is obviously important to share the bad news as well as the good. Individual physician-to-physician contact when there is a concern regarding patient care is a valuable source of information; it also demonstrates the commitment of the EMS system to quality patient care. EMS is the practice of medicine, and the responsible physician should desire as much input as possible about his patients.

As the ultimate patient advocate, the medical director can interpret the meaning and implications of QM data. There are many different reasons for "poor" performance as measured by an EMS system. The medical director can assist by putting the data in the appropriate perspective. This concept applies as well to the economic impact of system performance. In an environment of expanding missions, competing priorities, and decreasing revenues, the medical director is the most appropriate member of the partnership to provide this crucial perspective.

When performing system evaluation, too often the focus is on the negative—the non-performers, outliers, sentinel events and protocol violations. The importance of positive reinforcement should not be overlooked. As the "medical boss" of a system, recognition of excellence is a very powerful tool and a potent motivator. Unsolicited contacts regarding how well a patient was managed or how well a family member was treated dramatically demonstrate that the medical director is aware of what is going on, and cares enough to recognize the provider's efforts.

Research

Historically, very little emphasis has been placed on research in the EMS environment. Much of our clinical development has been a result of transferring applicable practices in a hospital or emergency department setting to the EMS world. Our past is replete with examples of adopting technology that was not tested in the field, protocols that were designed for a more controlled setting, and practices that, in retrospect, did not make good sense.

In contrast, modern medicine has evolved into an evidence-based approach to decision making. Much of what is done in EMS is not supported by good data, or is supported by data from a dissimilar environment. Fortunately, EMS research is no longer a newborn, but an infant. Medical development continues to expand the efforts to study the interventions using sound scientific methodology, accurate data collection and logical analysis. The medical director must approve any study conducted in the field. The field environment is a challenging arena for research. Good ideas have to be operationally feasible. Often, it is the medical director who identifies an area in need of investigation while attempting to develop protocol where no good data exists.

Administration

Administration is the least understood, often most uncomfortable, and unquestionably the most underemphasized role of a medical director. While it is not a separate entity or responsibility, administration should be an integral part of the medical director's everyday practice. Administration requires good business practice and an organized, consistent, accountable approach to activities pertinent to one's job responsibilities. Physicians who are capable of becoming excellent managers have the opportunity to become good leaders and influence patient care through previously uncharted channels. Another important concept for an effective physician-administrator is the ability to develop consensus among the many stakeholders and to focus on the "big picture." The unique environment of EMS requires a comprehensive, dynamic series of professional relationships among the community, public safety agencies, hospitals, and the medical community. Influential physician medical directors have developed the ability to establish mutually beneficial relationships with the many entities involved in out-of-hospital care.

Public Health

EMS scholars have long debated whether an EMS system is predominantly a public *health* or public *safety* function. Those supporting a public health focus argue that an EMS system is, first and foremost, a healthcare delivery system. The primary mission is more aligned with the concepts and principles of health than any other model. Many alternative models of care promote delivery systems or primary care integration with an EMS system to provide more efficient, more appropriate non-urgent care or triage. The public safety camp, on the other hand, views EMS as the third leg of the three-legged stool of law enforcement, fire, and EMS.

Regardless of how one views the category most appropriate for defining EMS, there is a clear role for an EMS system in public health. In a discussion of the function of an EMS system in public health emergencies, McIntosh describes a plan developed for dealing with an epidemic alert.[22] In test situations, the plan extended the public health "surveillance net" further into the community, and enhanced the ability to properly isolate suspected cases until arrival at a definitive care facility. The recent rash of anthrax threats and cases in the United States has dramatically changed the relationship between EMS and public health. Many EMS systems, such as Austin, have developed integrated plans with public health for mass screening and prophylaxis in the event of potential bioterrorism events.[23] Traditional disease surveillance programs have expanded into dynamically monitoring EMS and emergency department patient volumes

as well as hospital diversion statistics as critical adjuncts to standard surveillance practices.

EMS, by design, responds to failures in disease and injury prevention. Public health problems, such as motor vehicle crash fatalities and intentional injuries, can be more effectively addressed through a multidisciplinary approach that includes a thoughtful and expanded role for EMS systems.

Summary

As with any profession, personality and professional ethics have a significant impact on the EMS physician's ability to function. The world of EMS is filled with strong egos, powerful personalities, and many hidden agendas. The medical director has a unique opportunity to develop a focus on patient care, not individual agendas. If the medical director is inclusive, truly informed, honest, and perceived as a partner, the potential for significant system-wide dedication to clinical excellence is great. If not, the most significant investments of time, energy and money usually lead to nought. Physicians with the dedication and passion to create clinically sophisticated healthcare systems by developing consensus among the many stakeholders will be successful.

Indirect medical oversight provides the entire infrastructure and framework to develop a comprehensive, clinically sound EMS system. Thinking of EMS as a "practice of medicine" is a useful tool for involvement in and the development of the system.

References

1. Holroyd BR, Knopp R, Kallsen G. Medical control: quality assurance in prehospital care. *JAMA.* 1986;256(8): 1027–1031.
2. Alonso-Serra H, Blanton d, O'Connor RE. National Association of EMS Physicians position paper: physician medical direction in EMS. *Prehosp Emerg Care.* 1998; 2(2):153–157.
3. Wydro GC, Cone DC, Davidson SJ. Legislative description of EMS medical direction: a survey of states. *Prehosp Emerg Care.* 1997;1(4):233–237.
4. Culley LL, Henwood DK, Clark JJ, et al. Increasing the efficiency of emergency medical services by using criteria based dispatch. *Ann Emerg Med.* 1994;24:867–872.
5. Neely KW, Norton RL, Schmidt TA. The strength of specific EMS dispatcher questions for identifying patients with important clinical field findings. *Prehosp Emerg Care.* 2000;4:322–326.
6. Snyder JA, Baren JM, Ryan SD, et al. Emergency medical service system development: results of the statewide emergency medical service technical assistance program. *Ann Emerg Med.* 1995;25:768–775.

7. Billittier AJ, Lerner EB, Tucker W, et al. The lay public's expectations of pre-arrival instructions when dialing 9-1-1. *Prehosp Emerg Care*. 2000;4:234–237.

8. Kellerman AL, Hackman BB, Somes G. Dispatcher assisted cardiopulmonary resuscitation. *Circulation*. 1989; 80:1231–1239.

9. Culley LL, Clark JJ, Eisenberg MS, et al. Dispatcher-assisted telephone CPR: common delays and time standards for delivery. *Ann Emerg Med*. 1991;20:362—366.

10. Clark JJ, Culley LL, Eisenberg MS, et al. Accuracy of determining cardiac arrest by emergency medical dispatchers. *Ann Emerg Med*. 1994;23:1022–1026.

11. National Heart Attack Alert Program Coordinating Committee Access to Care Subcommittee. Emergency medical dispatching: rapid identification and treatment of acute myocardial infarction. *Am J Emerg Med*. 1995; 13:67–73.

12. Delbridge TR, Bailey B, Chew JL, et al. EMS Agenda for the future: where we are: where we want to be. *Ann Emerg Med*. 1998;31:251–263.

13. American College of Emergency Physicians. Physician medical direction of emergency medical services dispatch programs (policy statement). *Ann Emerg Med*. 1999; 33:372.

14. Pointer JE. Experience and mentoring requirements for competence in new/inexperienced paramedics. *Prehosp Emerg Care*. 2001;5:379–383.

15. Pirrallo R. Establishing biennial paramedic experience benchmarks. *Prehosp Emerg Care*. 1998;2:335–336.

16. Rottman SJ, Schriger DL, Charlop G, et al. On-line medical control versus protocol-based prehospital care. *Ann Emerg Med*. 1997;30(1):62–68.

17. Holliman CJ, Wuerz RC, Meador SA. Decrease in medical command errors with use of a "standing orders" protocol system. *Am J Emerg Med*. 1994;12(3):279–283.

18. McErlean M, Raccio-Robak N, Bartfield JM, et al. Safe out-of-hospital treatment of chest pain without direct medical control. *Prehosp Disaster Med*. 1996;11(1): 16–19.

19. Cone DC, Kim DT, Davidson SJ. Patient-initiated refusals of prehospital care: ambulance call report documentation, patient outcome, and on-line medical command. *Prehosp Disaster Med*. 1995;10(1):3–9.

20. National Association of EMS Physicians, National Association of State EMS Directors, American College of Emergency Physicians Joint Position Statement: Voluntary Guidelines for Out-of-Hospital Practices. 2001.

21. National Association of EMS Physicians, American College of Emergency Physicians Joint Policy Statement: Role of EMS Physicians in EMS Education. 1997.

22. McIntosh BA, Hinds P, Giordano LM. The role of EMS systems in public health emergencies. *Prehosp Disaster Med*. 1997;12(1):30–35.

23. Standards of Care: Bioterrorism. Austin/Travis County EMS System, Austin, Texas. 2001.

27

Direct Medical Oversight

Barbara A. McIntosh, MD
Brian Schwartz, MD

Introduction

Direct medical oversight has been defined as "the clinical instructions, usually from physicians, or from specially trained medical personnel, to EMS field personnel."[1] However, this definition does not even begin to describe direct medical oversight in its entirety, since current practice varies from state to state and from EMS system to EMS system. What started simply as a system to provide contemporaneous medical instructions to paramedics has become a means of assuring a medical-operational interface and quality assurance tool.

Today the prototypical EMS system utilizes direct medical oversight as a means for all providers to have real-time contact with a physician for medical advice and formal orders beyond the standing orders of the protocols. Direct medical oversight (as opposed to indirect medical oversight) emphasizes real-time medical contact that occurs as the EMS provider is actively caring for the patient, allowing for a case-by-case "tailoring" of the treatment protocols and procedures for each patient.

Which level of EMS providers should be required to contact medical oversight? Where in the treatment protocols are they required to contact medical oversight? What level of healthcare provider is allowed to provide direct medical oversight? These are but some of the potential questions relating to the operation of direct medical oversight systems. Additionally, most systems also use direct medical oversight to perform functions that may be considered more operational/administrative than medical in nature (see table 27.1).

For example, in many systems contact with medical oversight is required for patients who want to refuse medical aid (RMA), to assess both the patient's mental capacity to refuse aid and to convince the patient to agree to treatment and transport. Direct medical oversight is also used in protocols concerning transport decisions, hospital diversion requests, triage out of the system, and pronouncement of death. Some systems have interposed physician contact as a quality assurance/tracking mechanism.

Clearly an evolution has taken place in direct medical oversight, because of both the evolution of EMS provider protocols and the blurring of lines among various levels of care. The evolution of direct medical oversight programs has also progressed as a result of EMS systems in different settings designing and implementing programs specific to their localities and needs. In short, the setting in which one chooses to develop and utilize direct medical oversight defines the direct medical oversight system. For example, in a setting where paramedics have less experience in critical decision making, direct medical oversight may play a large role; conversely, where medical oversight is comfortable with the abilities of providers, more can be done via protocol, with direct contact with physicians occurring under narrowly defined circumstances.

This chapter discusses the origins of direct medical oversight, examines key and controversial elements, highlights some current special uses in prac-

TABLE 27.1
Direct Medical Oversight Functions

- Medical orders
- Refusal of Medical Aid
- Transportation Destinations (specialty referral, extended transports)
- Medevac Authorizations
- Hospital Diversion Requests
- Triage Out of System (ambulance transport not necessary)
- Pronouncements of Death
- Quality Assurance Mechanism Management
- Other Situations (for example, patient discharge with community follow up)

tice, and attempts to predict the future of direct medical oversight.

Historical Perspectives

"Prehospital care is the provision of medical care in the field by non-physicians who, in many states, function under the extension of a physician's license."[1] Direct medical oversight is the direction via telephone, radio, or in person of prehospital providers at the scene by an authorized medical provider. Direct medical oversight offers a means of formalizing the legal responsibility for patient care.

In 1970, Nagel described a program implemented in Miami, which utilized remote medical oversight for mobile emergency medical care. The authors hoped that their model would "enable many communities to build upon existing rescue capabilities at modest cost while retaining the tradition of physician responsibility." The program presented "an emergency care development whose objective is to combine in-hospital physicians with field paramedic rescue units through telemetry-radio command systems. The goal of this method is a total systems approach in which diagnosis and oversight is the responsibility of the in-hospital physician while the treatment phase is carried out by skilled paramedic technicians from their mobile vehicle base."[2] It reported 131 cases where the system was used, including the first recorded successful remotely directed paramedic defibrillation. It should be noted that the in-hospital physicians were residents rotating through the emergency department who were trained in radio communication techniques and rode out on calls with the paramedics as an orientation to their practice.

The legal acceptability of remote physician oversight and protocol had been discussed at a conference, where it was noted that "if ordinary care and prudence were exercised, the legal risks were virtually nonexistent if a doctor accompanied a rescue unit, or the unit was dispatched to carry out the physician's specific instruction, or the unit was guided by telemetry or other communication permitting the doctor to diagnose, prescribe, and supervise from a distance."[3]

The authors concluded that while the techniques and technology that they used were not new, "what is novel and exciting for the future of emergency medical care is the combining of these techniques into one diagnostic and treatment system with great economy of the physician's time and utilization of

strategically located and specially trained rescue squads to minimize the time lag between the receipt of the alarm and the actual delivery of medical services on the spot. Important side benefits are retention of the age-old principle of physician responsibility and oversight, immediate availability in most communities, lower costs, and much expanded capability in terms of number and variety of emergencies which can be handled."[3]

As systems have evolved, direct medical oversight, which was traditionally provided from the field or a hospital setting by physicians, has become more varied in its applications. Contact may now be accomplished via land-line, cell phones, or radio, to a hospital or a centralized communication facility, and medical directions may be given by physicians, nurses, or even specially trained prehospital providers. Crews may transmit standard rhythm strips or twelve-lead electrocardiograms. There may be multiple facilities providing direct medical oversight in a region, each with differing capabilities. Destination decisions and hospital assignments may be considered administrative decisions requiring physician contact, as are refusal of medical aid situations. The various means by which direct medical oversight can been delivered are delineated in table 27.2. All types continue to be used by various EMS systems today.

As the use of direct medical oversight increased and more systems incorporated direct medical oversight, the need for ensuring quality and consistency of direct medical oversight became evident. In 1984, the American College of Emergency Physicians (ACEP) first issued the following guidelines for the provision of direct medical control:

- Base hospital supplies, equipment, and personnel for medical control should be located within the emergency department.

- All requests by rescue personnel for medical oversight should be promptly accommodated with an attitude of participation, responsibility, and cooperation while following established protocols.

- Cooperation with the regional EMS system in collecting and analyzing data necessary for evaluation will be assured.

- Patient confidentiality will be maintained.

- The direct medical oversight physician (DMOP) will issue transportation instructions and hospital assignments based entirely on objective

TABLE 27.2	
Direct Medical Oversight Types	
TYPE OF DIRECT MEDICAL OVERSIGHT	COMMENTS
Physician on scene	■ Some systems employ criteria to request on-scene physician presence ■ Provides orders and advanced procedures when needed ■ The ideal quality assurance and educational tool
Physician with mobile radios	■ Allows physician to attend selected calls ■ Usually fewer physicians involved improving consistency
Attending physician in ED or medical oversight center	■ Dedicated area within facility required ■ DMOP may be receiving physician ■ Less consistency due to varied physician involvement—more quality control of physicians required ■ Teaching opportunities for residents/students
Emergency medicine resident in ED or mobile	■ Important in EM residency curriculum ■ Direct or indirect supervision by faculty required
Physician surrogates—nurses, senior paramedics	■ DMOP ultimately responsible ■ Direct or indirect supervision by physician required

analysis of patients' needs and the facilities' capabilities and proximity. No effort will be made to obtain institutional or commercial advantage through the use of such transportation instructions and hospital assignments.

■ When the base hospital is acting as an agent for another hospital, information regarding the patient shall be given to that hospital in an accurate and timely manner.

■ Physicians at base hospitals should conduct regular case conferences involving the medical control physicians and EMS personnel. This identifies problems involving both groups and provides continuing education to correct them.[4]

Standing Orders vs. Direct Medical Oversight

There has been a national trend toward the use of comprehensive, preexisting medical protocols with more standing orders, and fewer direct medical oversight options. The effectiveness of this trend remains controversial. Whether medical options requiring direct medical oversight confer benefit beyond the use of protocols utilizing standing orders is questionable. Some prehospital physicians are uncomfortable without providing a direct medical order on every call;

others point to evidence that direct medical oversight is time-consuming, expensive, and inconsistent. Most systems utilize medical protocols that consist mostly of standing orders, with mandatory direct medical contact for those patient conditions that fall outside the scope of these standing orders; other systems require direct medical oversight contact on every call.

The resolution of this controversy is difficult. Outcomes are not well defined, nor easy to measure; and data are often problematic in accessing. Traditional outcome measures, such as mortality and morbidity, may not be affected by direct medical oversight. Types of calls that may benefit from direct medical oversight (for example, cardiac, pediatric), articulated in some studies, have not been evaluated critically.[5,6]

Triage and disposition decisions in some systems with regionalized trauma, pediatric, cardiac, and burn care services are often cited as indications for physician contact. This theoretically provides backup decision support for borderline or questionable cases, and allows physician notification of the receiving hospital.[5] The effectiveness of this practice has not been studied.

The evaluation of direct medical oversight versus the use of standing orders may be discussed under several categories, namely: outcome effectiveness, quality of performance, scene time, the question of necessity of any direct medical oversight, medical legal issues, patient refusal of care, and cost.

Outcome Effectiveness

Few studies have attempted to evaluate outcomes of medical contact versus standing orders, for the reasons outlined. In 1979, Hunt compared direct medical oversight with pure indirect medical oversight (standing orders) on cardiac arrest patients in Charleston, South Carolina. The resuscitation rate (restoration of pulse and blood pressure) and admission rate to hospital did not differ significantly between the two groups. This was a before-and-after study; unfortunately other differences between the groups existed, such as the institution of a new airway procedure.[7] In a study of direct medical oversight in a Philadelphia EMS system, Erder and Davidson noted that patient health status improved in 5.5% of those treated with direct medical oversight, compared with 3.2% treated without direct oversight. The outcome measure for "health status" was a change in level of consciousness; however, the measurement tool was not reported. Scene time was on average eight minutes longer for patients who received treatment under direct medical oversight, with obvious implications in trauma patients. A limitation of this study is that the number of critical patients was small, making it difficult to assess the impact of direct medical oversight on the health status of patients most likely to benefit. Inclusion rules for direct oversight were broad, minimizing the potential impact of physician orders.[5]

In neither study were the qualifications of physicians performing direct medical oversight described. This is clearly a prerequisite for studying effective patient management. In a previous edition of this text, Braun observed that: "To adequately test the hypothesis that direct voice control is beneficial a study must be conducted in an EMS system that guarantees and documents quality medical control. Then "critical medical cases" that are most likely to benefit from direct medical control can be carefully studied. Ideally the study design would be prospective and the runs randomized to direct or no direct medical control. A large study population would also be required, because the number of patients in which a change in outcome is expected is small under even the best of conditions. Conclusions about lack of impact (beta or type II error) cannot be safely made from small numbers."[1] This study still needs to be done.

Quality of Performance

Prehospital provider compliance with protocols has been shown to be significantly higher with standing orders than with direct orders. Klein et al reviewed 774 ambulance call reports and found that adherence to protocol was significantly less likely to occur with direct medical oversight than without, regardless of the training of the provider. Non-adherence was more likely to occur as the acuity of the patient's condition increased.[8] This suggests that as the complexity of the patient's condition increases, the ability to apply even a well designed protocol diminishes. Thus the need for direct medical oversight in selected critically ill patients.

Rottman conducted a prospective before/after series comparing direct medical oversight and protocol based care. They found that inappropriate treatment decisions occurred in 7.4% of direct medical oversight decisions and in 5.1% of protocol decisions (RR 1.5; 95% CI, 1.0 to 2.1). Subset analysis showed no pattern of inappropriate treatment in patients with chest pain or altered level of consciousness when providers operated under protocol. Treatment of patients with dyspnea improved with use of standing orders, with both furosemide and albuterol used more appropriately.[9]

Problems with quality of performance under direct medical oversight include communication inaccuracies, lack of prehospital qualifications of the physician, unfamiliarity with skill sets and conditions in the field, and inconsistency in physician style of practice. In one study, direct medical oversight error rates, as assessed by physician reviewers, numbered 4.4% of all calls, with the most common error being failure to address the possibility of hypoglycemia with altered level of consciousness.[10] On the other hand, a skilled DMOP can elicit information or findings that the provider may have neglected. Gauche found that when direct medical oversight contact was made, vital signs were more likely to be taken.[6] In addition, direct medical oversight offers the opportunity of real-time quality improvement with the interaction of providers and physicians.[5,8,11]

Scene Time

There are several studies that show that scene times decrease when prehospital providers do not initiate physician contact.[5,12,13] This reduction in scene time could have a positive impact on the patient care as long as the care provided remains appropriate. Moreover, system use is optimized, and there is potential cost saving. However, in some cases the extended scene time required for physician contact may be justified if outcome is improved.[5]

Is Direct Medical Oversight Necessary at All?

There are situations that cannot be covered by standing orders, and require direct medical oversight. Conditions such as congestive heart failure, severe respiratory distress, and hypotension of uncertain etiology may benefit from the expertise of physicians knowledgeable in prehospital care. Hoffman and Diamond noted, in separate studies, that small numbers of patients with abnormal vital signs such as hypotension required therapy that was unanticipated before discussion with a DMOP.[14,15] The outcomes of these interventions were not evaluated.

Interpretation of rhythm strips or 12-lead EKG may necessitate direct medical oversight contact. Some procedures (e.g., surgical airway management) have such limited indication that some medical directors require DMOP consultation prior to implementation. This does not address the issue of timeliness of such therapy.

Medical Legal Considerations

In many systems, direct medical oversight is legally required for some procedures, the most notable being field pronouncement of death. In the Province of Ontario, a patient is "presumed dead" if decomposition, decapitation, transection, gross rigor mortis, or charring is present, and no physician pronouncement is required. Otherwise, a patient is not legally dead unless pronounced by a physician. In the absence of a doctor on-scene, a direct medical oversight physician fulfills this role, if legislation allows. Evidence suggests that physician pronouncement at scene through providers prevents transport of cardiac arrest victims with no chance of survival to emergency departments, thereby saving resources, reducing unnecessary risk of injury to providers and citizens, and providing more compassionate care to families of patients.[16]

Patient Refusal of Care

When patients refuse transportation, the medical oversight physician may provide direction to providers on-scene, speak directly to the patient, document the circumstances on the physician log report, and help to determine patient capacity for informed consent or refusal. This allows for medical legal support in an area of potential risk and liability. Stark and Alicandro have shown that intervention by a direct medical oversight physician improves transport rate among patients who initially refuse care.[17,18] Burstein have suggested that the degree of assertiveness by DMOPs correlates with the ultimate decision of the patient to accept transport.[19]

When standing orders are utilized, the medical director who has authorized and signed them has ultimate medical legal responsibility for the patient's care. If direct medical oversight is utilized, the medical oversight physician assumes at least part of this risk.[12] Physicians participating in direct medical oversight should be aware of this accountability and ensure appropriate medical protective liability coverage.[20]

Cost

Direct medical oversight is costly.[14] It may increase scene time, reducing system optimization. It requires physician time, and can theoretically compromise care in the emergency department, if the physician is on duty at the time. Space and equipment are required.

Quality management (QM) is required for physicians to perform appropriate direct medical oversight. An essential component of a high quality prehospital system includes resources dedicated to recruit and educate medical oversight physicians in prehospital care, telemetry, communications equipment and language, geographical considerations, and field issues. Hoffman found that reducing the number of physician contacts significantly curtails base hospital costs.[14]

Systems will likely continue to provide a combination of advanced medical directives in the form of protocols with standing orders and medical options. Direct medical oversight is often most utilized at the onset of a program, to provide the costly but essential familiarization with the process for both providers and physicians. It can then diminish, as the system matures, to a point where up to 95% of patients will be treated via standing orders, with fewer specific indications for physician contact (see table 27.3). The

> ### TABLE 27.3
> #### Indications for Direct Medical Oversight
>
> - Critical medical cases (for example, congestive heart failure, complex overdose, severe respiratory distress, hypotension of uncertain etiology, acute myocardial infarction)
> - Management of conditions that fall outside protocols (based on paramedic expertise and judgment)
> - Transmission of information for specific decisions (for example, telemetry)
> - Medical legal issues (for example, pronouncement of death, patient refusal of transport, physician on scene)
> - Maximizing resources (for example, paramedic decision not to transport, field pronouncement)
> - Triage decisions

advantages of such a combination are consistency and cost efficiency of care and quality oversight, with the opportunity of providing specific treatments in complex or unusual cases.[5,12] Prospective research should be performed in order to delineate what these indications should be, based on outcome assessment, if possible. This will result in a safe, cost effective integration of direct and indirect medical oversight.

Qualifications of Direct Medical Oversight Providers

In the early days of direct medical oversight, the qualifications of the physician answering the radio/phone were variable. Ideally, the emergency department (ED) attending physician would be the person providing direct medical oversight but, in practice, the physician who was closest to the radio/phone often was the one who gave the orders to providers. Sometimes this was the resident rotating through the ED. Some systems dealt with the problem by developing separate direct medical oversight communications facilities, removed from the distractions of an ED, where a designated physician was solely responsible for providing direct medical oversight; however, many systems did not have the wealth of resources or sufficient call volume to make a separate facility practical.

Some systems dealt with the lack of continuous physician availability by using delegated providers, nurses, or paramedics, to handle incoming requests for medical oversight. As was noted in the prior edition of this textbook, "In 14 states it is legal for individuals other than physicians to provide direct medical oversight. Non-physician direct medical oversight is usually conducted by either Medical Intensive Care Nurses (MICNs) or paramedic communicators trained to direct prehospital field personnel. Typically, MICNs are not required to obtain immediate physician agreement before issuing orders, whereas paramedic communicators are. MICNs may or may not be required to obtain a physician signature on orders. Paramedic communicators are rarely permitted to operate independently; rather, they act as screeners, calling for physician assistance when field care beyond standing orders is needed. In most areas, paramedic communicators function primarily in other capabilities, such as quality control officers."[1]

As noted, the level of medical sophistication for required physician contact will often determine the level of medical personnel providing direct medical oversight. For example, if a prehospital system requires direct medical oversight contact for all instances where an advanced medical procedure is done, then it may be appropriate for MICNs or paramedics to handle the majority of the calls. Conversely, if a system has structured its protocols such that field personnel can do most interventions under standing orders (so that crews call direct medical oversight only when they have exhausted their standing orders or for a difficult case), then it may be prudent to have an experienced physician providing direct medical oversight. In these circumstances, indirect medical oversight decisions (i.e., when contact is required) will determine direct medical oversight operations.

A recent development which has affected decisions about direct medical oversight is the adoption, by many states, of stricter regulations involving controlled substance administration. The exact regulatory requirements vary from state to state, but the impetus of these regulations is to require direct physician involvement and documentation whenever a controlled substance is ordered. Thus, some states may require a licensed physician to directly order controlled substances for prehospital patients.

Being a licensed physician does not necessarily make one qualified to provide direct medical oversight. Dinerman suggested in 1981 that minimum qualifications for physicians providing direct medical oversight included: (1) experience in emergency medicine, (2) training in appropriate prehospital protocols, (3) knowledge of personnel skills and scope of practice, and (4) familiarity with regional critical care centers and resources.[21] In addition, DMOP should be acquainted with the unique situations encountered in the practice of prehospital medicine. This will help to develop a collaborative rapport with prehospital providers and will minimize medically sound but impractical physician orders.

An example of a system where the direct medical oversight system has evolved over time is New York City. Until recently, the majority of direct medical oversight was performed at the municipally run 9-1-1 system, at a regional communication center. Recently, there has been an increase in the number of facilities (mostly hospital base stations) requesting to become certified direct medical oversight facilities. The New York City Regional Emergency Medical Advisory Committee (REMAC) developed explicit criteria with respect to availability, qualifications, training, and certification of medical oversight physicians. The physician criteria parallel regional criteria for emergency department attending physicians. The process to become certified as a medical oversight physician involves submitting all appropriate documents and application, completion of a REMAC course including a written test for DMOPs, and completion of a required telemetry observation rotation where the applicant must successfully complete a preset number of direct medical oversight calls under the supervision of a certified direct medical oversight physician. In addition, there are requirements for ongoing participation in the regional prehospital system (i.e., CME, paramedic testing, riding with field crews, etc.).

Many other cities have specific training and education programs and requirements for direct medical oversight physicians, yet this is not a uniform requirement. In spite of recommendations by the National Association of EMS Physicians (NAEMSP) and other organizations to develop a standardized course for training physicians performing direct medical oversight, implementation has been difficult in locales with scarce physician resources and the requirement of additional training may discourage some physicians from participating. Also, the regional authority to mandate such a requirement varies from state to state, making the prospects for a uniform requirement slim.

Telemetry

Telemetry was defined by Pozen in 1980 as "the transmission of an EKG strip over one of eight dedicated ultra-high frequency (UHF) pairs from a paramedic-staffed ambulance to a medically staffed opera-

tion center."[23] Given that the early focus of prehospital care was to prevent death from acute myocardial infarction (AMI), treatment was initially aimed at the life-threatening arrhythmias associated with AMI, namely ventricular fibrillation and ventricular tachycardia. The early model for telemetry was based on the work done by Nagel in Miami, where the underlying assumption was that physicians diagnosed dysrhythmias through telemetry, and then directed the field personnel to treat them[2]. However, Pozen stated in 1977 that it was unclear whether or not this conferred a benefit to patient outcomes.[22]

Early studies on diagnostic accuracy rates of field personnel and the need for telemetry centered around issues of prehospital provider training, with many prehospital systems adopting telemetry requirements to serve as checks on newly trained paramedics, allowing them to consult with physicians on EKG interpretations. The underlying assumption in this scheme was that the physician interpretation was the "gold standard." Yet Pozen noted in his 1980 study that one reason physician consultation on telemetry might not be beneficial was due to misdiagnosis by the direct medical oversight physician. Although most medical oversight physicians had extensive emergency department experience, their backgrounds were varied. When telemetry strips from patient encounters were reviewed by a board certified cardiologist who was unaware of the patient's diagnosis or treatment, 35% were deemed to be incorrectly classified by the medical oversight physician and the paramedic. Even so, Pozen concluded that routine telemetry transmission was clinically and financially justified because it improved prehospital care by (1) improving diagnostic skills in recognizing potential cases of ischaemic heart disease, (2) increasing field personnel accuracy in interpreting rhythms, and (3) aiding in enforcing provider compliance with medical direction.[23]

Cayten in Philadelphia in 1985 performed an in-depth three-year controlled trial evaluating direct medical oversight with and without telemetry. Medical oversight contact was established after immediate lifesaving measures (CPR, defibrillation) were instituted. All ambulances utilized the same hospital base station, which was staffed by second-year internal medicine residents, supervised by an emergency department attending physician. The author concluded that, "Telemetry was not found to affect the abilities of paramedics to read EKGs in either test or field situations. Paramedics who used telemetry spent more time in the field with their patient than did paramedics who did not use telemetry. We found no statistically significant different effect of telemetry on survival rates of VF patients. Using matched EKGs, readings by base-station physicians were found to be more accurate than were those by paramedics."[24] In the accompanying editorial Stewart noted that the small number of telemetry transmissions studied did not preclude the utility of telemetry as a learning tool. He also stated that he did not believe that use of telemetry would affect the survival rate of patients in VF; rather, he believed telemetry had the most benefit to offer in rhythms like supraventricular tachycardia or atrioventricular blocks because correct identification of these difficult-to-interpret rhythms would influence therapy.[25]

The situation regarding the balance between the level of training of field providers and original goals of prehospital advanced care was best summarized by Braun in the prior edition of this text, who stated, "Telemetry and direct medical control evolved early as mandatory functions and were relatively efficient because field teams were fairly unsophisticated and minimally trained." Now, some EMS systems have field personnel with up to 2,200 hours of training, that operate in systems in which acute cardiac patients are a distinct minority. In systems using physician surrogates, direct medical oversight often is provided by individuals with levels of expertise no greater than that of the paramedics in the field. In such situations, direct medical oversight provides no more benefit than the opinion of another paramedic on-scene; this scenario renders telemetry optional, and useful only in select cases. Initially telemetry was designed for and applied to populations having a relatively high incidence of significant arrhythmias; it is currently applied to large populations with non-cardiac disease. This practice may result in a higher incidence of dysrhythmias that are clinically insignificant, which may increase the incidence of unnecessary and potentially harmful interventions."[1]

A new controversy regarding the use of prehospital telemetry has emerged with the development of portable monitors capable of performing 12-lead EKGs. Initial questions addressed training of field personnel in performing and interpreting 12-lead EKGs and the potential delays in scene time that could occur as a result of this new technology compared to the benefits obtained by providers having this additional information. Aufderheide observed that diagnostic quality 12-lead EKGs can be obtained in 70% of prehospital patients and that the incremental increase in on-scene time is only 3.9 minutes. They also noted that utilizing 12-lead EKGs versus single-lead telemetry resulted in an increase in the specificity of the direct medical oversight physician's working diagnosis from 68% to 95%, and the positive predictive value increased from 33% to 71% in patients with a discharge diagnosis of AMI.[26] The small increase in on-scene time has been contrasted with the overall net decrease in time to definitive treatment with thrombolytic therapy which has resulted from prehospital 12-lead EKG use.[27,28]

Quality Management for Direct Medical Oversight

There are two aspects to maintaining high quality direct medical oversight, namely the QM of the EMS providers and that of the physicians. The components of a QM program for EMS providers include:

- *Specificity and sensitivity of patches*—How often were base-hospital contacts unnecessary? How many times did the paramedic not patch when it was indicated?

- *Assessment of reporting technique*—Organization, completeness, accuracy, clarity.

- *Compliance with direct orders*—All requests for direct orders must be recorded by both the provider on the ambulance call report and the physician on a log sheet designed for this purpose; the documents should be matched and compared for paramedic compliance.

A system should be in place to perform reviews of taped calls to medical oversight physicians on a regular basis. Calls may be selected randomly by provider, or by physician. However, the latter method is subjective and based on the physicians' own levels of expertise.

Tapes may also be selected as part of a general call review or audit, based on chart reviews, or by specific condition or procedure audits. Feedback can be in the form of an interview or in writing. Individualized remediation may be appropriate in individuals with recurrent deficiencies. In general, however, an education program incorporating issues identified on tape reviews will yield the most constructive results. Peer review of tapes demonstrating both good and poor technique is an effective means of improving the appropriateness of medical oversight physician contact and patching skill.

Chart review or data-base analysis will help identify cases that should have resulted in direct medical oversight but did not ("false negatives," such as procedures or medications requiring direct medical oversight that were administered without physician contact). Education, remediation, and system improvement should be instituted as needed with follow-up to assess compliance.

Components of a QM for DMOPs include:

- inclusion of prehospital care and a module on direct medical oversight in emergency medicine residency programs;

- an orientation and education package to new emergency physicians involved in direct medical oversight, including the concept of delegation, direct and indirect medical oversight, local standing orders, skill sets, and triage issues;

- direct observation and coaching by the prehospital medical director of new physicians during patching;

- regular prehospital care rounds which include tape reviews; and

- direct medical oversight log sheet reviews, correlated with the ambulance call reports, to identify accuracy of reporting, and appropriateness of orders and of decision making.[7,17]

Areas of concern should be discussed with the physician involved. Prehospital care should form part of the DMOPs performance appraisal by the department chief or medical director. A position as an attending physician in an emergency department that provides direct medical oversight does not automatically qualify one to perform this form of delegation to providers.

QM of the direct medical oversight system must also be performed. Are there any conditions currently managed by direct oversight more appropriately dealt with by standing orders? Issues of consistency, cost-efficiency, legislation, and quality of care must be considered. Feedback from physicians, providers, receiving hospitals, and other similar prehospital systems as well as current literature should be obtained by the medical director in making these decisions,

and appropriate tracking mechanisms should be in place to evaluate the effects of these changes.

Special Situations

Research Applications

Direct medical oversight facilities may be utilized as research centers or quality control centers by interposing the requirement to contact medical oversight into designated protocols. The success of using medical oversight facilities for these roles will depend on several factors including the volume of calls handled by a facility, the staffing levels at a facility, the level of communications/operational interface available at a facility, and the ability to capture all medical oversight facilities used within a prehospital system. The rationale in using a medical oversight facility for research or quality control purposes rests in the fact there is an advanced level practitioner (ideally a physician) available to prehospital personnel 24 hours a day, who can serve as a resource in real-time patient care.

As an example, the 1994 PHASE study, which examined the survival rate of victims of cardiac arrest in a large urban center, utilized the telemetry control unit of New York City EMS. The facility was situated in the regional communications center and, as such, had access to the call dispatch and monitoring system citywide. Direct medical oversight was provided by a medical oversight physician and paramedics 24 hours a day. For the study, an additional dedicated paramedic was stationed in Telemetry to monitor all medical oversight contacts for cardiac arrests within the 9-1-1 system. The PHASE medics were trained to query the dispatch system for cardiac arrest calls in which patients were transported without medical oversight contact. Additionally, all field providers were asked to contact telemetry upon completion of a cardiac arrest call. By using this resource, the researchers were able to capture all of the cardiac arrest calls for the time period of the study.[29]

Medical oversight facilities can also be utilized for information collection and as a quality check when new protocols or protocol changes are enacted. For example, when a prehospital albuterol administration project was recently undertaken in New York City, one of the requirements for participating services was that EMT-B crews have access to direct medical oversight for any questions that may arise. Although participating providers administered nebulized treatments under standing orders, the requirement for direct medical oversight access allowed crews the option to consult with direct medical oversight if a question regarding treatment options arose. Similarly, in the province of Ontario, a "symptom relief" package of medication, including albuterol, epinephrine for anaphylaxis, and glucagon for hypoglycemia was introduced for EMT-B providers. In this way a "fail-safe" check was incorporated into new projects. Care must be taken, however, to ensure that a balance is struck between the addition of medical oversight contact as a quality safeguard and the potential increment to on-scene time and subsequent potential delay in implementation of definitive care.

Public Health/Domestic Preparedness Interface

Direct medical oversight can also be used as a resource in public health emergencies. The medical oversight physician/advanced provider can be interposed to function as an intermediary between the on-scene prehospital providers and responsible health agencies so that a patient or situation considered at risk may be evaluated and the appropriate precautions taken (and destination determined) before transport to the hospital. A detailed description of how such a system could be developed and implemented was described in a study from New York City. In 1994 there was an outbreak of pneumonic plague in India. In response to the threat of infected persons from endemic sites entering the country, the U.S. Public Health Service (PHS) established evaluation and quarantine facilities at selected international airports, including New York City. The local health department surveyed and identified hospitals with the requisite isolation facilities and NYC EMS was advised of the potential need to transport suspected cases from the airport PHS facilities to the designated hospitals. Utilizing the EMS citywide communication facility, a plan was developed whereby each time a unit was requested to stand by at the airport for a potential case, the designated receiving hospital was notified, so that a direct route to the isolation room was available to the crew, thus bypassing crowded EDs and patient areas, and chemoprophylaxis could be provided to the transporting crew. In addition, a bulletin was sent to all providers in the 9-1-1 system outlining signs and symptoms of pneumonic plague, travel history, and appropriate precautions to be taken by providers.

As the epidemic progressed, it became apparent, based on the incubation period, that an infected person could have entered the country before becoming symptomatic and might then present with generalized systemic symptoms. In response to this possible scenario, the plan was extended to use the EMS direct medical oversight physician as the screening physician. All DMOPs were briefed about signs and symptoms, incubation periods, travel history, and the need to identify and isolate suspected cases. Additionally, the physicians were provided with contact people within the health department to notify if a suspected case was encountered. This system extended the public health surveillance net further into communities, so that potentially infected persons were identified and appropriate precautions were taken before they arrived at a hospital. During the study period, no documented cases of plague were encountered; however, there were four suspected cases isolated pending work-up. Two of the four cases were identified at the PHS surveillance site and the others identified by the DMOPs.[30]

The addition of direct medical oversight in the prehospital phase to the public health surveillance system extended the safety net further into the community. This type of system can be useful in a biological agent surveillance scheme with extended incubation times to screen cases, especially in the early phases of an epidemic or outbreak. However, for the plan to be successful a system needs to be able to monitor all potential index cases, to have an operational interface with the possible receiving hospitals, and to involve all medical oversight facilities within the region. Ideally, the best system to implement this plan is one with a centralized communications and medical oversight facility.

Expanded Scope of Practice

It has been suggested that the future of prehospital care involves the integration of EMS into the full spectrum of healthcare, including participation in community health monitoring activities, increasing critical care skills and the formalization of non-transport options for providers.[31] The required skills for these activities will require a significant commitment of resources and education. The proper performance and monitoring of these skills mandate both indirect and direct medical oversight. Although it is clear that direct medical oversight is not likely to be the exclusive mode of physician oversight as it was during the initial development of prehospital care, there will still be a need for the DMOP to make medical decisions in selected patients.[14]

The incorporation of critical-care skill levels in curbside response and interfacility transfer is addressed elsewhere in this text. Suffice it to say, the complexity of patient problems requiring critical interventions necessitates more frequent contemporaneous involvement by the direct medical oversight physician. For example, infusion rates of vasoactive agents based on invasive monitoring often require the expertise beyond the scope of the most highly trained critical-care provider. Indeed, many emergency physicians who perform direct medical oversight do not have this critical-care expertise either, and qualifications for delegating physicians in these systems must be adjusted accordingly by the medical director. The disadvantage of increased on-scene times required for physician contact is outweighed by the advantage of specific therapy based on the individual needs of complex patients.[12] The incorporation of critical-care nurses into paramedic crews does not obviate the necessity of physician availability by phone or radio at all times for these patients.

One paradox of prehospital care is that often the most highly trained providers work in urban areas where there are shorter transport times to hospitals and consequently fewer prehospital interventions needed. In contrast, transport times in rural areas can be 40 minutes or longer, especially in those without access to air ambulance service. Ideally, time-dependent interventions such as thrombolysis should be administered in the field, requiring more interventions ordered by direct medical oversight, utilizing 12-lead telemetry.[32] In addition, longer transport times mean more patient status changes, which may not be covered by standing orders. More complex procedures such as rapid sequence intubation, in addition to requiring extra training and education, may mandate direct medical oversight in some prehospital systems.

Pronouncement of death through providers via direct physician contact should be considered in areas with longer transport times where legislation permits. The higher cost and risk to providers of futile resuscitations that occur in the back of ambulances over long distances should be evaluated in comparison with the education and legislation required that would enable field pronouncement in appropriate patients.[16]

There are many systems looking at new models of out-of-hospital care rendered by paramedics. Some of these models involve the assessment, treatment, and referral of patients to community services without transport to hospital. This practice has generally been referred to as "refusal of care," but with the evolution of managed care along with the increasing assessment skills of providers and the increasing confidence of the public in their abilities, a more proactive approach has been proposed.[33]

Direct medical oversight may be useful or essential for these and other areas of expanded scope of practice, including advanced assessment and non-transport options for such patient conditions as hypoglycemia, self-limited seizures, and stable supraventricular dysrhythmias.[34] Further evidence is needed of the safety, efficacy, and cost-effectiveness of these innovations before widespread implementation is recommended.

Summary

From the early days of out-of-hospital care by delegated providers when direct medical oversight was utilized as an all-inclusive form of medical oversight, to the current position as a more limited but essential component of the overall quality improvement of prehospital providers, direct medical oversight has evolved and adapted. Many prehospital systems continue to utilize direct medical oversight as an essential component in areas such as refusal of care, complex cases, critical care transport, triage decisions and for field pronouncement of death.

In 1994, Braun wrote: "Although telemetric data transmission from the scene has waned and the use of standing orders has waxed, the most significant recent trends are the shifts toward contemporaneous on-scene direct medical control and required contact in problem situations such as refusal of care."[1] While the former trend has not generally been borne out except in extraordinary circumstances such as disasters, the latter has served as one of the starting points for what is now termed "expanded scope of practice."[31] Discussion and differences in practice continue to occur. It is hoped that these differences will be resolved through evidence-based studies. The authors believe that the future of direct medical oversight will most certainly be tied to a new horizon of out-of-hospital care provided by prehospital providers as physician extenders in the community, consisting of public health initiatives, tailoring paramedic scope of practice to local community needs, and interacting with other healthcare agencies.

Given the requirement for some degree of direct medical oversight in most prehospital systems providing advanced level care, direct medical oversight resources will continue to function into the future. The best approach to optimizing the contributions from direct medical oversight systems is to consider direct medical oversight as an ever-present physician (or advanced provider) resource, which is flexible and dynamic. This valuable resource can be utilized and adapted by the system, and its role tailored to each system's unique needs. In this way, direct medical oversight will continue to be both a constant source of real-time medical oversight and a dynamic resource which innovative prehospital systems will utilize to help them meet the unique needs of their communities.

References

1. Kuehl A. Prehospital Systems and Medical Oversight (glossary). 3nd Edition, 2001.
2. Nagel E, et al. Telemetry-medical command in coronary and other mobile emergency care systems. *JAMA*. 1970; 214:332–338.
3. Bethesda Conference Report. *Amer J Cardiol*. 1969; 23:603–608.
4. Medical control of emergency medical services: an overview for emergency physicians. *Physicians* 1984 editorial.
5. Erder MH, et al. On-line medical command in theory and in practice. *Ann Emerg Med*. 1989;8:3, 261–268.
6. Gausche M, Henderson D, Seidel J. Vital signs as part of the prehospital assessment of the paediatric patient: a survey of paramedics. *Ann Emerg Med*. 1990;19(2):173–178.
7. Hunt R, et al. Standing orders vs voice control. *JEMS*. 1982;26–31.
8. Klein KR, et al. Effects of on-line medical control in the prehospital treatment of atraumatic illness. *Prehosp Emerg Care*. 1997;1(2):80–84.
9. Rottman S, et al. On-line medical control versus protocol based prehospital care. *Ann Emerg Med*. 1997;30(1): 62–68.
10. Holloman CJ, Wuerz R, Meador S. Medical command errors in an urban advanced life support system. *Ann Emerg Med*. 1992;21(4):347–350.
11. Holroyd B, Knoop R, Kallsen G. Medical control: quality assurance in prehospital care. *JAMA*. 1986;256: 1027–1031.
12. Pointer J, Osur M. Effect of standing orders on field times. *Ann Emerg Med*. 1989;18(10):1119–1121.
13. Gratton M, et al. Effect of standing orders on paramedic scene time for trauma patients. *Ann Emerg Med*. 1991; 20(12):1306–1309.
14. Hoffman J, et al. Does paramedic-base hospital contact result in beneficial deviations from standard prehospital protocols. *West J Med*. 1990;153:283–287.
15. Diamond N, Schofferman J, Elliot J. Factors in successful resuscitation by paramedics. *JACEP*. 1977;6(2):42–46.
16. Cheung M, Morrison LJ, Verbeek PR. Prehospital vs. emergency department pronouncement of death: a cost analysis. *Can J Emerg Med*. 2001;3(1):19–25.
17. Stark G, Hedges J. Patients who initially refuse prehospital evaluation and/or therapy. *Am J Emerg Med*. 1990;8:509–511.
18. Alicandro J, et al. Impact of interventions for patients refusing emergency medical services transport. *Acad Emerg Med*. 1995;2(6):480–485.
19. Burstein, et al. Refusal of out of hospital medical care: effect of medical-control physician assertiveness on transport rate. *Acad Emerg Med*. 1998;5(1):4–8.
20. Frew SA. Emergency medical services legal issues for the emergency physician. *Emerg Med Clin North Am*. 1990;8(1):28–34.
21. Dinerman N, Rosen P, Pons P. Medical control in prehospital care. *Current Topics II in Emergency Medicine*. 1981;7.
22. Pozen, et al. Studies of ambulance patients with ischemic heart disease: 1.The outcome of pre-hospital life-threatening arrhythmias in patients receiving electrocardiographic telemetry and therapeutic interventions. *Am J Public Health*. 1977;67(6):527–531.
24. Cayten C, et al. The effect of telemetry on urban prehospital cardiac care. *Ann Emerg Med*. 1985;14(10): 976–981.
25. Stewart R. When less is more: teflon and telemetry in the space age. *Ann Emerg Med*. 1985;14(10):992–994.
26. Aufderheide TP, Hendley GE, Woo J, et al. A prospective evaluation of prehospital 12-lead EKG application in chest pain patients. *J Electrocardiol*. 1992;24S:8–13.
27. Kereiakes DJ, Gibler WB, Martin LH, et al. Relative importance of emergency medical system transport and the prehospital electrocardiogram on reducing hospital time delay to therapy for acute myocardial infarction: a preliminary report from the Cincinnati Heart Project. *Am Heart J*. 1992;23:835–840.
28. Karagounis L, Ipsen SK, Jessop MR, et al. Impact of field transmitted electrocardiography on time to in-hospital thrombolytic therapy in acute myocardial infarction. *Am J Cardiol*. 1990;66:786–791.
29. Lombardi G, Gallagher J, Gennis P. Outcomes of out-of-hospital cardiac arrest in New York City: the PHASE study. *JAMA*. 1994;271(9):678–683.
30. McIntosh BA, Hines R, Giordano LM. The role of EMS systems in public health emergencies. *Prehosp Disaster Med*. 1997;12(1):30–35.
31. Delbridge T et al. EMS agenda for the future: where we are . . . where we want to be. *Prehosp Emerg Care*. 1998; 2:1–12.
32. Morrison LJ, et al. Mortality and prehospital thrombolysis for acute myocardial infarction: a meta-analysis. *JAMA*. 2000;283:2686–2692.
33. Bissell RA, et al. A medically wise approach to expanding the role of paramedics as physician extenders. *Prehosp Emerg Care*. 1999;3:170–173.
34. Socransky S, Pirrallo R, Rubin J. Out-of-hospital treatment of hypoglycemia: refusal of transport and patient outcome. *Acad Emerg Med*. 1998;5:1080–1085.

CHAPTER 28

On-Scene Supervision

Fernando L. Benitez, MD
Paul E. Pepe, MD

Introduction

Advances in science and medicine, coupled with recent technological developments, have provided us with the opportunity to further improve and expand our scope of practice in the prehospital setting.[1] At the same time, regardless of new developments and innovations, the evolving discipline of emergency medical services (EMS) also needs to maintain certain core principles of basic patient care. A key linkage between the exploration of advances and the safeguarding of basic patient care is medical oversight.[1-6] Therefore, as discussed throughout this textbook, expert physician supervision and accountability should be considered a key element of the EMS system.[7-15]

Today, most regional and municipal EMS programs contract with a physician or several physicians for medical oversight.[9,16-18] In many major metropolitan areas, multiple EMS physicians may be hired full-time, while in many other smaller areas, it remains a part-time or even a volunteer job.[16,19] In theory, these physicians are required to provide direct and indirect medical oversight, and to delegate the performance of medical acts to those professional EMS personnel who work under their respective licenses.[1,2,7,17,18,20]

In some venues, the medical community, and the public in general, also view an EMS response as an automatic referral to the designated EMS physician and, of course, his practice surrogates (the EMS personnel).[1] The nature of this referral is a public trust to care for that community's patients during the brief prehospital phase of their emergencies.[15] In essence, according to the intent of some statutes and EMS regulations, the accountable EMS physicians are ensuring the community that the EMS personnel will deliver the same quality of medical care that they would have directly rendered had they been at the scene themselves. As such, it would be the obligation of a physician assuming the responsibility of medical oversight for a system to ensure such quality.[1,2,16,21] In turn, the medical director can offer this level of quality to the community by following some simple basic principles of medical education.[22]

Basic Principles

Specifically, an aggressive, comprehensive, and quality-providing medical educational program combines "street-wise" didactics, expert clinical apprenticeship, and expert, ongoing, on-scene supervision.[5,6,16] Indeed, the classic principles of medical education, regardless of specialty, have always involved an apprenticeship approach. Didactics, basic skills, and clerkships may earn one a medical degree, but the apprenticeships of internship, residency, and fellowships under specialized physician mentors remain the ultimate keystones of clinical medical training.

Basic emergency medical technician (EMT-B) and paramedic education must not be considered different from basic medical education. Medical students, residents, and fellows would not be sent alone to perform medical diagnoses, treatment plans, and procedures before undergoing a rigorous supervised apprenticeship. It must be made clear from the start that all EMS providers also require such an apprenticeship, which should involve routine on-scene supervision and training from physician experts in providing all levels of prehospital care.[20,23] Therefore, it is incumbent upon the medical director to be competent in all of these settings, and to provide a span of mentorship that bridges these three components.[24,25]

Typically, however, most EMS training programs integrate "apprenticeships" by means of clinical rotations, some briefly in the hospital setting and others using "ride-alongs" with established EMS crews. Although this approach often brings students closer to certain hospital-based physicians, those physicians may or may not be EMS-oriented, let alone EMS-experienced. Also, the experience with these physicians is short-lived in that they do not maintain a long-term mentor-student relationship. Much of the primary education and prehospital apprenticeship for providers is provided mainly by non-physician EMS instructors. Often, these instructors are more field-oriented and street-wise than their physician directors. But, in turn, this leaves a significant gap in the key role of the accountable EMS physician supervisor. Therefore, the medical director should be intimately involved in establishing or modifying educational objectives, participating in classroom teaching, and providing direct field supervision in order to bridge this gap. This kind of activity is more significant today because of the rapid changes in technology as well as the advances and controversies in research.[1,26]

Medical-Legal Accountability

Field mentorship and supervision by expert, knowledgeable, street-wise physicians is not only an essential component of proper medical education, but it is also a means of providing improved medical-legal accountability for the medical acts delegated to the EMS personnel. In most states, medical direction of EMS systems is mandated by law.[12,17,21] Therefore, it is the responsibility of the medical director and his designees to oversee and scrutinize the EMS personnel as well as any operational aspect of the system that affects medical care.[1,2,5,11,13,22,26–29]

Quality Management

It is human nature to err. It can also be human nature to develop certain inappropriate habits, particularly when operating in a void without proper scrutiny or feedback. In EMS, it often requires direct field observation to identify such behaviors. That which appears to have been the provision of proper procedure, either by way of information recorded during radio communication or even by direct scrutiny on arrival at the emergency department, may not necessarily reflect improprieties at the scene. For example, a poor extrication procedure can be masked by subsequent meticulous spinal immobilization in the ambulance; a patient may even be walked to the stretcher and then immobilized. Whether done knowingly or through ignorance, the poor scene performance not only goes unnoticed, but often such behavior is reinforced by kudos given for the way the patient presents at the hospital. The accountable medical director, however, would not have provided care in this manner, had he been at the scene.

For all the above reasons, at one point or another, personal, on-scene experience and on-scene supervision of EMS personnel becomes a must for EMS physician duties and responsibilities. However, on-scene supervision can be a nebulous concept for those unacquainted with such activities. The purpose of the following discussion will be to help establish some reasonable guidelines and approaches to on-scene supervision of EMS.

Structure and Function

Logistics

To be successful, the medical director can be aided by a better understanding of the structure and specific approaches to field supervision. Each EMS jurisdiction has its own unique characteristics, depending on its location and the size of the system. EMS can be a difficult practice to maintain properly because of either extremely high caseloads and/or difficult geographical logistics.[5,19,30] Some medical directors oversee systems with a relatively small geographic area of coverage but are accountable for tens of thousands of patients monthly.[30] On the other hand, other directors may only be responsible for a few hundred annual cases, but these occur in territories covering tens of thousands of square miles.[19] The logistics involved in assuring proper field care of patients are unique for each system and for each case. Therefore, supervision in such varied settings will probably require a special knowledge of the particularities of the system and a high level of dedication from the supervising physician.

Looking at a theoretical gold standard, the ideal situation would be to somehow oversee and supervise all phases of patient care from dispatch to delivery of the patient at the emergency department. This ideal concept could be made analogous to what some anesthesiologists might do in their practice. For example, they may delegate patient care to the nurse-anesthetists, but they are intermittently providing direct supervision, oversight, and accountability for patient management; they are always available in difficult situations. Unfortunately, the reality in EMS falls short of the idealistic goal because of logistics and volume. The geographic boundaries and the vastly expanded caseloads make it impossible for the physician to directly oversee each patient encounter.

However, adequate quality of care and oversight can be accomplished in the majority of EMS systems if certain mechanisms for scene supervision are established. The first step in providing such supervision is to establish an appropriate structure for out-of-hospital oversight.

Structure

The structure of EMS response includes multiple considerations such as vehicles, communication hardware, safety, and medical care equipment, as well as appropriate attire/protective clothing issues. Whatever structure is chosen, the logistics of EMS response for the supervising physician must be predetermined and arranged in accordance with the local jurisdiction. The responding physician must adhere to these local ordinances to ensure a safe and appropriate response.

To accomplish the supervisory activities, the medical director should have direct, round-the-clock access to an emergency response vehicle, which should be clearly marked (and maintained) by the local authorities.[24] Given the unpredictable nature of emergencies, this approach allows for a timely, uninhibited, and authorized response in key situations, at any time of day or night and from any location, including home. The EMS physician must be trained in an emergency vehicle operation course (EVOC) and understand the limits of emergency vehicle operation, both statutorily and technically in certain weather and traffic conditions.

Although a physician response vehicle represents the ideal for scene response, it is not always a possibility, due to financial constraints and other local problems. In those cases, other alternatives must be considered. Such alternatives include "ride-alongs" accompanied by EMS system officers and/or supervisors, field training officers, or directly with ambulance personnel. Even in EMS systems where the medical director can gain access to an emergency response vehicle, routine "ride-alongs" with ambulance personnel are still vital to assess direct patient care by the EMS personnel while en route to the hospital, to evaluate patient transition at the hospital, and also to establish better rapport with individual EMTs and paramedics.

Unless there are no other options, responses in one's personal vehicle, with or without warning devices are discouraged. Automobile insurance coverage, personal liability, and public safety become confounding concerns of the EMS physician when using a personal vehicle. Today, most urban EMS systems provide response vehicles to their EMS physicians.

It is advocated that the novice EMS physician respond to as many calls as possible. This is especially important at the beginning of the medical director's term when he needs to reach out, meet with, and assess the capabilities of the EMTs and paramedics. In fact, a strong suggestion is not to use one's own response vehicle at first. Instead, the new EMS physician should become part of the system and establish relations by ride-alongs with officers and ambulance crews. Once the medical director's level of confidence and, reciprocally, that of the EMS personnel is built, the physician can progressively delegate more medical supervisory responsibilities to field supervisors, veteran paramedics, or field training officers. Still, the medical director should continue to respond, both in scheduled and unscheduled fashions.

It is obvious that not all calls require the medical expertise of a physician at the scene, but some specific situations may merit a routine dispatch or notification of the EMS physician (see table 28.1). These situations include, but are not limited to, multiple or mass casualty incidents; specialized rescue situations

TABLE 28.1
Examples of situations for which an EMS physician might be alerted for potential scene response by dispatchers
▪ Multiple/mass casualty Incidents
▪ Major vehicle collisions with entrapment
▪ Specialized rescue (heavy rescue, trench, confined space, water/swift water, vertical)
▪ Major airport alerts (airplane crash)
▪ Hazardous materials incidents
▪ Weapons of mass effect incidents
▪ Tactical, hostage situations
▪ Significant structure fires or major fire with victims
▪ Structural collapse with entrapment
▪ Anticipated difficult airways
▪ Difficult deliveries
▪ Need for field amputations
▪ Incident involving a complicated field termination of resuscitative efforts
▪ Mass gathering events
▪ Major political or media events
▪ Unusual medical situation (anatomical oddity or unusual home medical device).

(trench, water or swift water, vertical, and confined space rescue); major airport alerts; hazardous materials or weapons of mass effect incidents; significant structural fires and major fires with victims; major vehicle collisions (particularly those with trapped victims); structural collapse with entrapment; any hostage or extended tactical operation; anticipated difficult airways; complicated deliveries; complicated field termination of resuscitative efforts; or need for a field amputation. Also, the physician can be available on-scene (or on a standby basis) for any mass gathering events or any major incident that would attract political or media attention. Sometimes the EMS personnel may also need advice and direction for a medical oddity or unusual at-home medical devices. The purpose of such responses is not necessarily to assume charge of medical care activity, but rather to stand by and assist as a medical advocate and as a medical resource, as well as to gain valuable insight into scene logistics and dynamics. Such experiences improve subsequent quality assurance activities as well as the preparation of future didactic initiatives for the EMS personnel.

In some instances, however, the physician may need to be involved with scene control and direct patient care. This eventuality might occur if the EMS physician is the first to arrive on-scene. Also, the EMS physician may be useful in double-checking for missed injuries or overlooked victims at a multi-casualty incident, and looking for occult hazards while paramedics care for the most sick and injured. Hands-on care may also be inevitable in cases involving multiple victims or a severely injured individual when extra hands are necessary to expedite critical care and/or evacuation.

Although jurisdictional EMS physicians can give direct medical oversight at the scene that can expedite patient care, it must be remembered that they are more effective in the role of a teacher. Future quality is more likely to be guaranteed if the provider is first asked, "What do you want to do now?" Although they do provide expeditious direct medical oversight, direct orders are relatively ineffective as either an evaluation or teaching tool.

Since adequate communication among the responding units is key to every response, direct contact between the EMS physician and the dispatch center, field personnel, medical control center, other local authorities, and hospitals must be available at all times. This rapid communication access can be accomplished by means of mobile radios, mobile phones, mobile data terminals, or pagers. Either one (with the exception of the pager) or a combination of these systems will help to ensure adequate rapid access for communications.

Safety is also of prime concern. For this reason, if responding directly, the physician should not only have specific training in emergency vehicle operation, but also be familiar with the relevant policies and procedures of the jurisdictional authorities. For example, emergency lights and sirens do not provide for a permission to disregard all traffic regulations. Also, responders should possess the appropriate identification required by authorities, particularly to avoid a frustrating confrontation at the very moment a patient may need the physician's support and services. Again, to expedite access, this concept applies to vehicular identification as well.

The EMS physician must be cognizant of street hazards that are not present in an emergency department environment, such as traffic, fire, weather, down-wind hazardous materials, live weapons, cross-fire, explosion risk, and hostile crowds. The development of a "street sense" is the ability to recognize an unsafe scene and to prevent bodily harm to oneself and others.

The EMS physician who responds directly to the emergency scene should be equipped and prepared to deliver advanced emergency medical care. Emergencies are unpredictable, and circumstances may suddenly place the supervising physician closer to the scene than the responding units, especially when their arrival may be delayed as a result of high-volume, geography, traffic, or even unexpected mechanical problems. On occasion, physicians in emergency response vehicles may happen upon or be "flagged down" at emergency scenes, even prior to activation of the EMS system. Also, in the event of multiple casualty incidents, the responding physician may be involved in direct patient care while other personnel attend other victims.

Although usually unnecessary, the capability of the EMS physician to perform direct patient care in the field is still clearly essential. Aside from the unexpected situations previously mentioned, the physician's ability to provide excellent prehospital care under the same conditions as any paramedic may also become a key factor in establishing credibility with EMS personnel. For this reason, the medical director is also advised to become involved with, or at least very familiar with, specialized rescue system training such as extrication and heavy rescue, weapons of mass effect and hazmat, among others. This type of training helps the physician gain knowledge about the expectations and logistics of field operations, and it improves communication, cooperation, and teamwork between the rescuers and the physician. It also improves safety awareness.

Therefore, the EMS physician must be equipped with sophisticated medical capabilities. The physician should have readily available a monitor/defibrillator, airway management kit, oxygen delivery system with a bag-valve-mask, a medical kit stocked with IV-access supplies, scalpel, and drugs. These should include epinephrine, atropine, lidocaine, amiodarone, dextrose, nitroglycerine, furosemide, diazepam, and any combination of drugs for rapid sequence induction (RSI) intubation, as well as certain antidotes such as 2-PAM and cyanide kits (see table 28.2).

In addition to classic medical supplies, thought should also be given to items such as a fire extinguisher, a high-powered flashlight, flares, binoculars, foul weather clothing, rescue blankets, and communication equipment (table 28.2). Depending on potential needs and the EMS system design, equipment such as splints, immobilization devices, hazardous materials references, bulletproof vest, and other drugs could also prove useful. However, the equipment just catalogued might be considered a basic minimum inventory.

Dress is a matter of personal choice, but one should take into account that out-of-hospital medical care is performed in the streets, in private homes, and in public venues within full view of the lay public, other professionals, and (often) public officials and the media. Physicians involved in field response should be cognizant of the patient's and their relatives' sensitivities and expectations, particularly when entering someone's home. For example, wearing jeans may not convey the appropriate respect for certain individuals. On the other hand, the physician may be involved with high-risk rescue operations and the elements and hazards likely to be encountered (e.g., blood, vomitus, and sharp objects) must also be taken into account. The use of rugged clothing, protective head, eye, and ear gear, protective shoes or boots, and adequate personal protective equipment are always recommended. In addition, visibility on dark, rain-slicked streets should be considered. Reflective gear should be worn as required by the specific environment.

TABLE 28.2

Some suggested EMS physician equipment and drug inventory

- Monitor/defibrillator or AED
- Airway management kit with endotracheal tubes/laryngoscope
- Oxygen delivery systems
- Bag-valve-mask device
- Medical kit with IV-access supplies
- Drug pack with: epinephrine, atropine, amiodarone, lidocaine, dextrose, nitroglycerine, furosemide, diazepam, drugs for rapid sequence intubation, 2-PAM, cyanide kit;
- Scalpel, 4x4 gauze, tape
- High-powered flashlight
- Rescue blankets
- Communications equipment (radio, pager, cell phone)
- Identification (card/badge)
- Fire extinguisher
- Flares
- Binoculars
- Foul weather clothing
- Reflective clothing/vests
- Bullet-proof vests
- Splints/immobilization devices
- Hazardous materials manuals

On-Scene Functions

The function of the physician at the scene should be one of supervision and facilitation. It could involve helping the incident commander with the logistics of patient triage and management, but it should not involve the presumption of total control of a medical scene just because the EMS physician is the most highly-trained person there. Except in those cases in which the patient outcome truly requires direct intervention (either as a matter of assistance or to correct clear mismanagement of critical medical care), scene supervision should ideally be considered an educational feedback event. This philosophy stems from the concept that the EMS physician is not always there day-to-day, and that an important axiom in EMS is that "day-to-day routines should not be routinely changed," unless they are bad routines.

As an initial approach, the physician's scene activities should center on observation while offering assistance ("Can I be of any help to you?" or "What can I do for you?"). This approach not only helps to identify the priorities and delegation talents of the EMS personnel, but it also helps to diminish their anxiety about being scrutinized though it does not totally remove that discomfort. The physician should be willing to do any kind of menial task needed at the scene, from assistance with basic CPR to picking up packaging and other waste. Such courtesy and humility establish credibility and role-modeling, as well as a sense of empathy for the roles of others.

A benefit of being primarily an observer at the scene is that the physician may have better perspective by standing farther away from the victim than the EMS personnel. This gives the advantage of having a global view of the scene, as opposed to those at the side of the patient who are mainly focused on the patient. This global view also lets one visualize the actions of the providers as a team, and provides a different perspective of the logistics involved in the management of the patient. It provides for identifying other ways of approaching the needs of both the patient and the rescuers while helping to identify hazardous situations. The EMS physician would be looking after not only the welfare of the patient but also the welfare of the EMS personnel.

There are two caveats about "standing back" at the scene. One can be perceived as standing back "too far" and not being involved. Therefore, it is important for the EMS physician to ask, early on, how he or she can help. Again, one must recognize the dynamics of individual preferences. More secure paramedics may welcome the physician's presence while the more insecure might find it to be interference. In contrast, the *very* insecure might also want the doctor to "take over" altogether. This, in itself, is an important consideration in on-scene interactions with various personnel, particularly in terms of evaluation of the efficacy of the EMS system.

One difficulty, therefore, is the sociological version of the Heisenberg Uncertainty Principle. The physician's very presence changes the situation, so one cannot "measure" what is really there. As with Heisenberg's principle, to see things, one must introduce light, and the "light" affects the measurement. Despite Heisenberg, the physician who comes to the EMS scene in a covert fashion can also be seen as "spying," which may engender distrust and less candor between the physician and the EMS personnel. Therefore, the ultimate compromise is to come as a teacher, advisor, and resource.

Recognizing this key role of a teacher, occasionally on-scene activities should involve a "helpful tip" approach such as "Let me show you something," or an even less patronizing strategy, such as "Let's try something here" or "I'd like to try something differ-

ent, if that's okay with you." Speaking in the first-person plural also works well (i.e., "You know what we should try. . ."). However, such helpful tips should be given some time after establishing rapport with the providers at hand, or else they may also be seen as patronizing.

Timely corrective action, coupled with positive and constructive feedback and reassurance, helps to maintain the morale of the EMS personnel in those situations in which the physician finds a problem with the management. As is the case when dealing with any type of supervisee, the egos and sense of self-esteem of the EMS personnel are best dealt with through encouragement and by instilling a sense of pride in their work. An even more important incentive may be to invoke the virtues of patient care. Doing what is best for the patient is a great motivator for EMS personnel. For example, after taking a corrective action at the scene (e.g., recommending a repositioning of the endotracheal tube marker from 28 cm at the front teeth up to a more correct depth for the patient), one might later explain to the paramedic the rationale behind the corrective action while simultaneously expressing something like: "I also want *us* to look 100% on target when our patient arrives at the emergency department." Also, efforts should be made later to praise the medics publicly for everything that was done appropriately at that very scene. A simple letter commending the team in a job well done on such a difficult case is also a good way of providing positive feedback, and it can take the sting out of any on-scene critique of an individual issue. Of course, whenever possible, any on-scene critique should take place out of earshot of patients and colleagues, or should wait until after the event if immediate corrective action is not critical. When it is timely, however, there are certain ways to handle the situation.

For example, take the case of a patient who has been defibrillated successfully and has strong pulses, and the protocol now calls for an anti-arrhythmic. If the paramedic does not immediately remember to give the drug, the EMS physician shouldn't just order the anti-arrhythmic. Instead, he should ask, "What do you want to do now?" If the response is, "Let's package him up and transport," the next query might be more directed, such as "Don't we need to give a drug now?" This type of interaction is more apt to reinforce proper protocol next time than just ordering the drug. The Socratic approach (asking questions) always provides better cognitive reinforcement. Being a teacher is a key role of the medical director and this establishes role-modeling for other senior EMS personnel such as supervisors, field training officers, and the like.

Above all, EMS physicians must be role models, not only in terms of the medical actions to be taken, but also in terms of their behavior and their demeanor. Compassion and caring should always be paramount in the EMS physician's mind, no matter how difficult the patient or the situation, particularly when considering the fact that 90 to 95% of all EMS incidents largely involve reassurance and basic "caring." Such physician-like behavior (in the classic sense) may be the greatest teaching tool. In addition, EMS physicians must keep in mind that the example they set in providing professionalism and decorum may be needed when enthusiasm, compensatory humor, and "esprit de corps" occasionally become too fervent.

Ground Rules

In most states, the medical director is responsible for the medical actions undertaken by the EMS personnel in his jurisdiction. It must be understood by everyone at the scene (e.g., police officers, fire personnel, and, by default, EMS staff and their supervisors) that medical direction and medical accountability do rest with the designated medical director. Therefore, no doubt should exist as to clear jurisdiction in terms of medical care. Nevertheless, it should be understood that the physician is merely accountable for medical management of victims and not for other aspects of scene operations. Other aspects, like scene safety and security, rest with law enforcement officials, the fire department chiefs, or other responsible agencies.

It should be common knowledge that the medical director may show up at any given time, day or night, announced or unannounced. It should also be understood that, unlike intervening physicians, medical directors have unquestionable responsibility for the medical care rendered. Therefore, they have the capacity and right to change any protocol or issue any medical order in any given case. However, physicians who do so without explanation (either concurrent or subsequent feedback) risk confusion or even credibility. Also, EMS physicians who are not the designated medical director, particularly those in training, may not be totally authorized to assume the responsibility attributed to the system medical director. Therefore, prospective authorization or restrictions should be established by the designated system medical director.

Again, the on-scene physician should be extremely careful when correcting or modifying the actions of any personnel to avoid embarrassing individuals and, perhaps more importantly, to avoid liability for all involved by announcing that a particular action or procedure was not done correctly. For example, take the case of a patient shot near the spinal area of the midback while riding on a bus, who appears to be stable in condition. If the EMS personnel are observed to be preparing to walk the man off of the bus, it might be more advisable and more tactful to suggest that, "Why don't we set this man onto a backboard to make him more comfortable?"

Liability

The physician's presence at an emergency scene raises a number of medical-legal questions regarding liability and standard of care. Many states have enacted Good Samaritan laws or other legislation that may provide some protection from liability. At the same time, many of these statutes specifically exempt physicians, even when there is no expectation of remuneration. More importantly, if EMS is part of a physician's job responsibility, the intent of the Good Samaritan legislation may not apply. Therefore, a physician would certainly present a greater target for litigation, particularly if expected to deliver prehospital care. The EMS physician's presence can also raise expectations about the level of care that can be provided. Unsuccessful outcomes are probably less easily forgiven than when the care providers at the scene are non-physicians.

Still, these problems should not discourage EMS physicians from participating in field responses. Physicians can often perform an important role by directly communicating with the patient or family, and their personal presence often lends further credibility and decreases exposure for the EMS system. Indeed, an EMS physician's presence in someone's home could be considered a house call and, if handled properly, can be extremely rewarding for the physician, the patient, the family, and the EMS system as a whole.

Above all, experienced EMS physicians eventually diminish liability for themselves (as well as for their EMS systems) by developing a unique expertise and knowledge base that is difficult to match, particularly in any courtroom.

Field Supervisory Skills

Developing Credibility

Prospective EMS physicians must gain credibility both as health professionals and as teachers. Also, they need to appreciate the differences between in-hospital and prehospital emergency care. Those who do not have clear medical authority (i.e., resident physicians on an EMS rotation, or new EMS fellows) are most effective after they have become a familiar face to the EMS personnel, particularly in a teacher-student role. This activity usually sets up a level of training hierarchy and establishes credibility, especially if it is later balanced with firsthand knowledge of field logistics.

As discussed previously, in addition to their didactic teaching roles, prospective EMS physicians or even established medical directors need to establish credibility and rapport by active and frequent participation in all aspects of prehospital care. Again, such activities should be made in more of an assistance and educational capacity, at least at first. Medical authority is mostly earned, not just appointed.[24] In the streets, and especially in well-entrenched EMS systems, this goal may take months or even years to accomplish.

Delegating Field Supervision

EMS activities may peak and wane, but they never sleep and, although round-the-clock direct physician oversight is ideal, the EMS physician does have other responsibilities and also need to have some degree of rest. Therefore, when unable to provide supervision at given times, a medical director may delegate this responsibility directly to certain EMS personnel. In some settings direct medical oversight or supervision can be delegated to assistant medical directors, command center personnel, and/or, perhaps more feasibly, to shift supervisors. A small cadre of field supervisors who can effect coverage 24 hours a day on behalf of the medical director can serve as an excellent point of control, particularly in urban settings.

The use of veteran paramedics or field training officers as supervisory personnel who can regularly interact and learn directly from the EMS system medical director, both on-scene and didactically, is often an efficient approach to effecting more full-time field supervision. Through close interaction with these few individuals, an effective, manageable span of control can be realized, particularly if operating in a large geographic jurisdiction. However, this relationship still requires the key element of apprenticeship and close physician mentorship for these select individuals, especially in the actual patient-care setting. This may be achieved by routine "ride-alongs" with these specialized supervisory personnel. Frequent meetings to provide didactics, address questions, and discuss specific or difficult cases will also provide valuable information to and from the medical director.

In some EMS systems, field officers not only provide good medical care, but also possess good leadership skills. The day-to-day EMS personnel must have respect, both medically and personally, for such supervisors. Therefore, mechanisms to ensure that they possess such leadership attributes must be present in the supervisor selection process. In addition, if the responsibility of medical supervision is to be delegated, the basic principles of EMS systems must be clearly understood and appreciated by these direct agents of the EMS physician. In turn, such principles must be passed on to the field personnel at large.

They also are excellent persons to help in the design and implementation of research, particularly innovative clinical trials.[26]

How Much Field Supervision?

Predictable Performance

Exactly how much on-scene supervision is enough? In general terms, field supervision is sufficient when the EMS physician feels reasonably confident that each individual EMS provider could be trusted to readily and safely care for the medical director's own family. At the very least, supervision should continue until each provider's individual behavior and medical performance are assessed, tailored to provide quality of care, and readily predictable.

Again, one of the principles of EMS is to delegate care to others, with the understanding that the care rendered will be the same quality as if the physician delegating that care were delivering it personally.[1,5] Therefore, to feel comfortable with the achievements of this obligation, the physician should have shared a large sample of experiences with each of the individual providers operating under his supervision. If necessary, EMS personnel located in distant low-volume venues might be assigned to work directly in higher-volume areas for a period of time under the medical director's direct oversight.[19]

As with anything else, EMS field supervision and evaluation can at first be intensive and almost continuous. Eventually, however, the relative frequency may diminish, once trust or at least predictability is established. Nevertheless, intermittent spot checks should always be conducted to keep everyone "on their toes" and also to introduce new innovations. Many new procedures are often developed by providers in conjunction with their medical directors on-scene.

Back to Basics

For many, the excitement of rushing to the scene and providing emergent medical care to the acutely ill or injured can be very appealing. Nevertheless, one should make a conscious effort to remember that field supervisory activities should not be limited to the more "exciting" cases. In fact, a routine effort should be made to spot-check and observe the more "mundane" cases which make up 90 to 95% of responses. Medical care, no matter how basic, is still medical care.[20] Furthermore, those cases that do not involve clear-cut "life and death" actions may pose some of the most difficult decisions. Cases involving refusal or denial of service are perhaps the most compelling to supervise. Here, judgment and liability walk hand in hand. Providing a good example or delivering sound advice in such cases may, in some ways, prove to be the most important role of the physician. Most importantly, few things in EMS are more essential than the role-modeling of an EMS physician who finds it just as important to hold the hand of a frightened child or an elderly man with abdominal pain.

Summary

The entity of EMS is the practice of medicine. Ideally, the actual care provided by EMS personnel at each scene should be the same as that which would have been provided personally by the designated physician for the EMS system. To best guarantee this presumption and to best train prospective EMS personnel and assistant EMS physicians alike, medical directors must provide on-scene education, feedback, and personal example. Because improper actions cannot be determined solely by the conditions at the time of hospital arrival or by review of prehospital care records, scene supervision remains the true cornerstone of quality assurance.

Therefore, physicians must be prepared to provide regular on-scene supervision. To do so, physicians must also understand field conditions and priorities. They must be willing to establish their credibility by actively participating both in classroom training and in routine tasks in all scopes of the prehospital setting. Authority is earned, not just appointed. Whatever the mechanism, field response must be done in coordination with the policies and procedures of local jurisdictional authorities. Often, the use of carefully selected supervisors, who represent the medical director around the clock, can provide an efficient and effective instrument to realize a continuous, manageable medical chain of command.

References

1. Pepe PE, Bonnin MJ, Mattox KL. Regulating the scope of emergency medical services. *Prehosp Disast Med.* 1990; 5:59–63.
2. Corey E. Medical oversight: to ensure success in EMS systems, medical oversight and the medical director's role must evolve. *Emergency.* 1995;27(4):28–32.
3. Krohmer JR. The patient's best advocate. *JEMS.* 1997; 22(7):42–44.
4. Ferko JG III. Why EMS needs physicians. *JEMS.* 1987; 12(9):51–57.
5. Pepe PE, Stewart RD. Role of the physician in the prehospital setting. *Ann Emerg Med.* 1986;15:1480–1483.
6. Stewart RD. Medical direction in emergency medical services: the role of the physician. *Emerg Med Clin North Am.* 1987;5:119–132.
7. Krentz MJ, Wainscott MP. Medical accountability. *Emerg Med Clin North Am* 1990;8(1):17–32.
8. *American College of Emergency Physicians.* Emergency Medical Services Committee: medical control of pre-hospital emergency services. *Ann Emerg Med.* 1982;11:387.
9. Falk JL. Medical direction of emergency medical service systems: a full-time commitment whose time has come. *Crit Care Med.* 1993;21(9):1259–1260.
10. McSwain NE. Indirect medical control. In: Kuehl AE, ed. *EMS Medical Directors Handbook.* St. Louis: Mosby-Year Book; 1989.
11. Pepe PE, Copass MK. Prehospital care. In: Moore EE, ed. *Early care of the injured.* Toronto: B.C. Decker Inc.; 1990:34–55.
12. Racht EM, Reines HD. Medical oversight. In: Kuehl AE, ed. *Prehospital Systems and Medical Oversight.* St. Louis: Mosby-Year Book; 1994:181–185.
13. Subcommittee on Medical Control, Committee on Emergency Medical Services, National Research Council, Academy of Life Sciences: *Medical control in emergency medical services.* In: *Subcommittee Report, Conclusions and Recommendations.* Washington, DC: National Academy Press; 1981.

14. *American College of Emergency Physicians.* Medical direction of emergency medical services. *Ann Emerg Med.* 1998;31:152.

15. Alonso-Serra H, Blanton D, O'Connor RE. Physician medical direction in EMS. *Prehosp Emerg Care.* 1998; 2(2):153–157.

16. Pepe PE, Mattox KL, Duke JH. Effect of full-time, specialized physician supervision on the success of a large, urban emergency medical services system. *Crit Care Med.* 1993;21:1279–1286.

17. Wydro GC, Cone DC, Davidson SJ. Legislative and regulatory description of EMS medical direction: a survey of states. *Prehosp Emerg Care.* 1997;1(4)233–237.

18. Stone RM, Seaman KG, Bissell RA. A statewide study of EMS oversight: medical director characteristics and involvement compared with national guidelines. *Prehosp Emerg Care.* 2000;4(4):345–351.

19. Garnett CF, Hall JE, Johnson MS. Rural emergency medical services. In: Kuehl AE, ed. *EMS Medical Directors Handbook.* St. Louis: Mosby-Year Book; 1989.

20. Pepe PE. Medical direction in basic life support (editorial). *Emergency.* 1990;22:6.

21. Davis EA, Billitier AJ. The utilization of quality assurance methods in emergency medical services. *Prehosp Disast Med.* 1993;8(2):127–132.

22. Storer DL, Dickinson ET. Physician medical direction of EMS education programs: policy resource and education paper. *Prehosp Emerg Care.* 1998;2:158–159.

23. Polsky S, Krohmer J, Maningas P, McDowell R, Benson N, Pons P. Guidelines for medical direction of prehospital EMS. *Ann Emerg Med.* 1993;22(4):742–744.

24. Stewart RD, Paris PM, Heller M. Design of a resident in-field experience for an emergency medicine residency curriculum. *Ann Emerg Med.* 1987;16:175–179.

25. Hall WL, Nowels D. Colorado family practice graduates' preparation for and practice of emergency medicine. *J Am Board Fam Pract.* 2000;13(4):246–250.

26. Pepe PE. Out-of-hospital resuscitation research: rationale and strategies for controlled clinical trials. *Ann Emerg Med.* 1993;22:17–23.

27. ACEP. Medical direction for staffing of ambulances. *Ann Emerg Med.* 1999;34:421–422.

28. Poulton TJ, Kisicki PA. Medical directors of critical care air transport services. *Crit Care Med.* 1987;15(8):784–785.

29. Rinnert KJ, Blumen IJ, Gabram SGA, Zanker M. A descriptive analysis of air medical directors in the United States. *Air Medical Journal.* 1999;18(1):6–11.

30. Pepe PE, et al. Geographical distribution of urban trauma according to mechanism and severity of injury. *J Trauma.* 1990;30:1125–1132.

Education

Bruce J. Walz, PhD, NREMT-P

CHAPTER 29

Introduction

Of the many roles and responsibilities of the EMS Medical Director, perhaps none are as important as those related to education. Education permeates all aspects of EMS. Traditionally, education has been the prime change agent for EMS systems. Thus, it is important for the medical director to have a broad understanding of the role of education in EMS, the EMS education delivery system, and the importance of quality in EMS education.

The importance of the medical director's role in EMS education was formally recognized by the American College of Emergency Physicians (ACEP) and the National Association of EMS Physicians (NAEMSP) in a joint policy statement issued in 1997. According to this policy, the role of the physician medical director in EMS education is:

> To approve the medical and academic qualifications of the faculty, the accuracy of the medical content, and the accuracy and quality of medical instruction given by the faculty; to routinely review student performance and progress and attest that the students have achieved the desired level of competence prior to graduation; and
>
> To have a significant role in faculty selection and curriculum development, authority over presentation of medical content, and authority to assure that faculty teach established medical practices.

The roles and responsibilities put forth in the joint statement may now seem commonplace in many EMS systems and services. However, this had not always been the case. The role of the medical director in EMS, and EMS education in particular, has been evolutionary, following closely the increasing acceptance of education as an integral component of EMS.

Since the development of modern EMS in the early 1970s, education has played a pivotal role in defining the scope and delivery of EMS. The educational content of provider training courses has been the primary means of defining what knowledge and skills EMS providers needed to function in the field. Although organizations such as the American College of Surgeons and American Academy of Orthopedic Surgeons developed suggested training outlines and core content, many of the early curricula were "best guesses" of the curriculum designers. The development of EMS training was farther complicated by the need to combine the clinical bases of medicine with the technician-based approach of EMS. Even to this day, the paradox of EMS as medicine versus public safety continues to complicate the philosophical underpinnings of EMS education. However, the introduction of a more research based curriculum development process has bought about significant change in our approach to training EMS providers. Utilization of a practice analysis, development of a *National EMS Education and Practice Blueprint*, and recently, the *EMS Education Agenda for the Future: A Systems Approach* have served to give structure and direction to EMS education.

Perhaps the most important single aspect of modern EMS education is the utilization of a national standard curriculum (NSC). Reliance on a nationally developed and accepted curriculum is almost unique to EMS as opposed to traditional allied health education. In 1971, the first NSC was developed under federal contract from the National Highway Transportation Safety Administration (NHTSA). This NSC was the basic curriculum for the education of the Emergency Medical Technician—Ambulance. Subsequent NSCs were developed for EMT-Paramedic and EMT-Intermediate. The development of these NSCs had a number of effects on EMS:

- They provided a standard approach to EMS education which was universal in scope.

- They defined the scope of practice for the EMT.

- They guided the development of educational materials and training programs.

- They provided a "national focus" on EMS education as opposed to a regional, state, or institutional focus.

- They were prescriptive in that they not only provided educational objectives but also declarative material and recommended hours of instruction.

Unfortunately, the development of the various NSCs was not coordinated, so the educational approach for each level was different. This made it difficult for providers to move between levels. Additionally, no formal process existed for input from providers and communities of interest in the development and revision of an NSC.

As the various NSCs evolved and underwent revision, the need for a more systematic approach to curriculum development became evident. Concurrently, the need to define a vision for the future of EMS lead to the consensus document, *The EMS Agenda for the Future*. The *Agenda* identified 14 attributes of an EMS system, one being Education. Building on the framework presented in the *Agenda*, the EMS community has developed the *EMS Education Agenda for the Future: A Systems Approach*. The premise of the *Education Agenda* is based on the following *Attributes of the EMS Education System of the Future* presented in the *Education Agenda*:

- The EMS education system is national in scope while allowing for reasonable state and local flexibility;

- The EMS education system is guided by patient-care needs, is educationally sound, and is politically feasible;

- The components of the EMS education system are clearly articulated, with a lucid definition of their interrelationships;

- The responsibility and time frames for updating each of the system components are clearly delineated;

- The method of providing input to and participating in the outcome of each component is clearly defined with an established role for providers, administrators, physicians, regulators, educators, and others;

- The ongoing system evolution is guided by scientific and educational research and the principles of quality improvement;

- The EMS education system is stable enough and strong enough to outlive its architects, and exists independently of the current leadership of any national EMS organization;

- Physicians are primarily responsible for determining the medical content; regulators for determining regulatory issues, and educators for determining educational issues;

- The EMS education system supports multiple instructional methodologies.

Using the above list of attributes and coupled with a list of recognized assumptions, the *EMS Education Agenda for the Future: A Systems Approach*, was developed. The *Education Agenda* has five interrelated components:

- National EMS Core Content

- National EMS Scope of Practice Model

- National EMS Education Standards

- National EMS Education Program Accreditation

- National EMS Certification

The EMS medical director has a significant and vital role in each of these five components of EMS education. Although the *Education Agenda* is a recent and visionary document, historically EMS medical directors have always been involved to some degree in these or related areas.

Medical Director Involvement in Core Content

The core content will serve to provide the bases for all EMS education. Naturally, the medical director must have an understanding and even a working knowledge of the National EMS Core Content. Currently, the medical director must turn to the National Standard Curricula and the *National EMS Education and Practice Blueprint* to define the core content for EMS providers. Development of the core content will involve input from various sources. One prime source will be research. The medical director is in an ideal position to involve his or her service in either ongoing multi-service research projects or to conduct original, local research.

Through involvement in national EMS organizations, the medical director has a forum for input and information about the development and approval of the core content. Such information allows the medical director to be proactive, as well as to be a source of information about national trends in EMS education and practice.

Medical Director Involvement in EMS Scope of Practice Model

The National EMS Scope of Practice Model defines the national levels of EMS providers. The model not only defines the knowledge and skills needed for providers at each level, but entry-level competencies as well. Currently, the closest thing to a practice model is the *National EMS Education and Practice Blueprint*.

Familiarity with the model will allow the medical director to have a better understanding of how the National EMS Core Content will be delivered by EMS providers. The model will also help medical directors who deal only with one level of provider, for instance paramedics, better understand the roles of other providers such as EMT-Basics.

Perhaps most importantly, the practice model will provide a framework from which the medical director can establish the local scope of practice for EMS providers. This is especially helpful when there may be local resistance to certain skills or medications being provided in the field. The medical director will have a national consensus document to support his or her position. Conversely, field providers will have a document to support their request for additional skills or medications.

Medical directors are often asked to participate in the selection of students to attend EMS training courses. Because the practice model lists entry-level skills and knowledge, the medical director, and the selection group as well, have an established basis upon which to make decisions.

The medical director, working with the local educational team, can use information from the model to ensure that local training programs adequately address the needs of each provider level. Likewise, when new training courses or other training activities are submitted to the medical director for approval, the director can use the model as a "yardstick" for evaluation and approval.

Medical Director Involvement with the National EMS Education Standards

As mentioned above, the driving force behind EMS education and practice has been the National Standard Curriculum for each EMS provider level. The NSCs contain not only terminal learning objectives, but declarative material, suggested program structure, and contact hours. The prescriptive nature of these curricula lead to rigid and dogmatic training programs which often do not adequately address the needs or situation of the learners. In contrast, development of National EMS Education Standards consisting primarily of terminal learning objectives will allow greater programmatic flexibility and alternative delivery methods. However, with this flexibility comes increased responsibility on the part of the medical director to assure that educational programs adequately prepare students to function in the field. Again, working with the local educational team, the medical director will be able to use the standards as a comparison tool for local educational activities. The standards can also be used when evaluating textbooks and training materials. The medical director will also have a national consensus document to support the need for new or additional local training.

Medical directors often are asked to provide a final "sign-off" of students completing an educational program. This approval process may be for a recommendation to participate in national certification testing. It may also be the final examination to determine whether a student passes or fails. The standards provide a means for the medical director to identify valid criteria to use for his or her evaluation by utilizing the terminal objectives contained in the standards. Again, the use of a national standard provides credibility and defensibility for the director's final decision.

In the area of continuing education and ongoing evaluation, the medical director can use the standards to design or specify continuing education requirements for local field providers. For the medical director involved in the ongoing evaluation of certified providers' knowledge and skills, the terminal objectives of the standards provide a baseline for measurement and evaluation. When faced with a personnel issue, the medical director is able to utilize a nationally accepted standard to support his actions.

Medical Director Involvement in National EMS Education Program Accreditation

The national accreditation of EMS training programs remains controversial. In some states and regions programs are accredited locally. Regardless of the accreditation body, the process of accreditation provides a uniform measure of program effectiveness, and assures a minimum level of protection for the student and consumer. Through accreditation, an educational program shows that it meets at least minimum acceptable standards.

The role of the medical director in accreditation is two-fold. First and foremost, the medical director must assure that a program meets the clinical practice standards for accreditation and is teaching medically acceptable knowledge and skills. This assurance is usually accomplished by working with the local educational team and through review of lesson plans, textbooks, and class visits. The medical director also evaluates students against the national EMS education standards.

The second role of the medical director in accreditation is that of site visitor. Most accreditation processes require an on-site visit by a review team representing the accreditation body. Site visit teams usually consist of a program medical director and a provider educator. Together, the team assures that the institution is indeed meeting the minimum requirements for accreditation. By participating as a site visitor, the medical director is showing his or her support for the accreditation process. Additionally, site visits provide an opportunity for the medical director to see other programs, and experience different approaches to EMS education.

Medical Director Involvement in National EMS Certification

The idea of a single, national certification for EMS providers is also controversial. However, regardless if a program subscribes to national certification or state and local certification, the medical director has a significant role to play in the certification process.

The most basic role of the medical director in certification is the final "sign-off" of students to sit for examination. The medical director is required to attest to the student's completion of an approved educational program and at least minimal attainment of program standards' terminal objectives.

During the examination process, the medical director may be called upon to serve as the medical director for the examination process. In this role, the medical director usually has the final say in questions related to medical acceptability of student performance. The medical director may also serve as an evaluator for one of the practical testing stations. Stations usually tested are patient assessment or cardiac resuscitation.

Other Areas of Medical Director Involvement

In addition to the five areas discussed above, the medical director has other potential roles related to EMS education. These roles include:

Educator

A medical director may be called upon to actually instruct prehospital providers in a formal setting. Such educational activities can include teaching a new procedure, introducing a new drug, teaching a section of the core content, or even serving as the lead instructor for an entire training course.

Medical directors possess medical expertise, but not all directors are teachers. Medical directors must realize their limitations in this area. They must also understand those they instruct. The volunteer or career EMT-B is not a first year medical student. The educational model used in most U.S. medical schools is not suitable for training prehospital providers, especially those who cannot devote all their time and effort to EMS-related training.

To assist the medical director in his or her role as an educator, most systems have established the position of non-physician instructor. This position can be regulated by law or regulation. Non-physician instructors are usually peer instructors who have demonstrated mastery of the curriculum material and have completed formalized instructor training. Often nursing and allied health professionals serve in this role. Responsibility for course organization, administration, and student management is frequently handled by a non-physician instructor or program coordinator, thus freeing the medical director to concentrate on teaching-learning activities.

Education Manager

In addition to the opportunity to serve as an educator, medical directors may be required to fill the role of manager of education. This can be a complex and demanding task. Managing an educational program requires involvement across the spectrum of program planning, development, delivery, teaching, evaluation, testing, and overall administration. Unless specifically trained in educational administration, medical directors are wise to delegate this task to a non-physician administrator. Resources in even the smallest EMS systems usually include the hospital in-service coordinator, patient-education coordinator, local community organizations, fire or police department training staff, and local school system. A valuable resource in many locales is the community college. Affiliating with a college has many advantages, not the least of which is an established mechanism for delivery of educational programs. In addition, the community college adds the potential for providing college credit for EMS-related training, thus contributing to the professionalism of EMS. With the continued sophistication of EMS education, affiliation with an academic institution is becoming almost a necessity.

Although medical directors may delegate administration of EMS education, they are nonetheless responsible for the quality of education being delivered. It is important to establish a quality assurance mechanism for training. Directors must recognize that determining the quality of education and training is just as important and as difficult as evaluating field care. Again, consultation with a trained educator may be helpful in establishing a quality assurance approach. However, medical directors must not be misled by output statistics that may not reflect the outcome of the educational experience. Outputs are measures of how an educational program is functioning. Measures such as number of students completing, student contact hours, and mean final grade reflect the output or final product of the educational program. Outcomes, however, are more nebulous, and attempt to measure the impact of education on the EMS system. Changes in mortality and morbidity after conducting a training program for prehospital providers are examples of outcome measures. Outcome measures used to judge an educational program should be established before conducting the program, and should be of a measurable nature.

Preceptor

One of the more rewarding, and to some degree more challenging, roles of the medical director is that of preceptor. In this role, directors have a unique opportunity to not only precept other health professionals, but to grow professionally themselves.

Preceptoring is the process of working one-on-one or with a small group in a clinical setting. The medical director's role becomes that of coach or mentor, rather than that of teacher in the more general sense. Most physicians engage in some form of mentoring on a regular basis, such as explaining a procedure to a resident or showing paramedics a technique in the emergency department (ED), all examples of informal mentoring. A preceptoring program can benefit the preceptor as well as the student. It can also present many disadvantages.

Despite the disadvantages to preceptoring, if planned and executed properly, it can be a rewarding experience for both the preceptor and the student. To ensure success, it is important for the medical director to continually monitor the performance of the student and the preceptor. Students should not just be "dumped" into a unit or assigned to a prehospital provider, physician, or nurse without some prior interaction and a clear understanding of the preceptor's role.

The preceptor experience has the potential to be less controllable than a classroom or lab setting; it can also be less dependable. The case mix presented to the student usually cannot be prearranged, especially in the field setting or in an ED. Personnel changes such as sickness or work schedules may alter or change the preceptoring activity.

To ensure a quality experience, preceptors need to be committed and willing to participate. In addition, they should possess exemplary clinical skills and ability. A difficult aspect of preceptoring is dealing with the stressed or incompetent student in a crisis situation. A student who freezes in the middle of a cardiac arrest needs to be firmly but compassionately dealt with. Training in student counseling and evaluation techniques may also be required of the preceptor.

Clinical performance objectives should be established for the program. These not only add structure to the experience, but also serve as the basis for student evaluation. A simple skills check-off sheet may be used until formal objectives are available.

Skill Instructor

The medical director may be called on to provide not only didactic instruction but skills instruction as well. Teaching a skill usually involves the demonstration method of instruction. The concept underlying the demonstration method of instruction is whole-part-whole. The instructor presents the whole of the procedure or skill, then the individual parts of the whole, followed by a review of the whole again. This approach allows the student to develop the proper set necessary to master the skill. In addition, repeating the whole serves as a summary to reinforce the steps and key points presented.

As during lecture, students are passive during the demonstration, but unlike the lecture, hearing is not the only sense stimulated. The students must be able to both hear the instructor's explanation and see his actions. Thus, good visuals are an important part of the demonstration process; they can be achieved by good classroom set-up and design and proper class size. The use of "larger-than-life" equipment or cut-away models can also improve visibility.

Equipment used in the demonstration should be identical to that used in the field. Expended or outdated equipment may confuse the student. Asking the student to pretend or visualize something distracts from the psychomotor skill learning process. The instructor should also check that equipment for the demonstration is working properly and all necessary ancillary supplies are on hand. Unfortunately, when Murphy's Law strikes in education, it is usually during the most critical point of a demonstration.

Although instructors may be presenting a skill that they have performed numerous times before, practice and rehearsal are still necessary. As the experienced providers become accustomed to performing a skill, they unconsciously alter and change the procedure in subtle ways. They may also become "sloppy" and not follow the procedure as outlined or required. It may help to review a skill or procedure manual in preparation for the demonstration. Also helpful is demonstrating the technique to a colleague, asking them to provide feedback from a student's point of view.

Not only should teachers present the skill correctly, but they need to be sensitive to the motor and sensory aspects of the procedure and how best to relate them to the learner. Take, for example, teaching the placement of an IV catheter. It is easy to describe the site preparation, angiocath preparation, and approaches to vein cannulation; however, what is difficult to "teach" is the feel of entering the vein and advancing the stylet a short distance before moving the cannula. For the teacher, this may be an almost automatic response that is overlooked in demonstrating the skill, but it is a critical action for the student to master.

Another aspect of skills instruction that teachers need to be cognizant of is coupling of activities. As they become more familiar with a skill or procedure, they may subconsciously link or combine the small steps of a skill or procedure together. When the skill is taught, it is important to separate these connections so the student is exposed to the intricate nuances necessary to master the skill. The use of a skill flow sheet or performance check sheet is helpful to ensure that critical steps are clearly presented and explained.

It is important for the skills instructor to appreciate that students will exhibit various levels of mastery as they attempt to learn a skill. Limits on skills practice prelude the student from leaving the instructional experience at much more than the demonstration stage of skills mastery. Following a demonstration, the student will be motivated to practice. Ample opportunity and facilities should be provided for student practice and review.

Skill Evaluator

Related to the teaching of skills is the role of evaluator of skills competence. This role is most often fulfilled during the practical examination required for certifications, such as paramedic. As with any evaluation process, it is important that the evaluation be intimately related to the objectives. The condition and degree statements of a well written objective provide the criteria for the evaluation. The steps and related knowledge that are determined in the occupational analysis form the skills check-off list and sequence.

As with skills instruction, it is important to realize that the student is not an experienced master but essentially an imitator. It addition to a limited ability to perform the skill the student may be intimidated by the teacher or evaluator. Nervousness and sudden forgetfulness are common. A simple smile or statement acknowledging the student's stress will not alter the evaluator's objectivity but will put the student at ease.

Instructor Evaluator

As a manager of education, the medical director should evaluate instructors working in the local program. It is helpful to understand some of the characteristics of a good instructor.

The process of instruction is in essence a specialized form of communication; therefore, it is imperative that instructors effectively communicate with people and understand human behavior. A student-teacher relationship built on mutual understanding and respect is a tremendously positive aid to learning.

Enthusiasm and a sincere desire to teach are also necessary qualities of a good instructor. If an individual is forced to teach or does so without enthusiasm, the learning experience will be mediocre at best, resulting in a lost opportunity for the system. In some systems, residents are required to teach parts of prehospital provider training programs. If they are not skilled at teaching or just not interested, this needs to be addressed by the medical director. Regardless of the outcome, how instructors perceive their role transfers directly to students. Therefore, enthusiasm on the part of the instructor has a good chance of stimulating enthusiasm in the students.

Loyalty to the instructional program and the overall field of prehospital care is as necessary as any other trait in a good instructor. To teach effectively, instructors must believe in what they are teaching, and in their students. Mutual respect and support, just like enthusiasm, motivate the student; they also add credibility to the instructor.

Instructors need to be resourceful and creative. The great diversity of field provider levels and educational programs require instructors to be flexible and dynamic. Nothing can be more frustrating to EMT-B students than a physician giving a lecture from notes and visuals designed for third-year medical residents. The ability to adjust the level of instruction to meet the needs of the students and the system is a valuable asset in an instructor.

Related to resourcefulness and creativity is the need to show empathy and sensitivity toward students. In volunteer systems a student who is late to class because he was held at his job needs support and assistance, not chastisement. The instructor's ability to see the world through the student's eyes can go a long way toward making the educational experience rewarding for both.

To ensure the quality of instruction, the medical director must plan for not only instructor evaluation but also instructor selection and education. Either directly or through others, the director must arrange for continual instructor evaluation during instruction, as well as a postcourse review and critique

Education versus Training

It may be helpful for the medical director to have an appreciation for the difference between education and training. So far the terms training and education have been used synonymously in this chapter. This is the case in much of the popular education literature. However, there is a difference between the two terms. A common example of this difference is the cliche, "You train animals; you educate people." The connotation drawn from this is that training is something less desirable than education.

One of the simplest ways to discuss the difference between education and training is to look at the definitions of each term. *Education* is defined as:

The act of educating, teaching or training; the act or art of developing and cultivating the various physical, intellectual, aesthetic, and moral faculties; instruction and discipline; tuition; nurture; learning; erudition

Training is defined as:

Teaching and forming by practice; the act of one who trains; the process of educating; education; drill; course of exercise and regimen.

From these definitions the difference between education and training may not appear cut-and-dried, especially given that both definitions refer to the other term. Perhaps there is no significant difference in the dichotomy as used today. However, the common perception of education and training is that education is directed toward the whole person; it is a holistic learning experience. Training, on the other hand, is perceived as a structured means to bring about a set change in knowledge and skill level. Another approach to this idea is that one educates the whole person, and one trains the individual for a given task.

Using field provider education as an example, a training program would focus on the student mastering the knowledge base necessary for functioning at the provider level. Drill and exercise would be used to develop mastery of the skills needed by a field provider. In contrast, using the idea of education as a holistic approach, the student would learn the knowledge and skills necessary to function as provider and be exposed to the broader concepts and ideas of medicine. An educated field provider would have been required, for instance, to complete courses in anatomy and physiology, general chemistry, and psychology. The trained field provider may be equally qualified to perform the same skills as the educated provider, but without a broad understanding of the underlying principles.

Training is not bad or less desirable than education. Many situations lend themselves well to the training approach, whereas others may allow for more extensive education. System considerations, budget, personnel requirements and regulations, time, and instructional resources may all influence the degree to which EMS personnel are educated or trained. However, if the plan is to build lifetime career ladders for EMS professionals, then a lifetime of education makes the most sense.

Curriculum Development

To ensure a positive learning experience the instructor must be knowledgeable of the material presented, and present the material in an ordered and logical way. Nothing is more frustrating for students than an instructor or speaker who obviously knows the material but loses the class because of a disorganized or inappropriate presentation. Hence the role of curriculum in the educational process.

Of special interest to the medical director is the conflict between assessment versus diagnostic-based curriculum. Traditional medical education and, by default, prehospital education have been based on the idea that the student must arrive at a diagnosis to apply the appropriate treatment regime. Such an approach requires an extensive knowledge base and understanding of the underlying pathophysiology. Assessment-based education, in contrast, teaches the student how to react to specific signs and symptoms. For example, if presented with an overdose patient, diagnostic-trained EMS providers would conclude that they were dealing with an overdose and attempt to differentiate the type of overdose involved. They would have been trained to recognize signs and symptoms associated with narcotic overdose, tricyclics, amphetamines, and alcohol. The assessment-based providers would understand that there are different types of overdoses, but they would react based primarily on how the providers would assure a patent airway. If hypotensive, they would treat for shock. It is important for medical directors to understand that these two methods of patient management exist and to recognize a curriculum as belonging to one of the groups. Directors may be called on to select the appropriate approach for local training activities.

In EMS education medical directors have two options concerning curriculum. One is to use a prepared curriculum developed either by national consensus groups or a commercial vendor. The other option is to develop a curriculum. The latter can be a lengthy, complicated, and arduous task.

Prepared Curriculum

Prior to the adoption of the *EMS Education Agenda for the Future*, national standard curricula were developed for the various prehospital provider levels. The curricula not only included educational objectives, but limited declarative material. Though not specifically designed to serve as lesson plans, the curricula could be easily expanded to serve as a teaching outline. Now, the national standard curricula have been replaced by the National EMS Core Content that consists only of educational objectives. Thus, the instructor will have to either develop his or her own lesson plans or utilize commercially available plans provided by publishers of EMS education products. The utilization of commercial lesson plans or guides will most likely be the most efficient approach for the instructor.

EMS-related training programs other than the Core Curriculum such as ACLS, BTLS, PMTLS, and so on, are examples of prepared curricula. These programs contain complete teaching packages including lesson plans and audio-visual materials. The instructor need only review and customize the material prior to teaching.

Developed Curriculum

The development of instructional curricula can be an involved process—entire books have been written on the subject. However, there are times when medical directors may need to prepare a training program, a series of lectures, or even an entire course for which no prepared curriculum is available or suitable.

The curriculum development process consists of the following five steps: needs assessment, objective formulation, course development, course delivery, and evaluation. An overview of the five basic steps is presented. Medical directors contemplating the development of a course of instruction would be well advised to seek the assistance of an educator or instructional designer.

Needs assessment. The needs assessment is designed to answer the fundamental question, "What do the students need to know?" Through needs assessment, assessors determine what the students know and compare this with what they should know. This difference or "gap" will be filled by the educational activity that is being developed. For instance, in developing a course to take providers from the intermediate level to the paramedic level, it is assumed that the students already know the material covered in the intermediate curriculum. The new course will focus on material needed to fill the gap to the paramedic level.

A needs assessment should not only focus on the learner's needs, but it should consider organizational and environmental needs as well. At the organizational level the question, "What level when?" must be answered. Environmental needs are those related to the environment in which the prehospital provider will function.

There are many different approaches to a needs assessment. Consideration should be given to using an outside consultant to prevent biased results.

Formulation of objectives. Once the needs have been established, they can be translated into behavioral objectives. First the needs are screened against organizational goals and objectives, available resources, learner concerns, and environmental considerations. For example, consider a hypothetical plan to train EMT-Bs to intubate. This plan requires that the student perform the skill successfully on five live patients. If clinical sites or approved preceptors are not available to handle the number of projected trainees, then this need is not feasible, and an alternative approach must be found. Similarly, plans to train paramedics to perform an advanced surgical skill such as peritoneal lavage would most likely be screened out by environmental parameters.

After the needs are screened, they are grouped. For instance, all those related to airway are in one group, fluid replacement in another, and fracture management in a third. The needs in each group are then prioritized considering such factors as urgency, sequence, frequency, and course goal compatibility. Objectives are prepared from the needs using a three-step approach. First the specific behavior to be exhibited by the student is defined as an action statement. For example, "The student will be able to list the bones of the upper extremity." Next, any conditions under which this behavior must occur are identified. These conditions should be as realistic as possible. Continuing with the example above, we would add, "from memory and without assistance." If this were a skill, conditions such as "while using universal precautions" or "while functioning as a team of two and given a simulated patient" would be added as well. The final step in developing an objective is to list the degree of acceptable performance. Again, adding to our example, "to an accuracy of 70%." The complete objective would read, "The student will be able to list the bones of the upper extremity from memory and without assistance to an accuracy of 70%." For a skill the objective might read, "The student will be able to demonstrate application of a traction splint while working as a member of a team, using universal precautions and given a simulated patient and traction splint, within 10 minutes and to the satisfaction of the instructor."

Objectives are the backbone of an educational activity. Not only do they define what the student must know and do, but also provide a means to express a behavior on the part of the student that is measurable. For this reason, it is important to avoid terms such as "know" and "understand" when describing a behavior. Such words cannot be directly measured. What can be measured are terms such as list, identify, recite, order, describe, and state.

Course development. This intermediate step in the curriculum development process involves the actual formulation of the instructional events. To begin this process the developer arranges the behavioral objectives in logical groups. For example, objectives for an EMT-B course might be grouped into all objectives dealing with patient assessment, fracture management, burns, and so on. These groups are the major topics areas or units of instruction; they are the chapters of a textbook.

Next, the objectives in each group are prioritized. The needs assessment stage may have identified many needs, but not all of them can be met in one course or at one time. They are like a bulls-eye target; the bulls-eye is those objectives the student "must know." The next ring out is "should know," followed by "nice to know," and finally the outer ring is "related information." How far one is allowed to move

EDUCATION

off target is usually determined by the amount of time allotted for training.

Finally the objectives remaining in each group are arranged according to the teaching cycle. Objectives can be classified as belonging to one of the following three domains of learning: affective (attitudes), cognitive (knowledge), and psychomotor (skills). Affective information is presented first, followed by cognitive, and then any skill related to the knowledge. For example, to master application of a traction splint the student must first learn the importance of proper splinting (affective) and know the musculoskeletal system and the general concepts of splinting (cognitive) before practicing (psychomotor) the application. Once the objectives are prioritized and arranged, the instructional format for each unit can be determined.

Methods of instruction. Criteria for selection of the instructional method varies by the objective type, instructor preference, and resources. For instances, a verbal explanation of intraosseous infusion could be accompanied by slides and a demonstration using a training mannequin, or a cadaver. Each method is appropriate for a given time, class size, and resources. Many methods of instruction are available to the program developer and instructor.

After the methods of instruction are decided on, lesson plans for each unit are developed. This is essentially a process of "exploding" the objectives into teaching points and operations. The lesson plan is in essence an outline of the material to be presented during the course. It should not be too specific or it will become a textbook rather that a plan or guide. A common approach in education is "whole-part-whole." The instructor presents an overview of the entire subject or activity, and then moves to the various parts of the material, concluding with putting the parts together again as a whole. Mager and Beach describe five techniques to use when arranging lesson material as follows:

1. General to specific
2. By area of interest (cover topics the student is most interested in first)
3. By logic (build upward from a foundation)
4. By skill
5. By frequency (cover the skills most often used or needed first)

Instructors should consider lesson plans a "personal thing." The program developer may write a lesson "guide," but it only becomes a lesson plan after the instructor personalizes it. Individual instructors add notes, examples, illustrations, and stories as they prepare to present the material outlined in the guide.

The last task of the development process is the formulation of the student evaluation scheme. This stage, like those discussed previously, is based on the objectives. When each objective was written, a condition and degree were identified. This information is transformed into the student evaluation. For example, if an objective states that students will list something with an accuracy of 70%, then the appropriate evaluation is a written test question asking them to list the information. If the action word in an objective is "discuss," then students are evaluated either through oral questioning or short answer or essay questions. For objectives requiring demonstration, a skills test is appropriate, using the degree statement as the performance criteria.

Program delivery. This step involves the planning for the delivery of instruction. Program delivery activities include four items:

Scheduling—A workable schedule for delivery of the training must be set. Medical directors may have to consider restraints such as shiftwork, restrictions on overtime compensation, volunteers, and their own work schedule. In addition, state or regional EMS system recertification and testing deadlines may influence the scheduling of training programs.

Facilities—Where training takes place is as important as the training itself. Concerns need attention that seem extraneous, such as student travel, travel cost, availability of alternative sites, and need for special facilities such as laboratories, anatomy labs, and field sites.

The quality of the training site must be evaluated. Many institutions such as hospitals and fire departments have training facilities, but others do not. Will an ambulance have to be pulled out of the garage, folding chairs set up, and a sheet taped to the wall as a screen before material can be presented? Distractions such as radio calls or on-call students who have to suddenly leave class need to be addressed. Parking availability and facility passes need to be arranged. All these things must be evaluated before the actual training session. The medical director should visit the proposed training site before a class begins, to prevent any surprises.

Classroom arrangement—How students are arranged in the classroom can directly affect the learning experience. A group may require rearrangement of optimal teaching. If the class will be divided into small discussion groups, the seating arrangements must be changeable. Arrangements will also have to be made for skills practice space. Rearranging the classroom during a class takes time away from instructional activities.

All students must also be able to see and hear the instructor. When dealing with adults, visual and hearing changes can adversely affect the learning outcome. In addition, it is uncomfortable for adults to sit in desks designed for school children. If chairs are provided, students must be able to take notes or complete written exercises. The general environment, including comfortable temperature, classroom accessibility, and rest rooms, is also a concern.

Support materials—The development and selection of media to support a presentation could be the subject of its own book, and is beyond the scope of this chapter. Nonetheless, it is an important consideration when planning and delivering a program. Instructors cannot assume that every training location has a selection of audio-visual equipment; they should check in advance and be prepared to provide their own support. The rule to remember with visual aids is that they should support the message, not be the message.

Program Evaluation. Although listed as the last step, this is one of the first things the medical director and others involved in the program development process should address. The means and criteria for evaluating the educational experience should be decided early in the development process; thus, the criteria will be established and the evaluation will be continuous. Waiting until after the program is developed to design the evaluation criteria would be like conducting research and then writing the hypothesis.

After deciding which characteristics to evaluate, the developer must decide with which criteria the learning experience will be compared. This is the "what should be" established during the needs assessment. Next, evidence to support the evaluation must be chosen. For instance, effectiveness of a program could be measured by how many students passed the state certification examination. Student evaluations using rating scales could be developed to measure the quality of instruction.

Evaluation can be a useful tool only if the results are used constructively. Feedback mechanisms to allow change and revision of the program must be developed and implemented by the medical director-educator to improve the learning experience.

Adult Learning

The course development process is important; however, it is just as important for the medical director to understand the recipient of all this activity—the learner, and more specifically, the adult as a learner.

Much of the current literature on adult learning has centered around the work of Malcolm Knowles. Knowles is best known for his idea of andragogy, which is the art and science of helping adults to learn. This concept contrasts the more traditional approach of pedagogy or child learning. Inherent in andragogy are four basic assumptions that are of use to instructors of adults.

1. The adult moves from childhood dependency towards self-autonomy. In terms of education, children depend on the teacher and the school system to determine what they must learn. Adults, on the other hand, are capable of self-directed learning. Additionally, learning changes from a full-time "occupation" to a part-time exercise.
2. The adult possesses an increasing reservoir of experience that can be used as a learning resource. This experience is often used by adults to define "who they are." Therefore, it is important that the learner's reservoir of experience be tapped in the learning experience.
3. The adult's readiness to learn is directed to current developmental tasks or social obligations. For example, you are reading this chapter because you are examining your role as a medical director. You have decided that you are now ready to learn more about being a medical director.
4. The adult's orientation to learning changes from delayed application to immediate application. Adults engage in learning activities that are usually related to their current life situation and needs. Thus they seek education that is problem- or performance-centered.

These four basic principles of adult learning can be applied directly to EMS education. In planning an educational activity the learners should be involved in the planning process as much as possible. This input allows the learners to feel empowered and in control of their own learning experiences. Giving the learner choices is another way to provide autonomy in learning. For example, a lesson on abdominal trauma could be offered in both lecture format and as student-paced interactive computer learning program. Learners would be free to choose the activity with which they are most comfortable.

Asking students to share experiences or identify topics of interest based on their backgrounds provides an opportunity to use the students' reservoir of experience. Excessive "war stories" should be avoided, but such expressions allow students to integrate experience with the learning task. Methodologies such as role-playing and simulation exercises also make good use of learners' experiences.

Although a learner's reservoir of experience can be a useful learning adjunct, it can also be a barrier to learning. Adults pass all new material through a personal experiential filter. Thus, it may be necessary early in the course of learning activity to break down such barriers, allowing the adult to be more objective and free of preconceptions. This is especially true of the adult who has had a negative experience with compulsory education. Such individuals may claim that they cannot learn. Providing opportunities for early success will help overcome this preconception.

Readiness to learn is exemplified by the new recruit or employee. One of the developmental tasks challenging young adults is getting started in an occupation. Young persons selecting EMS as their occupation have an increased interest in learning about the profession. In contrast, they probably would show little interest in a course on planning for retirement.

The orientation of adults to early application of learning can be addressed by providing them with knowledge or skills that can be immediately applied. Many EMT-A courses provide time for the trainee to ride along on actual calls after they have completed the initial part of the course. This provides an opportunity for the learner to see immediate application of material presented in class. In addition, it provides a problem-centered learning environment that is conducive to adult learning.

Beyond the four basic assumptions of adult learning already discussed, Knowles also identifies superior conditions of learning. The medical director should keep the following points in mind when planning learning experiences for adults:

Conditions that Influence Learning by Adults

- The learners feel a need to learn.
- The learning environment is characterized by physical comfort, mutual trust and respect, mutual helpfulness, freedom of expression, and acceptance of difference.
- The learners perceive the goals of a learning experience to be their goals.
- The learners accept a share of the responsibility for planning and operating a learning experience, and therefore they have a feeling of commitment toward it.
- The learners participate actively in the learning process.
- The learning process is related to and makes use of the experience of the learners.
- The learners have a sense of progress toward their goals.

Adult Motivation

The needs that bring the adult to an EMS educational program are as diverse as the individuals themselves. Ranging from the firefighter who is being "made" to attend, to the first-year medical student who simply cannot get enough information fast enough, the mix and degree of students' motivations present the teacher with a complex and often insurmountable instructional challenge.

In an ideal institutional setting the teacher would be able to integrate the needs and goals of each student with the needs and goals of the content to be taught. Unfortunately, that idea presupposes that the teacher had the opportunity to assess the motivational needs of each student and has the skills, knowledge, and opportunity to tap into and reinforce students' needs throughout the course. Two fundamental realities of field provider education make this virtually impossible: large class size and the magnitude of student heterogeneity.

The ability to accurately assess a student's motivational needs requires individual interaction that is not easily performed in a class setting involving 20 or more individuals. While a teacher may assess the needs of a few students, because they are either patently obvious or through personal discussions, it is unlikely that the teacher can discover the individual needs of an entire class. Therefore, class size is a barrier to the effective teacher-initiated management of student motivation. The heterogeneity of most field provider class exacerbates this barrier. In the usual absence of any screening or selection process for determining participation, most EMS provider classes are comprised of students with diverse sets of skills, backgrounds, competencies, and needs.

The responsibility for motivated learning remains with the student and by default the instructor. The responsibility of the instructor is not only to be a content expert but also to be able to demonstrate a superior level of instructional effectiveness that supports the student's motivational framework. Therefore, the medical director must have a basic understanding of adult motivation.

No discussion of motivation is complete without mention of the work of A. H. Maslow. Maslow arranged human needs in hierarchial order, beginning with basic physiological needs, followed by social needs, and finally what he termed *"self-actualization."*

What Maslow's hierarchy means to the medical director-educator is that basic physiological needs such as room temperature, sound level, and setting need to be met before higher needs can be addressed. This is why the learning environment should be carefully considered. In addition, activities such as a friendly greeting for the learners, "ice breaking" exercises, and positive feedback help meet the psychological and social needs of the students.

The literature of adult education contains numerous theories of adult motivation; however, a few basic concepts are useful for the director involved in teaching adults. The following is a series of characteristics of adult healthcare professionals that affect motivation as it relates to continuing education in health care.

- Most health professionals are motivated to continue their learning.

- Health professionals seek knowledge that has an immediate and pragmatic application in their current situation.

- Participation in continuing education is strongly influenced by an individual's past experiences.

- Efforts to improve the conditions of learning can influence the outcomes of continuing education.

- The realities of the practice world require that the health professionals know how to continue learning, stay abreast of new developments, and adapt to new environments.

- Continuing education should support health professionals' natural desire to learn.

- Health professionals should be encouraged to accept the personal responsibility of learning.

Cross developed the chain-of-response (COR) model of adult participation in learning which shows that the decision to participate in a learning activity is influenced by a series of related positive and negative reinforcers. If the sum of the factors is positive, the individual is likely to participate. If it is negative, participation is doubtful. In traditional adult education, getting the learner through the door is a least half the battle.

Meeting life cycle needs is a basic tenet of adult motivational theory. This sequential approach to adult development speaks of predictable crises or stages that confront the adult through life. Resolution of each stage is necessary before the next stage can be addressed. One of the methods used by adults to meet these challenges is education. The adult focuses on learning activities that will help him or her through each crisis or stage.

Although a useful approach, stage theory has come under increasing scrutiny in contemporary literature. Many of the studies were based on small samples of mostly middle-class, married, white males. Only recently has research focused on females or on the effects of cultural norms on development. A prime question confronting stage theorists is whether movement between the stages is abrupt or fluid. Regardless of the theoretical basis, adult development is nonetheless an integral part of the complex phenomenon of motivation.

The question often asked is what to do about the student who does not want to be in a provider class. Unless the student was physically bound and dragged into the classroom, a conscious decision has been made to attend the class. The motivation may not be that desired, but nonetheless there is some motivating factor. Take, for instance, fire fighters who are told to take an EMT-B course. They may have no interest in EMS, having chosen the profession of fire fighting because of the excitement. However, if they do not complete the course, they will be terminated; thus they will not meet their goal in life at that time. The challenge to the educator is to determine what motivates them and use that knowledge to accomplish the learning objectives. In the fire fighters' case the instructor could use an example, such as talking about how they feel when responding to an alarm and relating their explanations to the affects of sympathetic stimulation. Everybody is motivated by something. Once that motivation is identified, it can be channeled into positive developmental change.

Disruptive Students

There may be adult learners who are unintentionally disruptive. These individuals often fit into one of the following stereotypes: (1) the sturdy battler who constantly challenges the leadership role of the teacher; (2) the friendly helper who attempts to have all the answers; and (3) the rigorous thinker who, if left uncontrolled, can force the entire class to unnecessary depths of understanding.

By using the basic natural direction of the disruptive student's interest the experienced educator can move the student and the class in the appropriate direction. For example, by turning over a degree of authority and responsibility to the "sturdy battlers," they become invested in the success of the educational exercise. Being asked to present a later exercise may satisfy the friendly helpers craving for attention and approval. The rigorous thinkers must be carefully evaluated. If they truly know the required material, they may be allowed to "test out" and pursue an independent study in an advanced, related area. If the rigorous thinkers do not really understand the material, then that fact must be dealt with by the teacher, and a specific effort must be made to appropriately motivate the student by raising his or her awareness that behaviorally a change is beneficial.

Screening Students

Related to the problem student and the role of motivation in learning is the almost taboo subject of student screening. In many EMS systems, especially those staffed by volunteers, restricting entry or denying training to any interested student is met with great resistance. However, the medical director must decide whether to allow unqualified or educationally challenged individuals to occupy space that may be better used. All too often, "problem classes" are associated with instructor or testing problems when the real cause is the students. By not addressing the student population directly, the system is doing an injustice to both the instructor and the student. Marginal or below-standard students take time and resources away from other, more capable students who have a higher potential to succeed and thus become an asset to the EMS system. Screening should be designed and used as a tool to assist the program director, instructor, and student. Job-specific and validated screening tests provide a baseline against which perspective students can judge their potential for success. In addition, testing provides a diagnostic profile of the class for the instructor. Testing should be job-related and cover all critical domains of learning. Thus, for most EMS training, psychomotor and cognitive testing will be used. However, because EMS involves close interaction with people, evaluation of the student's affective skills should not be overlooked. Testing may also identify advanced or superior students who can be "fast-tracked" in an accelerated course.

The Future

The future of EMS education looks to be very exciting. Implementation of the *EMS Agenda for the Future* has the potential to alter how and to whom we provide service. Coupled with the *EMS Education Agenda for the Future*, the delivery of EMS education becomes even more important. As the focus of education moves from a prescriptive national curriculum to a more autonomous accreditation-passed program, not only will the role of the educator change, but that of medical director as well. The medical director will have multiple opportunities for involvement in the educational process. But most importantly, the medical director will be the central focus for medical oversight.

The basic delivery of EMS education will also change dramatically in the future. We are now just starting to witness the effect of computer and communications technology on education. Delivery of education through distributed learning presents many opportunities and challenges to the medical director. The education of prehospital providers through distributed and virtual learning moves the student from the local classroom and local instruction to global-based learning. Anytime-anywhere learning is rapidly becoming a reality. As such programs develop and proliferate, the local medical director will play an increasing role in assuring quality through the educational process.

Advances in telemedicine and robotic medicine will also impact on the education of providers. Distributed learning was once thought to be limited to the instruction of knowledge. Now it is possible to teach psychomotor skills to providers at a remote location. Virtual reality is allowing students to experience reality in the classroom in ways never thought possible. Again, all of this technology will not lessen the role of the medical director in education but make it paramount to the success of such endeavors.

Summary

EMS medical directors spend years learning a great deal of material; they have a responsibility to share that knowledge with field personnel. Too often the physician has either not learned to teach effectively or has not applied those lessons to the educational task at hand. Educating prehospital providers is a fulfilling and uplifting experience that has the potential to affect the lives and well-being of many people. By understanding and appreciating the many facets of education in their role as both educator and manager of education, EMS physicians can better accomplish their ultimate goal to provide sound, professional medical oversight.

Quality Management

Joseph L. Ryan, MD

Introduction

The challenge of quality care is inherent to scientific medicine. To a great extent, the advancement of medical science results from the rigorous application of the principles of structured thinking to investigation. The physician scientist is well acquainted with this "scientific method" and the practitioner struggles to integrate "medical fact" into the vagaries of clinical encounters with patients.

Attaining a certainty that medical care provided in the field by physician surrogates is safe, compassionate, timely, consistent, appropriate, and cost-effective, and that it positively influences patient outcome, is a primary responsibility for the EMS medical director. This quality assessment and monitoring are basic to the successful provision of prehospital health care.

Structured thinking in medical quality assessment is well developed. The significant work of Donabedian articulated a conceptual framework for quality of care. In *Explorations in Quality Assessment and Monitoring*, Donabedian describes, in authoritative detail, the definitions of quality, the approaches to quality assessment, the criteria and standards for quality, and the methods and findings of quality assessment and monitoring. These principles form the basis for understanding the dimensions of quality in health care.[1]

Quality Assessment to Quality Assurance

Quality assurance (QA), in the sense of a warranty of quality (and therefore having to do with its causation), is a far more complex and difficult goal. The costs of poor quality, in any dimension, are enormous. Although extended effort has been applied to "assure" quality in medical practice, a crisis of credibility contests the ability to produce quality that is recognizable to patients, communities, and the nation. Quality assurance as healthcare policy has largely backfired in enabling good care, and represents a major cause of the crisis facing organized medicine in the United States.

QA functions of the healthcare system largely developed to retrospectively police the quality of medical care. Influenced by the increasing spectre of societal expectation and governmental oversight, QA as defined by the AMA, JCAHO, HCFA, and so on, evolved almost exclusively into utilization review and "terminal inspection" (the autopsy being the ultimate in terminal inspection). QA processes became mechanisms motivated to identify "offenders" failing to adhere to normative values for hospital stay, frequency of laboratory tests, and consultations. Physicians equated QA with trouble and responded with a practice of "defensive" medicine, which had become a preponderant influence on health care, and which resulted in an increasingly estranged patient and paranoid practitioner. The QA analysts maintained that the root cause of poor quality in health care was the problem of flawed people.

In 1989 Berwick characterizes the sad state of affairs in healthcare quality assurance as the *Theory of Bad Apples*:[2]

> . . . because those who subscribe to it believe that quality is best achieved by discovering bad apples and removing them from the lot. The experts call this mode "quality by inspection," and, in the thinking of activists for quality in health care, it predominates under the guise of "buying right," "recertification," or "deterrence" through litigation. Such an outlook implies or establishes thresholds for acceptability, just as the inspector at the end of an assembly line decides whether to accept or reject finished goods. They search for outliers—statistics far enough from the average that chance alone is unlikely to provide a good excuse. Bad Apple theorists publish mortality data, invest heavily in systems of case-mix adjustment, and fund vigilant regulators. Some measure their successes by counting heads on platters.

In this landmark article, Berwick presented the arguments for a different way of doing business.

Quality Assurance to Continuous Quality Improvement

In the early 1980s, many American industrialists recognized that the competitive edge the United States once enjoyed in world markets had been largely eroded by the Japanese. "Made in Japan," once a synonym for poor quality, was rapidly becoming the benchmark for comparison, and American products were not measuring up. The study of this phenomenal turn-about in Japanese industry led to a shocking realization: the manufacturing and production strategies that revolutionized Japan were invented by American industrialists in the early twentieth century and were generally ignored or forgotten at home.

The rediscovery of these *industrial* **Quality Management** (QM) strategies became a major focus of the vanguard of American manufacturing and service industries in the latter 1980s, and the pervasive feature of a new philosophy of management. The ideas of Shewhart, Deming, Juran, Fiegenbaum, Crosby, Drucker, Peters, Ishikawa, Taguchi, and Imai gained new recognition. Their philosophies have a wide variety of names: Statistical Process Control (SPC), Statistical Quality Control (SQC), Total Quality Control (TQC), Company-Wide Quality Control (CWQC), Total Quality Management (TQM) and Continuous Quality Improvement (CQI), each with its conceptual nuances and disciples. For purposes of this discussion, the broad group of these industrial concepts will be referred to as Quality Management (QM). Continuous Quality Improvement (CQI) is the predominant term adopted by authors to refer to the adaptations of these concepts to medical practice.

The general principles of QM, however, are best expressed in the work of W. Edwards Deming and Joseph M. Juran.[3] In Deming's "Fourteen Points," the fundamentally different way of doing business is described.[4]

The Red Beads

The relevance of Deming's work to medicine is readily seen in an experiment he used to illustrate the flaws in thinking about producing quality.[5] Although the experiment was not originally designed to describe healthcare delivery, the applied message is bitterly diagnostic of the ills of medicine. The parable of

The Fourteen Points— W. Edwards Deming

Point One:	Create constancy of purpose for the improvement of product and service
Point Two:	Adopt the new philosophy
Point Three:	Cease dependence on mass inspection
Point Four:	End the practice of awarding business on price tag alone
Point Five:	Improve constantly and forever the system of production and service
Point Six:	Institute training and retraining
Point Seven:	Institute leadership
Point Eight:	Drive out fear
Point Nine:	Break down barriers between staff areas
Point Ten:	Eliminate slogans, exhortations, and targets for the workforce
Point Eleven:	Eliminate numerical quotas
Point Twelve:	Remove barriers to pride of workmanship
Point Thirteen:	Institute a vigorous program of education and retraining
Point Fourteen:	Take action to accomplish the transformation

the red beads can be viewed as the plight of the healthcare industry with the physician as producer (the industrial worker) of health (the product).

A group of workers is given a box of beads; 80% are white and 20% are red (good and impaired health status). The workers' job is to make white beads (good health). They are given a paddle with 50 holes arranged in five rows of ten (the tools of medical care). Each is told at length of the importance of making white beads, the elaborate and rigid procedures to be followed, and the severe consequences of failing to produce the requisite quota of white beads. The workers then dip into the box and return a paddle filled with beads to be inspected (by the Utilization Review Committee) for the percentage of white beads produced. The workers are variously praised, exhorted, threatened, retrained, suspended, or dismissed for their production of red beads despite objections that the raw materials (health status) are flawed, as are the imperfect processes (medical care) by which they are forced to work.

The fundamental flaws of the "bad apple" strategies of QM for health care are plainly evident from this analogy. Although workers are held responsible and exhorted, intimidated, and coerced to produce white beads (health), they are ultimately unable to influence effectively the quality of raw materials or the processes on the line, which are designed to mitigate illness rather than produce health.

Industrial Quality Management Models Applied to Medicine

In 1987 the Harvard Community Health Plan hosted the first meeting of a group of 21 healthcare agencies and an equal number of industrial QM experts, to launch the National Demonstration Project on Quality Improvement in Health Care (NDP). As a reference point for the mainstream of the medical care establishment, this project can be considered the point of departure from traditional medical models of QA to the application of concepts of industrial QM concepts for healthcare delivery systems.

This experiment, funded by the John A. Hartford Foundation, was designed to answer this question: *Can the tools of modern quality improvement, with which other industries have achieved breakthroughs in performance, help in health care as well?*[6] The answer was a clear, if qualified, yes. Although the problems of health delivery systems are somewhat unique, the principles of QM hold great promise for revolutionizing and humanizing the pursuit of quality in health care.

Quality Management

Quite significantly, in 1987 a number of EMS systems had been utilizing concepts of QM to measure and improve clinical service provision for about 8 years.[7,8] **System Status Management** (SSM) developed in 1979 by Stout remains the most highly evolved and successfully implemented example of the concepts of QM in EMS.[9] This anticipatory ambulance deployment strategy, based on the pathophysiology of cardiac arrest and the mandate for equal access to care, is archetypical of patient-oriented service delivery.

In the **Public Utility Model** of EMS, Stout's concepts of EMS system design and operation were developed independent of influence from contemporary industrial quality theorists, and represent a parallel evolution of customer-centered QM for EMS systems.[10,11] The "Advanced SSM Workshops," developed by the Fourth Party, characterize the vanguard of current thought in quality improvement in EMS for system managers.[12]

Leadership for Quality

It is an unfortunate reality that rare opportunities exist for medical directors to define, a priori, the structure of the system they oversee. Typically, configurations of systems are inherited, having been designed by well intended but medically naive governmental committees with little input from prehospital practitioners. The genesis of the system is often tangential to the provision of emergency medical care. Rather, it may have been motivated to capture funding opportunities, to extend power bases, or to stunt free-market competition. Understanding the sometimes Byzantine political realities of a given system is paramount to the success of the medical director. The "system" at its worst lacks definition altogether. Definition and refinement of system configuration, however, are the foundations of effective quality planning.

The ability of the medical director to plan for quality is a prerequisite for effective system medical control. In general, state law and local ordinance grant the authority to direct. This authority is further defined in the contract between the medical director and the system. This contract should include a detailed description of the medical director's role in defining, monitoring, and modifying the configuration of the system and its attributes. It should describe the manpower, equipment, and funding necessary to fulfill the requirements of oversight of the system.

These elements are *fundamentally lacking* in most current systems. For example, the information management tools that enable any meaningful retrospective, let alone real-time, monitoring of quality of care remain primitive. The computerized information systems in the dispatch center (except for Emergency Medical Dispatching systems), while improving, remain provider oriented and not patient oriented in their data collection. For example, the prevailing definition of response time ends on the scene and not at the patient.

Davidson distinguishes authority from power in characterizing the ability of the medical director to be effective in his role.[13]

Power comes to the medical director through the careful exercise of authority and through the expertise that the medical director brings to the activity of EMS through his/her ability to negotiate the interests of all while serving as a consultant to everybody, thereby enhancing everyone else's ownership of issues and solutions. In this fashion, rather than serving as a single voice on high whose opinion is delivered, as if *ex cathedra,* the medical director serves at every opportunity in the role of physician expert, consultant, and educator, thereby facilitating and bridging the multiplicity of political interests into consensus.

Physicians have traditionally been recognized as "knowing what's best for their patients." In the development of EMS systems, however, this expertise has been inconsistently provided, recognized, and integrated into the processes of care. In many ways the mandates of medical authority have been seen as naive and unrealistic when applied to the prehospital environment since many of its proposals have no basis in scientific fact or are extrapolated from fundamentally different and controlled environments. There will be less acceptance of this paternalistic perspective in future medical care systems.

In experience, The NDP recognized the fact that involving doctors in quality improvement was difficult. Underlying barriers included availability, skepticism regarding appropriateness, relevance and helpfulness of these groups, and reluctance to share authority over aspects of care for which they viewed themselves as disproportionately accountable. "For doctors in the past decade or more, the word 'quality' has meant 'trouble.'"[14]

Industrial quality theory acknowledges that the key to creating a successful QM program lies in the consensus support and substantive commitment of leadership to the mission of quality. Deming recommends ". . . create constancy of purpose for the improvement of product and service, . . . adopt the new philosophy, . . . improve constantly and forever the system of production and service, . . . institute leadership, . . .and take action to accomplish the transformation."[3] Because of the unique and diverse relationships in the hierarchies of EMS systems, accomplishing these goals has been quite difficult. The medical director has a pivotal role in articulating an inarguable mission of quality in patient care for the system capable of catalyzing consensus among leadership in support of these goals.

Reconciling the Medical and Industrial Philosophies of Quality Management

The Juran Trilogy

Juran identifies three universal processes of management for quality. These are interrelated as shown in the Juran Trilogy diagram. Figure 30.1 shows graphically the relationship of time on the horizontal axis and quality deficiencies (cost of poor quality) on the vertical axis. The initial activity of QM involves quality planning. After processes are designed and tested

FIGURE 30.1.
The Juran Trilogy. (From Juran Institute, Inc., Wilton, Conn.)

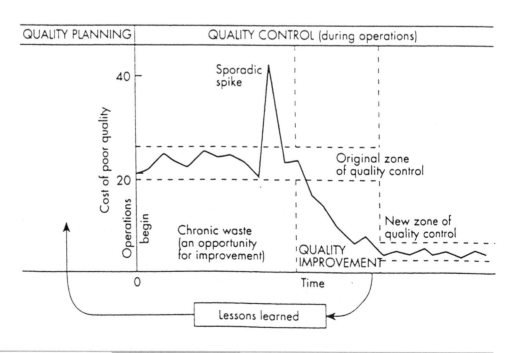

QUALITY MANAGEMENT

to meet customer needs, they are implemented on the production line. Quality control monitors, in real-time, assure the conformance of production processes in relation to product goals. The results of these monitoring functions are evaluated continuously by quality teams to discover production breakthroughs and reduce quality deficiencies—quality improvement (QI).

Structure/Quality Planning

Definitions

Donabedian defines structure as:

"... the relatively stable characteristics of the providers of care, of the tools and resources they have at their disposal, and of the physical and organizational settings in which they work. ... But the concept also goes beyond the factors of production to include the ways in which financing and delivery of care are organized. ... The basic characteristics of structure are that it is relatively stable, that it functions to produce care or is a feature of the environment of care, and that it influences the kind of care that is provided. ... Structure, therefore, is relevant to quality in that it increases or decreases the probability of good performance."[15]

He further notes:

"... as a means for assessing the quality of care, structure is a rather blunt instrument; it can only indicate general tendencies. The usefulness of structure as an indicator of the quality of care is also limited because of our insufficient knowledge about the relationships between structure and performance. It remains to be seen what improvement in specificity and sensitivity can be achieved by the development of more detailed, more condition-specific structural requirements."[16]

This concept illustrates a most telling difference between the medical and industrial philosophies of quality. Structure in an industrial sense (i.e., the design of products that meet customer needs and the organizations and mechanisms that produce them) is of paramount importance to the company. Through quality planning, problems in reliability and efficiency are recognized and eliminated from the production line before they ever appear. The effects of "getting it right the first time" in eliminating product failure and rework are monumental in industry, and have literally spelled survival from doom in the market for many companies. This has not been widely recognized in medical care. Due to the refusal of medical organizations to recognize the "85/15 rule" so well proven in industry, "... the potential to eliminate mistakes and errors lies mostly (85%) in improving the *systems* through which work is done, not in changing the workers (15%)." The systems are the responsibility of management.[17]

Donabedian		Juran
Observation		*Management*
Structure	←——→	Quality Planning
Process	←——→	Quality Control
Outcome	←——→	Quality Improvement

Juran on Quality Planning

Juran, in his book on leadership for quality, identifies a series of requirements for the transformation of companies into quality-driven organizations. These benchmarks serve well as a guide to the application of QM to EMS.

Quality Planning

Determine who the customers are
Determine the needs of the customers
Develop product features that respond to customer needs
Develop processes that are able to produce the features
Transfer the resulting plans to the operating forces

Engineering Quality by Design

Stout noted, "Of all the forces influencing an EMS system's ability to convert available dollars into clinical performance and response-time reliability, system design is by far the most powerful."[18]

Quality planning for EMS derives from a fundamental principle: the standard of care defines the system; the system does not define the standard of care. The transformation of EMS systems into quality-driven organizations (after Deming) requires the commitment of leadership and management to this constancy of purpose. There can be no "sacred cows" that escape scrutiny in the planning process.

Determine Who the Customers Are

The "customers" of EMS are the patients. Despite any sense among clinicians that this regard of the patient as customer inadequately expresses or even denigrates their unique relationship with the patient, considerations of this industrial concept of customers are enlightening.

Parallel to this concept of patients, industrialists recognize the consumers of their products as customers. However, the industrialist considers that the company has many more types of customers, both external and internal, than simply buyers of goods and services. Quality management defines their customer as anyone who depends on them.[19]

Therefore the customers of EMS services are not only patients, but also their families, their physicians and hospitals, the medical community, other public safety agencies, the community at large, and the governments of the geopolitical units in which the systems operate. These are referred to in QM jargon as "external customers."

A wide variety of interdependent processes exists within organizations, and each has its own internal suppliers and customers. The quality of any intermediate product in the manufacturing assembly line is dependent on the quality input of the up-line suppliers, the workers' own processes of production, and the workers' output as supplier to their down-line internal customers.

Industrial QM views each person in an organization as part of one or more processes. Each worker, through a number of individual tasks, receives the work of others, adds value to that work, and supplies it to other workers in the process. Therefore, each individual has a triple role—customer, processor, and supplier (fig. 30.2).[20]

It is worthwhile to extrapolate these views to problems in prehospital medicine. For example, the application of these concepts to the "chain of survival" from cardiac arrest yield striking insights. For example, the product of poor dispatch—failure in early notification and mobilization of resources—irrevocably impairs even the best of on-scene automatic defibrillation.

The methods to determine the customers of an EMS system are recognizably complex. Juran recommends the development of flow charts for the important processes of an organization to enable management to identify clearly the range of customers. This is useful for several reasons:

1. The development of flow charts provides the team with an understanding of the whole. Frequently, individuals understand their own parts of the puzzle but have little understanding of the interrelation of process elements.
2. Flow charts often identify customers previously neglected. The discipline necessary in preparation of the chart reveals most often internal customers with overlooked needs.
3. Most flow charts reveal sub processes or "loops" which are evidence of the rework of previous elements of the process. These are often chronic deficiencies in systems and are the targets of improvement planning.[21]

The flow chart is one of a number of basic tools used to clarify elements of QM. An example of a flow chart for an EMS system response to a cardiac arrest is illustrated in figure 30.3.

Determine the Needs of the Customers

In medicine there exists a confounding and destructive arrogance regarding the customer's needs. Patients have almost never been consulted to express their perspectives on the characteristics of quality health care. The liability crisis in medicine is the result in great part of the failure to recognize and appreciate this aspect of care. Patients can accept mistakes made in good faith; they are unable to accept being treated in a callous, dehumanizing, and uncompassionate manner.

FIGURE 30.2.
Juran's Triprol™ diagram. (From Juran Institute, Inc., Wilton, Conn.)

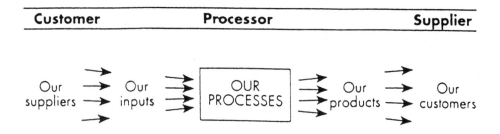

A Case of Sudden Death Found in Ventricular Fibrillation: an Algorithmic Analysis

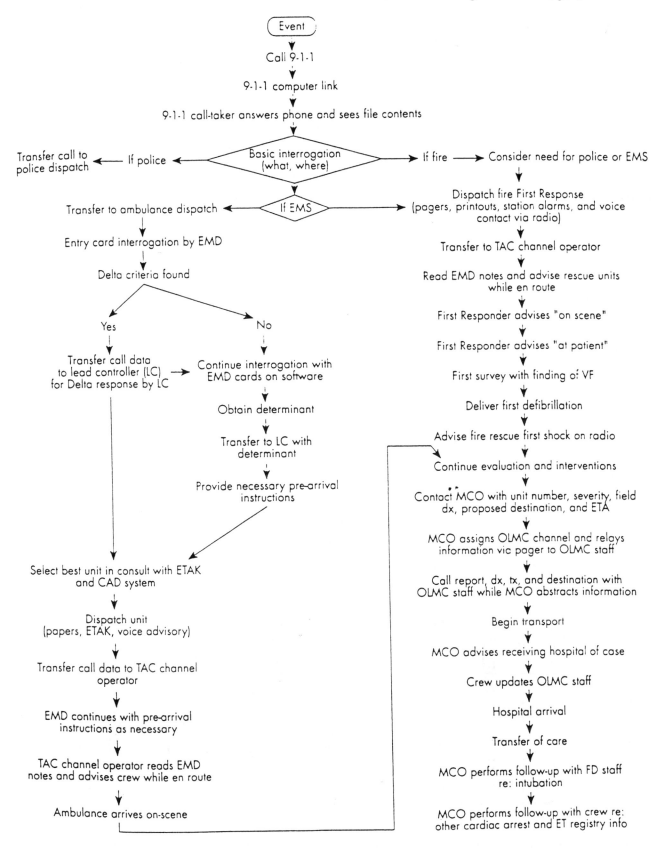

FIGURE 30.3. *A process flow chart for an EMS system's response to sudden cardiac death. (Courtesy Office of the Medical Director, Pinellas County EMS, Largo, FL)*

These problems have their parallels in industry. The manager's or engineer's view of a product often varies substantially from the consumer's. Ishikawa distinguishes the concepts of true quality characteristics from substitute quality characteristics.[22] The patient may perceive the answering of the 9-1-1 call within two rings, or the lack of need to repeat his complaint, as attributes of quality. The system recognizes these as aspects of a streamlined process to triage and responds in a timely and appropriate manner to the entire community. The reliability of this process in an individual encounter is a substitute quality characteristic for the consistency of call processing that matches demand to supply in the most timely and efficient manner for the needs of the public. Quality management in EMS requires leadership to seek out and incorporate these customers' perspectives. The role of the medical director is in part that of a "quality engineer." Detailed understanding of the scientific basis of medical practice is key to integrating the substitute and true quality characteristics of system goals into the quality planning process.

Cardiac arrest is the ultimate personal emergency. Although the paramedic's scope of practice is certainly broad-based, advanced life support (ALS) is fundamentally directed toward a knowledge base and psychomotor skills that resuscitate the patient in arrest. Understanding the pathophysiology of sudden cardiac death resolves to a small number of basic facts. Patients survive, practically speaking, only witnessed ventricular fibrillation. The key factors influencing their survival are the early provision of basic life support (bystander CPR) and definitive care (defibrillatory shock). This is illustrated graphically by Eisenberg (fig. 30.4).[23]

For the individual patient the definition of customer need in this worst case scenario is straightforward, and has been extensively addressed in medical literature. The requirement of a high level of reliability for the provision of equal access to definitive care for all the customers of an EMS service area should be the basic design feature of an ALS system. The needs of the customers of an EMS system are the standards of care for the system (i.e., the standards of care of the system are the derivative of the needs of the customers of an EMS system).

The reorganization of Emergency Medical Services in the city of Kansas City, Missouri in 1978–79 remains the best early example of the recognition and synthesis of these diverse customers' needs into the design of an EMS system.[16] As a result of public outcry over the tragic death of a police officer who exsanguinated after a 25-minute response by the EMS provider, and a general perception by the public of unequal access to services among neighborhoods, the city government obtained consultation to reconfigure the system. The requirements of this new system (the customers' needs) were straightforward, yet pro-

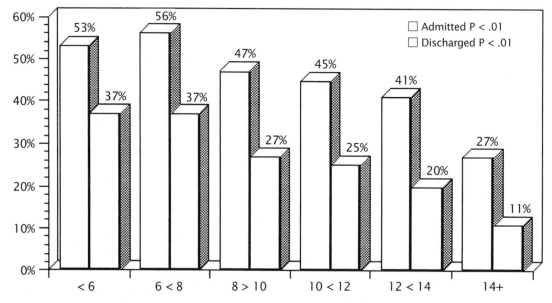

FIGURE 30.4. *The window of survivability of sudden cardiac death in the community describes a fundamental design feature of an effective ALS system.[23] Adapted from Eisenberg, M. et al: Clinics Emerg Med 1983; 2:13–25.*

QUALITY MANAGEMENT

foundly impacted the delivery of care. All 9-1-1 customers shall be afforded equal access to care for life-threatening emergencies as prospectively defined by emergency medical dispatch.

Develop Product Features that Respond to Customer Needs

According to Juran, every product feature should meet a certain set of minimum criteria. The feature should first meet the needs of the customer. Those needs include stated needs as well as perceived, real, and cultural needs. Second, the product feature should meet the needs of the supplier, including the needs of the internal customers. Next, the product feature should meet competition. Meeting the needs of external and internal customers does not ensure the customers will buy it—a competitor's product may be better or give better value. Meeting competition is an important criterion for developers. Lastly, product features should minimize the combined costs to both customers and suppliers. Each incurs costs relevant to the product and seeks to keep its own at minimum. The optimum for society is when price reflects actual costs and both are kept to a minimum.

The fundamental constructs of the reorganized EMS system in Kansas City were based on the standards of medical care defined by the consensus of community medical authority, the Emergency Physicians Advisory Board (EPAB) (the medical community-customer). The citizens of the community (the patient-customers) were to be afforded equal access to timely and appropriate Emergency Medical Services that met their needs with 90% reliability at the eight-minute interval (the lower specification limit of the product). This response time requirement applied to all council manic districts of the city, irrespective of the call density or difficulties in coverage. (Criterion #1—meet the customers needs)

The city government, through the creation of a trust entity in the public's interest, would have control over all necessary aspects of delivery of service. (Criterion #2—meet the needs of the supplier)

The Metropolitan Ambulance Services Trust (MAST), a type of public utility commission representing the governmental or civic customer, was created. It had several critical functions. It would (1) contract for the cost-effective provision of services by competitive bid for the market, in contrast to **in** the market (making it economically feasible by directly controlling costs); (2) award, through performance contract to a single provider, exclusive market rights to the community (like an electric or water company); (3) monitor performance requirements using objective criteria, through its own activities, and those of the EPAB; (4) exercise contractual recourse for failure to perform, including firing the contractor for breach if necessary. (Criterion #3—meet competition; Criterion #4—minimize combined costs)

Develop Processes that are Able to Produce the Features

In QM terms a process is a "systematic series of actions directed to the achievement of a goal." Process development refers to process design and evaluation, process selection, provision of facilities, provision of methods, and procedures for operation, as well as control and maintenance of the process.

SSM was developed out of necessity to provide the levels of coverage and response-time reliability that met the needs of system customers at an affordable cost. Consider the problem—most EMS systems seek to keep response times low and often appear to do, as average response times are within acceptable ranges. This concept is critically flawed, however, from the customer's perspective. All systems have a heterogeneous pattern of call density. By responding to those needs with ambulance placement, it is possible to reduce average response times by providing short responses to high call-density areas while sacrificing the lives of those in lower call-density areas (fig. 30.5).

However, using the principles of demand pattern analysis and peak-load staffing, equal access to care for patient-customers can be provided. These SSM systems are driven, in contrast, by a fractile response time requirement (e.g., an eight-minute response to life-threatening emergencies provided with 90% reliability over all subunits of a service area). This is known in QM as a lower control limit (LCL), or specification limit, for a process, and is a contractual requirement in many systems. The shift to this strategy in the Kansas City system resulted in a 35% increase in efficiency while affording the system equal access to care (fig. 30.6A–C).[24]

Transfer the Resulting Plans to the Operating Forces

The transfer of processes from the planners to the operating forces is necessary to confirm that theoreti-

Comparison of Response Time Performance for Two Communities

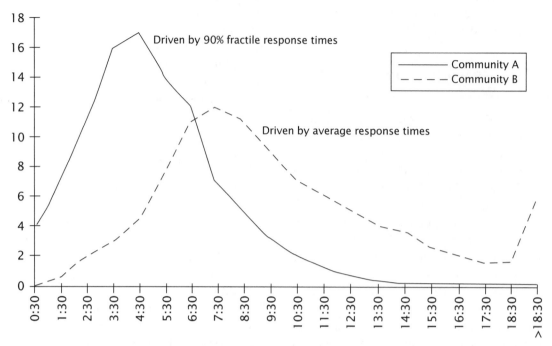

FIGURE 30.5. *The differences in emergency response time performance between these two communities are striking. The first (driven by fractile response time performance) clusters 90% of emergency responses within the eight-minute interval. The system driven by average response time performance has a much longer "tail". This design flaw severely limits the potential for survival from sudden cardiac death. (Courtesy The Fourth Party, Inc., West River, MD.)*

cal process capability can be accomplished on the production line. This commonly occurs through testing the process. This may involve dry runs, pilot tests, or simulations. It is important that these approximate the real world events that they seek to reproduce. Often these are cooperative projects of the quality planning team and selected line personnel. The interaction of these groups is extremely valuable in refining process capability.

Process/Quality Control

Definitions

Donabedian defines process as having to do with the characteristics of provider behavior in the management of health and illness.[15] Process deals with a set of activities between practitioners and patients. The observation of process is best done directly or secondarily by the study of documents of care.

Juran considers process from an operational viewpoint. The concept of control is one of "holding the status quo"—keeping a planned process in its planned state so that it remains able to meet the op-

erating goals. A process that is designed to be able to meet operating goals does not stay that way. Many events can intervene to damage the ability of the process to meet goals. The main purpose of control is to minimize this damage, either by prompt action to restore the status quo or, better yet, by prevention of the damage from happening in the first place.

The Controllability of Processes

If consistency and reliability are quality attributes of the processes of an EMS system, then strategies are required to assess and improve these features of care. There are obviously profound differences in machining ball bearings in a factory and delivering emergency care in the diverse and uncontrolled environment of the street. These are not conceptual differences, however, and should not cause one to reject, out of hand, the appropriateness of applying industrial process models to EMS. Rather, many emergency care processes can be controlled and are highly consistent and reliable in their production of quality care.

FIGURE 30.6. *Temporal (right) and Geographic (below) demand patterns are shown. By peak load staffing, the demand patterns for service are covered. © 1984 The Fourth Party, Inc. Used with permission.*

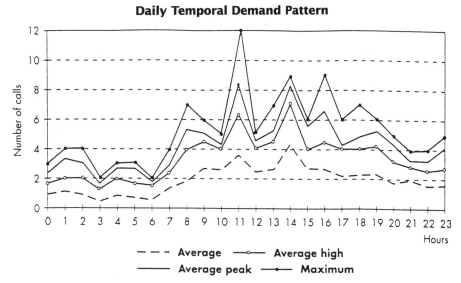

Daily Temporal Demand Pattern

- - - Average   —○— Average high
—— Average peak   —•— Maximum

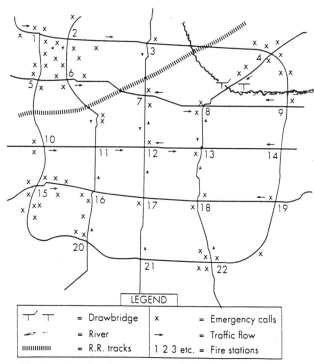

Demand Map for Hour 8

LEGEND

⊤ ⊤	= Drawbridge	x	= Emergency calls
	= River	→	= Traffic flow
▥	= R.R. tracks	1 2 3 etc.	= Fire stations

The train goes through town to the river several times a day. It travels under the interstates, but crosses both roads loading from post 6 to posts 7 and 11, and blocks traffic several times a day. The drawbridge opens on demand for commercial vehicles and on the hour for pleasure vehicles.

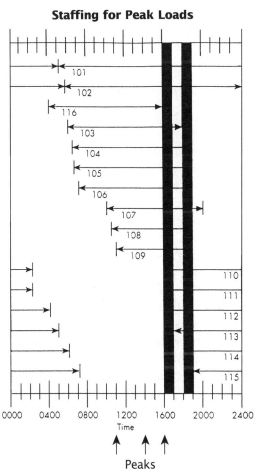

Staffing for Peak Loads

Peaks

The Control Pyramid

Control of processes exists at all levels. Nearly all effective control of EMS care is exercised by the workers. The controllability of processes is largely a function of self-control by individual EMS providers. Overlying this is a layer of managerial control provided directly by the communications center and indirectly by the administrative supervisors. This pyramid differs significantly from those described by Juran for industrial processes. The level of automated controls in EMS is relatively small compared to the level of control by the work force. Process control by management, communications, and field supervisors, usually at a distance, is also less (fig. 30.7).

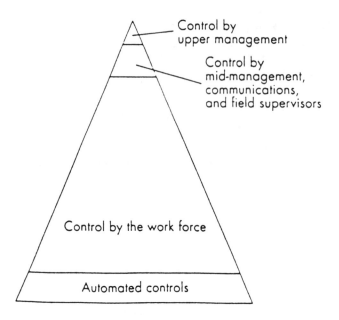

FIGURE 30.7. *The pyramid of control of EMS process. (Modified from Juran. 1993, OMD)*

The Concept of Statistical Process Control

Central to QM concepts of quality planning is the standardization of processes to increase their reliability and productivity. These standards are inherently quantitative, measurable, and suitable for statistical analysis. All measured processes exhibit elements of variation. The understanding of the distribution and patterns of variation in processes is a key feature of the industrial approach to quality control.

Variation in systems is attributable to the inherent randomness of the system (common causes) or to some specific event (special causes). The evaluation of any process first seeks to determine whether or not the process is stable.[25]

A stable process, one with no indication of a special cause of variation, is said to be, following Shewhart, *in statistical control,* or stable. It is a ran-

dom process. Its behavior in the near future is predictable. . . . A system that is in statistical control has a definable identity and capability. . . . In the state of statistical control, all special causes so far detected have been removed.

Statistical Process Control, as developed by Shewhart about 1924, refers to the application of analyses of the means, ranges, and standard deviations of a process quantifying its variability and randomness. These analyses are often represented and monitored using control charts that graphically illustrate the stability of processes and the common and special causes of variation (fig. 30.8).

Are the processes by which we provide medical care consistent (i.e., in statistical control or stable); are their behaviors in the near future predictable?

No, with a few exceptions, they are probably not stable. One need only review the medical literature to recognize that these concerns are almost never acknowledged or addressed in published research. Most typically, clinical trials in which the process was flawed are simply discarded from the sample, labeled incomplete, or eliminated from statistical analysis. Infrequently reported ranges and standard deviations for study groups indicate that these concepts are not widely recognized in scientific medicine.

Do we have examples of processes in EMS that are in statistical control as defined by QM?

Yes—There are a number of tracked system processes that appear to be in statistical control. These are predominantly in so-called high performance (HP) EMS systems: (1) reliability of preventative maintenance programs in production of critical failure-free miles for ambulances; (2) 90%+ reliability of eight-minute response time performance to life-threatening emergencies for HP systems; (3) 98%+ reliability for non-emergency response times for HP systems; (4) 98%+ reliability for 9-1-1 complaint

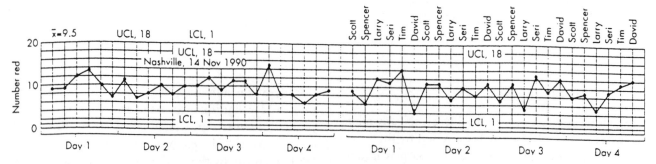

FIGURE 30.8. *A statistical process control chart for the Red Beads Experiment. It illustrates the sequence of production runs for each of the willing workers over a four-day period. The upper and lower control limits (UCL and LCL) are three standard deviations from the mean. (From Deming WE: The New Economics, 1993 MIT.)*

answering in PSAPs; (5) 95% reliability for correct dispatch determinant selection by dispatchers in Medical Priority Dispatch systems;[26] (6) reliability of synchronized time measurement in EMS communications centers.[i]

Juran's benchmarks for quality control are shown in the box below.

Quality Control

Evaluate Actual Product Performance
Compare Actual Performance to Product Goals
Act on the Difference

Evaluate Actual Product Performance

A significant problem arises during an attempt to evaluate "product performance" in the services provided. By what measures and with what tools is the quality of care in EMS evaluated? And in what areas of performance does it make sense to evaluate?

Eisenberg calls the system audit of cardiac arrest the "best outcome evaluation of an EMS system's performance."[27] The characteristics are (1) the event is important; (2) the event has a clear case definition; (3) the outcome is measurable; (4) the intervention is straightforward; (5) the intervention has an effect;

and (6) the event occurs frequently. Cardiac arrest is the ultimate personal emergency and serves as a benchmark of system performance.

The measures and tools for evaluation of EMS processes are problematic but improving.[28] It is nearly impossible to directly observe the process of care in a systematic way. Rather, dependence is on indirect observations (e.g., real-time through radio communications, or documents produced by the chain of internal processes). Significant progress has been made in the standardization of measurement and the exploration of new tools and technologies to refine field data collection.[29] Improvement in EMS systems is fundamentally dependent on the definition of essential data for field performance and the reliable methods for its retrieval. These methods will only be successful when field providers recognize their critical roles as clinicians/investigators. Such efforts to date have been ambivalent at best.

System Status Management was implemented first in Kansas City, Missouri, as a result of the reorganization of that EMS system. The performance of the system was measured on an ongoing basis through a number of statistical tools and was continually refined to equalize access to care and improve overall response times. Figures 30.9 and 30.10 illustrate actual measurements of performance improvement over the period from 1979 to 1982.

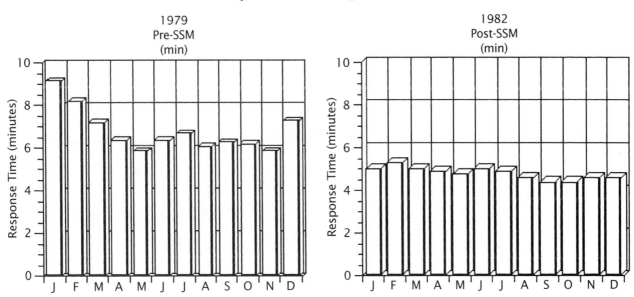

**Average Emergency Response Times
Kansas City, Missouri, EMS System 1979 & 1982**

FIGURE **30.9.** *Measurement of performance improvement from 1979 to 1982. (Courtesy Metropolitan Ambulance Services Trust, Kansas City, MO. 1984)* [24]

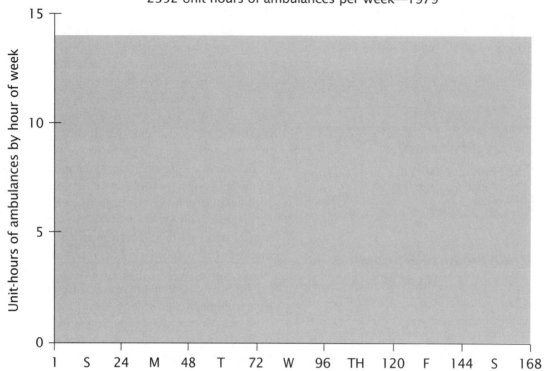

2352 Unit-hours of ambulances per week—1979

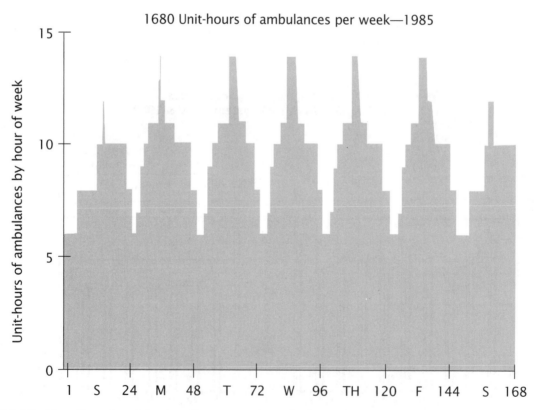

1680 Unit-hours of ambulances per week—1985

FIGURE 30.10. *The effect of peak load staffing on unit hour deployment. Source: Metropolitan Ambulance Services Trust, 1984.*[24]

QUALITY MANAGEMENT

The indirect but real-time observation of care has been used reliably in a number of systems. The unique vantage point of the EMS communications center provides the best practical "look" at overall system performance. This nerve center is equipped with a large array of "sensors" that can be utilized in quality control. An increasing number of computerized ambulance dispatching systems (CADs) is incorporating clinical features.[30] The Medical Communications Officer (MCO) collects a number of ongoing registries of clinical information and acts as an "umpire" to actuate the feedback loops for quality control. The Pinellas Cardiac Arrest Registry Data Set is shown (fig. 30.11).

Compare Actual Performance with Product Goals

The process of quality control, from an industrial perspective, requires the application of a familiar concept from physiology, (i.e., the feedback loop). Figure 30.12 illustrates this feedback.

The implementation of System Status Management was accomplished initially by hand and then computerized to run on a 48k Apple II computer. The CAD program informed dispatchers of historical demand patterns for service (system status plans). As calls were received and dispatched, their locations and time intervals were measured and recorded. Ongoing evaluation of this data produced subsequent refinement in system status planning. Although steady and significant improvements occurred in response time performance and efficiency, the 90% fractile performance goal was not achieved until 1982 (figs. 30.9, 30.10, and 30.13).

Act on the Difference

How system leaders and managers act on the differences between system goals and performance will ultimately determine the success or failure of QM in EMS. Davidson points out that there are two choices in management styles: first, to continue with the "bad apples" approach and close the loop through a cycle of fear, or second, to enter a pathway toward a model of participatory management which focuses attention on the system of work and not individuals.[31] Workers work smarter and not harder, having increased pride in their work with higher productivity, quality, and effectiveness.

Outcome/Quality Improvement

The third element of classical medical quality assessment theory is the analysis of outcome. Outcome as defined by Donabedian relates to changes in health status as a result of the effects of structure and process. It is the most significant of the three elements; however, it is also the most elusive.[15] Particularly in EMS, the direct association of the process of care and its relation to outcome is often difficult to ascertain.

Juran's benchmarks for Quality Improvement are described in the box below.

Quality Improvement

Establish the infrastructure

Identify the improvement projects

Establish project teams

Provide the teams with resources, training, and motivation to:
    Diagnose the causes
    Stimulate remedies
    Establish controls to hold the gains

Although conceptually the QM process begins with quality planning, the mandate for change is often more difficult. Just as most medical directors do not design the system in which they function, most systems are not quality-oriented organizations at that point either. QM authorities recommend beginning the cycle with a QI project that will catalyze the change.

Establish the Infrastructure

In *Kaizen, the Key to Japan's Competitive Success*, Imai contrasts improvement East and West in industrial organizations.[32] Western management, he notes, "worships at the altar of innovation." The solution to most problems lies in quantum leaps in the wake of technological breakthroughs. In Japan, alternatively, QM is subtle, gradual, but pervasive in the organizational culture. Kaizen, which means improvement, is an ongoing process involving everyone in the organization, both managers and workers. The Kaizen philosophy is not confined only to the workplace, but influences social and family life as well.

QM in EMS will most likely fail (as it has in many U.S. companies) if it is viewed as a quick fix to what is wrong. For example, the advent of automatic defib-

CARDIAC ARREST AND INTUBATION REGISTRY/FIELD DATA FORM

Get the following information (from the 9-1-1 CAD only) before calling the ED:

Date: _____ Co. Inc. # _____ SS Inc. # _____ MOD/MD: _____ Grid: _____

First arriving ALS unit: Agency: _____ Shift: _____ FD unit # _____ SS unit # _____

Dispatched: _____ On-scene: _____ Transp. time: _____ Hosp. arrival time: _____

Was "At-Patient" notification given in 9-1-1 notes? (circle one)   Yes = 1   No = 2   At-Patient Time: ____ OLMC Time: _____

Ask call-taker who was given pre-arrival: None = 0   EMS = 1   Bystander = 2   PD = 3   Nursing staff = 4   Family = 5   Other = 6

Call the ED and ask for the nurse in charge of patient care:

Who am I speaking with? _____   Can you confirm tube placement: (check one)   ○ Yes   ○
No
                                    (nurses name)

If yes, who confirmed tube placement? (read list to nurse) (check one)   ○ MD   ○ X-ray   ○ RT   ○ RN

Ask to speak to paramedic in charge of patient care:

Patient Type: ○ Adult   ○ Pediatric (0-17 yrs)   Run Type: ○ Medical   ○ Trauma

Intubation time: _____   Tube size: _____

# of attempts: (check one)   ○ 1   ○ 2   ○ 3   ○ >3

Intubation method: (circle one)   Orotracheal   Nasotracheal   Digital   TTJV

Major difficulty: (circle one)   None   Anatomy   Secretions/Vomitus   Trauma   Equipment failure
                        Foreign body   Environment   Patient position   Available light   Other_____

Equipment/Maneuvers used: (circle all that apply)   None   End tidal CO_2 Stylet   Cricoid pressure
                                Magill forceps   Transillumination   Other_____

Other airways used: (circle all that apply)   EOA   EGTA   OPA   Nasopharyngeal   Other _____

Intubation performed: (circle one)   On-scene   En route   ED

Reintubation because: (circle one)   Esophagus intubated   Dislodged   Other _____

Intubation successful: ○ Yes   ○ No   Medic ID# _____

                            If first medic unsuccessful, second medic ID#: _____

Was intubation performed with cardiac arrest? (check one)   ○ Yes   ○ No

If NO, complete box below: ▼   If YES, go to other side. → → → → → →
                        ▼
                        ▼

Name of MCO filling out form: _____   Reviewed by: (circle one)   D. Shepherd / M. Wallace
                        (REQUIRED)

FIGURE 30.11. *An EMS Cardiac Arrest Registry Data Entry Form. This form is used by communications center personnel to gather real-time information regarding cardiac arrests. The time and effort involved in tracking this important data is minimized by immediate follow-up. ©1982 OMD Used with permission.*

(continued)

Historical data:

Lead medic in charge of patient care: _____ ID # _____

Patient name: _____
                            (last)   (first)

DOB: _____   Age: _____ (if < 1 yr use 1)   Sex: (circle one)   M = 1   F = 2

Arrest witnessed by whom: (circle one)   No Witness = 0   EMS = 1   Bystander = 2   PD = 3   Nurse = 4   Family = 5   Other = 6

Time CPR initiated: _____   By whom: EMS = 1 Bystander = 2 PD = 3 Nursing Staff = 4 Family = 5 Other = 6
                                              (circle one)

Initial presenting rhythm:

What was the initial presenting rhythm with no pulse: V-Fib = 1   V-Tach = 2   Asystole = 3   Idiovent = 4   Other = 5 ____

If initial rhythm was VF/VT, was "First Shock" notification given in 9-1-1 CAD notes? (circle one)   Yes = 1   No = 2   Time:____

If no, ask medic the time of the first defibrillation/cardiovertion: _____

During the code, was there ROSC? (circle one) Yes = 1   No = 2   Time: _____   and/or
                          was there ROSV? (circle one) Yes = 1   No = 2   Time: _____

Circle the ROSC rhythm: N/A = 0   SR = 1   A-Fib = 2   1°HB = 3   2°HB-I = 4   2°HB-II = 5   3°HB = 6   Idiovent = 7   Other = 8

Blood pressure: _____   Pulse: _____   Resp: _____   IV access time: _____

Pt. Hx: None = 0   Cardiac = 1   COPD = 2   HTN = 3   Seizure = 4   Diabetes = 5   CVA = 6
            (circle one)

Patient outcome:

Ask the paramedic: Before arrest, was the patient experiencing CHF, cardiogenic shock, or chest pain or was the arrest
                     of unknown etiology? If yes, circle Cardiac = 1

                     OR

                     Before arrest, was the patient in cardiac arrest due to etiology of trauma, COPD, CVA, or other
                     condition? If yes, circle Non-Cardiac = 2

Hospital dest. #: H _____   Patient outcome: (circle one)   Died in ED = 1   Admitted = 2

Name of MCO filling out form: _____   Reviewed by: (circle one)   D. Shepherd / M. Wallace
                              (REQUIRED)

FIGURE 30.11. *Continued*

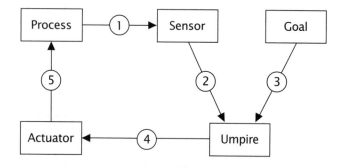

FIGURE 30.12. *Industrial Quality Control feedback loop. (1) Each process is equipped with various sensors, which quantify actual performance. (2) Those sensors are evaluated by an umpire who also receives information regarding the goals or standards for the process. (3) The umpire compares actual performance with the goals or standards and initiates an actuator if the process is out of range. (4) The actuator makes changes in the process to bring performance into line with goals. (From Juran Institute, Wilton, Conn.)*

rillators (a technological breakthrough) has had ambivalent success in improving outcome from cardiac arrest.

The transformation of organizations to this new way of doing business must be handled with care. Some organizations (such as the Public Utility Model Systems) are equipped with design elements that facilitate these concepts (Figure 30.14). For most, however, these elements are less clear. Identifying a project and selecting and organizing a quality team are the key steps.

Identify the Improvement Projects/ Establish Project Teams

These two steps are typically interrelated. At a strategic level, management identifies its agenda for improvement based on consensus and often with the special expertise of a quality engineer or external consultant. At an operational level, similar consensus building occurs to establish common ground for the initial improvement project. The choice is critical.

FIGURES 30.13. *System efficiency and cost as shown by improvements in unit hour utilization were large over the period of implementation of SSM. However, the goal of 90% fractile response time performance reliability was not achieved until 1982. Source: Metropolitan Ambulance Services Trust, 1984.[24]*

	1979 Pre-SSM	**1982 Post-SSM**	**Change (%)**
Emergency responses (yr)	14,600	16,126	+10
Average responses (wk)	281	310	+10
Unit-hours (wk)	2352	1680	−29
Unit-hour utilization ratio	.12	.18	+35

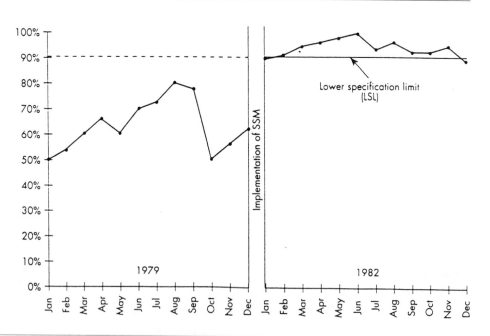

QM experts recommend a process that is significant both to management and to workers, one that has a relatively straightforward solution and will likely be a quick success to provide momentum for QM within the organization. The selection of the quality team reflects the cross section of management and workers who are necessary for the solution and who are interested in making a commitment to learn the process. Most EMS organizations cannot afford external consultants to facilitate the process. A useful and well-written guide to team building and working through projects is *The Team Handbook* by Scholtes.[33]

Resources, Training, and Motivation

Eastham has developed an excellent program for introducing the QM process to EMS organizations. Provider based Quality Assurance (PBQA) uses a form of nominal group process to define and prioritize QM issues. The program requires the support and commitment of leadership, and one individual must manage the program. By involving organizations from the ground up, the program increases the likelihood of early success and ongoing support. Eastham uses concepts of "just in time" training to enable team members to apply QM tools to practical problems within their organizations.[34]

Seven Statistical Tools

QM uses seven statistical tools to evaluate the causes of poor quality. They are key to managing systems by fact and are, in some cases, familiar concepts to medical directors.[35]

PROCESS FLOW CHART. As discussed in quality planning, the initial evaluation of processes through flow charts is revealing. A process flow diagram is a graphic representation of the sequential steps in a process. The actions of the team in constructing the chart often reveal hidden aspects of a process and hidden customers. By illustrating the interrelations of different elements, members of the team are afforded new perspectives of their area's effects on other parts of the flow (e.g., the 9-1-1 complaint-taker and the emergency medical dispatcher). Flow diagrams illustrate critical steps, locate process flaws, and graphically elucidate the sources of inefficiency and rework. Figure 30.3 illustrates the complex sequence of steps necessary to provide definitive care in cardiac arrest.

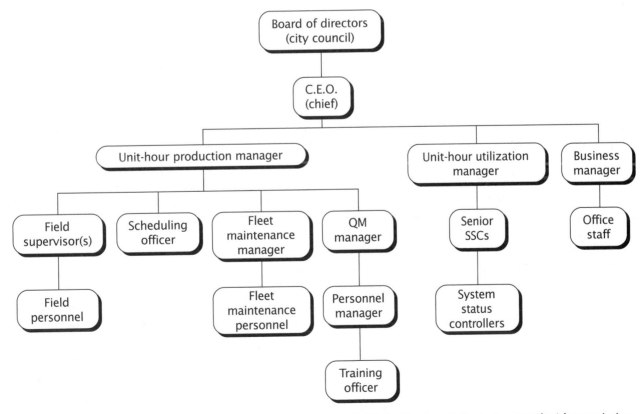

FIGURE 30.14. *Effective Organization in the SSM Environment. © 1989. The Fourth Party, Inc. Used with permission.*

CAUSE-AND-EFFECT DIAGRAMS. Ishikawa, cause-and-effect or "fishbone" diagrams categorize and display, in groups, theories about how and why processes fail.[13] They serve, as do flow diagrams, to build the team's understanding of each member's elements and of how individual perceptions of problems are often incomplete. They illustrate how the causes of problems are often interrelated. Ishikawa diagrams also point out the need for data points regarding elements of a process to quantify problems.

The fishbones relate associated elements using a number of conceptual threads. Often these are the "5 Ms" in manufacturing processes: men, machines, materials, methods, and measurements. In service industries the "5 Ps" are often used: patrons (external customers), people (internal customers), provisions (supplies), places (the work environment), and procedures (policies and protocols for work).

An Ishikawa diagram of causes of late responses and definitive care is illustrated in figure 30.15.[6]

CHECK SHEETS. In the evaluation of any process, the quantification of quality or defects is based on data. Check sheets organize necessary data elements efficiently to allow for collection. In a sense the EMS prehospital care report (PCR) is a check sheet. More often, these reports are matrices that allow the check-off of types of observations, thereby allowing quantification of the frequency of defects by type.

The Pinellas County EMS Report was developed over a 3-year period by a team of field clinicians and medical control staff; it is an example of the evolution to a structured computer-oriented field record for care (fig. 30.16). Computer software based on this data set enables the provider to create an electronic record using clipboard computers at the patient's side or in the destination hospital.

A monthly check sheet illustrates PCR documentation accuracy by paramedics (fig. 30.17). The goal is 100% accuracy by all personnel. The ambulance contractor is required by contract (a performance specification) to sample 30% of records using an explicit criterion review technique. The check sheet (a Microsoft Excel™ spreadsheet) is entered by field training officers instructed in the process. Summary data are published by the medic for review by all personnel.

HISTOGRAMS. A histogram is a frequency distribution chart of a process. The chart is a special form of line or bar graph that illustrates the variation of continuous data such as time, weight, size, or temperature. The histogram also illustrates the distribution of continuous data. Important concepts in the significance of these distributions are illustrated in the comparison of histograms of response times between an average response and a fractile response time-driven system (Figure 30.5).

RUN OR TREND CHARTS. These graphic tools illustrate changes in a process over time. In industry they are frequently used with quality control samples to track the changing performance of an operation on the assembly line. For example, they show the wear and loss of precision tolerances of a machine tool. There are many processes that are observable in EMS by use of trend charts (Figure 30.13).

PARETO CHARTS. Juran identified the concept of the "Pareto Principle" to separate causes of poor quality between the "vital few" and the "useful many."[37] By graphing the frequency of occurrence of defects by type from greatest to least, it is obvious where efforts should be prioritized to decrease defects. This concept is used to improve PCR documentation in cooperation with the ambulance contractor. This tool can be applied to a broad group of issues as a method of prioritization. The Pareto chart in figure 30.18 illustrates prioritization of causes of incomplete PCRs.

STATISTICAL PROCESS CONTROL CHARTS. A special application of the run or trend chart is the statistical process control chart or "control chart" (Figures 30.8 and 30.9). The concept of statistical control is discussed earlier in this chapter. The control chart illustrates the trends in control of processes and identifies graphically some common and special causes of variation. There are a number of specific types of control charts, each applicable to different data types. Typically a basic chart shows the variability of sample or population data around its mean, and a companion chart quantifies the variation in the range of the values. The control limits of a process represent standard deviations of the mean (Figure 30.19).

The control chart is by far the most powerful of the statistical tools because it describes not only the causes of variation but it also points in the direction of solutions. A detailed discussion of the use of this tool is noted.[34,35] Last, the control chart provides a method to hold the gains. Through sampling processes that are in control on an intermittent basis,

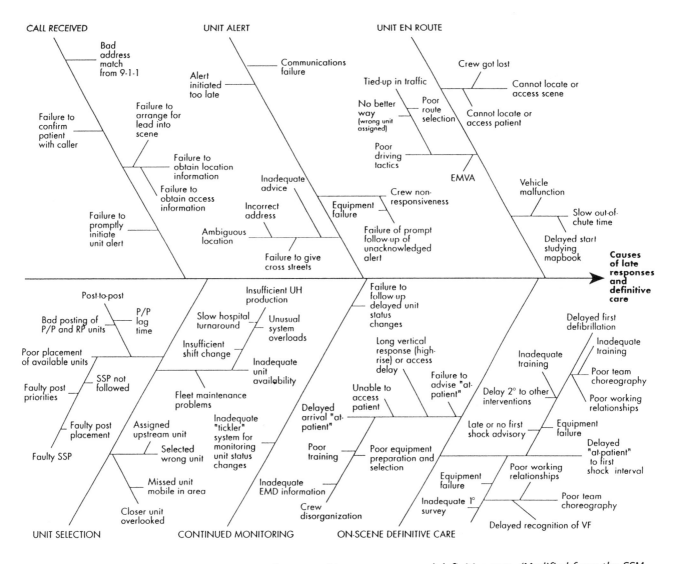

FIGURE 30.15. *A Cause-and-Effect Diagram of causes of late responses and definitive care. (Modified from the SSM Workshops; Courtesy The Fourth Party, Inc., West River, MD)*

evidence can be found for the slipping of processes that may be readdressed by quality teams.

Results

The influence of QM implemented in systems of prehospital care can be profound. Yet breakthroughs in quality are only the result of a diligent and relentless pursuit of optimization of the system. Experience with cardiac arrest survival illustrates these points.

Optimization of system design exists throughout the Pinellas EMS system. Established in 1986 as a public utility model system, it provides all prehospital care services to 1 million residents of Tampa Bay, Florida. The system responds to over 150,000 calls per year with fire service ALS First Responders and a single private ALS transport provider. An emergency response time interval (call received to unit on-scene of 6.5 minutes) is provided with 90% reliability through the use of SSM. A powerful SSM computer-aided dispatching system provides access to a wide variety of non-clinical performance data. MCOs monitor and track in real-time a broad group of clinical quality indicators from the EMS Communications Center.

Resuscitation is provided to more than 1200 field cardiac arrests annually. A paramedic-level emergency medical dispatch system and an aggressive community-wide CPR training campaign increased the frequency of bystander CPR from 11% to more than

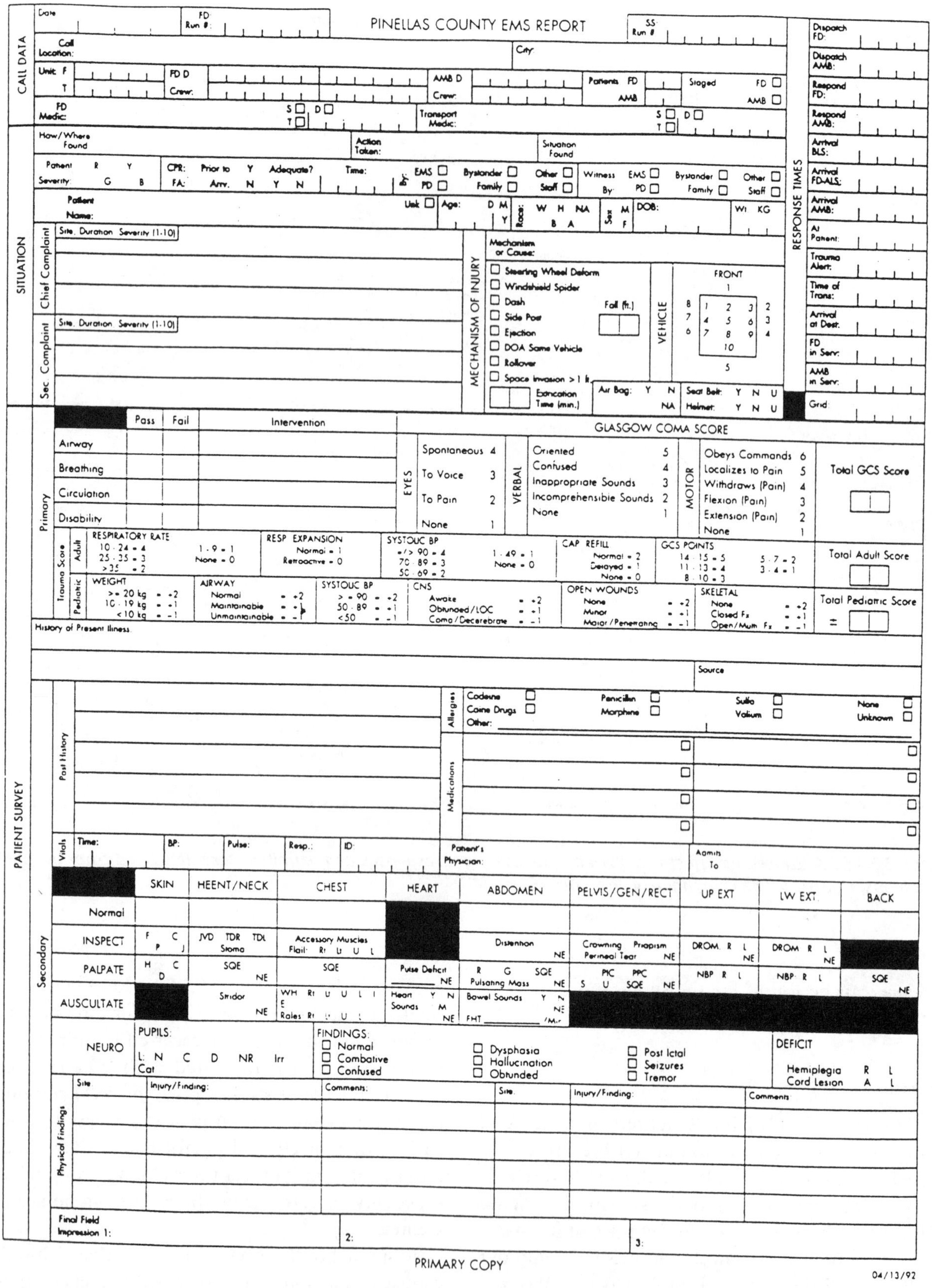

PINELLAS COUNTY EMS REPORT

CALL DATA

Date | FD Run #: | SS Run #

Call Location: | City:

Unit: F T | FD D Crew: | AMB D Crew: | Patients FD AMB | Staged FD ☐ AMB ☐

FD Medic: S☐ D☐ T☐ | Transport Medic: S☐ D☐ T☐

SITUATION

How/Where Found | Action Taken: | Situation Found

Patient Severity: R Y G B | CPR: Prior to Arrv. Y N | FA: Adequate? Y N | Time: | By: EMS ☐ Bystander ☐ Other ☐ FD ☐ Family ☐ Staff ☐ | Witness: EMS ☐ Bystander ☐ Other ☐ By: FD ☐ Family ☐ Staff ☐

Patient Name: | Unk ☐ Age: D M Y | Race: W H NA B A | Sex: M F | DOB: | Wt KG

Chief Complaint: Site, Duration, Severity (1-10)

Sec Complaint: Site, Duration, Severity (1-10)

MECHANISM OF INJURY

Mechanism or Cause:

☐ Steering Wheel Deform
☐ Windshield Spider
☐ Dash
☐ Side Post
☐ Ejection
☐ DOA Same Vehicle
☐ Rollover
☐ Space invasion > 1 ft.

Fall (ft.)

Extrication Time (min.)

VEHICLE: FRONT 1; 8 1 2 3 2; 7 4 5 6 3; 6 7 8 9 4; 10; 5

Air Bag: Y N NA | Seat Belt: Y N U | Helmet: Y N U

RESPONSE TIMES

Dispatch FD: | Dispatch AMB: | Respond FD: | Respond AMB: | Arrival BLS: | Arrival FD-ALS: | Arrival AMB: | At Patient: | Trauma Alert: | Time of Trans: | Arrival at Dest: | FD in Serv: | AMB in Serv: | Grid:

PATIENT SURVEY

Primary

	Pass	Fail	Intervention
Airway			
Breathing			
Circulation			
Disability			

GLASGOW COMA SCORE

EYES		VERBAL		MOTOR	
Spontaneous	4	Oriented	5	Obeys Commands	6
To Voice	3	Confused	4	Localizes to Pain	5
To Pain	2	Inappropriate Sounds	3	Withdraws (Pain)	4
None	1	Incomprehensible Sounds	2	Flexion (Pain)	3
		None	1	Extension (Pain)	2
				None	1

Total GCS Score

Trauma Score — Adult

RESPIRATORY RATE: 10-24 = 4; 25-35 = 3; >35 = 2; 1-9 = 1; None = 0
RESP EXPANSION: Normal = 1; Retroactive = 0
SYSTOLIC BP: =/> 90 = 4; 70-89 = 3; 50-69 = 2; 1-49 = 1; None = 0
CAP REFILL: Normal = 2; Delayed = 1; None = 0
GCS POINTS: 14-15 = 5; 11-13 = 4; 8-10 = 3; 5-7 = 2; 3-4 = 1

Total Adult Score

Trauma Score — Pediatric

WEIGHT: >= 20 kg = +2; 10-19 kg = +1; <10 kg = -1
AIRWAY: Normal = +2; Maintainable = +1; Unmaintainable = -1
SYSTOLIC BP: > = 90 = +2; 50-89 = +1; <50 = -1
CNS: Awake = +2; Obtunded/LOC = +1; Coma/Decerebrate = -1
OPEN WOUNDS: None = +2; Minor = +1; Major/Penetrating = -1
SKELETAL: None = +2; Closed Fx = +1; Open/Mult Fx = -1

Total Pediatric Score =

History of Present Illness

Source

Past History

Allergies: Codeine ☐ Caine Drugs ☐ Other: | Penicillin ☐ Morphine ☐ | Sulfa ☐ Valium ☐ | None ☐ Unknown ☐

Medications ☐

Vitals: Time: | BP: | Pulse: | Resp.: | ID: | Patient's Physician: | Admits To

Secondary

	SKIN	HEENT/NECK	CHEST	HEART	ABDOMEN	PELVIS/GEN/RECT	UP EXT	LW EXT	BACK
Normal									
INSPECT	F C P J	JVD TDR TDL Stoma	Accessory Muscles Flail: Rt U U L		Distention NE	Crowning Priapism Perineal Tear NE	DROM R L NE	DROM R L NE	
PALPATE	H C D	SQE NE	SQE	Pulse Deficit NE	R G SQE Pulsating Mass NE	PIC PPC S U SQE NE	NBP R L	NBP R L	SQE NE
AUSCULTATE		Stridor NE	WH Rt U U L I E Rales Rt U U L	Heart Y N Sounds M NE	Bowel Sounds Y N NE FHT /Min				

NEURO: PUPILS: L N C D NR Irr Cat | FINDINGS: ☐ Normal ☐ Combative ☐ Confused ☐ Dysphasia ☐ Hallucination ☐ Obtunded ☐ Post Ictal ☐ Seizures ☐ Tremor | DEFICIT: Hemiplegia R L; Cord Lesion A L

Physical Findings: Site | Injury/Finding: | Comments: | Site | Injury/Finding: | Comments

Final Field Impression 1: | 2: | 3:

PRIMARY COPY

04/13/92

FIGURE 30.16. *Data-oriented, structured prehospital call report. Note that nearly every field is designed to be drawn from forced-choice look-up tables. Only "history of present illness" and a section for remarks are designed to be free text. This design enables EMS data to be highly computerized and retrievable. (Courtesy Office of the Medical Director, Pinellas County EMS, Largo, FL)*

Treatment Protocol	1st	2nd	3rd	4th	PINELLAS COUNTY EMS REPORT	V/S	BP	Pulse	Resp	Skin	GCS	TS
						Meds	Dose	Route	Resusr	Change		
						ECG	Rhythm	Rate	Ectopy	Rate	Lead	

TREATMENT FLOW CHART

Time	Action	Performed By	Parameters
		2 MC	

(repeated rows, each with "2" and "MC" in Performed By column)

REMARKS

MISC

A.	B.	C.	D.	E.
Medical Control: MD MOD	Supplemental Sheets:	Abuse Registry ☐ Trauma Registry ☐	Blood Consent ☐ Telemedic ☐ Chapter ☐ 401	Refusal on Back ☐ Additional Sheets	No. of Refusals	FD AMB

TRANSPORT DATA

FD Y Ride In: N	Trans To:	Destination Address:	City	State	Zip	Odometer	Start: Stop:

| Hospital Selection: | Patient Choice ☐ Nearest Facility ☐ | Special Needs ☐ Diversion ☐ | Response Code: | BLS ☐ ALS ☐ | Standby ☐ Out of Town ☐ | Cancelled ☐ | Wait Time | Trans By: Unit # | Admitted: Y N |

| Moved to Ambulance: | Walked ☐ Carried ☐ | Chair ☐ Stretcher ☐ | Transport Position: | Prone ☐ Supine ☐ | Shock ☐ Sitting ☐ | Left Lat ☐ Recum ☐ | Oxygen Y Supplied: N |

BILLING

Patient Address:		City	State	County	Zip Unk. ☐	Patient Phone:
Patient SS #:	Medicare #:		Medicaid #:		Ambulance Member #
Guarantor Name: Last, First				Guarantor Phone #:
Guarantor Address:	City	State	County	Zip	Worker's Comp.: Y N	Hospice: Y N
Employer Company Name:				Employer Phone #:
Employer Company Address:	City	State	County	Zip

Reviewed By: FIRE	Reviewed By: TRANSPORT	Reviewed By: MEDICAL CONTROL

PRIMARY COPY

04/13/92

FIGURE 30.16. *Continued*

PARAMEDIC	PR#	FTO	Reports Complete (%)	Reports Complete (#)	Reports Incomplete (#)	Audit TOTAL
Paramedic 01	2194	VG	100%	9		9
Paramedic 02	2141	AB	100%	7		7
Paramedic 03	574	AB	100%	41		41
Paramedic 04	2043	VG	100%	7		7
Paramedic 05	943	AB	96%	49	2	51
Paramedic 06	2082	VG	96%	44	2	46
Paramedic 07	888	VG	94%	46	3	49
Paramedic 08	2027	NP	94%	45	3	48
Paramedic 09	2123	LP	89%	41	5	46
Paramedic 10	2143	AB	83%	40	8	48
Paramedic 11	496	AB	82%	41	9	50
Paramedic 12	1083	NP	81%	42	10	52
Paramedic 13	864	NP	79%	34	9	43
Paramedic 14	2084	AB	78%	25	7	32
Paramedic 15	2128	NP	76%	29	9	38
Paramedic 16	2171	VG	74%	26	9	35
Paramedic 17	835	LP	67%	33	16	49
Paramedic 18	2148	LP	67%	32	16	48
Paramedic 19	2156	AB	67%	28	14	42
Paramedic 20	754	NP	63%	30	18	48
Paramedic 21	354	LP	58%	25	18	43
Paramedic 22	2151	LP	57%	8	6	14
Paramedic 23	512	NP	54%	22	19	41
Paramedic 24	456	LP	50%	9	9	18
Paramedic 25	2152	NP	48%	19	21	40
Paramedic 26	500	AB	46%	19	22	41
Paramedic 27	2144	NP	42%	22	31	53
Paramedic 28	513	NP	41%	16	23	39
Paramedic 29	2183	LP	34%	10	19	29
Paramedic 30	764	AB	30%	3	7	10
COMPANY AVERAGE			78.67%	2699	758	3457

BREAKDOWN OF MISSING OR INCOMPLETE ITEMS (column headers): Run #, Name/date, Call ktn, Actn ktn, Sit fnd, Crew ID, Pt C/O, Meds, Allg, Past hst, Phys exm, Time assmt score, Final, Prtcl used, VS, Tx to chart, Rx meds to, Ma, Guar name, Addr and zip, Pt DOB, Soc Sec #, Insur info, Not legible, Repl missing, Tr rpt reg, Arr Requ.

Previous scores as of:

Date	Score
10/31/91	47.60%
12/05/91	62.00%
12/17/91	64.00%
12/31/91	68.69%
02/01/92	77.39%
02/15/92	76.42%
03/01/92	77.58%
03/16/92	77.91%

FIGURE 30.17. *A check sheet of causes of incomplete documentation of EMS PCRs. The use of a computerized check sheet (a spreadsheet) enables the data to be analyzed and reports generated efficiently. (Courtesy Wayne Ruppert, National Director of Quality Improvement, LifeFleet, Inc., 1992).*

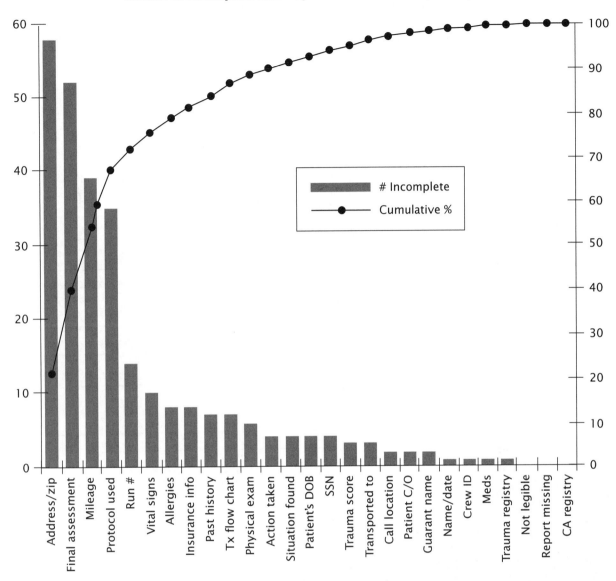

FIGURE 30.18. *Causes of incomplete PCR documentation in the first quarter of 1992. (Courtesy Office of the Medical Director, Pinellas County EMS, Largo, FL)*

50% in two years. The system anecdotally perceived itself as producing high quality care and a high survival rate from cardiac arrest.

Early in 1992 a cardiac arrest quality team was organized by the Office of the Medical Director (OMD) to implement an Utstein-style cardiac arrest registry. The team worked for several months constructing data collection and verification processes. Arrests were analyzed on a monthly basis, and reports were generated and refined (Figure 30.20). By June, reliable data showed the system had a survival rate for cardiac arrests of cardiac etiology of only 1.9%!

This realization was both shocking and confounding. The group began dissecting the problem. The process was described using a flow chart to identify the parallel and sequential elements, as well as internal and external customers (Figure 30.3). The elements of event reporting and data collection were recognized as integral to the process and were included in the flow diagram.

The causes of late responses and definitive care were listed and grouped into an Ishikawa Diagram, showing major process categories upon which to focus the team's attention (Figure 30.15). The branch

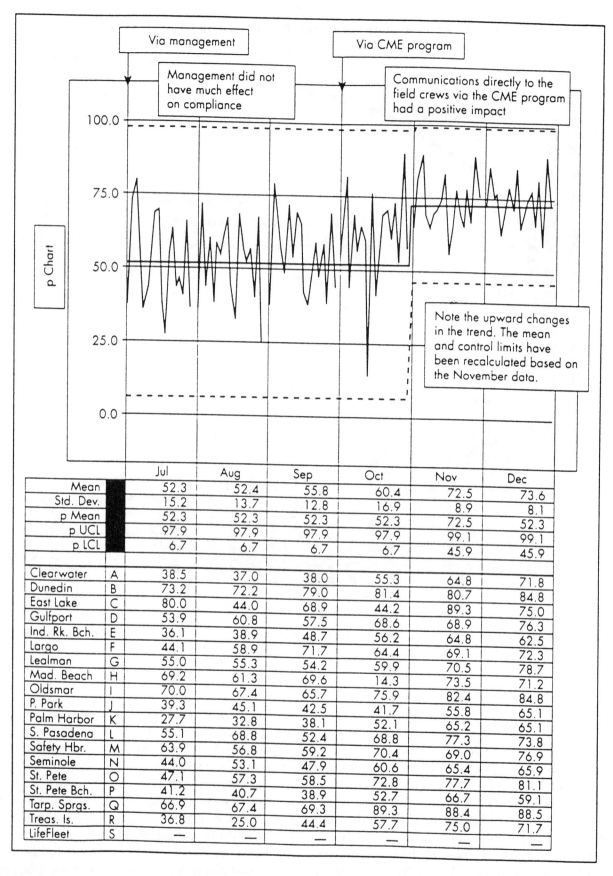

Via management

Management did not have much effect on compliance

Via CME program

Communications directly to the field crews via the CME program had a positive impact

p Chart

Note the upward changes in the trend. The mean and control limits have been recalculated based on the November data.

		Jul	Aug	Sep	Oct	Nov	Dec
Mean		52.3	52.4	55.8	60.4	72.5	73.6
Std. Dev.		15.2	13.7	12.8	16.9	8.9	8.1
p Mean		52.3	52.3	52.3	52.3	72.5	52.3
p UCL		97.9	97.9	97.9	97.9	99.1	99.1
p LCL		6.7	6.7	6.7	6.7	45.9	45.9
Clearwater	A	38.5	37.0	38.0	55.3	64.8	71.8
Dunedin	B	73.2	72.2	79.0	81.4	80.7	84.8
East Lake	C	80.0	44.0	68.9	44.2	89.3	75.0
Gulfport	D	53.9	60.8	57.5	68.6	68.9	76.3
Ind. Rk. Bch.	E	36.1	38.9	48.7	56.2	64.8	62.5
Largo	F	44.1	58.9	71.7	64.4	69.1	72.3
Lealman	G	55.0	55.3	54.2	59.9	70.5	78.7
Mad. Beach	H	69.2	61.3	69.6	14.3	73.5	71.2
Oldsmar	I	70.0	67.4	65.7	75.9	82.4	84.8
P. Park	J	39.3	45.1	42.5	41.7	55.8	65.1
Palm Harbor	K	27.7	32.8	38.1	52.1	65.2	65.1
S. Pasadena	L	55.1	68.8	52.4	68.8	77.3	73.8
Safety Hbr.	M	63.9	56.8	59.2	70.4	69.0	76.9
Seminole	N	44.0	53.1	47.9	60.6	65.4	65.9
St. Pete	O	47.1	57.3	58.5	72.8	77.7	81.1
St. Pete Bch.	P	41.2	40.7	38.9	52.7	66.7	59.1
Tarp. Sprgs.	Q	66.9	67.4	69.3	89.3	88.4	88.5
Treas. Is.	R	36.8	25.0	44.4	57.7	75.0	71.7
LifeFleet	S	—	—	—	—	—	—

FIGURE 30.19. *Statistical Process Control Chart (p chart) for EMS agency compliance with reporting of "At-Patient" times. (Courtesy Office of the Medical Director, Pinellas County EMS, Largo, FL)*

"on-scene/definitive care" was added in recognition of the unmeasured interval between the customary "response time," that is, the time between call reviewal and on-scene arrival, and the clinically important event, the delivery of the defibrillatory shock.

The cross-functional team developed and instituted a process to capture and integrate the measurement of "at patient" time (the time of first physical contact with the patient) and "first shock" time (the delivery of the first defibrillatory shock). The process was piloted by a single high-volume rescue unit and then instituted system wide.

The integration of this new process into the management of cardiac arrests was initially slow and problematic. The team reviewed causes of unreported and incomplete data. Process analyses or refinements and positive competitive reinforcement of performance were widely distributed to field personnel. Graphic representations of current performance and process goals, as well as improvements in cardiac arrest survival, were distributed and discussed at monthly CME seminars attended by all personnel (Figures 30.19 and 30.20).

In June of 1993 the system achieved a survival rate of 20% for cardiac arrests of cardiac etiology, a ten-fold increase in survival (fig. 30.22). This improvement is remarkable in that process goals for "at patient-first shock" intervals had not yet been achieved, that is, 90% reliability at the 1-minute interval and 100% reliability at the 2-minute interval.

Benchmarking

Benchmarking is the search for industry best practices. Industrial quality managers have used this method widely to compare their organizations to the best in class. Processes are selected for benchmarking and comparative companies are identified for study. These companies are often in other industries, but have demonstrated world-class practices. Package handling by Federal Express, for example, has been studied by many unrelated industries seeking to improve their own shipping processes.

Benchmarking has been used widely in healthcare CQI. The National Demonstration Project was an early example of collaboration between medical organizations and other industries to study key processes and learn. The Institute for Healthcare Quality has sponsored a number of Collaboratives focused on care processes.[36] Two among them have dealt with reducing waits and delays in the emergency department.

A taxonomy for benchmarking EMS operational performance was described by Stout in 1997.[37] He defines a broad group of key processes that may be measured by providers and used to compare performance across service types. Thus, private ambulance companies may compare their processes with those of public safety agencies or public utility models. He notes, "competitive value is the ultimate benchmark—a combination of quality and price that is at or near the best service attainable from any supplier for the money spent."

A fundamental tool for benchmarking clinical performance in EMS was described by the Utstein workgroup in 1991.[38] This document defined guidelines for uniform reporting of data from out-of-hospital cardiac arrest. For the first time a consensus of international clinical leadership enabled performance comparisons of EMS systems in this core area of ALS.

The Baldrige National Quality Award

In 1987 the U.S. Department of Commerce established the Baldrige National Quality Program through its National Institute of Standards and Technology.[39] The program describes a set of criteria enabling description and comparison of core values, concepts, and framework across organizations. Highly competitive prizes are awarded each year for best in class in the areas of manufacturing, service, small business, education, and health care. The program's greater value, however, has been in the fostering of organizational self-assessments—a national benchmarking standard to help companies improve performance practices, capabilities, and results. The program facilitates communication and sharing of best practices information among U.S. organizations of all types. The program is a working tool for understanding and managing performance and for guiding and planning opportunities for learning.

Many states and government agencies have adapted the program to enable quality competitions. At least one private EMS provider (Mercy—Las Vegas) has won its state quality award. The U.S. Fire Service and American Ambulance Association have used principles of the Baldrige criteria in their accreditation processes. The criteria form the core of a robust QM program at the EMS organizational level.

Quality to Value Management

Value is the relationship between quality and cost. Value management has become the "holy grail" of

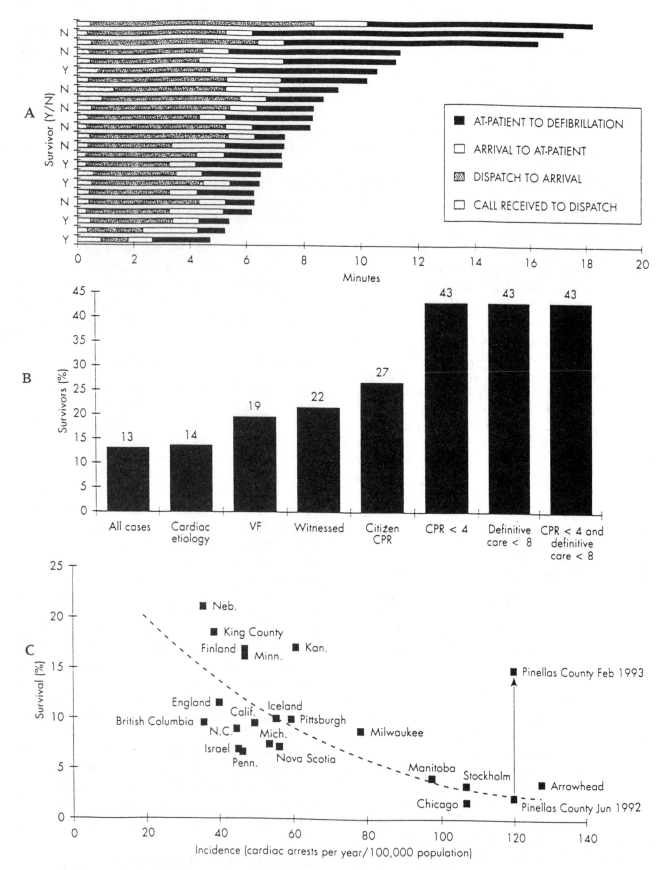

FIGURE 30.20. A, *Cardiac arrest response time intervals from call received to defibrillation (n-97).* **B**, *Cardiac arrest survival to discharge, Pinellas County EMS, Feb. 1993.* **C**, *Relationship of incidence and survival. (Modified from Becker L: Incidence of cardiac arrest: a neglected factor in evaluating survival skills. Ann Emerg Med 22:1, Jan 1993.)*

QUALITY MANAGEMENT

contemporary industrial QM philosophy. Value management theory holds that for industrial processes to yield value they must produce the highest quality at the least cost. Superlative quality is not competitive in the marketplace if it is not affordable to produce or buy.

$$V = Q/C$$

Healthcare quality theorists have recognized similar constraints. The HMO as a delivery model for care is the philosophical result of the pursuit of value in medicine. The still-predominant fee-for-service medical care system is one in which illness pays. Managed care is driven in principle by an economic model in which illness costs. The greatest value in managed care is theoretically achieved when the healthiest patient is created and maintained at the lowest cost. Evidence-based medicine seeks to define interventions that produce value, that is, measurable quality at affordable cost.

Defining value in health care is provocative.[40] Aside from the issues of health care as business, a fundamental conflict of interests exists between the clinician whose advocacy is the patient and the policymaker whose advocacy is the public health. The United States in the 21st century remains the only major nation without a national health policy. The prioritization of healthcare expenditures enacted by Oregon's voters—and dubbed "rationing" by its detractors—remains a controversial experiment.

The pursuit of value in health care has proven difficult. Execution of the managed care model has been, so far, flawed at best. The for-profit HMOs have repeatedly subrogated health status to shareholder value and short-term ROI (return on investment). The consolidation of the private sector has presented EMS with similar conflicts.

Emergency Medicine and EMS are foursquare in the middle of this debate. If the basic validity of the approach of QM to medicine, is accepted, a singular conclusion seems irresistible: the medical care system, focused on the treatment and mitigation of illness and injury, rather than the preservation of health, is fundamentally flawed in concept. As the "Humpty Dumpty repairmen" of health care, the system bears witness daily to the costs and limitations of putting the old egg back together again.

Whose interests are served, for example, by publicly funded basic science and clinical research in liver transplantation? The direct costs of a single liver transplant—whose beneficiary is an individual—approach $1M. What is the value, the "return on investment," of those funds when compared to the $1M in research, development, and distribution of hepatitis b vaccine to at-risk populations—only a few of whom could otherwise hope to be a recipient of a future transplant?

There is evidence that EMS is responding to the challenge. A growing body of work in EMS has looked at the questions of value.[40-45] Valenzuela and Spaite, in an excellent study, demonstrated the cost/benefit of resuscitation from sudden cardiac death.[46] EMS outcome studies have been divided, however, and are addressed elsewhere in this text. A disturbing group of studies has questioned the fundamentals: training, clinical interventions, provider skill levels, direct medical control, and system design.[47,48] Evidence-based EMS remains primitive but has been identified as a priority.[49]

A Public Health Perspective

The greatest opportunities to demonstrate future value in EMS are in the area of public health.[50-52] The role of an EMS medical director combines the clinical practice of medicine in the field with the management of a highly sophisticated organization responding to the emergency health needs of populations.

Emergency Medicine and the EMS system are considered to be the medical safety net of the community. Hospital and field practitioners are continually at the "scene of the crime" when the system fails. The capability for them to be intimate observers of the epidemiology of illness and injury is here; the problem is they don't do it.

Here is the potential. The EMS system provides what is perhaps the largest nascent laboratory that has ever been available to public health. It provides a platform to study, understand, and influence the health of communities for a broad spectrum of illness and injury.

EMS is the largest delegated practice of medicine. Importantly, paramedics and EMTs are afforded access to the community that is available to no one else. There is no other group in society that is able to walk into a stranger's home, unannounced and uninvited, and be welcomed. These field observers are capable of collecting data related to the cofactors of illness and injury, and are available in every community in the nation.[53,54] This challenge was recognized and addressed by the EMS agenda for the Future.[55] The principles of prevention and its role in improving community health have yet to be widely taught as a part of the core of EMS education.

Where to Start

A Leadership Guide to Quality Improvement for Emergency Medical Services Systems has been published by NHTSA.[56] This document was created by a national panel of experts representing the major stakeholders in EMS. The work uses the Baldrige Quality Program as a philosophical model for EMS organizations and is an excellent guide for governmental agencies and providers to use in creating QM plans.

The document addresses the seven key action areas contained in the Baldrige program with specific application to EMS issues (Figure 30.21).

This medical director has used a simple Quality Management Screen (QMS) as a starting point to identify key clinical performance strengths and weaknesses in several EMS systems. The tool is used by clinical supervisors to randomly sample EMS records from dispatch and the field for performance indicators in the areas of response time compliance, refusals of care, PCR completeness, protocol compliance, and outcome. The size and power of the sample may be adjusted to the workload of reviewers and the variation in the data. By counting the frequency of compliance and defects, the tool enables the organization to prioritize processes for improvement and measure the effects of change.

Compliance-to-protocol is a powerful performance indicator. The EMS clinical protocol is fundamentally a research protocol. In the laboratory, successful performance of the experimental process is prerequisite to relating the hypothesis to the conclusions. When the burette breaks, that particular trial must be excluded from the results. In like manner, a treatment protocol is the expert consensus of medical leadership translated into a scripted response to a clinical stimulus. The frequency of faithful execution of the experiment must be measured in order to conclude reasonably that improvements in clinical outcome are the result of care, and not due to chance or a better alternative provided, ad hoc, by thoughtful field personnel. The QMS provides a model for this analysis.

Becoming a Learning Organization

Deming's final admonition is to "take action to accomplish the transformation."[4] He views this as a never-ending quest to optimize the system that he called the "Shewhart Cycle" but has generally become known as the PDCA (plan-do-check-act) or Deming Cycle (Figure 30.23).[58]

The ultimate goal of this transformation is a fundamental change in the organizational culture. In *The Fifth Discipline*, Senge describes this as a *metanoia* or transcendence of mind; "becoming . . . learning organizations, organizations where people continually expand their capacity to create the results they truly desire, where new and expansive patterns of thinking are nurtured, where collective aspiration is set free, and where people are continually learning how to learn together."[58]

He notes that what will ultimately distinguish learning organizations from traditional authoritarian "controlling organizations" is the mastery of certain basic disciplines. Organizations that have mastered these disciplines are capable of producing robust quality in their processes of care (i.e., processes that are not only able to demonstrate benefit in the clinical laboratory but reliable quality in the street). "Quality is a virtue of design. The 'robustness' of products is more a function of good design than of on-line control, however stringent, of manufacturing processes."[59] The disciplines of the learning organization are personal mastery, mental models, shared vision, team learning, and systems thinking (the fifth

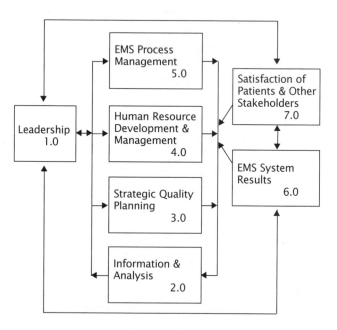

FIGURE 30.21. *The Seven Baldrige Categories From A Leadership Guide to Quality Improvement for Emergency Medical Services Systems, July 1997 (Courtesy NHTSA)*

QUALITY MANAGEMENT

discipline). This is what EMS is challenged to become.

Summary

Continuous Quality Improvement has been recognized broadly in medicine as the future of quality management. These concepts have been successfully applied in EMS systems for a number of years. Largely through the influence of Stout, there are a number of well established examples of CQI already up and running. EMS is challenged to transform itself and the mission of the organizations by letting go of "bad apples" approach and replacing it with principles of participative management that support the dignity and contribution of the providers.

For those in EMS, the true horizon lies beyond the foothills of quality management in the unexplored realms of ideas that may come to be called preventative emergency medicine.

On Beyond Zebra

Finally, while the processes of **health care** clearly resemble industrial processes and will benefit from efforts to understand their order and to control their variability, **health** ultimately may not. The homeostatic tether to existence resembles, not so well, Nature's systems of order, but rather, the dynamical systems of sensitive dependence on initial conditions . . . the systems of chaos.[60]

So now I know everything *anyone* knows
From beginning to end. From the start to the close.
Because Z is as far as the alphabet goes.

Then he almost fell flat on his face on the floor
When I picked up the chalk and drew one letter more!
A letter he never had dreamed of before!
And I said, *You* can stop, if you want, with the Z
Because most people stop with the Z
But not me!

In the places I go there are things that I see
That I *never* could spell if I stopped with the Z.
I'm telling you this 'cause you're one of my friends.
My alphabet starts where *your* alphabet ends!

On Beyond Zebra! Dr. Seuss

References

1. Donabedian A. *Explorations in Quality Assessment and Monitoring.* Vols 1,2,3, Health Administration Press; 1980 (vol 1), 1982 (vol 2), 1985 (vol 3).
2. Berwick DM. Continuous improvement as an ideal in health care. *NEJM.* 1989;320:53–56.
3. Garvin D. A note on quality: the views of Deming, Juran, and Crosby. *Harvard Business Review.* 1986;9-687-011:1–13.
4. Deming WE. Principles for transformation: 24–92. In: *Out of the Crisis.* Boston: Massachusetts Institute of

1. **Plan**—What would be the most important accomplishments of this team? What changes might be desirable? What data are available? Are new observations needed? If yes, plan a change or test. Decide how to use the observations.

2. **Do**—Carry out the change or test decided on, preferably on a small scale.

3. **Check/study**—Observe the effects of the change or test.

4. **Act**—Study the results. What did we learn? What can we predict?

5. Repeat step 1 with knowledge accumulated.

6. Repeat step 2 and onward.

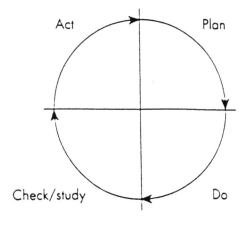

FIGURE 30.23. *The Shewhart Cycle. (From Deming, WE, Out of the Crisis, Cambridge, MA, 1986, MIT Center for Advanced Engineering Study.)*

Technology, Center for Advanced Engineering Study; 1986.

5. Walton M. *The Deming Management Method*. Perigee Books; 1986:40–51.

6. Berwick DM, et al. *Curing Health Care—New Strategies for Quality Improvement*. Jossey-Bass; 1991:xvi.

7. Stout JL. Measuring your system. *J Emerg Med Serv.* 1983;8(1):84–91.

8. Stout JL. How much is too much? *J Emerg Med Serv.* 1984;9(2):26–33.

9. Stout JL. System status management. *J Emerg Med Serv.* 1983;8(1):22–23.

10. Stout JL. Ambulance system designs. *J Emerg Med Serv.* 1986;11(1):85–89.

11. Stout JL. Wrestling with the big three policy issues. *J Emerg Med Serv.* 1989;13(6):79–81.

12. The Advanced SSM Workshops, The Fourth Party, Inc., 760 Crandell Rd., West River, MD 20778, (301) 261–9492.

13. Davidson SJ. Authority and Empowerment *in* The National EMS Medical Directors Course and Practicum, *emsAC* Foundation, 1989:9. (800) 637–0361

14. Berwick DM, et al. Curing Health Care—New Strategies for Quality Improvement. Jossey-Bass; 1991:151.

15. Donabedian A. Definitions of Quality and Approaches to its Assessment. Health Administration Press; 1980.

16. Personal communications with Overton, J; Authority Director, Metropolitan Ambulance Services Trust, 1982.

17. Scholtes PR. The Team Handbook. Joiner Associates Inc.; 1988:2–8. (800) 669–8326

18. Stout JL. System Design *in* The National EMS Medical Directors Course and Practicum, *emsAC* Foundation, 1989:2. (800) 637–0361

19. Ishikawa K. *What is Total Quality Control? The Japanese Way*. Prentice Hall Inc.; 1985

20. Juran JM. *Planning for Quality*. Juran Institute Inc. The Free Press, 1989:86–87.

21. Juran JM. *Leadership for Quality*. Juran Institute Inc. The Free Press, 1989:89–90.

22. Ishikawa K. The essence of quality control. In: *What is Total Quality Control? The Japanese Way*. Prentice Hall Inc.; 1985:46–49.

23. Eisenberg MS, Bergner L, Hallstrom AP. *Sudden Cardiac Death in the Community*. Praeger; 1984:55.

24. Ryan JL, Overton J. An Anticipatory Ambulance Deployment Strategy for A Large Urban EMS System (Abstract). University Association for Emergency Medicine, 1985.

25. Deming WE. *Out of the Crisis*. Boston: Massachusetts Institute of Technology, Center for Advanced Engineering Study; 1986:321.

26. Personal communications with Lifefleet Southeast, Mercy Las Vegas, Hartson/Medtrans San Diego, Medical Priority Consultants Salt Lake City, 1992.

27. Juran JM. *Juran on Leadership for Quality*. The Free Press; 1989:145.

28. Spaite DW, et al. Prospective evaluation of prehospital patient assessment by direct in-field observation: failure of ALS personnel to measure vital signs. *Prehosp Disaster Med.* 1990;5(4):383–388.

29. Proceedings of the Methodology in Cardiac Arrest Research Symposium, *Ann Emerg Med.* 1993;22:1.

30. Clawson J. *Pro QA (a Computer based Emergency Medical Dispatching System)*. Salt Lake City, UT: Medical Priority Consultants. 1998.

31. Davidson SJ. Closing the loop: discard the bad apples or continuously improve EMS? In: Swor RA. *Quality Management in Prehospital Care*, Mosby LifeLine; 1993:55–69.

32. Imai M. Improvement East and West. In: Kaizen. *The Key to Japan's Competitive Success*. New York: McGraw Hill; 1986:23–41.

33. Scholtes PR. *The Team Handbook: How to Use Teams to Improve Quality*. Joiner Associates Inc.; 1988.

34. Eastham JN. Assuring quality from the ground up. *J Emerg Med Serv.* 1991;16(5):48–59.

35. Juran JM. *Juran's Quality Control Handbook*. 4th ed. New York: McGraw Hill; 1988.

36. Institute for Healthcare Improvement, Boston, MA. http://www.ihi.org

37. Stout JK. Capture the Competitive Edge. *JEMS.* 1996;22(9):51–55.

38. Cummins RO, Chamberlain DA, et al. Recommended guidelines for uniform reporting of data from out-of-hospital cardiac arrest: the Utstein style. *Ann Emerg Med.* 1991;83:1832–1847.

39. Baldrige National Quality Program 2001. Criteria for Performance Excellence. http://www.quality.nist.gov

40. Doubilet P, Weinstein MC. Use and misuse of the term "cost effective" in medicine. *N Engl J Med.* 1986;314:253–256.

41. Garrison HG, Downs SM, et al. A cost effectiveness analysis of pediatric intraosseous infusion as a prehospital skill. *Prehosp Disaster Med.* 1992;7:221–226.

42. Valenzuela TD, Spaite DW, et al. Estimated cost-effectiveness of dispatcher CPR instruction via telephone to bystanders during out-of-hospital ventricular fibrillation. *Prehosp Disaster Med.* 1992;7:229–234.

43. Urban N, Bergner L, Eisenberg MS. The costs of the suburban paramedic program in reducing deaths due to cardiac arrest. *MedCare.* 1981;19:279–392.

44. Gough JE, Brown LH, et al. A comparison of outcomes research in emergency medicine and EMS. *Prehosp Emerg Care.* 1997;1:(4):292.

45. Macnab AJ, Wensley DF. Cost-benefit of trained transport teams: estimates for head-injured children. *Prehosp Emerg Care.* 2001;5:1–5.

46. Valenzuela TD, Spaite DW, et al. Cost effectiveness analysis of paramedic emergency medical services in the treatment of prehospital cardiopulmonary arrest. *Ann Emerg Med.* 1990;19:1407–1411.

47. Werman HA, Keseg DR, Glimcher M. Retention of basic life support skills. *Preshosp Disaster Med.* 1990;137–144.

48. Wuerz RC, Swope GE, et al. Online medical direction: a prospective study. *Preshosp Disaster Med.* 1995;10:174–177.

49. Judge T. A mosaic in transition: contemporary EMS in the United States: part 2. *Pre-hospital Immediate Care.* 1998;2:77–82.

50. Garrison HG, Foltin G, et al. Consensus Statement: The Role of Out-of-Hospital Emergency Medical Services in Primary Injury Prevention. Consensus Workshop on the Role of EMS in Injury Prevention. Arlington, VA, August 25–26, 1995. Final report.

51. Ogden JR, Criss EA, et al. The impact of an EMS-initiated, community-based drowning prevention coalition on submersion deaths in a southwestern metropolitan area. *Acad Emerg Med*. 1994;1(2):304.

52. Harrawood D, Gunderson MR, et al. Drowning prevention: a case study in EMS epidemiology. *JEMS*. 1994;19(6):34–41.

53. Hsaio AK, Hedges JR. Role of the emergency medical services system in region wide health monitoring and referral. *Ann Emerg Med*. 1993;22:1696–1702.

54. Krumperman KM. Filling the gap: EMS social service referrals. *JEMS*. 1993;18(2):25–29.

55. National Highway Traffic Safety Administration. *EMSAgenda for the Future*. DOT HS 808 411, Washington, DC, August 1996.

56. National Highway Traffic Safety Administration. *A Leadership Guide to Quality Improvement for Emergency Medical Services (EMS) Systems*. July 1997. Washington, DC. http://www.nhtsa.dot.gov/people/injury/ems/leaderguide

57. Shewhart WA. *Statistical Method from the Viewpoint of Quality Control*. Originally published 1939; reprinted Dover Publications; 1986.

58. Senge PM. *The Fifth Discipline: The Art and Practice of the Learning Organization*. New York: Doubleday Currency; 1990.

59. Taguchi G, Clausing D. *Robust quality*. Harvard Business Review. 1990; pp. 65–66.

60. Gleick J. *Chaos: Making A New Science*. Penguin Books; 1987.

Bibliography

Camp RC. Benchmarking The Search for Industry Best Practices that Lead to Superior Performance

Couch JB, ed. Health Care Quality Management for the 21st Century. Tampa, FL: American College of Physician Executives, 1991.

deBono E. *deBono's Thinking Course*. New York: Facts on File Publications; 1982.

deBono E. *The Mechanism of Mind*. New York: Penguin Books; 1969.

deBono E. *Sur/Petition: Creating Value Monopolies When Everyone Else is Merely Competing*. New York: Harper Business; 1992.

Eastes L, Jacobsen J, eds. *Quality Assurance in Air Medical Transport: The Association of Air Medical Transport*. Orem, UT: WordPerfect Publishing Co.; 1990.

Geisel TS (Dr. Seuss). *On Beyond Zebra!*. New York: Random House; 1955.

George S. *The Baldrige Quality System*. New York: John Wiley & Sons; 1992.

Goonan KJ. *The Juran Prescription*. New York: Jossey-Bass; 1995.

The Institute for Healthcare Improvement, Boston, Mass., www.ihi.org

Juran JM, Godfrey AB. *Juran's Quality Handbook*. 5th ed. New York: McGraw-Hill; 1999.

Juran JM. *Juran on Quality by Design*. New York: The Free Press; 1992.

The National Highway Traffic Safety Administration. Washington, DC, http://www.nhtsa.dot.gov

The Juran Institute, Wilton, Conn. http://www.juran.com

The National Institute of Standards and Technology: The Malcom Baldrige National Quality Award. http://www.quality.nist.gov

Ohmae K. *The Mind of the Strategist: The Art of Japanese Business*. New York: McGraw-Hill; 1982.

Osborne D, Gaebler T. *Reinventing Government: How the Entrepreneurial Spirit is Transforming the Public Sector*. New York: Penguin Books; 1992.

Pirsig RM. *Zen and The Art of Motorcycle Maintenance: An Inquiry into Values*. New York: Quill, William Morrow; 1974.

Polsky S, ed. *Continuous Quality Improvement in EMS*. Dallas, TX: American College of Emergency Physicians; 1992.

Swor RA, ed. *Quality Management in Prehospital Care*. National Association of EMS Physicians. St. Louis, MO: Mosby LifeLine; 1993.

Tenner A, DeToro I. *Total Quality Management: Three Steps to Continuous Improvement*. Reading, MA: Addison-Wesley Publishing Co.; 1992.

CHAPTER 31

Risk Management

Michael P. Wainscott, MD
David L. Morgan, MD

Introduction

In the practice of prehospital medicine the goal is to provide the best possible patient care. Many factors impact EMS patient care including primary training, medical supervision, and continuing education. Quality management (QM) is used to evaluate and improve patient care provided in an EMS system.

Prehospital risk management also enhances patient care and at times overlaps with QM. The term "risk management" traditionally implies that an adverse event has occurred and that actions are needed to mitigate damages to the patient, personnel, or institution.[1] Risk management in most EMS systems is a loosely defined mechanism for resolving patient care incidents, but it is important for this traditional view to be altered. Risk management includes not only a defined mechanism for managing patient care incidents, but in a broader sense, addresses multiple areas that facilitate improved patient care.

Prehospital risk management is a comprehensive mechanism for the identification, resolution, and disposition of medically related EMS incidents (adverse patient occurrences) including reporting, documenting, prioritizing, investigating, resolving, and defining disposition of those reported occurrences. It also includes the proactive assessment of other factors that affect patient care, including primary training, preemployment screening, medical supervision, continuing medical education, documentation, and patient expectations. These areas are the major focus of this chapter.

Components of Prehospital Risk Management

Many factors influence patient care. A comprehensive prehospital risk management program should take the following components into account:

Primary Training

Primary training of prehospital personnel has great impact on patient care. A solid foundation of knowledge, skills, and attitudes is necessary for EMS personnel to function effectively and provide consistent quality patient care.[2] An awareness of the quality of primary training institutions and used to educate EMS personnel is important. Factors such as curriculum, teaching techniques, methods of evaluation, and clinical training have important roles in the student's preparation for a role providing prehospital care. This knowledge is the responsibility of the EMS medical director, but EMS administrators should also be aware of this background. If the course medical director and the EMS medical director are different people, then communication between them is essential. EMS systems primary training is provided as part of the individual's employment, and this facilitates involvement of the system's medical director in the training process.

Preemployment Screening and Orientation

If a potential EMS field employee received primary training outside the EMS system, it is important for this individual to be assessed in terms of medical knowledge and patient care skills before being released to function independently in the field. As a prehiring assessment, many systems use a written examination that may include tests of basic knowledge such as reading and math. Other assessments that are used include EMS knowledge-based written and skills testing, physical ability testing, interviews, and psychological screening. Most systems have standard administrative procedures, such as background checks.[2]

New employees should receive a field orientation and evaluation before functioning as patient care providers. Orientation is provided in administration, operations, and medical areas, including protocols and field performance standards.

Medical Supervision

Assurance of quality prehospital health care is provided through the process of medical accountability.[3] The medical supervision of prehospital care is discussed extensively throughout this book. The vital role of the medical director in defining patient care standards, establishing protocols, approving the level of prehospital medical care that may be rendered by all individuals in the system, and impacting positively all the operational aspects that affect patient care cannot be overemphasized. In addition, the medical director should be directly involved in the risk management program.

Continuing Medical Education

Continuing medical education serves multiple purposes in an EMS system, including updating personnel on protocol changes, providing reviews, presenting medical information and technology, and evaluating knowledge and skills of field personnel. A number of studies have demonstrated deterioration of knowledge and skills in EMS providers. In 1980 Latman and Wooley demonstrated that Emergency Medical Technician-As (EMT-A) lost 50% of basic skills proficiency, and paramedics lost 61% of basic skills proficiency within two years of training.[4] In 1987 Skelton and McSwain reported a correlation between the amount of technical skill deterioration and increasing length of time from completion of the training program.[5] One role of continuing medical education is to evaluate and enhance knowledge and skills of field personnel.

Other roles of continuing education include updates on protocol changes, run reviews, and new medical information and technology. It also serves as a forum for EMS personnel to provide feedback regarding patient care. In 1990 Goldberg published a review of litigation in a large metropolitan EMS system and suggested that medicolegal continuing education could protect EMS systems and paramedics from future litigation.[6]

Documentation

The Joint Commission on Accreditation of Healthcare Organizations (JCAHO) requires that a medical record is established and maintained on every patient seeking emergency department care.[7] The JCAHO mandates certain elements be included in the record; other elements may be added to conform with state regulations and hospital requirements. In comparing this with the prehospital arena, it is apparent that documentation requirements for EMS patient records vary widely. Patient records are required for all transported patients, yet specific elements of the record are far from universal. A number of states have a standardized EMS patient record, but use of such a prehospital care report (PCR) may not be required.

Many systems maintain limited or no patient documentation if a patient is not transported. In 1992 Zachariah reported serious, even fatal, outcomes in patients not transported by EMS. Situations in which EMS personnel either denied transport (or mutually agreed with the patient not to transport by ambulance) were twice as likely to result in hospitalization than cases in which the patients declined transportation against the advice of the EMS personnel.[6] In 1990 Selden studied medicolegal documentation of prehospital triage and suggested that, rather than an abbreviated form or small section of the usual PCR, the release form (when a patient is not transported) must be at least as detailed as the usual incident report.[8]

In 1985 Solar reported on the 10-year malpractice experience of a large urban EMS system and stated that a properly completed PCR is the best defense against a malpractice allegation.[9]

Other important areas of documentation include the new employee's application, preemployment screening, and field orientation. Some systems document the new employee's knowledge of protocols. Written protocols governing prehospital care should be available to EMS personnel. Some states require the presence of protocols on ambulances. All aspects of patient care incident management should also be documented.

Quality Management

Quality management (QM) of the patient care rendered in an EMS system may identify actual or potential risks to patients and the system. This identification allows for the proactive management of such risks, and takes the EMS system out of the reactive mode of dealing with problems in patient care. The QM loop forms a continuous action loop, starting and ending with protocols and education. Documentation of variance from or compliance with protocols forms the basis for analysis of the quality of care delivered.[10] QM and risk management are closely linked.

Other Factors

Other incidents may occur in an EMS system that have potential impact on patients. If an ambulance is involved in an accident, the patient may receive injuries directly or have increased morbidity from a delay in transport. In 1992 Bowers reported on 182 session of alleged negligence involving prehospital care providers; 40% of the cases involved ambulance accidents (although some of these cases involved several identified categories of negligence).[11] This is compared with 42% of the cases that were related to negligence involving treatment or care. A provider who is injured while extricating a patient may no longer be able to provide patient care at the scene, potentially affecting patient care. Equipment malfunctions such as defibrillator failure may have direct bearing on morbidity and mortality for a patient. Steps should be taken to identify and address potentially preventable occurrences, such as special driver training programs and regular equipment checks.

Patient Expectations

The concept of patient expectations concludes the components of prehospital risk management. Locales, socioeconomic status, cultural influences, and many other factors play a role in a patient's expectations of the EMS system. It is important that patient expectations are taken into consideration. As a group, patients come to the healthcare system with basically realistic expectations. They expect that the healing professionals will treat them with dignity and regard their welfare as a principal concern.[12] When the expectation of the patient is different from that of the EMS crew, conflict may arise. Discussions with EMS personnel regarding potential patient expectations and responses to possible conflicts may have significant positive consequences for an EMS system.

In a study of 17,271 emergency department (ED) patients the first and third factors that patients perceive as reflecting quality care are physician courtesy and nurse courtesy. The other factors cited follow in order of importance: comfort of waiting area, satisfactory answers to patient questions, protection of privacy, acceptable waiting time for treatment, cleanliness of treatment area, and satisfaction with pain control.[10] Extrapolation of these findings to the prehospital area is logical.

In healthcare, patient satisfaction remains the major product. When expectations are not met, patients feel they are not getting their "money's worth." Anger can be expressed in many ways in this culture, and filing a lawsuit is one of them.[11]

Patient Care Incident Management

As a clearly recognized component of the healthcare system, EMS personnel are affected by the trend of increasing litigation. Over the 12-year period of Goldberg's review (1976 to 1987), claims made against the Chicago Fire Department EMS increased threefold.[5] Of the 60 lawsuits presented, 47% named a paramedic as a defendant and 3% named the medical director. As the direct medical oversight physician is increasingly recognized as a fundamental component of quality prehospital care, correlative potential liability will necessarily follow.[6] It is likely that oversight physicians will be named more often in lawsuits as time progresses.

In 1992 Bowers reported on the major categories of alleged negligence in 182 cases involving prehospital care services or providers (table 31.1). The category of "treatment and care" represented about 43% of the cases.[12] Goldberg reported 77% of the cases in his study involved alleged improper medical treatment.[6] It is important that the physician responsible for medical oversight grasps the full import of this information and responds by using an effective risk management system.

TABLE 31.1
Major Categories of Alleged Negligence Involving Prehospital Care Services or Providers

CATEGORY*	NO.	%=
Treatment and care	78	42.85
Ambulance accidents	73	40.10
Dispatch and transport	50	27.47
Training, staffing and administrative	41	2.52

From: Bowers MA: Negligence cases involving prehospital care providers and the implications for training, continuing education, and quality assurance, doctoral thesis, Ann Arbor, Mich, 1992, University Microfilm International.[11]

*In some cases, more than one category was identified and used in this table.

=Percent based on entire 182 cases.

Patient Care Incident

A patient care incident or occurrence is any situation where there is a concern or complaint regarding patient care. This concern or complaint may be related to the commission or omission of actions on the part of EMS personnel, bystanders, other prehospital personnel, physicians providing direct medical control, or others. These actions either affected or potentially affected patient-care and outcome of the situation.

At times, extenuating circumstances such as prolonged scene time may impact patient care, but could not have been prevented. Equipment failures, scene injuries to crew members, or accidents involving ambulances may impact patient care. The documentation and consideration of such problems are part of patient-care incident management.

Establishing a Comprehensive Mechanism

Establishing a comprehensive mechanism for managing patient-care incidents is an important aspect of a risk management program. This mechanism includes incident identification, incident investigation, investigation findings, indicated actions, documentation, and system impact. It is important that all are oriented to this mechanism, including field employees, supervisors, and senior level management.

Incident Identification

Incident identification occurs when a patient or other source expresses a verbal or written concern regarding EMS patient care. It also may result from an identified equipment failure or a crew's assessment of a difficult patient encounter such as a prolonged extrication.

Quality management studies and reviews may show areas that need improvement, such as success rate for initiation of IVs. The risk management program itself may identify trends in patient care incidents that indicate necessary systemwide intervention. It is important that a mechanism be in place to identify, document, receive information, and initiate the process for handling a patient-care incident.

Serious or Critical Patient-Care Incidents

Serious or critical patient-care incidents are occurrences that involve significant injury to a patient or impact negatively on patient care, morbidity, or mortality; they should be reported immediately. Usually the system has a chain of command for reporting incidents, and it is vital that this chain includes contacting the medical director.

Incident Investigation

Incident investigation is a uniformly applied, prearranged mechanism for investigating a patient-care incident. It includes a chain of command that identifies roles for all the players in the system and provides a routing mechanism for information and documentation obtained in the investigation. An investigation worksheet is a useful tool for the personnel investigating a patient-care incident. This worksheet contributes consistency to investigations and also serves as a reminder for necessary actions to be taken and items to be obtained. A list of critical checklist ingredients is shown in Table 31.2.

The personnel responsible for carrying out the investigation should be educated in this aspect of their work. These investigators should respond in a timely manner to patients or other sources expressing negative comments or concerns about patient care. Many complaints may be resolved quickly with the education of the person who calls or writes about some aspect of prehospital medical care. For example, a physician may be concerned because his patient was not brought to the appropriate hospital. Yet, when the EMS supervisor explains that the patient became critical, and it is the policy of the system to transport critical patients to the closest hospital, the physician gains a better understanding of the process, and the problem may be resolved. However, the supervisor should always document the incident.

Some EMS systems require receipt of a formal written complaint before initiating an investigation. This is short-sighted, and it profoundly limits the scope of risk management. Some systems have less formal requirements for when an investigation may be initiated; however, immediate documentation of all complaints and discussions is important.

EMS crew members involved in an incident should have the opportunity to respond verbally and in writing to a concern that is being investigated. These written incident reports serve as information sources and are a routine part of the investigation. Other individuals may be asked to make oral or written statements regarding the events surrounding an incident. For example, the ED physician who finds an endotracheal tube placed in the esophagus and notifies the EMS system should be interviewed by the investigator. Documentation of the interview is mandatory.

Any other information, tape transcripts, PCRs, and equipment pertinent to the investigation should be collected. These materials are then collated with the incident reports and other documentation to formulate the summary of the investigation. EMS administration and the medical director should evaluate this information through a formal process and make a disposition of the incident. Further discussions, interviews, or investigations may be necessary.

Patient privacy must be respected, and the PCR should be treated as a physician record. This is a logical extension of the premise that providers function under the delegated authority of the physician medical director. States such as Texas protect PCRs in the same fashion as hospital medical records. Any unnecessary written or verbal reference to an incident report or its contents lessens the confidentiality of the report, contributes to potential negative repercussions, and minimizes the resultant value of its completion.[13]

In most states the limits on discoverability of hospital incident reports are much better defined than for EMS incident reports. In general, prepare only a few copies of the report and define clearly who receives them. It may help to clearly mark on each incident report that it is being prepared for possible use by legal counsel. Because there may be multiple regulations and statutes involved, such as those protecting peer-review material, it helps to design the incident report and the risk management program with consultation from all appropriate medical, administrative, and legal entities.

All aspects of the investigation should be fair and involve due process for the employee, including the employee's prospective understanding of how the risk management program functions and how investigations are conducted. Some systems have review panels that include field personnel. EMS medical directors are the key individuals in the resolution of a patient-care incident; therefore, they should be made aware of the initiation of an investigation for minor incidents and be actively involved for more serious or critical incidents. Medical directors must have final authority on the evaluation of the clinical aspects of the incident.

Investigation Findings

Investigation findings are the conclusions from the investigation of a patient-care incident. Results of the investigation may show that the incident was related to safety factors, environmental influences, training, employee clinical performance, judgment error, equipment failure, product deficiency, vehicle operation, incomplete documentation, patient expectations, protocol problems, employee behavior, actions of other personnel, or medical control. These may be presented and indicated in the checklist (Table 31.2). The medical director must play an active role in evaluating investigation findings to determine appropriateness and accuracy.

Potential Investigation Findings

Results of the investigation may show that the incident was related to:

- Environmental influences
- Safety factors
- Training
- Employee clinical performance
- Employee behavior
- Judgment error
- Equipment deficiency or failure
- Incomplete documentation
- Patient expectations

TABLE 31.2

Incident Investigation Checklist

- Discussions with involved EMS crew members
  Name/date:
  Name/date:
- Documentation of discussions with EMS crew members
- Discussions with other personnel (patient, physician, etc.)
  Name/date:
  Name/date:
  Name/date:
- Documentation of discussion with other personnel
- Crew member incident reports
- Patient-care record (delete name and assign number)
- Other appropriate documentation
  Photographs
  Tape transcripts
  Direct medical oversight records
- Equipment or products causal to the incident

- Protocol or policy problems
- Actions of other personnel
- Direct medical oversight

Indicated Actions

Indicated actions depend on a number of factors, including seriousness of the incident from an administrative, medical, or media standpoint, system response to previous similar incidents or similar types of incidents, and the employee's long-term performance and disciplinary history. Indicated actions are administrative or medical. There is overlap at times, and communication between the administration and the medical director is essential.

Administrative actions usually fall into the generic classification of employee personnel actions. Medical actions generally fall into the categories of no action, policy or protocol revisions, product changes, remedial education, and corrective measures such as decertification. Remedial education actions include classroom education, clinical hospital education, testing, and supervised field preceptorship. Actions of an educational nature may also include systemwide training or retraining through continuing medical education. Potential corrective measures include counseling, probation, and decertification. The physician charged with medical oversight by contract has final authority on medical actions in response to patient-care incidents.

Generally, for an initial employee performance problem the employee receives some type of counseling and retraining that is specific to their needs. This process should be viewed as education-based rather than discipline-based, unless there are circumstances for which disciplinary measures are truly indicated. Even in the latter case the educational aspects must still play a vital role and represent a positive system response to a problem.

Documentation

Documentation of the investigation and resolution of patient-care incidents cannot be overemphasized; it facilitates a more complete and consistent understanding of the investigation and ensures fairness and due process. Decisions regarding documents to be used and to whom information may be disseminated should be defined by the risk management program.

Future Directions— Prehospital Medical Error

Medical error is a topic of an increasing body of literature and of increasing public awareness. In 1999, the National Institute of Medicine reported that medical errors kill from 44,000 to 98,000 Americans each year. For example, medication prescribing/dispensing errors kill an estimated 7,000 patients per year. Yet little literature exists on medical error in the prehospital setting.[14]

Medical error is what risk management programs seek to manage, and more importantly, to prevent. It is more than responding to errors or potential errors. It includes a response to studies that objectively evaluate or refine techniques used to treat patients. It includes a response to studies that seek to reduce error in patient care.[15]

In a study of CPR techniques using manikins, a high rate of error was noted for emergency healthcare providers (emergency medical technicians, firemen, emergency first responders, CPR instructors).[16] Though the application of this to the patient-care setting has limitations, it is a standardized technique that was monitored for adherence and found to have significant error rates. Recommendations were made to modify training programs. In a recent study of pediatric intubation, Gausche found that the addition of out-of-hospital endotracheal intubation to a paramedic scope of practice that already includes bag valve mask did not improve survival or neurological outcome of pediatric patients treated in an urban EMS system.[17] This study was done because of the difficulty associated with intubation of small children and because of intubation error, including unrecognized esophageal intubation. An EMS system risk management program should include a review of these types of studies. Changes to a particular EMS system may or may not be needed as a result, but the system should be aware of the studies.

One effective tool used by multiple industries to reduce error is already in place in EMS systems standardization. Examples of standardization in EMS systems include: protocols that guide patient care, consistency in the type and location of equipment used by EMS personnel, operational protocols that guide scene management, and dispatch protocols. And because of the "system" nature of EMS, prehospital care providers are in a unique position of being able to implement system-wide changes.

Leape stated that total quality management also requires a culture in which errors and deviations are regarded not as human failures, but as opportunities to improve the system.[14] The psychology and culture of hospital and prehospital providers will need to change if progress is to be made in reducing errors.

Summary

One major goal for the risk management program is to provide effective patient-care incident management so the incident becomes part of the overall QM program, and so it does not simply become an isolated circumstance with no system impact. Trends and patterns must be observed and interventions taken as necessary.

The goals for an EMS risk management program extend far beyond reactive management of patient-care incidents. A good program allows for the prospective management and evaluation of all the medical care provided in an EMS system; it considers factors and influences that may negatively impact patient care even before a patient care incident occurs. The program affects protocols, continuing education, training, pre-employment screening, medical oversight, and administration.

Change is facilitated through the identification of problems reactively and proactively; all personnel involved in the EMS system become part of the solution. The ultimate benefactors are the patients in the EMS system; their medical care improves through the changes and growth that result from the program.

In 1989 Valenzuela reported that less than 65% of emergency medicine residency training programs provided formal instruction in EMS risk management.[18] Both present and future EMS medical directors must become active, knowledgeable participants in prehospital risk management.

References

1. Krentz MJ, Wainscott MP. Medical accountability. *Emery Med Clin North Am.* 1990;8:17–31.
2. Cason D, Wainscott MP. Training and evaluation. In: Polsky SS. Continuous quality improvement in EMS. American College of Emergency Physicians; 1992.
3. Polsky SS, Weigand JV. Quality assurance in emergency medical service systems. *Emerg Med Clin North Am.* 1990;8:75–84.
4. Latman NS, Wooley K. Knowledge and skill retention of emergency care attendants, EMT-As, and EMT-Ps. *Ann Emerg Med.* 1980;9:183–189.
5. Skelton MB, McSwain NE. A study of cognitive and technical skill deterioration among trained paramedics. *JACEP.* 1977;6:436–438.
6. Goldberg RJ, Zautcke JL, Koenigsberg MD. A review of prehospital care litigation in a large metropolitan EMS system. *Ann Emerg Med.* 1990;19:557–561.
7. *National Emergency Room Survey: Quality of care monitor.* Park Ridge, IL: Parkside Associates; 1991.
8. Selden BS. Medicolegal documentation of prehospital triage. *Ann Emerg Med.* 1990;19:547–551.
9. Solar JM, et al. The 10-year malpractice experience of a large suburban EMS system. *Ann Emerg Med.* 1985;14:982–985.
10. Bukata WR. Emergency department medical record. In: Henry GL, ed.: *Emergency Medicine Risk Management: A Comprehensive Review.* American College of Emergency Physicians; 1991.
11. Henry GL. Patient expectations. In: Henry GL, ed. *Emergency Medicine Risk Management: A Comprehensive Review.* American College of Emergency Physicians; 1991.
12. Bowers MA. *Negligence Cases Involving Prehospital Care Providers and the Implications for Training, Continuing Education, and Quality Assurance.* Doctoral Thesis. Ann Arbor, MI: University Microfilms International; 1992.
13. Shanaberger CJ. Legal issues in medical control. In: Kuehl A, ed. *EMS Medical Director's Handbook.* St. Louis: The CV Mosby Co.; 1989.
14. Leape LL. Error in medicine. *JAMA.* 1994;272(23):1851–1857.
15. Corrigan J, Kohn LT, Donaldson MS, eds. *To Err is Human. Building a Safer Health System.* Washington, DC: National Academy Press; 2000.
16. Lieberman M, Lavoie A, Mulder D, et al. Cardiopulmonary resuscitation: errors made by prehospital emergency personnel. *Resuscitation.* 1999;42:47–55.
17. Gausche M, Lewis RJ, et al. Effect of out-of-hospital pediatric endotracheal intubation on survival and neurological outcome: a controlled clinical trial. *JAMA.* 2000;283(6):783–790.
18. Valenzuela TD, et al. Evaluation of EMS management training offered during emergency medicine residency training. *Ann Emerg Med.* 1989;18:812–814.

Legal Issues

Carol J. Shanaberger, EMT-P, JD
Spencer A. Hall, MD, JD

Introduction

Medical oversight in prehospital care is distinctly different from any other supervisory activity performed by a physician. Although it is acknowledged as an integral element of an EMS system, medical oversight has been a bit of a mystery to the law, the public, and the medical community.[1] Despite their immense responsibilities in providing medical control, medical directors were rarely defendants in litigation during the first 30 years of EMS. Although weakening, this trend continues.

There have been obvious improvements in the sophistication of EMS systems since the early days of "invalid coaches" staffed by "ambulance drivers," and a continued appreciation for "the speed with which the ambulances reach the sick and injured, bringing help that literally wrest the sufferer from the jaws of death, as the last flickering spark of life is leaving the body."[2] However, prehospital medical care is often misunderstood, and consequently the role of the medical director is often not understood by lawyers, citizens, bureaucrats, and even some physicians. As recently as 1989 an appellate court judge referred to an ambulance as a "medical taxicab" rather than a mobile intensive care unit.[3]

Ignorance and misperceptions affect medical directors. They face confusion, misconceptions and uncertainty in the day-to-day events of medical direction and in the legal crises that may erupt from those duties. The medical profession has had decades to develop standards and predictability in legal rulings involving medical malpractice. However, only recently has a patchwork of legal decisions involving EMS activities solidified sufficiently to provide some predictability. In a few states, trends are evolving about liability issues that help define responsibilities of systems or prehospital providers and interpret immunity statutes governing prehospital care. Medical directors may benefit from the few legal precedents established by other participants in this unique and developing area of medical care. However, any medical director, whether a novice or an expert, must keep in mind that there are many unresolved issues surrounding medical direction.

In most states, the birth of EMS, with its "call to arms" by countless physicians, paraprofessionals, and citizens, preceded the enactment of enabling legislation authorizing this unique delivery of medical care.[4] When federal highway grant funds were offered, every state eventually enacted EMS legislation to qualify; however, intense physician supervision was not necessarily mandated in these early statutes, many of which remain in effect more than three decades later.[5]

During the development of EMS systems, immunity from liability for the rescuer gradually became a focus of many state legislatures. It was assumed that immunity was a prerequisite for volunteer, that is, uncompensated, provider involvement in emergency response, although there was, and still is, no good evidence to substantiate this proposition.[6] In a 1978 appellate court ruling absolving from liability rescuers who failed to oxygenate a patient in cardiac arrest, the court reasoned that immunity laws were essential because of the difficulty in obtaining insurance and because unlimited liability could "be enough to drive many providers of ambulance service out of business and greatly discourage others from entering."[7] Immunity for the prehospital provider became common, and remains rooted in EMS law. Eventually laws were passed to protect the trained rescuer and professional paid responder, as well as the "Good Samaritan." Governmental immunity also became a strong shield from liability for the public agencies. Immunity for the Good Samaritan physician became commonplace, and immunity for the supervising physician was seen as early as 1976.

It is important that the medical director realize that medical oversight as a necessary component of a system has not been recognized with uniform enthusiasm in legislation. Although physician participation (often side by side with paramedic personnel) existed in the early mobile cardiac care units, legislative mandates for physician involvement varied tremendously from state to state. Physician involvement commenced only at the hospital door for the majority of volunteer basic life support units that covered the expanse of highways and hillsides across the country. Even as EMS passes into the 21st century, medical directors still are not required to supervise the medical care of many nonparamedic services, particularly in rural, nontransporting EMS services. However, the delivery of medical care in the prehospital setting has matured largely to the credit of many physicians willing to divide their medical practices between patient care in emergency departments or private practices and the care of patients miles from the hospital.

Despite the years of muted development of medical oversight, the silence of the courts regarding the role of the prehospital medical director has begun to change. Medical oversight will become increasingly recognized in the legal arena as a fundamental component of quality prehospital care, especially as medical directors become more active and more informed, some even having had fellowship training in EMS, and the level of care delivered by EMS providers becomes more complex. Potential liability is the inevitable corollary that shadows the development of responsibilities in medical oversight.

Sources of Accountability

The role of the medical director involves multiple and diverse responsibilities. Aspects of administration, medical care, personnel management, and education occupy the daily activities of the medical director in the oversight of an EMS system. Consequently, liability concerns are also multifaceted. As with any form of medical practice, physician conduct must conform to accepted standards of care. Sources that may provide some definition of those standards are discussed here.

Federal Law and Regulations

Although EMS is almost exclusively under state and local law as a health and safety concern, there are several areas of federal law that medical directors need to be aware of. If medical directors are part of the employment hierarchy, their actions may allow them to be named in lawsuits based on employment disputes. There are more of these occurring yearly.

Medical directors should recognize the newer definition of sexual harassment. Formerly, overt inappropriate action was required, now all it takes is the creation of "an oppressive or hostile work environment."[8]

There is a continuing tightening of safeguards against Medicare and Medicaid fraud and abuse. One of the areas being closely watched is the appropriate use of ambulance services, especially for transport. Physicians have been warned against easy certification of medical necessity for the use of ambulances when other avenues of transportation are available. Merely signing the medical necessity form stating the patient needed transport by ambulance could subject a physician to fines, damages, and civil monetary penalties under the false claims and Medicare fraud and abuse acts which have been targeted by government investigators, including FBI task forces, in recent years.[9,10] Now, new regulations for ambulance reimbursement have been drafted that state what are acceptable reimbursement levels for ambulances based on the condition of the patient.[11] Generally, the patient must demonstrate a need for advanced life support (ALS), such as abnormal vital signs or a need for medications in order to qualify for ALS reimbursement. Additionally, final rules from the Department of Health and Human Services clarify "medical necessity," provide minimum staffing levels for ambulances, and revise rules for physician certification of the need for ambulance transfer of patients.[12]

New federal rules promulgated as part of the Health Insurance Portability and Accountability Act of 1996 (HIPAA) require the protection of any information collected, in electronic or paper form, by a healthcare provider that may "relate to the past, present, or future physical or mental health or condition of an individual; the provision of health care to an individual;" and "identifies the individual; or . . . can be used to identify the individual."[13] These will require EMS services to examine their record keeping and consent procedures as well as those of the entities with which they commonly share information.

Civil Rights

A Federal 'civil rights' statute, 42 U.S.C. § 1983, provides that "Every person who . . . subjects, or causes to be subjected, any citizen . . . to the deprivation of any rights, privileges, or immunities secured by the Constitution and laws, shall be liable to the party injured in an action at law."[14] The effect of this brief passage is significant. Any individual who believes that another has acted against them in violation of any law may choose to sue in Federal court for a civil rights violation.

Civil rights claims usually include claims of due process and equal protection violations as well. The Fourteenth Amendment of the United States Constitution states, "No person shall be deprived of life, liberty, and the pursuit of happiness, without due process of law." This has been interpreted to provide a right for fundamental fairness requiring, at the minimum, "notice" and "an opportunity to be heard" before some right, such as a license, is taken away. Equal protection is the Constitutional requirement that similarly situated individuals are treated similarly—this is why discrimination lawsuits are civil rights questions as well.

These claims are significant for a number of reasons. State immunity statutes do not affect the ability of the plaintiff to sue and seek damages in federal court, and there are no federal immunities that apply to these types of cases. State damage caps, which may affect the maximum recovery in malpractice actions, do not apply. The successful plaintiff may recover punitive damages and attorney's fees. Often the individual charged does not have proper insurance coverage to indemnify them against the costs of the lawsuit. A few examples demonstrate why these "1983 actions" can be significant in prehospital care.

The decision of *Doe v. Borough of Barrington* was rendered in 1990.[15] It ruled that a city violated a citizen's rights because the city failed to train police officers about acquired immune deficiency syndrome (AIDS) and the need to keep confidential the identity of a person infected with human immunodeficiency virus (HIV). Reasonably extrapolated to EMS agencies, failure to train public employee prehospital providers about the transmission of AIDS and patient confidentiality may result in liability if medical treatment and confidentiality are not correctly managed because of ignorance on the part of the prehospital providers. New HIPAA requirements directly address these issues.

An obstetric patient argued that she had a constitutional right to direct a county ambulance to the hospital of her choice in *Wideman v. Shallowford Community Hospital, Inc.* The patient contended that when an ambulance transported her to a county hospital that was the direct medical control facility for the ambulance service, she was deprived of her "constitutional right to essential medical treatment."[16]

However, the appellate court held that there was no Constitutional right to prehospital treatment and transport to a facility of patient choice.

Medical directors may face Constitutional issues when a prehospital provider contests termination from employment based on due process. Grievance procedures that involve the qualifications of personnel may involve the medical director. Understanding due process may prevent unnecessary review proceedings. For example, in *Baxter v. Fulton-DeKalb Hospital Authority,* a federal court ruled on the due process claim of a paramedic who had been cleared of misconduct in a hospital investigation of field performance.[17] The medical director, who was employed by the hospital and supervised the paramedic who was employed by a public hospital, refused to reinstate the paramedic, even though the paramedic had been cleared of misconduct. The court ruled that the paramedic's claim against the hospital should not be dismissed because the hospital deprived the paramedic of due process by acquiescing to the decision of the medical director without holding a hearing.

A New Mexico physician found himself charged with federal civil rights violations after he withdrew medical oversight from two providers who were suing him for medical malpractice.[18] The providers claimed that they had a "right" to medical oversight just by virtue of being EMTs, and sued for civil rights violations. A significant problem for this physician was the fact that his malpractice insurance did not indemnify him for civil rights lawsuits.

A Kentucky physician was named as a defendant in a state lawsuit alleging violation of rights under the Family Medical Leave Act as well as for civil rights violations, because he withheld medical oversight for a paramedic in a delegated practice state.[19,20] The physician refused to extend medical oversight to the paramedic after the paramedic tried to return to work after treatment for alcoholism and depression; the medical director had a long list of prior complaints against this individual, unrelated to his illness, and was in the process of bringing them to the attention of the state licensing authority. The state case is pending. Again, the physician's insurance did not clearly cover the costs of his defense. This case is somewhat interesting because the plaintiff chose to bring it in state, rather than federal, court. A federal district court had already dismissed a related case brought by the same paramedic against an ambulance service, citing that the plaintiff had not proven his case under the Americans with Disabilities Act (ADA).[21,22] Individuals, such as this medical director, are not subject to the ADA unless they are an employer.

State Statutes and Regulations

Although the role of the medical director is complex, the statutory provisions that directly address the role are often brief. Each state statute has supplemental regulations concerning the responsibilities of medical directors to the EMS personnel they supervise or the EMS system in which they function. There are different regulatory structures and varying degrees of specificity in different jurisdictions.[23] For example, some state laws provide little more than a short definition of the medical director as a licensed physician responsible for the supervision and training of EMS personnel. Some regulations only state the responsibilities of the medical director in general terms, and it is assumed that the medical director will engage in certain supervisory activities. In other states, regulations identify the responsibilities of the medical director in detail. The Florida statute requires, for example, that the medical director "establish a quality assurance committee to provide for quality assurance review of all EMTs and paramedics under his supervision."[24] Medical directors are encouraged to ride with the ambulance services in Oregon.[25] In Washington, rules expressly provide that the "medical program director" is certified by the EMS regulatory authority and can be terminated for failure to perform the duties of the position.[26] Clearly, trends are emerging in the regulatory arena to abolish the "paper doc" and mandate quality supervision and involvement.

Increasingly, states are attaching qualifications to the role of medical director beyond mere state licensure to practice medicine. In Oregon the Board of Medical Examiners must review and approve an application for the position of prehospital medical director.[27] Board certification in emergency medicine, family practice, internal medicine, or surgery, or certification in both advanced cardiac life support (ACLS) and advanced trauma life support (ATLS), are required in Missouri.[28] Now that medical director training is available at the national level, certain states now require their medical directors to undergo certification.[29] New Mexico requires that new medical directors receive, within two years, either a nationally recognized EMS medical director course, a state approved course, or local orientation provided by a regional or state medical director.[30]

State regulations also cover the scope of practice, licensure, or certification, and training of prehospital personnel. Licensure differs from certification in that certification by a state only recognizes that an EMS provider has achieved a certain level of training, but does not confer any right to practice based on that training.[31] Notably, licensure by a state conveys a property interest which requires due process in any proceeding to take away that license. These are both different from the "verification" given by such training as Advanced Hazmat Life Support and ATLS which simply state a person has completed the education, but makes no representations about their ability to use the new skill. It is important to mention, however, that some states use "certification" inappropriately, such as when the provider is actually licensed—it is important to look at the underlying rights that go with the position.

At least one federal court has stated that state protocols, not the training of the EMT, dictate his duty.[32] In this case, a basic EMT who had ACLS training was faulted for not intubating a patient. Although he had been trained to do so in his ACLS class, intubation was not within his scope of practice, and therefore he did not have a legal duty to intubate.

State law determines the link between the medical director and the provider; whether the provider functions under the license of the physician, that is, delegated practice, or the provider has her own license and practices with physician supervision and control. The medical director must ensure that protocols delegate medical functions consistent with each prehospital care provider's certification and training. On more than one occasion an unwary medical director has conceded to a provider's request to perform a medical act not legally authorized by statute nor covered by that individual's training. Some skills are subject to extra reporting requirements. For example, EMT-Defibrillation (EMT-D) programs, or other special skills, may involve considerable reporting to the state agency, and documentation of skills proficiency. In addition, specific testing or training requirements may exist for registered nurses who function in the prehospital setting, such as flight medics who are often required to have significant critical care experience; the medical director should keep abreast of these regulatory provisions.

Another common regulatory provision is the prerequisite that the medical director provide written authorization for a provider to qualify for certification. Quite often the medical director signs a form, often the provider's license application, making a statement such as ". . . I understand that I am legally and professionally responsible for the directed medical actions of this EMT-Paramedic." This language is quite explicit and may impose significant legal responsibilities on the medical director. The medical director who makes a commitment on paper must ensure that the prehospital provider is capable and can practice with reasonable skill and safety. Available evaluation or risk management tools should be used. At the very least, documentation of proficiency or capability from reliable sources such as training institutions or employers should be provided.

Medical directors must be aware of these regulatory constraints that define and affect their role. They should not rely on an apparent lack of enforcement by the state regulatory authority to justify ignoring legally imposed responsibilities. A shortage of prehospital providers in a community should never be justification for authorizing practice by a person with serious deficiencies in skills or poor judgment. New medical directors are wise to contact state and local EMS offices early in their tenure to be sure that they are compliant with these matters. Veteran directors will hopefully have maintained communication channels that enable them to use regulatory agencies as a reliable resource.

In addition, the physician remains accountable to the state licensing board for his medical oversight functions. A recent Arizona case has held that a physician medical director for an insurance company who was engaged in making "medical decisions which could affect the health and safety of a patient or the public" was subject to the jurisdiction of the Board of Medical Examiners even though he did not have a physician-patient relationship with any patient.[33] Recently, several state legislatures have attempted to put this responsibility into statute.

There is now an attempt by the NAEMSP to provide a central registry, available on the Internet, for all state laws and regulations concerning EMS.[34] A central data bank will allow states and individuals to compare laws and possibly lead to more standardization.

Local Ordinances

The medical director will encounter additional layers of codifications in county and municipal government. City ordinances and county resolutions often target activities not addressed by state regulations. Such provisions can be very stringent and sometimes quite outdated. Although the sanctions imposed on ambulance services for violations are sometimes insignificant fines, misconduct may lead to revocation of an ambulance service permit to operate in the jurisdiction. These provisions may require proof of protocols, insurance, and proper staffing and may restrict the response activities of the ambulance service. Medical directors who give orders that conflict with local laws set their service up for trouble with the "city fathers." Local government politics can be a major source of consternation, and seemingly minor infractions can seriously complicate community relationships.

County attorneys and plaintiff lawyers scrutinize the "black letter law" of these various codifications and hold the physician accountable to the "letter of the law" and the "spirit of the law" as circumstances warrant. The medical director must know and operate within these legal statutes, regulations, and codes. Sound legal advice should be sought if there is a question of interpretation or application, preferably before a legal conflict has materialized. Competent private counsel, city and county attorneys, and state regulatory boards can provide valuable guidance in medical director decision making.

Arguably, medical directors have a moral obligation to try to influence the regulatory framework that controls them. Unworkable, or senseless, bureaucracy may be as much of an impediment to the proper delivery of prehospital care as is a lack of trained personnel.

Immunity Laws

Some states have statutes that provide immunity from liability for acts performed by medical directors as long as they act in good faith or in a non-reckless manner.[35] The medical director immunity laws may, therefore, give a medical director a sense of comfort that the courts will forgive some misjudgments in medical control activities. These statutes have not yet been the subject of review at the appellate court level. However, the responsibilities of the medical director remain unchanged, and only the payment of damages is avoided; the medical director may still be responsible for attorney fees and court costs. Immunity laws are also venue-specific; state immunity is good only in state courts; if the complaint involves a federal question, there is no immunity in the Federal court system. There may be an ongoing tendency for courts to limit sovereign immunity.[36]

Immunity statutes for EMS providers have successfully shielded providers from liability for simple negligent conduct, but providers typically still remain accountable for "grossly negligent or reckless" conduct.[37] For example, Washington paramedics were sued when a patient died after arrival at a hospital with an esophageal intubation.[38] They received immunity under Washington law, however, because "there [wa]s absolutely no evidence in the record to suggest that the paramedics acted without good faith."

SOVEREIGN IMMUNITY. Often EMS services are run by a governmental subdivision such as a county or municipality. These generally benefit from sovereign immunity which greatly limits actions for which governmental, that is, sovereign, agencies may be sued. Lawsuits generally require gross, or willful, negligence, although in some states specific instrumentalities of the alleged negligence, such as the use of an automobile, may allow lawsuit. For example, a county and city ambulance service was sued by a patient who was allegedly rendered quadriplegic during a difficult extrication from a canyon.[39] All of the defendants were found to be immune from lawsuit under a sovereign immunity statute. Although the statute stated that immunity did not apply to the negligent use of "equipment," the Court determined that this did not include the rescue equipment used. Similarly, sovereign immunity has shielded municipalities from lawsuits for accidents involving ambulances.[40] Recently, however, a Tennessee court found that prehospital providers were "health care practitioners" because they were licensed under state law, and as such were specifically exempted from the state tort claims act which read "No claim may be brought against an employee or judgment entered against an employee for damages for which the immunity of the governmental entity is removed by this chapter unless the claim is *one for medical malpractice brought against a health care practitioner. . . .*"[41,42]

The sovereign immunity of the U.S. government is controlled by the Federal Tort Claims Act which, on its face, seems to allow federal employees to be sued on the same basis as private individuals.[43] Federal employees do have further protection, however; an additional section of federal law exempts *any claim based upon an act or omission of an employee of the Government, exercising due care, in the execution of a statute or regulation, whether or not such statute or regulation be valid, or based upon the exercise or performance or the failure to exercise or perform a discretionary function or duty on the part of a federal agency or an employee of the Government, whether or not the discretion involved be abused.*[44] The boundaries of the Federal Tort Claims Act have been examined in a recent California case where the National Park Service and two of its providers were sued for failure to have neither the proper equipment nor training for proper c-spine immobilization and CPR.[45] The court determined that any decision as to the training level of providers and what equipment they were provided was a discretionary function and therefore immune from lawsuit. On the other hand, the proper delivery of care at this scene was not a discretionary function and could be heard at trial.

Although medical directors have yet to specifically benefit from sovereign immunity, lawsuits against EMS providers have been dismissed based on sovereign immunity, and without liability of a provider it would be impossible to derive liability against their medical oversight physician.

GOOD SAMARITAN STATUTES. Such statutes are another possible source of immunity for the medical director, though they are more likely to be of benefit in limiting his direct liability from actions at a scene than by preventing indirect liability by giving immunity to the actions of the providers. These are quite variable from state to state, so no blanket statements are possible.[46] In general, however, good Samaritan statutes usually are written to protect a physician, although others, such as providers, are sometimes included; California, for example, protects nurses, prehospital providers, fire fighters, or anyone attempting to aid a choking victim at a restaurant. They usually apply to actions rendered "at the scene of an emergency," which has been limited to the roadside in some jurisdictions and expanded to hospital rooms in others.[47,48] They usually require that the care rendered is gratuitous and delivered in "good faith." The statutes vary in their protection, some offer complete immunity, while others just excuse ordinary negligence.[49,50] A medical director should understand the limitations of his state Good Samaritan statute, and how it might apply to medical direction activities. Not surprisingly, ACEP has made a policy statement supporting Good Samaritan legislation.[51]

A recent decision in Maryland temporarily extracted Baltimore firemedics from their state Good Samaritan statute because the city billed for their services and allowed a suit against a paramedic for an alleged esophageal intubation.[52] This was overturned on appeal; the court based the decision on another specific fire company immunity act and did not specifically address the Good Samaritan issue.[53]

Recently, a limited federal Good Samaritan law was passed. The Aviation Medical Assistance Act of 1998 immunizes qualified individuals from liability in state or federal court unless they are guilty of "gross negligence or willful misconduct" in their response to an in-flight medical emergency.[54]

Court Decisions

Case law is a source of law in which a written decision by a judge, or panel of judges, interprets statutes or the applicability of legal principles to a case. Often referred to as common law, these rulings can determine the merit of a plaintiff's negligence claim or interpret a statute. For example, in recent years, interpretations of the working of immunity statutes and what conduct constitutes "gross negligence" have abounded. However, because of varying facts from case to case, varying interpretations from state to state, and passing years between the date of the incident and a court ruling, case law is sometimes an ineffective educator. Often, though, it is all we have.

Court decisions in one state are not binding on any other state; however, the discussions of issues in state case law reveal the success or failure of legal theories proposed by plaintiffs, thereby highlighting the kinds of conduct that attract the attention of judges and juries. Courts also often look to see how other jurisdictions have handled new legal theories and are sometimes persuaded by their reasoning. An awareness of the legal arguments by plaintiffs seeking recovery from EMS agencies and prehospital providers can guide the medical director in areas where acceptable protocols and negligent conduct have not been well defined. Specific areas of EMS case law important to the medical director are discussed further below. In areas where there is little law directly on point, analogous situations serve to show current legal reasoning.

Remarkably, few legal decisions have discussed medical oversight or implicated the medical director in allegations of providers' misconduct. One of the few negligence actions that addressed the role of the medical director resulted in a ruling adverse to the medical director. In Florida, an appellate court upheld a jury verdict against a medical center, because the EMS medical director failed to properly supervise, train, and instruct the paramedics.[55] A 5-year-old female patient was assessed at her home by paramedics who decided no emergency medical care was needed; the young patient died hours later of congestive heart failure. The EMS medical director admitted that there was no written protocol for "how to take a history or how to distinguish between an emergency and non-emergency situation," or for taking pediatric vital signs. Instead, the medical director depended on the paramedics' prior schooling and experience to provide the necessary guidance. The jury concurred with the plaintiff's contention that the medical director was responsible for developing procedures "and deviated from the standard of care by not having established such written procedures."[56] Protocols addressing, or simply forbidding, nontransports might have protected the system and the medical director.

Areas of Liability

The roles played by the medical director require that discussion of potential liabilities be separated into two general categories: professional and administrative. The professional role encompasses most of what is thought of as the traditional role of the medical director. This includes delivering and supervising patient care. The liabilities for the medical director in the professional role are those of negligence, and common professional liability insurance often provides protection. The administrative role is less clearly defined. Because medical oversight is necessary for employment of a provider, decisions on the part of the medical director about withholding medical oversight effectively become employment decisions. Often, disgruntled former employees will find ways to blame the medical director for this. Additionally, a medical oversight physician may be placed in a position where he deals with reimbursement issues for the service. This may expose the physician to liabilities for false claims/fraud issues. The significant feature of administrative liability is that traditional professional liability insurance does not apply in these areas. Most of the subsequent discussion will address medical director liabilities in the professional role, often where it is derived from actions/inactions of the providers.

Absent any judicial interpretation of the duties for proper medical oversight, the legal claims against medical directors that will prove successful for a plaintiff attorney can only be surmised. The relationship of the medical director to the prehospital provider is unique, although there are similarities to the relationships between nurse and physician or physician assistant and physician.[57] Extrapolating from these medical professional relationships and from general medicolegal principles, a few theories are worth noting. These legal theories are some of the pathways by which a medical director can be linked to liability. No doubt there will be other theories proposed by inventive plaintiffs' attorneys.

The areas of liability may be direct, where the medical director personally fails in a duty, or indirect, where the medical director bears the responsibility for someone else's lapse.

Direct Liability

FAILURE TO PERFORM RESPONSIBILITIES. The clearest source of liability is a negligent act committed by the medical director. This could be a simple malpractice action for treatment rendered at the scene of an accident by a medical director who rides along with the ambulance, but is more commonly a failure in other areas. Through statute and regulation, medical directors are obligated to perform certain tasks, such as providing direct medical oversight, establishing protocols, and auditing the performance of field personnel. Despite many variations among EMS systems and state laws, standards of conduct in medical control for the medical director have taken shape. Expert testimony by other medical directors is usually necessary to give substance and shape to the professional duties of colleagues when litigation arises. A malpractice action against a medical director could be a valid cause of action if the plaintiff can establish the requisite elements of malpractice including duty, breach, proximate cause, and damages. This was successfully argued in the case of *Tallahassee*, discussed previously.

NEGLIGENT SUPERVISION. A claim of negligent supervision requires proof of a duty to supervise and a failure to do so that causes harm to another person. Negligent supervision might be argued if the medical director failed to take action to correct deficiencies such as (1) the medical director observes a paramedic with poor intubation technique; (2) a supervisor of an ambulance service reports a series of patient care incidents involving a paramedic who verbally abused patients; or (3) the medical director fails to establish medication protocols consistent with current standards of medical practice, thereby letting the paramedic exercise unfettered discretion in the field. If a physician fails to act on knowledge, whether acquired from direct observation, field audits, patient complaints, or other sources, that a provider is lacking in skills or is practicing in a dangerous manner, the physician is duty-bound to remove, restrict, or otherwise prevent the prehospital provider from continuing to render substandard care. This responsibility would likely be shared (although not necessarily equally) with the provider's direct employer. This duty to supervise arises from the statutory role of medical directors, as well as by virtue of the medical director's delegation of medical practice. It may be clarified in the medical director's contract. A jury would likely view medical directors, with their superior training and their authority to have taken corrective action, to be culpable because of failure to exercise their lawful authority. Although errors in judgment regarding the capabilities of a particular prehospital provider can still occur, negligence claims against medical directors are less likely to materialize if the physician is active, informed, and involved.

Until recently, "no court in the country has heretofore held a private physician liable for injuries suffered by an individual whom he has never treated, never met, and never agreed to treat."[58] This has changed. North Carolina has found a non-traditional physician-patient duty formed between a physician and a patient seen only by residents the physician had contracted to supervise.[59] Although the reasoning in this case has been criticized, extending this to medical director liability for patients seen by EMS providers he contractually supervises is a possible expansion of this legal theory.[60] There are several recent cases that follow the same theory. A Missouri surgeon agreed to be on-call for the emergency department (ED) at the same time he was attending a medical conference out of town. A patient was injured in an MVA and the delay in obtaining surgical treatment for her due to the absence of the surgeon led to complications. A Missouri Court of Appeals determined that even in the absence of a traditional physician-patient relationship, public policy and the foreseeability of harm to patients supported finding a duty on the part of the on-call surgeon.[61] An Arizona Court of Appeals has recently determined that a physician had a duty to a patient he had never seen nor treated just be providing an informal, or "curbside," consultation about an EKG.[62] The court determined that the consultant physician was in the best position to prevent future harm to the patient by giving correct advice, no matter how informal the request. Again, extending this reasoning to creating a duty on the part of a medical oversight physician is not difficult.

Medical directors usually do not have complete control over the employment or membership of a prehospital provider in an EMS agency. However, active involvement in the personnel aspects of an EMS service is important because the skills and judgment of prehospital care providers directly affect the quality of patient care. The authority of medical directors to determine who may practice under their license was the focus of a ruling from the state of Minnesota, *County of Hennepin v. Hennepin County Association of Paramedics and Emergency Medical Technicians.*[63] A county paramedic who was a member of a union had been terminated by the county because of patient-care related conduct. After a hearing for reinstatement, an arbitrator ruled that the paramedic should be reinstated. The case was appealed and the testimony of the medical director was important because he had stated that he could neither trust the paramedic nor be certain that the paramedic would perform safely and appropriately even if on probation. The appellate court ruled that the medical director could not be forced to authorize the paramedic to work under this medical license. The unique relationship of medical directors extending their license to the paramedic could "impose potential tort and disciplinary liability on the medical director for actions of unfit paramedics." Therefore the medical director may exercise "medical judgment" to decide who should or should not work as a paramedic, according to the *Hennepin County* decisions. It was noted that the paramedic could have been assigned to a position not involving direct patient contact.

If an employer such as a fire department fails or refuses to impose restrictions, the medical director's ability to invoke conditions on the scope of practice of a prehospital provider may seem complicated. Medical directors are not forced to continue extending their services, or license, to a prehospital provider employed by an uncooperative agency, whether in a paid or volunteer service, if that provider has demonstrated incompetence in patient care. The employer hopefully would be persuaded to follow the medical director's recommendations for remediation. Such scenarios can be quite divisive and are best averted by being addressed before they occur, such as at the time of contract negotiation. For example, the author's contract stated that he "may after reasonable investigation, limit, suspend, or withdraw medical control (oversight) from any EMT."

The medical director should remember that EMS is fundamentally the provision of health care. At least one jurisdiction has determined that following a protocol is "following the instructions of the physician."[64] Medical oversight should be just that—responsible oversight of patient care. No medical director should allow individuals to function under his oversight without an ability to completely supervise and, if necessary, limit their action. This oversight extends to direct medical oversight contact with prehospital providers. Every radio contact between physician and provider is a potential source of liability. Failure to treat these interactions seriously and appropriately document them, may result in problems.

Indirect Liability

Another type of liability that the medical director should be aware of is indirect liability. This legal doctrine provides that the negligent conduct of one person is imputed to another person because of the relationship between the two. The common phrase "Let the master answer," or the Latin *respondeat superior,* exemplifies vicarious liability where an agent's actions are ascribed to whoever gave him the authority to act. The "master" (employer) is accountable for the actions of the employee even if the employer's conduct is faultless, as long as the employee was acting within the scope of his employment and presumably benefitting the employer. This form of liability is not new to the medical profession. It has been the source of liability for physicians in situations in which the physician was considered "the captain of the ship." This doctrine evolved when hospitals generally were immune from liability as charitable or governmental institutions; the negligence of the nurses was not imputed to the institution but rather was imputed to the surgeon.[65] It was reasoned that because the nurse functioned under the direct control and supervision of the surgeon, the injured patient could seek compensation from the surgeon even if the surgeon committed no act of carelessness.[66] This legal theory has eroded over the years, however, in response to the increased independent professional responsibility assumed by nurses and other members of the healthcare "team" and increased liability imposed by the courts on hospitals.[67]

The theory of indirect liability has rarely surfaced in EMS case law; it may have very limited applicability in the prehospital scenario, as there is often not the direct economic benefit to the physician that is required. Of course, it is to the medical director's advantage that this principle not apply. Although the term "direct medical oversight" may seem to create a claim of vicarious liability, actual over-the-shoulder supervision is not typically involved in the relationship between the prehospital provider and the medical director. The element of control is diminished in the context of contact only through radio and protocols. A Florida case has held that an emergency room cannot be held liable for the promulgation of protocols which led to alleged negligent triage.[68]

The factor of control is pivotal in existing cases involving nurses acting on physicians' orders. Applied to EMS, this principle necessitates scrutiny of the extent of control the physician exercises over the particular action of the prehospital provider, the authority of the medical director to exercise control over the prehospital provider at the particular time, and the prehospital provider's skill and training in the specific medical act. Just as the nurse usually has independent professional and dependent medical functions when acting on a physician's orders, it is likely that the courts would examine the latitude of the prehospital provider's medical functions. The administrative medical director or an indirect medical oversight physician can clarify responsibilities and authority through frank discussion and written agreements that occur before any controversies arise.

System Concerns

By definition, EMS is a network of resources and therefore medical directors must construe their role and responsibilities jointly and cooperatively with the other components and players in the EMS system. Modern EMS is often tainted with antiquated principles that define structures by political boundaries rather than patient needs. Medical directors rarely have an opportunity to implement the system of their choice; they are usually saddled with a machine that is in terrible need of repair, functioning suboptimally, and probably not up to code. Nonetheless, medical directors' responsibilities cannot be shirked; certainly they are no less accountable, and perhaps over time even more so, if they acquiesce to the unabated continuation of problems in their system.

System problems such as regionalization, patient destination, and the use of paramedics or aeromedical transport can cause a damaging ripple effect in an EMS system. Competing agencies can compromise patient care if coordination and cooperation are not

promoted by the medical director, who often has to remind everyone that appropriate patient care, rather than turf and egos, is the important factor. These politico legal battles are among the most vociferous and most costly. Often, problems are the result of parochialism, competition for patients, or simply ignorance. Medical directors often can be instrumental in correcting the errant habits and customs of a system, although it may take years of patience, debate, and befriending; if they do not make the effort, both they and the system are destined to fail.

Entire EMS systems, not just individual providers, are increasingly under legal scrutiny. Although medical directors usually are not identified as the negligent defendant in these cases, they are not simply an unwitting appendage to the system. They should be the quarterback of all EMS resources. Medical directors should have their position in the system command structure defined by contract and implemented in standard operating procedures (SOPs). Dealing with fire department, or other, personnel who are used to using chains of command is facilitated by this definition. There should be no hesitation when the medical director appropriately assumes medical control of a scene. The following system concerns can become less daunting when addressed with protocols and policies founded on and driven by the principle of optimal patient care.

Dispatch

Structured and prioritized emergency medical dispatch (EMD) has become the standard of care in most areas; the widespread use of commercial EMD products has both fueled this expansion and established a standard of care. Although dispatchers are often not EMTs, they are providing medical information and services as part of an EMS system, and they usually are required to have medical oversight. Their actions may potentially implicate a medical director. The medical director bears the responsibility to ensure that the dispatch protocols and procedures are reviewed and updated at least as often as patient-care protocols. This is especially true if protocols are obtained 'off the shelf' from a commercial source—they should be reviewed and modified to ensure compliance with local protocols as well as provision of proper patient care.

It is not clear what, if any, liability might be claimed against dispatchers who work for 3-1-1 lines, which are becoming common in large metropolitan areas to accept calls that are not emergencies. They will still likely receive some emergency calls; and these dispatch centers should have protocols in place to mandate call transfer to an appropriate emergency dispatch center.

Lawsuits have occurred over the issue of dispatch; and while none have yet implicated medical directors, they are worth reviewing. The suits have generally been based on dispatchers sending ambulances to the wrong address, or delay/not sending one when needed.[69,70] The results of these cases have been mixed, but usually the dispatch agency has escaped liability. There are two reasons for this. The first is sovereign immunity which was discussed above.

The second theory blocking these lawsuits is somewhat more complex and has to do with the concept of duty. Governments, and their agents such as dispatchers, have a general duty to provide basic, or "essential," public services such as police, fire, and EMS to their citizens. This duty is owed to the population as a whole, not to specific individuals. Unless a court can find that a public service has established a "special duty" toward a specific individual, that individual may not sue for negligence. The key to finding a special duty is finding that a "special relationship" has formed that includes the open assumption by the municipality to act on behalf of an injured party, knowledge on the part of the municipality's agents that inaction could lead to harm, direct contact between the agents and injured party, and the injured party's justifiable reliance on the municipality's help.[71] For example, a call to a dispatcher, by someone with a headache who was advised to try aspirin and was later found to have a stroke, was not sufficient to establish a special duty, where a series of two phone calls to another dispatcher was.[72,73] Special duty has not been clarified in all states, and is more likely than other theories to vary between jurisdictions. New York and the District of Columbia, for example, have a series of cases discussing special duty, while in New Mexico the public duty/special duty distinction has been eliminated by statute.[74]

A recent lawsuit from Chicago addressed both of these issues.[75] A patient dialed 9-1-1 requesting assistance for an asthma attack. The dispatcher indicated help was on the way, but did not keep the patient on the phone until the providers arrived. When the providers arrived, no one answered the door. The EMS personnel made no attempt to enter the apartment. The patient was found dead in the apartment the following morning. The city was sued for failing to keep the caller on the phone until help arrived, and for failure to either attempt to open the apartment or to use force to enter it. An appeals court initially found that the city had sovereign immunity from lawsuit as well as a defense under the special duty exemption, but this was overturned on appeal.[76] The court specifically noted that conduct that is beyond the level of a paramedic's training is not immunized, while conduct that merely deviates from a paramedic's training and constitutes negligence is subject to immunity unless it is willful and wanton. In the presence circumstance, the court noted that the paramedics' failure to attempt to open the unlocked door may have been a gross violation of the department's "Try Before You Pry" policy.

Interestingly, many municipalities routinely make forced entrances on homes to which they are called, preferring to pay for a broken window or door, rather than face criticism for not finding a patient *in extremis*. On the other hand, in late 1999, a Florida paramedic was shot in the chest as he attempted to make entry into a locked apartment which he thought held a disabled woman who had dialed 9-1-1; he had inadvertently entered the wrong apartment.

Special duty has also been addressed in federal court. In Virginia, a federal district court determined that a municipality had no "special relationship" with plaintiffs in a fire rescue case that would support a claim brought under 42 U.S.C. §1983.[77] The Court specifically noted that "not every death that results from the state's failure to act is a deprivation under the Fourteenth Amendment. Before an omission that leads to a death is actionable under the Fourteenth Amendment and §1983, the Constitution must recognize an underlying duty on the part of the state to act."[78]

Response

How a fire department staffs rescue units or uses medical personnel to respond to a medical emergency is as much a medical decision as is the choice of intravenous solutions. Optimal patient care is sacrificed by the poor placement of ambulances, the lack of coordination of tiered responses, and many other political, emotional, and business factors. Medical directors must study objectively the components and agencies within their systems; the goal of quality patient care must dictate system management decisions.

Ambulance response should be timely. A Honolulu jury awarded nearly $2 million against the City for a two-hour delay in ambulance arrival.[79] It is important to recognize, however, that even when the ambulance response is appropriate, patients often perceive that it took too long.[80]

The type of response needed is worth exploring. It is imperative that the service, with the help of the medical director, develop clear and appropriate guidelines for the use of lights and sirens in emergency responses and transfers. Accidents involving emergency vehicles represent more than half the claims paid by insurers of EMS systems.[81] Some providers do not even have an adequate knowledge of ambulance traffic laws.[82] Insurers often recommend special training for drivers of emergency vehicles, to protect both EMS personnel and their patients; medical directors are in a unique position to support this training.

An example of a system failure is *Brooks v. Herndon Ambulance Service, Inc.* The care of a patient was compromised when an EMT-A unit responded to a call. The patient, a student in a gym class, began seizing and then arrested.[83] The ambulance that received the call had difficulty finding the address, equipment malfunctional on-scene, and finally the ambulance broke down en route to the hospital with the patient. Ten minutes from the school was a fire department with a paramedic unit that was never notified. Modern EMS will not tolerate such provincialism and uncooperative practices.

Volunteer systems are not immune to attack. Many communities depend on the willingness of individual, uncompensated volunteers to respond to emergencies. However, such EMS services still must meet the same minimum standards as paid services. The volunteer spirit and contribution must not compromise patient care. A promise to provide EMS through the formation of a fire department or fire protection district supported by public funds creates obligations irrespective of the uncompensated status of the responders or the absence of charges to the patient. The duty for these providers to act reasonably is not altered by their gratuitous services. For example, a volunteer fire department with so few providers that there are no adequately staffed ambulances to respond to a call may invite liability if the delay in response was avoidable. This issue was raised in a Virginia case where a volunteer rescue service repeatedly had a shortage of personnel during early morning hours. The dispatcher was not notified of this problem and as a result did not request the assistance of a neighboring agency until the local rescue service

failed to acknowledge the requests.[84] Unless medical directors are actively involved in these aspects of an agency, the care rendered in the field may be less than optimal, thus inviting legal complications. Medical directors must show prehospital personnel how such operations endanger or compromise patient care. They can encourage other options to be considered by the service and perhaps lead efforts for system-wide improvement that had not yet been recognized as necessary by the community. Mutual aid arrangements and insistence that only qualified personnel accept patient-care responsibilities are examples of the input the medical director may offer to minimize legal risk.

The issue of several appellate court decisions has been the inappropriate use of personnel and equipment; liability has generally been defeated only because of the protections of immunity laws. For example, in *Malcolm v. City of East Detroit* fire fighters trained only in first aid were dispatched to care for a man complaining of chest pain, while available EMT-A fire fighters stayed at the station.[85] The patient arrested and the fire fighters attempted to ventilate with a bag-valve mask, although the patient was aspirating. The jury decided the city's action was willful and wanton, and therefore immunity protections did not apply. However, the judgment of $500,000 was vacated by the state Supreme Court, which gave an expansive interpretation to the governmental immunity statute.[86] The message is that although the law may excuse substandard care from monetary damages, scrutiny and evaluation of EMS resources must still be pursued by the medical director of the system.

Scene Handling

Besides the delivery of medical care, there are other scene issues the medical director should consider. These include the use of incident command (IC), and scene safety. While neither of these is directly a medical concern, they have an impact on the efficient delivery of patient care.

Mass casualty incidents are a scene of confusion. There needs to be a command and control structure in place to ensure that appropriate use of resources is accomplished. A recent New Mexico lawsuit charged municipal, county, and private EMS agencies with negligence in failing to discover the body of a driver who had been thrown 200 feet from an accident scene.[87] Plaintiffs alleged that the agencies had failed to implement a proper incident command structure (allegedly required in their SOPs) which might have required a search; the court disagreed, finding for defendants. There are federal requirements for the use of IC in all hazardous materials incidents,[88] and NPFA 1500 requires fire departments to establish written procedures for IC.[88,89]

Scene safety should be a concern for the medical director. Texas paramedics began applying a backboard and c-collar in the middle of an intersection to a patient who had been ambulatory for 10–15 minutes after an accident. They were forced to abandon the patient, still strapped to the board, when a vehicle careened into the intersection, ultimately running over the patient. The appeals court found that sovereign immunity did not apply.[90] The paramedics' attention to their own, as well as their patient's safety, would have prevented this tragic error. The United States Fire Administration has recognized that scene management is of primary importance in decreasing injuries for all types of emergency personnel.[91]

Destination

The wrath of the courts has surfaced in decisions addressing the destination policies of EMS systems. When transport of a patient is not dictated by medical concerns and the patient's best interests, or is hindered due to nonmedical reasons, juries have been harsh in their verdicts. In *Hospital Authority of Gwinnett County v. Jones,* the plaintiff convinced a jury that the transport of a patient who had sustained serious burn injuries was dictated by consideration of potential economic gains for the receiving hospital. The jury awarded punitive damages against the hospital in the amount of $1.3 million and $5000 against the ambulance service. A burn facility was approximately 15 to 20 minutes away by helicopter, and the defendant hospital was closer by ground. Rather than transporting the patient directly to the burn facility by the helicopter already en route to the scene, the patient was brought to the defendant hospital by ambulance, thereby necessitating another transfer of the patient to the burn facility. Arrangements for this second transport caused further delay. When lifting off from the hospital enroute to the burn facility, the helicopter crashed, killing the pilot and crew but sparing the patient. The helicopter landing area had been used for years but was not approved by the Federal Aviation Administration. The jury returned its verdict with an additional powerful message, "We the jury find that there should be more stringent regulations of the ground and air ambulance services in the state of Georgia."[92]

The authority of the patient to direct the ambulance to a specific hospital poses troubling issues. A state court found no liability against a direct medical oversight physician who advised EMT-As to comply with a patient's preference to be transported to a Level II hospital.[93] The providers had assessed the patient's injuries and felt that transport to a Level I facility was more appropriate. However, the patient's stated preference was honored, consistent with a protocol approved by the regional EMS authority. The patient died from a ruptured aneurysm while awaiting treatment at the Level II facility. The father's claims against the physician and hospital providing direct medical oversight were dismissed because the father failed to produce evidence that the patient would have survived the injury at the Level I facility. This state court ruling emphasizes the need for protocols that reflect sound medical principles; these are defensible even when patient outcome may not be optimal.

The issue of hospitals placing themselves on diversion or bypass has begun to be addressed by the courts, and should influence how service protocols deal with the issue. In an early federal case, a hospital on bypass was found to have established a duty to a patient in an ambulance when they established radio contact with the ambulance to tell them to divert.[94] The hospital escaped liability for simple negligence under an immunity statute. A related case from Maryland, however, supports bypass, stating that hospitals have no duty to accept persons when they are unable to treat them.[95] There is a potential complication for hospital-owned ambulances. The Consolidated Omnibus Budget Reconciliation Act of 1985 (COBRA) included the Emergency Medical Treatment and Active Labor Act (EMTALA), which requires hospitals to screen any and all individuals presenting to the emergency department for an emergency medical condition or active labor, and to stabilize their condition before transfer. "Coming to the emergency department," the action that triggers COBRA, includes just being in a hospital-owned ambulance.[96] COBRA does allow hospitals to refuse patients after radio communication if they are formally on diversion, but this applies only to ambulances not owned by the hospital. There has been a recent case that considers "coming to the emergency room" to apply to an ambulance in radio contact with the hospital heading toward the hospital, but this may be an aberrant decision.[97]

Failure to Transport

Emergency responses in which the patient is not transported can seem like wasted effort. In some systems, these ambulance encounters consume time and resources; they constitute a significant patient population the medical director never sees, yet may still be responsible for.[98] These calls are a medicolegal quagmire involving issues of patient autonomy, consent, medical assessment, and ill-defined legal duties. Patients denied transport or convinced by field personnel to forgo ambulance transport have been a source of numerous claims and case law.[99] Research indicates that a significant number of individuals who refuse transport are eventually seen by physicians, and a high number of patients who are refused transport by EMS personnel are eventually admitted to hospital.[100,101]

This area of liability may become more visible as some ambulance services began pre-transfer patient assessment.[102] Under this practice, paramedics determine if a patient needs ambulance transfer to an emergency facility, or if an alternative form of transportation, such as a medical taxi, may be used. This practice is being prompted by HMOs and other insurers, which save money when they only have to pay an evaluation fee rather than the fee for EMS transfer. Interestingly, insurance companies support this practice, because their liability exposure is greater when emergency vehicles are actually in operation transporting patients than for the smaller number of claims they may receive for inappropriate transfer refusals.

When field personnel are called to a scene and do not transport a patient because they discover no medical reason for the patient to be taken by ambulance to the hospital, questions of liability are raised quickly if the patient suffers deterioration or demise. If the patient refuses the transport despite apparent medical need, the questions focus on whether patient refusal was "informed"; the medical profession requires that refusal of treatment be informed refusal.[103] Informed refusal requires that the competent patient be informed of her diagnosis, the recommended treatment and alternatives, and what is likely to happen if treatment is refused. Claims of liability in either case depend on the following two factors: (1) the thoroughness or accuracy of the prehospital field assessment, and (2) the adequacy of the prehospital communication with the patient about the findings of the assessment and the need for medical treatment.

The principle of consent is well known to the practicing physician. It is established that adults of sound mind have the right to refuse medical treatment, even if the refusal of treatment may result in death.[104] Refusal of transport is complicated by the fact that there are indications in EMS that there is no Constitutional right for a patient to be transported to the hospital by a governmental EMS agency.[105] In addition to outright refusal, there is some indication that the patient may insist on transport to a hospital less qualified to provide necessary emergency care.[106]

Several issues make "no-transport calls" troublesome. To minimize the risk in these situations, short of transporting every patient, the medical director must understand the legal pitfalls inherent in the protocols or absence of protocols for these calls. First, although it is repeatedly impressed on EMS providers that they cannot "diagnose" illness, they are often directed by protocol to determine whether a patient is mentally "competent," a determination which is both a diagnosis and arguably a legal conclusion.[107] Second, prehospital providers have only basic training in assessing mental capacity or lucidity to evaluate a patient's ability to refuse treatment. Typically, they are instructed to ask only simplistic, routine questions about orientation such as "awake, alert, and oriented times three." This training is insufficient for evaluating mental status and providing information to patients for purposes of informed refusals. Third, there is no clear standard of the validity of mental status evaluations made outside the clinic or hospital environment.[108] These cases are further complicated by the lack of established legal standards regarding what constitutes informed refusal in the prehospital environment, to what extent consent is warranted for transport, and to what extent the duty to establish consent or refusal can be delegated by the medical director. Medical directors should make certain that their protocols are based on sound medical, rather than economic, grounds.

Another important issue is the scope of informed consent in the prehospital environment. Decades of case law in medical malpractice regarding the principle of consent involve patients seen in doctor's offices and hospitals, but the field environment is different. It may therefore be unrealistic to assume that the physician's duty to obtain informed consent or informed refusal applies to the prehospital provider, particularly given the dearth of training in EMS for this task, and EMT's current poor record of informed consent practices.[109]

Similarly, there have been no judicial interpretations of the relationship between a patient contacted in the field and a prehospital provider or the medical director. Although arguably a physician-patient relationship is created in both cases, there are several cases which suggest that direct contact between a physician and patient is necessary for this to occur. A telephone call, for example, is not usually sufficient.[110] Similarly, there is no judicial statement that the prehospital provider must contact the base station to terminate the patient relationship in a no-transport situation. However, sound medical oversight dictates that the medical director consider direct medical control essential, or that very clear and precise protocols be in place if the patient prehospital provider relationship is terminated without such supervision.

Factually, legal cases involving nontransport often involve glaring deficiencies in the assessment performed by the EMS provider; often, they reflect lack of discipline by the providers in adherence to protocols.[111] Liability can befall prehospital providers who leave the patient in the field without thorough and adequate assessment; medical directors may be responsible if they fail to provide sufficient protocols that detail the circumstances under which patients may be left in the field.

DENIAL OF AMBULANCE TRANSPORT. *Wright v. City of Los Angeles* expounded on the paramedic duty to assess in a costly incident of failure to transport.[112] Police summoned EMS personnel for a man found lying on the sidewalk. He appeared to have been involved in an altercation. The paramedic did only a cursory assessment and decided ambulance transport was not necessary; he advised the police officers that the patient could be checked by a physician before booking. In fact, the patient was in sickle-cell crisis. The court held that if the paramedic had conducted an examination consistent with the standard of care, he should have been able to determine that the patient was in need of immediate treatment. There was no contact with the direct medical oversight for approval of the nontransport; the paramedic testified that he "saw no symptoms indicating such a call was necessary."[113] Minutes after the paramedic left the scene the patient arrested and died. The paramedic thought that the patient was simply intoxicated. The court found that the failure of the paramedic to provide "even a scant amount of care" was an "extreme departure from the standard of care for a paramedic in such a situation." Governmental immunity therefore did not shield the defendant from liability in this state court ruling, because the conduct was deemed grossly negligent. Although the medical director was not implicated in *Wright,* the case exemplifies how direct medical oversight might have averted a death and a costly lawsuit.

The medical director should evaluate the substance of the prehospital provider's radio report when any request is made for a nontransport disposition. Although the prehospital provider has the best direct view of the patient's situation, the direct medical oversight physician may have the medical expertise to evaluate the complications or implications of the patient's signs and symptoms; therefore, the need for consultation and careful supervision is certainly warranted. The medical director should also carefully monitor radio contacts and ensure that all physicians providing direct medical oversight know the protocols for nontransport situations.

An example is provided in *Green v. City of Dallas,* which involved paramedics who failed to transport a 35-year-old male patient complaining of chest pain.[114] Because of the patient's age, the fact that he was on no medications, and the observation that he was exhausted from playing basketball, the paramedics reasoned that the pain was not cardiac in nature. Five minutes after the crew departed the man arrested; the ambulance was sent back to the scene, but the man could not be resuscitated. The city avoided liability only through sovereign immunity.

The decision in *Hialeah v. Weatherford* demonstrates that the time between the EMS contact with the patient and patient demise need not be brief to establish proximate cause.[115] In this case, the patient died 24 hours after the ambulance crew left. The patient's wife had called for assistance; the prehospital providers observed her husband lying naked and stuporous when the ambulance arrived. The ambulance crew refused to transport the man, despite his wife's requests. The patient was transported 24 hours later when his wife again called for an ambulance; he died shortly afterward. The court held that there was sufficient evidence of proximate cause between the failure of the first crew to transport and his death more than 24 hours later, notwithstanding the wife's delay in requesting an ambulance the second time.

A delay of transport due to prolonged scene time (20 minutes for someone with chest pain) was determined to be a cause of loss of a decedent's chance of survival and resulted in a jury award of damages against the paramedics involved in a case from Louisiana.[116]

Patient Refusal

Sometimes a patient adamantly refuses transport, although the EMS crew feels transport is necessary. These cases are troubling for the prehospital providers who feel that it is in the patient's best interest to receive medical care. In addition, some prehospital providers have been instructed by medical directors who would rather take the risk of forced transport than leave an injured patient. Therefore, transport is accomplished so a physician can evaluate the patient and establish informed refusal in the controlled setting of the ED. It can be argued that transport is warranted because the patient is unable to give informed refusal if, for example, circumstances or injuries appear to impair their ability to comprehend the risks and consequences of refusal. On the other hand, an adult of "sound mind" is allowed to refuse medical treatment; patients have the right to make medical treatment decisions that may result in deterioration and even death.[117]

Often a friend or relative has summoned the ambulance and wants the patient transported. Liability claims may still be argued against the EMS agency. In *St. George v. City of Deerfield Beach* an ambulance was summoned by a visitor of a man found bleeding extensively from a tooth extraction.[118] The paramedics failed to transport the man who was "obviously drunk and bleeding, but he absolutely and continually refused examination or treatment." The visitor called 9-1-1 a second time about 20 minutes later, but the dispatcher refused to send an ambulance. The appellate court rejected the defendant's motion to dismiss, ruling that sovereign immunity did not apply. Additionally, the court determined that the service owed a "special duty" toward the patient based on the repeated phone calls (*vide supra*).

An interesting area of patient refusal arises in the context of children. Some states possess specific statutes which allow consent for medical treatment, and therefore refusal, to individuals as young as 14, but they often poise a dilemma.[119] Frequently, ambulances are dispatched for a minor driver involved in an MVA who does not need, nor want, transport. It is important to have protocols in place to deal with this situation.

TRANSPORT AGAINST WILL. Transport against the patient's express desires, particularly if restraints are used, may constitute false imprisonment. The pivotal issue is whether the detention of the patient is justified under the circumstances.[120] There is some legal authority for a physician to forcibly restrain a person in need of treatment by virtue of a qualified privilege.[121] In any event, deprivation of a person's liberty is always a serious and risky matter.

The big area where a flurry of lawsuits have occurred has been in the area of deaths from individuals who have been restrained. These "in-custody death" cases have mushroomed in recent years and are often coupled with civil rights claims.[122] These will require services to closely scrutinize any restraint policies they may use.

A few states have statutes that provide legal authority for peace officers to direct EMS personnel to take a person to a hospital, if it reasonably appears that medical treatment is needed. Such statutes usually require the peace officer or transporting personnel to act in "good faith" to gain the protections of immunity.[123] In other states, the statute may allow EMS personnel this authority on their own. New Mexico allows transport upon a "good faith judgment" by the EMS provider that it is needed.[124] These types of statutes provide both authority and legal protection in the unwilling transport situation; however, medical oversight is no less important and may be evidence of "good faith." The medical director must understand the circumstances under which such laws may be used. Consultation with local law enforcement may be vital for the effective application of protective custody efforts. Immunity was not available for paramedics who forcibly took an allegedly suicidal patient to a Wyoming hospital against her will, although they were acting under the state's valid emergency detention statute.[125] The "reasonableness" of their actions, carrying the patient, naked, uncovered, and handcuffed, to the ambulance, was left for the jury to decide. In a similar circumstance, the city of Louisville was forced, after an unsuccessful appeal, to go to trial to determine if their actions of transporting a patient to the hospital and inserting an IV against her will constituted false imprisonment and battery.[126]

Many EMS agencies and medical directors require that the provider contact direct medical oversight in every patient refusal encounter. This is useful only if the quality of the contact is not superficial. The EMS provider must be thorough, accurate, and honest in their report to the physician. The physician must be diligent in listening, questioning, and evaluating the soundness of the information. The medical director must tailor the protocol for patient refusals according to the EMS system and the prehospital providers' skill and experience. Quality supervision by a medical director thereby diminishes claims of negligent failure to transport or patient abandonment.

DOCUMENTATION OF THE REFUSAL. Careful patient assessment and instructions or advice regarding refusal of treatment must be documented. The documentation on the prehospital care report (PCR) should unequivocally demonstrate an assessment adequate for an informed decision regarding the need for transport. Liability might arise for the medical director who fails to review retrospectively cases of nontransport or patient refusal to identify deficiencies in assessments or information provided to patients.

The use of releases, waivers, or other such documents that the patient signs in the field has limited legal merit for several reasons. First, courts frown on documents that attempt to deprive a person of recourse to the courts through such language as "release of liability." Therefore as a matter of public policy, these documents are construed against the party placing them in use. Some state court rulings have rejected the medical professional's efforts to contract away potential liability for negligent medical treatment.[127] Release from liability for negligent care has also been rejected when the patient has little choice in where these services may be obtained.[128] Many of these forms are written in nearly incomprehensible legalese, which further invalidates their use. Therefore documents purporting to relieve the prehospital provider from liability might be invalid. Second, "promise not to sue" language in these documents does not preclude the necessity of obtaining an "informed refusal" of treatment and transport from the patient.

Obtaining a patient signature may be beneficial for simply demonstrating the patient's physical and cognitive abilities. Such a document may be appropriate if used as a written acknowledgment by patients of their voluntary refusal of treatment. It may serve as a testimonial of the efforts made to educate and persuade the patient to be transported. However, such forms should be supplemented with appropriate documentation of the patient's physical and mental condition as assessed by the prehospital provider. The document should reflect attempts to warn the patient of the risks of delaying treatment and alert the patient that the prehospital provider may not be aware of the full extent of the injuries.[129] The medical director should not permit a release form to be used until it has been evaluated by legal counsel. Well reviewed forms may be available from the insurance agency that provides liability coverage for the ambulance service.

Management of Nontransport Calls

1. The medical director must understand that these are potentially the area of greatest exposure and liability for a service, and the medical director.

2. The medical director should have an accurate understanding of local and state laws regarding patient rights, and the circumstances, if any, under which a physician may authorize or direct treatment and transport without the consent of the patient.

3. The medical director must ensure adequate training is provided to prehospital providers on specific techniques for evaluating mental status in the field.

4. Protocols should be guided by optimum patient care, rather than economic benefit to any entity.

5. Protocols must be appropriate for the prehospital providers' respective skill and experience levels, and should be reviewed periodically by the medical director and altered as needed.

6. Contact with direct medical oversight, if not required, should be encouraged in all cases in which a patient is not transported. Moreover, contact with direct medical oversight should not be an empty formality; it should be a true consultation.

7. Ongoing review and audit of radio reports, prehospital care reports (PCRs), and follow-up patient contact to evaluate the quality of field releases and patient refusals are imperative.

8. All use of restraints and any transport against a patient's will should be reviewed by the medical director.

9. A review by competent legal counsel of the release form is recommended, and if the release form used by the EMS agency is of questionable legal merit, then the medical director should prohibit its use.

FIGURE 32.1

Transfers

Interhospital transfers have evolved as one of the more lucrative profit centers for ambulance services. Transfers generally mean non-emergent use of ambulances; for many prehospital providers these patient contacts seem less exciting and less deserving of their medical skills. For example, these calls could include the "routine transfer" of a debilitated nursing home patient to and from a clinic appointment, a neonate in an incubator, or the cardiac patient with multiple intravenous lines infusing medications. Obviously, transfers can be as diverse and critical as 9-1-1 calls, and clearly require the attention of a medical director.[130]

A variety of problems can arise in the management of transfers. For example, the "transfer car" may be staffed with less experienced personnel, which can create patient risk should the unexpected occur. In addition, research shows that physicians may fail to use the appropriate level of skill for the patient's medical condition and, more importantly, fail to stabilize patients adequately before transport.[131] Transfers are often initiated by persons unfamiliar with EMS systems and ambulance service management. Transfer orders are often written by physicians who are unaware of current scopes of practice of the transporting personnel. This is evidenced by the requesting party directing the non-emergent response of the ambulance; it is also evident in the reimbursement problems that arise when the transport destination is based on physician convenience. Transfers can also be a source of liability for physicians and hospitals if a patient is unnecessarily put at risk because of the transfer. Efforts to decrease transport problems have led to the creation of patient transfer guidelines by certain critical care organizations, medical directors should ensure that their protocols are consistent with these.[132]

The case of *Morena v. South Hills Health System* involved the limited paramedic resources of the City of Pittsburgh.[133] One issue of the case was whether paramedics were negligent in not accepting an interhospital transfer of a gunshot victim. The paramedics had responded and transported the patient to the nearest hospital. The patient then required transport to another facility where a trauma surgeon awaited. At that time, the City of Pittsburgh had only four paramedic ambulances for emergencies; private ambulances handled non-emergent interhospital transports. A nurse asked the paramedics to handle the transfer, but she did not explain that the transfer was an emergency that the unit was authorized to accept. Consequently, according to the protocols the paramedics declined the transfer; the surgical treatment had to be delayed until the transfer was ultimately completed. "Due to this shortage of vehicles it was the policy of the service to not make interhospital transfers," the court noted. The court deferred to the policy and held that the duty of the emergency ambulance service was completed upon transporting the patient to the nearest facility; absent knowledge that the transfer was of an emergent nature, there was no basis for negligence in the paramedics' refusal to accept the transfer. The message from this is that ambulances in an EMS system should not be used or viewed as an unlimited resource, and sound policies are defensible.

With the enactment of federal legislation that regulates interhospital transfer of patients in COBRA, planning and preparation for transfers became serious business.[134] The law may actually protect prehospital providers from being "dumped on," as well as create more paperwork for EDs. COBRA only pertains to the transfer of "unstable" patients and mandates that any transfer be "effected through qualified personnel and required transportation equipment."[135] The law may also affect destination policies, because the patient must be transported to a qualified facility. The law can impose significant burdens on small ambulance services, which the medical director should attempt to limit. For example, in rural systems the need to transport an unstable patient to a higher level of care may be valid. However, the service may have only minimally trained personnel available and a limited number of ambulances. Nonetheless, "qualified personnel and transportation equipment" must accompany the patient. It becomes imperative that the medical director educate hospital staff about the transport capabilities of the ambulance service for transfers. The medical director should also be careful that "convenience transfers" do not misuse ambulance resources, exposing the rest of the EMS system to risk. Additionally, political and economic decisions should not dictate the movement of patients. One court considered it egregious to refuse ambulance service to a patient because of political interests. A hospital that refused to allow use of its ambulance unless the patient was brought to its facility (where the patient's attending physician did not have privileges) supported a verdict for outrageous conduct in *DeCicco v. Trinidad Area Health Association*.[136]

The medical director must vigilantly ensure that an ambulance service accept transfers only if adequately trained crews are available. This may entail careful examination of individual skills and prospective identification of specific medications that the prehospital provider may monitor. He must also keep the Medicare reimbursement regulations on staffing levels in mind. In addition, there may be need for cooperative arrangements between the hospital nursing staff who accompany the patient in the ambulance and the ambulance personnel. The respective responsibilities of nursing personnel and the EMS crew should be clarified before transports are initiated. There should be no question of responsibilities in the back of a moving ambulance with a critical patient dependent on the attendant care givers assigned to the transfer.

Ambulance services have also come under increased scrutiny in recent years from government efforts to stem fraud and abuse. Many services have found themselves liable for large fines when they have submitted bills to Medicare for ambulance transfer of patients from home to dialysis centers when the patients were ambulatory and could have traveled by van or taxi. For example, in a recent case, the former owners of an ambulance company agreed to pay $2.25 million in damages and penalties for fraudulent ambulance claims submitted to Medicare and Medicaid after they had been found guilty of fraud in earlier criminal proceedings.[137]

Documentation

Paperwork has been the bane of existence for many medical professionals otherwise skilled in the provision of patient care. Training in this critical area has been largely overlooked, and improvement has been dependent on retrospective audits. Poor documentation has persisted, and prehospital providers tend to believe that prehospital care reports (PCRs) are either an insignificant part of the medical record or routinely ignored by hospital healthcare providers. Lack of immediate feedback and tolerance of poor report writing by emergency department staff and medical directors undermine documentation efforts. Documentation is one of the first things reviewed by plaintiff attorneys, and sloppy illegible PCRs reflect poorly on the service, regardless of the quality of care delivered, when made four feet tall and placed before a jury.

The PCR is a measure of accountability for the EMS provider, just as the medical record substantiates the hospital healthcare providers' patient care. The PCR should reflect the quality of patient care and assessment. Adherence to protocols should be evident in the PCR. Although the medical director

may audit every PCR to monitor their emergency care performance, lower-level EMTs have less training and are often less experienced both in patient care and documentation. Therefore their PCRs warrant greater efforts toward improvement of report writing skills. Many medical directors supervise providers who run just a few calls each month; thus, each PCR should be reviewed and used as an opportunity for improvement.

The PCR has another important function. It documents the severity of the patient's illness as a justification for reimbursement. Any exaggeration of a patient's condition done in order to increase the reimbursement for that patient transfer may be fraud; and if the PCR is submitted to the federal government for payment of a Medicare claim, it may be Medicare fraud and abuse, a violation of the false claims act, or both.[138,139] The former is investigated by the Office of the Inspector General of Health and Human Services, the latter by the Department of Justice. A medical director's approval of a fraudulent PCR many implicate him in the violation.

Patience and persistence by the medical director can lead to improved PCR preparation and patient care. The medical director should develop useful PCR formats and discourage forms that impede quality documentation. Every PCR should address unique aspects such as scene factors or observations, patient positioning when first encountered, the apparent mechanism of injury, scene interventions, and extrication difficulties. Documentation of responses to interventions, justifications for interventions or for failures to treat, and the condition of a patient upon arrival at the emergency department are also important on the PCR. The medical director should take a proactive role in the quality management efforts of documentation.

Finally, legibility remains a critical factor in the usefulness of documentation. The medical director should insist on legible PCRs; only if the information in the PCR is legible can it be useful to subsequent healthcare providers, quality improvement efforts, and possible legal proceedings. New computer-based paperless systems may help improve PCRs by providing a standard legible report format as well as creating a data base for the service.[140]

Equipment

To some degree the skills and capabilities of EMS providers have been confounded by equipment or more precisely the compulsion to employ equipment in the "technical imperative."[141] The issue of proper equipment and procedures in EMS is compounded by the lack of significant evidence-based research on what works—many policies and procedures are, unfortunately, anecdote-based. From the insistence to dispatch a helicopter when rational assessment would obviate the expense and expedite patient care, to the forceful plunge of a 14-gauge angiocath when an 18-gauge would suffice, the use and abuse of medical equipment has been an implicating factor in many claims and lawsuits. Aided by the use of poorly drafted treatment protocols, the technical imperative has caused endotracheal tubes to be forcefully pushed into airways rather than deferring to oropharyngeal airway and bag valve mask ventilation. Although there is some evidence that surgical cricothyrotomy may have some efficacy in the field, there is still a concern that this procedure may be over used.[142,143] Besides being more risky for the patient, the use of advanced skills often contributes to precious time being consumed on-scene where rapid transport of a trauma patient is actually warranted. Medical directors should be the source of authority for the use of equipment, procedures, and protocols because they will be responsible for the consequences attributable to misuse of equipment.

At least one court has ruled that the equipment that is carried on an ambulance and used in patient care is a matter of "medical judgment."[144] The medical director should impress on providers that new equipment, as well as skills, must have a demonstrated capability to improve patient care to be implemented. There is an aphorism that may be appropriate: "Be neither the first nor the last to use a new medication or procedure." Medical directors should consider the legal protective measures listed in Figure 32.2 below for equipment usage by the personnel under their supervision.

Contracts

The role of the medical director is complex and demanding. The physician newly recruited as a medical director can benefit from predecessors and peers. One of the lessons to be learned is that accepting a position of responsibility for an EMS system and all patient care rendered within that system should be preceded by a frank and detailed discussion of everyone's roles and responsibilities. The job is more manageable if medical directors have clear and unequivocal authority to accomplish the tasks with which they are charged. A contract in which the medical direc-

Equipment Usage Protective Measures

1. Exercise authority in the selection and implementation of equipment such as defibrillators, drugs, and restraints.
2. Require skills check-off with new equipment and procedures through direct observation of each EMS provider to ensure proper use. Ensure their continuing skills by field observations or regular testing.
3. Implement clear, concise protocols that facilitate appropriate use of the equipment, and review the protocols periodically.
4. Remove hazardous or ineffective equipment and outdated skills from use or disallow their use if problems are not corrected.

FIGURE 32.2

tor's responsibilities and authority are delineated and agreed on is not an unreasonable formality; it is simple sound business practice.

Medical directors must acknowledge the fact that they are accountable regardless of how much time they devote to medical oversight and regardless of the number of field personnel practicing under their license. Medical directors must also realize the risks, the means, and the goals of the position and not hesitate to address these factors before accepting the position. Moreover, accepting the responsibility without any authority is an invitation for frustration, as well as risk. It is important to also recognize limitations that exist in the EMS system and negotiate the means and resources necessary to meet the goals of the job. For example, medical directors may insist that the fire department assume certain responsibilities in training and documentation and that practice restrictions invoked by the medical director be honored. They might insist that a coordinator position be established or equipment upgrades be made. If a private ambulance service has a contract with a city and has promised certain response times or other guarantees, potential medical directors must evaluate whether they can accept the constraints of that performance contract before they become the medical director for the ambulance service.

It is likely that the medical director has implied authority to impose certain restrictions and standards despite the absence of a formal written contract; he may accomplish some goals by using written protocols or establishing a quality improvement program with performance standards. In most states, medical directors extend their medical license to EMS providers as physician extenders, at least at the paramedic level. Inherent in that extension is the authority to exercise medical judgment in matters including who can function under their license. This was recognized in *County of Hennepin v. Hennepin County Association of Paramedics and Emergency Medical Technicians*. A state court ruled it a matter of medical judgment for medical directors to determine who can function under their license; the employer or the paramedic union could not force the medical director to accept a paramedic the medical director felt was incapable of practicing with reasonable skill and safety.[145]

Although many physicians have malpractice insurance coverage that may extend to certain of their activities as a medical director, they are unlikely to have coverage for all potential liabilities. Many of the insurance companies that provide insurance to ambulance services have begun offering secondary insurance policies that cover a physician for potential liabilities that may arise from his duties as a medical director.[146] Secondary insurance policies step in only when the primary insurance, usually malpractice, does not cover an event, or the policy limits of the primary policy have been exhausted. This is in the interest of the insurance companies who know that having a medical director will improve the quality of the service rendered by the ambulance service and therefore reduce insurance claims. If this si not available, the medical director needs to find a source that will protect him for these duties which are often classified as administrative, rather than the usual patient care, duties.

There is no standard contract, but there are certain minimum issues any contractual arrangement should address and are listed in Figure 32.3. Prospective medical directors should carefully scrutinize the EMS agencies' strengths and weaknesses, the political tone and community support for EMS, and other factors that may effect their goals. The detail and complexity of the contract will differ if it is an understanding between the medical director and each EMS provider rather than between the medical director and the county commissioners or a municipality.

The substance of the contract may differ, depending on the agencies, the patient populations, the training and staffing of the prehospital providers, and the different needs for immediate and long-range goals for quality improvement measures. The medical director's role must be formalized, because many systems consist of multiple management heads with

---

Minimum Provisions of Contracts

1. Responsibilities of both parties must be clearly delineated. For example, the medical director likely will be responsible for creating protocols, and the service agency is responsible for distribution of protocols to all prehospital providers.
2. The authority to fulfill the responsibilities must be provided. For example, the medical director should be allowed to impose education requirements and practice restrictions on any EMS provider who demonstrates inadequate performance. His position in the chain of command must be made clear—the medical director is in charge of anything which affects patient care.
3. The medical director should have a clear understanding of the person or entity to whom he is responsible. At the same time, it must be understood that the medical director is at all times a patient advocate.
4. The terms of payment, duration of the contractual arrangement, and the recourse for nonperformance by either party should be delineated.
5. The details of insurance coverage for the medical director should be provided.
6. The medical director must have the authority to participate in all aspects of the EMS system that affect patient care including dispatching, information about all patient complaints, equipment selection, and review of all contracts that may impact the medical director's responsibilities.

FIGURE 32.3

decision-making authority spread amongst fire chiefs, company owners, city managers, and medical directors. Medical directors must identify the correct party or parties with whom they must negotiate. A contract with the city health department may be meaningless if the city fire department chief has unbridled discretion regarding who is hired, what level of providers are dispatched to certain medical emergencies, and whether attendance at continuing education sessions is mandatory.

Summary

The role of the medical oversight physician is complex and time-consuming. It is a mixture of medicine, law, administration, public relations, and engineering. Careful delegation of tasks to field coordinators and hospital staff alleviates the burden quantitatively but does not lessen the physician's responsibility qualitatively. The benefit of interactions with field personnel is not merely for risk management. Medical directors who exercise and practice meaningful medical oversight gain by knowing their system and its people, understanding its operations, and participating in its improvement. Passivity or acts of omission such as failure to provide protocols, failure to discipline, or failure to implement quality management audits place medical directors at great legal risk, and deprive prehospital providers and the community of the expertise and leadership which good medical oversight should provide. Medical oversight is seldom hazardous unless the medical director serves only by signature. The days of passive and uninformed medical oversight are hopefully passing. Risks arise when the EMS physician fails to keep informed of accepted standards of prehospital medical practice, confuses politics or economics with good patient care, and acquiesces to inappropriate or inept actions by EMS providers. Through development of system-wide protocols, quality management systems, and personnel policies, the medical director should be secure.

Legal hazards and pitfalls are nothing new to the emergency physician, who is constantly presented with the unexpected, vagaries of caring for strangers, community pressures, and unrecognized sacrifices. The delivery of prehospital medicine is as complex and uncertain as emergency medicine, perhaps more so. Despite the medically and legally uncharted territories in prehospital care, the apparent variations and questions of duty in all aspects of medical oversight rely on the basic principles of medical practice—paramount concern for patient care and professionalism in the delivery of health care. The EMS medical director has a unique opportunity to serve innumerable patients, prehospital providers, and EMS systems in a challenging and evolving arena.

References

1. Policy Statement, American College of Emergency Physicians—Medical Direction of Emergency Medical Services. *Ann Emerg Med.* 1998;31(1):152. *All aspects of the organization and provision of emergency medical services require the active involvement and participation of physicians.*
2. *The Ambulance in American Cities* (editorial). *J. American Medical Assoc.* 1987;28:36–37.
3. *Kowalski v. Gratopp,* 442 N.W.2d 682, 1989.
4. Page I. *The Paramedics.* Morristown, PA: Backdraft Publications; 1979
5. *Highway Safety Program Standard Number 11: Emergency Medical Services.* 23 CFR 1205.4, Nov 14, 1968.
6. Norris JA. Current status and utility of emergency medical care liability law. *Forum.* 1980;15:377–405.
7. *Anderson v. Little & Davenport,* 251 S.E.2d 250, 1978.
8. *Harris v. Forklift Systems Inc.,* 114 S. Ct. 367 (1993). Reviewed in: Flaherty M, Shoemaker D. Supreme court eases proof for sexual harassment cases. *EMS Insider.* 1994;21(1):2–3 and Stecklel MH. New sexual harassment concerns. *EMS Insider.* 1998;28(10):2.
9. The pertinent part of the False Claims Act (31 USC 3730) reads: *Any person who—(1) knowingly presents, or causes to be presented, to an officer or employee of the United States Government or a member of the Armed Forces of the United States a false or fraudulent claim for payment or approval; (2) knowingly makes, uses, or causes to be made or used, a false record or statement to get a false or fraudulent claim paid or approved by the Government; (3) conspires to defraud the Government by getting a false or fraudulent claim allowed or paid; . . . is liable to the United States Government for a civil penalty of not less than $5,000 and not more than $10,000, plus 3 times the amount of damages which the Government sustains because of the act of that person.*
10. The pertinent part of the Medicare law dealing with fraud (42 USC 1320a) reads: *Any person (including an organization, agency, or other entity, but excluding a beneficiary, as defined in subsection (i)(5) of this section) that —(1) presents or causes to be presented to an officer, employee, or agent of the United States, or of any department or agency thereof, or of any State agency, a claim that the Secretary determines—(A) is for a medical or other item or service that the person knows or should know was not provided as claimed, (B) is for a medical or other item or service and the person knows or should know the claim is false or fraudulent, . . . shall be subject, in addition to any other penalties that may be prescribed by law, to a civil money penalty of not more than $2,000 for each item or service. In addition, such a person shall be subject to an assessment of not more than twice the amount claimed for each such item or service in lieu of damages sustained by the United States or a State agency because of such claim. In addition the Secretary may make a determination in the same proceeding to exclude the person from participation in the programs under subchapter XVIII of this chapter and to direct the appropriate State agency to exclude the person from participation in any State health care program.*
11. Federal Register: September 12, 2000, 65(177):55077–55100 As this chapter goes to press, negotiations are continuing between HCFA and representatives of the EMS community regarding the details of this issue.
12. *Federal Register.* January 25, 1999; 64(15):3637–3650.
13. *Federal Register.* December 28, 2000; 65(250):82461–82829.
14. The full statute reads: *Every person who, under color of any statute, ordinance, regulation, custom, or usage, of any State or Territory or the District of Columbia, subjects, or causes to be subjected, any citizen of the United States or other person within the jurisdiction thereof to the deprivation of any rights, privileges, or immunities secured by the Constitution and laws, shall be liable to the party injured in an action at law, suit in equity, or other proper proceeding for redress.*

15. 729 F. Supp 376, 1990.
16. 826 F.2d 1030, 1987.
17. 764 F. Supp 1510, 1991.
18. *Atwater v. Caruana,* United States District Court of the District of New Mexico, No. CIV 96-1218JP. The case was settled before a decision was made by a judge on the merits of the action.
19. 29 U.S.C. § 2601.
20. *Hagan v. Anderson et al.,* Anderson Circuit Court, Commonwealth of Kentucky, No. 98-CI-00259, complaint filed 23 October 1998.
21. *Hagan v. Anderson,* United States District Court for the Eastern District of Kentucky, No. 99-11, filed August 3rd, 2000.
22. 29 U.S.C. § 706(8)(D).
23. See, for example, Wydro GC, et al. Legislative and regulatory description of EMS medical direction: a survey of states. *Prehosp Emerg Care.* 1997;1(4):233–237.
24. Florida Public Health Law 401.265.
25. Board of Medical Examiners. Oregon administrative rule 847-35-025.
26. Washington statute RCW 18.71, WAC 246-976920, revised 1990.
27. Board of Medical Examiners. Oregon administrative rule, Ambulances and Emergency Medical Personnel, 847-35-020(2).
28. Missouri Rule, 19 CSR 30-40.160, updated Feb 25, 1995. A requirement for Pediatric Advanced Life Support is pending.
29. NAEMSP provides a 7-hour course at least twice yearly.
30. § 9.3.2, 7 NMAC 27.3, Medical Direction for Emergency Medical Services, 1996.
31. 1977 US Department of Health, Education and Welfare Report, Credentialing Health Manpower.
32. *Fullmer v. USA,* U.S. 10th Circuit Court of Appeals, No. 97-4136, http://laws.findlaw.com/10th/974136.html.
33. *Murphy v. Board of Medical Examiners of the State of Arizona (BOMEX),* 95-0327 and 1 CA-CV 95-0182 (Consolidated), filed 7-15-97. Arizona Supreme Court denied cert.
34. It is available on their website: <http://www.naemsp.org/>
35. For example, Washington, RCW 18.71.215 provides that: *The Department of Health shall defend and hold harmless any approved medical program director, delegate, or agent, including, but not limited to, hospitals and hospital personnel in their capacity of training EMS personnel for certification or recertification, provided that their acts or omissions were committed in good faith in the performance of their duties.*
36. A review of immunities is available at 16 ALR5th 605, Liability for Negligence of Ambulance Attendants, Emergency Medical Technicians, and the Like, Rendering Emergency Medical Care Outside Hospital.
37. See, for example *Malone v. City of Seattle,* 600 P.2d 647, 1979.
38. *Marthaller v. Kings County Hospital,* Court of Appeals of the State of Washington, No. 41288-4-I, filed 29 March 1999.
39. *Sadler v. New Castle County,* 524 A.2d 18, 1987.
40. *McIver and Gentry v. Smith and Forsyth County,* North Carolina Court of Appeals, No. COA98-1039, filed 17 August 1999 (slip opinion).
41. *Mooney v. Sneed,* Supreme Court of Tennessee, No. W1997-00089-SC-R11-CV, filed October 13, 2000.
42. Tenn. Code Ann. § 29-20-310(b) (Supp. 1999).
43. 28 U.S.C. §1326 allows *claims against the United States, for money damages, accruing on and after January 1, 1945, for injury or loss of property, or personal injury or death caused by the negligent or wrongful act or omission of any employee of the Government while acting within the scope of his office or employment, under circumstances where the United States, if a private person, would be liable to the claimant in accordance with the law of the place where the act or omission occurred.*
44. 28 U.S.C. § 2680.
45. *Fang v. U.S.,* U.S. 9th Circuit Court of Appeals, March 31, 1998, http://laws.findlaw.com/9th/9656800.html.
46. Frey V. The scope of Good Samaritan legislation. *Medical Trial Technique Quarterly.* 1994;40:159–169.
47. Arizona, for example, in *Guerrero v. Copper Queen Hospital,* 537 P.2d 1329, 1975.
48. California, for example, in *McKenna v. Cedars of Lebanon Hospital,* 155 Cal.Rptr. 631, 1979.
49. Alabama, Colorado, Georgia, Utah, Washington, and Wyoming. Frey V. The scope of Good Samaritan legislation. *Medical Trial Technique Quarterly.* 1994;40:169.
50. For example Arizona, Ariz Rev Stat Ann § 32-1471, provides that: *Any health care provider licensed or certified to practice as such in this state or elsewhere, or a licensed ambulance attendant, driver or pilot as defined in § 41-1831, or any other person who renders emergency care at a public gathering or at the scene of an emergency occurrence gratuitously and in good faith shall not be liable for any civil or other damages as a result of any act or failure to act to provide or arrange for further medical treatment or care for the injured persons, unless such person, while rendering such emergency care, is guilty of gross negligence.*
51. American College of Emergency Physicians. Good Samaritan protection. *Ann Emerg Med.* 2000;635–640.
52. *Chase v. Mayor and City Council of Baltimore,* May 26, 1999, No. 677, Court of Special Appeals of Maryland. See also Fogelson RJ. Legal immunity dwindles for EMS providers. *EMS Insider.* 1999;26(10):6.
53. *Mayor and City Council of Baltimore, et al. v. Sharon E. Chase,* July 27, 2000, No. 77, Court of Appeals of Maryland.
54. Public Law 105-170 §5(b). This includes "any person who is licensed, certified, or otherwise qualified to provide medical care in a State, including a physician, nurse, physician assistant, paramedic, and emergency medical technician."
55. *Tallahassee Regional Medical Center, Inc. v. Meeks,* 543 So.2d 770, 1989.
56. *Tallahassee Regional Medical Center, Inc. v. Meeks,* 560 So.2d 778, 1991.
57. Gore CL. A physician's liability for mistakes of a physician assistant. *J. Legal Medicine.* 2000; 21(1):125–142.

58. *Mozingo v. Pitt County Memorial Hospital*, 415 S.E.2d 341, 347 (N.C. Sup. Ct. 1992).

59. *Mozingo v. Pitt County Memorial Hospital*, 415 S.E.2d 341 (N.C. Sup. Ct. 1992) For a good review of this case, see Sharon M. Glenn, *Liability in the Absence of a Traditional Physician-Patient Relationship: What Every "On Call" Doctor Should Know: Mozingo v. Pitt County Memorial Hospital*, 28 Wake Forest L. Rev. 747 (1993).

60. *Rivera v. Prince George's County Health Department*, 649 A.2d 1212 (Md. App. 1994) and Sharon M. Glenn, *Liability in the Absence of a Traditional Physician-Patient Relationship: What Every "On Call" Doctor Should Know: Mozingo v. Pitt County Memorial Hospital*, 28 Wake Forest L. Rev. 747 (1993).

61. *Millard v. Corrado*, Missouri Court of Appeals Eastern District, No. ED75420, Filed 14 December 1999 (slip opinion).

62. *Diggs V. Arizona Cardiologists, Ltd.*, Arizona Court of Appeals Division 1, 1 CA-CV 99-0508, filed August 8th, 2000.

63. 464 A.2d 578, 1990.

64 *Falkowski v. Maurus*, 637 So. 2d 522, 1993.

65. Holder AR. *Medical Malpractice Law*, 2nd ed. New York: John Wiley & Sons; 1978.

66. *Tonsic v. Wagner*, 329 A.2d 497, 1974.

67. Reviewed in Furrow BR, et al. *Health Law*. St. Paul: West Publishing Co., 1995 (7):2.

68. *Ramirez v. University of Miami*, 1999 Fla. App. Lexis 10731; 24 Fla. Law W. D 1871.

69. *De Long v. County of Erie*, 457 N.E.2d 717, 1983.

70. *Johnson v. District of Columbia*, 580 A.2d 141, 1990.

71. *Cuffy v. City of New York*, 513 N.Y.S.2d 372, 1987.

72. *Wanzer v. District of Columbia*, 580 A.2D 127, 1990.

73. *St. George v. City of Deerfield Beach*, 568 So.2d 931, 1990.

74. *Schear v. Board of County Commissioners*, 687 P.2d 728, 1984.

75. *American National Bank & Trust Co. of Chicago v. The City of Chicago*, No. 1-97-1212, Appellate Court of Illinois, First Judicial District, filed 24 July 1998.

76. *American National Bank & Trust Co. of Chicago v. The City of Chicago*, Docket No. 86215-Agenda 14-November 1999, Supreme Court of Illinois, filed August 10, 2000.

77. *Estate of Morgan v. Mayor and City Council of Hampton, Virginia*, 1996 U.S. Dist. Lexis 519 (E. D. Va.)

78. Ibid., footnote 5, quoting *Jackson v. Byrne*, 738 F.2d at 1446.

79. *Cooper v. City of Honolulu*, 1st Cir. Ct. (Haw. 1992).

80. Harvey AL, et al. Actual vs. perceived EMS response time. *Prehosp Emerg Care*. 1999;3(1):11–14.

81. Steve Forry, VFIS/AIS, personal communication.

82. Whiting JD, et al. EMT knowledge of ambulance traffic laws. *Prehosp Emerg Care*. 1998;2(2):136–140.

83. 475 A.2d 1319, 1985.

84. *Overman v. Occoquan, Woodbridge, Lorton Volunteer Fire Department*, District Court, 90-42A, 1990.

85. 447 A.2d 860, 1989.

86. *Malcom v. City of East Detroit*, 468 N.W.2d 479, 1991.

87. *Otero v. City of Albuquerque, et al.* CV 94-10501, Second Judicial District Court, County of Bernalillo, New Mexico. The case is on appeal.

88. 29 CRF §§ 1910.120 and 1926.25.

89. Chapter 6.1, 1992.

90. *Borrego v. City of El Paso*, TC# 92-10222, County Court at Law No. 4, El Paso County, Texas. The Texas Supreme Court denied cert.

91. USFA/FEMA. *Firefighter Fatalities in the United States in 1997*. 1998:31.

92. *Hospital Authority of Gwinnett County and Gwinnett Ambulance Services Inc v. Jones*, 386 S.E 2d 120, Supreme Court of the State of Georgia, Brief of Appellee, 1989.

93. *Smith v. Medical Center East*, 585 So.2d 1325, 1991.

94. *Johnson v. Univ. Of Chicago*, 982 F.2d 230, 1992.

95. *Davis v. Johns Hopkins Hospital*, 585 A.2d 841, 1991.

96. 42 C.F.R. § 489.249(b) **Comes to the emergency department** *means, with respect to an individual requesting examination or treatment, that the individual is on the hospital property (property includes ambulances owned and operated by the hospital, even if the ambulance is not on hospital grounds). An individual in a nonhospital-owned ambulance on hospital property is considered to have come to the hospital's emergency department. An individual in a nonhospital-owned ambulance off hospital property is not considered to have come to the hospital's emergency department, even if a member of the ambulance staff contacts the hospital by telephone or telemetry communications and informs the hospital that they want to transport the individual to the hospital for examination and treatment. In such situations, the hospital may deny access if it is in "diversionary status," that is, it does not have the staff or facilities to accept any additional emergency patients. If, however, the ambulance staff disregards the hospital's instructions and transports the individual onto hospital property, the individual is considered to have come to the emergency department.*

97. *Arrington v. Wong*, United States Court of Appeals for the Ninth Circuit, Opinion No. 98-17135, Filed January 22, 2001.

98. Selden BS, et al. The "no-patient" run: 2,698 patients evaluated but not transported by paramedics. *Prehosp Disaster Med*. 1991;6(2):135–142.

99. From Handler H: Vice President, The American Agency, 1988, and Forry S: Director of EMS Programs, VFIS/AIS, 1997.

100. Sucov A, et al. The outcome of patients refusing prehospital transportation. *Prehosp Disaster Med*. 1992; 7(4):365–371.

101. Zachariah BS, et al. Follow-up and outcome of patients who decline or are denied transport by EMS. *Prehosp Disaster Med*. 1992;7(4):359–364.

102. Albuquerque providers paid to evaluate: transport unnecessary for reimbursement. *EMS Insider*. 1998; 25(11):8.

103. *Canterbury v. Spence*, 464 F.2d 772, (cert denied 409 US 1064) 1972.

104. *Schloendorf v. Society of New York*, 105 N.E. 92, 1914.

105. *Salazar v. City of Chicago*, 840 F.2d 233, 1991.

106. *Smith v. Medical Center East*, 585 So.2d 1325, 1991.

107. Kaplan K, et al. The clinician's role on competency evaluations. *Gen Hosp Psychiatry*. 1989;11:397–403.

108. Zun L. A survey of the form of the mental status examination administered by emergency physicians. *Ann Emerg Med*. 1986;15:916–922.

109. Abbott JL, Birnbaum G. Current Practices of Emergency Health Service Providers in the Acquisition of Informed Consent. Unpublished data from presentation at ACLM annual meeting, March 2000.

110. *St. John v. Pope*, 901 S.W.2d 420, 1995.

111. Holroyd B, et al. Prehospital patients refusing care. *Ann Emerg Med*. 1988;17:957–963, and Selden BS, et al. Medicolegal documentation of prehospital triage. *Ann Emerg Med*. 1990;19:547–551.

112. 268 A.2d 309, 1990.

113. Ibid.

114. 665 S.W.2d 567, 1984.

115. 466 So.2d 1127, 1985.

116. *Ambrose v. New Orleans Police Department Ambulance Service*, 627 So2d 233, 1993.

117. *Lane v. Candura*, 376 N.E.2d 1232, 1978.

118. 568 So.2d 931, 1990.

119. Reviewed in §19.01[3][c] *Statutes Permitting General Consent to Treatment*, in Treatise on Health Care Law (Matthew Bender, 1996). For example, Alabama allows consent at 14, Oregon at 15, Kansas at 16, etc.

120. *Wideman v. DeKalb County*, 409 A.2d 537, 1991.

121. *Blackman v. Rifkin*, 759 P.2d 54, 1988.

122. W.A. Maggiore, personal communication.

123. Florida statutes, Section 396.072(1), 1979.

124. §24-10B-9.1 NMSA 1978.

125. *Moore v. Wyoming Medical Center*, 825 F.Supp 1531, 1993.

126. *Mistelle Cathey v. City of Louisville, Joseph Schiess, and Lee Schmid*, 1999 Ky. App. LEXIS 108.

127. *Threadgill v. Peabody Coal Co.*, 526 P.2d 676, 1974.

128. *Vasquez v. Board of Regents, State of Florida*, 548 So.2d 251, 1989.

129. Shanaberger CJ. Why releases don't work. *JEMS*. 1988; 13:47–49.

130. Policy Statement, American College of Emergency Physicians—Medical Direction of Interfacility Patient Transfers. *Ann Emerg Med*. 1998;31(1):154.

131. Martin G, et al. Prospective analysis of rural interhospital transfer of injured patients to a referral trauma center. *J Trauma*. 1990;30(8):1014–1019.

132. Guidelines for the transfer of critically ill patients. *Critical Care Med*. 1993;21(6):931–937.

133. 462 A.2d 680, 1983.

134. 42 U.S.C. 1395dd.

135. 42 U.S.C. 1395dd(c)(2).

136. 573 P.2d 559, 1977.

137. *United States v. Gieger*, S.D. Miss, No. 3:97214cvLN, 9/24/98.

138. 42 USC 1320. This states (in part): *Any person (including an organization, agency, or other entity, but excluding a beneficiary, as defined in subsection (i)(5) of this section) that—(1) presents or causes to be presented to an officer, employee, or agent of the United States, or of any department or agency thereof, of any State agency (as defined in subsection (i)(1) of this section), a claim (as defined in subsection (i)(2) of this section) that the Secretary determines— (A) is for a medical or other item or service that the person knows or should know was not provided as claimed, . . . shall be subject, in addition to any other penalties that may be prescribed by law, to a civil money penalty of not more than $2,000 for each item or service (or, in cases under paragraph (3), $15,000 for each individual with respect to whom false or misleading information was given). In addition, such a person shall be subject to an assessment of not more than twice the amount claimed for each such item or service in lieu of damages sustained by the United States or a State agency because of such claim. In addition the Secretary may make a determination in the same proceeding to exclude the person from participation in the programs under subchapter XVIII of this chapter and to direct the appropriate State agency to exclude the person from participation in any State health care program.*

139. 31 USC 3730, which states: *any person that—(2) knowingly makes, uses, or causes to be made or used, a false record or statement to get a false or fraudulent claim paid or approved by the Government; . . . is liable to the United States Government for a civil penalty of not less than $5,000 and not more than $10,000, plus 3 times the amount of damages which the Government sustains because of the act of that person.*

140. Big EMS Systems Go Paperless . . . pen-based computing comes of age. *EMS Insider*. 1998;25(11):1,3–4.

141. Rosen P, et al. The technical imperative: its definition and an application to prehospital care, *Topics Emerg Med*. 1981;79–85.

142. Jacobson LE, et al. Surgical cricothyroidotomy in trauma patients: analysis of its use by paramedics in the field. *J Trauma*. 1996;4(1):15–20.

143. Fortune JB, et al. Efficacy of prehospital surgical cricothyrotomy in trauma patients. *J Trauma*. 1997; 42(5):832–838.

144. *Lyons by Lyons v. Hasbro Industries and Arrow Medical Services*, 509 N.E.2d 702, 1987.

145. *County of Hennepin v. Hennepin County Association of Paramedics and Emergency Medical Technicians*, 464 N.W.2d 578, 1990.

146. Steve Forry, VFIS/AIS, personal communication.

CHAPTER

33

Ethical Issues

James G. Adams, MD

Introduction

EMS providers frequently use ethical skills: when dealing with people who refuse needed care, when dealing with difficult situations near the end of life, when facing issues of confidentiality and conflict.[1] Decisions of high impact are demanded, even though the questions are more than medical or scientific. These are complicated human challenges, and solutions might seem unclear. To ease the route to problem solving, understanding the principles that underpin proper decision-making is required.

Aristotle believed that ethics is a real-world, rough and tumble business. He believed that ethical debate should be undertaken by those on the line, those making the tough decisions. Nowhere is this truer than in out-of-hospital care.[2] This chapter will provide insight into some of the more common ethical dilemmas that occur in the out-of-hospital setting, and provide some debate, along with routes to resolution.

Familiarity with prevailing laws, guidelines, statutes, and regulations is essential, but may be inadequate for many situations. Importantly, the ethical duty of emergency caregivers may exceed the requirements of the law. There is no clear legal obligation to understand patients' concerns or to ease patients' fears, for example. There is no law that requires kindness and compassion. There is no statute that mandates honor and integrity. There is no legal obligation to act with courage. Yet these are the characteristics that have led to the success of the emergency medical system. These qualities, in addition to technical skill, have led the public to trust and respect emergency medical services. Further, the law cannot generally answer ethical dilemmas for us. When a patient refuses care, for example, the person must have sufficient decision-making capacity to do so. The assessment of decision-making capacity is a medical judgment, so ethical and clinical information is key. These ethical decisions must be made quickly, given the limited time available. The EMS providers in the field must have this skill and expertise. Professionalism and ethics are also required in order to maintain high levels of respect, honor, and trust. The public has a high regard for EMS not only because of clinical ability, but because that ability is exercised according to strong ethical standards.

Refusal of Treatment and Transport

Case 1

A 30-year-old male was shot in the left lower abdomen. The paramedics noted a tense, rigid abdomen. The patient refused placement of an IV line and said he did not want to go to the hospital, while intermittently yelling, "The Iceman got me" and thrashing and rolling in obvious discomfort.

DISCUSSION:

Our modern ethical framework emphasizes patient autonomy, which is the ability of the patient to make reasoned decisions regarding his or her own body. It is well accepted that any patient has a right to refuse care, even care that is needed to sustain life and health. Yet this patient's refusal is intuitively illogical to the caregivers because it is made without reason. Despite the strong presumption that patients have the right to refuse care, there are conditions that must be met in order for a person to exercise autonomy. First, the patient must have sufficient information about the medical condition. Second, the person is to understand the risks and benefits of the options. Finally, the person has to be able to use the information to make a decision that is in keeping with their goals, wishes, and values.[3,4,5] This patient meets none of the criteria. The EMS providers on the scene instinctively understood this. They moved him over to the gurney, despite his thrashing, and transported him to the hospital.

The EMS providers confronted an ethical choice between the patient's right to self-determination (autonomy) and their obligation to provide patient care (beneficence). The EMS providers, along with society and the legal system, have an overriding interest in the preservation of life and health. In this scenario, the obligation to attempt to care for the patient must take precedence over the patient's possibly irrational attempt to self-determination. As a general rule, the EMS providers must make every reasonable attempt to provide for the best interest of the patient, limited only by the reasoned wishes of the patient with intact decision-making ability.

As the patient was moved to the gurney, he continued to yell erratically "I was shot," then he would curse. He yelled for everyone to get away from him. Then he would express disbelief by yelling, "no way," and "get out of here." He pulled his arms away whenever the EMS providers attempted to obtain vital signs or place an IV, so these were not accomplished. After the patient was stabilized in the ED, he admitted that he had acted "out of his head."

Case 2

EMS responded to the scene of a woman who fell, hit her head, and appeared to sustain a short period of unconsciousness, according to bystanders. The patient was found to be staggering down the street, refusing any intervention. Her staggering gait made her appear intoxicated. In a nearby locked car, presumably the patient's, needles were evident. The patient adamantly and violently refused care and continued to walk away.

DISCUSSION:

As in the prior case, medical professionals must make determinations of decision-making capacity when a patient refuses important medical care. Did this patient appear to possess sufficient information and understanding to make a reasoned decision? This patient appeared to the EMS providers to lack the capacity to make any form of rational decision. This patient violently and clearly refused treatment and transport, but she fulfilled none of the requirements to indicate that the decision was even minimally informed. Based upon the obligation to promote the health and well-being of the patient, the EMS providers should use reasonable means to safely evaluate this patient. If the potential for violence is great, the police might become involved to assist in restraint and transport of the patient. Commonly, the police will

not become involved unless a crime has been committed. The EMS providers themselves have no ethical obligation to place themselves at risk to accomplish the evaluation. They do, however, have an obligation to do their best to attempt to provide for the safety of this individual. Impatience, frustration, or prejudicial judgments should not interfere with responsible care for the individual.

In general, a direct medical oversight physician (DMOP) should be contacted when a patient's refusal of care could result in harm. When the patient does not appear lucid or is uncooperative, the DMOP can help ensure that maximal safe attempts are made to evaluate and care for the patient, including requesting peace officer assistance. When a patient does have intact decisional capacity, a satisfactory conclusion can often be reached when the DMOP discusses risks of refusal.

It should also be noted that the term "decision-making capacity" is used in this chapter, but not competence. Competence is usually reserved for legal determinations of sanity. This means that the terms "competent" or "incompetent" should not be used to describe patients' cognitive abilities, but "capacity" can be.

It was recognized that this patient had significant impairment in her decisional capacity. The EMS providers were able to engage the patient, who appeared to have no purposeful intent to her wandering. The patient put up modest resistance when confronted. The EMS providers were calm, obviously caring, but firmly told her, "you have to be checked." She was found to be markedly hypoglycemic. The needles in her car were for insulin, which she took without food that morning. After treatment, she was calm, pleasant, and thankful.

Case 3

A 68-year-old man called the paramedics because of crushing substernal chest pain. The medics found him diaphoretic and in acute distress. A single sublingual nitroglycerin provided some relief. He refused to go to the hospital, however, until his wife returned from shopping. He understood that the delay could risk his life.

DISCUSSION:

This patient appeared lucid but also appeared to be making a dangerous decision. He did seem to have sufficient information, understanding, and reasoning. The EMS providers understood that, technically, they could have him sign a refusal and get back into service, but this did not seem right to them. They explored the patient's reasoning in more detail, not necessarily through a legal obligation, but because of their ethical concerns. As the case unfolded, it was discovered that the patient had a large sum of money in the dresser drawer that he wanted to give his wife. He was afraid that his son, who was addicted to drugs, would otherwise take the money. Once this issue was identified, a resolution was achieved as the money was secured for the wife and the patient was transported.

Appropriate care of this patient was facilitated by making the effort to discuss the patient's reasons for refusing care. Given the significant medical concerns, efforts were properly made to explore the patient's reasoning. The EMS providers also might contact medical oversight, or even the patient's family physician or another relative, given the potential seriousness. If the patient has intact decisional capacity, fully understands the risks, and otherwise meets the criteria necessary for an informed refusal, the EMS providers are not to force transport. Legal consultation might be sought when such high-risk non-transports occur, but it is the rare service that has such resources available; however, legal consultants will not make the medical decisions. The medical professionals need the ethical skills and good judgment.

Another challenge must be discussed, namely, how to transport a physically able person who lacks decisional capacity and who also is resisting transport. Although this was not the circumstance in this instance, the problem frequently arises. It is worthy to note that most states have statutory support for the involuntary transport of a person in only three circumstances: (1) patients with psychiatric crisis who are formally declared to lack capacity, (2) those patients with other legal declarations of incompetence, and (3) those patients who have committed a crime. Adherence to these legal guidelines and clear policies is important in order to minimize the impact of allegations of assault and battery or kidnapping. In any circumstance, it is always necessary to ensure good judgment and careful documentation of the patient's decisional capacity.

Case 4

EMS was called for a 70-year-old woman with a history of COPD and acute worsening of shortness of breath. Upon arrival, the EMS providers found her in significant respiratory distress. Her pulse was 120 and her blood pressure was 95 systolic. A modest amount of oxygen was applied and an aerosolized albuterol treatment was administered. The treatment provided some relief. The patient subsequently refused transport to the hospital. The family demanded that she be taken to the ED. The daughter said, "You have to take her to the hospital. She could die."

DISCUSSION:

Should the EMS providers allow the patient to refuse further therapy and risk her death? Although the patient seemed to understand the risks, the paramedics still worried that it was wrong not to take her to the ED. They also wondered about their duty to the family, the caretakers, who strongly and emotionally urged that she be taken to the emergency department.

The first determination that must be made is whether the patient has intact decisional capacity. If she has information, appreciates the consequences of her decision, including the risks and benefits, and is able to come to a reasoned decision, then her wishes should generally be honored. It is up to those on the scene to explore the patient's reasons for refusing care. It is also prudent to involve the DMOP when danger is present. It is not necessary that danger be removed, however. Nor must the caregivers agree with the patient's decision. The refusal does not have to be reasonable according to our personal standards, but it does have to be reasoned according to the values of the patient.[6]

This patient, in her home hospital bed, with home oxygen and nebulizer machine, emphatically refused to be transported. She said that of the past 160 days, she had spent 117 in the hospital, according to her careful count. She said that she knew she did not have long to live and preferred to die at home. She accepted the warning that this episode could worsen and she might die. She further noted that it was the family, not her, who called the EMS providers and it was they who were having difficulty dealing with the situation.

Does this argument clarify the obligation to the patient? In the end, the patient was judged to possess full capacity to make this decision, the family was counseled that ambulances would return if the patient should change her mind. The DMOP was notified, and the family was further advised to call the patient's physician. The patient was not transported. The family members were not happy, but they understood that the EMS providers could not transport the patient against her will. The discussion with the patient was documented in detail, including the fact that the patient had sufficient information, understanding, and reasoning. Evidence of her capacity was described, at the encouragement of the legal consultant who was also involved.

Withholding Resuscitation Attempts

Case 5

A 67-year-old woman "passed out" in a restaurant. EMS providers found her in ventricular tachycardia. Her husband reported that she had metastatic lung cancer. Full resuscitation attempts were initiated. After two defibrillation attempts the patient had electrical cardiac activity, but no pulse. The husband then produced a "Living Will," which was officially notarized and signed by the patient, a physician, and her attorney. After being presented with the document, the EMS providers called the DMOP to ask if they should cease resuscitation attempts.

DISCUSSION:

It has long been recognized that patients have the right to limit resuscitation attempts in the event of cardiopulmonary arrest.[7,8,9] When a Do Not Resuscitate (DNR) order is established according to authorized guidelines, then resuscitation should be withheld. Guidelines are meant to assure patient identity, validity of the wish to not undergo resuscitation attempts, and applicability for the specific circumstance. Every state has some relevant legislation, directive, or EMS policy governing DNR orders outside of the hospital.[9] Most states have a specific DNR document that must be completed. If the person has not completed a directive that is officially recognizable, then resuscitation attempts should usually proceed until the circumstances are clarified.

Living wills are not applicable unless they contain a DNR provision that conforms to acceptable policy. Any person can have a living will that specifies wishes in the event of a terminal or hopeless condition, so they are often not relevant during an emergent crisis. This patient's living will had no DNR provision, so it only presented distraction and confusion. The EMS provider should not attempt to interpret complicated documents at the time of crisis. This is the reason that easily recognizable systems have been set up in most states. If DNR provisions are to be recognized, they must be simple and clear.

Some patients might have a legally designated healthcare proxy. The proxy has the right to make healthcare decisions for the patient. As in the case of living wills, a clear, recognizable, legally applicable DNR directive must still be present. At the time of crisis, when immediacy is required, it is difficult to assure validity of the proxy.

Ethically, if the patient's informed wishes are known with certainty, then we should attempt to honor those wishes. If there are any doubts, then resuscitation must proceed. The reasons to err on the side of treatment are obvious. The patient might have a reversible condition for which the document would not apply. Family members might be expressing their wishes instead of the patient's. Even patient identity might be confused. It must be certain that the patient wishes the specific care to be withheld at that moment. This complicated challenge cannot be met at the instant of crisis unless a clear and recognizable directive allows a presumption of certainty.

Terminating Resuscitation

The previous case also signals concerns about termination of resuscitation outside the hospital. Some patients would not want resuscitation attempts or transport under any circumstance. For other patients, resuscitation attempts would be medically futile, so there is no good argument for initiating or continuing care. This medical logic does not address the ethical concerns, however. It is proper to consider the family, the setting, and the current situation when termination of resuscitation attempts is considered.

In the case presented, the patient was rapidly moved to the ambulance and taken to the emergency department. If a genuine DNR provision had been present, it still seems improper to pronounce a patient dead in a restaurant. The family would need a place to grieve, so a proper judgment could be made to transport the patient. Others may not fully understand the challenges outside of the hospital, yet the EMS providers should remain confident in good judgment. In the home, families seem to be satisfied with termination of resuscitation.[10] Termination of resuscitation attempts without transport to the hospital can be appropriate with sound medical decision making and good policies. Adequate physician participation, cooperation of the coroner and police, and sound legal guidance are also important.

Case 6

An 83-year-old woman was found by paramedics to be asystolic after she suffered a cardiac arrest. The family watched her stop breathing suddenly and they called the EMS providers immediately. The patient was cachectic, in a home hospital bed set up in the living room. The family presented a paper to the paramedics, signed by a physician, noting that the patient was not to be resuscitated in the event of cardiac arrest. The family called 9-1-1 because they were frightened and did not know what else to do.

The EMS providers believed that the directive was indeed the patient's. The family confirmed identity. The patient and her physician had apparently signed the directive within the prior six months. The family repeatedly confirmed that the patient did not want any attempted resuscitation. The note did not conform to state law, however, but was written on a hospital progress note.

DISCUSSION:

This patient's directive was not legally valid, but it still seemed to the EMS providers that the proper ethical response was to withhold resuscitation attempts. No resuscitation was undertaken. The police were notified that the patient was dead on arrival (DOA) and the case was documented not as DNR, but as DOA. They circumvented protocol by overlooking the fact that this was a witnessed cardiac arrest and the technical requirements of the law were not met. Was this proper?

A primary ethical rule is that presumption that life and health must always be preserved, maintained, or restored, if possible. One means to overrule this presumption is medical futility, but there is little scientific guidance to identify futility determinations. The only other way that resuscitation attempts are properly withheld is when there is absolute evidence of patient wishes to the contrary. This is ideally done through a valid DNR order. This usually, but not always, requires the diagnosis of a terminal or hopeless condition. Both decisions must be carefully and conservatively made.

A decision to withhold resuscitation can therefore never be a spontaneous decision by the family. This must be considered before any crisis, ideally by the patient herself, or at least according to the patient's values. The role of the EMS provider is not to make judgments about the validity of documents, the prognosis of the patient, or the appropriateness of resuscitation. If no written document of assured validity and applicability exists, then full resuscitation must be attempted. All of this is meant to promote the interests and the wishes of the patient. In this circumstance, it seems that the ethically proper action was carried out even though the documents did not meet the legal requirements.

Primary care physicians and patients are often not aware of the legal requirements for out-of-hospital DNR orders. The EMS provider and command physician must therefore respond to the evidence at hand, erring on the side of attempted resuscitation. Ethically, it is proper to honor the clear and certain wishes of the patient, but some directives will not be legally valid. This dilemma is not likely to go away anytime soon.

Case 7

An elderly woman was found in cardiac arrest in her home. Her daughter had called 9-1-1. As resuscitation attempts were begun, the patient's husband, obviously distraught, emphasized that the patient had a "tumor." He believed that nothing should be done. He was emphatic, tearful, and obviously caring. He knew that his wife's heart had stopped and he believed that she would not have wanted it started again. The tumor had already caused enough anguish; and he wanted his wife to find peace. He believed that God had called her.

DISCUSSION:

According to the principles established in the prior cases, there is insufficient evidence to withhold resuscitation attempts, even though the EMS providers heard persuasive information arguing otherwise. Although the husband's anguished pleas were compelling, the medical command physician encouraged them to continue and to transport the patient. It was not clear that the wishes represented the informed and reasoned wishes of the patient. Further, no paperwork was present. Ethically, care can be withdrawn at a later time once the patient's desires are confirmed.

Resuscitation attempts were continued on the way to the emergency department. In the hospital, her medical records were reviewed and her primary physician was contacted. The "tumor" was a large lipoma on her back. The patient had been considering surgical removal and had obviously not understood when told it was benign.

This case illustrates the reason that decisions to withhold care must be carefully made. Uncertainties of patient understanding can complicate decisions. Cases of mistaken patient identity, alternative family agendas, even attempted homicide, have led or almost led to inappropriate restrictions of care. Only clear evidence of the well informed, well reasoned, carefully considered wishes of the patient are sufficient. Outside the hospital, in the midst of crisis, only indirect evidence is often available, which must meet high standards of validity.

Triage Decisions

Case 8

While responding to a call for "a lady who sat on broken glass and is bleeding," EMS providers encountered a motor vehicle accident. There were people with obvious injuries and no police or rescue squads were yet present. The EMS providers had no more information about the patient who sat on the glass. Calls were just coming in regarding the current accident scene.

DISCUSSION:

Should the paramedics stop at the new scene, where they are sure their assistance is needed? Under what circumstances does the obligation to a second patient supersede the obligation to the original patient who requested aid? Most EMS systems have worked out procedures for such circumstances. Efficient dispatch is required to rapidly prioritize calls. For the individual EMS provider, however, a sense of conflict might persist. This ethical dilemma surrounds allocation of scarce resources.

Allocation and rationing decisions should not be made on an ad hoc basis. Some principles should be applied. Someone should make the decision with a view of the entire scope of needs. This presumes that the individual units proceed under the assumption that their obligation is to the original call. They can report the events unexpectedly encountered and ask for a change in prioritization. Proper allocation of resources cannot be done at the level of the individual caregiver. It requires decisions to be made by someone who can assess the entire set of circumstances. The obligation of the EMS provider, then, is to provide information and expect further instruction.

If an immediate and life threatening need is apparent, such as severe active bleeding or acute airway obstruction, it would be reasonable to stop to render aid. Allocation of resources demand justice and fairness. The original patient may have a life-threatening injury or may have a trivial problem. The only way to assure proper prioritization is through sophisticated crew coordination and insight into the full scope of patient needs.

Confidentiality

Case 9

A 32-year-old male in a motor vehicle accident was transported to the regional trauma center. His vital signs were stable and his sensorium was clear. The EMS providers did not smell alcohol but asked if he had been drinking or taking drugs. The patient admitted to "a beer or two" and "a little cocaine" about 30 minutes before the accident. The patient said, "Don't tell anyone" and the EMS providers said, "Don't worry about it." At the trauma center the police asked the EMS providers if the patient had been drinking. The response would likely have determined whether the police would have requested a serum alcohol level and would have pursued a "driving under the influence" investigation.

DISCUSSION:

Physicians have the ethical and legal obligation to maintain the confidentiality of patient information. EMS providers share this duty. Caregivers learn information about a patient only because of their privileged position. Personal information is obtained, secrets are learned, in order to provide for the person's health and well-being. In order to maintain trust and therefore the position as honored caregiver, this information must not be divulged to those who do not share the direct obligation to the patient. This obligation extends to all that have access to information in the normal course of care, including secretaries and nurses as well as EMS providers and physicians.

A dangerous conflict can arise when the personal values of the caregiver are offended and the patient seems to deserve punishment. The caregiver must avoid blaming or condemning patients, since it interferes with the primary obligation. In this case, simple, unemotional cooperation with police might seem reasonable, except for the fact that this also undermines the role of those charged to provide care. It is entirely reasonable for the peace officers to conduct their usual investigation. It is not reasonable for the EMS provider to act as a surrogate peace officer, since the integrity of the EMS provider could be lost as society learns that information cannot be safely shared with out-of-hospital caregivers.

While the duty to the patient seems logical, what about the duty to society? The EMS providers might believe that they have a duty to ensure the driver receives just punishment. Again, the EMS providers only learned sensitive information because of their role as caregivers. They undermine themselves and their role by using the information for anything but the patient's interest. They should professionally defer from involvement in issues outside their scope of practice, including the notoriously unreliable predication of legal intoxication. The police can easily gather such important information by exercising their usual and customary authority. When society determines that an interest overrides individual rights, then laws are passed that require reporting, while indemnifying the person who reports. For example, suspected child abuse, elder abuse, and public health threats are to be reported, based on laws that supersede the obligation of confidentiality.

Case 10

EMS providers responded to a call for a child who "fell down." Upon arrival, a 5-year-old with multiple bruises and contusions on three extremities was encountered. The EMS providers felt these injuries were inconsistent with the stated history. The EMS providers did not mention their concerns to the parents. After the EMS providers evaluated the child, the parents refused transport. Conflict arose because the EMS providers wanted to protect the child by transporting him to the hospital, where social services agencies would become immediately involved. The EMS providers felt that there was an imminent threat to the child's health. Should they insist on transporting this child?

Discussion:

Every state has legal requirements to report suspected child abuse because society holds that the interest of the child takes precedence over the obligation of confidentiality between. However, this does not mean that all obligations are lost and parents turn into an adversary. There is little benefit, and potential danger, in getting into a conflict or altercation with the parents. In virtually all jurisdictions, social service agencies are available to investigate, whether the child is taken to the hospital or not. As always, the approach should be underpinned by caring, by the obligation

to provide for the best interests of the child, and by an understanding that the parents might need help as well. The EMS provider is not the legal system and is not in a position to make judgments or final determinations, but only to help such determinations proceed.

Astute observation, avoidance of impulsive judgments, and knowledge of legal requirements would limit the conflict in most situations. While the EMS provider can say little with certainty, the clear concern should prompt a call to the on-line physician or dispatch, which can assist in contacting social service agencies. If there is immediate threat to the child, social service supports and the police can often intervene. If a high level of conflict is not present, but danger to the child possible, the EMS provider can work with medical oversight and social services to determine how to proceed. Emotions must not rule. Thoughtfulness must guide, and well informed concerns can help ensure calm action.

Case 11

A city police official suffered a cardiac arrest while at work. EMS providers arrived, initiated resuscitation, and transported the patient to the nearest hospital. The media arrived and asked the EMS providers for information. Should the EMS providers speak to the media? How much should they say? Is the duty to keep confidence different when caring for a public official?

Discussion:

The EMS provider has an ethical obligation to protect confidentiality of information and privacy of the person. Talking to anyone who does not share this obligation violates this ethical rule. When high visibility people are involved, the intense interest generates many questions. In an attempt to be helpful, some caregivers provide small amounts of personal information. Even this technically violates the patient's interests. The patient should be the one to determine what information is shared, by whom, and when. Systems that can provide this level of confidentiality are regarded with esteem.

The best policy is to designate a spokesperson for the EMS who is experienced in media relations, especially regarding patient confidentiality. Media relations are not generally a core skill of the EMS provider and should not be taken lightly. Such information could have consequences for the patient's family, friends, colleagues, and others. Political or social effects can result from seemingly inconsequential comments. There is significance in assuming responsibility as spokesperson for the system, so casual comments are ill-advised.

Case 12

A television crew wishes to accompany the EMS providers in order to videotape events of interest. Patient consent will later be obtained from selected patients. If a patient consents, the care will be shown on a national television program. The video of those who do not consent will be destroyed.

DISCUSSION:

This has been a common scenario in many busy emergency medical services as popular television shows have been developed out of the drama of real-life situations. The ethics of this practice is currently being called into question, however. The American Medical Association states that only patients who can consent should be filmed. Videotaping patients who cannot prospectively consent is held as a violation of patient privacy.[11] The Society for Academic Emergency Medicine has adopted a substantially similar policy.[12] Ongoing debate about the filming of patients is likely to continue.

Truth-Telling

Case 13

EMS providers responded to a 78-year-old patient with severe abdominal pain. The family stated that he had recently been diagnosed with stomach cancer but did not know it. Should such secrets be kept?

DISCUSSION:

There is a general duty to be honest with patients. The only exception to this duty is when a patient has an overriding desire or interest not to know the truth. These exceptions are uncommon but are encountered by every level of provider.[13] These patients may be of different cultures or they may simply want to hear bad news. The fundamental presumption is that only the patient himself can determine what is right. This generally requires full information, unless their interest is clearly best served by not knowing.

What is the duty of the EMS provider in this case? What if the patient asked about his illness? Is avoiding the truth the same as deception? Since the EMS provider does not have insight into the complex reasons for the deception, it is not possible to know. In this case, the EMS providers have little knowledge of the medical history, and know few details about his background, the family, the patient's values, or the psychosocial implications of such information. This is too much to sort out in the short time outside of the hospital. It is probably not necessary to sort it out. Conversations about chronic medical conditions can easily be deferred. The EMS providers can professionally and appropriately focus on initial stabilization of the immediate issue, the abdominal pain.

Personal Risk

Case 14

EMS providers arrived at a scene where a man reportedly was "beat up and bleeding." He was inside a tavern, where bystanders were shouting and screaming at each other. A person spotted the ambulance pull up and ran to the unit yelling, "my man's hurt in here, come on in and help him." Police were not on the scene.

DISCUSSION:

How much risk should the EMS provider assume? Should the EMS provider enter the tavern without police assistance? EMS providers' duties to patients are sometimes constrained by safety concerns. The extent of responsibility of the paramedics to patients and others is sometimes unclear, and presents ethical conflict. The provider must evaluate the safety of the scene and make a judgment. The provider must not be encouraged to take risks in the name of bravado or heroism. Assistance of peace officers should be enlisted. The immediacy of the friend's request makes the providers feel pressured, but does not change the ethical obligation. There is no requirement to be a battlefield medic and put oneself in harm's way to rescue people in the midst of conflict. A safe scene, preventing additional casualties, is a fundamental premise of civil EMS. This does not mean the EMS providers can avoid all danger and prevent all risk. One must only minimize risk and calculate reasonable actions, avoiding situations for which one is not trained.

Training

Case 15

Paramedics attempted resuscitation of an 88-year-old cardiac arrest victim. Efforts were discontinued after

35 minutes. One of the paramedics asked if anyone would mind if he extubated and re-intubated the patient to practice.

DISCUSSION:

It is imperative that the paramedics develop and maintain procedural skills, including intubation, to expertly care for patients. During out-of-hospital care of patients, it is not appropriate to deviate from the accepted procedures. To maintain skills, standards of training must be in place, and continuing education should be available, as needed. In order to practice on recently deceased patients, family consent is generally required.

Asking for family permission is not widely discussed in the out-of-hospital setting because of the obvious and substantial difficulties. The AMA notes that the teaching of life-saving skills should be the culmination of a structured training sequence rather than random training opportunities. This is especially challenging for those who are able to perform life-saving skills rarely and require every opportunity to ensure skill maintenance. According to the AMA, a person with authority must consent prior to using the deceased patient for training purposes.[14] Given the current ethical climate, it is reasonable for all medical professionals to abide by such guidance. In the case above, the senior EMS provider said that it was not appropriate to reintubate the patient.

Treatment of Minors

Case 16

A 14-year-old patient called the paramedics because she had severe lower abdominal pain. Her blood pressure was 95/70 and her pulse was 90. The paramedics wished to initiate an IV line and transport her to the ED, but wanted to know if parental consent was required first.

DISCUSSION:

As a rule, the consent of the parent or legal guardian is required for the care of a minor, but there are a few exceptions. State laws designate emancipated minors who do not need parental consent. These would generally include minors who are financially and functionally independent. In addition, minors who seek care for pregnancy-related problems or sexually transmitted diseases are usually considered emancipated. Another exception to the requirement for consent is the "emergency exception," which allows care neces-

sary to prevent mortality or serious morbidity when the patient is unable to provide consent.[4] Usually when this exception is invoked, the illness is obvious and the situation grave. It is clear that there is sufficient basis to provide important care to a person who is incapacitated or in serious need. This patient did not meet either of these criteria with certainty, so debate still existed regarding how to proceed.

A third principle that might apply is that of the "mature minor." An adolescent has some decision-making capacity, even if legal limits exist. This patient makes a reasonable choice in requesting care. In the absence of parental presence, a reasonable presumption can be made that the minor's health could be at risk without simple stabilizing maneuvers and medical testing. Since the risks of initial evaluation are minimal, care could proceed as the guardians are contacted. This request of a mature minor might help provide some basis for initial care, but it is insufficient to proceed completely without parental consent. A supporting principle is that of presumed consent. A reasonable-person standard suggests that the potential seriousness of the medical problem would lead most individuals to proceed with stabilizing care and basic evaluation. Important care can therefore be justified, since the health of the minor could be at risk. The legal and ethical principles are surprisingly unhelpful in such cases. Since the patient's medical condition is not known, absolute guidance is not offered. It is up to the EMS provider and DMOP to focus attention on the potential consequences of delayed care. It can be legitimately argued that delayed care could result in serious consequences, so one must err on the side of providing necessary care. Transporting the patient for definitive evaluation at the ED seems of relatively smaller consequence and smaller risk.

Acting in the best interest of the patient, according to the needs of the patient, especially with a minimal chance of harming the patient, will help minimize conflict. Invasive procedures should be avoided or deferred, if possible, until parental consent is obtained. If there is a risk of death or permanent disability, however, care might proceed under the emergency exception to consent. It is important to request parent or guardian permission before treating non-emancipated minors, but essential emergency care should never be withheld when the delay could present harm to the patient. Important needs must be met, while attempts are undertaken to contact the responsible adult, especially if a minor's life is at risk. Less urgent issues must wait for the parent's permission.

Coercion of Uncooperative Patients

Case 17

Paramedics arrived at the scene of a single motor vehicle accident and encountered an obviously intoxicated, unrestrained driver who had been ejected from the vehicle. The patient was thrashing and cursing. The paramedics attempted unsuccessfully to calm the patient. The patient attempted to punch one of the paramedics. The team of paramedics held down the patient's arms and legs and forcefully told him that if he didn't calm down they would give him medicine to paralyze him and would put a plastic tube down his throat to breathe for him. The patient became cooperative enough for the paramedics to proceed with the evaluation, immobilization, and rapid transport.

DISCUSSION:

Technically, the EMS provider committed assault by threatening the patient. Operationally, the EMS provider felt he was doing what was needed in order to provide important care. Still, holding the patient down may have been battery. Are these actions ever justified to ensure compliance? Does the severity of the patient's illness affect the justification? What limitation should be placed on paramedics' ability to "convince" patients to submit to care? Usually there are less aggressive means to encourage care and, very often, agitation is a sign of a medical rather than interpersonal pathology. This patient was clearly in need of medical evaluation, but there are many problems with using threats or violence to deal with violent patients. The incident can escalate, causing more problems. Calm restored by establishing rapport works best. This is true for everyone, including intoxicated patients and those with psychiatric disease. The better way to achieve needed compliance is to couple a caring approach to clear, firm boundaries. At the same time, quiet visibility of other EMS providers or police can help convince the patient. After all, the goal is to take care of the patient and he should be reminded of this fact in a caring, if matter-of-fact manner. Third, if the incident goes awry, suspicions of threats and violence on the part of the EMS provider are difficult to resolve. Displays of combative behaviors on the part of the EMS provider are more difficult to forgive. The EMS provider's action should never be punitive, can never be excessive, and must provide for the best interest of the patient. Hostility,

impatience, or impulsive reaction on the part of the EMS provider is not beneficial. A deliberate, reasoned, decisive action is important and effective. Genuine excellence is usually coupled with authority and imperturbability, not anger or violence.

Research

Case 18

When patients were encountered with tonic-clonic seizure activity, the EMS providers were asked to administer a drug of uncertain identity, then collect data as part of a research project. The EMS providers were told that the vials contained either diazepam, lorazepam, or placebo, but they could not know which was being administered. Coded labels were used instead of the name of the drug. If a patient was at high risk for a major complication, open-label diazepam could be administered. The EMS provider was to document the clinical status of the patient every five minutes.[15] People not involved in the study asked if it was ethical to be administering experimental drugs to patients who could not consent.

DISCUSSION:

One of the most important principles of our current culture is the right to individual self-determination. Proceeding with research on people who cannot offer consent is indeed ethically challenging. On the other hand, if research does not proceed, then it is not possible to make meaningful therapeutic advances for many emergency conditions. The dilemma, then, is how science can proceed without prospective informed consent. In order to address this concern, the Food and Drug Administration and the Department of Health and Human Services offered specific guidance for the protection of human subjects for emergency research.[16] These requirements include communication with the community at the time the research is proposed, and discussion with the patient, family members, and others close to the patient, as possible, when the research is carried out. The research should also entail minimal risk. Accountability to an independent oversight board is required during the course of the study. Ideally, patient safety, trust, and justice can be protected even as research proceeds on vulnerable patients.[17] In this case, initial detailed review and approval was carried out by at least three formal supervising agencies. An external advisory committee was then established, made up of experts not affiliated with the study, to periodically review the data during the course of the investigation. Additionally, a committee from the National Institutes of Health carried out annual monitoring. All adverse events and deaths were reported to these two monitoring boards, as well as the Institutional Review Boards of the destination hospitals. Extensive safeguards were in place because the research was proceeding without the most important protection of the interests of the individual subjects: their informed consent.

Summary

Issues of informed consent, refusal, and limitation of resuscitation highlight the important role that ethical decision making plays in out-of-hospital care. It is imperative EMS providers be educated to skillfully handle the patient who refuses care or the family that requests no CPR for their loved one in cardiac arrest. One cannot assume that all caregivers have the ability to identify conflicts, assess competing values, and make reasoned judgments, but this is what is required.[1,18] More extensive in ethics might better equip care providers to deal with these issues. Such education could promote appropriate, efficient, and optimal avoidance or resolution of conflicts. Physicians providing direct medical oversight must also have sufficient skills to handle the conflicts that may be asked to help resolve. Policy must also be developed to promote adequate resolution for difficult situations, such as refusal of care, DNR orders, and informed consent. Appropriate resolution of ethical conflicts will be promoted when the provider and medical oversight can identify the conflicts, and when effective policy is developed to provide a guiding framework.

References

1. Adams JG, Arnold R, Siminoff L, et al. Ethical conflicts in the prehospital setting. *Ann Emerg Med.* 1992;21: 1259–1265.
2. Robinson D, Garratt C. *Introducing Ethics.* New York: Totem Press; 1997:40.
3. Applebaum PS, Grisso T. Assessing patients' capacity to consent to treatment. *New Engl J Med.* 1988;319:1634–1638.
4. Beauchamp TL, Childress JF. *Principles of Biomedical Ethics.* 2nd ed. New York: Oxford University Press; 1983.
5. Grisso T, Applebaum PS. *Assessing Competence to Consent to Treatment.* New York: Oxford University Press; 1998: 31.
6. Ridley DT. Informed consent, informed refusal, informed choice: what is it that makes a patient's medical treatment decisions informed? *Med Law.* 2001;20:205–214.
7. Miles SH, Crimmins TJ. Orders to limit emergency treatment for an ambulance service in a large metropolitan area. *JAMA.* 1985;254:525–527.
8. *President's Commission for the Study of Ethical Problems in Medicine and Biomedical and Behavioral Research: Deciding to Forgo Life-sustaining Treatment: A Report on the Ethical, Medical and Legal Issues in Treatment Decisions.* Washington, DC: U.S. Government Printing Office; 1983.
9. Sabatino CP. Survey of state EMS-DNR laws and protocols. *Journ Law, Medicine, and Ethics.* 1999;27:297–315.
10. Delbridge TR, Fosnocht DE, Garrison HG, et al. Field termination of unsuccessful out of hospital cardiac arrest resuscitation: acceptance by family members. *Ann Emerg Med.* 1996;27(5):649–654.
11. *Report of the Council on Ethical and Judicial Affairs, American Medical Association.* Report 3-A-01. Adopted 2001.
12. Ethics Committee, Society for Academic Emergency Medicine, Lansing, Michigan, adopted 2001. Available at http://www.saem.org.
13. Munn S. Doc, I don't wanna know! Patient requested noninformed consent. *Amer J Roentgenol.* 2001;177(2): 473.
14. *Report of the Council on Ethical and Judicial Affairs, American Medical Association.* Report 5-A-01. Adopted 2001.
15. Alldredge BK, Gelb A, Isaacs SM. A comparison of lorazepam, diazepam, and placebo for the treatment of out-of-hospital status epilepticus. *New Engl J Med.* 2001; 345:631–637.
16. Office of the Secretary. Protection of human subjects: informed consent and waiver of informed consent requirements in certain emergency research: final rules. *Fed Regist.* 1996;61(192):51498–51553.
17. Adams JG, Wegener J. Acting without asking: an ethical analysis of the Food and Drug Administration waiver of informed consent for emergency research. *Ann Emerg Med.* 1999;33:218–233.
18. Welie JV, Welie SP. Patient decision-making competence: outlines of a conceptual framework. *Med Health Care Philos.* 2001;4(2):127–138.

CHAPTER 34

Political Realities

Norm Dinerman, MD

Introduction

The emergence and maturation of the specialty of emergency medicine has spawned and nurtured the development of prehospital care. In turn, prehospital care has become a subspecialty of its own, attracting a subset of emergency and acute care physicians whose focus of technical expertise and clinical acumen has been directed to the provision of care from the moment of system access to the arrival of the patient at the emergency department. The original EMS medical directors were those individuals fascinated by the possibility of extending "sophisticated" methodology to the patient at the scene.

Equally intriguing to them was the opportunity to provide this technical sophistication using individuals operating under the broad-based concept of "licensure-extension" of the physician. Not surprisingly, and by the very nature of prehospital care itself, those physicians attracted to this subspecialty of emergency medicine were captivated by the eclectic and unique attributes of medical practice in this complex arena.

They were soon faced, however, with daunting challenges concerning their own creativity in an equally complex arena, that of the political one. The multiple interfaces required of the medical director, within and outside the medical community, have created an especially challenging section of emergency medicine practice, where technical expertise by itself proves insufficient in creating a workable system. While the magnitude of this challenge is attractive for some physicians, the emotional energy required, and the intense, continuous interaction in the political arena may cause an abbreviated career for even the most innately passionate physicians. As with most areas of medicine, if not life itself, an "apprenticeship" is the means of conveying a "practice" from veteran to neophyte. The growth and development of training programs in emergency medicine have been slow to develop "fellowships" in prehospital care, however,

and our literature contains but few citations on formalized approaches.[1-6]

While there are numerous structures within which the medical director may work (full-time academic; full-time public safety with academic affiliation; part-time volunteer), none guarantees success. The skillful political behavior of the physician in his role ultimately determines the success of system function, and may even alter the administrative structure within which the physician resides.

Politics and economics are omnipresent forces with which the medical director must work as he attempts to craft and manage a prehospital care system. These "forces" are usually neither familiar, understood, nor embraced by individuals who originally entered the field of medicine in pursuit of the satisfaction derived from patient care. Many opportunities for frustration and disappointment thus await the unwary and idealistic physician who fails to acknowledge these forces, or is unable to master their elements. Similarly, those physicians who appreciate the "leverage" to be gained from an understanding of politics and economics will be rewarded by the growth and development of their systems. Some thoughts and perspectives are herein shared with the interested reader to enable a means of creatively employing these forces for the ultimate benefit of the patient, and the community.

For most physicians, the difficulty, indeed the resistance to comprehending the political climate in which prehospital care activities are crafted, is deeply seated. How many physicians entered medicine because of a love of politics and economics? These are not motivating factors identified on a frequent basis by anyone in medicine. In addition, there are few individuals who are able to provide an apprenticeship for the aspiring medical director that addresses the political realities requiring mastery.

Fewer still are the institutions which have committed to providing a formalized experience in prehospital care, not to mention a fellowship. Sadly, the attempted metamorphosis of the clinician into a political "statesperson" more often than not results in his transmogrification into a political dyslexic. The technical dexterity and intellectual prowess of the physician do not readily provide the interpersonal skills and tools for triumphing in the political arena. Further, the frequently misperceived position of physicians as "superior" to other members of the healthcare team seduces them into behaving as such with nonmedical individuals, with predictable and disastrous results. Political acumen must be forged slowly, over time, and with a mentor (an "Obewan Kenobe" of sorts) who nurtures the individual physician.

The disaffection for politics found inherently in most healthcare providers accrues perhaps to the physician's affiliation with the precepts of the "craftsman." As one of four "corporate types" defined by Maccoby in his book, *The Gamesman,* the craftsman experiences perhaps the greatest disparity between the reality and the ideal.[7] It is most difficult for this individual to juxtapose the desired medical goals of a "perfect" prehospital care system with the political realities found in any community. Friction between value systems surface. For most, the emotional cost produced by this paradigm discordance is high, and for some, too great to sustain a career of permanence in this aspect of practice of emergency medicine. In the pursuit of quality, however, the craftsperson is handicapped by the lack of a definition easily communicated to the political veterans in the community. Quality, as with style, class, poise, and pornography, tend to be attributes of human behavior which are recognizable, but poorly articulated. Political awareness is not usually found imbedded in the "genetic code" of the healthcare practitioner. At most, it remains a dormant gene which needs to be "turned on."

While many definitions of politics abound, it is based, practically speaking, on an attempt to engender, gather, manufacture, or express consensus. The relationship to the technically "ideal" system, at best, is viewed as oblique, from the perspective of the scientifically forged physician.

The genesis of EMS systems is not founded on logic and rationality. These attributes are not the legal tender in the political community. He who possesses the power or the money, and who "sleeps" with whom are more often the determining factors.

While the medical director may desire an arena devoid of political influences, this is as impossible to achieve as eliminating the vagaries of human behavior itself.

Case Studies

Examples of the influence of politics in medicine are ubiquitous but, many times, subtle. Even in the most academic aspects of prehospital care, such as the creation of medical protocols for providers (e.g., ACLS), the political process is operative. Most obviously, legislation to enact seat belt, helmet, and drunk driving laws must of necessity enlist widespread public support in the very citadel of the political process, the statehouse. Between these two extremes, political processes are operative to varying degrees. Examples include the following:

1. determination of hospital destination policy for ambulances;
2. trauma center designation;
3. creation of a combined (unified) communications center; and
4. participation of a hospital in the 9-1-1 system, emergency medicine residency, helicopter program, etc.

Specific examples of the use of the political process abound, but are difficult to scrutinize from a distance. They are known only by those involved in the creation of a specific program, and shared infrequently, and usually in confidence. Yet it is only through the process of sharing case studies that the "apprenticeship" process is actualized. Clearly, forums to achieve this are necessary, on a local and national scale. As an example, the unification of the Denver prehospital care system lacked the formalized participation of the fire department in 1979. A plan was drawn up to achieve such formalized control, and assure the competence of the firefighters, serving in their capacity as first responders. When presented to the fire chief, it was found unacceptable for a variety of reasons, not the least of which was the perception of power ceding to physicians at Denver General Hospital. This medical director then donned firefighter's clothes and, after direct observation and participation with firefighters in the provision of emergency medical care, designed a curriculum for first responders. This was joined with the course of the same title by the DOT, and gained acceptance within the fire service. More important, the educational process, and the creation of a more formal involvement of the fire service, were embraced by a sufficient number of city officials to encourage a "re-evaluation" of the position taken by the fire chief. Ultimately, a document prepared by the physician emergency medicine staff, and acceptable to the fire service, was issued as an executive order by the Mayor. The process took two years. While the process was cumbersome, the outcome has proven durable.

The emplacement of paramedic presence at Stapleton International Airport, and subsequently at Denver International Airport, provides another example of the political process in prehospital care systems design.[8] The growth of the population in Denver at the periphery of the city (the social epiphyseal plates of the community) produced an area of increasing demand for prehospital care services. As response times increased, complaints were heard from members of the city council whose constituents populated these areas. The support of council members was obtained through a citizen oversight council, to enable funding of a paramedic response unit on a golf-cart at the airport. The latter site was chosen because of its identified volume of calls (approximately 5% of system total), and the large number which were fraudulent, cancelled, or refused. By providing paramedic presence at the airport, triage could now be accomplished by system paramedics, reserving the need for ambulances to those who were both ill and willing to be transported. By encouraging the airport to financially support the endeavor, a public relations benefit could be realized, and the over-all system performance improved without additional cost to the fiscally strapped municipal hospital.

The citizen oversight council and the City Council were publicly praised for their insightful and creative address of a technically complex, operationally driven solution to the problem. The paramedic presence has been increased over the years, consonant with growth of the airport facility. By avoiding the obvious solution of increasing the number of ambulances serving the entire system, the over-all number of paramedics remained small (maximizing individual experience rate), and increased efficiency was gained. City ambulances were now available for more calls, as a unique solution for the airport population had been created. A byproduct of the new system was the more rapid availability of advanced life-support care at the airport to passengers and employees. Were this the initial objective of the project, it is highly unlikely that the Stapleton International Airport Mobile Paramedic Unit (SIAMPER) would have been emplaced, simply because most passengers at the airport do not vote in the councilmatic districts of Denver, since they are from out of state.

Power Blocs, Vectors and Pressure Points

The approach of the medical director who is new to the community must be one of openness, and great caution. While espousing an "ideal" system, it is well for the physician to identify the power blocs. Typically, they consist of a bouillabaisse of the following:

- Mayor/Council/Manager
- Fire chief
- Line firefighter
- Pre-hospital care providers
- Patients
- Taxpayers
- City attorney
- Regional EMS council
- State health department

Fundamental to appreciating the appropriate movement of a system is the need for the physician to understand the pressure points within it. This requires patience, a willingness to invest time with each of the above principles, and an ability to discern the history of the present situation. A pivotal mission for the physician advisor is to reframe, refocus, and redefine the agendas of others. Clearly, he must become intimate with the capabilities and desires of each of the provider groups and the position of government leaders, before attempting to choreograph a new system of prehospital care for the community.

If one visualizes the aforementioned "power blocs" as "political vectors" with magnitude (force) and direction, the objective becomes the exertion of pressure in such a way as to realign the vectors as parallel as possible toward the desired EMS agenda of the system.

Philosophy, Perspective, and Bias

Five political senses require mastery. They are as follows:

1. A sense of mission—yours, that of the specialty, and that of the institution—should first be defined, then amalgamated and articulated. It is also helpful to frame the efforts of the medical director not only as a practice champion and political choreographer, but as a genetic engineer as well. Indeed, the manipulation of the system is analogous to skillfully revising the "genetic code" of the prehospital care system of the community. While the object is to create a "superior high-performance species" of system, more resistant to the onslaught of political viruses, one never knows what will crawl out of the petri dish five years from now. The mission of the medical director is also that of a "steward" of the system. It is in this role as a "trustee," with a fundamental medical fiduciary responsibility to the patient, that the physician must speak most directly.

2. A sense of tradition—The history of the community and the service within it should be studied. This provides guidance in maneuvering around the political obstacles which have emplaced barriers toward development.

3. A sense of position—The position of the medical director within the organization, and the community, and the position of the service agency, should be acknowledged. In addition, prehospital care (EMS) may be "positioned" as technically within the practice of emergency medicine, operationally within public safety, and philosophically within public health. The ability of the medical director to articulate this categorization, and relate to each of the individuals who inhabit these three worlds, is important in determining over-all success.

4. Humor—invaluable, and to be perfected during the entire professional lifespan.

5. Timing—The introduction of new ideas and programs should take advantage of other changes being introduced into the institution, community, or agency.

Preparing Yourself

Goals of the organization, and the individual, require the achievement of excellence in five spheres: academic, operational, administrative, clinical, and community relations. The target audience of the medical director should be defined in the broadest possible context, that of other healthcare providers, citizens, and every other "customer" whom the medical director and his agency touches.

Understand the concept of "Political Darwinism": The political and economic topography define "reality." As the topography changes, you must adapt, or perish; in other words, "mutate or die." The individual who can seize upon innovative management and communication styles, and who is alert to changes in the "big picture," is able to adapt the needs of his/her agency to the vicissitudes of politics. Always keep reality squarely in your sights. Sadly, Darwinism is not pretty.

Distinguish between a politician and one who is "political." A politician is loyal to his constituency. A medical director is free to be loyal to the principles of sound clinical practice. The director's demonstrated "awareness" of the political climate in which he must work does not impugn his motives, however; nor should he be an apologist for his insight.

Systems evolve. The goal of system excellence will be well served, and the sanity of the medical director preserved, if he/she appreciates the glacial time frame within which change is accomplished. Perhaps the most for which any one individual can hope is to refine the system, in preparation for his successor to refine it still further. Yet another analogy is the "river" concept of individual efforts. Acute diversion of a river in one direction may beget spontaneous direction changes downstream for miles to come. Many, if not most of these distant changes are unforeseen.

Nurture your colleagues. Patients and issues come and go. Long after your colleagues have forgotten the reason for your anger, they will recall the unpleasantness of the interaction. Expressed alternatively, friends may come and go, but enemies accumulate. Your colleagues outlast the issues, and should be respected. Technical errors are more easily forgiven than those which are normative, or behavioral. Strive to develop an ethical, emotional, and behavioral gyroscope within you. Like its physical counterpart in navigation, a similarly stable operational perspective will allow you to weather the buffeting vicissitudes of system change with constancy of purpose, enabling accurate tracking toward the goal you and your colleagues have identified.

Attempt to create win-win solutions to problems. When this is impossible, ensure that both sides appreciate compromise.

Be the source, and you become the force. Too often, the goal of the medical director is to become the power broker in the community. By striving to become the "source," (i.e., the consultative resource to whom people turn for guidance), the medical director soon becomes the force for change.

Define quality in meaningful terms. Since the definition of "quality" is so elusive, choose those measurement parameters which are meaningful to the intended audience.

Every transport of a patient is a political statement.

Choose realistic mentors. Mentors who are great and flawed are more likely to be emulated than those who are perceived as great and perfect. The former are seen as "human," the latter, "god-like." We see some hope of improving upon the former, but are never able to reach the standards of the latter.

Observe why others fail. To be effective, one must have a good engine (innate talent), a good transmission (personality and communication skills), plenty of fuel in the tank (endurance), with a good set of windshield wipers to see where you're going. It also helps if you're on the most appropriate road. It's quite a waste to place a Ferrari on a jeep trail, and quite dangerous to run the jeep on the Autobahn. When colleagues fail, observe the reasons.

Develop a shared paradigm for your staff. Stress the provision of agency services with competence, compassion, class, creativity, and credibility.

Strive to develop a demeanor and countenance which reflects an academic, intellectual, and collegial approach to solving problems.

A special note of caution about bureaucracies is in order. Often, an adversary will remain camouflaged, if not silent and stealthy. While the demonstrative opponent is easy to identify if not to outmaneuver, the bureaucrat has proven more lethal to great ideas and system reform, if for no other reason than his resistance, persistence, and longevity. The bureaucracy will consume enormous amounts of energy on the part of the medical director. More reforms have been defeated in an attempt to navigate a bureaucratic quagmire than the withering verbal artillery of individual or collective opponents. Bureaucrats fundamentally perceive themselves as underappreciated, if not powerless. A bureaucrat, if provoked, can erect enormous obstacles, and subvert and condemn the most noble and meritorious ideas of the medical director, if only to demonstrate his power over the physician. Respect, acknowledgement, and interaction with the bureaucracy may not provide a dramatic victory but it will pave the way for one.

Principles of Action

Unlike the provision of police or fire suppression services, prehospital care is inextricably tethered to hospital healthcare politics and economics. Every transport of a patient is thus a political, and an economic statement. Institutional paranoia dictates that whoever controls ambulances controls the patients, and the revenue. Economically, ambulances thus become charged particles, to be gathered by some institutions and repelled by others, depending on their fiscal "force fields." Thus, stereotypically the trauma center may desire critically injured patients, regardless of insurance status (or despite the absence of third-party coverage), while the suburban community hospital may seek to avoid these patients in favor of the medically ill, and third-party reimbursed clientele. Into this economic maelstrom is placed the medical director, for whom none of this fiscal agenda is inherently germane, but in which the service he is to provide exists. Is it any wonder that such an individual perceives the political and economic topography as foreign, if not hostile? To steer an academically neutral course becomes an ordeal that has daunted many. No wonder the physician advisor feels like Harrison Ford slashing through the political and economic vegetation!

To be effective in an arena which is inherently unfamiliar to the physician, a number of principles of action are herewith submitted, as follows:

1. An understanding, if not a mastery of political judo is encouraged. As with its physical counterpart, the politically diminutive physician must understand the simple but effective maneuvers necessary to tumble opponents in the desired direction. The political agility of the medical director accrues from his allegiance to principles of medicine, and not to a political constituency or the egomaniacal forces of his opponent. With regard to adversaries, it is more effective to exploit their psychopathology than perseverate about it.

2. Before pushing the first domino, know where the last one falls. Do not be tempted by the seductively easy "win," unless you are aware of all the political connections of your opponents. Better to be one who sets up the dominoes than the one who pushes them. Natural political forces will cause one to fall eventually. The wise medical director will have spent years

establishing the desired direction in which they should fall, content that fate or circumstance will eventually tumble the first one.

3. The movements of the chess game are instructive. The pawn, slowly moving ahead, can become as effective as any other "chess piece." At any moment in time, the chessboard can be upset, moving all the pieces in different and unpredictable directions. For example, the regulatory bureaucracy may decree innovative torment for all, or a new mayor may be elected. Consider the illustrative case of the party switch of Senator Jeffords in June, 2001, as an example of the "upset chessboard" on a national level. Public officials rapidly acquire a global perspective of each piece on the chessboard, as well. Like the professional tournament athlete, consistent performance over time will usually create substantial success.

4. Covet identified problems. Complaints may be seen as "opportunities in drag." They permit creative manipulation of the system, and insight into behavioral issues which must be addressed. The medical director is a "problem solver," as much as any other single role he plays.

5. Identify the relationships among people. The prehospital care system within the community is a complex political eco-system, with myriad political connections among even the most far-flung members. A movement or alteration of the power at any end of the "pond" will move the "lily pads" at the other.

6. Become dispensable, but not openly so. As a wise physician administrator once demonstrated, place your finger in the middle of a glass of water. The finger represents your presence within the system, or institution. Remove your finger. Notice the hole that is left.

7. Learn to swim with sharks.[9] Thus:
   a. If bitten, do not bleed;
   b. Before recognizing another individual as a non-shark, ensure that you have witnessed docile behavior on more than one occasion;
   c. Rescue an injured swimmer with due regard for external and internal reasons for his incapacity, lest you succumb during the effort;
   d. Periodically give a known shark a forceful punch in the nose to remind him that you have some power.

8. Stage a crisis on your own terms. When a crisis looms, ensure that you orchestrate it to occur at such time that it will be optimal for you. For example, when funding for a poison center in the community was threatened by legislative inaction, the administrator notified the press that this clinical facility was about to lose its WATS line. This was timed for release shortly before Christmas, and coincident with public safety messages to parents concerning the potential poisonous nature of Christmas foliage. The legislature quickly authorized the funding before recessing for the holidays.

9. Be a political chameleon. It's helpful to have a full set of costumes to enable you to project a panoply of images, appropriate to the political moment.

10. Identify all the customers. Too frequently, only the patient is identified as the customer. Within any organization, however, internal and external customers must be satisfied. They are not necessarily direct supervisors of the medical director. Every individual within the system who must be satisfied, or at least acknowledged, should be identified, and never ignored.

11. As expressed in "In Search of Excellence." understand the business you're really in.[10] The medical director is a choreographer of care. The challenge is to rise above the technical image of the physician as a provider of care to only a single patient. In providing the choreography for the entire system, one cares for thousands of people, and influences the well-being of people far beyond the limits of a single individual. This becomes one of the strongest motivating factors for the craftsman to continue the quest for system improvement.

12. Project academic passion with political neutrality. In others words, craft the system to enable acknowledgement and allegiance to medical imperatives while achieving political equanimity.

13. Visible power is vulnerable power. The final decision maker enjoys the most ego-gratification and the least potential for long-term survival. The individual who is invisible and informal in the use of power is most insulated from assault, but will not enjoy adoration of the public, or the recognition from same. Strive

for a position between these two extremes, to enable a "low profile" but with a somewhat formalized power base.

14. Never satisfy a bureaucratic need completely. To do so will cause them to forget you. Partial solution enables an occasional reminder to the bureaucracy of your importance as a problem solver, and your inadequate funding.

15. Control the key factors, but not all. For example, the medical director must retain the power to sign off the eligibility of each paramedic to sit for recertification. The power to "hire and fire" is thus focused into an academic arena, rather than a political one.

16. Avoid the use of fear, embarrassment, anger, frustration, intimidation, and guilt. They are transparent and managerially myopic means of motivating behavior. They are also anti-academic, anti-intellectual, and anti-collegial.

17. Survival alone defines a certain success of design, and merits your respect. Individuals who have existed within a system for some time have evolved successful forms of adaptation. Do not ignore what may appear to be conservative postures, or clever camouflage.

18. Remain vigilant, but not suspicious. The latter is an emotionally draining posture with which to confront life.

19. Subject projects to the OREO analysis:
    a. Identify Opportunities
    b. Identify Resources
    a. Identify Expectations
    b. Identify Obstructions.

Sustaining the Drive

It is said in physics that all energy is devoted to overcoming friction and gravity. This is true of human behavior as well. The energy of the EMS medical director is expended on overcoming the resistance (friction) of the status quo in order to move the system to higher performance and greater accountability. The gravitational forces of tradition and bureaucracy exert profound influence to restrain new ideas. While there is no substitute for having the raw strength of merit, it is frequently, by itself, insufficient. Innovative tactics and strategies, coupled with endurance, prove more effective in the long term.

It is perilously easy to impugn the motivations of adversaries. More durable is to approach each individual or group with a respect for their position and an understanding of why a particular position is held (we all have religion, but we worship at different altars).

Publicity should be used advisedly, deliberately, and with due regard for the law of unintended consequences. The use of the media is worth mastering. As often as possible, give credit to others for the success of the system.

History belongs to the person of letters, the student of language, but most of all to the master of synthesis. The individual who can amalgamate the various resources of the community, and weave a tapestry involving many threads, will be the individual who contributes the most to any system. Remember that institutions, professions, and communities are platforms for your creativity. Respect them, and ensure that they are used wisely.

Each medical director must consider his own personal evolution. The goal should be to leverage your creativity at every opportunity. Assist not only a limited population of patients, but an entire community. In the process, contribute to the knowledge base of the specialty and assist an entire nation. Key to this personal evolution is the need to become "more than a physician."

To this end, the medical directors should consider acquiring the knowledge, skills, and abilities from other professions such as teaching and business, to augment his own innate talent. Such education may be acquired by either informal (apprenticeship) or formal (MBA acquisition) methods. Borrowing from other professions to augment the persuasive talents of the physician can be extremely powerful. Likewise, adding non-medical literature, such as the *Harvard Business Review* and the *Wall Street Journal*, will suggest a multitude of approaches which are effective in the non-medical venue of business and government, in which the medical director must forge his vision of the high performance EMS system.

System development and maturation are non-linear and anything but smooth. They do not follow the measured, predictable tempo of a Strauss waltz as much as that of a raggae rhythm.

The EMS medical director must be a seasoned clinician (practice champion) who is able to move beyond the bedside and choreograph the system. It is important to appreciate that the choreographer need not be the best dancer, but he or she must recognize who those individuals are.

Always have an exit strategy for yourself. The frustration of system choreography over the years may be lessened by identifying the myriad other venues in which your creativity can be expressed.

Be substantive. Figureheads soon become hood ornaments, and the first to be sacrificed when the system crashes.

Summary

Though politics and economics may appear abrasive to the physician, they act as sand within the oyster, which produces the pearl.

Remain professionally satisfied by performing meaningful work, identifying and placing yourself proximate to role models to emulate, keeping things eclectic, and capturing a childhood fantasy on a daily basis. Most of all, identify your own vision of the medical director to enable each of the above. Finally, know when your effectiveness has waned, and your tenure is drawing to a close. A timely, gracious, and dignified exit will nullify the harshest critics, and establish your accomplishments in the institutional memory of EMS.

References

1. Boyle MF, et al. Objectives to direct the training of emergency medicine residents on off-service rotations: emergency medical services. *J Emerg Med*. 1990;8(6): 791–795.
2. Dinerman N, Pons PT, Markovchick V. The emergency medicine resident as paramedic: a pre-hospital in-field rotation. *J Emerg Med*. 1990;8(4):507–511.
3. Otten EJ, et al. A four-year program to train residents in emergency medical services. *Acad Med*. 1989;64(5):275–276.
4. Stewart RD, Paris PM, Heller MB. Design of a resident in-field experience for an emergency medicine residency curriculum. *Ann Emerg Med*. 1987;16(2):175–179.
5. Swor RA, Chisholm C, Krohmer J. Model curriculum in emergency medical services for emergency medicine residencies. *Ann Emerg Med*. 1989;18(4):418–421.
6. Valenzuela TD, et al. Evaluation of EMS management training offered during emergency medicine residency training. *Ann Emerg Med*. 1989;18(8):812–814.
7. Maccoby M. *The Gamesman: The New Corporate Leaders*, New York: Simon and Schuster; 1976.
8. Cwinn AA, Dinerman N, Pons PT. Prehospital care at a major international airport. *Ann Emerg Med* 1988;17: 1042–1048.
9. Cousteau V. How to swim with sharks: a primer. *Perspectives in Biol and Med*. 1973;16(4):525–528. Also *Am J Nurse* 1960; Oct 1981.
10. Peters TJ, Waterman RH Jr. *In Search of Excellence: Lessons from America's Best Run Companies*, New York: Harper Collins; 1982.

Authorization and Empowerment 35

Theresa Hatcher, DO
James O. Page, JD

Introduction

While it may be an honor, it is also a significant challenge for a physician to be affiliated with an EMS agency. The purpose of medical oversight for out-of-hospital emergency services is to provide medical accountability to ensure all ill and injured patients receive medical care that meets or exceeds acceptable standards.[1] EMS medical directors are in a position that, when properly structured and implemented, provides them with the opportunity and authority to achieve improved patient care.[2] "Empowerment is the authority to make decisions within one's area of responsibility."[3] Empowerment is essentially the ability to effect change. This ability is both direct and indirect. The direct ability, more properly called authority, is what is established by the department's by-laws, rules, standard operating guidelines, etc. The medical director's authority is also set by state statute and regulations and will vary from state to state. County and municipal ordinances and their corresponding regulations may affect the medical director, but his authority also is established by contract or job description.[4–8] It is for that reason that physician medical directors need to be educated in these topics. They need to understand the impact these documents may have on their effectiveness.

Empowerment also is achieved indirectly. This aspect is dependent on the medical director's personality and his ability to operate in the organization and culture of a specific emergency service organization. There are many types of agencies providing EMS services, including private, volunteer, tax-based, and fire-based; they can function at city, county, regional, or state levels. So a woman functioning as the medical director for a city volunteer fire-based system may need a different management style to be effective than a male medical director who administers a regional system. Even the same physician functioning in each of those roles would have to handle the cir-

cumstances very differently. Therefore, in addition to using the direct tools of empowerment, the medical director must be familiar with the culture of the organization and be able to work within its constraints.

External forces also may be a factor. The presence or absence of an employee bargaining group with its own contract between a provider organization and its work force can substantially influence the effectiveness of the medical director. Personnel rules and turf issues between labor and management also can interfere.

In order for an agency to have effective medical oversight, there needs to be a supportive organizational structure. Empowered leaders must be able to set goals, make decisions, and solve problems within their area of responsibility. Working within state statutes and regulations, the agency can enforce physician empowerment in many ways. These items may need to be negotiated into a contract and include issues of salary; support staff; vehicles; access to resources, including phones, fax, computers, and turnout gear; and help with membership dues, subscriptions and continuing medical education. Spelling out these needs in detail also will help avoid conflict with other people in management positions.[9–15]

Empowerment will vary from state to state, department to department, and individual to individual. Working within already established statutory and organizational rules, it is the physician's responsibility to ensure his ability to effect change. Using the wrong approach, whether direct or indirect, usually will deter achievement of his goals. The written job description may provide the opportunity to outline and establish those mechanisms the medical director will need to meet the challenge of medical oversight.[16,17]

Preliminary to the creation or redesign of the job description, one must decide where the medical director fits operationally in the EMS organization. The role of the medical director is directly tied to the organizational structure. Is the medical director a consultant or is he to be involved operationally? If so, the extent of involvement in fire, rescue, transport and/or occupational medicine must be established. A need exists for a clarification of medical oversight vs. operational control. Several operational models are possible. Regardless of the model, the chain of command must be established and understood by all parties. The job description should be tailored to these responsibilities. The "paid" vs. "volunteer" status of the organization also may need to be considered. Restructuring the role of the medical director from being an advisor to being an operationally involved medical director is frequently a political as well as structural process. Most systems fall in between, but the operationally involved medical director is the ideal for which to strive. Such a medical director can truly influence policy and serve as an effective agent of the medical community.

Two general approaches exist for enlisting the services of a medical director: (1) to contract with the medical director or (2) to make them an officer or employee of the organization. If the contract approach is used, it is recommended that both an employment contract and an accompanying separate job description be utilized. The contract can set the length of service and specify how the medical director is to be rewarded or compensated for the time, skills and assets he brings to the organization as outlined in the job description. Depending on the model used, the employment contract may be with a university, hospital or clinic, private physicians' group, or an individual physician. When an organization uses multiple physicians, more than one physician may serve in a medical oversight capacity, especially if the department is large or encompasses more than one function, as in fire, rescue, transport, occupational health, etc. Their duties may be shared, separate, or overlap. If the second option is selected (officer or employee of the organization), a change in by-laws or a resolution by elected policy-makers may be needed to incorporate the job description into the organization. This is a reasonable approach for a volunteer organization where the medical director is a non-funded position. When there is monetary compensation to the medical director, an employment contract is more desirable. With either model there should be an option for the medical director to delegate certain responsibilities, but not the ultimate oversight. Physicians may also want the option to delegate duties and responsibilities to other appropriate individuals, such as nurses, paramedics, and physician assistants.

Titles may be chosen to reflect positions and responsibilities: medical director, fire surgeon, fire medical officer, or occupational medicine specialist. Credentials of a jurisdictional or commercial ambulance service medical director may need to be approved by the regional or state office respectively, or by the State EMS Office. Legal review is also recommended before the execution of any contract or the adoption of the new job description.[18,19]

There should be a formal process for appointing the medical director. As an example, one volunteer fire department in a mid-western state designates the fire chief, rescue chief and assistant chief of operations as the appointing authorities; and appointment of the medical director is accomplished by a majority vote of these individuals. Tenure is set for three years. There should also be a periodic review process to evaluate the performance and effectiveness of the medical director. Provisions can be added for suspension of the medical director's position or status with the organization, subject to procedural due process.

Appendix I is a model agreement between an EMS agency and the medical director. This model agreement is comprehensive in scope and may be useful for EMS agencies to use as a reference in developing contracts and job descriptions for the medical director. Appendix II is a model job description for a fire based EMS medical director in the state of Nebraska.

Summary

It is important that medical directors be sufficiently empowered to ensure that medical care meets or exceeds acceptable standards. Empowerment is achieved through both direct and indirect means. To be effective, medical directors must understand these principles and, when necessary, utilize them to enable change.

References

1. The Physician Medical Director. *The Five Points of Medication Direction.* Iowa Department of Health, July 17, 1996.
2. Kuehl A. *Prehospital Systems & Medical Oversight.* St. Louis: Mosby; 1994:267.
3. Leming RS. Preparing and empowering the Fire Services Leaders of the 21st Century. *The Voice.* 1996;25(6):16.
4. Position Description for EMS-MD for Lincoln, Nebraska.
5. Medical Director's responsibilities as listed by Omaha Fire Department.
6. Qualifications for EMS-MD, State of Iowa Department of Health.

7. EMS-MD position description for Multinomah County, Oregon.
8. EMS Director for Howard County, Maryland, request for proposal.
9. Policy statement, Medical direction of Prehospital Emergency Medical Services, approved by ACEP Board of Directors, October 1992.
10. Air Medical Committee. *Medical Director for Air Medical Transport Programs*. NAEMSP position paper; 1995.
11. Medical Direction Agreement, State of Maryland.
12. Wydro C, Cone DC, Davidson SJ. Legislative and regulatory description of EMS medical direction: a survey of states. *Prehosp Emerg Care*. 1997;4:233.
13. Serra HA, Blanton D, O'Connor RE. Physician Medical Direction in EMS. Position paper of NAEMSP. *Prehosp Emerg Care*. 1998;2(2).
14. Virginia Operational Medical Director Notebook.
15. Walker R. Qualification and Training of the Air Medical Director. *Air Medical Physicians' Handbook*. 1993(7):1.
16. Medical Support for the Fire Service. Current Priorities and Roles of Physicians. Proceedings of the Symposium with Recommendations to US Fire Administration and NFA.
17. Department of Health, Division of Health Standards and Licensure, Comprehensive Emergency Medical Services System Regulations. State of Kansas. Craft 1998.
18. Hall SA. Potential liabilities of medical directors for actions of EMTs. *Prehosp Emerg Care*. 1998;2(1):76.
19. Page J. Whose license is it anyway? *JEMS*. 1999;(21)92.

Appendix I

Model Agreement

This Agreement is between <u>(name of medical director)</u> ("Medical Director") and <u>(name of agency or entity that is contracting for medical direction)</u> ("EMS System"). By entering into this Agreement, the parties agree to be bound and obligated by its specific terms and conditions, as defined and described in this document. Any changes, amendments, addenda or attachments to this Agreement must be in writing and signed by both parties.

I. Term of Agreement

This Agreement shall become effective on the date of its execution and shall remain effective for <u>(period of time)</u> unless terminated <u>(for cause)</u> <u>(for any reason)</u> by either party, subject to ninety (90) days written notice. This Agreement may be renewable if the parties so desire.

II. Title, Rank and Status

A. Medical Director shall hold the official title and rank of "Medical Director" in the EMS System's formal organization.
B. Medical Director shall serve as an agent of the <u>(local)</u> <u>(regional)</u> medical community for the benefit of <u>(customers)</u> <u>(patients)</u> served by the EMS System. To accommodate these responsibilities, Medical Director shall have a direct reporting relationship with <u>(title of the administrative head of the organization)</u> and shall possess authority to communicate directly with any person or persons that provide, supervise, manage, or direct emergency medical care on behalf of the EMS System.

III. Operational Authority

A. Medical Director shall have authority to observe and monitor the availability and quality of emergency medical care <u>(and transportation)</u> provided by the EMS System and its agents, representatives, members and employees.
B. Medical Director shall have primary authority and responsibility for developing the EMS System's training, treatment, and medical transportation policies, subject to budgetary limitations, state and federal regulatory requirements and constraints, and labor agreements between the EMS System and its employees and/or members.
C. If, in the discretion of Medical Director, an administrative policy, procedure or practice of the EMS System requires altering or amending in order to assure the availability and quality of service, Medical Director shall have immediate, unrestricted access to <u>(title of the administrative head of the organization)</u> in order to report on the needed alteration(s) or amendment(s) and to recommend alternatives.
D. Medical Director will serve as the EMS System's representative to the <u>(local)</u> <u>(regional)</u> medical community and the medical community's representative to the EMS System.
E. Medical Director shall be considered a member of the EMS System's executive leadership staff and shall be included in all meetings and policy discussions relating to the availability and quality of

emergency medical care (and transportation) provided by the EMS System.

F. The operational authority of Medical Director shall be articulated to every agent, representative, member and employee of the EMS System, and that authority shall be defined and described in the organization's rules and regulations, manual of operations, or similar policy documents.

IV. Responsibilities

A. Medical Director shall be responsible to the EMS System for:

1. Developing and maintaining in accordance with applicable statutes, regulations, and current standards for emergency medical care (and transportation), comprehensive protocols, policies and procedures to guide and direct EMS personnel in their contact with and care for patients in the delivery of emergency medical care (and transportation) services.

2. Observing and monitoring the availability and quality of emergency medical care (and transportation) provided by the EMS System and its agents, representatives, members and employees.

3. Making regular reports to (title of administrative head of the organization) on the clinical performance of the EMS System.

4. Reporting to (title of the administrative head of the organization) on needed alteration(s) or amendment(s) to the EMS System's administrative policies, procedures and practices.

5. Designing, implementing and overseeing a continuous quality improvement program that focuses on prospective measures and participative review and analysis of system performance.

6. Representing the EMS System to the (local) (regional) medical community and responding to questions, criticisms, concerns or complaints from physicians, surgeons and/or hospital personnel about the performances, policies or practices of the EMS system and its agents, representatives, members and employees.

7. Whenever requested by (title of the administrative head of the organization), responding to questions, criticisms, concerns or complaints from citizens (including patients) about the performances, policies or practices of the EMS system and its agents, representatives, members and employees.

8. Participating with the (title of the administrative head of the organization) in investigations and decisions regarding disciplinary actions related to performance, behavior, aptitudes or fitness for duty of any member or employee of the EMS System that provides patient care or medical transportation services.

9. Attending all meetings of the EMS System executive leadership staff where items or topics to be discussed or deliberated fall within the purview of the Medical Director's interests and responsibilities.

B. The EMS System shall be responsible to Medical Director for:

1. Providing reasonable opportunities and access to observe and monitor the availability and quality of emergency medical care (and transportation) provided by the EMS System and its agents, representatives, members and employees.

2. Subject to budgetary constraints and availability of personnel resources, providing clerical assistance and personnel necessary to conduct ongoing evaluation of the EMS System's clinical performance and continuous quality improvement processes.

3. Providing reasonable opportunities and personal access to (title of the administrative head of the organization) for purposes of making regular reports on the clinical performance of the EMS System and on needed alteration(s) or amendment(s) to the System administrative policies, procedures and practices.

4. Providing reasonable opportunities and access to emergency operations, reports and records, and agents, representatives, members and employees of the EMS System for purposes of conducting a comprehensive continuous quality improvement program.

5. Providing timely notice of all meetings conducted by or participated in by representatives of the EMS System where items or topics to be discussed or deliberated fall within the purview of the Medical Director's interests and responsibilities.

6. Official recognition of the Medical Director's status as a member of the EMS System's executive leadership staff.

7. Providing or establishing an official radio title or designation to identify Medical Director in

electronic communications conducted on the EMS System voice and data transmission networks.

8. Providing a cellular telephone and pager for official use by Medical Director in performance of the duties and responsibilities specified in this agreement.

9. Providing private office space and office equipment, including a computer terminal, for official use by Medical Director in performance of the duties and responsibilities specified in this agreement.

10. Providing protective apparel and equipment for use by Medical Director at the scenes of emergency incidents.

11. Providing Medical Director with employee status for purposes of workers compensation insurance coverage.

12. Providing insurance or formal indemnification of Medical Director against claims, suits, and judgments of liability for all acts or omissions that are within the course and scope of duties and responsibilities that are specified in this agreement.

13. Providing an official automobile, to be maintained by the EMS System and equipped with required audible and visible warning devices, for use by Medical Director in performance of

the duties and responsibilities specified in this agreement.

V. Compensation

As consideration for the services rendered by Medical Director under this agreement, EMS System shall pay Medical Director the annual amount of $_____.

VI. Indemnification

EMS System agrees to indemnify and hold harmless Medical Director from any and all loss and expense, including but not limited to legal fees and other costs incurred by Medical Director in defense of any claims or suits related in any way to any alleged acts or omissions by EMS System, its agents, representatives, members and employees, during all periods covered by this agreement, plus that period of time thereafter which may be covered by any applicable statutes of limitation.

_____
(representative of EMS System)   (date)

_____
(Medical Director)   (date)

Appendix II

EMS Medical Director for Fire-Based Service

The Emergency Medical Service Medical Director (EMSMD) oversees all medical aspects of both fire and rescue divisions. The EMSMD will hold responsibility and ultimate authority of medical oversight of both structure and operations, including both direct and indirect medical oversight. The EMSMD will also oversee occupational health of the department.

(1) Licensing and Education:

a. He/she must be an approved licensed physician who is active in emergency medicine or primary care. He/she is to be familiar with state statutes relating to the Uniform Licensing Law, the Emergency Medical Services Act, the Trauma Act, as well as the rules and regulations pertaining to the above. He/she

should also be familiar with the state's Mandatory Reporting Regulations, and the Federal Controlled Substances Act.

b. Current state and federal controlled substance regulations must be maintained for the service program location. He/she will register and manage all controlled substances that are used in accordance with state and federal statutes and regulations. All substances must be kept current and have appropriate authorization signatures to demonstrate accountability. He/she will assure comprehensive record keeping and security measures for controlled substances which will be evaluated on a monthly basis

c. He/she will oversee Emergency Medical Services (EMS). He/she will allow Advanced Life Support (ALS), Automatic Defibrillator

(AD) and Emergency Medical Technician (EMT) medicine to be practiced under his/her medical license. This will be done in compliance with all state laws, rules and regulations.

d. He/she should maintain at least minimum knowledge levels for the EMSMD through continuing education. It is recommended that he/she have completed training in:
   1. Firefighter I
   2. Hazardous Materials (HAZMAT) operational level
   3. Incident Command System (ICS)
   4. Critical Incident Stress Debriefing (CISD)
   5. Other instruction as suggested by the Fire Chief.

(2) Authorization and Empowerment:

a. He/she shall maintain liaison with other physicians including other local medical directors and local emergency department physicians, and attend regional, state, and national meetings.

b. He/she is to interact with regional, state and local EMS authorities to ensure standards, needs and requirements are met and resource utilization is optimized.

c. He/she is to provide liaison with County Health Board and State Advanced Care Board.

d. He/she is to promulgate public education and information in the prevention of emergencies.

e. He/she is to collaborate with officers on a procedure for the management of complaints involving EMS.

f. He/she should be involved with budget planning and financial management on any matters involving the EMS.

g. He/she is to be involved in department Standard Operating Guidelines (SOG) and policy development as it relates to the EMS.

h. He/she shall oversee all EMS and Occupational Health issues and policies and is to be ultimately accountable to the Fire Chief.

i. He/she may appoint supervising physicians and physician surrogates.

(3) Occupational Medicine:

a. He/she should have knowledge of Occupational Safety Health Administration (OSHA) regulations, as well as occupational health and safety committee regulations (as described in National Fire Protection Association (NFPA) Standard 1500).

b. He/she is to be involved in operational and safety protocols and procedures as it pertains to EMS.

c. He/she is to be involved in policy regarding preventive health, infection control, vaccines, exposures, risk reductions and mitigation of all hazards.

d. He/she is to be notified of hazmat and body fluid exposures ASAP.

e. He/she is to be involved in injury and illness policies and be notified of line-of-duty injuries and death ASAP.

f. He/she is to be involved in "public health" surveillance, accessing risks to fire/EMS personnel. He/she is to be the liaison with the Health Department and collaborate on issues of public health.

g. He/she is to be involved in medical and physical requirements of new personnel, periodic exams, evaluations for disability and return to work.

h. He/she is to be involved in development of a wellness program.

i. He/she is to be involved in CISD.

(4) Direct Medical Oversight:

Also called "on-line", base station", or "immediate" Medical Director is the contemporaneous physician in charge of a field provider. The communication may be via radio, telephone or actual contact of a physician on scene. This function of communication between the provider and responsible oversight physician may be delegated to a medical oversight surrogate or use of standing orders and/or protocols.

a. He/she should be notified, as soon as possible, of all child births in the field, all multiple casualties, prolonged extrications, and multiple alarm fire calls for the opportunity to respond and provide direct medical oversight.

b. He/she may be involved in medical monitoring and rehab and treatment of personnel at incident scenes at his/her discretion.

c. He/she may be notified of other calls at the discretion of scene command or at the request of the EMSMD.

(4) Indirect Medical Oversight:

Also called "off-line", or "project" Medical Director is defined as the physician who is responsible for the ultimate medical accountability and appropriateness of the entire departmental system including overall system design implementation (protocol development) and evaluation (quality management).

a. Prospective:

1. He/she will review and approve protocols and standing orders of local EMS for all EMT-A, EMT-B, EMT-A/D, EMT-I and EMT-Ps with the option to amend or adjust to meet specific needs thereof.
2. He/she will review functions of First Responders.
3. He/she will be available to coordinate continuing education, identify goals and meet requirements.
4. He/she may be involved in discussions regarding ambulance and fire equipment, supplies and operations.
5. He/she should be involved in discussions regarding EMS communications including dispatch and hospital communications.
6. He/she should be involved with local and regional EMS for disaster and mass casualty planning.
7. He/she should be involved in coordination of activities such as mutual aid and hazmat exposures.

b. Retrospective:

1. He/she will evaluate the competence of each EMT-A, EMT-B, EMT-A/D, EMT-I and EMT-P to operate a recording monitor/defibrillator in accordance with subpart 010.04.
2. He/she will oversee a quality assurance program including evaluation of EMS personnel.
3. He/she may provide individual consultation and written evaluation of each at his/her discretion.
4. He/she will provide counseling to specific individuals if inappropriate care is rendered. This is to be followed with targeted instruction and follow-up. He/she may withhold or qualify privileges as deemed necessary.
5. He/she should be involved in disciplinary proceedings involving EMS.

Section Four

Michael Gunderson

There are many different groups who work with or are affected by EMS. It is important for EMS medical directors and administrators to understand how these groups fit into the overall system—at a local, state, and national level. The chapters within the Perspectives section will look at these stakeholder groups and explore what they offer and expect from EMS— ranging from the federal government to the spouse of an EMS medical director. Insights on these perspectives will better equip the medical directors to anticipate their needs, find "system" solutions, balance their sometimes competing interests, and perhaps to reach a better balance in their own personal and professional lives.

CHAPTER 36

ED Interaction with Prehospital Providers

Suzanne K. Elliott, MD
James M. Atkins, MD

Introduction

The most important role that prehospital providers perform is that of treating and transporting patients to the hospital. EMS personnel must rely on their own training and intuition prior to bringing patients to the emergency department (ED). The transition between field and hospital treatment is critical, and something that ED personnel must treat with attentiveness and respect. EMS providers serve as an emergency physician's eyes and ears in the prehospital environment, and ED personnel should consider these providers as extensions of the emergency care team. These dedicated individuals can provide a wealth of information to ED staff, if allowed to give their input. The following sections describe the optimal interaction between prehospital providers and the ED staff.

Taking Reports

While not all EDs give direct medical oversight, many take reports from en route vehicles. Radio and telephone communication directly links the prehospital providers with definitive hospital care. Transmitting concise and accurate information is something that takes confidence and practice. It is important to remember that talking "over the air" and organizing a report for the ED can be an intimidating process. Not all personnel have experience with this, and may initially give too much or too little information. A new provider may talk excessively and without a break in transmission, perhaps reading all twenty medications a patient is taking, including over-the-counter bowel preparations. A gentle reminder to be brief and concise should be made privately to the provider when he arrives in the department. Faulty reports such as this should not be corrected on the radio where other agencies are listening. Be patient and do not pass judgment if a report is fragmented or the ambulance crew sounds frazzled. Just as an emergency room can be chaotic, frequently a scene can be crazy as well, with multiple casualties or hysterical family members. The crew members may be busy trying to diffuse a situation or calm bystanders, and deserve a little slack.

The American College of Emergency Physicians states that ED personnel must respond "to all requests for medical guidance promptly and with an attitude of participation, responsibility, and cooperation while following established protocols." ED staff who give direct medical orders over the radio must be expected to have knowledge of system protocols, and order medical options in a direct and concise fashion. If a protocol exists for IV Valium, do not confuse a squad by ordering rectal Valium. Prehospital providers are not physicians, and need to have clear instruction when confronted by a difficult patient or scene. Any new physician should be required to take a direct medical oversight course, and be aware of what they can realistically expect from EMS personnel. House staff rotating through the ED need to be knowledgeable on policies and procedures concerning prehospital care providers before attempting any interactions.

Prehospital personnel may also ask for instruction on where to take a patient. EMTALA dictates that hospital designation is directed with a facility's capabilities and proximity in mind. ED nurses and physicians must avoid placing EMS personnel in an awkward position, and instead give direct and objective transport instructions. If a hospital is the only healthcare facility in the area, this will not be an issue. If one of multiple facilities, the system protocols for transport should be familiar to the ED staff giving direction. For example, a critically injured, hypotensive trauma patient would be directed to the Level I trauma facility, while an asthma exacerbation would go to the nearest facility.

Accepting Patients

EMS personnel are an important link between scene and hospital. When a nurse or physician accepts care of a patient in the ED, they must encourage prehospital providers to give a brief report. Regardless of how critical a patient's condition, there is always time for a brief synopsis of the patient's status. This may occur while the crew is bringing the patient into a treatment room, or transferring the patient to a hospital stretcher. Frequently EMS gives valuable information regarding the scene, family, home life, or medical history, in addition to patient data such as signs or symptoms. A bent steering column with intrusion into the passenger compartment, or an apartment with human and animal excrement are important factors for the ED physician's treatment and disposition. Always listen carefully, and review the prehospital care report (PCR) as early as possible. Ideally, the PCR should be completed concurrent with patient care or, at least, shortly after the patient arrives.

When questioning prehospital providers about specific transports, the language of ED staff should be chosen carefully. Question a paramedic as if talking to a physician colleague, but use simpler dialogue when obtaining information from a basic EMT. The language skills and knowledge base not only vary from one training level to another, but are also different among individuals with similar training.

Feedback

Prehospital providers, depending on their level of skill, may or may not have a strong handle on the patient's problem and treatment. They may assume that an elderly woman with a history of congestive heart failure is tachypneic from this condition, when she is actually hyperventilating because of her anxiety. Feedback on such cases is a critical component of the prehospital-ED interface. Complimenting an ambulance crew on their assessment and treatment skills of a truly hypoxic patient in heart failure appropriately will make them feel that they have played an important role in a patient's care. This holds especially true with the volunteer prehospital provider. It may be equally important to point out to paramedic staff that fully examining a diabetic would have revealed the cellulitis causing a patient's tachycardia and hot, dry skin.

Another area of importance for feedback involves transport and scene times. Field personnel, while providing transition between the scene and emergency department, must remain focused on getting the patient to definitive care. It is easy to lose this focus in the heat of the moment. Picture arriving on the scene of a high-speed roll-over MVA, and finding a screaming teenager ejected twenty feet from her vehicle. On approaching this patient you realize that her femur is folded at a funny angle beneath her, obviously fractured. You would like to spend time calming her, performing a history and physical, starting intravenous lines, and so on. In truth, however, this is a load-and-go situation, as the patient has potentially life-threatening injuries. Additional information can be obtained in the back of the ambulance, as well as initiating both psychological and medical interventions. Extended scene times in similar situations are dangerous, and prehospital providers may need this reinforced. On the other hand, a forty-five minute extrication time may make delay unavoidable. Periodic review and discussion of scene and transport times should be part of the feedback loop.

While it is optimal to give people immediate feedback, this is not always feasible. Each institution should initiate a system for feedback on every patient through written notes to squads, patient case reviews, or other mechanisms. This process should be a collaborative and ongoing effort between prehospital providers and emergency department personnel.

Training and Case Review

A vital link between the ED staff and prehospital providers can be maintained via training and case review. It is a well known fact that clinical skills deteriorate over time, so that periodic refreshers are essential. Even basic points such as head positioning for bag valve mask ventilation or endotracheal intubation can be forgotten. Supervised training in the ED can be used to reiterate such points. Squads perform "in house" training regularly, but need physician interaction as well via lectures and case review. Lectures can be squad-specific, or district-wide as in case review. Case reviews can be condition- or symptom-specific (trauma, shortness of breath, chest pain) or more general. Another specific review that deserves mention is critical stress debriefing. This usually follows a stress or anxiety provoking call, and may include cases such as child abuse, suicide, or mass casualty incidents. Many times both prehospital providers and emergency department personnel can benefit from joint discussions. The prehospital providers should be allowed to give input and interact amongst themselves and ED staff at such training sessions. All of these interactions are required toward continuing medical education credit for EMS re-certification, and help foster better communication and rapport.

ED observation time can be a great opportunity for prehospital providers to learn and build a good relationship with staff. Much of their initial patient assessment and treatment skills are obtained in the ED. Periodic refresher rotations through the ED allow staff to become comfortable with the care these providers render in the field. If allowed at individual institutions, prehospital providers may demonstrate skill proficiency in front of their physician and nurse peers. While such activities have great educational value, they can be very intimidating for field personnel. Be supportive and encouraging!

Recognizing System Problems

Occasionally problems will arise that are not specifically the fault of EMS or the hospital, but need to be addressed so as not to affect patient care. When such problems are recognized, they must be dealt with expediently. EMS personnel frequently have to wait for a nurse or physician to assume patient care, and they need to know that seeking out the charge nurse if they have another call is expected. Similarly, with construction of a new ED facility, plans must be implemented for diversion, alternative parking, or patient drop-off. EMS needs for space for equipment exchange, PCR completion, and drug replacement must be addressed. If a cardiac arrest is called in the ambulance and the patient taken directly to the hospital morgue, a plan must be in place for signing the body in and notifying the medical examiner. System problems should be taken care of promptly so that EMS providers are not placed in an awkward position or made to look incompetent in front of the patient or the family.

Summary

In summary, ED staff need to be open and receptive to prehospital providers. From volunteer to career professional, these people work diligently to deliver definitive prehospital emergency care. Good rapport and interaction with local medical oversight and the ED staff help EMS providers in their delivery of health care, and also encourage behaviors that they can emulate. The patient is the one who ultimately benefits when providers are allowed to do their job in a healthy, fostering environment. The care delivered to patients in the field is a direct reflection of the training received, and the emergency department should play an active role in this experience.

Nurses

Beth Lothrop Adams, MA, RN, EMT-P
Peggy Trimble, MA, BSN

Introduction

The history of nursing is replete with examples of nurses providing care outside the environs of a hospital. From the days of Florence Nightingale to the present day, nurses have found the opportunity to contribute to the health care of the communities where they lived and worked, as well as the armies they supported and served. The earliest days of modern emergency medical services relied on nurses for staffing, alongside a physician, the "collapse services" rushing aid to the victim of acute myocardial infarction.[1] Soon after the development of the mobile coronary care unit came the National Academy of Sciences and National Research Council report on trauma deaths.[2] The military experience in Vietnam provided trained trauma experts in the form of recently discharged military medical personnel.[1] When the then-newly developed Department of Transportation (DOT) training standards for paramedics blended coronary and trauma care, nurses were often called upon to bridge the gap for these experienced trauma care technicians by assisting the EMS physician with the necessary training. Since that time, nurses have been and continue to be instrumental in the initial and ongoing education of prehospital providers.

Then, as now, the administrative demands of system development, implementation, and maintenance exceed any one person's abilities and endurance. Soon, nurses with their broad-based education and team leadership skills were augmenting the physician in this area as well. In those early days, there was no abundance of educated, experienced field personnel to assist the burdened medical director with program and system development. Boyd in Illinois and Cowley in Maryland relied heavily on nurses to build their state EMS systems.[3] Trauma nurse coordinators and nurses in EMS system administration were implemented in these states. These nurses participated in system design, as well as in developing applications, formulating designation criteria for trauma centers, and educating other providers.

Overview

Today, in many parts of the United States and the world, nurses work closely with physicians, government agencies, and field personnel to establish and maintain systems. As EMS continues to evolve and mature, it is both reasonable and appropriate to develop systems that maximally utilize the capabilities of all members of the multidisciplinary team. As such, nurses contribute expertise in skills such as (1) communicating with and coordinating the efforts of many disciplines to address patient or system issues; (2) applying organizational skills for the management of multiple endeavors at a variety of levels (for example, patient or family, interdepartmental, interagency, interhospital); and (3) focusing on the well-being of the patient or family as the goal of EMS. These skills are foremost goals of professional nurses' education and experience bases.

TABLE 37.1
Nursing Associations with Interest in EMS
American Association of Critical Care Nurses
American College of Nurse Midwives
American Practitioners for Infection Control
Association of Rehabilitation Nurses
Association of Operating Room Nurses
Emergency Nurses Association
National Association of Orthopedic Nurses
National Flight Nurses Association
Nurses Association of the American College of Obstetrics and Gynecology
Organization of Nurse Executives
Society of Post Anesthesia Nurses
Society of Trauma Nurses

The maturing system should examine potential contributions from nurses for three reasons. First, a system includes responsibilities ranging from prevention through rehabilitation. When seen as a system that includes multiple high-risk populations (trauma, burns, cardiac, high-risk maternal and neonatal, behavioral, and toxicology), the value of a professional nurse as a member becomes clear.[4] Much of the work of EMS is well matched to the skills of the nurse; professional education and guided experiences acquired during many nurses' careers have even developed some EMS areas of concentration into specialties. For example, patient and family teaching principles readily adapt to community efforts in prevention, fund raising, system access and awareness, legislation, lobbying, and staff work for special projects.

In addition to the skill match of professional nurses to EMS needs, nurses are often the largest provider group in a system. Professional nursing organizations such as the American Association of Critical Care Nurses (AACN), the Emergency Nurses Association (ENA), and the Society of Trauma Nurses (STN) can be valuable allies when EMS efforts are underway locally or nationally. Nursing associations with EMS interests are listed below. Often, nurses access many networks by collaborating with professional organizations and interacting in the patient-care delivery system of many health care agencies. This enhances the value of nurses as members of the management structure because these networks and organizations are natural vehicles for communication. They provide a mechanism for systems to address such collaborative work as data collection, special projects, quality management, and policy and protocol development and dissemination, as well as problem solving. A nurse-to-nurse process often works best here. Even when the process calls for a non-nurse lead, the partnership with nursing adds a dimension of patient and professional sensitivity possibly not present otherwise.

As a third consideration for the inclusion of nurse leaders in EMS, the phase of the system beginning when the patient reaches the hospital and phases that follow need to be included and addressed by the system. To date, the in-hospital phase has lagged behind the prehospital phase in system development and formalization. Nursing staffing shortages, hospital diversion policies, overcrowding, reimbursement, and societal issues continue to challenge systems in their efforts to ensure not only that the high-risk patient gets to the right place at the right time but that the hospital and staff there will be able to care for the patient in spite of other competing and confounding demands. The in-hospital and post-acute-care settings are familiar territory for nurses. Additional progress in system management could occur when nurses address issues of resource allocation, organization of the care environment, and critical communication linkages.

The role of nurses within a system is dependent on several variables including (1) state or local laws, (2) the director, (3) the type of agency or system, and (4) economics—especially supply and demand.[5] To address legal aspects first, existing state and local laws govern the scope of practice for registered nurses (RNs) in all states. To date, no states have laws that allow the independent licensure of field personnel. In contrast, RNs are independently licensed and must legally function according to the Nurse Practice Act in their states. As one example of legally integrating the traditional nurse-physician relationship into prehospital care, some system medical directors have delegated the responsibility for direct medical oversight to nurses within a framework of standing orders or indirect medical oversight protocols.[6] This is not a great departure from the advanced role coronary care nurses have accepted in managing Advanced Care Life Support (ACLS) situations using medical protocols in an in-hospital setting. In some systems, failure to implement this nursing role would significantly limit the availability and delivery of prehospital care.

The second variable influencing the role of the nurse in EMS is the director; the director establishes and promotes the vision for a system. Whether this vision includes an interdependent, multidisciplinary team directly determines the inclusion or exclusion of the nurse in a recognized, legitimized role. Often the experience of the director influences the selection of vision and paradigms supported. Those directors who have experienced collaborative practice with professional nurses value the enhanced delivery of care because of such firsthand knowledge. For others, this model represents a departure from strongly held beliefs, an element of risk-taking, and perceived loss of control. The continued inclusion of this chapter in this book is for visionary risk-takers who recognize the potential for system enhancements that professional nurses offer.

The successful medical director must be intimately and actively involved in all aspects of the system from administration and education to standard setting, quality assurance, and research. Yet no one person can or should provide all that a system may need. Collaborative, collegial relationships with nurses have strengthened systems by enabling directors to maximize their time and efforts. For example, verifying that providers' educational requirements for entry and recertification are met can be a Herculean task and, as such, may necessitate delegation to a nonphysician training coordinator if the medical director is to fulfill any other obligations and responsibilities.

As a third variable, the type of agency or system affects the extent of nurses' participation and involvement. Systems with an aeromedical component often use nurses in partnership with other patient-care experts as caregivers on the flight team. Although it seems that a hospital-based prehospital service is more likely to employ nurses in a variety of roles, Houston and Seattle (both fire-based systems) use nurses in prehospital response. The Houston system created the role of prehospital nurse clinician, which serves as a model for other systems.[7] The New York City system used nurses as an integral part of dispatch as early as 1979.

Lastly, although it might be a matter of medical preference to use physicians and experienced paramedics to fill all roles and functions within a system, economic pressures, availability of qualified practitioners, and especially standards of care in many parts of the country may necessitate sharing the responsibility with nurses or other non-physicians. As examples, the burden of delivering prehospital emergency care in rural America often cannot be borne by a limited number of available physicians and field personnel.

Education and Training

According to demographic information provided by the National Association of EMS Educators (NAEMSE) only 315 members (20%) identified themselves as RNs, including 107 (6.9%) who identified themselves as RN/EMT-P. However, it should be noted that only 67% of the membership provided information about their credentials on their membership applications.[8]

Broad-based nursing education provides a sound framework of knowledge that, when coupled with the appropriate clinical experience and certain personal attributes, well equips the nurse for a role in EMS education throughout the continuum. In addition to required nursing process and skill courses, nurses complete course work in anatomy and physiology, cardiology, medicolegal aspects, microbiology, ob-

stetrics, pathophysiology, pediatrics, pharmacology, and psychology. Although all of this coursework may not translate directly to the delivery of prehospital care, the depth of knowledge such a background provides is very beneficial in training. This is particularly true with the expanded content in the 1999 Emergency Medical Technician-Paramedic National Standard Curriculum.[9]

It is not sufficient to merely know as much about a given topic as one's student. To teach successfully, one needs a broader depth of knowledge, as well as the ability to convey complex medical concepts in an easily understood manner. For nurses this capability often results from formal training and experience in providing education to patients and families in a clinical environment. Hence, the experienced nurse is often an experienced educator prior to entering EMS. These teaching skills can be applied at many points along the continuum. Prevention initiatives in the community, fund-raising addresses to contributors, interagency continuing education, and multidisciplinary training programs are only a few examples.

In the prehospital arena the global patient perspective, which is the essence of nursing, is a valuable adjunct for the education of prehospital personnel. Physician educators often focus on history, diagnostics, and disease; providers tend to be more task-oriented. This orientation can limit the ability to adapt when patient complaints or physical findings fall outside defined parameters. Patient management problems often have psychosocial aspects, or fall under the "interpersonal relationship" category. Nurses who impart their skills to other providers extensively address these processes. Nurses are well prepared to blend the two perspectives—the priorities of the "golden hour" and the patient's overall status and chief complaints that extend beyond it.

As the spectrum of technical skills required of prehospital personnel continues to expand, initiation of therapeutic modalities in the field necessitates a working knowledge of infusion pumps, oximeters, and other monitoring devices, as well as the ability to calculate dosages and prepare drugs for infusion. Experienced nurses are a valuable resource for training others in the set-up, maintenance, and troubleshooting of such equipment, and they can relate the patient responses to the technology in training programs. This allows for application rather than the "cookbook" approach.

Clinical experience is an essential component in the educational process for all levels of prehospital personnel. Ideally patient interaction in the clinical setting should take place in the field environment under the direct supervision of an experienced preceptor. However, the reality is that many systems cannot support such experiential activities and utilize a variety of in-patient and emergency department settings to augment field training in order to provide a well grounded clinical experience.

Previous prehospital curricula focused on a specified number of hours in a variety of designated clinical environments as part of the student experience.[10,11] EMS curricula revisions over the past decade were based on the National EMS Education and Practice Blueprint, as well as the EMS Education Agenda for the Future, consensus documents commissioned by the National Highway and Traffic Safety Administration and widely endorsed by EMS and EMS-vested organizations.[12,13] A new perspective has replaced minimum hours with competencies. For instance, the 1994 EMT-Basic National Standard Curriculum requires a minimum of 5 patient interview/assessment experiences.[14] The 1999 Paramedic National Standard Curriculum specifies minimum competencies for psychomotor skills and patient encounters across the span of life with the associated special needs of unique populations (such as obstetric, psychiatric or trauma patients) as well as a variety of pathologies (such as chest pain, syncope, or respiratory distress).[9]

It is advantageous to have a nurse who is familiar with EMS facilitate, coordinate, and supervise student clinical experience. Often, nurses design clinical training activities that maximize student experiences most likely to result in skill mastery needed for care in the field. Nurses easily interact with the various departments and facilitate student adjustment in the hospital environment, having worked within that milieu themselves. Acceptance by hospital staff is most frequently negotiated on a nurse-to-nurse basis, as is the approval and implementation of the clinical programs.

For patient populations that do not originate at the roadside or in similar prehospital environments but rather enter EMS at the interhospital level, the interhospital link is paramount. Nurses are often key policy or protocol supporters, educating and coaching staff. Packaging the patient for transport and transmitting vital information to the transport team are roles that the community hospital nurse usually performs. A system that attends to the education outreach for these nurses will see an impact on care and transfer compliance.

Nurses in many systems have become experts in specific clinical aspects of EMS. Trauma registries, high-risk neonatal transport, communicable disease management, and patient support groups are examples. These nurses are the best educators for sharing their expertise, regardless of the learner population. As EMS challenges continue and systems evolve, resources should be identified and applied appropriately. Enlisting the educational support of nurses from organizations such as the Association of Practitioners for Infection Control (APIC) to educate prehospital providers about principles of self and patient infectious disease protection, cleaning of equipment, and regulation compliance are examples of nurse partnerships in EMS that reduce cost, improve patient care, and increase provider competency through education and training.

Quality Management

Realizing that quality management (QM) is the *sine qua non* of the present and future of any system, it is imperative that the medical director has a pivotal role in all aspects of QM. In most systems, virtually all prehospital care is rendered under the medical director's license. Even for aspects of the system that are not delegated medical tasks, QM remains the framework for assessing areas for improvement, and ensuring that the system is attaining the goals that the public entrusted it to meet. Once standards are established, it seems unrealistic and imprudent use of physician resources for the medical director to perform the routine, day-to-day monitoring activities. This is particularly true in large systems in which such an undertaking would be a great burden, or those in which the medical director role is an additional duty for a practitioner. The logical conclusion is to delegate such monitoring to nurses or other non-physicians. Collectively, nurses are known for their attention to detail and, as such, are well suited for QM monitoring activities if they are knowledgeable of the existing practice standards. Because the scope of nursing practice differs from that of prehospital care, it is beneficial if not essential that the nurse have EMS training and field experience, if they are to be perceived as credible auditors of prehospital care by field personnel.

Many systems have capitalized on the willingness of nurses to cross agency and geographic barriers to address patient-care issues. If a nurse is in the system QM model, the identification and facilitation of these opportunities for improvement are more readily evident. In concept and in implementation, the QM aspect of most systems is rudimentary. It is an excellent match of work to nurse talents. Including nurses may add significant momentum to further develop this important but difficult aspect of EMS.

Administration

The role of management is to enable the workers to do their job. Although this demands that an administrator know and respect the job to be done, it does not require that they have done the job. The qualities that enable nurses to be successful contributing members of the EMS community as educators or QM coordinators also stand them in good stead as administrators. Communication and organizational skills, the nurse's work experience in a professional environment, and the resultant understanding of legal issues and regulatory agencies are valuable assets for any administrator.

Although the domain of the agency may limit the potential for nurses to move into administrative positions (particularly in a fire-based system), other systems have vast potential for including nurses in administration.[7]

In Maryland, for example, nurse administrators manage the high-risk neonatal and high-risk maternal programs; also they are responsible for budget, protocols, and QM. In many states, nurses administer grants. Most trauma systems include nurse coordinators on the management staff. The tables that follow provide an inventory of trauma nurse coordinators' responsibilities. Research projects are another example of nurse management skills put to good use, because this concept is another part of the profession's fundamental education.

Patient Care

Even now controversy persists regarding the legal and professional practice requirements for nurses delivering care in the prehospital environment. The National Association of Emergency Medical Technicians (NAEMT) maintains that nurses practicing in the prehospital setting may be certified as EMTs only after completing the appropriate DOT standard curriculum.[15] ENA members formally developed their own National Standard Guidelines for Prehospital Nursing Curriculum that combined the emergency nursing focus with the national standard paramedic

curriculum.[5] Additionally the ENA scope of practice document includes the prehospital arena as a part of the emergency nursing environment.[16]

State boards of nursing are researching the scope pf practice issue. The 1988 joint statement from the ENA and National Flight Nurse Association opposed the necessity for dual-licensure for nurses opting to practice in the prehospital environment, and recognized state boards of nursing as the regulatory agency for all aspects of nursing practice.[17] In 1993, a national survey regarding the regulation of prehospital nursing practice by state EMS agencies, revealed that 44 of 50 states offered no certification in prehospital nursing, while the majority required certification to practice on an EMS unit.[18]

Nursing education makes it possible for nurses to readily grasp the scope and content of paramedic course work, but does not prepare students for all the technical skills or the reality of delivering patient care outside of a controlled environment. On the other hand, requiring nurses to duplicate components of their education creates a barrier to entry for areas where additional advanced life support personnel are needed. Another problem is that the regulation of nursing practice by entities other than state boards of nursing potentially violates the state regulations.

Even when prehospital certification is not required, many nurses find that EMS training and certification facilitates their acceptance and ability to relate to others in prehospital care. Taking into account state or local statutes, the required training should depend on the role to be filled and the EMS director's preference; if the individual is to function as a prehospital provider, competence must be equivalent to that of peers.

The prehospital patient-care environment should incorporate the physician-extender role of the EMS provider and acknowledge that high-quality patient care depends on a collaborative, interdependent effort and mutual respect among caregivers. This model does not dilute the medical director's authority; it supports it. Prehospital care personnel interact regularly with physicians; they interact with nurses daily in extended care facilities, clinics, and emergency departments. In a mature system, prehospital providers benefit from exposure to the comprehensive patient perspective of nurses, the scientific perspective of physicians, and the technical expertise that experienced EMTs and paramedics provide. In such a model the team concept is essential for effective patient care.

Clinical functions in the prehospital arena may include direct patient-care responsibilities as an ALS crewmember, or as mobile intensive care nurses (MICNs), flight nurses, or preceptors. Probably the most evolved nursing clinical role in EMS systems is that of trauma nurse coordinator. Beachley discussed this role, which began in some states as long ago as 1971.[3] Although the position is used in many systems today, variations in organizational structure and job descriptions exist. See table 37.2 for a sample role functions.

Unlike the care given by physicians who move throughout the hospital environment with the patient, nursing care traditionally is delivered based on unit assignment. Specialty units (e.g., operating, recovery, and critical care) should be considered a part of the EMS system. The nurse providers on such units should be adequately connected to the system and prepared to provide the appropriate care for the specialty populations—adults, children, or neonates—in the acute care hospital. The trauma nurse coordinator is a logical choice as the organizational connection among these specialty areas.

At the University of California-Davis Medical Center, the trauma nurse practitioner position is being explored in an effort to provide service where workload exceeds available trauma physician staff. This model has been used successfully for many years in the postoperative through rehabilitative phases of care for neurotrauma patients in the Maryland system. Likewise, the National Children's Hospital in Washington and The Johns Hopkins Hospital Children's Trauma Center in Baltimore use nurse specialists to coordinate care from the acute hospital, to rehabilitation, and to home.[19]

The public criticism that EMS systems save lives but provide inadequate follow-up must be addressed. Existing home healthcare and rehabilitation services should be recruited into the EMS system continuum just as acute care hospitals and rescue squads were recruited in the earlier days of system development. Where gaps exist, they can be filled by implementing

TABLE 37.2				
Trauma Nurse Coordinator Role Functions				
RESEARCH	**CLINICAL PRACTICE**	**EDUCATION**	**CONSULTATION**	**ADMINISTRATION**

Data collection	Clinical rounds	Inservice
		  New equipment
		  New protocols
			Develops protocols	Implementation of protocols and standards

Trauma registry	Patient care follow-up	Orientation to team roles	Liaison with community EMS council	Change agent

Identifies and monitors specific investigations with the trauma population	Applies primary and secondary assessment and interventions based on ATLS guidelines for trauma resuscitation	Continuing education
		Trauma nursing course
		  ATLS
		  ACLS
			Liaison with prehospital care providers	Preparation of trauma program reports

Initiates nursing research for trauma	Formulation or supervision of written care plans for trauma patients	Outreach
		  Prehospital
		  Nursing
		  Public
			Participation in planning and ongoing management of multi-disciplinary programs	Preparation and management of trauma or trauma program budget

Interprets and communicates recent nursing innovations and research findings	Integration of team approach to trauma	Role model for other		Staff for trauma management committee

Translates relevant scientific knowledge into trauma nursing practice	Monitors nursing care of patient through the trauma care continuum	Role model for other trauma nurses through demonstration	Consults with discharge planners
			  Rehabilitation
			  programs
			  Special support
			  services
			  Home care
			  Medical staff
				Monitors effectiveness of trauma program through QM activities

Experiments with new patient care modalities and practice models	Patient advocate within trauma system	Trauma patient care conferences		Initiates corrective action measures for problems identified in trauma programs
	Gives feedback to nursing staff of referring hospitals			Marketing trauma programs
				Legislative activities

From: Beachley M, Snow S, Trimble P, Developing trauma care systems: the trauma nurse coordinator. *J Nur. Adm.* 1988;18(7):34.

plans developed as part of a system that best serves the patient. For example, specialty follow-up clinics may need to be created. Nurses are predominant caregivers and administrators in home health services and rehabilitation agencies. A nurse coordinator or administrator who facilitates communication and bridges patient connections across agencies at the "back door" of the system can improve not only continuity but also outcome of patient care.

For a number of patients and their families, community support groups serve an important role during recovery in re-establishing healthy behaviors. Nurses have been instrumental in establishing these groups for trauma, burn, and cardiac patients, and in conducting the programs. Although not the motivating factor for organizing, such groups often take on the role of system supporters, lobbying for services, backing prevention legislation, and educating their own communities.

Support Staff

An experienced nurse with a good understanding of the prehospital environment and the EMS system is a valuable resource. Although specific roles may vary from system to system, depending on the availability of other resources and the agency needs, nurses are often comfortable with an ombudsman role. They are trained to deal with the psychological needs of caregivers and patients, as well as the integration of research and clinical practice. The wide array of support roles filled by nurses attests to the flexibility their education and training give them to address patient care via many different avenues. Such roles may include infection control, peer counseling, critical incident stress debriefing, research and public relations, and participation in advisory groups and disaster planning. Their ability as professionals to move throughout agencies and across disciplines is unmatched.

Summary

The optimal role for nurses in prehospital systems is aggressively debated. Recommendations range from the traditional to the innovative. Certainly, some aspects of EMS are better suited for nursing involvement than are others. Although controversy exists regarding preparation for roles, consensus exists in many areas. Licensure as an RN alone is not sufficient for successful integration of the nurse into EMS, just as licensure itself is not the only qualification for a physician to serve as an EMS medical director. Although the role of nurses may not be as clearly defined as that of the field provider or medical director, nurses contribute to the delivery of EMS care throughout our country on a daily basis.

If one accepts the premise that critical care begins in the streets, then it is reasonable that nurses continue to be part of that team, along with all the other prehospital providers. Each member brings a unique perspective and expertise to the delivery of patient care. If systems accept the mission to serve the critically ill and injured, based on a continuum of care, nurses will continue to be valuable assets in areas where specialized nursing care is required (for example, critical care transport), where interagency interface is important (e.g., development of protocols and policies), or when skilled educators are required (e.g., interosseous infusion education and community prevention efforts).

One of the challenges that has always faced EMS innovators is how to progress in spite of constrained resources. The nurse talent in EMS is to a great extent untapped. EMS systems have made major strides. Perhaps the 21st century will be remembered as the era in which EMS recognized the potential for exponential growth from its collaboration with nursing. Models already exist but others must be developed.

EMS has a history of attracting the innovative practitioner. Opportunities for expanding and improving systems abound. Nurses have responded to EMS in small numbers, considering the population available. The ability of EMS leaders to mobilize nursing support is directly proportional to their abilities to include nurse leaders in the organization and to practice collaboratively.

References

1. Stewart R. Historical perspectives. In: Rousch, W, ed. *Principles of EMS Systems.* Dallas: American College of Emergency Physicians; 1989.
2. Mustalish AC, Post C. History. In: Kuehl, AE, ed. *Prehospital Systems and Medical Oversight.* National Association of EMS Physicians, St. Louis: Mosby; 1994.
3. Beachley M, Snow S, Trimble P. Developing trauma care systems: the trauma nurse coordinator. *J Nursing Admin.* 1988;18(7,8):3442.
4. Boyd D. The conceptual development of EMS systems in the United States. II. *Emerg Med Serv.* 1982;11(2):26–35.
5. Emergency Nurses Association. *National Standard Guidelines for Prehospital Nursing Curriculum.* Des Plaines, IL: 1991.

6. Moore HS. MICNs: who can help? *J Emerg Nursing.* 1987;13(6):325–327.

7. Lyle NA. Prehospital nurse clinician: job description and evaluation tool. *J Emerg Nursing.* 1989;15(6):365–369.

8. Adams B. Personal correspondence with Diane Ohm of National Association of EMS Educators, 2001.

9. US Department of Transportation, National Highway Traffic Safety Administration. *Emergency Medical Technician-Paramedic National Standard Curriculum.* 1999.

10. US Department of Transportation, National Highway Traffic Safety Administration. *Emergency Medical Technician-Ambulance National Standard Curriculum.* 1984.

11. US Department of Transportation, National Highway Traffic Safety Administration. *Emergency Medical Technician-Paramedic National Standard Curriculum.* 1985.

12. US Department of Transportation, National Highway Traffic Safety Administration. *National EMS Education Agenda for the Future.* 2000.

13. US Department of Transportation, National Highway Traffic Safety Administration. *National EMS Education and Practice Blueprint.* 1993.

14. US Department of Transportation, National Highway Traffic Safety Administration. *Emergency Medical Technician-Paramedic National Standard Curriculum.* 1994.

15. National Association of Emergency Medical Technicians. *Role of the Registered Nurse in the Prehospital Environment.* Official position statement; 1990.

16. Emergency Nurses Association. *Position Statement: Scope of Emergency Nursing Practice.* Des Plaines, IL: 1999.

17. Emergency Nurses Association and National Flight Nurse Association. *Joint position statement: role of the registered nurse in the prehospital environment.* Des Plaines, IL: 1988.

18. Johnson RI, Childress SE, Harron HL. Regulation of prehospital nursing practice: a national survey. *J Emerg Nursing.* 1993;19(5):437–440.

19. Spisso J, et al. Improved quality of care and reduction of house staff workload using trauma nurse practitioners. *J Trauma.* 1990;30(6):660–665.

CHAPTER 38

Volunteers

Joseph J. Fitch, PhD

Introduction

Volunteerism is a tradition that dates to colonial times. As the United States transformed from an agrarian to an industrial society, the concept of "neighbors helping neighbors" continued to flourish. However, as the nation became a more mobile, motorized society, cities and suburbs replaced family farms and villages. Volunteering for the local ambulance corps or rescue squad became a socially accepted way for individuals to continue the volunteerism tradition.

As society moves toward the twenty-first century and into an advanced information-based environment, EMS volunteers are becoming an increasingly endangered species. In this chapter the strengths and weaknesses of volunteer organizations are reviewed, the special sensitivities needed for working with volunteers outlined, and the benefits of the continued involvement and development of volunteer squads emphasized.

A Changing Environment

Volunteer rescue squads make a significant contribution to health care in America. The heaviest concentration of independent volunteer ambulance corps (often referred to as rescue squads) is in the Northeast region of the country. However, EMS volunteers are found as part of volunteer fire departments in most parts of rural America. According to a study published by *Firehouse* magazine, 65% of the nation's EMS providers are volunteers, supplying EMS service to more than 30% of the population.[1]

Outside the Northeast, volunteers most frequently provide care to lower population density areas. These areas would otherwise be underserved; because of low call volumes, it would not be cost effective to operate a career service. In recent years, many volunteer squads have been negatively impacted by changes in rural society. As rural areas became more suburbanized, with access to cable television and other "advancements," the lack of discretionary free time has drained the pool of available volunteers. The Congressional Office of Technical Assistance (OTA) in a comprehensive study of rural health care called the volunteer drain "one of the most salient problems confronting rural EMS systems." According to the OTA report, many rural programs lack specialized providers and resources, operate with inadequate tranportation and communications equipment, and are not part of a regional system.[2,3]

The volunteer drain is not limited to the rural area. Urban and suburban areas have been hit especially hard. For example, in a 1990 study of America's largest cities, only three of the largest 200 cities reported EMS service being provided by volunteers. The state of Pennsylvania, which has long been an area in which EMS volunteerism flourished, reports major declines in recent years. Pennsylvania statistics indicate that five years ago volunteers represented 90% of those involved in EMS, but only 40% are involved today. Squads are closing, using paid personnel, or being absorbed by either public or private ambulance services.[3]

There are a number of reasons for that phenomenon. Volunteer agencies typically relied heavily on young, single members. That group is getting smaller. According to the U.S. Department of Labor's Bureau of Statistics, there is a declining pool of 18–24 year olds. Members of that age group are moving into the entry-level job market, and many must work two jobs. Many cannot afford to live in the communities in which they grew up. The cultural norms of the "twentysomething" generation also impact volunteer agencies. Popular literature has characterized that group as members of the "me generation." Fewer individuals see the value of volunteering. Similarly, potential volunteers who are "thirtysomething" are often deeply enmeshed in careers. Many married volunteers are part of two-career households. Children, the pressures of balancing two careers, and the availability of leisure activities reduce the time available for volunteering.

There are a number of additional reasons for declining EMS volunteerism. They include commuter lifestyles, concerns about Acquired Immune Deficiency Syndrome (AIDS), and training requirements. Several decades ago most workers lived in the community in which they worked. Employers permitted individuals to leave work, enabling an occasional ambulance call to be answered as part of the employer's civic responsibility. In our commuter society, this practice declined because often neither the employer nor the employees have strong community ties. The fear of AIDS and other infectious diseases make some individuals reluctant to enter the health profession, and most likely this fear also negatively influences those who consider volunteering.

Increased training and continuing education requirements are the reasons most often cited as barriers to volunteerism in EMS, in recent studies conducted by Fitch & Associates. Being a volunteer has changed from a "club" atmosphere to one requiring a continuing commitment to competence. Twenty-five years ago, anyone could stop by the station and become a volunteer with an evening or two of training. Today, it requires at least 110 hours to become an Emergency Medical Technician-Basic (EMT-B) and, depending on local requirements, 500 to 1000 hours of training to become a paramedic. With the evolution of paramedics as the minimum standard of care for urban and suburban areas, increasing training requirements have compounded the problem for volunteers.[4] Not only is it harder to find volunteers, but they now must obtain and maintain a higher standard of training than was required in the past. The standard should not be lowered or exceptions granted for volunteers because competence is required; increased training opportunities and flexible scheduling are better options to reduce the perceived barriers.

Volunteer organizations throughout America are in transition. They must either meet expanding care expectations with fewer resources or categorically resist change, ultimately resulting in their organizational demise. Communities desiring to maintain volunteerism can work with squads to include them in progressive EMS systems without denigrating care. It takes time, energy, and patience; however, the rewards for both the volunteers and the community can be great.

The city of Richmond is a good example of such an approach. Richmond embraced those local squads willing to make the commitments to provide predictable, sophisticated prehospital care and to become an integral part of the system. Parts of Richmond had been served by volunteer rescue squads for more than 30 years. When the city undertook a complete redesign of its fragmented EMS system in 1989, special attention was paid to providing opportunities for volunteer participation. The city required that participating squads meet all citywide requirements established by the medical control board, including providing advanced medical service and responding to life-threatening emergencies within 8 minutes 90% of the time. Richmond is the only public utility model EMS system that has an active volunteer component.

The squads initially resisted change and exerted considerable political pressure to continue a tiered system. Once the medical community made it clear that level of care was not a negotiable item, the squads were given an ultimatum to comply with the standards or cease operations. To facilitate compliance, the city provided new medical equipment, advanced training, and daytime staffing during the transition period to facilitate the training process. The system has been functional since 1990.

Positive Factors

There are a number of common positive descriptors that can be associated with excellent volunteer ambulance services. They include a variety of attributes, some of which are discussed here.

Tenacity, Desire, and Confidence

Many volunteer services survive because of the sheer will and perseverance of key members. In any group there are those who are halfheartedly involved, those who are committed, and a few who are passionately committed. It is this last core of individuals who have a true love for EMS. Their passion comes from a deep desire to serve. In the best volunteer agencies the passion and commitment are patient-centered rather than internally focused on the squad. Confidence is another common descriptor of successful squads.

Flexibility and Willingness to Experiment

The limited size of most volunteer services often makes them more flexible than either business or government. By their very nature, volunteer squads can often be more responsive than business or government in meeting the needs of a specific neighborhood or community. Volunteer organizations understand that there are many ways to attack a problem, some of which may not be practical for other entities. The best volunteer services are on the cutting edge of care and technology issues, and are always willing to experiment with equipment or procedures that may better serve patients. For example, volunteer Cypress Creek EMS in Houston was among the early groups to use monitor-defibrillator-external pacemaker systems and a computer-aided dispatch system. Forest View Volunteer Rescue Squad in Richmond was part of a multi-site epinephrine study. Numerous volunteer squads have been at the forefront of advancing prehospital care.

Access to Private Funds and Volunteer Labor

Volunteer ambulance services are positioned to receive funds from practically every philanthropic source, ranging from the largest institutional donor to individual neighbors. Local corporations and individuals like giving to volunteer rescue squads because they see the results at work in the community, and they may need service at some point in the future. Volunteer labor, when effectively harnessed to meet the clinical, operational, and administrative needs of the squad, provides unique advantages because volunteers provide EMS service at a fraction of the cost of private and government operations.

Community Spirit

The very act of beginning a volunteer EMS group has the potential to develop a valuable community force, not just for emergency health care but across the breadth of society. The Bedford-Stuyvesant Volunteer Ambulance Corps, located in an area of Brooklyn heavily populated by minorities, was recognized by President Bush in 1991 as part of the 1000 Points of Light program. The organization serves as a community educational and organizational focus, in additional to its EMS role. Another volunteer squad to receive the 1000 Points of Light award was Sun City Center (Florida) Emergency Squad Number 1, which has no member younger than 57 years old and answers 6,000 calls each year. It provides van transfers for those who do not require an ambulance and a wheelchair exchange for the retirement community that it serves.

Challenges

There are also several common challenges faced by volunteer ambulance services. These challenges include the following.

Lack of Clarity About Goals and Purpose

Many volunteer ambulance services cannot articulate the reason they exist. Other than stock phrases such as "providing care to our community," when asked hard questions about local needs, program delivery, and community response, many squads reveal glaring holes in their organizational methodologies. Like many voluntary organizations, rescue squads often believe that their survival, no matter how difficult or necessary, is their purpose. The worst believe that it is their right to preserve their "club" no matter what the consequences for the patient or the community. Volunteer organizations may resist improvements in the local EMS system simply because it is not to their organizational benefit. In sum, squads must adequately meet patient needs before attempting to meet the needs of the rescuers.

Ineffective Leadership

Many volunteer services lack leaders with strong management skills. Some squad leaders shun the notion that they must be strong leaders by saying, "we're just volunteers." Leaders are elected. In many cases elections are based on popularity rather than competence. Management shortcomings in volunteer squads are often masked by sacrifice, avoidance, or ignorance of the problem. Many organizations appear to be in better shape than they actually are. Most members join a volunteer rescue squad to provide care not to get bogged down in administrative matters. Leading and managing a volunteer organization requires additional skills, and it is often difficult to attract and promote individuals prepared to provide the nurturing leadership necessary for long-term success.

Insufficient and Undependable Financial Support

The fiscal life of volunteer ambulance services has been increasingly difficult in recent years. While the fund-raising techniques have become more sophisticated, the competition for donations has also increased. Squads often rely heavily on individual donors, and they are expending more effort raising funds than in the past. Most members do not enjoy asking for money. A common refrain is, "That's not the reason I joined; I want to save lives." As fiscal pressures increase, a number of squads have had to delay both equipment replacement and facility repairs; some have simply folded. The billing of consumers and insurance carriers remains a foreign concept for many squads. It is often equated with becoming a private ambulance service rather than recovering the costs necessary for the squad's survival.

Public Invisibility

Most members of the public are oblivious to EMS, until they need help. The needs of the local volunteer rescue squad are not usually a high priority of the average citizen. Squads often fail to state adequately their needs for fiscal support, leadership resources, and line personnel. Even those who have been provided service by a volunteer ambulance squad quickly forget among the cacophony of other societal activities. In many areas, EMS is regarded as a jurisdictional responsibility; users may not recognize the degree of volunteerism involved in the specific area.

Working With Volunteers

Encouraging a volunteer agency to maximize its strengths and minimize its weaknesses to benefit its patients and its members is not an easy task. One volunteer organization that is working to accomplish those goals is Cypress Creek EMS. Cypress Creek uses both career and volunteer staff, and operates five advanced-level units in a 250-square-mile area that borders Houston. The following ideas for working with volunteers were offered by Cypress Creek's former executive director.

Focus on Need and Pride as Motivators

Volunteers are motivated by need and pride. The more the need to provide a service, the greater the desire from the volunteer. A person must be needed to perform work for free. The less the perceived need for the volunteer, the more incentive programs are necessary to keep up the membership. Although some organizations are looking at pension plans and merit systems for regularly riding members, the primary reason volunteers perform is pride in their job. Perks are good, but they are also an indication that volunteers are not getting satisfaction from their

work and need more reinforcement. Need brings in the volunteers; pride and job satisfaction keep them.

Recognize the Time Required for Training

It is increasingly difficult for a volunteer to commit the time necessary for learning and practicing the level of medical expertise required. Most EMS organizations, especially those providing sophisticated prehospital care, require more training, certifications, and continuing education than ever before. The more the medical capability expands, the more time commitments are necessary from the volunteer provider to obtain training and demonstrate proficiency.

Hold Volunteers to the Same Standards as Paid Personnel

Volunteers must be held to the same standards as paid personnel or the volunteer feels less professional. There cannot be two standards of care. Although it may be more difficult and require more time for a volunteer to maintain higher levels of training, by achieving those standards the volunteer feels as professional as any paid provider. This includes strict adherence to local and state motor vehicle laws as they apply to ambulances.

Limit Turnover

The reason a volunteer leaves an organization is usually a change in personal priorities such as children or a new job. Volunteers and paid personnel do not "burn out" in the same way. Paid individuals usually demonstrate stress and burnout symptoms that can be addressed, whereas volunteers may have no sign of burnout or problems before leaving the organization. Internal organizational politics, clashes of personalities, or loss of need and pride in the organization are other reasons volunteers leave. Internal strife is usually tied to either a lack of direction or weak leadership in the organization. People working together for a common goal are usually too busy attaining the goal to worry about power struggles.

Avoid Comparing Volunteers with Paid Personnel

Volunteers are very sensitive about being compared to paid professionals. They want to be treated and perform at the same or a higher level than paid personnel. Always using paid personnel as positive examples or using phrases such as "You're just a volunteer," should be avoided. Never refer to only the paid providers as "professionals."

Focus Competitive Energy on Personalized Service

The attitudes and approaches of volunteers to patients are often excellent. This is one area where competition between paid and volunteer personnel may be healthy. Paid personnel should be challenged to provide the same high levels of personalized service as the volunteers. The medical director should direct energy toward improving the level of personalized service given by both the volunteer and paid staff.

Educate Rather than Test for Competency

Volunteers have a natural desire to do their best. Instead of testing their abilities, as is common for paid personnel, educate! The volunteers need support in attaining the goals that are set. If the goal is for volunteers to be proficient in CPR, then they should be trained on the procedures and allowed the opportunity to reach that goal. Assure that the volunteers also accept it as their goal. If the volunteers buy into the goal, they will be working to accomplish their goal, not someone else's. Spend incentive dollars on education, not perks like coffee cups, license plate holders, and beer blasts.

Facilitate Information Dissemination

Because volunteers do not work with the organization every day, they must have a clear and direct avenue to receive information and direct their concerns and questions. Clear-cut operations procedures are essential. The chain of command is very important; everyone must know who is responsible for correcting problems and effecting change. This clarity of authority also decreases the problem of getting the run-around about a problem. One person must have the responsibility and authority of leadership.

Provide Specific Goals

Volunteer organizations require a better mission statement than "to provide emergency medical care." They need direction toward obtainable goals. Once a major goal such as a new building or an award has

been achieved, the group may stagnate. Certification in a higher level of care is an example of a short-term goal for a member. There also needs to be clear and consistent long-term goals for the organization. This is particularly important since many volunteers are not exposed to the organization on a daily basis, and the leadership in many volunteer agencies can change with the popular vote of the membership. The organization should establish long-term goals that do not change with the whims of the new administration.

Put the Right Person in the Right Job

Good field providers are not necessarily good fundraisers. However, volunteers have the advantage of being experts in other fields of work that can be useful to the organization. Tap members for both medical and operational expertise. Volunteers are eager to help in areas they understand but shun areas that are unfamiliar, such as asking for funds or discounts. It may be helpful to designate a group or an individual specifically for that difficult or unusual task.

Summary

Volunteerism in America is changing. To continue to be an effective force in EMS, volunteers need to embrace rather than resist enhanced levels of care and other advances in providing service. Special care must be taken by medical directors to recognize the strengths and limitations of volunteer squads. In many suburban and rural areas, volunteers are strategically located to work with the EMS system and the medical director to bridge geographic or organizational service gaps.

References

1. McNally VT. A history of the volunteers. *Firehouse*. 1986;11:49–50.
2. Congress of the United States, Office of Technology Assessment. *Rural Emergency Medical Services*. Special report, OTA-H-445,1985.
3. Ornato J. The need for ALS in urban and suburban EMS systems. *Ann Emerg Med*. 1990;19:151–155.
4. Keller RA. EMS in the United States. *JEMS*. 1990;15:79–80.

Bibliography

Allison EJ, et al. Specific occupational satisfaction and stresses that differentiate paid and volunteer EMTs. *Ann Emerg Med*. 1987;16:676–679.

Bachman JW. The good neighbor rescue program: utilizing volunteers to perform cardiopulmonary resuscitation in a rural community. *J Fam Pract* 1983;16:561–566.

Carter HR. Is the volunteer fireman an endangered species? *Rekindle*. 1985;14:12.

Congress of the United States, Ofice of Technology Assessment. *Rural Emergency Medical Services*. Special report, OTA-H-445, 1985.

Daily RC. Understanding organizational commitment for volunteers: empirical and managerial implications. *Journal of Voluntary Action Research*. 1986;15:19–31.

Division of Medical Science, National Academy of Science-National Research Council. *Accidental Death and Disability: The Neglected Disease of Modern Society*. Washington, DC: The Council; 1966.

Drucker PF. *Managing the nonprofit organization*. New York: Harper-Collins; 1990.

Gilbertson M. The volunteer crises. *JEMS*. 1988;13(6):6–7.

Gora JG, Newerowicz GM. *Emergency Squad Volunteers: Professionalism in Unpaid Work*. New York: Praeger Publishers; 1985.

Hudgins E. Volunteer incentives. *JEMS*. 1988;13(6)58–61.

Karter MJ Jr. Taking the measure of the fire service. *Fire Command*. 1985;52:17.

Keller RA. EMS in the United States. *JEMS*. 1990;15(1):79.

McNally VP. A history of volunteers. *Firehouse*. 1986;11(3):49.

Miller A. The new volunteerism. *Newsweek*. 1988;111:42–43.

Ornato J, et al. The need for ALS in urban and suburban EMS systems. *Ann Emerg Med Serv*. 1990;151–155.

Perkins KB, Metz CW. Note on commitment and community among volunteer firefighters. *Sociological Inquiry*. 1987;57(3):117–121.

Perkins KB. Volunteer fire departments: community integration, autonomy, and survival. *Human Organization*. 1987;46(4):82–85.

Smith DH. Altruism, volunteers, and volunteerism. *Journal of Voluntary Action Research*. 1981;10:21–36.

Swan TH. Keeping volunteers in service. *JEMS*. 1988;13(6):50–54.

Swan TH. Recruiting EMS volunteers. *JEMS*. 1986;11(6):50–54.

Spouses

Gina Eckstein, BA

Being an EMS Medical Director entails a unique set of challenges and demands. Naturally, these demands have a profound impact on a medical director's spouse and children. When my husband became the medical director of the Los Angeles City Fire Department, I realized that children's dreams do come true. Where else could one carry a radio, dress like a firefighter, drive a car with lights and sirens and have the opportunity to save lives on a daily basis?

I was thrilled for my husband when he was selected as the medical director of LAFD. I knew that he had always wanted such a job since he was a paramedic in New York City. He loves the action, the fast pace, the administrative challenges, the interactions with so many people, and the ability to potentially impact four million people. However, I soon realized that such a position comes with a price.

After attending a number of EMS conferences with my husband, I have found that as the wife of a medical director I have many things in common with the spouses of other medical directors. The most obvious one is that we all hate the radio! It has become our spouse's security blanket that continuously whispers descriptions and outcomes of shootings, stabbings, and the most horrific accidents known to man. We sometimes fantasize the many ways in which we can destroy their toy. We could always give it to the dog to chew on or throw it into the nearest swimming pool. To them, it is a form of relaxation to hear the crackling noises screeching from the radio. To the rest of us, the tragedies we hear are more than just incidents; there are people suffering and we feel it deeply. We visualize the incident, the injuries, and the families involved. To us it is a reminder of how fragile life can be. To our spouses, listening to the radio is a way of staying in touch with what is going on in the field, noting ways of improving the system, and, most importantly, always being ready to go to the major incidents with lightning speed. That is why our spouses don't seem to understand why we would prefer not to listen to the radio during dinner or quiet moments alone.

Our spouses are always on call. Running a close second to the most disliked "medical director gadgets" are the pagers and cell phones. If a large incident unfolds, so many people page them that they begin to sound like a one-man band. They are more likely to leave home without their wallet than without their pagers. I can never truly plan an outing or an evening without having some concern that my husband will be paged and go from a nice dinner one minute to being in his response car going to an incident the next.

While this can make for a very unsettling existence, I have learned to live with it. Even if we plan to go out, there is always that possibility he will decide to respond to an incident along the way. Once we were headed out to a rare evening out, chatting along the way. However, I underestimated the fact that even though my husband may seem to be giving me his undivided attention, the background noise of the radio is ever present. Before I knew what was happening, my husband interrupted our conversation to inform me that we were responding to a multi-victim traffic accident on the freeway. A few minutes later, after travelling for a few miles along the right shoulder past the gridlocked traffic I was sitting in the fast lane of the freeway surrounded by fire trucks, ambulances, and police cars, with an overturned auto nearby. He told me to stay in the car to be safe, and even reminded me that we were parked in front of a ladder truck for additional protection. However, by the time he returned from assisting with the patients, I had the beginnings of a severe migraine from staring at flashing strobe lights for twenty minutes. I really couldn't get angry at him, since I realized that he was there for the right reasons. However, the question of priority, that is, "the job" versus his family, is one that persists.

As I'm sure all medical directors have explained, he has told me that in the event of a major incident such as an earthquake, he will first assure the safety of our family and will then have to respond to the command post. I guess I can't help but feel a sense of jealousy, but at the same time I understand the commitment and the dedication.

There is no such thing as a typical day. Each moment is a race against time to arrive at the next meeting or incident. How do they remember which outfit to wear? Scrubs? Suit? Turnouts? The truth is this job attracts a wonderful breed of human beings with a lot of testosterone. They are brilliant, and sensitive, yet they crave the roughness of being out on the field, searching through debris to find a buried, but breathing person.

I remember the day of the bank shoot-out in North Hollywood, which was broadcast live on national television. My husband was listening to the radio when the incident started. He shouted "I'm going to an incident" and before I knew it I heard the sirens outside. I ran to the television and froze at what I saw. There were an unknown number of gunmen surrounding a bank, carrying enough armor and weapons to kill scores of people. The scene was not secured and my husband was on his way there! As I rubbed my pregnant belly, I prayed that all would be fine and that he would return safely. Within minutes, I saw his car parked near the fire engines during a live news report. My husband was actually with the first

ambulance crew to enter the bullet-ridden bank, checking for casualties. Luckily he got out safely.

One of the prerequisites for being a medical director should be either to live in Washington, D.C. for a few years or to get a master's degree in political science, since politics are such a significant part of the job. Juggling between the needs and desires of the paramedics, the medical community, the firefighters, and the unions can be a most daunting challenge. Despite my husband's efforts to listen to everyone's concerns, it seems that many people will not be happy with change, even in the interest of saving lives. Setting new policies or enforcing old ones necessitates that a medical director quickly develop some very thick skin. As spouses, we must encourage them to stay focused on their mission to serve the best interests of the community at large, even if a decision will not be popular with the paramedics or medical colleagues.

While most people flee danger, a medical director is usually attracted to it, mostly to help save lives. There have been times when I know my husband will be late for dinner when I turn on the television news and see him at an incident rendering aid or giving a live update on a victim's prognosis. I tell the kids "Look, there's daddy, say goodnight." While his job sometimes forces us to change our plans, we feel such pride in what he is doing to better the medical system in which he works. So what if he gets to have a little fun too? I guess it just comes with the territory.

40

State Office

Bob Bailey, MA

Introduction

Since the passage of the federal EMS act of 1973, every state and territory has established a state EMS office; the location and the function vary from state to state. Most state offices are located within the Department of Health or some variation, such as Health and Human Services. Some are located in public safety and a few operate under free-standing Boards such as in Kansas, Minnesota, and Kentucky.

The role of state offices also varies. Some have comprehensive responsibilities for all aspects of EMS, including trauma and injury prevention, in addition to the traditional roles of most that include training, licensure, continuing education, communications, and other oversight functions. State offices vary in the number of personnel they have to fulfill their roles and responsibilities. Staffing levels range from 3 to greater than 80 personnel. Generally, the larger the state office, the broader the roles and responsibilities.

Virtually every state has a regulatory role to ensure that the EMS laws and the rules and regulations are enforced. This regulatory role may vary but generally includes certification or licensure of EMS personnel, organizations, and vehicles. It may include designation of trauma centers or other specialty care centers. Compliance investigations to ensure that EMS personnel are properly trained and functioning within approved scope of practice, vehicles are properly equipped and staffed, and medical directors are properly credentialed are common responsibilities of EMS offices.

As the lead regulatory agency for EMS in a state, the EMS office can be a tremendous asset to medical directors. They can assist medical directors in understanding the various EMS laws and regulations and ensure that medical directors are aware of their responsibilities and liabilities. Often the EMS office can assist the local medical director in EMS personnel compliance issues. Many states offer medical director courses that provide local medical directors with a clear understanding of their roles and authority, and the specifics regarding EMS rules for their particular state. It is important for medical directors to meet their state EMS representatives and work collaboratively with them.

According to the March 2000 membership list of the National Association of State EMS Directors (NASEMSD), 22 states have a state EMS medical director. The majority of these positions are part-time positions. In most cases, a practicing physician who has a contract with the state EMS office to function in that role fills the position of state EMS Medical Director.

Most state legislation has historically required that local Advanced Life Support (ALS) agencies or programs have a medical director to provide oversight of the ALS activities. More recently, many states are also requiring medical oversight for all levels of prehospital care providers or organizations. In some cases, this applies even to emergency medical dispatch programs. Some states also have a structure requiring regional medical directors; the roles and responsibilities of those positions are generally defined in state legislation or rules and regulations. Other chapters in this text describe the roles and responsibilities of local medical directors.

The purpose of this discussion is to relate the traits/attributes of successful medical directors at the local, regional, and state level from the perspectives of the state EMS Director and the state EMS medical director.

Local Medical Directors

State EMS Directors must enforce state laws and rules and regulations regarding EMS activities. They see first-hand those local programs that are successful and those that are struggling. A successful local medical director is usually a sign of a successful program; the following are some of the crucial attributes.

Clinical Competence

A successful local medical director has to be much more than a good clinician, although that is a must if he is to have the support and respect of the EMS field personnel. He must be current on new trends and technologies in prehospital care, and have the personality to be accepted as part of the team by the field personnel. The medical director must get in the street to see what it is really like. He must be part of the training, medical oversight, and quality management (QM). While some of these activities can be delegated, successful medical directors usually stay involved at all levels of medical oversight.

EMS Advocacy

The medical director must take an active role in promoting and improving the local EMS system. This may mean appearing before the city council or county board of commissioners to educate them on issues affecting EMS, including budget issues impacting EMS. It may mean educating people one-on-one about the importance of a quality local EMS system. It may involve educating the local EMS director on the importance of including the medical director in all issues pertaining to patient care, competence of personnel, and reward and discipline of personnel regarding quality of care.

Political Awareness

An understanding of the political process, how decisions are made, and how resources are allocated is a critical attribute of the medical director. Today the successful local medical director not only understands the political process but also participates to bring about needed changes and enhancements to the local system. The simplistic position that "the physician knows best" does not necessarily work. Educating the politicians to the importance and necessity of a sound EMS system in terms that underscore that it is in their and their constituents' best interest, generally yields better results. However, this takes time and effort. The medical director who realizes the importance of this effort and does not view setbacks as personal attacks is much more likely to be successful in achieving meaningful change.

Objectivity

Many times local EMS medical directors find themselves pulled into issues with organizations with different agendas. The issues may be between paid and volunteer agencies, commercial services and fire service agencies, EMS and police, or any of a number of other combinations. In areas with multiple receiving hospitals, disagreements often occur among those receiving hospitals. The ability to function as a facilitator without being considered aligned with one group is critical to effective functioning as an EMS system medical director. The abilities to remain objective to all perspectives and to remain an advocate of the patient and the system, are traits that successful medical directors must possess.

Understanding State Requirements

The successful medical director does not rely on second-hand information regarding what is required and accepted by the state EMS office. The medical director must have first-hand knowledge of those requirements and the parameters of local EMS programs. This knowledge ensures that local enhancements are within state law. Often local medical directors will disagree with state requirements and feel that they are not restrictive enough or that they are too restrictive. As an advocate for EMS, the local medical director should enter into discussion with the state EMS director and state EMS medical director to ensure that the state understands the local system. He should also advocate change at the state level to better meet both the system and patient needs of the locality.

Consensus Building

Usually, constructive and long-term change can only occur through consensus-building. The successful local medical director is aware of this and continually strives to build consensus. In order to do this effectively, the medical director must understand the needs and perspectives of the various players within the system. He must develop credibility and be able to educate the various players on the importance of working together to make improvements. Finally, each player in the system will need to understand that consensus-building not only addresses global needs but ultimately will address their individual needs as well.

Regional Medical Directors

Most successful regional medical directors possess similar traits to those addressed above. However, the roles and responsibilities of regional medical directors not only differ from those of local medical directors but may also vary from region to region, and certainly from state to state. Regions within states may be established legislatively or via rules, or the regions may reflect natural patient referral patterns and may have "evolved" over time.

Generally, regional medical directors are involved with broader issues, and interact more frequently with other EMS physicians. A regional medical director may or may not have any real "authority" over local medical directors. Generally, they are expected to ensure (or at least advocate for) quality and consistent delivery of care within a multi-jurisdictional area (the region). Additional attributes are the following:

Credibility among Peers

It is essential that a regional medical director possess current knowledge and skills to be deemed credible by the local medical directors. This is especially important if the regional medical director has compliance responsibilities over local programs and medical directors.

Public Speaking

The regional medical director often speaks before groups of colleagues, hospital personnel, governmental officials, politicians, EMS providers, and the public. While one-on-one communication skills are still important, the regional medical director should be a successful public speaker who can leverage his position to influence, develop consensus or diffuse potentially harmful confrontations.

Physician Advocacy

While the regional medical director is still an advocate of EMS, he must also be, and be perceived by his peers as, an advocate of the physicians providing medical oversight. This advocacy is important, since regional medical directors interact more frequently with regional councils, the state EMS office staff, as well as the legislature and licensing boards.

State Medical Directors

As might be expected, a successful state medical director requires similar traits to those possessed by local and regional medical directors. As a state EMS medical director, the physician finds himself or herself engaged in statewide system development activities, rule promulgation, state level program oversight, enforcement, advocacy, planning, and many other activities, usually as a part-time contracted position. The state EMS medical director is in a role to educate other medical directors and to serve as a resource to facilitate medical oversight activities at local and regional levels.

In an informal survey of 22 state EMS Directors who, according to the March 2000 National Association of State EMS Directors Directory, have state EMS medical directors, several additional attributes are common to those who were seen as successful. Some of those attributes are discussed below.

Easily Approachable

State EMS staffs need to feel comfortable in approaching the state EMS medical director with issues and concerns. This is important, since most state EMS medical directors are contracted on a part-time basis, are not considered full-time state employees, and are rarely in the office more than one or two times a week. If office staff, the EMS director, training director, trauma coordinator, or other staff do not feel comfortable approaching the state EMS medical director, or do not feel he is "accessible," they simply will find alternative avenues to obtain direction and answers. Being perceived as unapproachable has significant negative impact on the state EMS medical director.

Understanding Process and Constraints

The successful state EMS medical director understands the political process for bringing about change as well as the constraints of the state EMS offices. For example, if a state department is opposed or indifferent to an external EMS initiative, most EMS directors cannot speak their true feeling or be supportive of a bill, since they must abide by the position of the department or the governor's on bills or issues impacting state government. Alleviating this problem is part of the rationale for establishing freestanding state EMS boards or commissions such as those in Minnesota, Kansas, and Kentucky. The state EMS medical director who understands the constraints is less likely to be at odds with the state EMS staff or the executive branch over issues that the state staff may personally support but not publicly support as government employees. The state EMS medical director can also often serve as a liaison among the state EMS office and local and regional EMS agencies, as well as state medical organizations.

Teamwork

Successful state EMS medical directors practice teamwork. A close working relationship between the state EMS director and state EMS medical director is critical to ensure a clear understanding of roles and responsibilities, to send consistent messages to the EMS community and general public, and to consistently and fairly enforce laws, rules and regulations. In addition, the state EMS medical director will be in a better position to work cooperatively with local and regional medical directors, if the relationship within the state office is close.

Objective Listening Skills

The state EMS medical director serves in a unique position. In most cases, he is not a state employee. In some cases, he is not truly regarded as "part of the staff." By the same token, he is no longer considered by his peers as "one of them." In combination with many of the other traits already listed, the ability to listen objectively to all parties is crucial to the state EMS medical director in order to effectively carry out the role. The state medical director is usually the first person that state EMS office staff will go to if they have a problem that they want a "doc" to solve. He is also normally the first person contacted at the state office by physicians who seek information or change. The ability to listen objectively to everyone, and to process fact from fiction without preconceived ideals

are important traits in successfully performing the state EMS medical director function.

Credibility among Peers

A successful state EMS medical director is recognized among his peers as being clinically competent, current in new EMS skills and trends, knowledgeable in street level care, EMS inititatives, and future directions, and aware of current laws, rules and regulations.

Without peer credibility the state EMS medical director will be unable to deal effectively with the medical community. The state EMS medical director should be functioning in a facilitative position for all of the constituents with whom he or she interfaces.

Patient Advocacy

While everyone in EMS should be a patient advocate, the state EMS medical director is in a position to bring meaning to those words. He should be a voice of reason during internal state office deliberations. Since most state EMS medical directors are contracted for only one or two days a week, they can bring a fresh perspective to internal deliberations. State EMS staff who have to work within the bureaucracy every day sometimes lose sight of the patient focus. By the same token, the state EMS medical director is in a unique position to educate peers of the importance of comprehensive medical oversight and ways to accomplish it.

Summary

Successful EMS medical directors at the local, regional, and state levels have many traits in common. They are people-oriented. They have excellent communications skills. They are not caught up in their own importance. They have a passion that drives them to make a difference.

CHAPTER 41

Federal

Jeffery Michaels, EdD

Introduction

A wide variety of federal government support is currently available to state and local EMS systems. A number of departments and agencies provide direct funding to state or local systems through grant programs, and others provide technical assistance in the form of practice guidelines, educational curricula, community outreach programs, and reference materials. This chapter presents an overview of the types of federal resources now obtainable, and indicates how these services may be accessed. While not a comprehensive account, the resources described are representative of the range of federal support for EMS, and are offered to assist EMS medical directors or administrators in their search for resources to maintain or improve system operation.

With the quantity and diversity of EMS resources available through federal sources, the World Wide Web is a particularly effective tool for identifying the most appropriate or current resource to meet a specific need. Each of the federal agencies offering EMS assistance maintain extensive web sites, with links both to other agencies and to non-government sources.

System Development Funding

Federal funding opportunities for EMS system development reflect the varied services EMS provides in the community. For example, funding for EMS as a component of the healthcare delivery system is available through a Department of Health and Human Services (DHHS) primary care block grant. Funding for EMS as a transportation safety intervention is offered through the Department of Transportation, and funding for an EMS contribution to domestic emergency preparedness is supplied by the Federal Emergency Management Agency and the Department of Justice.

The primary source of information regarding federal funding opportunities for EMS is the *Catalog of Federal Domestic Assistance* (CFDA), a government-wide compendium of federal programs, projects, services, and activities which assist or benefit the American public. The CFDA includes funding programs that provide assistance or benefits to states, territorial possessions, counties, cities, domestic profit or non-profit corporations, institutions, or individuals. Program information is cross referenced by functional classification (Functional Index), subject (Subject Index), applicant (Applicant Index), deadline(s) for program application submission (Deadlines Index), and authorizing legislation (Authorization Index). For each program, the catalog includes a program description, types of available assistance, eligible applicants, matching requirements, authorizing legislation, and application deadline dates.

The CFDA is published annually in two editions. The first edition, usually published in June, includes current Congressional action regarding funding program legislation. An update, usually published in December, reflects completed Congressional action on the President's budget proposals, and legislation as of the date of compilation.

The CFDA is available on the web at *http://www.cfda.gov/* or from the Government Services Administration (GSA). The catalog is available in hardcopy, high-density floppy diskettes, and CD-ROM. The CD-ROM includes the complete catalog and a search engine with an on-line tutorial. To order a copy of the CFDA, contact:

Federal Domestic Assistance Catalog Staff (MVS)
General Services Administration
Reporters Building, Room 101
300 7th Street, SW
Washington, DC 20407
Telephone: (202) 708-5126
Toll-Free Answering Service: 1-800-669-8331

Another source of information on sources of federal funding for EMS development is offered by the U.S. Fire Administration (USFA). *The Guide to Funding Alternatives for Fire & EMS Departments* reviews over 170 local, state, and federal resources including grants, loans, donations, reimbursements, technical assistance, training, and information resources. A guide to developing and writing grant proposals is also included. This document is available through the USFA online catalog at *http://www.usfa.fema.gov/usfapubs*.

The Heath Resources and Services Administration (HRSA) EMS for Children (EMSC) Program publishes an overview of potential funding resources for pediatric EMS initiatives. *Meeting the Needs of Children: A Guide to Funding EMSC Projects* includes a list of funding sources and information on writing grant applications. This document and a variety of other information concerning funding for EMSC-related system development is available from the EMSC web site at *http://www.ems-c.org/funding*.

While primarily a source of funding for service reimbursement rather than system development, The Center for Medicare and Medicaid Services (CMS) is an essential resource for many EMS systems. Of particular interest are the descriptions of Medicare payment services located at *http://www.hcfa.gov/medicare/payment.htm*.

Research Support

Financial support for EMS-related research is offered on at least an occasional basis from a number of agencies. The Centers for Disease Control and Prevention's (CDC) National Center for Injury Prevention and Control (NCIPC) supports injury prevention and control research on priority issues, especially those identified in national policy documents such as *Healthy People 2010*. Current CDC research funding opportunities can be viewed at *http://www.cdc.gov/od/pgo/funding/grantmain.htm*.

Support for health services research is also available from the Agency for Healthcare Research and Quality (AHRQ). The AHRQ focuses on healthcare organization, delivery, financing, utilization, patient and provider behavior, quality, outcomes, effectiveness, and cost. The agency evaluates both clinical services and the system in which these services are provided, and provides information about the cost of care, as well as its effectiveness, outcomes, efficiency, and quality. The agency also conducts studies of the structure, process, and effects of health services for individuals and populations, addressing both basic and applied research questions, including fundamental aspects of both individual and system behavior and the application of interventions in practice settings. A review of current research priorities can be found at *http://www.ahrq.gov/*.

The National Institutes of Health (NIH) fund a wide variety of healthcare research in pursuit of their mission to uncover new knowledge that will lead to better health. The NIH Extramural Research Program supports the research of non-federal scientists in universities, medical schools, hospitals, and research institutions throughout the country and abroad; helping in the training of research investigators; and fostering communication of medical information. Information about NIH funding opportunities can be found at *http://grants.nih.gov/grants/*.

The National Highway Traffic Safety Administration (NHTSA) supports research which is consistent with the *EMS Agenda for the Future*. Current examples include EMS outcomes research, preventable mortality studies, and educational research. An overview of current research efforts can be found at *http://www.nhtsa.dot.gov/people/injury/ems/*.

Several federal agencies have provided or are developing guidance regarding priority EMS research directions. Consensus EMS research agendas are being developed by NHTSA and the HRSA EMSC program. The NHTSA *National EMS Research Agenda* was initiated in response to a priority recommendation of the consensus strategic planning document, the *EMS Agenda for the Future Implementation Guide*. The Research Agenda is being developed by an interdisciplinary group of EMS researchers, facilitated by the National Association of EMS Physicians (NAEMSP). Information is available at the NAEMSP web site *http://www.emermed.uc.edu/ResearchAgenda*, or the NHTSA site at *http://www.nhtsa.dot.gov/people/injury/ems/*.

To encourage research on pediatric EMS topics and direct researchers to sources of funding, the EMSC organized a federal interagency committee, composed of representatives of HRSA, AHRQ, the NIH, and the CDC, to develop a joint program announcement. The completed EMSC research guidance will be available through *http://www.ems-c.org/funding*.

In addition to funding and direction, a range of federal information resources are available to support EMS research. NHTSA maintains the Fatal Analysis

Reporting System (FARS), containing detailed information on every fatal motor vehicle crash in the nation, and the General Estimates System (GES) which consists of a nationally representative sample of injury crashes. Information regarding access to these databases is available from the NHTSA National Center for Statistics and Analysis at *http://www.nhtsa.dot.gov/people/ncsa*. NHTSA also sponsored the establishment of the *Uniform Prehospital Data Set*, a collection of 80 data points and definitions developed by consensus among EMS researchers. These prehospital data elements can be reviewed at *http://www.nhtsa.dot.gov/people/injury/ems*.

The National Center for Health Statistics (NCHS) publishes a range of data on vital events as well as information on health status, lifestyle and exposure to unhealthy influences, the onset and diagnosis of illness and disability, and the use of health care. Information concerning access to this data is available at *http://www.cdc.gov/nchs*.

The AHRQ maintains a number of databases useful for EMS-related research. For example, the Health Care Expenditure Survey (HCUP) consists of a number of administrative longitudinal databases, including state-specific hospital-discharge databases and a national sample of discharges from community hospitals, as well as powerful, user-friendly software that can be used with both HCUP data and with other administrative databases. The Medical Expenditure Panel Survey (MEPS) is a nationally representative survey that collects detailed information on the health status, access to care, healthcare use and expenses, and health insurance coverage of the civilian noninstitutionalized population of the United States and nursing home residents. Further information on these databases is available at *http://www.ahrq.gov/*.

The CDC wonder provides a single point of access to a variety of CDC reports, guidelines, and numeric public health data. For the anonymous user (general public), CDC Wonder provides access to more than thirty numerical databases and document collections. Or by registering, users can access additional resources specifically intended for public health practitioners. CDC Wonder is located at *http://wonder.cdc.gov/*.

The CDC NCIPC is also coordinating a national effort to develop uniform specifications for data entered in emergency department patient records. The *Data Elements for Emergency Department Systems (DEEDS)* are intended for use by individuals and organizations responsible for maintaining record systems in 24-hour, hospital-based emergency departments throughout the United States. The current DEEDS data specifications are located at *http://www.cdc.gov/ncipc/pub-res/deedspage.htm*.

Another overview of federal data sources is available in FedStats at *http://www.fedstats.gov*. FedStats is maintained by the Federal Interagency Council on Statistical Policy, and facilitates access to data from more than 70 federal agencies.

Strategic Planning

A number of federally-supported initiatives have combined the thoughts of public and private sector into jointly supported statements of healthcare direction and priority. For example, *Healthy People 2010* is a national health promotion and disease prevention initiative coordinated by the DHHS, Office of Disease Prevention and Health Promotion, that brought together government agencies at all levels along with nonprofit, voluntary, and professional organizations, businesses, and individuals to lay out objectives for improving the health of all Americans. *Healthy People 2010* includes objectives which relate to EMS care, and can be viewed at *http://www.health.gov/healthypeople/*.

In 1999 the Institute of Medicine (IoM) published a status report and recommendations concerning the national injury problem. *Reducing the Burden of Injury: Advancing Prevention and Treatment* is a milestone in injury control analysis with far-reaching implications for EMS. The document is available from the National Academy Press at *http://www.nap.edu*.

The *EMS Agenda for the Future* is a consensus vision for the future of the nation's EMS system, developed by NHTSA and HRSA with broad input from the EMS community. First published in 1996, the EMS Agenda was followed by an Implementation Guide in 1998 and a number of specific derivative planning activities, including the *EMS Education Agenda for the Future*, a *National EMS Research Agenda*, and a *Trauma System Vision*. These documents reflect the perspectives of the full range of EMS stakeholders, and provide common directions for system growth. These documents can be viewed at the NHTSA EMS Division web site at *http://www.nhtsa.dot.gov/people/injury/ems/*.

HRSA's EMSC Program maintains a Five Year Plan which lays out specific objectives for improving EMS for pediatric populations. The Five Year Plan is developed by the EMSC National Resource Center's National Steering Committee with extensive peer input, and is consistent with the objectives of the *EMS Agenda for the Future*. The *EMSC Five Year Plan* can be viewed at the EMSC web site, *http://www.ems-c.org/products*.

Tools and Resources

Federal agencies offer an assortment of resources for facilitating the management of EMS system operations, including curricula and instructional aids, equipment and operational guidelines, and materials for community outreach programs.

Educational Resources

NHTSA develops and maintains the National Standard Curricula for EMS providers. In addition to their use as instructional tools, these curricula are often used by states to define the scope of practice for EMS providers. NHTSA currently maintains the National Standard Curricula for First Responders, Basic, Intermediate and Paramedic Emergency Medical Technicians, Emergency Vehicle Operators, Emergency Medical Dispatchers, EMS Instructors, and Air Medical Crews. To complement the National Standard Curricula, NHTSA provides a number of specific instructional aids, such as administrative guides for implementing the Intermediate and Paramedic curricula.

NHTSA also provides specific training opportunities to state EMS Offices, including one day courses on EMS Information Systems (EMSIS), covering the fundamentals of data collection and utilization, and Quality Improvement For EMS Systems, introducing methods for applying the Malcolm Baldrige Quality Program to EMS systems and evaluating system progress. For further information on these courses contact the NHTSA EMS Division at (202) 366-5440.

The HRSA EMSC Program offers a range of educational tools covering basic pediatric EMS issues and many specific topics. The *Teaching Resource for Instructors in Prehospital Pediatrics* (TRIPP) is a comprehensive source of prehospital pediatric knowledge, containing a range of didactic and clinical information, from educational methodologies and teaching skills to issues concerning children with special health care needs and injury prevention. A list of available curricula and instructional tools on specific pediatric topics can be found at the EMSC web site, *http://www.ems-c.org/education*.

The US Fire Administration's (USFA) National Fire Academy conducts specialized training courses and management programs on EMS-related topics in a concentrated, residential setting at its Emmitsburg, Maryland headquarters. On-campus programs target middle- and top-level fire officers, fire service instructors, technical professionals, and representatives from allied professions. Any person with substantial involvement in fire prevention and control, EMS, or fire-related emergency management activities is eligible to apply for Academy courses. Students can also attend resident courses within their geographical region through the Academy's off-campus, Regional Delivery program. Through a cooperative working relationship with state and local fire training systems and the four branches of the Armed Services, the Academy Train-the-Trainer Program provides opportunities for fire service personnel to participate in courses at the state and local level. Additional information on the National Fire Academy is available at *http://www.usfa.fema.gov/nfa/aboutnfa*.

Operational Guidelines

Federal resources for EMS operations range from comprehensive system reviews to targeted guidelines for specific aspects of systems operations or development. Assistance in evaluating the comprehensive effectiveness of a state EMS system is available through the NHTSA EMS System Assessment Program. This peer review process involves a site visit by a team of national EMS experts who systematically assess the status of the state system according to a set of established standards. The team completes their review and recommendations while on site. States find the initial assessment and subsequent reassessments to be useful in prioritizing system enhancements. For further information concerning the NHTSA EMS System Assessment Program, contact the NHTSA EMS Division at (202) 266-5440.

NHTSA also provides recommendations for specific system aspects such as the *Guidelines for Medical Directors,* which offers advice for educating and preparing local EMS medical directors, and the *EMS Education Agenda for the Future* that proposes priorities for improving the competence of EMS students.

The EMSC Program offers a self-assessment tool, the *EMSC Needs Assessment Tool and Resource Supplement,* intended for use with planning grants or by systems interested in evaluating their current EMS/EMSC system. A complementary *Resource Supplement* supplies information concerning issues that may be raised by a needs assessment. The EMSC Program also provides a number of specific guidelines such as the *Pediatric Equipment and Supplies for Basic Life Support and Advanced Life Support Ambulances*, which lists essential and desirable pieces of pediatric equipment and supplies for Basic Life Support (BLS) and Advanced Life Support (ALS) ambulances. These documents are available on the EMSC web site, *www.ems-c.org*.

The NIH National Heart Lung and Blood Institute (NHLBI) offers guidance for a number of EMS-related operational issues, including those that affect rapid response to acute myocardial infarction, such as EMS staffing and equipment, 9-1-1 system design, and EMS dispatching. These resources are available at the web site of the NHLBI National Heart Attack Alert Program, *http://www.nhlbi.nih.gov/about/nhaap*.

Summary

Increasingly, EMS systems are involved in health promotion and injury prevention as well as emergency response, and this area is well supported by federal agencies. A variety of traffic safety materials suitable for use by EMS personnel are available from NHTSA. Program materials addressing safety belt and child safety seat use, impaired driving, pedestrian and school bus safety, and motorcycle and bicycle helmet use are located at *http://www.nhtsa.dot.gov/people/injury*. Advice on implementing local community outreach programs is available from the NHTSA Safe Communities web site at *http://www.nhtsa.dot.gov/safecommunities*. Injury prevention materials designed specifically for EMS organizations, including the *EMS PIER Manual* (Public Education, Informa-

tion, and Relations), the *SAFE Manual* (Safety Advice from EMS), and the *First There-First Care Bystander Care Program* are listed at *http://www.nhtsa.dot.gov/people/injury/ems/products.htm*.

Pediatric injury prevention materials are a primary focus of EMSC Program. The EMSC offers a guide to developing pediatric injury prevention programs, *Preventing Childhood Emergencies: A Guide to Developing Effective Injury Prevention Initiatives, 2nd Ed.* and several specific program resources, including the *Injury Prevention for Children with Special Health Care Needs Resource Guide*. These materials are available through the EMSC web site, *http://www.ems-c.org/injury/frameinjury.htm*.

The CDC (NCIPC) National Center for Injury Prevention and Control provides detailed information on a variety of injury issues, including unintentional injuries such as falls, motor vehicle crashes, and drowning, as well as intentional injuries such as suicide and youth violence. For each issue, the NCIPC offers research findings, statistical overviews, program evaluations, and resource references. These resources may be found at *http://www.cdc.gov/ncipc/ncipchm.htm*.

Both public information and corresponding healthcare provider information on a comprehensive range of health issues are available from the NIH. The NIH web site, *http://www.nih.gov/health/* provides links to specific NIH Institutes with extensive outreach program resources, including public service ads, Awareness Month information, patient information, and prevention strategies.

The nature of EMS requires that providers be prepared with knowledge and skills from an extraordinarily wide range of technical topics. Fortunately, there is a corresponding array of resources, both federal and non-federal, for the EMS provider to turn to for assistance.

Leadership and Team Building

Mike Taigman, EMT-P

Introduction

A leader has been defined as someone you choose to follow, to a place you wouldn't go by yourself. One of the hard lessons for many medical directors is the realization that being the medical director does not automatically mean that they are a leader. The front line employees in the current generation of EMS providers are not impressed with positions, titles, or degrees. In order to gain followership, medical directors must build their platform on a foundation of vision, commitment, communication, compassion, trust, integrity and inspiration.

In 1998, psychologist Daniel Goleman published what may be the most important book on leadership in the last century, *Working with Emotional Intelligence*.[1] Dr. Goleman and his colleagues, David McClelland and Richard Boyatzis, have collected a staggering amount of management science and analyzed it to discover what factors make the difference among average leaders, very successful leaders, and leaders who derail. They found that top executives who fail shared two traits. They were rigid, unable to adapt their style to changes in the organizational culture, or they were unable to take in or respond to feedback about traits they needed to change or improve. They couldn't listen or learn. They also had poor relationships, being too harshly critical, insensitive, or demanding, so that they alienated those they worked with.[1]

The very successful leaders and managers shared a mix of what Goleman and his colleagues have come to call Emotional Competencies. These competencies are clustered into five groups: Self-Awareness, Self-Regulation, Motivation, Social Awareness, and Social Skills. The self-awareness cluster contains competencies like emotional self-awareness, having an accurate self-assessment, and having a strong sense of one's self-worth and capabilities. Self-regulation is focused around managing one's internal states, impulses, and resources. Self-control, trustworthiness, conscientiousness, adaptability, and innovation are all part of self-regulation. Motivation involves having a drive for achievement, commitment to align with the goals of the group or organization, initiative, and optimism. Social awareness involves having empathy, an ability to recognize feeling in others, an ability to develop others, a bias toward service, an appreciation for the value of diversity, and awareness of the political landscape of a group. Social skills are focused around inducing desirable responses in others. This involves influence, communications, conflict management, being a change catalyst, building bonds, collaboration, cooperation, and team skills that create group synergy in pursuit of collective goals.

The information detailed in the book *Working with Emotional Intelligence* should be of particular interest to physicians in leadership positions. Much of their work is based in neuro-anatomy, and is validated using methods of scientific inquiry similar to what is used in clinical research.[1]

Feedback

Management author Ken Blanchard says, "Feedback is the breakfast of champions." In the world of prehospital EMS, feedback from the medical director is the breakfast, lunch, dinner, and midnight snack of good clinicians. The results of a 25-year research study involving over 80,000 managers found that the answers to these six questions determine employee turnover rate, a key factor in employee satisfaction.[2]

1. Do I know what's expected of me at work?
2. Do I have the materials and equipment I need to do my work right?
3. Do I have the opportunity to do what I do best every day?
4. In the last seven days, have I received recognition or praise for good work?

5. Does my supervisor, or someone at work, seem to care about me as a person?
6. Is there someone at work who encourages my development?

Medical directors who are skilled at interpersonal communications can have a powerful impact on the retention and satisfaction of clinicians in their system. No matter how scientific and academic the conversation, the vast majority of a message that is received during an interaction with another human being is emotional. Albert Marabian researched interpersonal communications in the early 1970s. He found that of messages people receive, 7% are made up of the words they use, 38% of their tone of voice, and 55% of their body language. Therefore, how one communicates has a greater impact than what is actually said. The phrase "I love you" leaves one impression when it is delivered from a sarcastic angry person and another when it is shared in loving passion. When kindness and caring are communicated, even negative feedback can be perceived positively by the receiver.

Replace "constructive criticism" with "useful feedback." The term constructive criticism is an oxymoron. Construct means to build; criticize means to tear down. When constructive criticism is provided, receivers are torn down; when that happens, they are not likely to improve their performance. It is very difficult to improve effectiveness when one is feeling down. Also, people react to criticism by becoming defensive and are likely to become more firmly entrenched in their belief system. On the other hand useful feedback is like a gift that can be used to improve the future. Useful feedback is a powerful relationship-building tool.

A couple of linguistic constructs can improve the chance that a receiver will actually be able to integrate feedback without becoming defensive. The first is to construct feedback in the form of an "I statement." An "I statement" comes across as a request for assistance. Almost everyone in EMS likes helping people, since it's a useful way to engage their energy. Effective "I statements" have four parts: your emotional state, their action, your interpretation of their action, and a request. For example, "I get frustrated when you bring in patients with only their head immobilized to the back board, because my interpretation is that you don't understand the damage that can occur if your have to roll the patient to clear their airway. My request is that whenever you immobilize a patient's spine that you secure their head, shoulders, chest, and hips to the board." Another trick for pro-

viding effective feedback is to replace the word "but" with the word "and." "You are a really good EMT but, ..." has a much different impact than, "You are a really good EMT and . . ." When most people hear "but" used like this, it sends the message that everything said before the word is a lie and it signals that an attack will be immediately following the word. Immediately a psychological defensive wall flies up. Of course, what this wall blocks is the very message that was to be delivered in the first place. When people hear a compliment followed by "and" their ears tend to perk up expecting more good news. "You are really a good paramedic and if you were more aggressive with your airway management this patient would not be hypoxic." When they hear useful feedback tied to a compliment, they are more likely to put the message to use.

Most customer service literature suggests that people treat others the way they have been treated. Medical directors who are kind and caring in their interaction with paramedics are likely to have paramedics who are kind and caring toward their patients. Conversely, paramedics who have been abused are more likely to become abusive. How paramedics feel when they leave an interaction with their medical director has a direct impact on the way their next few patients are treated.

Similarly, meaningful feedback should be provided in private. Even if the feedback is not likely to embarrass or stress the receiver, it should be given in private. This approach increases respect for the leader; it also is more effective, as demonstrated in the following case. A medical director dressed down a paramedic in front of the emergency department staff and the patient; the paramedic had made a potentially dangerous mistake. Following the interaction, the physician felt that he had been effective in his communication. He also felt that it was an added benefit for the rest of the staff to hear the feedback, so they would not make the same mistake. However, all the paramedic and the staff who witnessed the event could focus on was what a jerk the medical director was. They felt that he acted innappropriately, and they totally missed the feedback he provided. The general consensus was that in the future they needed to be more careful not to get caught.

A similar situation occurred in another city. However, this medical director chose to wait until the patient was cared for and his anger had lessened. He then asked the paramedic to step into a private room to discuss what had happened. After the physician communicated his concern in the form of an "I statement" he asked the paramedic how she perceived the situation, and she was allowed to explain her thought process and decision making. Only then did the medical director point out the cognitive flaws and provide remedial education. After the interaction the medical director felt that he had been effective in communicating the message; more important, the paramedic felt the medical director really cared about the treatment that patients received. Feeling supported, the paramedic provided as many of her peers who would listen with the details, so they would not make the same mistake. Now, paramedics in this system bring their mistakes to their medical director before he hears about them from another source. In addition, he is regularly sought out as a consultant for retrospective review and advice about challenging calls.

It is important that the field personnel provide a reality check for the medical director. The reality, that medical directors care enough to ask how they are doing and then listen to the feedback, builds both their position and the team.

EMS team members generally have positive intentions; however, those intentions may be difficult to discern. Few providers wake up in the morning thinking, "I wonder how many patients I can harm today?" If the provider has a positive intent during a discussion, then education and information will probably solve the problem. If providers do not have a beneficial motive for their incorrect actions, they may have chosen the wrong profession.

Protocols

Rules, regulations, policies, protocols, and procedures have strengths and limitations. Very little of the strength resides in the written document. The ability of a policy or protocol to guide and improve care comes from the process of their preparation, implementation, and daily use. Protocols need to be flexible and dynamic in their ability to evolve and adapt with the changing needs of the system. Ideally, changes in the protocols should be driven by scientific research, and choreographed by the local practice of medicine. Provider involvement in the development and implementation of protocols is essential. Protocols are best followed when providers understand the rationales supporting them; one of the best ways to understand them is to participate in their creation.

The education in the implementation phases of protocol revisions is critical to the ability of clinicians to use the protocols successfully in the care of patients. Communication and education about the new information are best accomplished with an eye toward developing new competencies in clinicians. The most effective systems use multiple mechanisms (classes, newsletters, audio education, computer-based training) to ensure that everyone practicing in the system understands and can activate the new information. It is an absolute mistake to deliver a new protocol in every mailbox and expect instantaneous compliance. The effectiveness of training can be assessed at four possible levels:

1. *Level 1:* Post-training participant satisfaction assessment. This is designed to fine-tune the delivery mechanism for training to best meet the needs of the learner.
2. *Level 2:* Knowledge retention assessment (post-training test). This is designed to see how well students remember the information that is presented in our training programs.
3. *Level 3:* Behavior change assessment. This is designed to see if the new knowledge translates into a change in action by crews when taking care of patients.
4. *Level 4:* Clinical outcome assessment. This is the most difficult level of training effectiveness assessment and can only be accomplished in certain clinical conditions.

The primary weakness of protocols is the inability of anyone to write a protocol for good judgment. Systems attempting to promulgate protocols that account for every variable of the EMS equation have paradoxically produced huge monoliths that are essentially incomprehensible, impossible to remember, and ineffective in supporting good clinical care. The key is to use protocols as guidelines; thus, everyone in the system is playing variations from the same sheet of music.

A "values-based" leadership style is more effective than a "rules-based" style. Since the practice of prehospital clinical care is an extension of the practice of the system's medical director, everyone practicing under his or her license should know the medical director's values. It influences the decisions made and actions taken by prehospital care providers if their medical director believes that the only real stabilization of patients occurs in the emergency department, or if they believe that whenever possible, patient choice should drive clinical decision making. In most systems, the only time the policy manual, protocol manual, or union contract is consulted by management is when something did not go well.

A core problem with management by rules is that it allows people to quit thinking. All providers know of cases in which the supervisor intensely studies the rulebook until something that fits the situation at hand is found. Instantly, the supervisor relaxes when the rule that applies is located. If unsuccessful in the search for a rule, the supervisor quickly begins the process of writing. The results of these endeavors in reactionary rule making are often ridiculous. The following are a few real life examples: "Starting June 15th there will be no slouching in the ambulance," and, "Forthwith employees are required to follow the following eight-step process for washing their hands after every patient contact or handling of equipment. Violators will be subject to the progressive disciplinary process." "All employees are required to adhere to everything in the Book-O-Memos." (This book has every memo written in the organization since 1981; it is expanded to four volumes, and is full of contradictory information.) EMS leaders and medical directors who rely only on memos and addenda to the protocol manual for leadership rarely get their messages to the team.

Some rules do help lead and build the EMS team. The key to developing a new rule effectively is to avoid overreacting to the current situation. A good strategy is to write the new rule or protocol and lock it away for 30 days. If at the end of the waiting period it still makes sense to implement, put it in place. Many leaders who use this strategy find that 80% end up in the shredder. There are some protocols that must be implemented immediately. A successful medical director knows which problems are best addressed with immediate protocol revision, and which are not.

Star Care

An organization should be led with a simple set of values and principles, that is, a shared paradigm. Paramedic and author Thom Dick wrote such a set of guiding principles, which has been adapted widely since its introduction at BayStar Medical Services in San Mateo County, California in 1990. Personnel use this "Star Care" checklist to ensure they cover all the important aspects of each call. Medical directors and system leaders use the checklist to evaluate programs, policies, protocols, and improvements in their systems.

- Safe—Were my actions safe for me, my colleagues, other professionals, and the public?
- Team-based—Were my actions taken with due regard for the opinions and feelings of my co-workers, including those from other agencies?
- Attentive to human needs—Did I treat my patient as a person? Did I keep the patient warm? Was I gentle? Did I use the individual's name throughout the call? Did I tell the patient what to expect in advance? Did I treat the patient's family and friends with the kind of respect that I would have wanted to receive myself?
- Customer accountable—If I were face-to-face right now with the customers I dealt with on this response, could I look them in the eye and say, "I did my very best for you"?
- Reasonable—Did my actions make sense? Would a reasonable colleague of my experience have acted similarly under the same circumstances?
- Ethical—Were my actions fair and honest in every way? Are my answers to these questions?

One of the challenging parts of using the Star Care system is deciding if a particular action was or is ethical or not. An easy way to get through this difficulty is to imagine how you'd feel if what you are about to do were to be featured as the headline story in tomorrow's newspaper. If you and the people in your system would be proud of the article, it is probably an ethical decision. If not, then it's probably not.

This Star Care checklist is printed on wallet-sized cards and carried by everyone in the system. It provides a very simple yet powerful method to recognize, reward, and reinforce strong performance. It also provides a template to work through any improvement opportunities. Incidentally, this checklist may be reprinted if credit is given to Thom Dick and BayStar.

References

1. Goleman D. *Working with Emotional Intelligence*. New York: Bantam; 1998.
2. Buckingham M, Coffman C. *First, Break All the Rules*. New York: Simon and Schuster; 1999.

CHAPTER 43

Media

Paul E. Pepe, MD, MPH
Linda L. Pepe
Robert Davis

Introduction

As a medical expert for the emergency medical services (EMS) system, the EMS physician often is called upon to render an opinion about medical care or about medically related aspects of EMS operations and training. Many times they must do so in a public forum, such as a city council meeting, or in interviews with the news media. In addition, as a local medical leader of a community public service, the EMS physician may also become a reliable, recognized or readily accessible source of medical information for the public.

The purpose of this chapter is to provide EMS physicians and their colleagues with certain tools that can help them to optimize their public speaking and, in turn, their effectiveness in delivering important public communications. More than ever before, with the various evolving challenges to EMS such as diminishing healthcare resources or the threats of bioterrorism, the skill of public speaking becomes a critical function for those practicing emergency medical care, both in the in-hospital and out-of-hospital setting.

Assumptions

The recommendations made in this chapter are stated with the consideration of some basic assumptions. Those assumptions are that the EMS physician/public speaker is the appropriate spokesperson and that he or she has received clearance from his or her supervisor or applicable public information officer (PIO). Likewise, in cases involving specific patients, one should also make sure that the patient/patient's family has been advised of any public comment. In principle, they should be apprised of and agree to the anticipated statements to be made, as well as the likely answers to probable media questions concerning the patient's situation, especially those that may

go beyond the typical disclosures that conventionally fall within the "public domain." While non-specific public information such as: "a 43-year-old man received a gunshot wound to the abdomen and is in critical condition" may be public domain, it is still generally wise for the public speaker to prepare the related parties for the information to be disseminated.

Most patients, and families in particular, are very reluctant to have *any* information disclosed whatsoever. Therefore, it is helpful to point out to them that, in most "media-worthy" events, the media will report "something" and that the proactive physician spokesperson may be best able to help control and minimize the impact of whatever information eventually is disclosed to the public. It is important to recognize that, analogous to a chewing puppy pulling even harder on a sock when the sock is being pulled away, the more one withdraws from the media, the harder they may look into the issue. If they sense an attempt to conceal facts, they are more apt to pursue them further.

In that respect, no matter what public-speaking endeavor one encounters, it is key that the EMS physician approach the situation as a sincere patient advocate first and foremost. Self-promotion, insincere advocacy, or indiscriminate information dissemination soon becomes obvious to the news media personnel, colleagues, and other patient advocates. Recognizing and appreciating these ethical and sociological concepts, one can become a much more effective, sought-after, and long-lived public speaker. Those seeking good "PR" will be seen as self-serving and not public servants. Those sincerely seeking patient advocacy, first and foremost, will be seen as true public servants and, in turn, good "PR" will ensue naturally.

The Challenges of Bite-Speak

One of the more common public communication challenges of modern life has been the task of finding the right "sound bite." With the evolution of mass-media network teams, worldwide Internet communications, and highly reactive information management systems, a massive amount of information is available to be delivered to millions of people. With the expanding availability of information and information sources, and with a growing competitiveness among news organizations as well as a "fast-food" society that prefers "get-to-the-point" news, individual news stories are, more and more, becoming "bullets" of information. In addition, the news media is a business. Air time or columns of print must be trimmed and "budgeted." The success of *USA Today*, for example, is in part due to their "economies of scale," both in terms of circulation and "efficiencies" of individual articles. Likewise, *CNN Headline News, MSNBC*, and the like are examples of the societal demands for bulleted information.

Even locally, the typical half-hour television (TV) news program is actually only 10 to 15 minutes of news, once one excludes commercials, weather, and sports. To deliver 20 or more news pieces within that half-hour broadcast, the news producer for that show must keep each story extremely short. Also, stylistically, most network affiliates will still run at least two or three "packages" per show, even during a late evening broadcast. A package usually is a more extended taped story provided by a reporter. Typically, the package often is introduced by the involved reporter with a "live shot" from some site or from a desk in the newsroom, followed by the main videotaped story and, in turn, a departing live closure from the reporter, who may engage in some parting chat with the broadcast anchor. While a package can run longer, it may be as short as 90 seconds and it still needs to include the story set-up, graphics, and several interviews, as well as the live introduction and closure. Therefore, this may leave only a few seconds for each of the individual interviews.

In addition, if a third or more of the news time is dedicated to packages, then each of the many other news pieces will be even shorter. Therefore, the other 15 (or more) news items may be presented in much less than a minute (e.g., 15 to 30 seconds) in formats such as a "voice over," in which an anchor reads the narrative while videotape is run; or a "voice over with a sound bite," in which a short interview with a relevant person is inserted. The bottom line is that interviews must be only seconds long, particularly if there is a need for a "pro-con" format. In fact, based on the previous discussion, one could have been in-

terviewed by a reporter for five minutes, but an expected sound bite length, once it is aired, be it radio or TV, would be seven to ten seconds. In turn, one should choose one's words wisely and economically, and most importantly, stay on focus.

Live interviews may be longer and may often run for 2 or 3 minutes, be it TV or radio. Nevertheless, typically one can expect 2 to 4 questions. While the answers may not have to be limited to the 10-second sound bite, they still should be relatively brief, because listeners often fatigue in terms of attention span when the answers get lengthy (>20 seconds). Brevity and bullets do it best. Take, for example, this heat illness prevention tip: "One—Wear light-weight, light-colored, loose-fitting clothing; Two—Stay in well-ventilated areas, even if in-doors; Three—Drink lots of water; and Four—Avoid Alcohol."

While brevity and "bullets" are necessary for media interactions, they are just as applicable to other public-speaking settings. For example, city council interactions may only allow for a minute's communication in a less structured presentation. Therefore, one must be prepared to get to the point directly or present relevant arguments cogently and briefly. This should not be a surprise to anyone who has sat through lengthy city council or legislative sessions in which hours of tedious comments are made and attention spans grow shorter and shorter throughout a long day of "listening." Therefore, the sound bite may not just be a "necessary evil," but also an important communication format in which one is challenged to make a point, without short-changing accuracy in order to achieve the communicative objective.

Sound Bite

Most public communications of an EMS physician are informational, but some may also need to address a point of contention. In the former case, a simple three-part format may be effective, while a different strategy may be needed for an argumentative position. For example, if called to comment on a new helmet ordinance for youthful bicycle riders, the medical public speaker is more effective if he or she can anticipate the opposition's point of view. In theory, the pros of the proposed ordinance already should have been articulated and disclosed. Generally, these have been cited in previous briefings. Therefore, it would be less effective to focus on the "informational" sound bite (i.e., "90% of all serious head injuries to children can be prevented by bicycle helmets"). Rather, one might want to focus upon defusing the opposition with a "counter-argument" sound bite.

In the case cited, the EMS physician may first want to ascertain the opposition's arguments from someone like an aide of the councilmember supporting the ordinance. If it turns out that the "con" arguments consist of "we can't impose a financial impact upon families" or "we can't interfere with one's freedom of choice," then the public speaker (at the council meeting or in interviews with the media) should recognize these concerns and, when appropriate, even address them somewhat sympathetically. For example, in the public statement to be made, the EMS physician might say "When I first heard about this ordinance, it seemed that it would be unrealistic because, even though the expense is small, you are still forcing a cost upon families. *But*—as I really looked into it more and more, I became convinced that it makes tremendous sense, both medically and economically."

That alone could be the "sound bite" (main statement) for the city council. In fact, more than likely, it will invite further factual comment for the inquiring council or, subsequently, the media. The follow-up then can be the "informational" sound bite in which the medical expert states: "The data are clear: 90% of all serious bicycle-related head injuries in children can be prevented by the children wearing a bike helmet—it's one of the best 'vaccinations' against injury that we have—and for every dollar we spend, we save two dollars or more in healthcare costs."

The media may or may not include the last part of this statement, but they may still use the information as part of their own narrative. Likewise, at the city council meeting, there probably is just enough time to include all of these remarks. In the end, the obvious points are addressed, but so are the counter-arguments if they are prioritized and discussed initially.

Two other points should be made about this particular statement to the city council. The issues about cost, though important in helping to defuse the opposing position here in the council meeting (or similarly in a hospital board room), may not be ripe for the media sound bite. The media know that the public may not relate to "cost savings" as much as safety, and so they may not use that initial statement about the ordinance making economic and medical sense. For them the informational sound bite is most important. Nevertheless, in this setting, where "freedom of choice" and "taxation" anxieties are circulating, the challenge has to be anticipated and politely pre-empted to help to salvage the undecided council votes.

The other point to be made is the issue of what to say on each side of the "but" in a statement. Take, for example, the verdict yielded by the judge on a typical prime-time TV drama. The judge always says something like, "The acts committed here were unconscionable and go against every ethical substance in my body. BUT, the laws are clear in terms of the procedures for proper evidence collection and these procedures simply were not followed. Therefore, I am bound to rule in favor of the defendant." The counter-argument starts with the sympathetic statement for the state (and victims/victims' families of the crime being judged). However, the true crux of the statement comes with the phrases following the "but." Similar considerations can be seen in day-to-day personal interactions. Take, for example, statements like: "I'm very sorry I snapped at you. I apologize, *but* I've been under a lot of pressure lately"; or "Oh, I really would have loved to come, *but* I've already have something scheduled for that evening." Both of these statements might be seen as insincere or, at best, polite responses when one considers what phrases come after the "but." Juxtaposed, the statements come cross more sincerely: "I'm sorry—I've been under a lot of pressure lately—*but* that's no excuse to snap at you. I apologize"; and "Oh—I have already have something scheduled for that evening—*but* I would have really loved to come." Therefore, in the counter-argument sound bite, keep this in mind.

As with the counter-argument sound bite, the "informational" part of the public speaking has to be succinct as well. As stated previously, a three-part format might be recommended. First, the sound bite starts with a definitive word or phrase such as "Absolutely!" or "There's no doubt about it!" or (as in the previous example) "The data are clear." Then there is a short core explanation such as: "90% of all serious head injuries . . . . etc." Finally a parting resolve (which may or may not be cut by media editors) would be provided such as: ". . . it's one of the best 'vaccinations' against injury that we have!"

If one measures the elapsed time for such a sound bite, it should be about 10 seconds or so. Take, for example, another sound bite about cardiopulmonary resuscitation (CPR). If asked whether or not it is important for everyone to learn CPR, the EMS physician might respond: "Absolutely! (opening exclamation) There's no way a professional rescuer can routinely get to your loved ones in the four or five minutes in which permanent brain damage can occur when their heart stops beating (core explanation), so it's up to each one of us to be prepared to save our families" (parting resolve). That sound bite is just about 10 to 12 seconds, if executed well. The video editors may cut the parting resolve, but if said immediately, enthusiastically, and with sincere advocacy, it will most likely stay in the final cut.

A minor variation on this theme is to first answer the question asked during the opening exclamation. For example, if asked "Is it important for everyone to learn CPR?" the answer might be, "Absolutely! It's *critical* for everyone to know CPR . . . etc." This is truly stylistic, but this approach can be highly effective in terms of reinforcing one's point, depending on the question. Still, just using "Absolutely!" can work if the question is clear, particularly if brevity is needed.

Finally, when the interview drifts, the EMS physician should keep it on track. An interviewer may ask: "What about the chance of getting AIDS or some other infectious disease?" The interviewee should stay on the mark and state that: "Keep in perspective: 70 to 80% of the cases requiring CPR occur in and around the home—and another 15% in the workplace—it's going to be a family member or friend you will need to save!" (note: <10 seconds). The suggestions here are not only to remind the audience that one's own family members are the most important persons to teach CPR to (your main point overall), but also to avoid repetition of the question if it involves words that might flag a concern.

Print Versus Electronic

The majority of people get most of their news information from the electronic media (radio and TV). Therefore, learning how to deal with the electronic media should become part of the EMS physician's repertoire of expertise. However, printed media can be of benefit as well, in that a permanent, easy-to-transmit copy can be reproduced and disseminated or scanned into a transmissible computer file that can be shown in presentations. Also, print media often drive electronic coverage in trend reports. TV and radio assignments editors and researchers often tear out stories from newspapers or download printed reports from Internet-based newspaper reports which capsulize information to give their reporters for follow-up.

That also means that print stories can also give EMS physicians the opportunity to shape a story better, or even rapidly catch up on the issues being ex-

amined, because someone already has distilled the latest information and gotten the interviews directly from the researchers. Print stories give sources (prospective interviewees) more than just a sound bite to assimilate their reactions to the subject at hand. Also, the tear-outs or print-outs can be filed away for future use or sent on to potentially interested parties. In addition, important reports that relate to, or impact upon, your own operations can be sent along to appropriate managers. Likewise, positive stories about the EMS system can be sent as an "objective" (i.e., someone else's) viewpoint about performance to bosses, city officials, and other "stakeholders," including the EMS personnel themselves.

One potential downside of print media, however, is that the reporters typically paraphrase the interviewee's comments because they are taking shorthand notes (unless they are directly recording it). In contrast, with electronic media, the words that come out are the interviewee's actual words. Although they may be taken out of context, they will still be the actual words.

To that end, it is not entirely inappropriate at the end of the interview to ask the print media reporter to call you back (after writing the story) to hear the quotes that might be used and to check them for accuracy (and also to see if he or she really got the point that needed to be emphasized). First, this means that the EMS physician must be readily available at the "on deadline" time for the possible "read-back." Second, when doing so, the interviewee has to understand that not all print reporters are entirely receptive to this request. Therefore, it is best to understand that such a request should be done in the spirit of the interviewee's limitations, not the reporter's (e.g., "I know I talked fast—do you want to go over any point now or call me back later after you've had a chance to assimilate all of this stuff?—In fact, I'd love it if you call me back so I know what to expect—also you can double-check your facts with me if you want").

One also should budget time in an interview session to go back over anything that might need more detail. It would be advisable to be patient and ask if the reporter would like to go over his/her notes to see if anything needs to be discussed in more detail, or modified. This suggestion is reasonable because most interviewees do provide their facts and comment rather rapidly. Therefore, in addition to being available for deadlines, one should also switch gears with print reporters (talk more slowly) and reiterate certain points if they are key. Reporters want to get it right, but deadlines are unforgiving.

Ten Rules

Whether delivering a live radio interview, a state legislature address, or a taped TV video, there are ten easy but key axioms to keep in mind that should guide one's approach to each public-speaking event. These "ten golden rules" can be itemized as follows:

Rule #1: Always Tell the Truth and Do It in a Ten-Second Sound Bite

Information is highly regarded, but false information is scorned and never forgotten by the media, the public, public officials, and even one's colleagues. Credibility is the EMS physician's most important asset.

Sometimes, however, a fine line must be negotiated between the "truth" and the "whole truth." For example, there are ethical issues, and even governmental security issues, that must be taken into consideration. In the case of a famous person's sudden illness, the media always want to know why the celebrity was rushed by ambulance to the hospital. This becomes an ethical concern. Aside from the family's or patient's reluctance to have anything said to the media (patient confidentiality issues), there is also the concern that information that gets out through indiscreet persons will not be accurate, or will lead to inappropriate speculation. Therefore, a balance may be struck, and the EMS physician may be the person to do so. Since something needs to said, it is best done by a credible, patient-oriented spokesperson who can tell the truth but also knows where to draw the line on disclosures.

Take the case of the celebrity who has probable gastrointestinal bleeding heralded by melena and severe hypotension, but also accompanied by transient ischemic electrocardiographic changes. The media, knowing only that the patient was rushed to the hospital after EMS received a "man down" call, may want to know if there was foul play or if the person had something serious like a heart attack or stroke. If the patient/family concedes to saying "something" to the media, the preliminary public report might be more generic (i.e., "He's having some type of abdominal pain and they will be running a few standard tests to try to figure out what's going on"). However, if the media still specifically ask about the "heart attack" issue, one could reply (in this particular case): "We don't have any evidence of his having a heart attack at this time, but as we do with everyone else, we will consider all possibilities and we'll make sure that we rule that out." In this case, for example, not mentioning the ischemic changes (which are prob-

ably only transient) avoids embarrassing detail and unnecessary speculation. At the same time, one's credibility is still maintained in case of the unlikely possibility that the patient's cardiac enzymes eventually do indicate myocardial infarction. Some reporters may push harder and ask what tests are being done; one should be prepared for that possibility, but the answer can also be followed with a generic statement: "I'm not aware of all the specific tests at this time (assuming that is true), but I know he's in the best of hands and they'll be doing all the appropriate things." So the truth, but not necessarily the whole truth, is being discussed due to patient confidentiality issues.

On the other hand, sometimes aggressive disclosure, either by the patient, or by a physician with the patient's permission, is also the best way to go. Take the case of U.S. President George Bush's pretzel-swallowing incident. Much of the original flurry of media attention was rapidly defused by full disclosure and even assertive humor about the incident over the next day or so. In that case, the President's physician was immediately responsive and gave full disclosure about the incident, the care provided, and the prognosis. At the same time, the President is a very special case and such disclosure may not always be appropriate for other persons, even those of great celebrity. As discussed previously, full disclosure is not always necessary.

Likewise, there are other considerations regarding full disclosure, such as governmental security issues. For example, one must be cautious about releasing what plans are in place for dealing with terrorists. Once again, there is a fine line between the making of statements that assure the public that protective strategies are in place and statements that give away important security information. For example, one might state that there are multiple well-placed caches of chemical antidotes, but still not disclose their whereabouts.

Regardless of the issue, one must always tell the truth and always maintain credibility. If a reporter suddenly calls to inquire about an anonymous report from a hospital regarding a missed endotracheal intubation by EMS personnel, it is important to give a response. However, even if the preliminary information sounds like some grave error was made, it is still reasonable to simply state, "If such a thing did occur, you can be sure that we will be looking into this aggressively." In fact, giving too much detail generally is inappropriate and unfair to the "accused" in terms of due process until the formal investigation is done.

Again, these same caveats are important for the medical "expert" at town hall meetings, civic groups, and other public locations. In addition, be it for city council or the media, it is important to keep one's truthful comments to the "ten-second sound bite," or at least be as cogent and brief as possible in the applicable situation. Thus, there is a challenge to the EMS physician to convey the disclosable information as succinctly as possible.

Rule #2: Respond Quickly and Accurately (Even if Initially in the Dark) and Become an Available, Familiar, and Helpful Resource

When you are contacted by the media, rapid response is important. Most reporters are on some deadline. In case an assistant to the EMS physician answers the phone and takes the message from the media, it is important for the assistant to find out if there is such a deadline. But whether or not a deadline exists, the reporter may still "shop around" to rapidly confirm an interviewee, even if the EMS medical director was the first choice. Although busy, it is important for the prospective media interviewee to be flexible enough to make some impromptu appointment time or get the media another good source right away. In that respect, the EMS physician is seen as the immediate, helpful, and familiar resource to go to in the event of an urgent situation. The same is true if it is a public official calling.

Being flexible and available is important in terms of future relations with the media or the public officials, be it to soften the hit when a negative situation occurs or, more importantly, to collect some "brownie points" in the event that the EMS physician may eventually need help as well. It is no promise, but if the EMS system needs help with an injury-prevention program or to promote a new lifesaving campaign, it is always good for the EMS physician to have established responsiveness with the media or at city hall when the tables are turned.

More importantly, when the media (or council-member) calls about the negative story such as the alleged missed intubation, it is important to respond quickly and accurately, even if in the dark. All the media may need is a quick sound bite to meet a deadline for the 10 P.M. broadcast or tomorrow's paper, such as: "I can't confirm that this has really happened yet, but you can be sure that we will be looking into this aggressively." First of all, this is the fair thing to do in terms of the due process for the "accused" EMS personnel. Also, by the time the matter is formally investigated, the story usually is no longer as appealing to the media. This is because it may be long forgotten or it will no longer be "news" regardless of the outcome of the investigation. Therefore, the quickly delivered sound bite, ("we'll be investigating it aggressively") on the night of the event may be all that is ever required. Most importantly, by responding rapidly, the EMS physician is seen by both the media and the public as a trusted public servant who is very responsive and concerned. The public's trust and the public's safety will be maintained—and that is the key point of the media inquiry in the first place.

In turn, in negative situations, the EMS physician will get a fair shot and not be as susceptible to the "ambush" interview. While it does not grant immunity from attack, being a reliable, familiar resource will be an attribute taken into account under these circumstances. Therefore, it is also wise for the EMS physician to build relations with local media, particularly assignment editors and producers at electronic media (radio and TV) stations or their counterparts at print media organizations. While one can schedule elusive appointments with these busy people, the best way for EMS physicians to gain the familiarity with the media or city officials is to do their EMS job well, to establish proactive programs such as injury prevention activities and CPR-AED programs, and to have a high visibility at EMS scenes.

In the end, it is always key for EMS physicians to make themselves readily accessible to those entities that represent the public. It is important to establish your first interactions as positive interactions and not adversarial ones. Responding quickly and accurately, and being a helpful, reliable, and eventually familiar resource is the best mechanism to accomplish that goal.

Rule #3: Be a Human Being and Act Like One and Talk Like One

In addition to being "available, responsive, and truthful" (in short sound bites), perhaps the most important axiom to follow is to be a human being. The EMS physician is ostensibly credible to the public just by having the medical degree and the position of EMS medical director. Specifically, the EMS physician does not need to use terms such as "cerebral infarction" or "COPD," nor does he or she need to wear a suit specifically for the spot media interview. When contacted by the media, rapid response is more important—as is realism. If the prospective speaker is in a scrub shirt at work, that is the way to give the interview. In fact, this image is probably preferred to an image of a detached physician in a suit with books in the background (unless it is a pure medical information piece on a more esoteric subject). Language-wise, the EMS physician can use terms like "ventricular fibrillation" as long as it is immediately defined. For example, one might say, "One out of five people who will die today, will die from sudden ventricular fibrillation, an unexpected and abrupt short-circuiting of the heart's electrical system," or, "We think that Officer Carter has a pulmonary contusion—essentially a bruise in the lungs—that is giving him some breathing problems." At the same time, words like "suffer" and "sustained" are too colloquial and even inappropriate, as in, "He *suffered* a heart attack." After all, the medical community is supposed to keep you from "suffering."

When providing an interview, it is also important to avoid visual and auditory distractions, both in the background and on one's person. Dangling earrings or wild hairs can be very distracting. Multiple colors or flashy nametags can also take away from the point of the interview, the sound bite itself. Chewing gum or fidgeting with some object can also be annoying, as is looking around aimlessly. Sometimes a simple, symbolic prop can be reasonable, such as a steadily held stethoscope or walkie-talkie. Likewise, a background with an ambulance (outside the emergency department), a chest x-ray (inside the emergency department), or a lit-up dispatch office display map can be effective, as long as the background is not flashing or busy with movement.

More important than what one wears is what his or her demeanor exudes. Nothing is more engaging in an interview than comfort and enthusiasm. Even in a serious, "negative" story, a sense of sincerity and vivacity still appeals to viewers and listeners. Likewise, in a print media story where a demeanor would not seem to be portrayable, many reporters may still comment on (or reflect) your enthusiasm in their final copy.

Most importantly, the key approach here is to do something similar to what the physician might do with patients when giving them informed consent. When necessary, and in applicable situations, a healthcare practitioner might say, "If this was my mom, this is exactly what I'd advise her to do." Simi-larly, the EMS physician may be able to use this same technique in the sound bite or public comment. For example, "Knowing CPR is critical. As a father, I can't think of a more important thing to know for the protection of my children—it's one of those things we all need to know." This statement emphasizes that, while the medical expert may be a physician, he or she is also a family person with whom the average person can identify. It also takes advantage of an important human motivator, even for the often inattentive and unmotivated male viewer who *does* see himself as the "protector" in the family. It also says that CPR is something that all of us (not just healthcare workers) need to know for the sake of our families. In other words, from the basic human being's point of view, it is a basic social obligation. Bringing this subject down to the level of one dad's own advice to himself makes it more effective for the target audience.

In fact, considering what one would do for one's own family or loved ones not only is an effective sound bite, but it is smart in terms of establishing credible policy and procedure, or in decision-making day-to-day. If a policy or position is good enough for the responsive, available, truthful, and enthusiastic EMS physician and his or her own family members, then public trust is better gained. Comments such as, "If this had been my own daughter, I would have wanted the paramedics to have done the same thing," provides a very cogent opinion. Likewise, "Persons will be entered into the study on an even-odd (every other) day basis—whatever way the cards fall—if it's my son who's in a car wreck on an 'even-numbered' day, the so-called 'control' day, he will get the usual treatment we always provide—and if the incident happens on an odd-numbered day—the 'different approach' day—then he'll get the study drug. It's a flip of a coin—and no matter who it is—your family member or mine—everyone gets a 50-50 chance of getting either our current standard of care or the new approach."

Not only does this approach make the concerns more palatable, but it is ethically the correct thing to do. Moreover, if the EMS physician is sincerely willing to enter herself/himself or a beloved family member into a study according to its rules (be it control or study arm), that probably handles 90% of any ethical concern that most regulators would have, let alone the public at large.

Rule #4: The Glass is Half-Full on Issues and Half-Empty on Individual Patients

Most people do not want to hear pessimistic things. It is more appealing to stress an optimistic perspective, even if stating the same facts. For example, if asked: "Doctor, isn't it true that if we don't get this new lifesaving equipment, over the next year many people will die unnecessarily?" The best reply is: "Absolutely! If we can get this new equipment, many lives will be saved." Therefore, in this "negative" interrogatory ("... many people will die ...."), one would not use the direct "repeat the question" approach for the opening exclamation of the reply. Instead, one would use the reciprocal.

"The glass is half-full" approach is much preferred to the "sky is falling" approach. At the same time, the media, and particularly managing editors, still want to "sell papers." They know that a compelling headline in the newspaper or alarming break tease tends to get attention. In fact, despite what one says during the interview, the statements may still seem to be turned around when the morning paper headline says, "Many Will Die Unnecessarily Without New Device." Hopefully, your quote or sound bite within the article or news broadcast will still reflect the proactive position: "Many more lives can be saved."

In contrast, when speaking about an individual patient, one should avoid terms like "stable" unless that is the unequivocal situation. A person with a gunshot to the abdomen should not be billed as "stable" just because the blood pressure and heart rate are currently "normal." Media statements should always anticipate the potential for complications like: "Anytime someone is shot in the abdomen—we consider it a critical situation because of the possibility of severe internal bleeding and infections—fortunately now, he's in the best of hands—this is where I'd want my family member taken with this kind of problem—we'll let you know how he does!"

In this case, if the patient was declared as stable and then dies unexpectedly from an insidious iliac vessel injury, it looks very worrisome. However, if it is made clear that all abdominal gunshot wounds should be considered critical, an unexpected death will not necessarily be seen as "unanticipated" whether talking to the family, the media, or anyone else. On the other hand, if the patient goes on to survive the critical injury, it makes the trauma center and EMS system look good, and appropriately so. Obviously, this is inappropriate if the patient has a small laceration, but whenever doubt exists about complete stability and no risk for serious problems, then a "glass is half-empty" approach is a little more appropriate.

Rule #5: Make Others Look Good and You Will Look Good

Complimenting others is extremely important, even when the interviewee was the main person involved in some successful situation. For example, if the EMS physician arrived on a scene first and single-handedly resuscitates someone in an unusual circumstance, it is still recommended to give credit to the EMS personnel for the save. They will look good and, in turn, will appreciate you for your generosity. But also, in the long run, the medical director of an admired service looks good because of the reputation of his or her EMS personnel.

Likewise, if the EMS personnel save a young boy awaiting a heart transplant who suddenly goes into ventricular fibrillation, they should make sure to state that "all of the credit needs to go to the dad who did CPR" even if the dad wasn't doing the greatest CPR. It not only shows sensitivity, but it also tells the public that CPR is important. It is already clear that the paramedics had to have done some of the lifesaving. Therefore, saying "we were just doing our job and wouldn't have been able to do anything without the dad's actions" portrays humility and professionalism—it makes the EMS persons look like they've "been there before."

Conversely, when bad things happen, the "buck stops here" approach is just as appropriate. The leadership should say, "This is my responsibility and I will be handling it." Even though people understand that the "boss" was not directly responsible for the unfortunate incident, a medical director or EMS chief who portrays a great sense of responsibility for the incident helps to inspire public confidence that the problem is being taken very seriously and being dealt with accordingly.

Rule #6: Provide A Good "Hook" and Suggest A Simple Valuable Lesson

What catches the public's attention is a simple "take-home" point or something that gains their sympathy. A good approach is to use willing persons as examples, such as the person who survived because of CPR or the trauma victim who is now fully rehabilitated. Kids and animals, either as subjects, or as adjuncts to the story always work well. Establishing re-

MEDIA

lations with interesting survivors is important to do proactively. Many patients are extremely grateful or already innately willing to help with public health initiatives. However, the key word here is "willing." Referring the media directly to patients or former patients is inappropriate and, in addition, care must be taken to not take advantage of the "doctor-patient" relationship and place patients in uncomfortable positions, either through overt solicitation or their own internal perceptions of pressure ("I guess I owe it to my lifesavers, even if I don't feel like doing this"). Many times, this is a good situation for involvement of the PIO for the EMS system or applicable receiving hospital. They can be of great assistance and provide a buffer for the doctor-patient relationship.

With or without attractive, willing subjects, however, it is still important to make a simple "take-home" lesson regarding the situation being discussed. For example, in a school bus crash involving another vehicle (in which an automobile driver is killed outright), one might want to catalog the number and age of school bus children injured (i.e., "twenty-four 2nd, 3rd, and 4th graders"), the types of injuries (various minor injuries) and where the children are being taken (five different area hospitals). However, an important "hook" is to recognize that, although the crash was bad enough to kill the driver of the car outright, an infant in the child safety seat in the back passenger area of the car was still totally intact. If possible, one might even do the interview at the scene with the child's car seat in the background or nearby, and talk about the child surviving.

Likewise, in a heat wave, one can provide a textbook account of heat exhaustion, heat stroke, and other esoteric "doctor" information. However, it is much better that a simple, valuable lesson be prioritized for the limited sound bite time. Therefore, it is prudent to focus on "take-home" tips to prevent heat illness.

Nevertheless, while preparing for the interview, one can provide some relevant background information to the reporter, emphasizing that prevention and treatment of dehydration are the key issues. One can also state preliminarily that, classically, the very young and the very old are considered to be the most susceptible to heat illness because of their inability to sense a problem with heat or to fend for themselves (getting out of the heat or getting fluids). However, it is then important to note that a large number of the serious heat illness cases (in fact, the majority in some communities) involve the "weekend warriors," young healthy adults who work in super-cooled environments all week who then suddenly exert themselves out in the environment on a weekend day (e.g., playing tennis, jogging, doing yardwork, working in the attic).

Again such preliminary background statements are probably relevant to setting the stage for the interview, but, most importantly, one should be focused on providing useful recommendations in the actual interview itself. As mentioned previously, in the example of heat illness, a few quick prevention tips can be provided in "bullets": *first*, wear the three L's of "light-weight, light-colored, and loose-fitting" clothing (most body heat is eliminated around the head and neck, in particular); *second*, stay in well ventilated areas, even if indoors (for example, it is very typical for those working in poorly ventilated attic areas to get heat illness); *third*, drink lots of water (enough to keep you going to the bathroom if possible); *fourth*, avoid alcohol (because it can dehydrate you further and inhibit your ability to sense a problem with the heat); and *fifth*, use a "buddy system" when you plan to exert yourself or be out in the heat for a period of time (the first symptom can be wooziness or frank disorientation, and having someone else there can help).

Rule #7: Give Them Simple Statistics and Graphics

The "take-home" points are easier to take home if one uses simple statistics and graphics. For example, in the heat illness prevention interview, one could supply the media personnel with ready-to-run, short, bulleted graphics (displayed sequentially, as in a computerized slide presentation) to accompany your narrated tips:

- Light-Weight, Light-Colored, Loose-Fitting Clothing
- Stay in Well-Ventilated Areas
- Water, Water, Water
- Avoid Alcohol
- Use the Buddy System

Actually, this list is relatively long. Generally, three lines of graphics is the preferred length, but the use of fewer words (with capitalized first letters) allows for faster reading of the information. The idea here is that your sound bite will match this graphic and that it will be shown simultaneously with your interview. This works especially well in a live interview because it gives them some structure and helps you to control the focus of the interview. Therefore, providing such bullets by e-mail or fax can be very useful.

In other situations, it is *how* you say things that can capture attention. Saying that "there were 25 million EMS incidents in the U.S. last year" may be less effective than saying, "every other second, there is a call for EMS across the United States." A stroke "every 50 seconds" may be more powerful than "600,000 a year." Simply said, "The simpler the statistics, the stronger the impact." Also, showing simple graphics such as a bar graph with progressively increasing sizes over time can say more than a sound bite (clearly, a picture is worth a thousand words).

It is key to remember that such graphics may only be shown for 5 to 7 seconds (or less). Experience has shown that it takes at least 3 to 4 seconds for a person to recognize and cognitively appreciate an image. At the same time, that image may fatigue within a few seconds more, so the timing of the duration of the graphics and images need to be compatible with that type of schema. Likewise, in graphic computer presentations, similar considerations must be kept in mind. Instead of showing all of the slide elements at once, each line should be introduced in sequential order, one at a time, in short order.

Rule #8: Stay on the Mark and Remember the Three R's of Repetition, Redundancy, and Reiteration

After all is said and done, it is up to the EMS physician to get a finite distilled piece of information across to the public. As discussed before, if the point is to get everyone to learn CPR and the interview gets off the mark onto the "hazards of mouth-to-mouth," it is the job of the interviewee to get back on track and remain focused on the point to be made. Even as an interview setting goes along, it is not inappropriate to repeat and reiterate the same point, particularly if it is not a live interview. In a live interview, repetition is a little annoying, but in the majority of other situations (such as a taped interview session with a reporter from which a sound bite will be extracted), reiteration is actually encouraged because it may come out better on a second or third try and it will continue to reinforce your main point.

Likewise, if one is saying to the reporter that the glass is half-full and the reporter comes back and asks if that means that the glass is half-empty, the EMS physician must stay on the mark and not relent. If necessary, he or she must be repetitive and stay on the mark.

Rule #9: Don't Trust Anyone and There Is No Such Thing as "Off the Record"

EMS physicians (or anyone for that matter) should assume that anything that comes out of their mouth or is transmitted on their e-mail, be it stated confidentially or not, will appear in print tomorrow. That caution does not apply only to conversations with media personnel. EMS physicians should recognize that their own employees, colleagues, supervisors, or supervisees may covertly tape-record personal conversations or understand that any joke, including those thought to be told in the privacy of a phone call or e-mail, is subject to dissemination. Even the act of confidentially disclosing something in one's own home may at times place a loved one in a position to inadvertently express sentiments or information that needed to be kept discreet. As a public servant, the EMS physician should maintain a public trust and he or she should always assume that any verbal or written statement, made under any circumstance, could become public record.

Therefore, one should not ask to be "off the record" unless the interviewee wishes to test the reporter's discretion. The term "off-the-record" (OTR) is a flag. One should always question what OTR means. Some reporters mean that they will not repeat the information at all, while others mean that they can use the information without saying the source. Oftentimes the EMS physician can disclose something OTR and find that the OTR statements are still broadcast or printed using statements like, "However, certain officials within the EMS section still tell Channel 9 that. . . ." Therefore, it is best not to provide OTR information and those wishing to maintain absolute discretion should not trust anyone.

Rule #10: Anticipate the Worst and Expect the Mediocre

Oftentimes, rookie reporters, full of enthusiasm, are sent out to quickly get an interview about a subject with which they are completely unfamiliar. Particularly when one must discuss a complicated subject that the EMS physician has studied for years (e.g., tiered deployment systems or waiver of informed consent to study participation), it becomes difficult to reduce it all to a sound bite, or an accurate print statement. As hard as they may try to understand, the reporter may not be able to grasp, let alone accurately distill, a relatively abstract and multi-faceted concept in a short period of time.

More concerning sometimes is the fact that, even if the interview goes well, the audience may not get the message, or at least retain the specific message. One should be prepared for statements like, "Hey, saw you on channel 11 last night (when you were actually on channel 8)—you looked really good." But when asking "Oh good—which one was that—what was it about?" one should not be surprised when the reply is, "I can't remember—it was about some emergency thing—but you looked good!" At least, in this case, the viewer got the "good" vibe. Sometimes, it can also be "I guess there was some kind of problem."

Another problem is the print story headline or the electronic media "lead-in" (the news anchor's introduction of the story) or "break tease" ("When we come back . . ."). These "headlines" set up the upcoming story. Even if the reporter fully grasps the concepts and writes a wonderful piece, the headline, written by an editor who wants to catch the reader's eye or simply "didn't get it," may say something that is perceptibly negative. Take, for example, a story written to say that despite a great group of well trained EMS personnel, the EMS system survival rates are low because bystanders are infrequently performing CPR. The point of the story, of course, was to encourage bystander CPR, but still the editor might write "Paramedic Survival Rate Low" for the headline. Naturally, this will give the wrong impression despite a wonderful text below. Likewise, for a break tease, the anchor may state, "When we come back from our break—a new program to save lives may itself need resuscitation." In this case, a negative impression may be made despite an ensuing balanced story by the reporter.

Therefore, one should anticipate the worst of an interview, and, at best, expect the mediocre in terms of its ultimate effectiveness. In turn, one should not take it personally when the broadcast or printed output falls short of the mark. EMS physicians cannot always get their expert knowledge across in a matter of minutes and, at best, a mediocre representation of their key points may occur. On the other hand, some-times the point does get across, especially if the speaker is given the chance to come back and speak again. Therefore, this realization makes it more incumbent upon the EMS physician to become a responsive, familiar, helpful resource and to become extremely adept at preparing and producing those sound bites and printed bullets for the various potential subjects about which he or she will be asked to speak.

Summary

EMS and trauma systems are in the public domain. Even if the EMS is managed by a private ambulance service or the trauma center is a private hospital, they both come under public scrutiny (be it media or public officials). EMS and trauma care are part of a public trust largely because, whoever the patient is, access to 9-1-1 and trauma care are considered to be the same. EMS is an expected public service, and often tax dollars or governmental subsidy are a large part of the operation. In turn, the EMS physician must be prepared to deal with that public trust when it comes under question.

In addition, by virtue of the very nature of the business, the circumstances involving emergencies can be very volatile and emotional for families and patients alike. Furthermore, EMS is in the fishbowl. Most EMS activities occur in the public domain in situations accessible to cameras, microphones, and public observation. Even the emergency department and its ambulance bay may be the part of the hospital most easily viewed by and adjacent to the outside world. The EMS physician must therefore recognize that media interactions are very likely at one time or another (if not daily in some venues).

Also, when the killer heat wave comes to town or the "flu" is filling up ambulances and emergency departments, the EMS physician may be the person who can best address the media questions. Knowing about drownings, skating injuries, hypothermia, choking, strokes, graduated driver licensing, gunshots, bioterrorism, food poisoning, and a myriad of other topics must all be part of the EMS physician's repertoire.

Some may consider the media "friend"; some "foe." In fact, for the EMS physician, use of the mass media can be a powerful tool for effecting mass public education (i.e., regarding CPR, injury prevention, etc). Public speaking through the media can also have a major societal impact, if not a life-saving effect, in major disaster incidents such as in a possible bioterrorism event. Therefore, becoming an effective and trusted public communicator is an important aspect of the job for an EMS physician.

Again, the recommendations made in this chapter do not in themselves guarantee effectiveness. It takes experience and lots of it. Like an advance cardiac life support (ACLS) algorithm, the ten axioms provided in this discussion establish a working guideline for success based on the experience of others. Just as the clinician needs to practice the ACLS algorithm over and over again, the public speaker needs to practice public speaking repeatedly, using the axioms outlined here. Individual EMS physicians may also want to explore and research their own styles of public speaking, based on their own experiences. Regardless of the pathway taken, the EMS physician must follow the general principles of truthfulness, accessibility, reliability, and down-to-earth focused statements as outlined in this chapter.

While making oneself always available to the media or public officials can be painstaking and even very uncomfortable when it involves a problem, the payoff is worth it. Being an effective public communicator is not only good for the public's health and for advocacy for the EMS system, but it is also a large component of leadership. The EMS physician who always puts patient care first, and who can articulate it responsibly and cogently, will have achievements and will become widely recognized as a knowledgeable public advocate. Particularly when one needs to be persuasive in terms of gaining more resources for the EMS system, effective communication is essential. As the ever-wise Obi-Wan Kenobi of EMS, Dr. Norman Dinerman, always reminds us: "Be the source and become the force." As outlined in this discussion: Be a patient advocate, be a front of information, be a public communicator—be worthy of public trust.

Appendix

National EMS Related Associations and Federal Agencies

Air Medical Physician Association (AMPA)

383 F Street
Salt Lake City, UT 84103
Phone: 801-408-3699
Fax: 801-408-1668
www.ampa.org

AMPA Mission Statement

The Air Medical Physician Association is a unique association comprised of physicians and professionals involved in medical transport who are committed to promoting safe and efficacious patient transportation through quality medical direction, research, education, leadership, and collaboration.

Air and Surface Transport Nurses Association (ASTNA)

9101 E. Kenyon Avenue, Suite 3000
Denver, CO 80237
Phone: 800-897-NFNA (6362)
Fax: 303-770-1812
www.astna.org

ASTNA Mission Statement

The Air and Surface Transport Nurses Association (also known as National Flight Nurses Association) is a nonprofit member organization whose mission is to represent, promote, and provide guidance to professional nurses who practice the unique and distinct specialty of transport nursing.

American Association of Poison Control Centers (AAPCC)

3201 New Mexico Avenue, Suite 310
Washington, DC 20016
AAPCC does not manage poison exposure cases.
Phone: 202-362-7217
For poisoning emergencies, call 1-800-222-1222.
www.aapcc.org

AAPCC Mission Statement

The American Association of Poison Control Centers (AAPCC) is a nationwide organization of poison centers and interested individuals. It provides a forum for poison centers and interested individuals to promote the reduction of morbidity and mortality from poisonings through public and professional education and scientific research. It also sets voluntary standards for poison center operations.

American Ambulance Association (AAA)

1255 Twenty-Third Street, NW, Suite 200
Washington, DC 20037-1174
Phone: 202-452-8888
Fax: 202-452-0005
www.the-aaa.org

AAA Mission Statement

The American Ambulance Association promotes health care policies that ensure excellence in the ambulance services industry and provides research, education, and communications programs to enable members to effectively address the needs of the communities they serve.

American College of Emergency Physicians (ACEP)

ACEP maintains offices in both Dallas, Texas and Washington, DC.

National Headquarters:
1125 Executive Circle
Irving, TX 75038-2522
Phone: 800-798-1822
Fax: 972-580-2816
P.O. Box 619911
Dallas, TX 75261-9911

DC Office:
2121 K Street, NW, Suite 325
Washington, DC 20037
Phone: 800-320-0610 or 202-728-0610
Fax: 202-728-0617
www.acep.org

ACEP Mission Statement

The American College of Emergency Physicians (ACEP) exists to support quality emergency medical care, and to promote the interests of emergency physicians.

American College of Osteopathic Emergency Physicians (ACOEP)

142 E. Ontario Street, Suite 550
Chicago, IL 60611
Phone: 312-587-3709; 800-521-3709
Fax: 312-587-9951
www.acoep.org

ACOEP Mission Statement

The ACOEP exists to support quality emergency medical care, promote interests of osteopathic emergency physicians, support development and implementation of osteopathic emergency medical education, and advance the philosophy and practice of osteopathic medicine through a system of quality and cost-effective healthcare in a distinct, unified profession.

American College of Surgeons (ACS) and the Committee on Trauma (ACS-COT)

633 N. Saint Clair St.
Chicago, IL 60611-3211
Phone: 312-202-5000
Fax: 312-202-5001
www.facs.org

ACS Mission Statement

The American College of Surgeons, as an association of surgeons, is dedicated to promoting the highest standards of surgical care through education of and advocacy for its Fellows and their patients. The College provides a cohesive voice addressing societal issues relating to surgery.

The American College of Surgeons supports programs and policies which ensure patients access to high-quality, effective care provided by appropriately prepared and well-qualified surgical specialists of their choosing. Such care is to be delivered in a system that provides maximum safe-guards for patient safety. Since 1913, the American College of Surgeons has initiated programs that have protected patients both in and out of the hospital. The American College of Surgeons will work with interested and qualified parties to provide patients with the maximum safety in a system that puts patient welfare first.

ACS-COT Mission Statement

Through its Committee on Trauma, works to improve the care of injured and critically ill patients—before, en route to, and during hospitalization. Conducts training courses in emergency care for ambulance personnel; sponsors courses for the management and prevention of injuries for trauma specialists as well as for physicians who do not treat trauma victims on a regular basis; and works to encourage hospitals to upgrade their trauma care capabilities. Maintains a voluntary verification/consultation program for trauma centers.

Objectives: To improve all phases of the management of the injured patient including prehospital care and transportation, hospital care, and rehabilitation; to prevent injuries in the home, in industry, on the highway, and during participation in sports; to establish and implement institutional and systems standards for care of the injured; to provide education to improve trauma care; and to cooperate with other national organizations with similar objectives.

American Heart Association (AHA) and the Emergency Cardiovascular Care Committee (ECC)

American Heart Association National Center
7272 Greenville Avenue
Dallas, TX 75231-4596
Phone: AHA: 1-800-AHA-USA-1 or 1-800-242-8721
ASA: 1-888-4-STROKE or 1-888-478-7653
www.americanheart.org

AHA Mission Statement

The American Heart Association is a national voluntary health agency whose mission is to reduce disability and death from cardiovascular diseases and stroke.

www.cpr-ecc.org

AHA-ECC Mission Statement

The National ECC Committee is composed of volunteers with expertise in science, education, business, and administration. Through its four subcommittees—Basic Life Support (BLS), Advanced Cardiovascular Life Support (ACLS), Pediatric Resuscitation (PEDS), and Program Administration (PROAD)—the National ECC Committee prepares scientific and educational guidelines for emergency cardiovascular care. These include the Guidelines 2000 for Cardiopulmonary Resuscitation and Emergency Cardiovascular Care: International Consensus on Science (Guidelines 2000). The ECC guidelines are updated after each ECC guidelines conference and used in developing the courses (BLS, ACLS, and PALS) offered through the AHA ECC Training Network and those of many other national and international organizations.

American Medical Association (AMA)

515 N. State Street
Chicago, IL 60610
Phone: 312-464-5000
www.ama-assn.org

AMA Mission Statement

To promote the science and art of medicine and the betterment of public health.

American Public Health Association (APHA)

800 K Street, NW
Washington, DC 20001-3710
Phone: 202-777-APHA (2742)
Fax: 202-777-2532
www.apha.org

APHA Mission Statement

APHA is an association of individuals and organizations working to improve the public's health and to achieve equity in health status for all. It promotes the scientific and professional foundation of public health practice and policy, advocates the conditions for a healthy global society, emphasize prevention and enhances the ability of members to promote and protect environmental and community health.

American National Red Cross (ARC)

430 17th St., NW
Washington, DC 20006
Phone: 202-639-3685
Fax: 202-434-4886
www.redcross.org

ARC Mission Statement

The mission of the American Red Cross is to provide relief to victims of disasters and help people prevent, prepare for, and respond to emergencies.

American Society for Standards and Testing (ASTM)—F30 EMS Committee

100 Barr Harbor Drive
West Conshohocken, PA 19428-2959
Phone: 610-832-9585
Fax: 610-832-9555
www.astm.org. (go to F30 committee)

ASTM Mission Statement

To be the foremost developer and provider of voluntary consensus standards, related technical information, and services having internationally recognized quality and applicability that promote public health and safety, and the overall quality of life; contribute to the reliability of materials, products, systems and services; and facilitate national, regional, and international commerce.

Committee F30 on Emergency Medical Services
Staff Manager: Scott Orthey, 610-832-9730

F30 EMS Committee Overview

Committee F30 on Emergency Medical Services was formed in 1984. F30 meets twice a year, in May and October, to develop and update documents relevant for quality emergency medical service. The committee, with current membership of approximately 99, currently has jurisdiction over 50 standards, published in the Annual Book of ASTM Standards, Volume 13.01.

Association of Public Communications Officials (APCO) International

World Headquarters
351 N. Williamson Blvd.
Daytona Beach, FL 32114-1112
Phone: 386-322-2500; 888-APCO-911;
  888-272-6911
Fax: 386-322-2501
www.apco911.org

APCO International Mission Statement

Foster the development and progress of the art of public safety communications by means of research, planning, training and education;

Promote cooperation between towns, cities, counties, states, and federal public safety agencies in the area of communications;

Represent its members before communications regulatory agencies and policy-making bodies as may be appropriate; and

Through its efforts strive toward the end that the safety of human life, the protection of property and the civic welfare are benefited to the utmost degree; and

Aid and assist in the rapid and accurate collection, exchange and dissemination of information relating to emergencies and other vital public safety functions.

Association of Air Medical Services (AAMS)

110 North Royal Street, Suite 307
Alexandria, VA 22314-3234
Phone: 703-836-8732
Fax: 703-836-8920
www.aams.org

AAMS Mission Statement

AAMS is dedicated to promoting, supporting and representing transport medicine through: Education & Information, Advocacy, Standard Setting and Member Services.

Centers for Disease Control and Prevention (CDC)

1600 Clifton Road
Atlanta, GA 30333
Phone: 404-639-3311
Public Inquiries: 404-639-3534; 800-311-3435
www.cdc.gov

CDC Mission Statement

To promote health and quality of life by preventing and controlling disease, injury, and disability.

Continuing Education Coordinating Board for Emergency Medical Services (CECBEMS)

5111 Mill Run Road
Dallas, TX 75244
Phone: 972-387-2862
Fax: 972-716-2007
www.cecbems.org

CECBEMS Mission Statement

CECBEMS will serve as the recognized leader for continuing education in EMS, promoting its evolution and growth through development of continuing education standards, encouragement of innovative learning solutions, the support of continuous learning opportunities and the assurance of optimal learning experiences to better prepare all EMS providers for their professional challenges.

Citizen CPR Foundation

PO Box 911
Carmel, IN 46082
Phone: 317-843-1940
Fax: 317-843-1831
www.citizencpr.org

Citizen CPR Foundation Mission Statement

The mission of the Foundation is "to strengthen the Chain of Survival." The Foundation has three primary co-sponsors: the American Heart Association, the American Red Cross and the Heart and Stroke Foundation of Canada. The primary "products" of the Foundation are its biennial conference, now called the "Emergency Cardiac Care Update," and the quarterly newsletter, Currents in Emergency Cardiovascular Care.

Commission on the Accreditation of Ambulance Services (CAAS)

1926 Waukegan Road, Suite 1
Glenview, IL 60025-1770
Phone: 847-657-6828
Fax: 847-657-6819
www.caas.org

CAAS Mission Statement

The Commission on Accreditation of Ambulance Services was established to encourage and promote quality patient care in America's medical transportation system. Based initially on the efforts of the American Ambulance Association, the independent Commission established a comprehensive series of standards for the ambulance service industry.

Commission on Accreditation for EMS Professions (CoAEMSP)

1248 Harwood Road
Bedford, TX 76021-4244
Phone: 817-283-9403
Fax: 817-354-8519
www.coaemsp.org

CoAEMSP Mission Statement

The CoAEMSP currently provides accreditation services for paramedic programs. Its primary goal is to foster a partnership with educational programs in continuous quality improvement. The secondary goal is to certify that a program meets the standards of quality that are approved by its sponsoring organizations.

Commission on the Accreditation of Medical Transport Services (CAMTS)

PO Box 1305
Anderson, SC 29622
Phone: 864-287-4177
Fax: 864-287-4251
www.camts.org

CAMTS Mission Statement

Professionals involved with air medical services and ground interfacility transport services strive to provide the highest possible quality to their constituents.

The Commission on Accreditation of Medical Transport Systems is dedicated to assisting these professionals in offering a quality service. The Commission offers a program of voluntary evaluation of compliance with accreditation standards which demonstrates the ability to deliver service of a specific quality.

The Commission believes that the two highest priorities of an air medical or ground interfacility transport service are patient care and safety of the transport environment.

By participating in the voluntary accreditation process, services can verify their adherence to quality accreditation standards to themselves, their peers, medical professionals, and to the general public. Professionals involved with air medical services and ground interfacility transport services strive to provide the highest possible quality to their constituents. The Commission on Accreditation of Medical Transport Systems (CAMTS) is dedicated to assisting these professionals in offering a quality service. The Commission offers a program of voluntary evaluation of compliance with accreditation standards which demonstrates the ability to deliver service of a specific quality. The commission believes that the two highest priorities of an air medical or ground interfacility transport service are patient care and safety of the transport environment. By participating in the voluntary accreditation process, services can verify their adherence to quality accreditation standards to themselves, their peers, medical professionals and to the general public.

Congressional Fire Service Institute (CFSI)

900 Second Street, NE, Suite 303
Washington, DC 20002
Phone: 202-371-1277
Fax: 202-682-FIRE (3473)
www.cfsi.org

CFSI Mission Statement

To educate members of Congress on issues that make a difference for the emergency services. As a policy institute, CFSI's mission is in educating and forming partnerships. Throughout the year, it conducts a number of educational programs for Congress to sensitize them to the fire service. It offers basic firefighter training programs, fire extinguisher training programs, and special briefings. It prepares briefing papers on specific fire-related topics. It also provides certificates of recognition that members of Congress can present to fire and EMS personnel in their respective Congressional districts for length of service, valor and other achievements.

Emergency Nurses Association (ENA)

915 Lee Street
Des Plaines, IL 60016-6569
Phone: 800-900-9659
Fax: 847-460-4003
www.ena.org

Emergency Nurses Association Mission Statement

To provide visionary leadership for emergency nursing and emergency care.

Emergency Medical Services for Children (EMSC) & EMSC National Resource Center (EMSCNRC)

111 Michigan Avenue, NW
Washington, DC 20010-2970
Phone: 202-884-4927
Fax: 202-884-6845
www.ems-c.org

EMSC Mission Statement

EMSC is a national initiative designed to reduce child and youth disability and death due to severe illness or injury. Its goals are to ensure that state-of-the-art emergency medical care is available for all ill or injured children and adolescents; that pediatric services are well integrated into an emergency medical services (EMS) system; and that the entire spectrum of emergency services, including primary prevention of illness and injury, acute care, and rehabilitation, are provided to children and adolescents. A federal grant program supports state and local action.

The EMSC Program supports two resource centers—the EMSC National Resource Center (NRC), located in Washington, DC, and the National EMSC Data Analysis Resource Center (NEDARC), located in Salt Lake City, UT. NRC provides support and assistance to states on a variety of topics, operates a clearinghouse, and provides information to professionals and the public. NEDARC specializes in providing assistance on data collection and analysis. The EMSC web site provides additional information: www.ems-c.org

EMSC is primarily supported and is jointly administered by the Maternal and Child Health Bureau of the U.S. Department of Health and Human Services' Health Resources and Services Administration (http://www.mchb.hrsa.gov or www.dhhs.gov) and the U.S. Department of Transportation's National Highway Traffic Safety Administration (www.nhtsa.gov).

Federal Emergency Management Agency (FEMA)

500 C Street SW
Washington, DC 20472

FEMA's National Emergency Training Center
16825 South Seton Avenue
Emmitsburg, MD 21727
Phone: 800-238-3358
www.fema.gov

FEMA Mission Statement

To reduce loss of life and property and protect our nation's critical infrastructure from all types of hazards through a comprehensive, risk-based, emergency management program of mitigation, preparedness, response and recovery. FEMA is an independent agency of the federal government with offices in Washington, DC; Emmitsburg , MD; and with regional offices in 10 states.

HHS-USPHS-Office of Emergency Preparedness (OEP)

National Disaster Medical System
12300 Twinbrook Parkway, Suite 360
Rockville, MD 20857
Phone: 301-443-1167 or 800-USA-NDMS
Fax: 301-443-5146 or 800-USA-KWIK
In addition to its main office in Rockville, MD, OEP has Regional Emergency Coordinators located in the ten Federal regions. To contact an Emergency Coordinator located in your region, please click on the appropriate section of the map in the Contacts section of the website.
www.oep-ndme.dhhs.gov

OEP Mission Statement

OEP is an office within the U.S. Department of Health and Human Services and has the Departmental responsibility for managing and coordinating Federal health, medical, and health related social services and recovery to major emergencies and Federally declared disasters including:

Natural Disasters
Technological Disasters
Major Transportation Accidents
Terrorism

Working in partnership with the Federal Emergency Management Agency (FEMA) and the Federal interagency community, OEP serves as the lead Federal agency for health and medical services within the Federal Response Plan. OEP also directs and manages the National Disaster Medical System (NDMS) a cooperative asset-sharing partnership between HHS, the Department of Defense (DoD), the Department of Veterans Affairs (VA), FEMA, state and local governments, private businesses and civilian volunteers. OEP is also responsible for Federal health and medical response to terrorist acts involving Weapons of Mass Destruction (WMD).

International Association of Fire Fighters (IAFF)

1750 New York Avenue, NW
Washington, DC 20006-5395
Phone: 202-824-1588 (Dept. of Public Relations
 & Publications)
Fax: 202-737-8418
www.iaff.org

IAFF Mission Statement

The International Association of Fire Fighters is an AFL-CIO affiliated labor union representing more than 240,000 professional fire fighters and emergency medical personnel in the United States and Canada. IAFF members protect more than 85 percent of the lives and property and are the largest providers of prehospital emergency medical care in the U.S.

International Association of Fire Chiefs (IAFC)

4025 Fair Ridge Dr., Suite 300
Fairfax, VA 22033-2868
Phone: 703-273-0911
Fax: 703-273-9363
www.iafc.org

IAFC Mission Statement

To provide leadership to career and volunteer chiefs, chief fire officers and managers of emergency service organizations throughout the international community through vision, information, education, services and representation to enhance their professionalism and capabilities.

International Rescue and Emergency Care Association (IRECA)

PO Box 13527
Charleston, SC 29422-3527
Phone: 800-221-3435
www.ireca.org

IRECA Mission Statement

The International Rescue and Emergency Care Association's mission is to be the preeminent provider of technical and specialized rescue and emergency medical services education and training, with the incorporation of shared ideas and experience by our collective global rescue and emergency medical services community.

National Academies of Emergency Dispatch (NAED)

139 East South Temple, Suite 530
Salt Lake City, UT 84111
Phone: 800-960-6236 (USA); 801-359-0996 (Int'l.)
www.naemd.org

NAEMD Mission Statement

To advance and support the Emergency Dispatch professional; to ensure citizens in need of emergency, health and social services are matched safely, quickly and effectively with the most appropriate resource.

National Association for Search and Rescue (NASAR)

4500 Southgate Place, Suite 100
Chantilly, VA 20151-1714
Phone: 703-222-6277
Fax: 703-222-6283
www.nasar.org

NASAR Mission Statement

The National Association for Search and Rescue is a self-supporting, nonprofit association whose primary goal is to aid in the implementation of a total integrated emergency response, rescue and recovery system.

National Association of Air Medical Communication Specialists (NAACS)

P.O. Box 3804
Cary, NC 27519-3804
Phone: 1-877-396-2227
www.naacs.org

NAACS Mission Statement

The National Association of Air Medical Communication Specialists is a not-for-profit professional organization whose mission is to represent the air medical communication specialist on a national level through education, standardization and recognition.

National Association of Emergency Medical Technicians (NAEMT)

408 Monroe Street
Clinton, MS 39056-4210
Phone: 800-34-NAEMT; 601-924-7744
Fax: 601-924-7325
www.naemt.org

NAEMT Mission Statement

The mission of the National Association of Emergency Medical Technicians, Inc. is to assure a professional representative organization to receive and represent the views and opinions of prehospital care personnel and to thus influence the future advancement of EMS as an allied health profession. NAEMT will serve its professional membership through educational programs, liaison activities, development of national standards and reciprocity and the development of programs to benefit prehospital care personnel.

National Association of EMS Educators (NAEMSE)

700 North Bell Avenue, Suite 260
Carnegie, PA 15106
Phone: 412-429-9550
Fax: 412-429-9554
www.naemse.org

NAEMSE Mission Statement

The mission of the National Association of EMS Educators is to promote EMS education, develop and deliver educational resources, and advocate research and life-long learning.

National Association of EMS Physicians (NAEMSP)

PO Box 15945-281
Lenexa, KS 66285-5945
Phone: 913-492-5858; 800-228-3677
Fax: 913-541-0156
www.naemsp.org

NAEMSP Mission Statement

The National Association of EMS Physicians is an organization of physicians and other professionals who provide leadership and foster excellence in out-of-hospital emergency medical services.

National Association of EMS Quality Professionals (NAEMSQP)

Project Manager, Southeastern Regional Trauma
  and Emergency Network
New Hanover Regional Medical Center
2131 N. 17th Street
Wilmington, NC 28401
Voice: 910-343-2599
www.naemsqp.org

NAEMSQP Mission Statement

To promote quality improvement in Emergency Medical Services.

National Association of State EMS Directors (NASEMSD)

111 Park Place
Falls Church, VA 22046-4513
Phone: 703-538-1799
Fax: 703-241-5603
www.nasemsd.org

NASEMSD Mission Statement

The National Association of State EMS Directors supports its members in providing vision and leadership in the development and improvement of EMS systems and national EMS policy.

National Collegiate EMS Foundation (NCEMSF)

NCEMSF
210 River Vale Road Apt#3
River Vale, NJ 07675-6281
Tel: 208-728-7342
Fax: 208-728-7352
www.ncemsf.org

NCEMSF Mission Statement

The National Collegiate Emergency Medical Services Foundation's (NCEMSF) purpose is to support, promote, and advocate Emergency Medical Services (EMS) on college and university campuses. The Foundation is committed to the advancement of existing response groups and assisting in the development of new response groups. The Foundation provides a forum for the exchange of ideas of campus-based emergency response issues. To these ends, the Foundation is committed to scholarship, research and consultancy activities and to creating a safer environment on college and university campuses.

National Council of State EMS Training Coordinators (NCSEMSTC)

111 Park Place
Falls Church, VA 22046-0587
Phone: 703-538-1794
Fax: 703-241-5603
www.ncsemstc.org

NCSEMSTC Mission Statement

The purpose of the Council shall be to promote the training of Emergency Medical Services personnel based on sound educational principles, current medical knowledge and practice. The Council will seek the standardization of nationwide training curricula; certification/recertification policies and procedures; the reciprocity of certification from state to state; and the public recognition and trust of prehospital EMS personnel health care providers.

National Emergency Number Association (NENA)

Dept. 911
PO Box 182039
Columbus, OH 43218
Phone: 614-741-2080; 800-332-3911 (toll free)
Fax: 614-933-0911
www.nena.org

NENA Mission Statement

NENA's mission is to foster the technological advancement, availability, and implementation of a universal emergency telephone number system. In carrying out its mission, NENA promotes research, planning, training and education. The protection of human life, the preservation of property and the maintenance of general community security are among NENA's objectives.

National Emergency Medical Services for Children (EMSC) Data and Analysis Resource Center (NEDARC)

615 Arapeen Drive, Suite 202
Salt Lake City, UT 84108-1226
Phone: 801-581-6410
Fax: 801-581-8686
www.nedarc.org

NEDARC Mission Statement

To help Emergency Medical Services (EMS) agencies and Emergency Medical Services for Children (EMSC) projects develop their own capabilities to formulate and answer research questions and to effectively collect, analyze, and utilize EMS data.

National EMS Pilots Association (NEMSPA)

110 N. Royal Street, Suite 307
Alexandria, VA 22314
Phone: 703-836-8930
Fax: 703-836-8920
www.nemspa.org

NEMSPA Mission Statement

We the National EMS Pilots Association will help the air medical industry prosper safely and will enhance the delivery of health care. We will provide the leadership necessary to establish operation and safety standards, a forum for dissemination of knowledge and the guidance to formulate positive change in our profession.

National Fire Academy (NFA)

USFA
16825 S. Seton Ave.
Emmitsburg, MD 21727
Phone: 301-447-1000; 800-238-3358
www.usfa.fema.gov/nfa

NFA Mission Statement

Our mission is to reduce life and economic losses due to fire and related emergencies. The training and educational programs offered through the NFA help us achieve this mission. Through its courses and programs, the National Fire Academy works to enhance the ability of fire and emergency services and allied professionals to deal more effectively with fire and related emergencies.

National Fire Protection Association (NFPA)

1 Batterymarch Park
PO Box 9101
Quincy, MA 02269-9101
Phone: 617-770-3000
Fax: 617-770-0700
www.nfpa.org.

NFPA Mission Statement

The mission of NFPA (formerly the National Fire Protection Association) is to reduce the worldwide burden of fire and other hazards on the quality of life by developing and advocating scientifically based consensus codes and standards, research, training, and education.

National Highway Traffic Safety Administration—EMS Division (NHTSA)

400 7th St., SW
Washington, DC 20590
Phone: 888-DASH-2-DOT (888-327-4236);
    202-366-0123
www.nhtsa.org/people/injury/ems

NHTSA Mission Statement

What is the Mission of The Emergency Medical Services Division? The National Highway Traffic Safety Administration's (NHTSA) mission is to save lives, prevent injuries and reduce traffic-related health care and other economic costs. The goal of NHTSA's EMS Division is to develop/enhance comprehensive emergency medical service systems to care for the injured patients involved in motor vehicle crashes. We are proud of the fact that improving EMS systems for the highway crash patients has a positive effect on all patients.

National Native American Emergency Medical Services Association (NNAEMSA)

C/o Ak-Chin Fire Department
42507 W. Peters & Nalls Rd.
Maricopa, AZ 85239
Phone: 520-568-2258
Fax: 520-568-0023
www.heds.org/nnaemsa.htm

NNAEMSA Mission Statement

To support the efforts of all EMS, rescue, and public safety organizations who provide services on Native American and Alaska lands. It is clearly understood by the NNAEMSA that strong support of these agencies will result in significant improvements in the quality of patient care to all people within each EMS service district. The provision of the highest quality service to Native American and non-Native American people alike is the highest priority of the members and the officers of the National Native American Emergency Medical Services Association.

National Registry of EMTs (NREMT)

Rocco V. Morando Building
6610 Busch Blvd.
P.O. Box 29233
Columbus, OH 43229
Phone: 614-888-4484
Fax: 614-888-8920
www.nremt.org

NREMT Mission Statement

The National Registry of Emergency Medical Technicians (NREMT), registers emergency medical services providers from across the nation. The NREMT is a not-for-profit, non-governmental, free-standing agency led by a Board of Directors comprised of members from national Emergency Medical Services (EMS) organizations or with expertise in EMS systems.

National Safety Council (NSC)

1121 Spring Lake Drive
Itasca, IL 60143-3201
Phone: 630-285-1121
www.nsc.org

NSC Mission Statement

The National Safety Council, founded in 1913 and chartered by the United States Congress in 1953, is the nation's leading advocate for safety and health. Our mission is "to educate and influence society to adopt safety, health and environmental policies, practices and procedures that prevent and mitigate human suffering and economic losses arising from preventable causes."

National Volunteer Fire Council (NVFC)

1050 17th Street, NW, Suite 490
Washington, DC 20036
Phone: 202-887-5700 or 1-888-ASK-NVFC
Fax: 202-887-5291
www.nvfc.org

NVFC Mission Statement

The NVFC shall represent the volunteer fire and emergency medical services in national legislative, regulatory and standards making matters; Provide a national voice for the volunteer fire and EMS service; Promote the welfare of the volunteer fire and EMS service.

Society for Academic Emergency Medicine (SAEM)

901 N. Washington Avenue
Lansing, MI 48906-5137
Phone: 517-485-5484
Fax: 517-485-0801
www.naemt.org

SAEM Mission Statement

The Society for Academic Emergency Medicine's (SAEM) mission is to foster emergency medicine's academic environment in research, education, and health policy through forums, publications, inter-organizational collaboration, policy development, and consultation services for teachers, researchers, and students.

Society of Trauma Nurses (STN)

PMB 193
2743 S. Veterans Parkway
Springfield, IL 62704
Phone: 217-787-3281
Fax: 217-787-3285
www.traumanursesoc.org

STN Mission Statement

The Society of Trauma Nurses is a membership-based, non-profit organization whose members represent trauma nurses from around the world. STN is the sole sponsor of Advanced Trauma Care for Nurses, an educational course held in conjunction with ATLS, and the publisher of the Journal of Trauma Nursing. An annual one-day educational conference, Trauma Nursing: Critical Issues is held each March in Las Vegas preceding Trauma and Critical Care Conference.

State and Territorial Injury Prevention Directors Association (STIPDA)

2141 Kingston Court, Suite 110-B
Marietta, GA 30067
Phone: 770-690-9000
Fax: 770-690-8996
www.stipda.org

STIPDA Mission Statement

STIPDA's mission is to promote, sustain, and enhance the ability of state and territorial public health departments to reduce death and disability associated with injuries. STIPDA accomplishes its mission by disseminating information on state-of-the-art injury prevention and control policies and strategies.

Wilderness EMS Institute (WEMSI)

Center for Emergency Medicine of Western
   Pennsylvania
230 McKee Place, Suite 500
Pittsburgh, PA 15213-4904
Phone: 412-578-3203
www.wemsi.org

WEMSI Mission Statement

The Wilderness Emergency Medical Services Institute is a project of The Center for Emergency Medicine of Western Pennsylvania and The Appalachian Search and Rescue Conference.

WEMSI's mission is to improve medical care for people remote from the Emergency Medical Services system. It works for improved Wilderness EMS in three ways: teaching; research; and directly providing Wilderness EMS services.

World Association for Disaster and Emergency Medicine (WADEM)

1930 Monroe Street, Suite 304
Madison, WI 53711-2077
Phone: 608-263-2069
Fax: 608-265-3037
www.wadem.medicine.wisc.edu

WADEM Mission Statement

The World Association for Disaster and Emergency Medicine is an international, humanitarian association dedicated to the improvement of disaster and emergency medicine. Fostering international collaboration, the organization is inclusive, culturally sensitive, unbiased, ethical and dynamic in its approach. While individual members are active in field operations, the organization remains non-operational, fulfilling its mission through:

1. Facilitation of academic and research-based education and training;
2. Interpretation and exchange of information through its global network of members and publications;
3. Development and maintenance of evidence-based standards of emergency and disaster health care and provision of leadership concerning their integration into practice;
4. Coordination of data collection and provision of direction in the development of standardized disaster assessment and research and evaluation methodologies;
5. Encouraging publication and presentation of evidence-based research findings and scientific publication and international conferences and congresses.

Mark Henry, MD

Introduction

MS systems serve populations, one patient at a time. Preparing for that one patient involves many aspects of the public, all coming together in an effort to match medical resources and expertise with the patient's needs in time to make a difference.

The patient is the focus, central to any medical operation. Most of the time the patient doesn't call EMS; someone else does on his or her behalf. The principles of autonomy and informed consent are no less operative in the field than they are in the operating room, even though we seldom ask for formal written consent to proceed. Yet patients may be brought to the closest hospital, transferred, or transported directly to a specialty center, bypassing local hospitals, sometimes at considerable distance by air. Our patients' informed consent is founded entirely on their belief that our treatment and transport decisions are in their best interest and based on data or knowledge which justifies their trust.

At the scene, physicians, by their nature and oath, will want to help. Integrating their talent at times when they are needed, and declining their offers when they are not, is a skill that speaks to the maturity and grace of the medical director as well as the medics at the scene. The location of the emergency does not dictate one's ability to assess, treat, and be of help. Likewise, emergency medical technicians and paramedics can be of great value to patients within the hospital, but their knowledge and skill do not stop at the door. EMTs state certifications, state education license restrictions, and labor union protestations are balanced by hospital manpower needs and patient demands in this unsettled ground. Mutual respect for each other's role and ability is enhanced by engaging these issues in the public interest, rather than with personal rancor or self-interest.

Likewise, there are patient populations at the extremes of age with their own EMS agendas. Both pediatric and geriatric patients have champions who advocate that more attention and resources be focused on the young and old. Emergency medicine as a young medical specialty has never been defined by age. Ensuring that EMS meets the needs of all patients is a basic goal, advanced by paying attention to our colleagues who look closely at different patient populations. Indeed, while we decry inappropriate use of our service, unmet need remains, measured and perhaps best articulated by patient advocacy groups who remind us of the work still ahead.

Some treatment modalities used first or primarily in prehospital care have found widespread use; others have receded. Advances in technology and engineering led to AEDs, whose benefit was first tested and proven with EMTs and are now found in settings as diverse as hospitals and airports. Other prehospital treatments, such as PASG, once advocated with enthusiasm to elevate blood pressure, have seen limitation in their use as randomized trials questioned their benefit.

In the course of medical operations, the medical director of EMS has a unique viewpoint of the healthcare system, as the following chapters attest. Consent and refusal, balancing patient need with patient demand, matching patients with the right treatment, the right hospital, the right mix of people, all in *emergency* time, will test one's mettle. Amidst so many advocates, opportunity abounds; the sagacious medical director will gather support, forge alliances, and move ahead to advance the care of individual patients and the public's health.

Refusal of Medical Assistance

Larry Mottely, MD, MPA

Introduction

This chapter discusses the application of the informed consent process to a subset of emergency patients: those patients treated by EMS providers who are not yet physically at the hospital and therefore not yet evaluated by a physician. The role of the concept of "informed refusal" as an integral part of informed consent is discussed and applied. "Denial of aid" and "no transport" are briefly discussed, and "refusal of medical assistance" (RMA) is discussed at length. This theoretical discussion is translated into a policy statement addressing the issue of patient restraint, which has been the focus of increasing debate (Appendix A).

In 1982, The President's Commission for the Study of Ethical Problems in Medicine: *Making Health Care Decisions*, analyzed the topic of informed consent after Congress identified "concerns about the relationship between patients and healthcare providers." The Commission concluded that "shared decision making" would be the "ideal for patient-professional relationships that a sound doctrine of informed consent should support." It also indicated that the ideal would not be reached if primary reliance were placed on the courts; the concern with the legal system was related to "the likelihood that an expansion of the existing law could control ever more minutely the relationships of patients and healthcare professionals."[1] Table 44.1 summarizes the findings of the commission concerning shared decision making in informed consent.

Informed consent promotes and protects the medical autonomy of the individual in medical decision making. It allows for information exchanged between patient and provider to help the patient to make an educated decision about their medical options. The contemporary concept of autonomy has intellectual roots in 17th-century political philosophy and legal roots in even older English common law.[2]

TABLE 44.1
The President's Commission for the Study of Ethical Problems in Medicine and Biomedical Research findings and conclusions on the subject of shared decision making in informed consent included:

1. Although the informed consent doctrine has substantial foundations in the law, it is essentially an ethical imperative.
2. Ethically valid consent is a process of shared decision making based on mutual respect and participation, not a ritual to be equated with reciting the contents of a form that details the risks of particular treatments.
3. A universal desire for information, choice, and respectful communication about decisions—for all patients, in all healthcare settings.
4. Informed consent is based upon the principle that competent individuals are entitled to make healthcare decisions based upon their own personal goals. However, the choice is not absolute.
5. Healthcare providers should not ordinarily withhold unpleasant information simply because it is unpleasant.
6. Patients should have access to the information that they need to help them understand their conditions and make treatment decisions.
7. Improvements in the relationship between healthcare professionals and patients must not come primarily from the law but from changes in teaching, examination, and training of healthcare professionals.
8. Family members are often of great assistance to patients in helping them understand information about their condition and in making decisions about treatment. Their involvement should be encouraged to the extent compatible with respect for the privacy and autonomy of individual patients.
9. To protect the interest of patients who lack decision-making capacity, decisions made by others should, when possible, replicate those that patients would make if they were capable; when not feasible, the decisions of surrogates should protect the patient's best interests. |

In 1914, Supreme Court Justice Cardoza stated, "every human being of adult years and sound mind has a right to determine what shall be done with his own body."[3]

In 1960, the case of *Natanson v. Kline* established that physicians had an "obligation to disclose and explain in simple language" the risks and complications of a procedure.[4] This was further expanded in 1972 by *Cobbs v. Grant*, which ruled that the patient's right of self-decision is the measure of the physician's duty to reveal. "That right can be effectively exercised only if the patient possesses adequate information to enable an intelligent choice. The scope of the physician's communication to the patient, then, must be measured by the patient's need, and that need is whatever information is material to the decision."[5]

A dilemma arises when a patient is unable to make an informed decision and yet wishes to refuse medical treatment. When can EMS personnel transport a patient to the hospital against his will? How can providers minimize both their liability for assault and battery and their liability for abandonment and/or a wrongful death. In 1989, when confronted with this situation, "err on the side of over-treatment and assault and battery, as opposed to abandonment."[6] Today, that same legal reasoning may be fraught with much more potential liability.

In order to deal with this dilemma, it is essential to have medical oversight develop policies that provide guidance for providers as to how to deal with a patient who refuses treatment and/or transport to a medical facility see appendix B. Prehospital providers and physicians must have a clear understanding of the medical and legal issues involved with patients refusing treatment and/or transport to a medical facility. Training for EMS physicians and providers should include reasons "why patients refuse transport, the management of patients refusing transport including specific policies and procedures and interpersonal relationships with these patients, medicolegal implications of patients signing out against medical advice, and explanations as to the absolute necessity of complete and accurate documentation."[7]

Competency and capacity are terms that are often used synonymously in the handling of patients who refuse treatment, yet they have very different meanings. Competence is a legal test and can only be determined by a judge in the courtroom. Determining whether a patient is competent involves a three-step process that assesses whether a patient (a) can comprehend and retain relevant information, (b) believes the information, and (c) can weigh the information in the balance and arrive at a choice.[8]

The capacity of a patient, however, can be established by a medical provider in a hospital, in an ambulance, or on the street and is used as a presumptive determination of a patient's competence. "In an emergency, when a patient does not wish to cooperate with evaluation and there is substantial indirect evidence of the impairment of the patient's capacities (based on information from caregivers and relatives and on the patient's other behavior), it is appropriate to conclude that the patient would probably be found incompetent by a court."[9]

A determination of whether a patient possesses capacity is required before a patient can be allowed to sign a refusal of treatment form or be taken against their will to the hospital. Establishing capacity necessitates a conversation between the provider and patient. Ultimately, the question that must be answered by the provider is: Does the patient understand the nature of his medical condition and the potential consequences of refusing treatment and/or transport to a hospital? "The proper assessment of decision-making capacity involves the integration of multiple functions, including the absence of deficits in cognition, judgment, understanding, choice, expression of choice, and stability. . . . Each component is interrelated, interdependent, and necessary to understand the whole. Together, the six components are needed to understand the whole."[10]

It is essential to realize that the patient's decision-making ability or capacity is what actually must be scrutinized by the medical provider, not their ultimate decision. The patient must be able to make his own decision and understand the consequences of that decision. The patient is legally allowed to make what the medical provider would characterize as the "wrong" medical decision. Disagreement with the provider does not necessarily constitute a lack of capacity. The seemingly illogical choices of a patient must be respected even if the patient cannot be convinced to change their decision, if the patient possesses capacity.

In *Lane v. Candura*, an elderly patient who had developed gangrene of her lower leg refused to allow an amputation of her leg even after that recommendation by her attending physicians. The Court ruled that "the irrationality of her decision does not justify a conclusion that Mrs. Candura is incompetent in the legal sense. The law protects her right to make her own decision to accept or reject treatment, whether that decision is wise or unwise."[11]

Specific departmental policies should be followed, depending on whether or not a patient is considered to possess capacity (appendix B). Development of these policies should include input from a medical director, administrative staff, legal counsel, and local law enforcement, as well as members of the community. It is important to determine whether laws exist regarding the issue of refusal of treatment in the out-of-hospital setting and to recognize whether regulations or guidelines have been promulgated by state regulatory agencies.

In New Mexico, state law has existed since 1993 that allows emergency medical technicians who are acting in "good faith" and under medical oversight to transport to an appropriate medical facility a patient who is unable ". . . of making an informed decision about his own safety or need for medical attention and is reasonably likely to suffer disability or death without medical attention. . . ."[12]

In 1997, a nationwide survey was performed to determine the percentage of EMS systems that used a formal refusal-of-transport policy, and to establish their adequacy in preventing potential litigation. Eighty-three percent of the nation's 100 largest EMS systems required that a determination of a patient's "competence" be performed and documented. Establishing a patient's competence most frequently included patient orientation, lack of alcohol intoxication, clear speech, comprehension of the nature and severity of the illness or injury, and comprehension of the risks and benefits of the procedure. Seventy-eight percent of the systems surveyed allowed providers to obtain a patient's refusal unsupervised. Only 15% required contact with a direct medical oversight physician (DMOP).[13]

"ACDC" is a mnemonic that can be used to summarize the elements of informed consent. It stands for "a substantially *autonomous* authorization by a *capable* individual to whom adequate information has been *disclosed* and who *comprehends* that information in terms of the nature, risks, benefits, and alternatives to the procedure."[7] Determining whether an individual comprehends the information that is being explained to them should involve the notion of a "sliding scale" standard. Drane suggests that this sliding scale should be adjusted to mirror the risks and potential dangers associated with the patient's treatment decision. "The more probable or serious the risks posed by the patient's decision, the more strin-

gent the standard of capacity required."[14] Under the Drane standard, acceptance of a refusal of EMS transport to a hospital, an extremely high risk, would therefore require convincing evidence of the patient's capacity to make an informed decision.[14]

The amount of time allocated to the important issues of consent, patient autonomy, and decision making during provider training is minimal, and not enough for the responsibility routinely thrust on prehospital personnel. To legal authorities, prehospital personnel have a limited scope of training traditionally restricted by the following underlying assumptions: the prehospital care provider responds to, assesses, and stabilizes to the extent possible in the prehospital phase, then transports the patient to a higher level of medical care, specifically a physician. Law and rulings have generally failed to address the nature of the relationship between the patient and prehospital provider. This confusion is not unusual; in some states, the professional registered nurse (RN) may have an independent relationship with a patient, while in others the RN relationship is dependent upon the attending or personal physician of the patient. This is an important issue when evaluating termination of the relationship in the field and the patient's refusal of medical assistance. At least one federal court ruling held that the care of a physician's assistant who treated and discharged a patient without the patient or patient's chart ever having been reviewed by a physician was below the standard.[15]

A widely held assumption exists that all patients coming into contact with prehospital care providers will be seen by a physician before being released. Clearly this does not occur in practice. While there are innumerable factors and circumstances in patient encounters in the field, there are essentially three types of no-transport situations (quadrants B, C, and D of table 44.2). Each has its own underlying or contributing factors, and each has its own legal implications. Similarly, each may have a different remedy to be addressed by the medical director in a protocol for the prehospital providers. As seen in table 44.2, the patients in quadrant A fit the underlying assumption, that, those patients who desire to be transported to the hospital and EMS desires to transport them to the hospital.

Patient Refuses Transport and EMS Disagrees (B)

The most complex quadrant of the matrix (table 44.2) is quadrant B. This is the true refusal of medical as-

TABLE 44.2		
Matrix of Patient Transportation Decision		
	PATIENT DESIRES TRANSPORT?	
	Yes	No
EMS DESIRES TO TRANSPORT — Yes	A: Transport	B: Refusal of Medical Assistance
EMS DESIRES TO TRANSPORT — No	C: Denial of Aid	D: No Transport

sistance (RMA). In these instances, the EMS providers believe the patient has or may have a medical problem that requires immediate evaluation or treatment. The patient, however, refuses to go to the hospital.

This area is fraught with danger to both the patient and the prehospital care provider. The RMA form typically contains language indicating that the patient was advised to go to the hospital and that he understands the possible consequences of the decision not to go to the hospital, which may include death. A key statement in such a document is the explicit assertion that the EMS provider did advise the patient to go to the hospital and that the patient understands the risks if he does not go.

Patient Desires Transport and EMS Disagrees (C)

The magnitude of misuse of ambulance resources for medically unnecessary ambulance transport varies widely. It appears to be greatest in the larger cities and least in the rural areas. "The refusal of EMS to transport is the single most common complaint."[16] Attempts to rectify this situation by refusing ambulance transportation on the basis of provider assessment at the scene are fraught with liability. Publicly owned or operated EMS services, including contracted services, have a duty to aid victims of accidents or other emergencies. It is likely that private and volunteer services have a similar duty, once they have responded. Should the patient have an adverse outcome it would become virtually impossible to justify the failure to treat and transport the patient.[17] Additionally, the argument can be made that the failure to treat and transport the patient constitutes a diagnosis by a prehospital provider that is more properly reserved for a physician.

Therefore, if a disagreement about the necessity for transport arises between the patient and the providers, the DMOP should decide whether the patient requires transport. Although this leads to overuse of the ambulance and even tolerates abuse of the system, it minimizes the risk of inappropriately denying ambulance transport to an ill patient. It is clear that such a system of medical decision making is more practical in a paramedic system with direct medical oversight than in a system that commonly does not have a mechanism for field personnel to contact the DMOP. Nevertheless, when there is direct medical oversight, as there is in virtually all paramedic systems, it is clear that the failure to transport a patient without such contact is a potentially serious liability.

Patient Refuses Transport and EMS Agrees (D)

Assume that EMS is called to the scene of an automobile accident where the person involved in the accident does not initiate the call. Neither the victim nor the EMS crew identifies a serious injury or any injury at all, and the victim refuses transportation to the hospital. The EMS crew may ask the patient to sign a statement on the prehospital care report (PCR) indicating that the patient does not wish to be transported to the hospital; often the only printed form for the patient to sign when he declines transportation to the hospital is the RMA form.

Often, because of misplaced faith in the value of an RMA, the result is that the patient is asked to sign a statement that neither the patient nor the provider believes to be true. Should this patient have problems subsequently, it would be difficult to reconcile the findings on the PCR (which should indicate no injury) with the statement on the RMA that indicates that the patient is at risk by not going to the hospital.

Similarly, if the patient was advised to go to the hospital, then legal counsel might ask why more aggressive procedures were not put into effect. Clearly, if neither the patient nor the EMS providers believe the patient is in need of immediate transportation to the hospital, the patient should be asked to sign a statement to that effect rather than an RMA statement. It may be appropriate to provide such patients with follow-up care sheets in the event signs or symptoms do present.

If patient care is initiated, if only the taking of vital signs, and/or the patient is reassured "that he is

OK," clearly all bets are off. Unless there is a formal procedure to "triage out" such patients the legal exposure is significant.

Desire for a Specific Hospital

Patients often request transport to a particular hospital, such as the hospital of their personal physician. It is equally common for EMS provider agencies to have a policy requiring transport to the closest hospital. Two good reasons for such a policy include keeping units within their service districts and emphasizing the importance of transporting patients to the nearest appropriate hospital. However, there are also valid reasons to comply with the desires of the patient. It is usually in the best interest of an individual patient if the continuity of care can be maintained by a physician who knows the patient and who has ready access to the patient's prior records.

A reasonable compromise can often be reached between these two alternatives. Some large EMS providers have adopted two rules. The first rule, often known as the "10-minute rule," allows the prehospital providers to transport a stable patient to the hospital of patient choice if it is no more than 10 minutes further than the nearest hospital. This eliminates the vast majority of complaints, since most patients are reasonable and do not request transportation long distances in an acute situation. Under the second rule, in the instance where the prehospital care providers feel that there is a potentially life-threatening problem, the DMOP is contacted and advised of the patient's condition; he may then authorize the patient to be transported elsewhere if the patient would otherwise refuse EMS transport or if there is a compelling argument.

Specialty Referral Center Candidates

Trauma and other specialty referral centers present a unique problem. When field personnel identify a specialty referral candidate, such as a trauma patient, who expresses a desire to go to a hospital other than the designated trauma center, the situation becomes a conflict between the best medical judgment of the provider and desires of the patient. A strong case can be made that the trauma patient cannot make an informed judgment in the prehospital setting. If the patient is brought to a nontrauma center and dies at the hospital, the case could be made that the patient did not have the capacity to make such a decision and that the provider should not have complied with the patient's wishes. If, on the other hand, a patient is brought to a trauma center against his will and does survive, the patient would be filing suit against EMS for saving his life.

The provider should act as would a reasonable and prudent provider in that community; that is, to act in the best medical interests of the patient, reflected in written trauma treatment protocols. Therefore, it is a reasonable course of action to transport defined trauma patients to trauma centers even though the patient may object, as long as he does not physically resist (Appendix C). Caroline also emphasizes the necessity of both informed consent and informed refusal.[18]

Informed Refusal

The leading case addressing the issue of informed refusal is the California case of *Truman v. Thomas*.[19] In that case the California Supreme Court held that a physician had a duty to warn a patient of the dangers involved in refusing to undergo a diagnostic test. In the Truman case, the physician had repeatedly requested his patient submit to a diagnostic test. The patient had refused, to the point that the physician ultimately refused to prescribe any further medication until she underwent the test. The physician went as far as informing the patient's pharmacist of his decision, but because he had not specifically delineated to the patient the risks of refusing the test, the physician was held liable when the patient was ultimately found to have inoperable cancer.

Before *Truman v. Thomas*, the controlling doctrine had been *Cobb v. Grant*, which required that a physician divulge "to his patient all information relevant to a meaningful decision process."[5] The interpretation in the Cobb case and subsequent cases applied only to patient consent for a procedure. If the patient did not undergo the procedure, the assumption—until Truman—was that the doctrine did not apply. Subsequently, a New York Court delineated the decision rule that the law would assume that the patient would have acted "as a reasonable person would have acted if he knew all pertinent information."[20] A California court further extended the liability to physicians who simply refer a patient to a specialist for possible treatment.[21]

All these cases refer to Cobb for its seminal elucidation of this doctrine. Cobb has the following essential postulates:

- The knowledge of the physician and the knowledge of the patient are not in parity.
- Adults exercise control over their own body with the right to determine what treatment is acceptable.
- Consent to treatment must be informed.
- Because of the nature of the physician-patient relationship, the physician has a special obligation to the patient.[5]

In Truman, the court found the concepts of "informed consent" and "informed refusal" to be "indistinguishable." The courts have recognized certain exceptions to the rule of informed consent. One of the principal exceptions is the emergency situation when the patient lacks capacity. Rozovsky delineates two conditions for such an exception to apply.[22] First, the patient must be incapacitated and unable to reach an informed judgment. This limitation "may be attributable to an injury . . . shock, or trauma. . . ." Second, "a life-threatening or health-threatening disease or injury that requires immediate treatment is present," where delay would mean death or impairment.[23]

Patient Refuses Transport Requested by Family

In some instances a family member or concerned bystander calls EMS, but the patient does not share the concern and refuses transportation to the hospital. This is a classic double bind. If there is a bad outcome, the family may sue if the patient is not transported, yet the patient may sue if he is transported against his will. If in the judgment of the crew there is no evidence of acute or life-threatening problems, then they may explain the situation to the caller and utilize an RMA form (preferably witnessed by the caller and the police), while offering to return should the patient change his mind. If there is a substantial risk of further deterioration, the situation becomes much more complex. In such an instance, EMS providers should take some or all of the following steps:

1. The EMS crew attempts to persuade the patient to accept transportation.
2. The EMS crew enlists the aid of the family in persuading the patient.
3. The EMS crew asks the Police Department's assistance in persuading the patient to voluntarily go to the hospital.
4. An EMS supervisor responds to the scene in an additional attempt to persuade the patient, as well as to provide documentation by a person of supervisory rank.
5. The EMS crew calls direct medical oversight and, preferably on a recorded line, the physician talks directly to the patient. One study has shown that, even if the patient has resisted all entreaties up to this point, 40% of the patients acquiesce and accept transportation to the hospital when the DMOP so requests.[24]

If the patient continues to refuse, the physician will have the opportunity to determine if the patient is alert and oriented, and has the "capacity" to make a reasonable and knowledgeable RMA. The physician can then reasonably authorize the prehospital care providers to discontinue their efforts, if all reasonable steps in the interest of patient care have been taken. On the other hand, if in the physician's judgment the patient does not have the capacity to make such a decision, the physician should enlist the aid of the Police Department to authorize involuntary transport of the patient to the hospital. In many jurisdictions, only a peace officer may legally do this.

A tape-recorded system provides positive documentation of the number of times that the patient was requested to go to the hospital and that the patient knowingly chose not to be transported. It may also provide documentation that the patient refused to speak to the physician or EMS crew, and that the patient had capacity to make an informed judgment.

Patient Restraint

"Some systems routinely and forcibly transport and sometimes treat resisting patients against their will with or without law enforcement assistance. Although this practice has been warned against by both physicians and EMS legal counsel, it continues unabated."[28]

In 1999 in a wrongful death and unlawful imprisonment suit (*Shine v. Vega*), the Supreme Court of Massachusetts ruled that a competent adult patient has the right to refuse medical treatment, even in a life-threatening situation.[26] The case in question occurred in 1990 when Katherine Shine, a lifelong asthmatic, developed an asthma exacerbation while staying with her sister in Boston. Her sister convinced her to go to the emergency department where she wanted only to be treated with oxygen and refused other treatment. Shine and her sister had attempted to leave the emergency department and were detained by a physician and security guard. Shine was placed in restraints and eventually intubated. She was discharged two days later. Her family testified that the experience had traumatized her and caused her to avoid obtaining hospital treatment during a subsequent exacerbation in 1992, which caused a delay that eventually led to her death. The Shine family sued the hospital and the attending emergency medicine physician for negligence, assault and battery, false imprisonment, emotional distress, civil rights violations, and wrongful death.

The Superior Court Judge had ruled in favor of the physician and hospital after an argument had been made that Shine had faced a life-threatening emergency and the physician therefore did not need to consent to proceed with treatment. The jury had been instructed that "no patient has a right to refuse medical treatment in a life-threatening situation." This decision was appealed and eventually overturned by the State Supreme Court which held that a doctor could care for a patient without consent only when a life-threatening condition exists and the patient is either unconscious or otherwise incapable of giving consent. The case was sent back to the lower court so that a new jury could reexamine the suit.[26]

The issue of false imprisonment has been contested recently in the case of *Cathey v. The City of Louisville*.[27] Louisville Emergency Medical Services were called on February 21, 1997, to treat a 19-year-old woman, Mistelle Cathey. It was reported that she had a syncopal episode while working at the hotel where she was employed as a housekeeper. Prior to the arrival of EMS, Cathey had regained consciousness but was hysterical, according to witnesses. A paramedic, convinced Cathey to have her vital signs taken and noted that her blood pressure was low and her breathing was fast. Cathey became upset again upon seeing a police officer in the doorway and screamed for him to leave. The paramedic instructed Cathey that it was important that she go to the hospital for further evaluation and treatment, as he felt she had passed out and had abnormal vital signs. Cathey stated that she did not wish to go to the hospital.

Eventually the paramedic, with the help of a police officer, restrained Cathey, placed her in the ambulance, and inserted an intravenous line into her arm on the way to the hospital without her consent. Cathey sued with claims of false imprisonment and battery. The case was originally dismissed by the Circuit Court. The court recognized that the paramedic had used his own judgment to decide that Cathey needed further treatment and was unable to completely consent to such treatment because he observed behavior that he considered to be bizarre and inappropriate. The court decided that it "cannot substitute its judgment of the paramedic who was on the scene and witnessed the behavior."[27] The paramedic and his partner were recognized to be acting under the statutory privilege found in Kentucky Statutory Law (503.110-(4)). The statute considers that:

The use of physical force by a defendant upon another person is justifiable when the defendant is a doctor or other therapist or a person assisting him at his direction, and:

(a) The force is used for the purpose of administering a recognized form of treatment which the defendant believes to be adapted to promoting the physical or mental health of the patient; and

(b) The treatment is administered with the consent of the patient or, if the patient is a minor or a mentally disabled person, with the consent of the parent, guardian, or other person legally competent to consent in his behalf, or the treatment is administered in an emergency when the defendant believes that no one competent to consent can be consulted and that a reasonable person, wishing to safeguard the welfare of the patient, would consent.[28]

The case was appealed by Cathey and the Court of Appeals of Kentucky felt that "while there is evidence which casts doubt upon Cathey's ability to make a rational decision at the time the paramedics chose to restrain her, that evidence merely creates a fact issue which must be resolved by a jury."[27]

In Massachusetts, no legislative mandate existed until September of 2000 to allow out-of-hospital providers to restrain patients. A revision at that time in the EMS laws for the state included the following paragraph:

Subject to regulations and guidelines promulgated by the department, an emergency medical technician may restrain a patient who presents an immediate or serious threat of bodily harm to himself or others. Any such restraint shall be noted in the written report of said emergency medical technician. (Chapter 111c, section 18)

"Department" is defined in this paragraph as the State Department of Public Health, which is the parent organization for the Massachusetts Office of Emergency Medical Services (OEMS). OEMS is responsible for regulating the provision of prehospital emergency medical services in accordance with Massachusetts General Laws. At present time no regulations or guidelines involving patient restraint have been developed by OEMS to guide local EMS departments. OEMS had suggested that each local EMS system develop their own policy and procedure regarding the restraint of patients in the out-of-hospital setting. Appendix B provides an example of such a system policy and protocol for the management and restraint of dangerous patients.

Summary

Although the concept of informed consent is well established in medicine, the concept of informed refusal is often more germane. When there is disagreement between patient and crew over the need to transport, access to direct medical oversight is essential. Should a field unit agree with the patient that transport is not required, the "traditional" RMA form is *not* appropriate; a second form and procedure should be developed stating the crew agrees that transport is not required and has informed the patient of their opinion. Of course the system would have tremendous exposure if the providers were wrong.

The medical director should ensure that both the EMS personnel and DMOP oversight have an understanding of their duties and obligations in the various "no transport" situations. This includes a familiarity with the assessment abilities of the prehospital providers, applicable state and local laws, transport times, call volume, and number of available ambulances and supervisors. Patients whose medical condition is immediately life-threatening should be taken to a medically appropriate treatment facility, even if they express a desire to be treated elsewhere. Appendix C contains a sample destination policy for trauma patients. EMS systems should strongly consider promulgation of a formal restraint policy developed as outlined above.

References

1. United States President's Commission for the Study of Ethical Problems in Medicine and Biomedical Research. United States G.P.O. Washington, D.C., 1982.

2. Meisel A, Kuczewski M. Legal and ethical myths about informed consent. *Arch Int Med.* 1996;156:2521–2526.

3. *Schloendorff v. Society of New York Hospital*, Court of Appeals of New York, 211 N.Y. 125. April 14, 1914 decided.

4. *Nathanson v. Klein*, Supreme Court of Kansas, 187 Kan. 186; 354 P.2d676. August 5, 1960 filed.

5. *Cobbs v. Grant*, Supreme Court of California. 8 Cal 3d 229; 502 P.2d1; October 27, 1972 decided.

6. Goldstein AS. EMS and the Law. Bowie, MD: Brady 1983.

7. Holroyd B, et al. Prehospital patients refusing care. *Ann Emerg Med.* 1998;17:957–963.

8. Biegler P., Stewart C. Assessing competence to refuse medical treatment. *Med J Australia.* 2001;174:522–525.

9. Appelbaum P, Grisso T. Assessing patients' capacities to consent to treatment. *New England J Med.* 1988;319: 1635–1638.

10. Thewes J, et al,. Informed consent in emergency medicine. *Emerg Med Clinics N A.* 1996;14:245–253.

11. *Lane v. Candura*, Appeals Court of Massachusetts. 6 Mass. App. Ct 377; 376 N.E.2d 1232; May 26, 1978 decided.

12. New Mexico State Law. Emergency Transportation Statute, 24-10B-9.1. Laws 1993, Chapter 161,§ 11.

13. Weaver J, et al. Prehospital refusal of transport policies: adequate legal protection? *Prehosp Emerg Care.* 2000;4: 53–56.

14. Miller S, Marin D. Assessing capacity. *Emerg Med Clinics N A.* 2000; 18:233–242.

15. *Polischeck v. United States*, US District Court for Eastern Pennsylvania, 535 F. Supp. 1261. April 1, 1982 decided.

16. Proceedings of the First National Conference on Medical-Legal Implications of Emergency Medical Care, 1976.

17. *Green v. City of Dallas*, Court of Appeals of Texas, 665 S.W. 2d 567, January 25, 1984 decided.

18. Caroline N. *Emergency Medical Treatment: A Text for EMT-As and EMT-Is.* Boston: Little, Brown; 1991.

19. *Truman v. Thomas*, Supreme Court of California, 611 P.2d 902, June 9, 1980 decided.

20. *Crisher v. Spak*, Supreme Court of New York, 471 N.Y.S. 2d 741, November 10, 1983 decided.

21. *Moore v. Preventive Medicine Medical Group, Inc*, Court of Appeals of California. 178 Cal. App. 3d. 728, March 11, 1986.

22. Rozovsky F. Editorial. *Defense Law J.* 1984;33:579.

23. Codified e.g. in Ga. 88-2905 (1971).

24. Kuehl A. Personal communication, New York, 1986.

25. Ayres R. Legal considerations in prehospital care. *Emerg Med Clinics N A*; 1993;11:853–867.

26. *Shine v. Vega*, Supreme Judicial Court of Massachusetts, 429 Mass. 456, 709 N.E. 2d58, April 29, 1999 decided.

27. *Cathey v. The City of Louisville*, Supreme Court of Kentucky, 1999. S.C. 0930-D, June 7, 2000 entered.

28. *Ky. Re v. Stat.* (KRS) 503.110(4)(b). Effective July 1, 1982.

Appendix A

Policy and Procedure

Subject: Patient Consent and Refusal

I. ABILITY TO REFUSE TREATMENT OR TRANSPORT

A. A patient has the right to refuse treatment and/or transport when he/she meets the following criteria:

1. The patient is 18 years of age or an emancipated minor; and
2. The patient understands the nature of his/her medical condition and the potential consequences of refusing treatment and/or transport to a hospital.

B. A patient may not refuse treatment and/or transport if:

1. The patient does not understand the nature of his/her medical condition or the potential consequences of refusing treatment and/or transport to a hospital; or
2. The patient is under the age of 18, unless a parent or guardian who understands the nature of his/her medical condition and the potential consequences of refusing treatment and/or transport to a hospital refuses treatment or transport.

C. Patient refusal—the patient possesses decisional capacity

Emergency Medical Technicians (EMTs) and paramedics shall perform the following when managing a competent patient who refuses treatment or transport:

1. Ask the patient directly if he/she wants to go to a hospital;
2. If there is an illness or injury, inform the patient of the need to receive treatment and/or go to the hospital or the potential consequences of not receiving treatment and/or going to a hospital;
3. Obtain the patient's signature on the EMS Patient Refusal Authorization Form. In the case of a minor patient, the parent or guardian's signature should be obtained; and
4. Document all findings on the Patient Care Report (PCR);
5. If the patient or legal guardian refuses to sign the form, the EMT shall write "Refused To Sign" on the line for the patient's signature.

II. PATIENT REFUSAL—THE PATIENT LACKS DECISIONAL CAPACITY

EMTs and paramedics shall perform the following when managing a patient who does not understand the nature of his medical condition or the potential consequences of refusing treatment and/or transport to a hospital:

1. Where time permits, request the assistance of the field supervisor and the police department;
2. Where time permits, the EMT shall notify direct medical oversight, describe the situation, and request permission to transport the patient against the patient's will;
3. If direct medical oversight states that transport is necessary, explain to the patient that a doctor has ordered that the patient be transported to the hospital and that if the patient still refuses transport, the EMTs will carry out the order of the doctor;
4. Document all findings on the PCR;
5. EMTs may restrain a patient who presents and immediate or serious threat of bodily harm to himself, EMS personnel or others, preferably with the assistance of the police, and shall document any such restrain in the PCR;
6. If restraint is necessary, EMTs shall complete a Patient Restraint Report.

III. PATIENT REFUSAL AUTHORIZATION FORM

The EMTs and paramedics shall complete and submit the Patient Refusal Authorization Form with a completed PCR whenever a competent patient refuses to be treated or transported to the hospital:

1. The patient, parent, or legal guardian shall initial the appropriate box and sign the form on the designated signature line;
2. If the patient or legal guardian refuses to sign the form, the EMT shall write "Refused To Sign Form" in place of the patient signature and shall secure the signature of any witnesses if possible.
3. A patient in the custody of any law enforcement or other agency who refuses transport shall initial the appropriate box and sign the form on the designated signature line. If the patient refuses to sign the form, the EMT shall write "Refused To Sign" in place of the patient signature. The police officer or other person in charge of the patient shall sign the Patient Refusal Authorization Form on the designated signature line and write in his badge number or employee number on the form.
4. Both EMTs shall sign the Patient Refusal Authorization Form.

APPENDIX B

Policy and Procedure

Subject: Patient Restraint

I. PATIENT RESTRAINT

A. The physical restraint of a patient is a last resort and should be utilized only after other approaches have failed. Establishing a rapport with the patient or removing the patient from the environment may alleviate the need to restrain;

B. The restraint of a patient shall be performed in accordance with the Managing The Dangerous Patient Protocol;

C. The type and method of restraint used to restrain a patient must be approved by the Bureau of Professional Standards;

D. When restraint of a patient is necessary, EMTs and paramedics shall complete a Patient Restraint Report.

Training Protocol

Subject: Protocol For Managing the Dangerous Patient

II. PURPOSE

The purpose of this protocol is to establish uniform guidelines for managing a patient who presents an immediate or serious threat of bodily harm to himself, EMS personnel, or others in the immediate area. The goal of managing a patient exhibiting violent behavior is to prevent further harm to the patient, EMS personnel, or bystanders.

III. PROCEDURE

A. General Guidelines
1. In order to standardize the control exercised with patients, EMS personnel should adhere to a progressive scale of the use of restraint referred to as the Use of Control Continuum. Nothing in this Protocol prevents EMS personnel from rapidly escalating to a particular level of the Use of Control Continuum or choosing a level from the outset which most appropriately meets the needs of the patient.
2. When restraint of a dangerous patient is necessary, EMS personnel shall use the least invasive technique as appropriate to the situation and increase the level of restraint progressively, as necessary for the particular patient.
3. EMTs and Paramedics shall not approach a violent patient until the situation has been declared safe by the responsible law enforcement agency.

4. Law enforcement authorities are responsible for identifying and engaging violent persons. They are responsible for restraining or otherwise containing such persons and searching for and securing weapons before referring a patient for medical evaluation and treatment.

5. EMS personnel shall never attempt to restrain persons with homicidal capacity. Personnel must immediately leave the area when faced with persons armed with firearms, edged weapons, or other life-threatening weapons.

6. If a violent situation develops and leaving the immediate area is impossible, EMS personnel may restrain a patient before law enforcement personnel arrive, if the patient presents an immediate or serious threat of bodily harm to himself, EMS personnel, or others in the immediate area.

7. A patient shall be closely monitored for signs of potentially negative affects of any restraint applied, including respiratory compromise or circulatory impairment. A patient's restraints shall be checked for such compromises and documented on the Patient Restraint Report, at five (5) minute intervals.

8. A patient may exhibit violent behavior due to an underlying medical condition. Such a patient may be restrained before law enforcement personnel arrive at a scene, if the patient presents an immediate or serious threat of bodily harm to himself, EMS personnel, or others in the immediate area.

9. Patients actively exhibiting muscle contractile or tonic-clonic seizure-like activity shall not be restrained. Instead, the incident area shall be cleared and the patient shall be supported and padding placed around the patient to minimize potential for injury until the tonic-clonic activity subsides or the patient receives medical intervention.

10. Patients shall not be transported in the prone position or held in the prone position after the application of restraints.

11. No form of restraint shall be applied so as to constrict diaphragmatic breathing or the normal expansion of the chest cavity.

12. EMS personnel shall not remove restraints from a patient during transportation. Changing the type of restraint might be appropriate from a hard mechanical restraint to a softer form of restraint, depending on the condition of the patient.

REFUSAL OF MEDICAL ASSISTANCE

13. A restrained patient shall be carried on a wheeled cot, scoop stretcher, stairchair, or backboard.

B. Definitions
   1. "Physical restraint" means the application of EMS approved restraints using the least invasive method necessary.
   2. "Control Continuum" means that when restraint is necessary, EMS personnel shall begin by using the least invasive technique and increase the level of restraint progressively, as necessary for the particular patient. The least number of points of control shall be used to meet the objective of effectively controlling the patient. Nothing in this Protocol prevents EMS personnel from rapidly escalating to a particular level of the Use of Control Continuum or choosing a level from the outset that most appropriately meets the needs of the patient.

C. Restraint of Patients
   1. Restraint of a patient is appropriate if either of the following two conditions are present:
      a. A patient has a medical or psychiatric condition and demonstrates behavior that presents an immediate or serious threat of bodily harm to himself, EMS personnel or others in the immediate area; or,
      b. A person authorized by (insert local law) such a licensed physician, qualified psychologist, psychiatric nurse/mental health clinical specialist or a police officer has ordered the patient to be restrained for medical reasons.
   2. EMS personnel shall use the control continuum as in Section D when restraint of a patient is necessary.

D. Restraint Devices
   EMS Personnel shall only use the following approved restraint devices:
   1. soft roller bandages;
   2. leather restraints;
   3. webbed straps to augment limb restraint devices and stabilize patients on back boards, wheeled cots, scoop stretchers, and stairchairs; and
   4. Trilock© restraints.

E. Anticipated Restraint Situation
   The following procedure shall be followed during a predetermined restraint situation:
   1. Law enforcement personnel and Dispatch Operations shall advise EMTs that a patient restraint situation may exist. A field supervisor shall be dispatched to the scene.
   2. As resources allow, law enforcement personnel and EMS personnel shall develop and implement an action plan for managing a dangerous patient, including, if necessary, patient restraint.
   3. A field supervisor and law enforcement personnel shall be present during the restraint process whenever possible.
   4. A wheeled cot, backboard, scoop stretcher, or stairchair shall be brought to the patient's side or to the immediate area.
   5. EMS personnel shall explain the restraint process to the patient and provide the patient with the opportunity to choose transportation without restraint, if it would not compromise the safety of the patient, EMS personnel, or others in the immediate area.
   6. If a patient requires restraint, EMS personnel shall restrain patients using the control continuum.
   7. Soft gauze roller bandage or leather restraints, when available, shall be the preferred method of appendage restraint. The Trilock© restraint device shall be an alternative method, depending on the condition of the patient and reasonable expediency.
   8. Patients shall be secured to transfer devices in a sitting (stair-chair), supine, a scoop stretcher, or a right/left lateral recumbent position only.
   9. A continuing dialog shall be maintained with the patient to communicate that everything possible is being done to ensure the patient's safety.
   10. If the Trilock© restraint device has been applied, the patient shall be transferred to soft roller gauze restraints or leather restraints as soon as feasible.
   11. EMS personnel must document the choice of restraint on the Patient Restraint Report.

F. Unanticipated Restraint Situation
   1. A field unit shall notify operations that a violent situation exists and exit from the situation if possible.
   2. If the life or safety of any EMS personnel is threatened or in any danger, the standard "Ambulance In Trouble" response shall be initiated.
   3. Dispatch Operations shall confirm that law enforcement personnel are responding.
   4. Dispatch Operations shall dispatch an EMS field supervisor who shall coordinate the restraint effort, if timely.
   5. All other applicable elements of the Patient Consent and Refusal Policy or the Managing the Dangerous Patient Protocol apply.
   6. If a patient must be restrained before the arrival of additional resources, EMS personnel shall use the appropriate restraint device.
   7. EMS personnel must document the circumstances regarding their use of a restraint on the Patient Restraint Report.

G. Restraint During Transportation
1. The EMT/Paramedic driver shall bring the vehicle to a safe stop and assist the EMT/Paramedic-Patient Care provider.
2. If the life or safety of any EMS personnel is threatened or in any danger, the standard "Ambulance In Trouble" response shall be initiated.
3. If necessary, the patient shall be appropriately restrained using gauze, leather restraints, or the Trilock© restraint device prior to resuming transport.

4. All other applicable elements of the Patient Consent and Refusal Policy or the Managing the Dangerous Patient Protocol apply to this situation.
5. EMS personnel shall document the circumstances regarding their use of a restraint on the Patient Restraint Report.

Appendix C

Trauma Destination Policy for the New York State Department of Health

As always, the Department's first concern is to ensure the best care for each patient while protecting the right of the patient to choose the provider of that care, or indeed, to choose not to accept care at all.

It is essential that such a decision by a patient be an informed decision. Informed consent is a guiding ethical and legal principle of medical care that the Department vigorously supports.

It is axiomatic that a patient cannot make an informed judgment unless he fully understands the risks and benefits of the course of treatment suggested by the provider. In the major trauma patient, this is often not possible. A number of factors interfere with this normal process of informed consent. First, the patient's injuries may result in an alteration of the patient's mental status. Such an alteration may result either directly from an injury to the head, or indirectly due to injury to other areas of the body resulting, for example, in shock or extreme pain. Obviously, a patient with an altered mental status is unable to make an informed judgment, nor is the prehospital provider trained to determine the patient's capacity to do so.

Secondly, the time constraints required to effectively treat trauma patients are extreme. Effective trauma care is measured in minutes. The nationally recognized principle of the "golden hour" of trauma care requires that optimum patient care can be achieved if the patient reaches definitive trauma center care as expeditiously as possible. The time required to list and explain the benefits of the various transport alternatives in a meaningful manner would prevent the patient from receiving this optimal care.

Third, and perhaps most important, informed consent requires that the patient be informed of the suggested and alternative courses of action, and the risks and benefits of each. Yet, in the prehospital setting, the provider is a certified EMT, not a licensed physician. The scope of training of an EMT does not include knowledge of the complications, alternatives, or even the likely outcome of a particular course of action, much less the range of likelihood of reasonably known complications. Thus, since the information needed to make an informed judgment in the prehospital setting is unavailable, an informed judgment—by definition—cannot be made.

In the absence of informed consent, the provider should follow the course of action of a reasonable and prudent EMT. Such course of action is clearly laid out in the New York State Emergency Medical Service BLS protocols. All EMTs are required to follow these protocols.

Finally, it is important to remember that the decision made by the EMT is the hospital destination. Once at the appropriate hospital, the patient will be cared for by a physician, who can accurately determine the capacity of the patient to make an informed judgment and provide the information necessary for that informed judgment to be made. For these reasons, it is the position of the Department that trauma patients, as defined in the New York State Emergency Medical Service BLS protocols, be transported in accordance with those protocols, even if the patient objects.

Physicians at the Scene

Robert Bass, MD
Jon Krohmer, MD

Introduction

It is not uncommon for EMS personnel to encounter a non-EMS system physician at the scene of an emergency response. This physician may be a true bystander who has come upon the incident, or may be a private physician who has an established relationship with the patient. The interaction of physicians in the field with EMS personnel can create a great deal of confusion, especially when trying to define medical authority and responsibility for patient care. If a patient is seriously injured or ill, this confusion, coupled with the stress of the situation, can lead to emotionally charged confrontations. Such confrontations rarely benefit patient care.[1] For this reason, it is important that prehospital care systems prospectively develop policies that address the interaction of field providers with bystander or private physicians who are on-scene. The role of the on-scene direct medical oversight physician (DMOP) is not addressed here.

Defining the Problem

Although there are no clear data that describe the incidence of such encounters, they are not infrequent. In one survey in 1991, paramedics from five urban areas reported an average of 3.4 encounters with physicians on-scene within the previous year.[2] Likewise, although it would seem self-evident that the expertise of a physician present at the scene would improve the quality of field management, there are little empirical data demonstrating such a benefit.[3] There are no data available to suggest that on-line medical direction is of benefit in certain groups of patients who are critically ill or injured, and who require treatment beyond or in deviation from protocols.[4] At the present time, it can only be assumed that field physician intervention might have similar benefits.

Many field personnel have a negative perception of their interactions with physicians in the field, and believe that such encounters benefit patient care in relatively few cases. A number of factors contribute to those perceptions, including a feeling by paramedics that physicians do not understand their roles. According to some paramedics, physicians in the field frequently insist on intervening because they assume that EMS providers have little if any training.[2]

There are a number of theoretical reasons why a bystander physician might benefit patient care. The physician may have greater training or medical knowledge than EMS personnel or may be capable of performing procedures that the EMS providers cannot. This may be more likely in a rural environment where provider training is often more limited. Depending on their specialty, training, and experience, the physician may be more skilled in certain interventions. If the physician has an established relationship with the patient, his knowledge of the patient's history and problems may be of benefit. Additionally, field expertise aside, physicians have a legitimate interests in the management of patients transported from their offices.[3]

On the other hand, there are times when a bystander physician may be a significant liability. Unless physicians are trained or experienced in prehospital care, critical-care medicine, or emergency medicine, they may not, in fact, be as knowledgeable or as skilled as the EMS providers in field care of ill or injured patients. In addition, the physician may be unfamiliar with prehospital interventions, the principles of emergency evacuation and transport, or the unique legal issues of the prehospital environment. As an example, an internist or cardiologists might be alarmed by the immediate transport of a hypotensive blunt trauma victim before the placement of intravenous lines, since this is contrary to their understanding of the management of medical emergencies. In one dispute recently publicized by the media over a similar issue, a persistent bystander physician was handcuffed by police to keep him away from the resuscitation area. At scenes where safety is an issue, physicians who are not familiar with field hazards may detract from patient care by distracting field providers who must ensure that the physician does not become of victim.

Bystander Physicians

The role and responsibility of a bystander physician is not always easy to define, and may vary greatly depending on the circumstances. In general, the following three varieties of interaction between a bystander physician and EMS providers can be described:

1. The physicians turns over care of the patient to EMS.
2. The physician turns over care of the patient to the EMS, but offers advice and assistance.
3. The physician directs and/or provides patient care (the intervener physician).

Most bystander-physician encounters result in the physician turning over the patient to the EMS providers, with perhaps an offer of assistance or advice. In such circumstances the EMS providers proceed with their evaluation and treatment according to protocol. Often, while EMS personnel are assessing the patient and initiating care, a physician will offer advice and suggestions for continued care. This type of intervention potentially benefits the patient. In such cases, physicians and EMS personnel working as a team can most likely provide for the best outcome for the patient.

In most cases, bystander physicians usually do no more than an assessment and provide first aid, and the patient is turned over to the EMS personnel for further care and transportation. Unless the physician has directly intervened (performed an invasive procedure or directed patient care) or is needed for continued care or advice beyond the scope of the EMS providers, the physician need not accompany a patient to the hospital. Whenever a bystander physician decides to intervene, direct medical oversight should be contacted and approval for such intervention obtained.[4]

Problems may arise when an intervening physician who is not familiar with prehospital care deviates from either established protocols or recognized standards of prehospital care. Whether intentional or inadvertent, such deviation creates a potential legal problem that should be resolved by direct medical oversight. A position statement by the American College of Emergency Physicians (ACEP) holds that even if a bystander or private physician is on-scene, direct medical oversight should remain ultimately responsible for patient care. In the event of a disagreement between the DMOP and on-scene physician, the EMS providers obviously should take orders from the DMOP.[5]

Private Physicians

In the case of an on-scene private physician, the ACEP position[5] is that EMS providers should defer to the orders of a private physician desiring to continue to direct patient care. In this situation, the private physician assumes responsibility for the patient's care. EMS providers with concerns about the quality or appropriateness of the care being rendered should contact direct medical oversight and ultimately defer to the DMOP.

Patients who are in a physician's office may have had diagnostic procedures and/or therapeutic interventions initiated before the arrival of EMS. In such cases, everything possible should be done to maintain the appropriate continuity of care. This may involve the physician or members of the physician's staff accompanying the patient during transport to the hospital, particularly if the EMS system is not capable of providing the level of care that the patient received in the office.

At the other extreme, EMS providers may find patients in a medical office who require critical interventions that have not been initiated. This situation is exacerbated when EMS providers are orders by a physician or nurse not to do anything except transport the patient. In such cases, a rapid evacuation to a more neutral environment where protocols can be initiated and direct medical oversight consultation can be obtained is in order. Confrontations rarely improve outcome. The best approach to this situation is for EMS providers to maintain a professional and composed attitude and try to exit the office as quickly as possible. Careful documentation in the prehospital care report of all of the events after such encounters is important.[4]

Office calls can be expedited by developing office response protocols, which specify office addresses and any other idiosyncracies of access, the entrance at which an employee will be awaiting the crew, and the arrangements that will be made for clinical management in the office. These protocols may be stored in the computer database at dispatch where they are immediately available. Such protocols improve not only response times and access but also the relationship among physicians and paramedics.

Medical Authority

In developing guidelines that address physicians at the scene, EMS services should consider any relevant state or local laws, rules, or regulations that define the authority of such physicians, whether bystander or private.

NAEMSP and ACEP believe that the ultimate authority for medical care delivered by an EMS provider rests with the medical oversight of the EMS system. Prehospital care is viewed as the delivery of health care by the physician medical director through the use of EMS providers. EMS providers are therefore viewed as agents of the medical director rather than of the physician at the scene. Medical directors in turn delegate to other physicians the authority to provide direct medical oversight. Therefore, such physicians should have the authority to override on-scene physicians if necessary. The potential liability of the system, the medical director, and DMOPs should be considered before delegating an on-scene physician to assume direct medical oversight.

Guidelines for Physicians at the Scene

In developing guidelines, it is important to consider the various roles that a physician at the scene may assume. When an on-scene physician does nothing more than transfer care of the patient to EMS or offer advice and assistance, patient care continues as with any other call, according to EMS protocols. Any further intervention should be based on protocol or authorized by direct medical oversight.

Physicians who intervene should be properly identified, since EMS incidents have been known to attract individuals posing as physicians. If the physician is not known to EMS providers, the physician should be asked to provide proof of state medical licensure. In some circumstances, it may be helpful to know the physician's specialty certification, as well as his or her prehospital and critical care experience. When relevant, such information should be relayed to direct

medical oversight to assist with decision making. Whenever possible, the DMOP and the on-scene physician at the scene should speak with one another. On-scene physicians should be told that they will be required to document any orders given or procedures performed, and that it may be necessary for them to accompany the patient to the hospital.

When a DMOP approves the intervention by an on-scene physician, the EMS providers should be immediately notified. Such notification should delineate the degree of authority that has been granted to the physician intervener. At any point that the providers believe that the care being rendered deviates from standards, is not appropriate, or goes beyond what was authorized, direct medical oversight should be immediately notified. Physicians who give orders, perform procedures, or assume full medical responsibility generally should accompany the patient to the hospital. However, this decision should ultimately be the responsibility of the DMOP. On-scene physicians who offer only assistance with the implementation of protocols need not necessarily accompany the patient. In those cases, to avoid a potential claim of physician abandonment, the patient should be stable and in no obvious need of further physician intervention. In cases where a physician has assumed full medical responsibility, especially where interventions have been initiated, the physician should accompany the patient to the hospital. Physicians who refuse to do so speak to the DMOP and should be warned that refusal to accompany the patient might be interpreted as abandonment or a violation of state laws on medical practice.

When an on-scene physician gives orders or performs procedures, they should provide written documentation on the patient-case record, including their name, license number, office address, and telephone number. Ideally, this information should be obtained whenever physician is on-scene, regardless of their role.

EMS systems guidelines should also address the procedure to be followed when providers are unable to establish contact with direct medical oversight. In such cases, state laws and the best interests of the patient should be considered. In a rural environment with limited EMS provider capability, when a physician who is well known to the EMS providers offers assistance, it would be unreasonable to deny the patient such intervention. At the other extreme, in the urban situation where sophisticated prehospital care is available with short transport times, EMS providers without immediate communications, when confronted with an unknown bystander physician intervening in a potentially harmful way, may wish to decline politely the offer of assistance and expeditiously place the patient in the unit for transport. Guidelines governing such situations should be prospectively issued and must take into consideration local circumstances, as well as all applicable laws and regulations.

Several EMS agencies have developed information cards for bystander physicians that delineate important points for the physician contemplating intervention (Appendix A). In addition to thanking the physician for volunteering assistance, they briefly summarize the legal authority directing the EMS providers and list the options for intervention. There should be a clear indication that assumption of responsibility for patient care or use of special expertise will either probably or definitely require a commitment to accompany the patient tot he hospital.[6] The information cards may be intimidating and should not be used simply to deter or delay physician intervention, especially when it would be beneficial. In New York City, physicians wishing to assume management of patient care must also sign a separate document (Appendix B).

Summary

On-scene physicians may fulfill various roles in conjunction with EMS providers. Any involvement beyond first-aid-level assistance should be approved by direct medical oversight. In most situations, the ultimate medical authority for EMS providers is the EMS medical director, who may delegate responsibility to on-line physicians. EMS agencies should develop guidelines for addressing the issues related to the on-scene physician, including the distinctive concerns of private physicians and office calls. The potential liability to the EMS agency should be considered before authorizing bystander physicians to intervene.

References

1. Vost A. Physician intervention at the scene: another point of view. *JEMS*. 1989;14:60–67.
2. Mellick LB, et al. Paramedic perceptions of the on-scene physician. *Prehospital and Disaster Medicine*. 1991;6:331–334.
3. Dickinson ET, Schneider RM, Verdile VP. The impact of prehospital physicians on out-of-hospital nonasystolic cardiac arrests. *Prehosp Emerg Care*. 1997;1(3):132–135.
4. Erder MH, Davidson SJ, Cheney RA. On-line medical command in theory and practice. *Ann Emerg Med*. 1989;18:261–268.
5. American College of Emergency Physicians. Control of advanced life support at the scene of medical emergencies. *Ann Emerg Med*. 1984;13:547–548. Reaffirmed by ACEP in 1997.
6. Smith M. Hello . . . I'm a doctor. *JEMS*. 1992;17(5):37–38.

Appendix A

Examples of Non-solicited Medical Intervention Cards and Signature Form

New York City Physician Information Card

Thank you for your offer of assistance. Please be advised that these Emergency Medical Technicians are operating under the authority of the State of New York and under protocols established by the NYC 9-1-1 Emergency Medical Service System. These EMTs may also be New York City certified Paramedics who are operating under the authority of a medical control physician and standing medical orders.

To avoid confusion and to expedite patient care, no individual should intervene in the care of this patient unless the individual is:

1. requested to by the attending Emergency Medical Service Personnel, or
2. authorized by the medical oversight physician, or
3. is capable of delivering more extensive emergency medical care at the scene.

IF YOU ASSUME PATIENT MANAGEMENT, YOU ACCEPT RESPONSIBILITY FOR PATIENT CARE UNTIL THE ATTENDING EMERGENCY MEDICAL SERVICE PERSONNEL OR MEDICAL OVERSIGHT PHYSICIAN ACCEPTS THAT RESPONSIBILITY. THIS WILL REQUIRE THAT YOU ACCOMPANY THE PATIENT TO THE EMERGENCY DEPARTMENT.

Assumption of Patient Management Statement

"I, _____, license # _____, have assumed authority and responsibility for patient management in the case to which this document refers.

I understand that in order to do this I must accompany the patient, in the ambulance, to the Emergency Department. I further understand that all EMS patient-care protocols must still be followed."

_____
Signature

_____
Date   Time

_____
Witness: EMS Member

_____
Witness: PD Officer, if present

Tacoma-Pierce County Washington Physician Information Card

THANK YOU FOR YOUR OFFER OF ASSISTANCE. This EMERGENCY MEDICAL SERVICES team is operating under Washington law and policy established jointly by the EMS Medical Director of Pierce County and the Tacoma-Pierce County Health Department. The EMS team is functioning under the command of the base-hospital physician.

The Pneumatic Anti-Shock Garment

Paul E. Pepe, MD, MPH

Introduction

Over the past three decades, the traditional consensus for managing trauma patients found to have low blood pressure following injury has been to presume internal hemorrhage and then attempt to restore normal systemic blood pressure.[1-3] The rationale for this approach has been to ensure and maintain vital organ perfusion while awaiting definitive surgical intervention and hemostasis.[1] The two modalities most widely used to achieve this goal have been: (1) rapid intravenous infusions of isotonic crystalloid or colloid solutions (normal saline, lactated Ringer's albumin or hetastarch); and (2) the use of the pneumatic antishock garment (PASG), also known as military antishock trousers (MAST).[1-22]

Several animal studies from the 1950s and 1960s largely formed the basis for this approach.[8,15,18,22] Researchers found that animals with severe hemorrhage had a greater likelihood of survival when they received both blood and isotonic fluid as resuscitative interventions when compared to those receiving blood alone. Animals that were untreated generally died or sustained irreversible organic damage. In addition, the researchers often found that restoration of blood pressure to or toward normal would be associated with an improved outcome. Among other ramifications, the results of these studies led to the concurrent standard treatment of wounded soldiers in Vietnam by battlefield medics. Eventually, with the development of modern emergency medical services (EMS) and paramedic programs, this treatment was transferred to the streets of the United States and other western societies by the 1970s.

Almost simultaneously, the PASG was developed as a modification of the jet aviator G-suit.[7,10,14] Recognizing its well studied effect of inducing increased peripheral vascular resistance, the PASG was designed to help with normalization of blood pressure in the face of post-traumatic hypotension.[9,23,24] It also had the theoretical advantage of providing a potential tamponading effect for underlying injuries with active bleeding.[15] By the 1980s, the PASG and aggressive IV fluid resuscitation had become standard of care for all trauma patients with signs or symptoms of hemorrhagic shock.[1-5,16]

Special Rationale for the PASG

The main rationale for the PASG is that it functions as a noninvasive device that can elevate systemic arterial blood pressure (SABP) by increasing peripheral vascular resistance.[13,24] It also has been suggested that the PASG may provide a tamponade effect that could curtail bleeding from sites underlying the inflated garment.[15] Although different in physical design, previous experimental models of circumferential wraps in small animals seemed to support this concept.[15]

Starting in 1970 reports began to tout the effectiveness of the PASG. However, many of these reports were based on small, non-randomized studies or anecdotal reports; most of these papers reported that patients sustaining post-traumatic hemorrhage would arrive at the hospital with elevated SABP levels after application of the PASG and, therefore, the patients were deemed to be in better condition.[20,23,25] The PASG became so widely accepted that by the 1980s the American College of Surgeons Committee on Trauma had made them a standard of care for trauma patients with signs or symptoms of shock and a SABP < 100 mm Hg, or *any* trauma patients with a SABP < 80 mm Hg.[1,2] Soon afterward, the PASG was required as standard ambulance equipment in two-thirds of the 50 U.S. states.[19,26]

Re-evaluation of the PASG

Although there was widespread empiric acceptance of the PASG by the mid-1980s, there still were no prospective studies that had ever proven scientifically the effectiveness of the PASG in terms of patient survival. The first prospective trials of the PASG conducted in Houston, actually indicated a potentially harmful effect. As compared with controls, patients with penetrating chest injuries, particularly those with penetrating cardiac injuries, had increased mortality with prehospital application of the PASG.[27-30] Potential explanations for this increased mortality were two-fold. One proposed cause was the time spent applying the PASG, delayed definitive surgical intervention.[31,32] Specifically, some studies found that it took two to three minutes longer at the scene to apply the PASG.[30,33] The second potential explanation for increased mortality was that the increased peripheral vascular resistance from the PASG further compromised cardiac output in cases of cardiac tamponade.[29,33]

Along with the trends toward increased mortality rates, other complications from the PASG were reported. Compartment syndromes developed in previously normal lower extremities.[28,30] In addition, several investigators began to raise the issue that the increased blood pressures resulting from application of the PASG actually accelerated uncontrolled hemorrhage.[27,30]

Meta-Analysis of Clinical Studies of PASG

Cumulatively, a number of retrospective studies conducted in the late 1980s from the EMS systems of Denver and San Francisco, as well as further prospective trials from Houston, all indicated worse patient outcomes with use of the PASG.[30,33,34] After publication of these studies, leaders in the field collectively began to warn against the use of the PASG, particularly in patients with penetrating chest injuries.[28,30,35] The standard prehospital provider textbooks since the 1970s recommended against the use of PASG for head and chest wounds and recommended the device for abdominal and lower extremity bleeding.[5,36]

Results from the prospective clinical trials in Houston found no significant benefits of the PASG in patients with penetrating abdominal injuries.[27] Based on experimental studies, it had been hypothesized that patients with major vessel injury in the abdomen would benefit the most from the PASG through a tamponade effect.[15,25] In these clinical trials, however, patients with both arterial and venous major vascular injuries trended toward decreased survival. Specifically, when the subset of 104 patients with large vessel involvement (e.g., inferior vena cava, renal vein, hepatic artery) was examined, survival rates were 49% for the PASG group and 65% for the control group.[27] In contrast, survival rates for patients were approximately 90% for all patients with solid organ, abdominal wall, or bowel injuries, with or without PASG application. This trend reinforced the hypothesis that hemorrhage from a distinct vascular injury is exacerbated by elevations in SABP, and even if tamponade does occur, this potential benefit is outweighed by the detrimental effects.

Before accepting the results of these prospective and retrospective studies, there are some issues that must be considered. First of all, the prospective PASG trials generally included patients with penetrating truncal injuries, and they were conducted in urban systems with short transport times.[27-30] The authors themselves issued caution in terms of applying the results of these studies to more suburban or rural settings, or to patients with blunt injuries. Also, in most patient subsets, statistical power for "worse outcomes" was not achieved. However, the trends were usually apparent; more importantly, advantages to PASG use were not demonstrated.

Subsequently, a multi-center, retrospective review from New York failed to demonstrate significant improvements for patients with blunt injuries.[35] These researchers did suggest, however, that in a select subset of severely hypotensive patients (SABP <50 mm Hg), patients may benefit from prehospital application of the PASG, despite an average of five additional minutes spent on-scene in the group using the garment.[37] Nevertheless, these conclusions were drawn following selective retrospective data analysis. In addition, the accuracy of prehospital blood pressure measurements with such severely hypotensive patients may be suspect, therefore limiting the validity of the study findings. A 1995 prospective randomized trial of the PASG in blunt injury patients in Kansas demonstrated no advantage to its use.[38]

Explaining the Negative Effect of PASG

At first, the trends for worse outcomes in certain subsets of trauma patients were somewhat surprising. Intuitively, one would expect that a PASG trial would demonstrate either a beneficial effect or offer no benefit at all; a detrimental effect for penetrating abdominal injuries was not anticipated.[27] One explanation could be a flaw in the study design, but the prospective trials of PASG for penetrating abdominal injuries turned out to have well-matched control groups with regard to demographic data and severity of injuries. Aside from the unblinded nature of the trial, there also were neither problems with study compliance nor other confounding variables.[27]

More recently, other hypotheses have arisen. In addition to trends toward worse patient outcomes in some of the subgroups of patients who received the PASG, particularly those with major arteriovenous injuries, there were two other important differences between the control and PASG groups. Patients who received the PASG had on-scene times prolonged by a few minutes, presumably because of application of the garment. This additional time spent in the field could be important for moribund patients or in patients with cardiac injuries, but presumably not for all others.[31,39–41] However, the other difference between the PASG and control patients was a marked elevation in SABP among those patients who had prehospital PASG application.[27] The elevation in SABP was consistent with findings of the previous retrospective studies and of the intitial anecdotal reports that supported the widespread use of the device. Based on traditional wisdom, most clinicians might anticipate that elevation of blood pressure in the face of presumed hemorrhatgic shock would be of benefit, and would improve patient outcome.[1–3,8] Recent studies, however, may explain why higher blood pressures do not always translate into better patient outcomes.[42–49]

Rapid elevation of blood pressure and restoration of perfusion to the vital organs are believed by most clinicians and researchers to be beneficial *after* hemorrhage is controlled. However, there is growing evidence that elevation of blood pressure *before* achieving adequate hemostasis may be detrimental.[42–50] While the original animal studies that laid the groundwork for fluid resuscitation usually involved controlled hemorrhage models,[8,18,22,42–49] more current studies have examined the effects of raising blood pressure during uncontrolled hemorrhage. In these studies, treatment with IV fluids prior to control of hemorrhage resulted in increased mortality rates, especially if blood pressures were elevated beyond mean SABP > 40 mm Hg. Possible mechanisms responsible for worse outcomes include hydraulic acceleration of ongoing hemorrhage as a result of the elevated systemic blood pressure, mechanical dislodgement of active soft clot formation, and dilution of existing clotting factors from administration of large volumes of IV fluids.[42] Clinical research has supported this

hypothesis. A large, prospective, controlled clinical trial comparing immediate prehospital and emergency department (ED) IV fluid resuscitation with fluid resuscitation delayed until arrival in the operating room was conducted in Houston in the early 1990s.[50] Patients in the immediate resuscitation group had higher mortality rates, along with higher rates of postoperative complications, compared with patients in the delayed resuscitation group. The study concluded that rapid administration of IV fluids prior to control of hemorrhage resulted in worse outcomes. One could speculate a similar result with the PASG, particularly when considering the clear discrepancies observed between vascular injuries versus solid organ injuries discussed previously.

Current Recommendations for the PASG

To summarize the previous sections, despite the elevation of the systemic arterial pressure with prehospital application of the PASG, the garment appears to increase mortality, particularly in patients with penetrating injuries. Thus, the device generally is not recommended for patients with gunshot or stab wounds. In addition, no clear evidence exists for their use in blunt injury cases at this time. Some EMS systems recommend the use of the PASG as a pneumatic splint for suspected pelvic fractures that might pose a risk of life-threatening hemorrhage if left unstabilized.[51–54] Again, no clear evidence exists for this use and circumferential wraps may work just as well, with fewer accompanying complications.[53–59]

Some authors have recommended multiple other EMS applications for the PASG including use for aortic aneurysms and anaphylaxis.[52,54] In fact, in one review, the authors attempted to categorize PASG use in terms of levels of evidence for multiple circumstances including cardiac arrest and paraplegia.[54] Nevertheless, the conclusions were strained by a general lack of data; some supportive conclusions drawn in that analysis subsequently received critical reviews.[59]

Summary

There exist few reasons to support the PASG, at least as currently designed. The concept of circumferential wraps for stabilizing pelvic fractures or even for tamponade effect may still be valid, but remains generally unproven. Still open minds should not shut the door, however. Further research is indicated and, as usual, the sound medical judgment of the responsible, accountable EMS medical director should be held as the last word in every EMS sytstem.

References

1. American College of Surgeons Committee on Trauma. *Advanced Life Support (ATLS) Course.* Chicago: American College of Surgeons; 1981:17.

2. American College of Surgeons, Committee on Trauma. *Advanced Trauma Life Support Program for Physicians: Instructor Manual.* Chicago: American College of Surgeons; 1984:189–191, 201–203.

3. Shock. In: American College of Surgeons' Committee on Trauma. *Advanced Trauma Life Support Program for Physicians: Instructor Manual.* Chicago: American College of Surgeons; 1993:75–110.

4. Fowler RL. Shock. In: Campbell JE, ed. *Basic Trauma Life Support: Advanced Prehospital Care.* 2nd ed. Englewood Cliffs, NJ: Prentice-Hall; 1988:107–119.

5. Caroline NL. *Emergency Care in the Streets.* 2nd ed. Boston: Little, Brown; 1983:57.

6. Buchman TG, Menker JB, Lipsett PA. Strategies for trauma resuscitation. *Surg Gynecol Obstet.* 1991;172:8–12

7. Cutler BS, Daggett WM. Application of the G-suit to the control of hemorrhage in massive trauma. *Ann Surg.* 1971;173:511–514.

8. Dillon J, Lynch Q Jr, Myers R, et al. A bioassay of treatment of hemorrhagic shock. *Arch Surg.* 1966;93:537–555.

9. Gaffney FR, Thal ER, Taylor WR, et al. Hemodynamic effect of medical anti-shock trousers (MAST garment). *J Trauma.* 1981;21:931–937.

10. Gardner WJ, Storer J. The use of the G-suit in control of intra-abdominal bleeding. *Surg Gynecol Obstet.* 1966; 123:792–798.

11. Gold MS, Russo J, Tissot M, et al. Comparison of betastarch to albumin for perioperative bleeding in patients undergoing abdominal aortic aneurysm surgery. *Ann Surg.* 1990;211:482.

12. Griswold JA, Anglin BL, Love RT, et al. Hypertonic saline resuscitation: efficacy in a community based burn unit. *South Med J.* 1991;84:692.

13. Kaback KR, Sanders AB, Meislin HW. MAST suit update. *JAMA.* 1984;252:2598–2603

14. Kaplan BH. Emergency autotransfusion by medical pneumatic trouser: Disclosure of invention, logbook entry 21. Ft. Rucker, AL US Army Aeromedical Research Unit, 1971.

15. Ludewig RM, Wangensteen SL. Aortic bleeding and the effect of external counterpressure. *Surg Gynecol Obstet.* 1969;128:252–259.

16. McSwain NE. Pneumatic trousers and the management of shock. *J Trauma.* 1977;17:719–726.

17. Munsch CM, MacIntyre E, Machin SJ, et al. Hydroxyethyl starch: an alternative to plasma for postoperative volume expansion after cardiac surgery. *Br J Surg.* 1988; 75:675.

18. Shires T, Coln D, Carrico J, et al. Fluid therapy in hemorrhagic shock. *Arch Surg.* 1964;88:688–693.

19. Trunkey DD, Lewis FR: Current Therapy of Trauma 1984–85. Philadelphia, BC Decker, 1984, p 1.

20. Wayne MA, MacDonald SC. Clinical evaluation of the antishock trouser: retrospective analysis of five years of experience. *Ann Emerg Med.* 1983;12:342–347.

21. Westfal RE. *Paramedic Protocols.* New York: McGraw-Hill; 1997:86–108.

22. Wiggers Q. *Physiology of Shock.* New York: Commonwealth Fund; 1950:121–146.

23. Civetta JM, Nussenfeld SR, Rowe TR, et al. Prehospital use of the military antishock trouser (MAST). *J Am Coll Emerg Phys.* 1976;5:581–587.

24. Niemann JT, Stapczynski JS, Rosborough JP, et al. Hemodynamic effects of pneumatic external counter pressure in canine hemorrhagic shock. *Ann Emerg Med.* 1983;12:661–667.

25. LiIja GP, Batalden DJ, Adams BE, et al. Value of the counterpressure suite (MAST) in prehospital care. *Minn Med.* 1975;58:540–543.

26. Texas Department of Health: *9 Tex. Reg. 2823* (1984). Codified at 25 Tex Administration (ODE & 157.68).

27. Bickell WH, Pepe PE, Bailey ML, et al. Randomized trial of pneumatic antishock garments in the prehospital management of penetrating abdominal injuries. *Ann Emerg Med.* 1987;16:653–658.

28. Pepe PE, Bass RR, Mattox KL. Clinical trials of the pneumatic antishock garment in the urban prehospital setting. *Ann Emerg Med.* 1986;15:1407–1410.

29. Pepe PE, Wyatt CH, Bickell WH, et al. Use of MAST in penetrating cardiac injuries. *Chest.* 1986;89:452.

30. Mattox KL, Bickell WH, Pepe PE, et al. Prospective MAST study in 9-1-1 patients. *J Trauma.* 1989;29: 1104–1112.

31. Gervin AS, Fischer RF. The importance of prompt transport in salvage of patients with penetrating heart wounds. *J Trauma.* 1982;22:443–448.

32. Ivatury RR, Nallathambi MN, Roberge RJ, et al. Penetrating thoracic injuries: In-field stabilization vs. prompt transport. *J Trauma.* 1987;27:1066–1073.

33. Honigman B, Lowenstein SR, Moore EE, et al. The role of the pneumatic antishock garment in penetrating cardiac wounds. *JAMA.* 1991;266:2398–2401.

34. MacKersie RC, Christensen JM, Lewis FR. The prehospital use of external counter-pressure: does MAST make a difference? *J Trauma.* 1984;24:882–888.

35. Berendt BM, Van Niewerburgh P. Survival not improved by MAST use in ITEC trauma registry. *The ITEC Newsletter.* 1991;16:6.

36. Caroline WL. *Emergency Care in the Streets.* 1st ed. Boston: Little-Brown 1979.

37. Cayten CG, Berendt BM, Byrne DW, et al. A study of pneumatic antishock garments in severely hypotensive patients. *J Trauma.* 1993;34:728–735.

38. Chanf FC, Harrison PB, Beech RR, Helmer SD. PASG: does it help in the management of traumatic shock? *J Trauma.* 1995;39(3):453–456.

39. Copass MK, Oreskovich MR, Blaedogroen MR, et al. Prehospital cardiopulmonary resuscitation of the critically injured patient. *Am J Surg.* 1984;148:20–24.

40. Durham LA, Richardson RJ, Wall MJ, et al. Emergency center thoracotomy: Impact of prehospital resuscitation. *J Trauma*. 1992;32:775–779.

41. Karcj SB, Lewis T, Young S, Ho CH. Surgical delays and outcomes in patients treated with pneumatic antishock garments: a population-based study. *Am J Emerg Med*. 1995;13:401–404.

42. Bickell WH, Bruttig SP, Millnarnow GA, et al. Use of hypertonic saline/dextran versus lactated Ringer's solution as a resuscitation fluid after uncontrolled aortic hemorrhage in anesthetized swine. *Ann Emerg Med*. 1992;21:1077–1085.

43. Bickell WH, Bruttig SP, Millnarnow GA, et al. The detrimental effects of intravenous crystalloid after aortotomy in swine. *Surgery*. 1991;110:529–536.

44. Bickell WH, Shaftan GW, Mattox KL. Intravenous fluid administration and uncontrolled hemorrhage (editorial). *J Trauma*. 1989;29:401.

45. Capone A, Safar P, Stezoski W, et al: Improved outcome with fluid restriction in treatment of uncontrolled hemorrhagic shock. *J Am Coll Surg*. 1995;180:49–56.

46. Gross D, Landau EH, Assalia A, et al. Is hypertonic saline resuscitation safe in uncontrolled hemorrhagic shock? *J Trauma*. 1988;28:751–756.

47. Kowalenko T, Stem S. Dronen S, et al: Improved outcome with hypotensive resuscitation of uncontrolled hemorrhagic shock in a swine model. *J Trauma*. 1992;33:349–353.

48. Stem SA, Dronen SC, Birrer P, et al. Effect of blood pressure on hemorrhage volume and survival in a near-fatal hemorrhage model incorporating a vascular injury. *Ann Emerg Med*. 1993;22:155–163.

49. Stem SA, Dronen SC, Wang X. Multiple resuscitation regimens in a near fatal porcine aortic injury hemorrhage model. *Acad Emerg Med*. 1995;2:89–97.

50. Bickell WH, Wall MJ Jr, Pepe PF, et al. Immediate versus delayed fluid resuscitation for hypotensive patients with penetrating torso injuries. *N Engl J Med*. 1994;331:1105–1109.

51. Bruining HA, Eeftinck SM, De Vries JE, et al. Clinical experience with the medical anti-shock trousers (MAST) treatment of hemorrhage, especially from compound pelvic fracture. *Neth J Surg*. 1980;32;102–107.

52. Domier RM, O'Connor RE, Delbridge TR, et al. Use of the pneumatic antishock garment (PASG). *Prehosp Emerg Care*. 1997;1:32–35.

53. Fowler RL, Pepe PE, Lewis RJ. Shock evaluation and management. In: Campbell JE, ed. *Basic Trauma Life Support*. 3rd ed. Upper Saddle River, NJ: Prentice-Hall; 1995:111–124.

54. O'Connor RE, Domeier RM. An evaluation of the pneumatic antishock garment (PASG) in various clinical settins. *Pre Emerg Care*. 1977;1:36–41.

55. Pepe PE, Maio RF. Evolving challenges in prehospital trauma services. *Prehosp Disast Med*. 1993;8:25–34.

56. Ali J, Qu W. Fluid Electrolyte deficit with prolonged pneumatic antishock garment application. *J Trauma*. 1995;38(4):612–615.

57. Hauswald M. Misquotation on PASG. *Prehosp Emerg Care* 1997;1(4):297–298.

58. Connolly B, Gerlinger T, Pitcher JD. Complete masking of a severe open-book pelvic fracture by a pneumatic antishock garment. *J Trauma*. 1999;46(2):340–342.

59. Salvucci AA, Koenig KL, Stratton SJ. The pneumatic antishock garment (PASG): can we really recommend it? *Prehosp Emerg Care*. 1998;2(1):86–87.

60. Clancy MJ. Pneumatic anti-shock garment—does it have a future? *J Accid Emerg Med*. 1995;12(2):123–125.

C H A P T E R

Automated Defibrillators

47

James M. Atkins, MD

Introduction

The development of sophisticated microprocessors allowed the development of automated defibrillators which can either be implanted permanently or used as external devices similar to a standard defibrillator. The implanted forms are called automatic internal cardiovertors (AICD). Initially, the AICD had a battery/circuitry box in the abdominal wall; however, advances have markedly reduced the size and now they are often implanted under the skin near the clavicle. These devices will give a limited number of shocks. If a patient has an AICD in place, the prehospital personnel should treat the patient like any other patient, including defibrillation if needed. The only concern with the AICD is to assure that the defibrillator electrodes are at least 2 to 4 inches away from the battery/circuitry box. If an AICD should discharge while someone is touching the patient, the person might feel a small jolt, but this should not cause harm. The focus of this chapter will be on the external form of automated external defibrillators (AED), commonly called automatic external defibrillators.

Background

There has been a renewed emphasis on early defibrillation over the past several years. The 1986 American Heart Association (AHA) guidelines on cardiac resuscitation gave emphasis to the importance of time to defibrillation as a key determinate of success in resuscitation of individuals having suffered a cardiac arrest;[1] this importance was reemphasized in the 1992 AHA guidelines.[2] The 2000 AHA guidelines moved early defibrillation to the forefront by extending the use of the devices by non-traditional rescue medical personnel.[3]

The importance of early defibrillation has been emphasized in a number of publications.[1-15] Initially, early defibrillation only was performed by paramedics, nurses, or physicians. However, there were extreme logistical problems in the rapid delivery of defibrillation because of the limited number of these personnel in the prehospital environment. Both in King County, Washington, and Iowa, it was shown that EMT-B trained personnel could perform defibrillation with a minimum amount of additional training.[16-23] As there were 40 times as many EMT-Bs in the United States as paramedics, this allowed an expansion of the concept of early defibrillation. With the availability of AEDs the concept can be further expanded. Recently, the AHA has greatly enhanced the roles of AEDs.[24]

The AHA defined three levels of providers of AEDs. Level I providers include all of the trained BLS responders; this group includes EMT-Bs, police, firefighters, security personnel, airline flight attendants, and other first responder groups that are organized for response in public places. Level II responders include citizens at worksites or in other public places. Level III responders are families and friends of high-risk patients. There is scientific evidence supporting Level I responders; however, there is insufficient information about Level II and III responders. There is active investigation to evaluate the effectiveness of Level II and III responders.

There are training materials for automated external defibrillation in the AHA *Advanced Cardiac Life Support (ACLS) Provider Manual*, along with an instructor's guide and slides which include the concept of automated defibrillation.[15,25] The AHA has emphasized the chain of survival (fig. 47.1).[15] This chain includes four basic links: early access, early CPR, early defibrillation, and early advanced cardiac life support. Early access means prompt recognition of the problem and activation of EMS through 9-1-1. Early CPR encourages the bystander to perform CPR and recommends that first responders should also be-

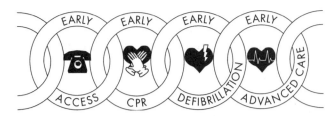

FIGURE 47.1. *The emergency cardiac care systems concept is displayed schematically by the "chain of survival" metaphor. (Adapted with permission from the American Heart Association.[14])*

gin CPR. Early defibrillation includes automated defibrillation by the first responders.

Automated external defibrillators have been shown to be an effective way of defibrillating patients.[16–23] Several systems have pointed out the critical nature of time in determining patient survival from cardiac arrest. In 1979 Eisenberg suggested that survival was 43% in *witnessed* cardiac arrests when CPR was begun within four minutes and defibrillation occurred within eight minutes; however, if CPR and defibrillation were delayed for 12 and 16 minutes respectively, survival was 0%.[26] Most unwitnessed arrests are not discovered for several minutes. For these reasons, witnessed cardiac arrests have a significantly better survival rate than unwitnessed cardiac arrests. The shorter the response time, the greater is the chance of long-term survival. In 1986 Weaver showed early defibrillation in ventricular fibrillation was an important determinant of success.[27] Long-term survival from ventricular fibrillation was related to response time of a team with a defibrillator. Long-term survival was 37% for a 1 to 3 minute response time, 31% for a 4 to 6 minute response, 23% for a 7 to 10 minute response, and 14% for a greater than 10 minute response for patients in witnessed ventricular fibrillation. Very few systems could achieve such response times; and those that did rarely obtained high successful survival rates. However, with these goals in mind, AEDs have been developed that can accurately analyze the rhythm, charge the device, and deliver a shock to the patient. These automated devices have been used in a number of studies with both EMT-Bs and first responders. Several studies have shown that, with a minimal amount of training (4 hours), patients can be reliably defibrillated with these devices.

Recently the importance of time has been accentuated. Early defibrillation by airline personnel has shown that people on aircraft and in terminals can be saved with the use of AEDs.[28,29] Impressive results were obtained in three other settings. Resuscitation in gambling casinos by security officers in two different studies have shown remarkable results. In multiple casinos in the study by Valenzuela, as well as an unpublished study in Canadian casinos, resuscitation rates of 70% have been achieved when the victim is defibrillated in the first 3 to 4 minutes after collapse.[30] The same 70% survival results have been achieved in the Chicago airports in an unpublished study. One interesting finding in the Chicago airport experience was that most of the rescuers were not the trained security personnel, but rather bystanders who generally had some type of medical background. Thus, very high survival rates can be achieved in witnessed arrests in public places when there is equipment and trained personnel present.

Devices

There are several different variations of AEDs available. Some are fully automatic. When the "on" button is pressed the device will analyze the EKG, arm itself, shock, and then reanalyze and repeat the sequence if indicated. Other devices have additional features, making them more operator-dependent. Semi-automatic defibrillators have an "analysis button" that starts the process. The machine will then have a visual or auditory signal suggesting the patient be shocked. The operator then presses a "shock" button to defibrillate the patient. These latter machines are usually called semi-automatic or shock advisory types of automated defibrillators. Some devices also have the ability to change the energy delivered by pressing a button, while others do this automatically. Most new devices have programmed energy levels with an "on" button, an "analysis" button, and a "shock" button.

All of these devices have paste-on electrodes that must be applied before use. The device is turned on and then the electrodes are attached. The device will then check the electrode resistance. If the electrodes are not making good contact, the device will give a visual or verbal signal to check the electrodes, and the machine will be disabled from analyzing or shocking the patient until the electrodes are making satisfactory contact. Some devices will also look for variations in resistance due to patient movement or breathing; these devices will not activate if there are major variations in resistance.

Once the machine has checked the electrode contact, the EKG will be analyzed. The machines can reliably tell the difference between medium to coarse ventricular fibrillation and other cardiac rhythms. Once the machine has determined ventricular fibrillation, the defibrillator will be armed or charged. After charging the defibrillator, some older machines will automatically discharge, while newer devices will give a visual or verbal signal to press a button to shock.

Algorithms can be programmed into some AEDs; for example, some will automatically shock using an algorithm chosen by the medical director such as first shock 200J, second shock 200J, third and subsequent shocks 360J. Newer devices are usually biphasic instead of using the older monophasic defibrillation wave. Some biphasic machines deliver far less energy, but are equally successful in defibrillating victims. The machines will either record the timing of events and EKG strips continuously, or simply before and after the defibrillation. The reliability of the machines is very high; they are more reliable at determining ventricular fibrillation than most human operators. Human operators may not always shock the patient in ventricular fibrillation, or may delay shocking because they are unsure. Human operators occasionally shock artifacts. Studies in the past have shown that 10% of shocks by human operators are improper, due to misinterpretation of information. The reliability of automated defibrillators is greater than 96%.[16-23]

These devices have been shown to increase resuscitation rates in both rural and urban areas. The King County data and the Iowa data have shown improvement in resuscitation rates after introduction of AEDs.[16-22] In Dallas, the resuscitation rates in some fire districts tripled, to greater than 10% survival for all cardiac arrests and greater than 21% for ventricular fibrillation patients.[31]

The cost effectiveness in various applications varies with the number of potential victims for which a device is intended and the age of the potential victims. A device placed in a small office might never be used, although it can be argued that it provides protection in case an event occurs. Placing AEDs in public places can have a dramatic effect; however, 80 to 85% of cardiac arrests occur at home.

Other applications may prove more cost-effective, such as on a first responding fire engine. The physician director should look at the potential use of the device and the estimated expected survival rates.[16-23] For example, in a given community the ambulance takes seven minutes to get to an area of town, while the fire engine arrives in 3.5 minutes. This area averages nine cardiac arrests/year. Using the data from Seattle and King County, if paramedic ambulance defibrillation only were used, the expected survival would be one patient/year. The expected survival, if first responder defibrillation were used, would be two patients. Hence, an automated defibrillation program would be expected to save one additional life per year. Since the devices will be used over seven years, the cost per year would be $500, and the incremental cost of such a program would be $500 per life saved. Presumably, this would be a cost-effective program. In another scenario, a similar area has a cardiac arrest every seven years. That would mean that an additional life would be saved every 63 years. The cost of such a program might be $31,500 per life saved. And even that calculation does not consider ongoing educational costs or liability costs; although such costs appear to be minimal in most systems.

It may be cost-effective to place these types of devices in shopping malls, security offices, and non-nursing types of elderly care facilities. However, the costs of training and supervision, issues of medical oversight, liability, and cost-effectiveness must be determined before these types of programs are begun.

Medical Oversight

If a program appears to be feasible and has the financial support of the host agency, the physician director must carefully plan how medical oversight will be provided. Medical oversight normally has two elements: direct and indirect. Direct medical oversight by radio, telephone, or physician presence is not necessary with these devices. The device is making the decision; therefore, the physician cannot see how the device is making that decision and cannot reasonably determine whether or not to override the decision. Thus, comprehensive prospective and retrospective indirect medical oversight must be established.

Prospective indirect medical oversight starts with legislation. The use of these devices is controlled or restricted in many states by the various medical practice acts. The physician must comply with these laws. In most, if not all states, the laws have been changed to cover these devices, thanks in part to the lobbying efforts of the AHA. Once the legislative and/or regulatory authorizations are understood, the physician director must ensure that the proposed plan is in accordance with those laws and/or regulations.

The physician director must look at policies, procedures, and protocols. Automated defibrillator programs must have rigid protocols and policies in place. These devices must be used only in patients with a cardiac arrest. The safety of the device can be improved by making sure the device is only attached after it has been determined that there is a cardiac arrest. The protocols must consider all potential outcomes. For example, the patient may be defibrillated after the first, second, or third shock. The protocol must address what should be done in each eventuality. The protocols and procedures must address what is to happen if the device recommends no shock. If an error message is given by the machine, then the protocol must address how to handle the problem. Therefore, great care must be given in developing the protocol. If the personnel using the automated defibrillator turn over care to a different set of personnel for transport, policies must be in place for how these two teams interface. Weigel has performed a thorough study of automatic defibrillator policies.[31]

Other major areas of prospective indirect medical oversight are training and certification. The physician director must be actively involved in setting up the training and the certification of the personnel using the device. While these devices are very simple to use, the important lessons to learn are safety and the fact that errors can be made. Safety must be a major portion of the training. To ensure that the device does not inappropriately shock someone with a perfusing rhythm, the operator must understand that the device is never to be used except in a cardiac arrest. The other major area of safety is to make sure that no one is touching the patient or anything that can conduct electricity from the patient, such as metal or water. Since the devices are very quick, the operator must insure that everyone is clear before the device is activated. The operator also must insure that everyone stays clear until the device has finished the cycle and is in a safe mode.

The major difference between traditional protocols for defibrillation and AEDs in ventricular fibrillation algorithms is the pulse check. There are no pulse checks between shocks with an AED (fig. 47.2). During defibrillation with a manual defibrillator, the electrodes may come loose, causing an artifact to appear on the screen that can be misinterpreted as ventricular fibrillation. With an AED, analysis will not begin if the electrodes are loose and an error message will be given. A second reason not to perform pulse checks between shocks is that AEDs may recharge and shock a second time within five; it is possible that a person doing a pulse check might get shocked. Another major difference with automated defibrillators is that shocks are given in stacks of three shocks. Figure 47.2 contains the AHA recommended algorithm for use of an AED.[15] A sample course outline is also provided in the AHA instructors guide.[26]

Training should address all of the potential outcomes that can occur and also should teach all of the problems that can arise. These devices give error messages, such as "check electrodes," "tape inoperative," "no memory module" or "maintenance required." The student must learn the appropriate actions to respond to each of these warnings or error messages. Once the training is complete, the students must be certified in accordance with the state laws and regulations. Retraining is also needed. If the device is not used within three months, a one-hour refresher inservice improves performance.

Retrospective review is the other major area of indirect medical oversight. Retrospective indirect medical control includes review of the prehospital care report (PCR), review of the voice and EKG recordings, and statistical review. The PCR can give the important times involved. The primary goal is to have the patient defibrillated as quickly as possible. The secondary goal is to deliver the first three shocks within one minute, if appropriate. Therefore, the PCRs need to be reviewed to see what time delays occurred and to determine if the time delays were appropriate. Sometimes there are logical and acceptable reasons for delays, such as the patient could not be found or the patient did not have an arrest until the team had been on site for a period of time.

Review of voice and EKG tapes is another important method of retrospective indirect medical control. Safety and timing can be determined from the memory cartridge. The time delays may be quite different from what was reported on the PCR. Figure 47.3 shows an automated form of a PCR. Reasons for time delays may be determined by listening to what was actually happening. Safety also can be analyzed. For example, if cardiopulmonary resuscitation is identified on the EKG or voice tapes while the automated defibrillator is in an analysis, charging, or defibrillation mode, the team clearly needs re-education. These logs also can determine whether the device did its job appropriately. Rarely does the tape or module find a device error; frequently they find an operator error.

VENTRICULAR FIBRILLATION AND PULSELESS VENTRICULAR TACHYCARDIA[14]

**Arrest Witnessed by
Emergency Personnel**

↓

Check pulse—If no pulse

↓

Precordial thump

↓

Check pulse—If no pulse

**Arrest Before Arrival
of Emergency Personnel
(Unwitnessed)**

↓

Check pulse—If no pulse

↓

CPR until AED attached*

↓

Press analyze
Defibrillate, 200 J or energy recommended by manufacturer

↓

Press analyze
Defibrillate, 200–300 J or energy recommended by manufacturer

↓

Press analyze
Defibrillate, up to 360 J or energy recommended by manufacturer

↓

CPR × 1 minute, if no pulse

↓

Press analyze
Defibrillate, up to 360 J or energy recommended by manufacturer

↓

Press analyze
Defibrillate, up to 360 J or energy recommended by manufacturer

↓

Press analyze
Defibrillate, up to 360 J or energy recommended by manufacturer

↓

CPR × 1 minute, if no pulse

↓

Repeat set of three stacked shocks with up to 360 J or
energy recommended by manufacturer

↓

CPR × 1 minute, if no pulse

*The single rescuer with an AED should verify unresponsiveness, open the airway (A), give two respirations (B), and check the pulse (C). If a full cardiac arrest is confirmed, the rescuer should attach the AED and proceed with the algorithm.

If "no shock indicated" appears, check pulse, repeat 1 minute of CPR, and then reanalyze. After three "no shock indicated" messages are received, repeat analyze period every 1–2 minutes.

Pulse check is not required after shocks 1, 2, 4, and 5 unless the "no shock indicated" message appears.

If ventricular fibrillation recurs after transiently converting (rather than persists without converting), restart the treatment algorithm from the top.

In the unlikely event that ventricular fibrillation persists after nine shocks, then repeat sets of three stacked shocks, with 1 minute of CPR between each set.

FIGURE 47.2. *Algorithm protocol for using an automated defibrillator in ventricular fibrillation and pulseless ventricular tachycardia. (Adapted with permission from the American Heart Association.[14])*

HEART *AID 1000 RUN REPORT

User data

Date: _____ Arrival time: _____

Provider service: _____

Patient age: _____ Sex _____

Cardiac arrest etiology: _____ Cardiac _____ Non-cardiac

User name(s): _____

– –

Event summary

Time:	Status:
22:09:58	HEART*AID ON
22:10:03	ASSESSING
22:10:09	ASSESSING/CHARGING
22:10:17	SHOCK #1 - 200 J
22:10:21	ASSESSING
22:10:27	ASSESSING/CHARGING
22:10:35	SHOCK #2 - 200 J
22:10:35	MONITORING
22:11:35	MONITORING

Incident data

Date: 10-0   Start time: 22:09:58
Serial no.:   Alarm status:

22:10:03

22:10:09   ASSESSING/CHARGING

22:10:15   SHOCK #1 - 200 J

22:10:21   ASSESSING

22:10:27   ASSESSING/CHARGING

22:10:33   SHOCK #2 - 200 J

22:10:55   MONITORING

FIGURE 47.3. *Sample of an automated patient case record from the memory module of a Heart*Aid 1000 defibrillator. (Adapted with permission from Weigel, et al.* Automated Defibrillation.[26])

Statistical records are another key area of retrospective analysis. It is essential that the medical director knows whether the program is doing an acceptable job as compared to what other programs are doing nationally. Only by comparing local statistics to national statistics can the local program improve. All programs can be improved; it is the statistical comparisons that demonstrate how.

A method of periodically checking the AED is needed; this periodic check will vary depending on the type of device, the battery, and the frequency of use of the device. Devices that are used frequently should have daily or shift checks. Figure 47.4 illustrates a check form that was developed by the Food and Drug Administration.

Summary

An early defibrillation program with AEDs can greatly improve the survival from cardiac arrest. In

Operator's Shift Checklist for Automated Defibrillators

Date: _____ Mfr/Model no.: _____ Location: _____

Serial no. or Facility ID no.: _____

DIRECTIONS: At the beginning of each shift, inspect the unit carefully. If problems are noted, place an "R" (to refer to the "Remarks/Corrective Action" section) in the correct column. Note any problems or corrective action taken. Sign the form.

	1st Shift	2nd Shift	3rd Shift	Remarks/Corrective Actions
1. Defibrillator unit				
a. Clean, no spills, clear of objects on top				
2. Defibrillator pads				

a. Set of two present?
   b. Package sealed and ready for use?
   c. Expiration date appropriate?				

3. Cables				

a. Inspect for cracks, frays, broken wire
     (1) Defibrillator-to-pads cables
     (2) Defibrillator monitor leads, if applicable
     (3) Defibrillator-to-charger cables				

4. Supplies				

a. Carrying case
   b. Cassette tape
   c. Monitoring electrodes
   d. Alcohol wipes
   e. Razors
   f. Spare pads
   g. ECG paper
   h. Spare battery
   i. Manual override key
   j. Memory module, event card plus spare				

5. Battery				

a. Plugged into live outlet
   b. Spare batteries charging
   c. Full charge checked				

6. Indicators				

a. Monitor working
   b. Energy select working
   c. Charge light working
   d. Power-on display working
   e. Tape recorder working
   f. Memory module in/out
   g. Audible alarms: disconnected cables, charging, shock				

7. Charge/Display cycle				

a. Unit detects connected and disconnected electrodes
   b. Unit detects, charges, and delivers shock for "VF" x 3
   c. Unit increases energy level for 3rd shock
   d. Unit responds appropriately to non-shockable rhythms
   e. Manual override capability operable				

Directions: Please check the appropriate box below after each use of the checklist.				
1. No action required				
2. Minor problem(s) corrected				
3. Disposable supplies replaced				
4. Major problem(s) identified (OUT OF SERVICE)				

Signatures: ¹ _____ ² _____ ³ _____

FIGURE 47.4. *Sample of an operator's checklist for checking an automated defibrillator. (Adapted with permission from the Defibrillator Working Group of the Center for Devices and Radiological Health, Food and Drug Administration.)*

order to be effective, it must be well planned, with effective medical oversight. The AHA has recommended that every ambulance should be equipped with a defibrillator, and that the personnel should be trained to perform defibrillation.[2] Scotland has recognized the importance of early defibrillation by placing an AED on every ambulance; and they have reported improved survival.[32] Both the AHA and the National Heart, Lung, and Blood Institute National Heart Attack Alert Program have recommended the widespread availability of AEDs; this recommendation should become a reality.[2,33]

References

1. AHA Standards and guidelines for cardiopulmonary resuscitation and emergency cardiac care. *JAMA.* 1986;255:2841–3044.
2. AHA Adult advanced cardiac life support. *JAMA.* 1992;268:2199–2241.
3. Guidelines 2000 for cardiopulmonary resuscitation and emergency cardiovascular care. *Circulation.* 2000;102 (suppl I):1–384.
4. Atkins JM. Emergency medical service systems in acute cardiac care: State of the art. *Circulation.* 1986;74(suppl IV):4–8.
5. Cummins RO, Eisenberg MS, Stults KR. Automated external defibrillators: clinical issues for cardiology. *Circulation.* 1986;73:381–385.
6. White RD. EMT defibrillation: time for controlled implementation of effective treatment. *American Heart Association Cardiac Care National Faculty Newsletter.* 1986;8:1–3.
7. Atkins JM, Murphy D, Allison EJ Jr, Graves JR. Toward earlier defibrillation. *Emerg Med Serv.* 1986;11:70.
8. Eisenberg MS, Cummins RO. Defibrillation performed by the emergency medical technician. *Circulation.* 1986; 74(suppl IV):9–12.
9. Cummins RO. EMT defibrillation: national guidelines for implementation. *A J Emerg Med.* 1987;5:254–257.
10. Ruskin JN. Automatic external defibrillators and sudden cardiac death (editorial). *N Engl J Med.* 1988;319:713–715.
11. Cummins RO, Eisenberg MS. EMT defibrillation: a proven concept. *American Heart Association Emergency Cardiac Care National Faculty Newsletter.* 1984;1:1–3.
12. Cummins RO, Eisenberg MS, Moore JE, et al. Automatic external defibrillators: clinic, training, psychological, and public health issues. *Ann Emerg Med.* 1985; 14;755–760.
13. Newman MM. National EMT-D study. *J Emerg Med Serv.* 1986;11:70–72.
14. Newman MM. The survival advantage: early defibrillation programs in the fire service. *J Emerg Med Serv.* 1987;12:20–46.
15. Anderson M, Atkins JM, Austin D, et al. Automated external defibrillation. In: *Textbook of Advanced Cardiac Life Support.* Dallas, Texas: American Heart Association; 1990:287–299. (Included in copies of the textbook published after 1990 as well as a supplement available from the American Heart Association.)
16. Stults KR, Brown DD, Schug CL, et al. Prehospital defibrillation performed by emergency medical technicians in rural communities. *N Eng J Med.* 1984;310: 219–233.
17. Eisenberg MS, Copass MK, Hallstrom AP, et al. Treatment of out-of-hospital cardiac arrest with rapid defibrillation by emergency medical technicians. *N Engl J Med.* 1980;302:1379–1383.
18. Weaver WD, Copass MK, Bufi D, et al. Improved neurologic recovery and survival after early defibrillation. *Circulation.* 1984;69:943–948.
19. Eisenberg MS, Hallstrom AP, Copass MK, et al. Treatment of ventricular fibrillation: emergency medical technician defibrillation and paramedic services. *JAMA.* 1984;251:1723–1726.
20. Ornato JP, McNeill SE, Craren EJ, et al. Limitation on effectiveness of rapid defibrillation by emergency medical technicians in a rural setting. *Ann Emerg Med.* 1984; 13:1096–1099.
21. Stults KR. Planning, implementing and evaluating a successful EMT-D program. In: *EMT-D: Prehospital Defibrillation.* Bowie, MD: Brady Communications; 1985: 123–131.
22. Cummins RO, Eisenberg MS, Bergner L, et al. Sensitivity, accuracy, and safety of an automatic external defibrillator: report of a field evaluation. *Lancet.* 1984;11:318–320.
23. Cummins RO, Eisenberg MS, Bergner L, et al. Automatic external defibrillation: evaluations of its role in the home and in emergency medical services. *Ann Emerg Med.* 1984;13(2):798–801.
24. The automated external defibrillator: key link in the chain of survival. In: Guidelines 2000 for cardiopulmonary resuscitation and emergency cardiovascular care. *Circulation.* 2000;102(suppl I):60–76.
25. Cummins RO, ed. *ACLS Provider Manual.* Dallas: AHA; 2001.
26. Eisenberg MS, Bergner L, Hallstrom A. Cardiac resuscitation in the community: importance of rapid provision and implications for program planning. *JAMA.* 1979; 241:1905–1907.
27. Weaver WD, Cobb LA, Hallstrom AP, et al. Factors influencing survival after out-of-hospital cardiac arrest. *J Am Coll Cardiol.* 1986;7:752–757.
28. O'Rourke MS, Donaldson E, Geddes JS. An airline cardiac arrest program. *Circulation.* 1997;96:2849–2853.
29. Page RL, Joglar JA, Kowal RC, et al. Use of automated external defibrillators by a U.S. airline. *N Engl J Med.* 2000;343:1210–1216.
30. Valenzuela TD, Roe DJ, Nichol G, et al. Outcomes of rapid defibrillation by security officers after cardiac arrest in casinos. *N Engl J Med.* 2000;343:1206–1209.

31. Weigel A, Atkins JM, Taylor J. *Automated Defibrillation.* Englewood, CO: Morton Publishing; 1988.

32. Cobbe SM, Redmond MJ, Watson JM, et al. "Heartstart Scotland": initial experience of a national scheme for out of hospital defibrillation. *British Med J.* 1991:302:1517–1520.

33. *Proceedings of the National Heart, Lung, and Blood Institute Symposium on Rapid Identification and Treatment of Acute Myocardial Infarction, Issues and Answers.* National Heart, Lung, and Blood Institute, U. S. Department of Health and Human Services, Public Health Service, National Institutes of Health. 1991:1–157.

48

Pediatric

George L. Foltin, MD
Arthur Cooper, MD

Introduction

Modern EMS evolved in the 1970s because of the recognition in the 1960s that (1) trauma and sudden cardiac emergencies were the leading causes of death in this nation, and (2) largely volunteer, fire company-based rescue squads were not, by themselves, optimally prepared to meet this challenge. The physicians who first created EMS were trained chiefly in the adult-oriented specialties of surgery, internal medicine, cardiology, and anesthesiology.[1] Infants and children were cared for in the EMS system, but their needs were not specifically addressed, and deficiencies in their care were not recognized.[2] Yet pediatric patients comprise some 5% to 10% of prehospital transports, 30% of emergency department visits, 21% of all prehospital trauma care, and 12% of all in-hospital trauma care.[3]

Although EMS did not develop with a focus on the special needs of infants and children, the healthcare system, in its entirety, certainly did. Children's hospitals—specialized centers of excellence in pediatrics dedicated to the tertiary care of children with infectious, metabolic, and developmental diseases, cancer, congenital anomalies, and major injuries—have existed in this nation for well over a century. The current emphasis on such critical care of serious childhood illness, however, has led to increasing reliance on transport of sick and injured children to these centers, particularly in urban environments where access to primary care is shrinking.[4] Moreover, there is growing recognition that trauma, especially preventable injury, is the leading public health problem for children.[5] Together with the development of emergency medicine as a distinct specialty and pediatric emergency medicine as a distinct subspecialties, each with approved recognized residency and fellowship training programs and board certifications that have undeniably improved the quality of pediatric emergency care, and the increased emphasis on pediatric trauma care by trauma surgeons and pediatric surgeons, both in practice and during training, these factors fostered the development of Emergency Medical Services for Children (EMSC) in many parts of this country, which, in turn, led to major federal initiatives in EMSC, including legislation and funding, systematic analysis of the nation's strengths and weaknesses in EMSC by the Institute of Medicine (IOM), and development of specific plans to remedy the weaknesses it identified.[6,7] The EMS medical director, therefore, should be aware of EMSC as a well established component of the system, including the need, the cost, the sources for funding, and directions for further improvement.

History

Government Discovers EMS

Before the 1960s, prehospital emergency care was neglected in the United States. Public policymakers were largely ignorant of the fact that systems of emergency care, perfected by military surgeons during World War II and the Korean Conflict, had proven capable of substantial reductions in the morbidity and mortality from traumatic injury. Despite a nearly threefold increase in hospital emergency department visits from the mid-1950s to the mid-1960s, and presumably (although no reliable figures exist) a concurrent increase in the number of ambulance runs, prehospital and in-hospital emergency services continued to be provided by individuals with little, if any, formal training in trauma or cardiac care. Although professional organizations such as the American College of Surgeons and the American Academy of Orthopaedic Surgeons were beginning to address this problem, ambulances, when available, were rarely if ever properly equipped or staffed to handle even simple prehospital emergencies involving adults or children.

The revolutionary changes in EMS systems following the 1966 publication of the National Academy of Sciences (NAS) report, *Accidental Death and Disability: The Neglected Disease of Modern Society*, are now well known to the public, which has come to expect high quality prehospital emergency care as a basic health right.[8] What is rarely noted is that neither this landmark report nor the key legislative initiatives that resulted from it—the Highway Safety Act of 1966, the Emergency Medical Service Systems Act of 1973, and the Preventive Health and Health Services Block Grant Program of 1982 that ultimately replaced the EMS Systems Act—made special mention of the unique needs of infants and children in the emergency care system, even though neonatal care was regionalized under the EMS Systems Act. As late as 1986, reviews describing the enormous progress made in EMS during the past two decades failed to mention pediatrics as a specific component of EMS.[9]

EMS Discovers Pediatrics

Review of early efforts by EMS planners to address pediatrics reveals a well-meaning but inaccurate needs assessment. The special needs of infants and children were simply not appreciated. This is not to say that their needs were intentionally overlooked, since literature identifying that the epidemiology of prehospital problems in children is different from adults had not yet been published. However, this lack of knowledge gave rise to the false notion that children could be treated as little adults.

As a result, the original Department of Transportation (DOT) curriculum for "medical emergency technicians"—now called emergency medical technicians (EMTs)—did not accurately reflect the range of pediatric emergencies commonly encountered in the field, nor adequately emphasize the necessary skills.[10] Instead, the didactic pediatric component focused on illnesses and injuries that were irrelevant to field care, such as Reye's syndrome, and ignored many critical conditions that prehospital interventions could affect, such as respiratory distress and failure. Another area that most training programs lacked, and that many training programs still lack, is clinical time spent evaluating children in an emergency department or on a pediatric unit. Such "hands-on" experience allows the trainee to learn assessment of the pediatric patient from experienced child health professionals in appropriately child-centered environments.

Pediatrics Discovers EMS

The process of improving the pediatric components of systems was initiated at the local and state levels in various regions by interested members of the pediatric, surgical, and emergency medical communities during the late 1970s and early 1980s. In 1978 the pediatric community of Los Angeles noticed that EMS was not fully meeting the needs of children, and successfully lobbied for the formation of a multidisciplinary committee with representatives from regional pediatric organizations, the regional EMS agency, and the county health department. The committee developed guidelines for prehospital care of pediatric emergencies, a pediatric equipment list for prehospital care providers, a curriculum for the education of paramedics in pediatric emergencies, and a plan for integration of EMSC into the existing EMS system.[11] The Maryland Institute for Emergency Medical Service Systems (MIEMSS), a model for a successful and fully integrated EMS system, was one of the first systems to incorporate pediatric trauma specialty referral centers, leading other regions, notably Mobile, Alabama, New York, and Milwaukee,[12–15] to follow suit in incorporating EMSC in their systems through an integrated approach.

Recent literature describes the unique epidemiology of pediatric prehospital care and documents deficiencies in the approach to children in the accessing, education, equipping, and medical control of prehospital personnel.[11–14,16–23] Although the acuity level of pediatric prehospital problems is lower than that of adults—approximately 0.5% of transported children require tertiary care and 5% involve life-threatening or limb-threatening problems—children account for 5% to 10% of all ambulance runs.[24,25] The result is that the average provider rarely cares for critically ill or injured children, with the caveat that their pediatric skills are difficult to maintain. Although constant retraining could improve skill and knowledge retention, continuing education in prehospital pediatrics is not routinely available in many communities. Moreover, while much progress has been made in recent years—the addition of a substantial pediatric component in the 1994 revision of the DOT curriculum for original training of EMTs is perhaps the most notable example—appropriate protocols and equipment for pediatric prehospital care still do not exist in all communities, most often reflecting a lack of pediatric expertise in both direct and indirect medical oversight. It is therefore hardly surprising that prehospital providers and medical control physicians rate critical pediatric calls among their most stressful encounters.[26]

Government Discovers EMSC

Federal funding has been available for EMSC system development since 1985, through the EMSC Program of Department of Health and Human Services (DHHS). Projects were originally established in Alabama, California, New York, and Oregon to improve EMSC and integrate this care into existing EMS systems. Since that time, virtually all states and territories, and many medical schools, have received funding for EMSC. The EMSC projects have developed strategies, programs, and resources that are shared nationally and have provided expertise and outreach for surrounding states and regions through knowledge transfer and utilization (KTU) programs and cooperative ventures.[27,28] In 1991 national EMSC resource centers were established in Torrance, California (The National EMSC Resource Alliance, or NERA) and Washington, DC (The EMSC National Resource Center, or NRC), vastly increasing access by the rest of the nation to educational material, recent advances and expertise in medicine, legislation, and data collection. In 1993, the Institute of Medicine (IOM) published its landmark report, *Emergency Medical Services for Children*, which has served as the blueprint for national EMSC system development since that time.[6]

The current program is administered jointly by the Maternal and Child Health Bureau (MCHB) of the Health Resources and Services Administration (HRSA) and the EMS Division of the DOT National Highway Traffic Safety Administration (NHTSA), with the assistance of the EMSC National Resource Center (NRC) at the Children's National Medical Center in Washington, DC, and the National EMSC Data Analysis and Research Center (NEDARC) at the Primary Children's Hospital in Salt Lake City, Utah. EMSC consists of six phases of care and contains several of the elements addressed in the EMS Systems Act of 1973; however, it encompasses the entire spectrum of care for the child requiring emergency services and exists within the established EMS system. These phases of care may reside in one or more of the multiple independent agencies that comprise the EMS system. Since the previous edition of this text, the program has been expanded to embrace a wide variety of projects designed and competitively selected to enhance the efficacy of each of these six phases of emergency care (tables 48.1 and 48.2).

System Development

Improved outcome from prehospital intervention following cardiac arrest is an EMS success for adults, but not for children.[29] It has been suggested that because cardiac arrest is rare in pediatrics, a more appropriate benchmark of success in the prehospital care of critically ill and injured children is intervention in prearrest respiratory failure and shock situations.[14] Bystander cardiopulmonary resuscitation (CPR) and prehospital intervention have proved effective in pediatric near-drowning and foreign body aspiration.[18,30] There is also evidence suggesting the importance of prehospital care in pediatric trauma management, as 80% of childhood injury deaths occur before admission to the hospital, while EMS agencies are involved in the vast majority.[3,31]

TABLE 48.1

EMS Component	EMSC Phase
Manpower	Prevention
Training	System Access
Communications	Field Treatment
Transportation	Emergency
Facilities	Department
Critical Care Units	Treatment
Public Safety Agencies	Inpatient Treatment
Consumer Participation	Rehabilitation
Access to Care	
Patient Transfer	
Coordinated Patient Record-Keeping	
Public Information and Education	
Review and Evaluation	
Disaster Plan	
Mutual Aid	

TABLE 48.2

Projects Supported by Federal EMSC Program

EMSC National Resource Center (NRC)

National EMSC Data Analysis and Resource Center (NEDARC)

Partnership grants with all interested states and territories

Partnership grants with stakeholder organizations in EMSC

Targeted grants addressing specific issues in EMSC

Research network grants supporting multicenter trials in EMSC

Prevention and Access

Emergency and intensive care for critically ill and injured children are expensive in terms of personal anguish and societal cost.[32] Prevention has the best outcome and costs far less. The link between communities and EMS agencies can be strengthened by developing, improving, and supporting successful injury and illness prevention programs.[33] Prehospital providers are ideally situated to provide support for such programs, based on their first-hand knowledge of the devastating effects that ensue when primary prevention efforts fail.[34]

Much attention has been paid in recent years to improving the chain of survival for pediatric patients.[35] Key among these are preparation of children's caregivers and environments, at home, at the day care center, at school, at the athletic field, and at the pediatrician's or family physician's office, for life-threatening pediatric emergencies.[36] Equally important is recognition of the importance of the medical home in providing anticipatory guidance for parents regarding bona fide pediatric emergencies. Parents can also be taught CPR, recognition of serious injury and illness, when to call for help, and what to do until help arrives.[37]

Field Care

Models for field treatment of pediatric patients should be based on the epidemiology of childhood illness and injury, using outcome data to support the interventions performed. Cardiac disease is rare in children, and evidence does not demonstrate an improved survival that justifies the delay inherent in providing advanced life support (ALS) to children in the field, whether for status epilepticus, poisoning, or vascular instability from dehydration. This is not to suggest that children should be categorically denied ALS in the prehospital environment, or that on-scene decisions regarding the need for ALS are infrequently required, but rather that, as for the adult trauma patient, priorities must be established.[38] Thus, although the value of early prehospital intervention in pediatric patients is recognized, the majority of pediatric prehospital emergencies do not require ALS interventions—a fortuitous circumstance for children living in rural and frontier areas where ALS is not routinely available.

The majority of pediatric patients require only short-term interventions, and prehospital care, usually at a basic level, is a single, crucial link. Although an investment is clearly required for manpower and training, the cost of an inadequate pediatric EMS response is much higher for the society and the family.[20] Yet certain prehospital personnel—particularly those trained prior to 1994, when the revised EMT-Basic National Standard Cirriculum was first disseminated—still lack an adequate foundation in basic pediatric knowledge and skills, and few have sufficient exposure to critically ill and injured children to retain these capabilities over time.[17,19,39] Additionally, there are still some communities that have yet to acquire appropriate equipment for pediatric emergency care, despite the fact that a single ambulance can be outfitted for less than the cost of an automated external defibrillator.[40]

Systems in the process of developing their pediatric capabilities cannot expect field personnel to feel suddenly comfortable with pediatric patients. Rather, a system's pediatric capabilities evolve as field personnel gain experience with children. If EMS teachers impart a positive mindset, prehospital providers respond with an attitudinal change that persists even when technical skills do not. Constant reinforcement of pediatric skills, building on the similarity to adult skills while emphasizing the differences, is essential to this process, and a necessity for any system that plans to deliver appropriate pediatric care.

Modern EMS planning has evolved to the point that field care is initiated at the moment the caller makes contact with the dispatcher, through the use of pre-arrival instructions. Very little work has been done examining the provision of appropriate care for children by dispatchers either in their triage role of deciding level and urgency of response, or in their ability to provide pre-arrival instructions for pediatric emergencies. Anecdotal reports attest to successful outcomes in individual pediatric cases because of timely provision of pre-arrival instructions, but these "saves" obviously did not occur by chance.[41] The dispatchers involved had sufficient familiarity with CPR and airway clearing techniques to be able to describe them over the telephone to distraught and untrained caretakers and convince the callers that they could actually perform them.

Hospital Care: Emergency Services

Seidel and associates suggested in the early 1980s that the availability of a receiving hospital with expertise in pediatric care affects outcome as much as, if not more than, the quality of the prehospital care.[22] During these same years emergency physicians and pediatricians began to recognize that the education they had received in emergency pediatrics during residency training was inadequate.[42] These trends gave rise in the late 1980s and early 1990s to an increased emphasis on pediatrics in emergency departments nationwide, and led to the development not only of guidelines defining a minimum standard of pediatric care for hospital emergency departments by the American College of Emergency Physicians (ACEP), and the American Medical Association and the American Academy of Pediatrics, but also of postgraduate training and continuing education requirements in emergency pediatrics.[43,44] Experiments with voluntary consensus standards have also been successful in many locales, particularly southern California's Emergency Departments Approved for Pediatrics (EDAP) Program and New York City's 9-1-1 Receiving Hospitals System.[11,45]

Hospital Care: Critical Care and Trauma Centers

A statewide study in Oregon indicated that regionalization of care for critically ill and injured children can improve outcome, if these patients are properly triaged and quickly transferred to a tertiary center pediatric intensive care unit.[46] Population-based studies in New York, in Oregon, and in Pennsylvania showed that outcome is better among injured children cared for in trauma systems with pediatric expertise than in systems without such capability.[47–49] Review of the MIEMSS pediatric experience demonstrates that compliance with regionalization guidelines allows as many as 90% of children with potentially lethal injuries to be treated in a pediatric trauma center.[50] Still unresolved is the question of whether seriously injured children can be optimally managed in general or adult trauma centers, although preliminary observations suggest that if the responsible surgeons (1) are experienced in pediatric trauma care; (2) are committed to providing this care; and (3) practice in an environment where appropriate pediatric emergency, critical, and acute medical-surgical and nursing care services are readily available, outcome may be as good as in comparably staffed and equipped pediatric trauma centers.[51,52]

Systems Issues: Urban

Most large metropolitan areas possess adequate monetary and professional resources for pediatric prehos-

pital care. The chief obstacle to the development of EMSC in most cities was that their EMS systems developed without specific emphasis on pediatric illness and injury. Thus, it has sometimes been difficult for child advocates to convince the administrative and medical leaders of the systems to invest in EMSC, particularly if resources were scarce. However, in recent years, proficiency in management of pediatric prehospital emergencies has become the standard of care in this nation. Hence, EMSC now requires the same level of emphasis and resources as other branches of prehospital care with respect to education, equipment, medications, and direct and indirect medical control. Fortunately, urban environments are typically rich in pediatric resources, upon which the medical director can draw in supporting the pediatric components of a fully integrated EMS-EMSC system.

Systems Issues: Rural

Children who are injured or become suddenly ill in rural areas are among those least likely to benefit from an adequate EMS response because of the large, sparsely populated areas that rural systems must cover. The results of long distances, difficult environmental conditions, and rough terrain are often prolonged response and transport times. Life-threatening injuries occur infrequently at any given location in rural areas, but 70% of all highway fatalities occur on rural roads. Prehospital and hospital personnel working in rural settings manage children with injuries as serious as any in a regional trauma center, but far less frequently, and they are less likely to have adequate training in childhood emergencies—suggesting that special emphasis should be placed on continuing education in prehospital pediatrics, particularly in areas where ALS resources are scrace and aeromedical transport is not readily available.[53]

Medical Oversight

Every system has its strengths and weaknesses. The logical approach to system development is for the medical director to identify the latter and build upon the former. In this process, each component of the system is carefully reexamined, and its pediatric needs are fully assessed. Emphasis should be placed on basic skills, but the system should not deny any child advanced interventions if they are needed and can be provided.

Education and Training

Developing and maintaining the knowledge, skills, and attitudes necessary for pediatric resuscitation require no reorientation with respect to basic management principles, but do require reassurance that previously mastered adult knowledge and skills can be readily transferred to infants and children, provided that (1) differences in anatomy, physiology, disease spectrum, and patient assessment are understood; and (2) special pediatric resuscitation techniques that have been mastered are constantly reinforced. Numerous educational packages that meet these objectives have been developed under the auspices of the federal EMSC Grant Program, and are available through the EMSC National Resource Center.[28] Many locales have also adapted the American Heart Association and American Academy of Pediatrics Pediatric Advanced Life Support (PALS) course for prehospital ALS personnel, which was recently revised to include prehospital scenarios.[54] The American Academy of Pediatrics (AAP) has created the Pediatric Education for Prehospital Professionals (PEPP) course, in one- and two-day versions designed, respectively, for BLS and ALS personnel, based upon pilot programs originated by the California and Florida EMSC Projects.[55] The National Association of Emergency Medical Technicians (NAEMT) has done likewise through its Pediatric Prehospital Care PPC course.[56] Minimum standards for education and training of all prehospital emergency personnel, as defined by consensus Task Forces on Education and Training from the federal EMSC projects, are also available, and are now reflected not only in national standard curricula for prehospital providers, but also in national accreditation standards and national registration testing (tables 48.3 and 48.4).[20,57–62]

Courses that can be self-taught or separated into modules allow for wide dispersion of teaching materials. The latter approach has been successfully adopted by the PEPP course, the PPC course, and the New York State Pediatric Prehospital Care (PPCC) Course, which also was recently revised.[63] Greater use of telecommunications and computer technologies, such as the Internet, has also been advocated to permit the large number of rural providers in this nation to have access to training that traditionally has been centered at major teaching institutions. However, while such models of distance and distributive education may obviate the need for local instructors with respect to didactic education, local preceptors knowledgeable in pediatrics will still be required for laboratory, clinical, and field training, for all of which sophisticated instructor support resources have recently been developed.[64,65]

TABLE 48.3

Minimum Standards for BLS Education and Training in EMSC

Knowledge
  Anatomic and physiological differences
  Psychological and developmental issues
  Pediatric physical assessment
  Pediatric vital signs
  Spectrum of pediatric illness/injury requiring
    emergency care
  Principles of neonatal/pediatric resuscitation
  Recognition/management of pediatric respiratory
    distress/failure
  Recognition/management of pediatric shock/
    trauma
  Treatment of pediatric medical/surgical
    emergencies
      Burns
      Near-drowning
      Seizures
      Poisoning
  Recognition/reporting of child abuse
  Recognition/management of SIDS
  Critical incident stress debriefing
Skills
  Infant/child cardiopulmonary resuscitation
  Infant/child obstructed airway clearing maneuvers
  Infant/child airway/ventilatory management
  Pediatric vital signs determination
  Pediatric pneumatic anti-shock garment use
  Pediatric extrication and spine immobilization

TABLE 48.4

Minimum Standards for ALS Education and Training in EMSC

All of Table 48.3 plus . . .

Knowledge
  Need for endotracheal/nasogastric intubation in
    pediatrics
  Need for intravenous/intraosseus access in
    pediatrics
  Dosage/administration of drugs in pediatric
    emergencies
  Dosage/administration of fluid in pediatric
    emergencies
Skills
  Pediatric endotracheal/nasogastric intubation
  Pediatric intravenous/intraosseous access
  Pediatric defibrillation/cardioversion
  Pediatric needle thoracostomy/cricothyroidostomy

Direct Medical Oversight

Direct medical oversight may be provided by emergency medicine physicians, ideally those practicing at the pediatric ambulance receiving hospital. Large centralized systems may have a dedicated physician provide direct medical oversight for the entire system. In examining this component, medical directors must ensure that training of direct medical oversight physicians (DMOP) is sufficient to provide sophisticated medical input for field personnel caring for infants and children. Incorporating the knowledge of physicians who are knowledgeable in pediatric telephone triage and transport medicine, such as pediatric emergency medicine physicians and pediatric critical care physicians, proves especially useful in EMSC system development and operation. Finally, in developing protocols for direct medical oversight of pediatric emergencies, the crucial role of basic providers must not be neglected. The majority of prehospital medical care, particularly in rural areas, is provided by basic providers with the most limited pediatric experience and, therefore, the most acute need for medical guidance.

Indirect Medical Oversight

Because of the maturation of the specialty of emergency medicine and the subspecialty of pediatric emergency medicine, every medical director should expect at least one member of the local physician advisory council to have pediatric expertise. Ideally, this representative should be an emergency medicine physician or pediatrician with fellowship training and board certification in the subspecialty of pediatric emergency medicine. In New York City, this individual is an appointed representative from a citywide committee on EMSC. Such an arrangement ensures that pediatric implications of EMS protocols, procedures, policies, and planning are consistently addressed. It also provides a liaison to the pediatric community, which often has only a fragmentary understanding of the EMS system.

Evaluation and Treatment

Because of the infrequency of serious pediatric illnesses in the field and the unique presentations in comparison with adult illnesses, New York City pediatric BLS protocols have been developed for a core group of critical pediatric conditions, using directed assessments to facilitate timely interventions (table

48.5).[66] In the face of inadequate data to support prolonged scene time for pediatric prehospital interventions, several additional New York City ALS protocols were designed using an approach termed "conservative yet permissive (table 48.6)."[12,66] The approach is conservative in that maintenance of airway, breathing, and circulation; rapid transport to an appropriate facility; and keeping the child warm are the primary priorities. It is permissive in that paramedics have standing orders that allow intubation based on their judgment, if other methods of airway control, such as bag-valve-mask ventilation, are ineffective, with other paramedic interventions permitted either en route, or at the scene only if there is unavoidable transport delay.

Modification of this paradigm may be necessary where lengthy transport times are anticipated because of great distance from the field to the receiving hos-

TABLE 48.5
Regional Emergency Medical Advisory Committee of New York City
PEDIATRIC BASIC LIFE SUPPORT PREHOSPITAL TREATMENT PROTOCOLS
Care of the Newly Born Newly Born Resuscitation Pediatric Respiratory Distress/Failure Pediatric Obstructed Airway Pediatric Croup/Epiglottitis Pediatric Non-Traumatic Cardiac Arrest Pediatric Anaphylactic Reaction Pediatric Shock Child Abuse* Abandoned Infant*

*Covered under General Operating Procedures

TABLE 48.6
Regional Emergency Medical Advisory Committee of New York City
PEDIATRIC ADVANCED LIFE SUPPORT PREHOSPITAL TREATMENT PROTOCOLS
Newly Born Resuscitation Pediatric Respiratory Arrest Pediatric Obstructed Airway Pediatric Croup/Epiglottitis Pediatric Non-Traumatic Cardiac Arrest Pediatric Asthma Pediatric Anaphylaxis Pediatric Altered Mental Status Pediatric Status Epilepticus Pediatric Traumatic/Hypovolemic Shock Pediatric Traumatic/Hypovolemic Arrest

pital. Thus, when a long ambulance run is expected, investment of valuable time to further stabilize the patient before transport is more justifiable than when transport time is short. Yet the majority of prehospital providers in the nation are basic providers living in rural and frontier regions, while advanced providers are concentrated in the urban and suburban communities. Hence, protocols designed for remote areas may require intercept with sophisticated providers dispatched by helicopter, or specialized training in intermediate levels of care that permits providers with limited education in pediatrics to obtain definitive airway control and establish venous access before transport may be necessary. National model pediatric protocols, recently developed by the National Association of EMS Physicians (NAEMSP), will meet the needs of most regions for optimal prehospital pediatric care.[67] Systems that perform more sophisticated interventions on children have a responsibility to study the effects of their efforts, so that optimal pediatric approaches can be further developed.

Equipment and Medications

ACEP has published guidelines of minimum equipment needs for pediatric prehospital care at both basic and advanced levels.[68] The Task Force on Education and Training of the Federal EMSC Grant Program has also written guidelines, which were recently updated (tables 48.7 and 48.8).[69] Although medications required by children differ little from those needed by adults, drug dosages, for the most part, are determined on the basis of size. The use of color-coded tapes that key drug doses and equipment selection to body length has proved effective in the field, and is now standard equipment in most agencies.[70]

The actual cost of equipping systems for pediatric resuscitation is remarkably low. Because many services already have some of the equipment, meeting current recommended standards is relatively inexpensive. For systems that do not already have equipment, comparing the actual costs of obtaining this equipment with other fixed expenses may be illuminating.[40] As noted, a single vehicle can be fully outfitted for considerably less than the price of a single automated external defibrillator (AED).

Funding

There are approximately 25 million children seen in the emergency departments of the nation each year. In 1985, when the federal EMSC program began,

TABLE 48.7
Minimum Standards for Pediatric Equipment in BLS Ambulances
Pediatric stethoscope, infant/child attachments
Pediatric blood pressure cuffs, infant/child sizes
Disposable humidifier(s)
Pediatric simple/nonrebreathing oxygen masks, all sizes
Pediatric face masks, all sizes
Pediatric bag-valve devices, infant/child sizes
Pediatric airway adjuncts, all sizes
Pediatric suction catheters, all sizes
Pediatric Yankauer device
Pediatric extrication collars, all sizes
Pediatric extrication equipment (including infant car seat)
Pediatric limb splints, all sizes

TABLE 48.8
Minimum Standards for Pediatric Equipment in ALS Ambulances
All of the above, plus . . .
Pediatric endotracheal tubes, all sizes
Pediatric stylets, all sizes
Pediatric laryngoscope blades, all sizes
Pediatric Magill (Rovenstein) forceps
Pediatric intravenous catheters, all sizes
Pediatric intraosseous needles, all sizes
Pediatric nasograstric tubes, all sizes
Pediatric ECG electrodes
Pediatric defibrillator paddles, infant/child sizes
Pediatric dosage-packed medications/fluids
Pediatric dosage/volume wall chart
Mini-drip intravenous infusion sets

the cost for the emergency department care of children aged 0 to 14 years approximated $13.8 billion; from 1979 to 1987, there was a 25% increase in the number of children living in poverty, and from 1983 to 1988, there was a 13% decrease in the number of children with health insurance. Costs and the percentage of underinsured children has increased by half. Moreover, the death rate for children from preventable injuries is twice that of other industrialized countries, with a significant proportion due to violent crime.[71]

Certainly, public funds are best spent on prevention. However, when primary and secondary prevention fail, tertiary prevention, consisting of the prompt recognition of a pediatric emergency, a rapid response by trained emergency providers, and the early provision of definitive care, is necessary to avoid further deterioration. Few children actually require critical interventions at the scene or during transport, but all children with potentially life-threatening illnesses or injuries deserve an assessment sophisticated enough to determine the need for such interventions. Thus the question is whether to expect the same level of system performance for children as is expected for adults. If so, the marginal cost of preparing providers to meet the needs of infants and children is an investment worth many times the initial down payment. This is especially true in trauma, since the societal cost of a single childhood injury death estimated at $250,000 in 1986, when the most recent comprehensive study of injury costs in America was performed, has nearly doubled since that year.[72]

Controversies

Regionalization

Data now exist attesting to the efficacy of pediatric intensive care unit and pediatric trauma center care in improving the outcome of combined system trauma victims with severe closed head, torso, and multiple skeletal injuries,[46-48] and to a lesser extent, patients with life-threatening, non-traumatic illnesses. However, since few institutions possess the financial or professional resources to provide such a level of care to pediatric patients, the number of centers that provide care for either group of children is limited,[73] even in larger metropolitan areas where a full range of pediatric specialty services may be available at more than one institution. Nonetheless, referral of critically ill and injured children to centers providing comprehensive pediatric critical care is well established, and such children should undergo primary transport to these institutions wherever possible. However, because many seriously ill or injured pediatric patients are transported by parents or police, who may be unaware of differences among hospitals with respect to the level of pediatric expertise, every receiving hospital must be capable of initiating resuscitation and stabilization of children.

Many pediatric comprehensive care centers have established specialized teams for interfacility transport of critically ill and injured patients to their institutions that additionally provide a decisive advantage in an increasingly competitive medical marketplace. Yet pediatric interfacility transport is not risk-free, as adverse events such as plugged endotracheal tubes and loss of vascular access occur at nearly twice the rate during interfacility transport as in the pediatric intensive care unit, and ten times more frequently with non-specialized teams than with specialized teams.[74,75] At a minimum, transport providers must be capable of critical pediatric assessment and monitoring, and must be highly skilled in the techniques of pediatric endotracheal intubation and vascular access, as well as fluid and drug administration in critically ill and injured children.[76,77] Whenever possible, interfacility transport of such patients should be conducted by specialized pediatric transport teams staffed by physicians and nurses with special training in pediatric critical care treatment and transport.[78,79]

Triage Scores

Triage scores are potentially an important tool in pediatric prehospital care. However, to be useful, they must be valid, reliable, and practical.[80] Both the Trauma Score (TS) and Revised Trauma Score (RTS) have been used in the pediatric population as field trauma triage criteria.[81,82] Yet, neither of these scores is ideal, because both of them fail to account for the greater impact of severe closed-head injury in children on ultimate outcome. For this reason, the Pediatric Trauma Score (PTS) was developed, and has been prospectively validated for field use (table 48.9).[83-85]

The Pediatric Trauma Score appears to encourage safer triage practices, is acceptable for outcome assessment as well as field use, and carries the endorsement of the American College of Surgeons Committee on Trauma and the American Pediatric Surgical Asso-

TABLE 48.9			
PEDIATRIC TRAUMA SCORE	+2	+1	−1
Size (kg)	>20	10–20	<10
Airway	Normal	Maintained	Unmaintained
Systolic blood pressure (mm Hg)	>90	50–90	<50
Central nervous system	Awake	Obtunded	Coma
Open wound	None	Minor	Major
Skeletal trauma	None	Closed	Open-Multiple

ciation Trauma Committee.[86–88] However, the Pediatric Trauma Score has not consistently proven superior to other scores, particularly the Revised Trauma Score.[89,90] Moreover, it has been recently demonstrated that a Best Motor Response of 1 on the Glasgow Coma Scale, and a U (for Unresponsive) on the AVPU Score are more accurate predictors of mortality than any of the currently available triage scores.[91] Therefore, reliance on anatomic, physiologic, and mechanistic criteria for primary transport to a pediatric trauma center may prove to be equally useful (table 48.10).[92]

Airway Management

Endotracheal intubation is the accepted standard for the airway resuscitation of children in cardiopulmo-

---

TABLE 48.10

Indications for Transfer to a Pediatric Trauma Center

History of Injury
Patient thrown from a moving vehicle
Falls from > 15 feet
Extrication time > 20 minutes
Passenger cabin invaded > 12 inches
Death of another passenger
Accident in a hostile environment (heat, cold water)

Anatomic Injuries
Combined system injury
Penetrating injury of the groin or neck
Three or more long-bone fractures
Fractures of the axial skeleton
Amputation (other than digits)
Persistent hypotension
Severe head trauma
Maxillofacial or upper airway injury
CNS injury with prolonged loss of consciousness, posturing, or paralysis
Spinal cord injury with neurologic deficit
Unstable chest injury
Blunt or penetrating trauma to the chest or abdomen
Burns, flame, or inhalation

System Considerations
Necessary service or specialist not available
No beds available
Need for pediatric ICU care
Multiple casualties
Family request
Paramedic judgment
Severity scores
    Champion Trauma Score 12 or less
    Revised Trauma Score 11 or less
    Pediatric Trauma Score 8 or less

---

nary or respiratory failure or arrest and traumatic coma. Most ALS services nationwide have embraced prehospital pediatric endotracheal intubation for such critical patients and have developed educational programs designed to prepare ALS personnel to perform this intervention when necessary.[93] However, a recent, large, randomized, prospective study of prehospital pediatric endotracheal intubation failed to show a survival advantage for infants and children who were ventilated via an endotracheal tube placed by paramedics in the field versus those who were ventilated via bag and mask.[94] Moreover, subset analysis demonstrated a worse survival or neurological outcome for intubated patients with respiratory arrest, child maltreatment, and foreign body aspiration, and a slight trend toward a worse outcome in patients with severe head injury, although this latter result could not be confirmed by a retrospective study of the much larger experience reported to the National Pediatric Trauma Registry.[95]

One conclusion that could be reached from the above studies is that because prehospital pediatric endotracheal intubation appears to provide no survival advantage to critically ill or injured children, its role should be limited in rapid-transport urban EMS systems. However, although the prospective study described above was designed to compare prehospital pediatric endotracheal intubation, with which the subject paramedics had no prior experience, with prehospital pediatric bag-valve-mask ventilation, with which the subject paramedics had significant prior experience, the need for both interventions was infrequent enough that most of the paramedics involved had no opportunity to use either technique over the course of the study, raising troubling questions about the retention and application of these important skills in the out-of-hospital environment.[96] Therefore, other conclusions that could be reached from the above studies are either that endotracheal intubation and bag-valve-mask ventilation are skills that are both poorly retained and applied in the out-of-hospital environment, or that bag-valve-mask ventilation, when properly taught, reinforced, and applied, can obtain results that are comparable to those achieved by prehospital pediatric endotracheal intubation. In deciding which conclusions might apply to their own EMS systems, medical directors considering or reconsidering the use of prehospital pediatric endotracheal intubation must carefully weigh the advantages and disadvantages of the two approaches to airway management, particularly in terms of the far higher costs associated with training and retraining in prehospital pediatric endotracheal intubation versus the relatively infrequent need for its use.

Ventricular Tachydysrhythmias

Epidemiologic research in prehospital care has previously held that the incidence of ventricular tachydysrhythmias in the pediatric population is extremely low, representing no more than about 10% of all cases of pediatric nontraumatic cardiac arrest. However, recent evidence suggests that the true incidence may be double this number, up to 20%.[97] This evidence implies that the traditional emphasis on initial respiratory management in nontraumatic cardiac arrest may not be true for all pediatric patients. Therefore, novel strategies to address ventricular dysrhythmias in pediatric patients must be developed and applied, just as is the case for adult patients.

Both national consensus pediatric resuscitation guidelines[98] and the Food and Drug Administration (FDA) have historically recommended against use of the AED in young children, due to the lack of suitable pediatric devices. Although pediatric-capable AEDs are conceptually attractive, the faster and smaller waveforms observed in pediatric patients subjected to electrocardiographic (EKG) monitoring, until recently, had not been amenable to waveform analysis of sufficiently high sensitivity and specificity to support safe use of AEDs in children less than about eight years of age, or weighing less than approximately 25 kg nor had there been a commercially viable method of adapting adult defibrillators to deliver the low-energy shocks that are currently recommended for use in children. In 2001, a pediatric-capable AED that utilizes modified pediatric electrode pads and cables to deliver significantly lower doses of electricity (about 50 J) than are currently administered to adults (about 150 J) was marketed with the approval of the FDA, based in part upon new evidence that this device was able to detect normal and abnormal rhythms in pediatric EKGs with great accuracy, and treat them safely.[99,100] Population-based studies of pediatric cardiopulmonary arrest document a need for such a device, and preliminary data were clearly supportive enough of safe use of this new pediatric-AED capability to allow its endorsement by NAEMSP as well as the FDA. Because it has only recently been marketed, large scale clinical experience from which to measure the impact of this device on pediatric prehospital care and public access defibrilla-

tion (PAD) programs is not yet available. However, the growing recognition that ventricular tachydysrhythmias are not so rare in infants and children as once thought—coupled with the widespread publicity that has followed upon recent reports of commotio cordis in young athletes—suggests that their impact may well prove to be significant.[101,102]

Safe Transport

Ambulance patient transport involves both a different purpose and a different environment from automobile passenger transport. The ambulance patient compartment is open and large, contains numerous heavy pieces of equipment, and carries restrained patients and passengers and unrestrained providers in a wide variety of places and positions. However, in contrast to automobile passenger safety, formal standards are not yet developed regarding ambulance occupant protection. This unfortunate situation obtains despite the documented lethal hazards of ambulance crashes, which are ten times more common per passenger mile than automobile crashes.[103]

Yet, the risks associated with pediatric ambulance transport can be minimized through use of safe driving practices, and effective restraint of patients, passengers, providers, and equipment. Unfortunately, many commercially available restraint devices are ineffective, but are not known to be so because they have been subjected only to static testing at the laboratory bench rather than dynamic testing in a moving ambulance.[104] Fortunately, recent evidence suggests that safe restraint of a child occupant can be achieved through the use of a child safety seat when secured to the ambulance stretcher using two standard ambulance gurney belts.[105] Still, the most important step in ensuring safe transport of ill or injured pediatric patients is to ensure that all personnel, regularly follow the Do's and Don'ts recently promulgated by the NHTSA and the EMSC Program (table 48.11).[106]

Disaster Management

Disaster management in pediatrics remains in its infancy, judging from the dearth of published studies in this area prior to the late 1980s and early 1990s, when the first comprehensive reviews of pediatric disaster medicine appeared in the pediatric literature.[107–112] Review of the 1989 Avianca plane crash in Nassau County, NY, confirmed much of what little

TABLE 48.11

The Do's and Don'ts of Transporting Children in an Ambulance

DO drive cautiously at safe speeds observing traffic laws.

DO tightly secure all monitoring devices and other equipment.

DO ensure available restraint systems are used by EMTs and other occupants, including the patient.

DO transport children who are not patients, properly restrained, in an alternate passenger vehicle, whenever possible.

DO encourage utilization of the DOT NHTSA Emergency Vehicle Operator Course (EVOC), National Standard Curriculum.

DO NOT drive at unsafe high speeds with rapid acceleration, decelerations, and turns.

DO NOT leave monitoring devices and other equipment unsecured in moving EMS vehicles.

DO NOT allow parents, caregivers, EMTs, or other passengers to be unrestrained during transport.

DO NOT have the child/infant held in the parent's, caregiver's, or EMT's arms or lap during transport.

DO NOT allow emergency vehicles to be operated by persons who have not completed the DOT EVOC or equivalent.

---

was known, and provided valuable insight into the continuing state of ignorance. The Nassau County disaster plan, like all others nationwide even to the present, made no special provisions for triage and transport of critically injured children (PTS≤8) to appropriate facilities, and more than half were not taken to pediatric critical care or trauma centers. Moreover, scene was ineffective, transport times were extended, and field documentation of the extent and severity of pediatric injuries by the 50-some volunteer ambulance squads that participated was extremely poor.[113]

More recent literature has focused upon multiple casualty incidents resulting from motor vehicle crashes, natural disasters, and terrorist incidents. Bus accidents predominantly cause closed-head injuries, soft-tissue damage, and superficial lacerations, but may overwhelm local emergency departments unprepared to deal with such catastrophes.[114] Major hurricanes appear to result chiefly in open wounds, gastroenteritis, skin infections, and (to a lesser extent) hydrocarbon and bleach ingestions.[115,116] Building collapses following massive bomb explosions are associated with high fatality rates, due chiefly to lethal head and torso injuries as well as traumatic amputa-

tions.[117] This small but tragically growing experience has given rise to the development of thoughtful approaches to pediatric disaster planning efforts, as well as the dissemination of policy and practice guidelines from major professional organizations and experts in pediatric emergency and disaster medicine.[118-123] These trends will only intensify in the aftermath of the September 11, 2001 attacks on the World Trade Center in New York City and the Pentagon.

Legal Issues

Refusal of medical assistance (RMA) is one of the most vexing legal problems confronting the medical director. In situations that pose an immediate threat to life, the doctrine of implied consent is the basis for medical intervention, and supersedes other concerns.[124] In less urgent situations, only those individuals with full parental rights may decline to accept prehospital emergency medical care for a child once requested. However, in most jurisdictions the law protects emergency providers who proceed in good faith to render medical assistance to a child if they perceive a potential threat to life or limb, even when permission is denied by the child's legal guardian.

Somewhat less clear is the prehospital provider's responsibility in cases of potential child abuse, including medical neglect. The prehospital provider, of course, is obligated to treat and transport any child whose life or limb may be in jeopardy. If no such emergency exists, but abuse is believed likely, prehospital providers should request police assistance in consultation with a DMOP because, in most jurisdictions, peace officers are vested with the final responsibility for public intervention in private matters. Regardless of the outcome of any particular event, however, the provider is obligated to perform a brief visual survey of the immediate surroundings for evidence of abuse, in addition to the usual patient assessment, to carefully record all pertinent findings on the prehospital care report, to verbally transmit this information to the physician or nurse on duty at the hospital, and in states where legally mandated, to immediately report suspicious cases to duly constituted child protective officials or agencies. In cases of RMA, the provider must also communicate with other appropriate authorities, as well as the DMOP.

Presumption of Death

CPR is indicated when the emergency provider encounters an unresponsive, pulseless, apneic patient.

Prehospital providers often are permitted by protocol not to institute resuscitative measures in cases where there is rigor mortis, extreme dependent lividity, tissue decomposition, obvious mortal injury, or a properly executed Do Not Resuscitate order that conforms to the local laws. None of these is typically present in the death of a child. By contrast, the most common fatal illnesses encountered by prehospital providers in the field are sudden infant death syndrome and traumatic cardiac arrest following blunt injury.

It is well recognized that the outcome following unwitnessed asystolic cardiac arrest, the dysrhythmia universally associated with both the above conditions, is abysmal. This has led some authorities to suggest that neither time nor effort should be expended in attempting to resuscitate such children. Moreover, in some jurisdictions, sudden infant death calls are treated as potential crime scenes, precluding prehospital providers from touching or moving the victims. However, in both of the above situations, attempts at resuscitation of children are justified despite near certain futility. Distraught parents will know, at least, that everything possible was done to revive their young one. Similarly, distressed prehospital providers will be reassured that their failure to intervene did not contribute to the ultimate demise of the infant or child, thereby minimizing the psychic impact of the critical incident.

Summary

The recent successful projects to revise the EMT-B, First Responder, EMT-P, and EMT-I curricula had a strong pediatric focus. Pioneering EMS-EMSC systems have already examined intubation, intraosseous infusion, defibrillation, out-of-hospital pediatric cardiopulmonary arrest, and ability of dispatch operators to identify true pediatric emergencies.[15,94,97,125-132] There is evidence that resuscitation of children in the prehospital phase of care improves outcome. Separate works by Rivara and Quan demonstrate that control of the airway and provision of adequate ventilation are critical to survival of children suffering multiple trauma and near-drowning.[18,131]

Even so, more extensive studies are needed to determine which interventions will result in the most benefit for children in the prehospital setting. For example, intraosseous infusion has been suggested as a useful procedure in the prehospital phase of care to gain emergency vascular access to children. Studies demonstrate that this procedure can be used successfully in the prehospital setting.[126-129] However, studies demonstrating that intraosseous infusion improves outcome for children have not yet been performed.

The fact that EMSC is a new area of the EMS system makes it ideally suited to careful study. One must be careful not to deny advances in pediatric critical care, such as intraosseous infusion and automated external defibrillation, to children only because their value in the prehospital environment has not yet been unequivocally proven, because EMSC is still in the early stages. In these endeavors, the EMS medical director occupies the central role, when new treatments are developed and evaluated that ultimately may benefit adults, as well as children.

The promise EMSC holds as an integrating force for the EMS system as a whole may prove to be its most important future role. EMSC requires and typically commands the truly collegial participation of many providers from a broad range of medical, surgical, nursing, and prehospital disciplines. It cannot be separated from the system as a whole, and each component must work in concert with all other parts for the optimal outcome of the child and the family. In short, it is the ideal model for the comprehensive EMS and trauma care system envisioned by the EMS medical director.[35,132-134]

References

1. Boyd DR. The history of emergency medical services (EMS) systems in the United States of America. In: Boyd DR, Edlich RF, Micik S, eds. *Systems Approach to Emergency Medical Care.* Norwalk: Appleton and Company, 1983:1–82.
2. Cooper A, Barlow B, Davidson L, et al. Epidemiology of pediatric trauma: importance of population-based statistics. *J Pediatr Surg.* 1992;27:149–154.
3. Foltin G, Fuchs S. Advances in pediatric emergency medical service systems. *Emerg Med Clin N Am.* 1991; 9:459–474.
4. Knickman R, Smith D, Berry C. *Improving Ambulance Use in New York City: A Final Report.* New York: The Commonwealth Fund; 1989.
5. Ramenofsky ML. How can we address the differences in trauma versus illness systems? In: Haller JA, ed. *Emergency Medical Services for Children: Report of the Ninety-Seventh Ross Conference on Pediatric Research.* Columbus: Ross Laboratories; 1989: 51–57.
6. Committee on Pediatric Emergency Medical Services, Institute of Medicine, National Academy of Sciences; Durch JS, Lohr KN, eds. *Emergency Medical Services for Children.* Washington: National Academy Press; 1993.
7. EMSC five-year plan.

8. Committee on Trauma and Committee on Shock, Division of Medical Sciences, National Research Council, National Academy of Sciences. *Accidental Death and Disability: The Neglected Disease of Modern Society.* Washington: National Academy of Sciences; 1966.

9. Mustalish AC. Emergency medical services: twenty years of growth and development. *NY State J Med.* 1986;86:414–420.

10. U.S. Department of Transportation, National Highway Traffic Safety Administration. *Emergency Medical Technician: National Standard Curriculum.* 3rd ed. Washington: Department of Transportation; 1984.

11. Seidel JS. EMS-C in urban and rural areas: the California experience. In: Haller JA, ed. *Emergency Medical Services for Children: Report of the Ninety-Seventh Ross Conference on Pediatric Research.* Columbus. Ross Laboratories; 1989: 22–30.

12. Haller JA, Shorter N, Miller D, et al. Organization and function of a regional pediatric trauma center: does a system of management improve outcome? *J Trauma.* 1983;23:691–696.

13. Ramenofsky ML, Luterman A, Curreri PW, et al. EMS for pediatrics: optimum treatment or unnecessary delay? *J Pediatr Surg.* 1983;18:498–504.

14. Foltin G, Salomon M, Tunik M, et al. Developing pediatric pre-hospital advanced life support: the New York City experience. *Ped Emerg Care.* 1990;6:141–144.

15. Losek JD, Halim Hennes H, et al. Prehospital care of the pulseless, nonbreathing pediatric patient. *Am J Emerg Med.* 1987;5:370–375.

16. Anonymous. History of emergency medical services for children. In: Seidel JS, Henderson DP, eds. *Emergency Medical Services for Children: A Report to the Nation.* Washington: National Center for Education in Maternal and Child Health; 1991: 5–11.

17. Seidel JS, Hornbein M, Yoshiyama K, et al. Emergency medical services and the pediatric patient: are the needs being met? *Pediatrics.* 1984;73:769–772.

18. Quan L, Wentz WR, Gore EJ, et al. Outcome and predictors of outcome in pediatric submersion victims receiving prehospital care in King County, Washington. *Pediatrics.* 1990;86:586–593.

19. Seidel JS. Emergency medical services and the pediatric patient: are the needs being met? II. Training and equipping emergency medical services providers for pediatric emergencies. *Pediatrics.* 1986;78:808–812.

20. Anonymous. Education and training of professionals and the public. In: Seidel JS, Henderson DP, eds. *Emergency Medical Services for Children: A Report to the Nation.* Washington: National Center for Education in Maternal and Child Health; 1991: 49–62.

21. Luten R. Educational overview. In: Luten R, Foltin G, eds. *Pediatric Resources for Prehospital Care.* Elk Grove Village, IL: American Academy of Pediatrics Committee of the Section on Emergency Medicine; 1990: 16–24.

22. Seidel JS, Henderson DP, eds. *Prehospital Care of Pediatric Emergencies.* Los Angeles: Los Angeles Pediatric Society; 1987: 102–106.

23. National Highway Traffic Safety Administration. *Summary of Consensus Workshop on EMS Training Programs.* Washington: U.S. Department of Transportation; 1990.

24. Tsai A, Kallsen G. Epidemiology of pediatric prehospital care. *Ann Emerg Med.* 1987;16:284–292.

25. Seidel JS. The six T's of emergency medical services for children: triage, time, treatment, transportation, tertiary care, and training. In: Barkin RM, ed. Pediatrics in the emergency medical services system. *Ped Emerg Care.* 1990;6:72–77.

26. Cooper A, Foltin G. Pre-hospital personnel. In: Dieckmann RA, ed. *Planning and Managing Systems for Pediatric Emergency Care.* Baltimore: Williams and Wilkins; 1992: 333–342.

27. Luten R. Emergency medical services for children projects. In: Luten R, Foltin G, eds. *Pediatric Resources for Prehospital Care.* Elk Grove Village, IL: American Academy of Pediatrics Committee of the Section on Emergency Medicine; 1990: 71–76.

28. Human Interaction Research Institute. *Emergency Medical Services for Children Innovation Bank.* 3rd ed. Washington: National Center for Education in Maternal and Child Health, 1991.

29. Eisenberg MS, Bergner L, Hallstrom A. Cardiac resuscitation for the community: importance of rapid provision and program planning. *JAMA.* 1979;241:1905–1907.

30. Luten R. Access to optimal care. In: Luten R, Foltin G, eds. *Pediatric Resources for Prehospital Care.* Elk Grove Village, IL: American Academy of Pediatrics Committee of the Section on Emergency Medicine; 1990:1–15.

31. Gausche M, Seidel JS, Henderson DP, et al. Pediatric deaths and emergency medical services (EMS) in urban and rural areas. *Pediatr Emerg Care.* 1989;5:158–162.

32. Division of Injury Control, Centers for Disease Control. Childhood injuries in the United States. *Am J Dis Child.* 1990;144:627–644.

33. Barlow B. Building a safe community in transportation, traffic, safety, and health. In: Holst HV, Nygren A, Andersen AE, eds. *Proceedings of the Second International Conference, Brussels, Belgium, 1996.* Stockholm: Karolinska Institute; 1998:149–154.

34. Garrison HG, Foltin GL, Becker LR, et al. The role of emergency medical services in primary injury prevention. *Ann Emerg Med.* 1997;30:84–91.

35. Cooper A. The surgeon and EMSC. *Pediatrics.* 1995; 96:184–188.

36. Mansfield CJ, Price J, Frush KS, et al. Pediatric emergencies in the office: are family physicians as prepared as pediatricians? *J Family Pract.* 2001;50:757–761.

37. American Academy of Pediatrics Committee on Pediatric Emergency Medicine; Seidel JS, Knapp JF, eds. *Childhood Emergencies in the Office, Hospital, and Community,* 2d ed. Elk Grove Village, IL: American Academy of Pediatrics; 2000.

38. Foltin G, Pon S, Tunik M, et al. Pediatric ambulance utilization in a large American city: a systems analysis approach. *Pediatr Emerg Care.* 1998;14:254–258.

39. Simon JE. Current problems in the management of pediatric trauma. In: Haller JA, ed. *Emergency Medical Services for Children: Report of the Ninety-Seventh Ross Conference on Pediatric Research.* Columbus: Ross Laboratories; 1989: 11–15.

40. Cooper A, Welborn C, Foltin G, et al. Costs of equipping and training emergency personnel for pediatric resuscitation. *Ped Emerg Care.* 1991;7:385.

41. Marzulli J. EMS phone turned into lifeline: operator helped save baby. *New York Daily News,* December 6, 1991.

42. Ludwig S, Fleisher G, Henretig F, et al. Pediatric training in emergency medicine residency programs. *Ann Emerg Med.* 1982;11:170–173.

43. American College of Emergency Physicians: *Pediatric Equipment Guidelines.* Dallas: American College of Emergency Physicians; 1990.

44. Anonymous. Pediatric emergencies. In: American Medical Association Commission on Emergency Medical Services. *Guidelines for the Categorization of Hospital Emergency Capabilities.* Chicago: American Medical Association; 1989: 43–59. (Reprinted in *Pediatrics.* 1990;85:879–887.)

45. New York City 9-1-1 Receiving Hospitals Advisory Committee. *New York City 9-1-1 Receiving Hospitals Emergency Department Standards.* 5th ed (revised). New York: New York City Emergency Medical Services; 1991.

46. Pollack MM, Alexander SR, Clarke N, et al. Improved outcomes from tertiary center pediatric intensive care: a statewide comparison of tertiary and nontertiary care facilities. *Crit Care Med.* 1991;19:150–159.

47. Cooper A, Barlow B, DiScala C, et al. Efficacy of pediatric trauma care: results of a population-based study. *J Pediatr Surg.* 1993;28:299–305.

48. Hulka F, Mullins RJ, Mann NC, et al. Influence of a statewide trauma system on pediatric hospitalization and outcome. *J Trauma.* 1997;42:514–519.

49. Potoka DA, Schall LC, Gardner MJ, et al. Impact of pediatric trauma centers on mortality in a statewide system. *J Trauma.* 2000;49:237–245.

50. Marganitt B, MacKenzie EJ, Deshpande JK, et al. Children hospitalized for traumatic injuries in Maryland: statewide epidemiologic trends over 8 years. Presented at the Third Pediatric Critical Care Colloquium, Santa Monica, CA, October, 1989.

51. Knudson MM, Shagoury C, Lewis FR. Can adult trauma surgeons care for injured children? *J Trauma.* 1992;32:729–739.

52. Fortune JM, Sanchez J, Graca L, et al. A pediatric trauma center without a pediatric surgeon: a four-year outcome analysis. *J Trauma.* 1992;33:130–139.

53. National Highway Traffic Safety Administration. *EMS Services: Program Update.* Washington: U.S. Department of Transportation; 1989.

54. Zaritsky A, ed. *Textbook of Pediatric Advanced Life Support.* Dallas: American Heart Association, 2002.

55. Dieckmann R, Brownstein D, Gausche-Hill M, eds. *Pediatric Education for Prehospital Professionals.* Elk Grove Village, IL: American Academy of Pediatrics and Jones and Bartlett Publishers; 2000.

56. Markenson D, ed. *Pediatric Emergency Care.* Upper Saddle River, NJ: Prentice-Hall, Inc.; 2001.

57. Gausche M, Henderson DP, Brownstein D, et al. The education of out-of-hospital emergency medical personnel in pediatrics: report of a national task force. *Prehosp Emerg Care.* 1998;2:56–61.

58. United States Department of Transportation, National Highway Traffic Safety Administration. *Emergency Medical Technician-Basic: National Standard Curriculum.* Washington: United States Department of Transportation; 1994.

59. United States Department of Transportation, National Highway Traffic Safety Administration. *Emergency Medical Technician-Paramedic: National Standard Curriculum.* Washington: United States Department of Transportation; 1998.

60. United States Department of Transportation, National Highway Traffic Safety Administration: *Emergency Medical Technician-Intermediate: National Standard Curriculum.* Washington: United States Department of Transportation; 1998.

61. Commission on Accreditation of Allied Health Education Programs, Committee on Accreditation of Educational Programs for the Emergency Medical Services Professions. *Standards and Guidelines for Educational Programs for the Emergency Medical Services Professions.* Chicago and Beford: Commission on Accreditation of Allied Health Education Programs and Committee on Accreditation of Educational Programs for the Emergency Medical Services Professions; 2002.

62. Brown WE. Personal communication, January 22, 2002.

63. Fitton A, Cooper A, et al, eds. *Pre-hospital Pediatric Care Course Student Manual,* 2d ed. Albany: New York State Department of Health; 2002.

64. Foltin G, Tunik M, Cooper A, et al, eds. *Teaching Resource for Instructors of Prehospital Pediatrics.* New York: Center for Pediatric Emergency Medicine; 1998.

65. Foltin G, Tunik M, Cooper A, et al, eds. *Teaching Resource for Instructors of Prehospital Pediatrics, Advanced Life Support Edition.* New York: Center for Pediatric Emergency Medicine; 2002.

66. Bove J, Cooper A, et al, eds. *Regional Emergency Medical Advisory Committee of New York City Pre-hospital Basic and Advanced Life Support Treatment Protocols.* New York: Regional Emergency Medical Services Council of New York City, Inc.; 2001.

67. Mulligan-Smith D, O'Connor RE, Markenson D. EMSC Partnership for Children: National Association of EMS Physicians Model Pediatric Protocols. *Prehosp Emerg Care.* 2000;4:111–130.

68. Pediatric Emergency Medicine Committee and Emergency Medical Services Committee, American College of Emergency Physicians: *Minimum Pediatric Pre-hospital Equipment Guidelines.* Dallas: American College of Emergency Physicians; 1991.

69. Emergency Medical Services Education & Training Taskforce, Emergency Medical Services for Children Grant Program, Bureau of Maternal and Child Health Resources Development. *Summary of Education & Training Issues Survey Responses*. Rockville, MD: U.S. Department of Health and Human Services; 1988.

70. Luten RC, Seidel JS, Lubitz DS, et al. A rapid method for estimating resuscitation drug doses from length in the pediatric age group. *Ann Emerg Med*. 1988;17:576–581.

71. Anonymous. Financing emergency medical services for children: identifying resources. In: Seidel JS, Henderson DP, eds. *Emergency Medical Services for Children: A Report to the Nation*. Washington: National Center for Education in Maternal and Child Health; 1991: 143–154.

72. Rice DP, MacKenzie EJ, et al. *Cost of Injury in the United States: A Report to Congress*. Atlanta: Centers for Disease Control; 1989: 59.

73. Foltin G, Tunik M, Cooper A, et al. Regionalizing care for critically ill and injured children: coast to coast experience. Presented at the Annual Meeting of the Ambulatory Pediatric Association, Washington, DC, May, 1989.

74. Kanter RK, Boeing NM, Hannan WP, et al. Excess morbidity associated with interhospital transport. *Pediatrics*. 1992;90:893–898.

75. Edge WE, Kanter RK, Weigle CGM, et al. Reduction of morbidity in interhospital transport by specialized pediatric staff. *Crit Care Med*. 1994;22:1186–1191.

76. Smith DF, Hackel A. Selection criteria for pediatric critical care transport teams. *Crit Care Med*. 1983;11: 10–12.

77. MacNab AJ. Optimal escort for interhospital transport of pediatric emergencies. *J Trauma*. 1991;31:205–209.

78. American Academy of Pediatrics Committee on Hospital Care. Guidelines for air and ground transport of pediatric patients. *Pediatrics*. 1996;78:943–950.

79. Day S, McCloskey K, Orr R, et al. Pediatric interhospital critical care transport: consensus of a national leadership conference. *Pediatrics*. 1991;88:696–704.

80. Wesson DE, Spence LJ, Williams JI, et al. Injury scoring systems in children. *Can J Surg*. 1987;30:398–400.

81. Champion HR, Sacco WJ, Carnazzo AJ, et al. Trauma score. *Crit Care Med*. 1981;9:672–676.

82. Champion HR, Sacco WJ, Copes WS, et al. A revision of the trauma score. *J Trauma*. 1989;29:623–629.

83. Tepas JJ, Mollit DL, Talbert JL, et al. The pediatric trauma score as a predictor of injury severity in the injured child. *J Pediatr Surg*. 1987;22:14–18.

84. Ramenofsky ML, Ramenofsky MB, Jurkovich GJ, et al. The predictive validity of the pediatric trauma score. *J Trauma*. 1988;28:1038–1042.

85. Aprahamian C, Cattey RP, Walker AP, et al. Pediatric trauma score. *Arch Surg*. 1990;125:1128–1131.

86. Tepas JJ, Ramenofsky ML, Mollitt DL, et al. The pediatric trauma score as a predictor of injury severity: an objective assessment. *J Trauma*. 1988;28:425–429.

87. Anonymous. Pediatric trauma care. In: American College of Surgeons Committee on Trauma. *Resources for Optimal Care of the Injured Patient 1999*. Chicago: American College of Surgeons; 1999:39–42.

88. Harris BH, Barlow BA, Ballantine TV, et al. American Pediatric Surgical Association: principles of pediatric trauma care. *J Pediatr Surg*. 1992;27:423–426.

89. Kaufmann CR, Maier RM, Rivara RP, et al. Evaluation of the pediatric trauma score. *JAMA*. 1990;263:69–72.

90. Nayduch DA, Moylan J, Rutledge R, et al. Comparison of the ability of adult and pediatric trauma scores to predict pediatric outcome following major trauma. *J Trauma*. 1991;31:452–458.

91. Hannan E, Farrell L, Meaker P, et al. Predicting inpatient mortality for pediatric blunt trauma patients: a better alternative. *J Pediatr Surg*. 2000:35:155–159.

92. Anonymous. Prehospital trauma care. In: American College of Surgeons Committee on Trauma. *Resources for Optimal Care of the Injured Patient 1999*. Chicago: American College of Surgeons; 1999:13–17.

93. Stratton SJ, Underwood LA, Whalen SM, et al. Prehospital pediatric endotracheal intubation: a survey of the United States. *Prehosp Disast Med*. 1993;8:323–326.

94. Gausche M, Lewis RJ, Stratton SJ, et al. Effect of out-of-hospital pediatric endotracheal intubation on survival and neurological outcome: a controlled clinical trial. *JAMA*. 2000;283:783–790.

95. Cooper A, DiScala C, Foltin G, et al. Prehospital endotracheal intubation for severe head injury in children: a reappraisal. *Sem Pediatr Surg*. 2001;10:3–6.

96. Glaeser P. Out-of-hospital intubation of children. *JAMA*. 2000;283:797–798.

97. Moygazel C, Quan L, Graves JR, et al. Out-of-hospital ventricular fibrillation in children and adolescents: causes and outcomes. *Ann Emerg Med*. 1995;25:484–491.

98. American Heart Association Subcommittee on Pediatric Resuscitation. Part 10: pediatric advanced life support. In: American Heart Association Committee on Emergency Cardiovascular Care, in collaboration with the International Liaison Committee on Resuscitation. Guidelines 2000 for cardiopulmonary resuscitation and emergency cardiovascular care: international consensus on science. *Circulation*. 2000 (Suppl 1);102(8):I–291–I–342.

99. Gurnett CA, Atkins DL. Successful use of a biphasic waveform automated external defibrillator in a high-risk child. *Am J Cardiol*. 2000;86:1051–1053.

100. Cecchin F, Jorgenson DB, Berul CI, et al. Is arrhythmia detection by automatic external defibrillator accurate for children? *Circulation*. 2001;103:2483–2488.

101. Sirbaugh PE, Pepe PE, Shook JE, et al. A prospective, population-based study of the demographics, epidemiology, management and outcome of out-of-hospital pediatric cardiopulmonary arrest. *Ann Emerg Med*. 1999; 33:174–184.

102. Markenson DS. The use of automated external defibrillators in children. *Prehosp Emerg Care*. (in press).

103. Kahn CA, Pirrallo RG, Kuhn EM. Characteristics of fatal ambulance crashes in the United States: an 11-year retrospective. *Prehosp Emerg Care.* 2001;5;261–269.

104. Levick NR, Winston F, Aitken S, et al. Application of a dynamic testing procedure for ambulance pediatric restraint systems. *Soc Automotive Engineering Australasia.* 1998;58:45–51.

105. Levick NR, Li G, Yannaccone J. Biomechanics of the patient compartment of ambulance vehicles under crash conditions: testing countermeasures to mitigate injury. *Soc Automotive Engineering Australasia.* 2001;2001-01-73.

106. National Highway Traffic Safety Administration/Emergency Medical Services for Children/Health Resources and Services Administration. *Do's and Don'ts of Transporting Children in an Ambulance: Fact Sheet.* Washington: National Highway Traffic Safety Administration/ Emergency Medical Services for Children/Health Resources and Services Administration; 1999.

107. Stalcup SA, Oscherwitz M, Cohen MS, et al. Planning for a pediatric disaster—experience gained from caring for 1600 Vietnamese orphans. *N Engl J Med.* 1975; 293:691–695.

108. Myers GJ, Colgan MT, Van Dyke DH. Lightning-strike disaster among children. *JAMA.* 1977;238:1045–1046.

109. Irani SF, Mahashur AA. A survey of Bhopal children affected by methyl isocyanate gas. *J Postgrad Med.* 1986; 32:195–198.

110. Cyr C. Multivictim emergency care: a case study of organophosphate poisoning in 67 children. *J Emerg Nurs.* 1988;14:277–279.

111. Leonard RB. Role of pediatricians in disasters and mass casualty incidents. *Pediatr Emerg Care.* 1988;4:41–44.

112. Holbrook P. Pediatric disaster medicine. *Crit Care Clin.* 1991;7:463–470.

113. Van Amerongen R, Fine J, Tunik M, et al. System response to a disaster: the pediatric perspective. *Pediatrics.* 1993;92:105–110.

114. Wass AR, Williams MJ, Gibson MF. A review of the management of a major incident involving predominantly pediatric casualties. *Injury.* 1994;25:371–374.

115. Quinn B, Baker R, Pratt J, et al. Hurricane Andrew and a pediatric emergency department. *Ann Emerg Med.* 1994;23:737–741.

116. Damien F, Atkinson CC, et al. Disaster relief efforts after Hurricane Marilyn: a pediatric team's experience in St. Thomas. *J Emerg Nurs.* 1997;23:545–549.

117. Quintana DA, Jordan JB, Tuggle DW, et al. The spectrum of pediatric injuries after a bomb blast. *J Pediatr Surg.* 1997;32:307–311.

118. Carley SD, Mackway-Jones K, et al. Delphi study into planning for care of children in major incidents. *Arch Dis Child.* 1999;80:406–409.

119. Mackway-Jones K, Carley SD, et al. Planning for major incidents involving children by implementing a Delphi study. *Arch Dis Child.* 1999;80:410–413.

120. American Academy of Pediatrics Committee on Pediatric Emergency Medicine. The pediatrician's role in disaster preparedness. *Pediatrics.* 1997;99:130–133.

121. American Academy of Pediatrics Committee on Psychosocial Aspects of Child and Family Health. How pediatricians can respond to the psychosocial implications of disasters. *Pediatrics.* 1999;103:521–523.

122. American Academy of Pediatrics Committee on Environmental Health and Committee on Infectious Diseases. Chemical-biological terrorism and its impact on children: a subject review. *Pediatrics.* 2000;105:662–670.

123. Henretig F, Cieslak TJ. Medical progress: biological and chemical terrorism. *J Pediatr.* (in press).

124. Lazar RA. *EMS Law: A Guide for EMS Professionals.* Rockville, MD: Aspen Publications, 1989.

125. Pointer JE, et al. Clinical characteristics of paramedics' performance of pediatric endotracheal intubation. *Am J Emerg Med.* 1987;7:364–366.

126. Smith RJ, Keseg DP, Manley LK, et al. Intraosseous infusion by prehospital personnel in critically ill pediatric patients. *Ann Emerg Med.* 1988;17:491–495.

127. Miner WF, Corneli HM, Bolte RG, et al. Prehospital use of intraosseous infusion by paramedics. *Ped Emerg Care.* 1989;5:5–7.

128. Seigler RS, Tecklenburg FW, Shealy R. Prehospital intraosseous infusion by emergency service personnel: a prospective study. *Pediatrics.* 1989;84:173–177.

129. Fuchs S, LaCovey D, Paris P, et al. A prehospital model of intraosseous infusion. *Ann Emerg Med.* 1991;20: 371–374.

130. Losek JD, Hennes H, Glaeser O, et al. Prehospital countershock treatment of pediatric asystole. *Am J Emerg Med.* 1989;7:571–575.

131. Rivara FP, Maier MV, Mueller BA, et al. Evaluation of potentially preventable deaths among pedestrian and bicyclist fatalities. *JAMA.* 1989;261:566–570.

132. Ramenofsky ML. Emergency medical services for children and pediatric trauma system components. *J Pediatr Surg.* 1989;24:153–155.

133. Barkin R. The system and training. In: Barkin R, ed. Pediatrics in the emergency medical services system. *Ped Emerg Care.* 1990;6:72–77.

134. Haller JA. Toward a comprehensive emergency medical system for children. *Pediatrics.* 1990;86:120–122.

Geriatric

Héctor M. Alonso-Serra, MD, MPH

Introduction

I t is a well-known phenomenon that with the aging of "baby boomers" the United States population will see a dramatic increase of elder citizens. For the purpose of this chapter we will define the geriatric or elder population as those 65 years of age or older. We will define the "oldest-old" as those persons 85 years and over. In November 2000 the geriatric population was estimated to be close to 35 million, making up 12.6% of the total population of the United States. Current projections from the Census Bureau indicate that by the year 2025 this segment of the population will increase to over 62 million, making up 18.5%, which is a relative growth of 47%. Not only will older people be increasing in number and proportions, but they will also be living longer. Figures 49.1 and 49.2 allow a comparison of the population pyramid for the United States in the year 2000 with the projected pyramid for the year 2025.

One of the most worrisome implications of this rapid aging of the population is its impact on a fragile healthcare system. Of course, as part of this healthcare system, EMS will also have to adapt to

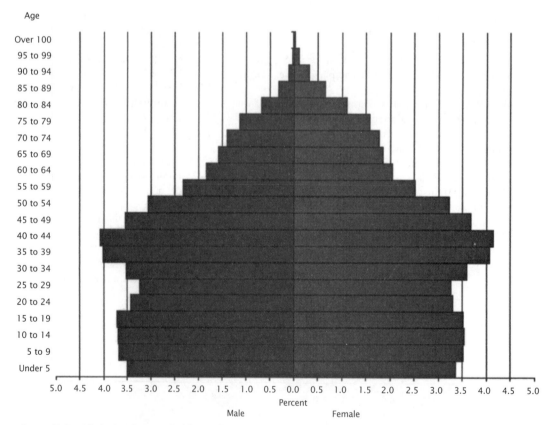

FIGURE 49.1. Resident Population of the United States as of July 1, 2000.

Source: National Projections Program, Population Division, U.S. Census Bureau, Washington, D. C. 20233

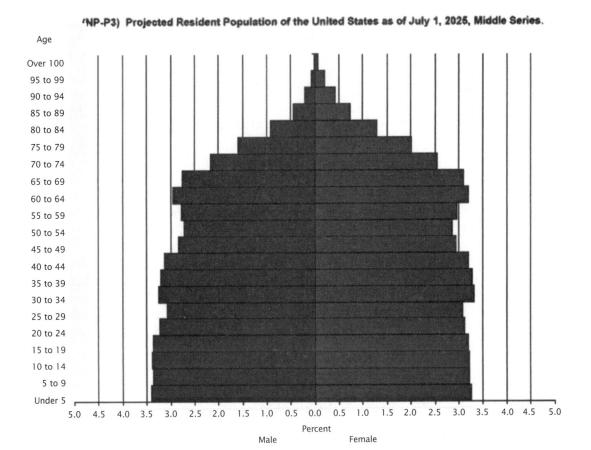

(NP-P3) Projected Resident Population of the United States as of July 1, 2025, Middle Series.

Source: National Projections Program, Population Division, U.S. Census Bureau, Washington, D. C. 20233

these changes and be ready to respond to a potentially significant increase in the demand for EMS. There are few population-based studies that define and characterize the use of EMS by the elderly population in different regions of the country.[1-5] All these studies described a higher utilization rate by the elderly and may be used as a platform to foresee the implications of an aging society on the demand for prehospital emergency medical care. McConnel and Wilson showed that the pattern of utilization associated with age by the citizens from Dallas was found to be tri-modal, with rates rising geometrically by age for individuals aged 65 and over.[5] Compared to the age group from 45 to 64 years of age, rates of EMS utilization for the oldest-old were 3.4 times higher for total EMS incidents, 4.5 times higher for emergency transports, and 5.2 times higher for incidents of a life-threatening nature. The observed age-associated increase in utilization was due primarily to medical conditions rather than incidents arising from trauma. This age-associated pattern of increased rates of EMS utilization seemed to be related to the high prevalence of medical conditions and high incidence of acute episodes affecting the elderly population. Dickinson found not only that geriatric patients used EMS more frequently, but they also had a higher utilization of more advanced resources and more prolonged scene times than younger patients.[4]

Based on population projections and reports of higher rates of utilization of EMS by elder patients, it seems that systems will indeed face an exponential increase in the demand for prehospital emergency care. Analyzing the pattern of EMS use by geriatric patients has obvious implications for system design. The nature of the geriatric patient's complaints will also be helpful in the allocation of resources and in the dictation of the type and frequency of continuing education programs for providers who will be required to treat these older and presumably sicker patients.

Just as pediatric and obstetric patients are known to have differing physiology and unique requirements for evaluation and treatment, the elderly patients' altered physiology dictates a specialized knowledge with the skills to provide for their needs. This chapter is designed to discuss some of the unique characteristics of our elderly patients that have implications for the delivery of prehospital emergency medical care. A general knowledge and understanding of these issues is important to help medical directors and EMS leaders improve the quality of care given to our elder population, as well as to provide guidance to EMS systems on how to better serve our communities' needs.

Assessment

The initial assessment of a geriatric patient by EMS must be directed to identify the presence of potentially life-threatening problems that may require immediate intervention for stabilization. This three part assessment usually requires less than one minute to complete, and should be based on the traditional "ABCs" as with any other patient. The "geriatric ABCs" may present some distinctive circumstances, different from that of younger adults, which merit a brief discussion.

Airway

Anatomically, the geriatric airway differs from the typical adult airway in a number of ways. The patient may be edentulous, having dentures in place. Teeth can be quite brittle and fracture easily. Well-fitting dentures make bag-valve-mask ventilation easier and more effective; however, all loose-fitting or partial dentures should be removed. The mouth may not open very wide, and immobility of the cervical spine, especially at the atlanto-occipital joint, may make visualization of the glottis difficult or impossible. When using rapid-sequence induction or "medication assisted intubation," in the elderly, the priming dose of nondepolarizing neuromuscular agent before succinylcholine may abolish ventilation and airway reflexes completely. In addition, because the elderly are more sensitive to most induction agents, the doses of barbiturates, benzodiazepines, and etomidate should all be reduced approximately 30% to minimize the risk of cardiac depression and hypotension. Doses of opiates and lidocaine should also be reduced. The doses of neuromuscular blocking agents should not be reduced.[6]

Breathing

Initial diagnosis of the cause for respiratory distress can be difficult because of coexisting disease and overlap of presentations. Differentiation between primary pulmonary disorders—asthma, chronic obstructive pulmonary disease (COPD), pneumonia, and pulmonary embolism—from cardiac failure and pulmonary edema can be difficult, especially in the prehospital setting. The list of drugs which the patient is taking can be more helpful than a physical examination in suggesting the cause of respiratory failure to prehospital personnel seeking guidance in the field.[6]

Withholding oxygen in a patient with COPD for fear of abolishing respiratory drive and inducing a respiratory acidosis is unfounded, especially if the patient is hypoxemic. If concern for CO_2 retention exists, a Venturi mask should be used in conjunction with a pulse oximeter to provide the necessary inspired oxygen concentration to keep saturation between 85% and 90%. If hypercarbia and a decline in mental status ensue, assisted ventilation or endotracheal intubation will need to be used. A Venturi mask is favored over use of a nasal canulae, because it provides a more precise method of oxygen delivery and does not vary depending on whether the patient is primarily mouth or nose breathing.[6]

Circulation

The initial approach to the geriatric patient in shock begins with the rapid intravenous access and appropriate use of resuscitative fluids in all patients without obvious signs of volume overload. Although aggressive fluid resuscitation may result in cardiogenic pulmonary edema in patients with limited cardiac reserve, repeated 250 mL fluid boluses, with special attention to physical examination signs, should prevent significant volume overload. Causes for shock and hypotension in the elderly are numerous, and include sepsis, dehydration, cardiac failure, and blood loss from gastrointestinal bleeding or trauma.[6]

Once the patient has been stabilized, the initial assessment is followed by focused and continued assessment. The patient's medical history and physical exam should yield more detailed information about the chief complaint. Continued assessment includes a more detailed physical examination and a continued reevaluation of potential life threats.[7] The focused and continued assessment of the elderly can be more complex than for other age groups. Older patients often have more than one chronic medical condition that may be contributing to the acute event. The patient himself may have a poor understanding of his medical conditions and history, and frequently there is no reliable family available. The complexity of the medical history and the difficulty in communication may be secondary to the disease and the common physiologic changes of aging. A detailed discussion of physiologic changes of aging is beyond the scope of this chapter, but in another section we will discuss some of the most obvious changes that may have a role in the prehospital assessment of an elder patient.

If the patient's condition is stable, prehospital providers should attempt a detailed focused assessment to identify subtle medical or social conditions that may be contributing to the chief complaint. This is of paramount importance to patients who present frequent calls to EMS. The chief complaint can be trivial, with the patient failing to report important symptoms or circumstances, possibly because the elderly patient is threatened by the thought of hospitalization and the resulting loss of independence.[8] Due to these considerations, older patients may refuse transport, and paramedics may be falsely reassured that the patient is stable and doesn't need further evaluation. In a study by Moss of prehospital patients who signed out against the medical advice of field paramedics, it was found that seven of ten patients who re-accessed EMS within 48 hours after refusing transport were older than 65 years old. The study also described that these patients' illnesses were of greater severity on their second evaluations, and concluded that geriatric patients appear to have a propensity to re-access paramedics by way of 9-1-1 and should be aggressively encouraged to be transported to a medical facility.

The provider's visit to the home can be the only opportunity to collect "in-vivo" information from the patient's environment that may be contributing to the present event or even to prevent future complications. Prehospital providers can be trained to look for: general cleanliness and living conditions; availability of food and water; potential hazards in the home such as loose carpeting, loose stairs, or loose floor boards; possible signs of physical abuse or neglect; and so on. If any worrisome situations are identified, they should be notified to the ED personnel, as well as reported to local authorities. In many cases, prehospital care providers report conditions in the home that are unsafe. These are later corrected and have probably prevented countless potential accidents.[8]

Communication with the elderly may also be difficult. Prehospital providers should make an effort to establish a good rapport. They should be encouraged to address the elderly with respect and avoid epithets such as "Grandma." Questions should be asked slowly, one at a time, and with simple wording. If the patient uses eyeglasses, a hearing aid, or dentures, these articles should be utilized to enhance communication. When possible, the providers should keep themselves at eye level with the patient in a lighted area to establish eye contact. If the patient is severely impaired (e.g., disoriented, blind, and/or deaf) gentle physical contact through touch may be the only means of communication to reassure the patient. If there are family members or friends available at the scene, they may be able to provide valuable information; communication with them at all times is very important.[8]

Physiologic Changes

The skin gradually becomes dry, transparent and wrinkled. Photoaging (the product of chronic sun exposure) produces 90% of the cosmetically undesirable changes in skin.[10] Skin of the elderly is thinner and fragile, and prehospital personnel must handle the patient with extreme care to avoid bruising and tearing.

The eye's anatomy suffers significant changes with aging. The iris becomes more rigid, yielding a smaller, more sluggishly responsive pupil. As a result, the older patient requires more time to adjust to light changes in order to ambulate safely. There is also an increase in cataract formation. The presence of a cataract may also contribute to the decreased ability to discriminate between colors of similar intensities, which can affect the elderly ability to distinguish between medications. Depth perception may also be diminished, putting the elderly at risk to falls.[10,11]

Hearing may be dulled due to atrophy of the external auditory canal and drying of the cerumen, with an increased probability for impaction. Different pathophysiologic processes commonly produce diminished hearing, especially of high-pitched sounds. Speaking loudly, which actually distorts sounds, does not solve the communication problem; rather, speaking slowly in a normal tone at the patient's level gives the patient a chance to hear without distortion and to read lips.[10,11]

The respiratory system undergoes changes that contribute to the higher rate of infections, increased likelihood of hypoxia, and decreased maximum oxygen utilization in the elderly. Lung elasticity and elastic recoil are decreased as a consequence of changes in collagen and elastin. As a result, the thorax expands, which causes increased work of breathing, primarily in expiration. Lung function decreases, resulting in a decrease in oxygen uptake. The cough reflex is diminished and less vigorous, and mucociliary clearance is slower and less effective. This means that the elderly have a diminished ability to clear secretions.[10]

In the cardiovascular system it is very difficult to distinguish disease from age-related changes. The high prevalence of hypertensive heart disease and coronary artery disease may confound the results of studies of age-related cardiovascular changes. As age increases, cardiac output and heart rate drop as a consequence of a markedly decreased response to catecholamine stimulation and to sympathetic nervous system stimulation. The left ventricle becomes thickened and more rigid, and there is a gradual rise in both systolic and diastolic blood pressures. The impact of these changes may be minimal to the person at rest, but they markedly decrease the ability to compensate during events of increased demand.[10]

Despite major changes in the anatomy and function of the kidney with age, the renal system maintains a homeostasis of fluids and electrolytes remarkably well unless it is challenged. Age-related changes may contribute to impairments in volume regulation. Maximum urine osmolality decreases, and achievement of maximum osmolality is delayed (inability to concentrate the urine). Thus, even in times of fluid depletion, the amount of water excreted in the urine is higher, with a higher predisposition for dehydration. On the other hand, it is much more difficult for older persons to excrete a water load, a condition which also predisposes them to hyponatremia. There is also a decrease in glomerular filtration and renal blood flow that increases the risk for toxicity of toxins processed in the kidney.[10]

Changes in the gastrointestinal system begin with atrophy of the salivary glands, which may make difficult the processing of food. Older persons chew food less effectively, even with intact teeth. As a result, older people keep food in the mouth longer and swallow larger pieces of food. The older person's swallowing is less coordinated, increasing the risk of aspiration. Functional changes in the small and large intestines include slowed transit due to impaired motility. Elders have frequent problems with food absorption and constipation. The mass of the liver decreases with age, and hepatic blood flow decreases 10% per decade. These changes result in a higher risk for toxicity with toxins and medications metabolized by the liver.[8,10]

At the central nervous system, the brain atrophies significantly with normal aging. Blood flow to the brain decreases 20% and significant alteration in cerebral autoregulation occurs. As a result of these changes, the patient may experience memory impairment, decreased complex learning, slowed psychomotor skills, slowed reflexes, decreased pain perception, decreased sense of equilibrium, and decreased perception of touch and temperature. Many of these changes contribute to the increased incidence of falls and risk of injuries in the elderly.[8,10,11]

Muscles undergo changes with aging, but these changes vary widely from one person to another. Different muscle groups in any individual also age differently. Overall, from age 30 to 80, muscle mass decreases in relation to body weight by about 35%; this results in loss of strength and range of motion. With age, water content decreases in tendons and ligaments, and tensile strength decreases. Body collagen turnover, and thus the rate of remodeling of the tendons and ligaments, also decreases with age. The results are stiff, less flexible, joints with arthritis which contribute to an increased risk of falls. Finally, there is a decreased total skeletal muscle weight and osteoporosis of some bones. Hip injuries are more frequent in this population than in any other age group.[8,10,11]

Abuse

Elder abuse is part of the epidemic of domestic violence in the United States. A 1991 report from the House Select Committee on Aging suggested that between 1 to 2 million adults older than 60 years are abused in the United States each year.[12] The National Elder Abuse Incidence Study (NEAIS) estimated that a total of 449,924 elderly persons, age 60 and over, experienced abuse and/or neglect in domestic settings in 1996.[13] Of this total, only 16% were reported to Adult Protective Services (APS) agencies. One can conclude that over five times as many new incidents of abuse and neglect were unreported than those that were reported to and substantiated by APS agencies in 1996.

Although described since 1975, elder abuse still receives significantly less attention than spouse abuse and child abuse.[14] The House Select Committee on Aging reported that funding for protective services was equivalent to $45.03 per child, versus $3.80 per geriatric resident.[12] Overall, elder abuse is even more difficult to detect than child abuse, since the social isolation of some elderly persons may increase both the risk of maltreatment itself and the difficulty of identifying that maltreatment. Approximately a quarter of elders live alone; many others interact primarily with family members and see very few outsiders. Children, in contrast, never live alone and are required by law to attend school.[13] For the elderly, a visit to the doctor or healthcare facility may be one of the few interactions of these citizens with the outside world. Consequently, healthcare professionals have an important responsibility to identify and act upon suspected cases of elder abuse. Surveys of practicing emergency physicians revealed that only 27% had elder abuse protocols available, versus 75% for child abuse, and that emergency physicians were not confident in identifying or reporting geriatric victims of abuse or neglect.[15,16] Another survey, this time of prehospital personnel, showed that EMTs also lack a complete understanding of their role in the identification and reporting of elder abuse.[17] Yet, emergency departments and EMS systems could have a big impact in the identification of victims of abuse. Prehospital personnel have the unique opportunity to witness actual living conditions and family interactions when responding to house calls.

Definitions

One of the problems in collecting data on elder abuse has been the lack of standardized definitions. Terms vary among researchers, and usage is not consistent in the laws of different states. Even the age at which a person is considered elderly, usually 60 or 65 years, is debated. EMS systems should use similar definitions and terminology when reporting to, and communicating with, other state and federal agencies dealing with elder abuse. The NEAIS provided the following categories and definitions of domestic elder abuse, neglect, and exploitation.[13]

Physical Abuse

Physical abuse is the use of physical force that may result in bodily injury, physical pain, or impairment. Physical abuse may include, but is not limited to, such acts of violence as striking (with or without an object), hitting, beating, pushing, shoving, shaking, slapping, kicking, pinching, and burning. The unwarranted administration of drugs and physical restraints, force-feeding, and physical punishment of any kind also are examples of physical abuse.

Sexual Abuse

Sexual abuse is nonconsensual sexual contact of any kind with an elderly person. Sexual contact with any person incapable of giving consent also is considered sexual abuse; it includes, but is not limited to, unwanted touching, all types of sexual assault or battery such as rape, sodomy, or coerced nudity, and sexually explicit photographing.

Emotional Abuse

Emotional abuse is the infliction of anguish, emotional pain, or distress. Emotional or psychological abuse includes, but is not limited to, verbal assaults, insults, threats, intimidation, humiliation, and harassment. Other examples include treatment of an older person like an infant, isolation of an elderly person from family, friends, or regular activities, and the display of a "silent treatment."

Neglect

Neglect is the refusal or failure to fulfill any part of a person's obligations or duties to an elder. Neglect may also include a refusal or failure by a person who has fiduciary responsibilities to provide care for an elder (e.g., failure to pay for necessary home care service or failure of an in-home service provider to provide necessary care). Neglect typically means the refusal or failure to provide an elderly person with such life necessities as food, water, clothing, shelter, personal hygiene, medicine, comfort, personal safety, and other essentials included as a responsibility or an agreement.

Abandonment

Abandonment is the desertion of an elderly person by an individual who has assumed responsibility for providing care or by a person with physical custody of an elder.

Exploitation

Financial or material exploitation is the illegal or improper use of an elder's funds, property, or assets. Examples include, but are not limited to, cashing checks without authorization or permission; forging an older person's signature; misusing or stealing an older person's money or possessions; coercing or deceiving an older person into signing a document (e.g., contracts or wills); and the improper use of conservatorship, guardianship, or power of attorney.

Self-Neglect

Self-neglect is characterized as the behaviors of an elderly person that threaten his own health or safety. Self-neglect generally manifests itself in an older person's refusal or failure to provide himself with adequate food, water, clothing, shelter, safety, personal hygiene, and medication (when indicated). For the purpose of this study, the definition of self-neglect excludes a situation in which a mentally competent older person (who understands the consequences of his decisions) makes a conscious and voluntary decision to engage in acts that threaten his health or safety.

The signs and symptoms of the seven kinds of abuse and neglect are summarized in table 49.1.

Identifying and Reporting Elder Maltreatment

Physical abuse/neglect should be suspected by EMS providers when there are repeated EMS calls, evidence of a lack of follow-up with medication recommendations, poor hygiene, conflicting reports between caregiver and older person, unexplained delay in seeking treatment for injuries, previous unexplained injuries, injuries inconsistent with medical findings, and a history of being "accident prone."

Psychological abuse/neglect may be difficult to identify during a short prehospital intervention and transport. Prehospital providers should be alert to signs and symptoms of psychological abuse such as frequent unexplained crying or an unexplained fear of a particular person by a patient. More detailed signs and symptoms of abuse and neglect are presented in table 49.1.

The American Medical Association recommends that doctors routinely ask geriatric patients about abuse.[18] When possible, prehospital personnel can take advantage of the transport time alone with the patient to ask about abuse. Questions should be direct and simple and asked in a nonjudgmental and non-threatening manner. The patient and the caregiver should be interviewed together and separately in order to detect disparities prior to any diagnosis of abuse. Accurate, objective documentation of the interview is essential.

Prehospital providers should be aware of risk factors that put elders at risk for being victims of abuse/neglect. Women are disproportionately represented as victims. In APS reports, women represent 60 to 76% of those subjected to all forms of abuse and neglect.[13]

A substantial proportion of the victims of neglect is the oldest old (over 85 years old). Older people who have difficulty performing activities of daily living (ADL) are more often neglected. Demented patients who cannot perform ADLs sustain more physical abuse. Overall, our oldest old are abused and neglected at two to three times their proportion of the elderly population.[13] It is not clear whether ethnic background affects risk for abuse, but there seems to be a higher rate of reported cases among African Americans. Only small proportions of Hispanics and other minorities are reported to APS.[13] Increased financial exploitation occurs in those who live alone, whereas more verbal and physical violence affects those living with someone.[14]

It is also useful to be aware of the characteristics and risk factors of the abusers. Males are more preponderant among perpetrators of abuse and neglect. Perpetrators are also younger than their victims (60% under age 60). Relatives or spouses of the victims commit most domestic elder abuses. Up to 90% of abusers are related to the victims, and adult children are the largest category of abusers.[13]

The abuser is frequently dependent upon the elderly for financial or housing support. Such dependence is often due to underlying problems on the part of the caregiver such as alcoholism, legal difficulties, psychiatric disease, and deviant behaviors. The older adult who is highly dependent upon the caregiver for personal care may also escalate the stress level of the caregiver ("caregiver stress hypothesis").[14]

Unfortunately, prehospital personnel infrequently report elder abuse. Two different surveys of prehospital personnel documented that, although they frequently recognize possible victims of elder abuse, they do not report the majority of these cases to the authorities.[17,19] Reasons for not reporting included (1) uncertainty about which authorities take reports, (2) unclear definitions of elder abuse, (3) lack of awareness of mandatory reporting laws, and (4) lack of anonymity.[17] Those who participated in an audio-visual training program that focused on elder abuse expected this material to change the way they would evaluate elderly patients in the future.[19]

EMS medical directors must be aware of local laws and regulations as well as the role of local authorities and available resources for follow-up of the victim's situation. This information can be shared with prehospital providers by protocols and training sessions. Knowledge by prehospital personnel of the above-mentioned definitions, signs, symptoms, and risk factors is instrumental in the prevention and manage-

TABLE 49.1

Signs and symptoms of abuse and neglect*

Type of Abuse/Neglect	Signs and Symptoms
Physical Abuse	■ Bruises, black eyes, welts, lacerations, and rope marks ■ Bone fractures, broken bones, and skull fractures ■ Open wounds, cuts, punctures, untreated injuries, and injuries in various stages of healing ■ Stains, dislocations, and internal injuries/bleeding ■ Broken eyeglasses/frames, physical signs of being subjected to punishment, and signs of being restrained ■ Laboratory findings of medication overdose or under utilization of prescribed drugs ■ An elder's report of being hit, slapped, kicked, or mistreated ■ An elder's sudden change in behavior ■ A caregiver's refusal to allow visitors to see an elder alone
Sexual Abuse	■ Bruises around the breasts or genital area ■ Unexplained venereal disease or genital infections ■ Unexplained vaginal or anal bleeding ■ Torn, stained, or bloody underclothing ■ An elder's report of being sexually assaulted or raped
Emotional/ Psychological Abuse	■ Emotional upset or agitation ■ Extreme withdrawal and non-communication or non-responsiveness ■ An elder's report of being verbally or emotionally mistreated
Neglect	■ Dehydration, malnutrition, untreated bedsores, and poor personal hygiene ■ Unattended or untreated health problems ■ Hazardous or unsafe living conditions (e.g., improper wiring, no heat or no running water) ■ Unsanitary or unclean living conditions (e.g., dirt, fleas, lice on person, soiled bedding, fecal/urine smell, inadequate clothing) ■ An elder's report of being neglected
Abandonment	■ The desertion of an elder at a hospital, nursing facility, or other similar institution ■ The desertion of an elder at a shopping center or other public location ■ An elder's own report of being abandoned
Financial or Material Exploitation	■ Sudden changes in a bank account or banking practice, including an unexplained withdrawal of large sums of money by a person accompanying the elder ■ The inclusion of additional names on an elder's bank card ■ Unauthorized withdrawal of funds using an elder's ATM card ■ Abrupt changes in a will or in other financial documents ■ Unexplained disappearance of funds or valuable possessions ■ Provisions of substandard care or bills unpaid despite the availability of adequate financial resources ■ The provision of services that are not necessary ■ Discovery of an elder's signature forged for financial transactions or for the titles of the elder's possessions ■ Sudden appearance of previously uninvolved relatives claiming rights to an elder's affairs and possessions ■ Unexplained sudden transfer of assets to a family member or someone outside the family ■ An elder's report of financial exploitation
Self-Neglect	■ Dehydration, malnutrition, untreated or improperly attended medical conditions, and poor personal hygiene ■ Hazardous or unsafe living conditions (e.g., improper wiring, no indoor plumbing, no heat or no running water) ■ Unsanitary or unclean living quarters (e.g., animal/insect infestation, no functioning toilet, fecal/urine smell) ■ Inappropriate and/or inadequate clothing, lack of necessary medical aids (e.g., eyeglasses, hearing aid, dentures) ■ Gross inadequate housing or homelessness

*U.S. Department 98

ment of elder abuse. Once identified, these patients must be offered emergency stabilization as needed and referral for follow-up by authorities.

Trauma

The combination of their increased longevity with our highly mechanized society puts the older population at greater risk for trauma exposure.[20] As discussed in this chapter, the elderly are predisposed to injury partly because of age-related deterioration in hearing and sight. Additionally, poor coordination, imbalance, and weakness further reduce the older person's ability to cope with injury hazard.

The injured older patient consumes a disproportionate amount of healthcare dollars. Although they constitute only 12.6% of the population, they consume one-third of all trauma healthcare resources.[20] Elderly patients are more likely to be hospitalized than are younger patients, and their hospital stays are often longer and more complicated. Despite the greater use of resources, elderly patients maintain a higher mortality rate when compared with younger cohorts matched for Injury Severity Score (ISS). Trauma is the seventh leading cause of death in patients over 65 years of age. This increased mortality is largely a reflection of diminished physiologic reserve associated with the aging process.[20]

Injury to the elderly is most commonly the result of falls, motor vehicle accidents (MVA), and pedestrian injuries. Thermal injuries and assaults are also quite common.[21-23] Multiple studies have shown that for a given injury's severity, mortality is higher in older victims.[6,24] Others have shown that pre-existing illness greatly increases mortality independent of disease severity. Pre-existing disease and age impact outcome sufficiently to recommend that triage patients with advanced age or significant medical illnesses be transported directly to trauma centers.[6] In spite of these recommendations, a recently published abstract reported that seriously injured elderly patients are not accessing trauma center care.[25] To improve outcomes for the injured elderly, EMS systems and their medical directors must be conscious of the needs of these patients, and should include age in prehospital protocols as a criteria for transport to the trauma center.

Falls are the most common cause of trauma in the geriatric population.[21] Ground level falls, at the patient's residence and during daily activities, tend to prevail, whereas falls from heights are uncommon.[26] Of all elderly emergency department patients who sustain a fall, 20% to 25% of these people are dead within twelve months.[8] In some cases, death is due to trauma from the fall or complications in the treatment or recovery. However, death is usually not from the fall itself but from complications of underlying medical conditions.[27] Providers at the scene of a fall should look for environmental factors that may have contributed to the fall, to try to prevent future falls.

Resuscitation

Prehospital providers frequently respond to the scene of a critically ill geriatric patient. If the patient is found to be on impending arrest or even in full cardiopulmonary arrest, the decision of whether to initiate aggressive life-sustaining treatments, such as endotracheal intubation or cardiopulmonary resuscitation, is a very difficult one. Prehospital protocols requiring aggressive treatment and resuscitation of every patient without consideration of premorbid condition, prior expressed wishes, or consultation with available family will cause unnecessary hardships on patients and families who already have come to terms with a patient's illness.[6] It may also put the EMTs at unnecessary risk for different occupational injuries characteristic of emergency transports, such as motor vehicle crashes, needle sticks, and the like. Unfortunately, prehospital providers are frequently called to scenarios where this information is simply not available and the family's understanding of the patient's condition is not clear. On the other hand, failure to initiate resuscitative efforts based exclusively on the patient's age, without knowledge of premorbid condition of the patient's and family wishes, is ethically and medically unjustified. Although cardiopulmonary arrest in the elderly usually carries a bad outcome, the same is also true for younger patients. Several studies have documented that age alone is a poor prognostic indicator. Reports from the prehospital setting indicate that geriatric patients with witnessed cardiac arrest, early CPR, and initial rhythm of ventricular tachycardia or ventricular fibrillation, had the same chances for successful resuscitation and return to pre-arrest functional state as their younger cohorts had.[6,28-30] Likewise, elderly patients who have an unwitnessed arrest and those whose original rhythm is a systole, or a pulseless electrical activity, rarely survive, and probably should not receive resuscitative attempts.

Each case must be evaluated individually, taking into account the patient's current condition, past medical history, and available documentation of patient's and family's wishes. A national survey of prehospital providers demonstrated that experienced providers withhold resuscitative efforts more often in futile situations, and that most providers would honor official state-approved advance directives.[31] Protocols with guidelines on when to withhold and/or cease prehospital resuscitation efforts must be available to prehospital providers, and must be in compliance with state laws and regulations. It is also desirable that direct medical oversight be readily available for real-time consultation by field personnel responding to unusual cases. EMS systems that frequently respond to institutions at high risk for this type of scenario, such as nursing homes, should have pre-arranged agreements with such institutions on how to proceed in this situation.[32,33]

Prevention

The following quotation is from the document "EMS Agenda for the Future."[34] In its section about prevention, the document describes "where we want to be" in regard to EMS and prevention in the future:

> EMS providers receive education regarding prevention principles. EMS systems and providers are actively engaged in injury and illness prevention programs. These are based on local needs, addressing identified injury and illness problems. EMS systems also maintain prevention-oriented atmospheres that emphasize safety and well-being for their own workers. They enhance their ability to document the circumstances contributing to illness and injuries. Such information is shared with other community resources to help attenuate injury and illness risk factors.[34]

Active involvement of EMS in prevention is a goal established by Delbridge et al in the "EMS Agenda." Several other authors have published and studied the different roles EMS can assume in this field.[35-37] Some of these activities have already been initiated by EMS systems in different parts of the country. Gerson, in 1992, used paramedics to identify elderly patients who needed referral to social agencies due to environmental, social, or medical problems.[38] Wofford, in 1994, presented his work using computerized EMS data to identify and maintain a surveillance system of elderly patients at risk of falls.[39] Seamon published an article about the use of a video program to enhance paramedics' knowledge of how to recognize cases of elder abuse.[19] These are only a few examples of how EMS systems can utilize their personnel and resources to offer preventive services to the elderly in their communities.

Summary

A National Association of EMS Physicians' position statement on medical oversight states that medical directors should demonstrate leadership in illness and injury prevention, through promulgation of injury and illness prevention programs, education of out-of-hospital personnel in principles of prevention, collaboration with other healthcare providers and authorities on prevention, collection and analysis of data identifying risk factors that contribute to injury and illness, and promulgation of public education in the prevention of injuries and illness.[40] The geriatric population is certainly a section of our population in much need of good prevention programs that may help them fully enjoy the last stage of their lives.

References

1. Meador SA. Age related utilization of advanced life support services. *Prehosp Disaster Med*. 1991;6:9–14.
2. Wofford JL, Schwartz E, Byrum JE. The role of emergency services in health care for the elderly: a review. *J Emerg Med*. 1993;11:317–326.
3. Wofford JL, Moran WP, Heuser MD, et al. Emergency medical transport of the elderly: a population based study. *American J Emerg Med*. 1995;13:297–300.
4. Dickinson ET, Verdile VP, Kostyun CT, et al. Geriatric use of emergency medical services. *Ann Emerg Med*. 1996;27:199–203.
5. McConnel CE, Wilson RW. The demands for prehospital emergency services in an aging society. *Soc Sci Med*. 1998;46:1027–1031.
6. Milzman DP, Rothenhaus TC. Resuscitation of the geriatric patient. *Emerg Med Clin North Am*. 1996;14:233–244.
7. Goodkoontzc G, Race SM. Focused and continued assessment. In: Pons P, Cason D, eds. Paramedic Field Care: A Complaint-Based Approach. American College of Emergency Physicians. St. Louis, MO: Mosby-Lifeline; 1997:326–342.
8. Hogan TM. *Geriatric Emergencies: An EMT Manual*. Turlock, CA: MedicAlert; 1996.
9. Moss ST, Chan TC, Buchana J, et al. Outcome study of prehospital patients signed out against medical advice by field paramedics. *Ann Emerg Med*. 1998;31:247–250.
10. Taffet GE. Age-related physiologic changes. In: Reuben DB, Yoshikawa TT, Besdine RW, eds. Geriatric Review Syllabus: A Core Curriculum in Geriatric Medicine. New York: American Geriatric Society; 1996:11–24.

11. Storer DL. Geriatric Assessment. In: Pons P, Cason D, eds. Paramedic Field Care: A Complaint-Based Approach. American College of Emergency Physicians. St. Louis, MO: Mosby-Lifeline; 1997:357–367.

12. Subcommittee on Health and Long-Term Care of the Select Committee on Aging House of Representatives. *Elder Abuse: A Decade of Shame and Inaction.* Washington DC: US Government Printing Office; 1990.

13. US Department of Health and Human Services' Administration on Aging and the Administration for Children and Families. *The National Elder Abuse Incidence Study.* Washington DC: US Government Printing Office; 1998

14. Kleischmidt KC. Elder abuse: a review. *Ann Emerg Med.* 1997;30:463–472.

15. McNamara RM, Rousseau E, Sanders AB. Geriatric emergency medicine: a survey of practicing emergency physicians. *Ann Emerg Med.* 1992;21:796-801.

16. Jones JS, Veenstra TR, Seamon JP, Krohmer J. Elder mistreatment: national survey of emergency physicians. *Ann Emerg Med.* 1997;30:473–479.

17. Jones JS. To report or not to report: emergency services response to elder abuse. *Prehosp Disaster Med.* 1995; 10(2):96–100.

18. American Medical Association. *Diagnostic Treatment Guidelines on Elder Abuse and Neglect.* Chicago, IL: American Medical Association; 1992;4–37.

19. Seamon JP. Identifying victims of elder abuse and neglect: a training video for prehospital personnel. *Prehosp Disaster Med.* 1997;12:269–273.

20. Mandavia D, Newton K. Contemporary issues in trauma: geriatric trauma. *Emerg Med Clin North Am.* 1998;167: 257–274.

21. Evans R. Trauma and falls. In: Sanders AB, ed. Emergency care of the elder patient. Beverly Cracom Publications; St. Louis: 1996.

22. United States Department of Health and Human Services: *A Profile of Older Americans.* Washington DC: American Association of Retired Persons and the Administration of Aging; 1994.

23. Rehm CG, Ross SE. Elderly drivers involved in road crashes: a profile. *Am Surg.* 1995;61:435.

24. Knudson MM, Lieberman J, Morris JA, et al. Mortality factors in geriatric blunt trauma patients. *Arch Surg.* 1994;129:448.

25. Lane PL, Sorondo B, Kelly JJ. Elderly trauma patients—are they accessing trauma center care? *Acad Emerg Med.* 2000;7:564–567.

26. Kudisch HG, King MB, Perdrizet GA, et al. Environmental factors related to falls in elderly patients presenting to the emergency department. *Acad Emerg Med.* 2000;7:576–581.

27. Meldon SW, Reilly M, Drew B, et al. Trauma in the very elderly: a community based study of outcomes at trauma and non-trauma centers. *Acad Emerg Med.* 2000;7:568–575.

28. Wuerz RC, Holliman CJ, Meador SA, et al. Effect of age on prehospital cardiac resuscitation outcome. *Am J Emerge Med.* 1995;13:389–391.

29. Longstreth WT, Cobb LA, Fahrenbruch CE, et al. Does age affect outcomes of out-of-hospital cardiopulmonary resuscitation? *JAMA.* 1990;264:2109–2110.

30. Bonin MJ, Pepe PE, Clark PS. Survival in the elderly after out-of-hospital cardiac arrest. *Crit Care Med.* 1993; 21:1645–1651.

31. Marco CA, Schears RM. Prehospital resuscitation practices: a survey of prehospital providers. *Acad Emerg Med.* 2000;7:411–417.

32. Dunn PM, Schmidt TA, Carley MM, et al. A method to communicate patient preferences about medically indicated life-sustaining treatment in the out-of-hospital setting. *L Am Ger Soc.* 1996;44:785–791.

33. Sosna D, Christopher M, Pesto M, et al. Implementations strategies for a do-not-resuscitate program in the prehospital setting. *Ann Emerg Med.* 1994;23:1042–1050.

34. Delbridge TR, Bailey R, Chew JL, et al. EMS agenda for the future: where we are . . . where we want to be. EMS Agenda for the Future Steering Committee. *Ann Emerg Med.* 1998;3:251–263.

35. Kinnane JM, Garrison HG, Coben JH, Alonso-Serra HM. Injury prevention: is there a role for out-of-hospital emergency medical services? *Acad Emerg Med.* 1997;4:306–312.

36. Garrison HG, Foltin G, Becker L, et al. The role of emergency medical services in primary injury prevention. *Prehosp Emerg Care.* 1997;1:156–162.

37. MacLean CB. The future role of emergency medical services systems in prevention. *Ann Emerg Med.* 1993;22: 1743–1746.

38. Gerson LW, Schelble DT, Wilson JE. Using paramedics to identify at risk elderly. *Ann Emerg Med.* 1992;21:688–691.

39. Wofford JL, Heuser MD, Moran WP, et al. Community surveillance of falls among the elderly using computerized EMS transport data. *Am J Emerg Med.* 1994;12: 433–437.

40. Alonso-Serra HM, Blanton D, O'Connor RE. Physician medical direction in EMS. *Prehosp Emerg Care.* 1998;2: 153–157.

Air Services

Douglas J. Floccare, MD
Daniel G. Hankins, MD

Introduction

A solid understanding of the fundamentals of air medical transport can allow EMS medical directors to have a profound impact on effective utilization of these services by their programs. While most direct interaction between ground EMS and air EMS providers will occur as a result of scene medevac responses, the medical director must also consider the role that emergent interhospital air transport plays in the local and regional system of care.

Goals of Air Medical Transport

The primary goal of air medical transport is to give patients who are not in proximity to emergent medical care the same chance of survival as those patients to whom the care is immediately available. The expectation should be to "level the playing field" as opposed to having patients "do better." An effective air medical transport should either decrease the time to a needed emergent medical intervention, decrease the out-of-hospital time for a potentially unstable patient, or both. Air transport also provides the opportunity to match experienced, high-level caregivers with specific patients' medical needs.

Brief History

Transportation of sick and injured patients is documented to have occurred by fixed-wing aircraft as early as 1915, approximately 12 years after the Wright brothers' first flight. While the helicopter was developed during World War II, it was not routinely utilized for patient transport until the Korean War. Patients at that time were strapped to stretchers outside of the aircraft, so that while rapid evacuation to a field hospital could be accomplished, no medical care could be provided while enroute. With the Viet-nam War came the use of the large, powerful UH-1H or Huey helicopter that could carry both patients and caregivers inside. Army medics provided stabilization during evacuation to forward field hospitals, and the lowest mortality rate of any major sustained conflict to that time was achieved. In 1970 Cowley partnered with the Maryland State Police and obtained a National Highway and Traffic Safety Administration grant to purchase a Bell Jet Ranger helicopter to transport trauma victims to the Shock-Trauma unit at the University of Maryland Hospital, the first civilian unit of its kind.

In 1972, the first hospital-based helicopter program was initiated at St. Anthony's Hospital in Denver, Colorado. The focus of this program was to provide interfacility transport of critically ill patients, but scene medevac response was also performed. As of 1978 there were nearly twenty new helicopter services initiated across the United States, the majority of them run by individual hospitals. By 1992 the number of air medical programs in the United States had grown to more than 220.

Helicopter vs. Fixed-Wing

The decision to transport via rotor-wing or fixed-wing aircraft depends on a number of factors, most importantly speed, distance, and weather. Helicopter flights tend to be for shorter-distance, more time-dependent emergent flights, while fixed-wing flights tend to be longer-distance, less emergent flights. Fixed-wing aircraft generally take longer to get mobilized for flight as opposed to the 7- to 10-minute launch time for most rotor-wing aircraft (300 knots or better vs. 150 knots), but they must land at an airport, rather than at a scene or medical facility. The speed advantage is further negated because of the need for ground transportation to and from the airport at each end of the trip. While fixed-wing aircraft have limited usefulness in truly emergent time-dependent medical flights, they may play a role in certain emergent situations that would normally be handled by helicopter.

Fixed-wing aircraft can fly under weather circumstances that many rotor-wing aircraft cannot. Many more medical fixed-wing aircraft are equipped and staffed to launch into poor visibility instrument flight rule conditions than are rotor-wing aircraft. Icing conditions are better dealt with in fixed-wing aircraft because the technology for de-icing the leading wing edge is more advanced and more widely available than in helicopters. The biggest advantage for fixed-wing aircraft is one of distance. While the flight radius of a medium sized rotor-wing aircraft used for medical transports is in the 150- to 200-mile range, the range for fixed-wing aircraft is dependent on the size of the plane, and can be trans-oceanic. There are many rural areas that are outside the range of helicopter transport and must rely on fixed-wing aircraft for patients who require flight.

Helicopter Operation

Basing

Hospital-based helicopters tend to view their mission as servicing patients who require rapid transport to their hospital or group of hospitals. There is generally not a perceived obligation to transport any patient not coming back to their center, although many programs will agree to perform transports to other centers on an as-available basis. Nationally, hospital-based programs tend to do more interhospital transports (65–70%) than scene responses (30–35%), although there are programs in which this is reversed. Public service programs tend to view their mission as providing for the emergency helicopter needs of any patient in their geographic area. Many public service programs will have missions that extend beyond medical care, to include areas such as search and rescue, law enforcement, and firefighting. Public service programs tend to transport to the closest center that is appropriate for the patient's medical needs, and generally perform a higher percentage of scene response than interfacility transport.

Helicopter basing is heavily influenced by the program type, program mission, and lack or presence of other air programs in the area.

Many programs operate a single helicopter out of their home hospital. An advantage to this approach is that it allows crew members to stay connected to the medical environment for things such as refreshing clinical skills, attending clinical/educational meetings, and performing patient follow-up. It also allows a high public profile for the helicopter. A major disadvantage, however, is that it tends to result in helicopters being located in urban areas, not near the patients who need to be transported.

Many programs with more than one aircraft, and some programs with a single aircraft, will have bases that are remote from the home hospital. A major advantage of this is that it tends to place helicopters closer to the patients who need them. Sometimes this will be used as a competitive edge over other air programs in the same area. Often these satellite bases are located at airports, freestanding heliports, or, on occasion, smaller hospitals. This may provide challenges to refreshing clinical skills, attending clinical/educational meetings, and performing patient follow-up.

An approach used more often by public service programs, aircraft are strategically based in an attempt to have no region of a coverage area be without a timely response. The obvious advantage of this approach is that all persons receive coverage. In addition to the same disadvantages associated with satellite basing, however, geographic basing often requires location of some aircraft in areas where call volume is inadequate to cover operational expenses if supported through patient billing.

Staffing

The majority of helicopter programs fly with a crew of two medical providers (93%) with a small number using either one medical provider (3%) or three medical providers (4%). The most common medical crew configuration is one flight nurse and one flight paramedic (67%). Less commonly used configurations are flight nurse/flight nurse (8%), flight nurse/flight physician (5%), flight paramedic/flight paramedic (5%), flight paramedic only (<2%), and flight nurse only (<1%).

A handful of programs limit themselves to solely interfacility transport, and do not utilize personnel with prehospital training. The majority of programs that perform any scene response have a crew that includes either a flight paramedic or a flight nurse who has been cross-trained as a paramedic. Some air medical programs utilize supplemental staff with unique clinical skills on specific transports of patients with special medical needs. Depending on the space and lift capabilities of the particular aircraft, they may either take the place of one of the regular crew members, or come aboard as a third caregiver. Some examples of personnel who may be used in this fashion would include perfusionists, respiratory therapists, neonatal transport nurses, pediatric transport nurses, and intensivists.

FAA Regulations

The Federal Aviation Administration (FAA) strictly governs air operations in the United States under Title 14 of the Federal Code. The two parts of the Federal Aviation Regulations (FARs) that have the most bearing on air medical services are Parts 91 and 135. FAR Part 91 deals with "General Operating and Flight Rules," which apply to all aircraft flying in this country. FAR Part 135 encompasses "Commuter and On-Demand Operations and Rules Governing Persons on Board Such Aircraft." These regulations basically govern such things as pilot rest and training, rules to follow in different kinds of airspace, rules for VFR (visual flight rules) and IFR, and aircraft maintenance. All aircraft that transport passengers "for hire" are required to operate under Part 135 FARs. Federal and state governmental operators are exempt from FARs Parts 91 and 135, although many choose to voluntarily comply with Part 91 regulations.

Part 135 Operators

A hospital or other entity that wishes to bill for providing air medical transport must decide whether to obtain their own Part 135 certificate or work with an air vendor that has Part 135 status. If a hospital acquires its own Part 135, the hospital must buy or lease the aircraft and hire the pilots and mechanics, as well as hire and train the medical crew. Many hospital administrators have neither the resources nor the expertise to do this. An aircraft vendor, on the other hand, may have a number of aircraft under its umbrella, an arrangement which provides both expertise and efficiency of aircraft usage. This vendor may be a local air operator or a national multi-programmed vendor. The vendor assumes the responsibility for providing aircraft, pilots, and mechanics, as well as such things as a back-up aircraft when maintenance must be done. Inability or unwillingness of the vendor to comply with the contract terms can make possession of a Part 135 more advantageous, because of ultimate control over both the medical and the flight aspects of the program.

Funding

It is very expensive to establish a rotor-wing air medical service. Typical medevac helicopters cost three to five million dollars each. In addition to medical crew, the program must hire and maintain four to six pilots per aircraft and one to two mechanics per aircraft, and must stock a parts inventory that in large programs can exceed one million dollars in value. In many cases special crew quarters, hangar facilities, and fuel storage systems must be leased or built. The need for back-up aircraft during downtime periods for the primary aircraft must also be considered. The independent operation of an air medical program by a single hospital is a significant undertaking. The attraction of leasing a ship through a vendor is strong. The vendor can then take the risks and responsibilities of the flight aspects of the program. This greatly reduces the initial investment by the hospital, but results in a greater overall long-term cost.

The primary funding source for hospital-based helicopters is revenue from patient billing. While patients may receive ground EMS at no cost or be billed up to several hundred dollars, the typical charge for a hospital-based helicopter transport will start at several thousand dollars in order to cover expenses. Insurance reimbursement for these bills varies markedly from state to state. Because of these expenses, in some instances multiple medical centers have joined to form consortiums to either run their own Part 135 program or to contract with an aircraft vendor. This approach brings less of a financial burden to each of the participating consortium members, since each partner bears only a portion of the costs. The development of a consortium can be challenging, however, because of competition, old rivalries, and suspicions among the potential partners. Such a design will not succeed everywhere, but the great expense of establishing and maintaining a helicopter air medical service may force consortium-building in many areas of the country because of trends in medical-care cost-cutting. Public safety agencies, such as police and fire departments, may provide medevac coverage on a local, regional, or statewide level. These programs typically do not bill patients, but rather are supported directly by tax revenues or by special funding sources, such as surcharges on motor vehicle registrations.

Industry Safety and Credentialing

Most states license air ambulances as ambulances, but states have no jurisdiction over the aviation aspects of programs, since this is a federal area of oversight. Safety has always been a prime concern of the air medical industry. One of the main thrusts of the FARs is safety. In spite of these precautions, the industry had a plethora of accidents in the 1980s. Concerns led to a number of individuals in various air medical disciplines to form a group called "Priority One" to look at standards for industry safety. Out of this process emerged the Commission on Accreditation of Air Medical Services (CAAMS) that was to devise voluntary standards involving medical care and safety for the air medical industry. CAAMS was conceived as an organization of organizations. The first meeting of CAAMS occurred in 1990, with seven organizations participating: the National Association of EMS Physicians (NAEMSP), the American College of Emergency Physicians (ACEP), the Association of Air Medical Services (AAMS), the National Association of Air Medical Communications Specialists (NAACS), the National EMS Pilot's Association (NEMSPA), the National Flight Nurses Association (NFNA), and the National Flight Paramedics Association (NFPA). CAAMS eventually became the Commission on Accreditation of Medical Transport Systems (CAMTS) because of the trend toward integration of air and ground transport modalities, with many services incorporating ground, rotor-wing and fixed-wing transport service into their offerings. Currently, CAMTS has 14 participating organizations and has accredited about 90 air medical and ground services. CAMTS only accredits ground services associated with critical care air services. The two major thrusts in the CAMTS standards, now in their fourth edition, are quality medical care and excellence in program safety. Additional information is obtainable at the CAMTS website at <http://www.camts.org>.

Integration of Air Medical Services

Air transport must be able to be viewed as an upper tier of the system. It should be able to be applied to a select small percentage of patients according to predetermined criteria in a rapid fashion. The degree to which a helicopter program can be integrated successfully into local and regional systems is highly dependent upon the extent to which scene response is viewed as a primary mission. It is unlikely that a hospital-based program will become an effective component of the EMS system, if scene response is viewed as something that only can be performed when there are no interfacility transports. A public service pro-

gram will be unable to integrate effectively with EMS if medical missions are viewed as taking a back seat to law enforcement.

Dispatch Criteria

The EMS system should have criteria guiding the use of air transport. Model criteria for air medical response have been developed in position papers by NAEMSP. Protocols are most readily developed for trauma, but can also be written for medical indications such as acute myocardial infarction or stroke when the patient is not in proximity to an appropriate care facility. There must be a clear method for requesting a helicopter, and the helicopter dispatch center must be able to provide rapid information regarding availability and estimated time of arrival. The helicopter must be prepared to respond quickly with information that is initially limited to location, number of patients, and nature of call.

Communications

Once enroute to the scene, the aircraft must be able to maintain communication with its dispatch center, the care providers at the scene, and the providers setting up the landing zone. EMS agencies must preplan with local air programs which frequencies will be utilized, and whether special links must be set up for duplex or digital radio systems. A radio frequency reference list for all agencies in the region must be maintained aboard the aircraft, as well as in the dispatch center.

Landing Zones

All agencies within the system must have a clear understanding of the landing zone requirements of the local air medical service. While there may be subtle differences among programs, in general they will want a firm, level surface, approximately 100 feet by 100 feet, without adjacent obstructions or loose debris. Ground personnel will need to secure the landing zone and prevent onlookers or vehicles from approaching the aircraft.

Training

In order to effectively integrate air medical services into a region, all ground EMS providers should receive at least basic, concise training as to when to request air transport. They should know what information is needed to request their local air carrier, and how to relay the request quickly. It is essential that ground crews are trained how to safely establish and maintain a landing zone, and that only trained personnel come in close proximity to the aircraft.

Trauma Scene vs. Interfacility Transport

The goal of an EMS system should be to transport major trauma victims directly to a center designated for trauma care. The avoidance of taking rural victims of major trauma by ground into the local non-trauma-center hospital is often dependent on rapid helicopter response. Better integration of air medical services allows for reliable scene response and decreases the need for interfacility transfer of trauma patients. Even with effective integration, however, there will always be patients who are best served by first going by ground to the local hospital because they are too unstable to wait for a helicopter or because the weather does not allow for safe flight. It is important for the EMS system to have access to effective interfacility helicopter transport once the patient has been stabilized or the weather has cleared.

Medical Challenges

There are some trade-offs made for the ability to fly up to 180 miles per hour in a straight line to the receiving medical facility. While there is much care that can be performed while in flight, helicopters are not simply "flying ICUs" as some may believe.

Space

Unlike some large military helicopters that can accommodate six or more patients, space is often quite limited in the aircraft used for civilian medevac operations. Access to the patient is highly variable depending not only on the model of helicopter, but also on the configuration of the medical interior of each individual aircraft. Some interiors place the patient so that they may be accessed only from the waist, or sometimes the chest, up to the head. Other configurations may allow total body access, but leave little room beyond the patient's head for airway management. Most medevac helicopters in use today have enough space for at least two caregivers and two patients, but there are still some in operation with room for just one provider and one patient.

Weight

Unlike ground transport, the weight of the medical equipment, the providers, and the patients must be considered prior to every call. The weight and size of medical equipment can factor heavily into which brands are selected and how much is carried. For example, while a ground ambulance may routinely carry a large steel oxygen cylinder with a supply that is limitless for the average transport, a helicopter may carry only small cylinders, composite cylinders, or liquid oxygen, each with their own special logistical issues. Certain models of ventilators, intra-aortic balloon pumps, extracorporeal membrane oxygenators, and other medical devices may be readily adapted for use in ground interfacility transport, but may be too bulky and heavy for use on a helicopter.

Hearing

A running helicopter creates a very noisy working environment, both while coordinating the loading of a patient, and while providing care in flight. All necessary medical history must be obtained before loading the patient, as conversation will be difficult in flight. Breath sounds must be evaluated before transport, as auscultation on board will not be fruitful without the use of an amplified electronic stethoscope wired into the aircraft intercom system.

Lighting

Lighting can be an additional challenge in providing medical care aboard a helicopter. While an ambulance driver generally is unaffected by what goes on in the patient-care area, the pilot of a helicopter can have his night vision affected by the light necessary to provide patient care. It is therefore necessary to illuminate the patient-care area with less distracting red lighting or blue lighting at night, or to pull a heavy curtain to separate the cockpit from the helicopter service area. In the daytime, the large helicopter windows that allow for operational visibility also allow large amounts of sunlight to enter the patient-care area, and can make viewing of medical monitoring equipment very difficult. Direct sunlight can also affect the function of certain medical equipment, such as the infrared sensor for certain end-tidal carbon dioxide monitors. Unlike ground ambulances, patients aboard helicopters can also develop "flicker seizure" by having sunlight shine directly through the moving rotor blades into their eyes, causing a strobelight-like stimulation and subsequent generalized seizure activity.

Electronic Medical Equipment

Electronic medical equipment must be evaluated for the effects of radio frequency interference (RFI) and electromagnetic interference (EMI) before it can be used safely aboard an aircraft. The general public has grown accustomed to commercial airlines restricting the use of portable electronic items in order to prevent untoward effects on aircraft navigational equipment and electronic switching devices. The interference from a device that is plugged into the aircraft inverter power supply or is actively delivering electricity to a patient can be substantially greater. For example, there are no transcutaneous pacing units certified for use in flight, and therefore patients with a high potential need for transcutaneous pacing should not be transported by air if there is a chance the aircraft may encounter bad weather and need to use its navigational instruments.

Testing must also be performed to determine whether specific electronic medical devices are susceptible to malfunction as a result of RFI or EMI. There are many sources of interference in the ground and air EMS environment that are not present in a hospital environment. As an example, when transcutaneous pacing began to move to the prehospital setting in the mid-1980s, it was found that certain pacing units that had been working well in the hospital would suspend pacing if an EMS portable radio were keyed in proximity to the patient. A device that is reliable inside a hospital may require special internal shielding for use on board an aircraft.

Physiologic Issues

Patients with air emboli or decompression sickness should routinely be flown at the lowest altitude that the pilot can safely maintain, which is generally at 500 to 800 feet above ground level (AGL) given favorable terrain and weather. Since most scene medevacs will be accomplished at altitudes of 1,000 to 2,000 feet AGL, there usually is little physiologic effect of altitude in most patients. This issue may warrant more consideration in high altitude areas, and in areas where the patient must be transported over mountains. Also, if bad weather necessitates sudden reliance on navigational instruments, the pilot may

need to climb an additional 1,000 to 3,000 feet to utilize instrument flight rules (IFR).

Strong and gusty winds can lead to considerable problems with motion sickness for both the patient and crew. This can be compounded if the weather is hot and the aircraft is without optimal air conditioning. While motion sickness may affect even the most seasoned flight crew, it can often be an issue for supplemental flight crew brought along for the needs of a specific patient. On days of high turbulence, prophylactic anti-emetic administration should be considered for patients. As with any medication, anti-emetic use by the flight crew must be in accordance with the appropriate regulatory and occupational medical oversight.

Operational Challenges

The EMS medical director should have insight into the environmental factors that can affect the ability of an air medical program to support ground EMS operations.

Visibility

With certain limited exceptions, timely scene medevac response requires the pilot to be able to fly to the scene under visual flight rules (VFR). In most EMS helicopter operations, this requires at a minimum a visibility of at least one mile with a cloud ceiling of at least 500 feet. Many programs utilize higher minimums in the interest of maximizing safety. While many EMS helicopters are equipped with navigational instruments that allow the pilot to fly safely under IFR when the visibility is poor, this has limited utility for scene response because it generally requires that the aircraft return to an airport. It is a tremendous safety feature, however, in the event the aircrew should inadvertently fly into bad weather and can no longer navigate by sight.

Freezing Precipitation

Anticipate rotor-wing aircraft to be grounded during periods of freezing precipitation. Rain itself generally does not prevent scene medevac response as long as visibility minimums are met. Freezing rain, sleet, and wet snow, however, can accumulate on the rotor blades and cause the aircraft to lose lift.

Ambient Temperature

The ambient temperature can have a significant impact on the maximum weight that a helicopter is able to carry. The higher the temperature, the less dense the air, and consequently the harder the engines must push the rotor blades to achieve the same amount of lift. The impact of temperature on lift is magnified at high altitude, where the air density is already low. Each pilot, at the start of his or her work shift, calculates the maximum weight of fuel, cargo, and passenger weight the aircraft can carry on that day. In certain air medical operations, temperatures greater than 90°F may prohibit the transport of two patients or may limit the amount of fuel that is carried.

Landing Surface

Recent weather may impact where local EMS can set up a landing zone for an inbound helicopter. Light, powdery snow will result in a "white-out" effect as the aircraft nears the ground, and will require location of a plowed area. Recent prolonged rains may result in the need to utilize a paved surface, as dirt and grass surfaces may be too soft. This is more often problematic for helicopters with wheels, as opposed to aircraft with landing skids on which the weight is more diffusely spread. Recent drought conditions may result in excessive dust clouds and much dried plant matter as loose debris. In addition, if flares are used to mark the landing zone, they can be blown over by tail rotor wash and result in brush fires.

Hazardous Materials

Unlike most ground ambulance drivers, helicopter pilots are enclosed in the same small air space occupied by the patient, and are at risk for exposure to any fumes coming from the patient or the patient's clothing. In addition, should a pilot begin to be affected, there is not the opportunity to "pull over" alongside the road. Patients who are contaminated with hazardous materials should not be transported by air. Patients who have been completely decontaminated may be appropriate for air transport, but the challenge is how to verify that decontamination has in fact been complete. This includes not only external decontamination, but also consideration of whether the patient may be off-gassing substances from the lungs.

Special Capabilities

The local EMS medical director should have an awareness of the special capabilities of the air medical services in their area. Some of these capabilities may already be available and only need be remembered when a unique situation presents itself. Others may require specific preplanning, training, and purchase of equipment in order to be utilized. Others yet may be beyond the scope or mission of the local air provider. The medical director should have knowledge of the types of special services that helicopters can provide, and evaluate whether these capabilities should be cultivated with the air medical providers in the local area.

Difficult Access Areas

Helicopters can be of great assistance for patients who are difficult to reach or remove from a remote area. Hikers and hunters may become ill or injured a great distance from a roadway. Rural roads may be inaccessible long after a big snowstorm. Island inhabitants may be inaccessible due to rough or frozen waters. These instances can readily be handled by most any air medical program, provided a suitable landing zone can be established in proximity to the patient.

Aerial Rescue

Hoist operations may be invaluable in dealing with a patient in a difficult access area where a landing zone cannot be established. Special equipment and training are required on the part of the local air medical service. Hoisting is most often used to remove a patient from a dangerous, precarious, or time-critical situation, but on occasion may also be the only means of inserting rescuers to access the patient.

Aerial Reconnaissance

Visualization of an incident scene from the air may provide important information as to the size of the event, the number of resources needed and the best route for responding units to gain access. In regional disasters such as flash flooding and earthquakes, aircraft can locate imperiled persons who are not yet patients, and can alert responding units to impassable roadways.

Search

Helicopters can be utilized effectively to assist ground EMS in locating patients in unusual situations. Some examples would include an overturned boat with persons swept downstream, a severely crashed vehicle found on an isolated stretch of road at night with evidence of bleeding and no patient, a young child or an Alzheimer's patient missing in cold weather, or a report of a person possibly fallen through the ice. Hunters and hikers may call from the woods via cell phone to report a serious injury or illness, but may be unable to provide an exact location. On occasion these patients are only located by staying on the line and telling the 9-1-1 center when they hear the helicopter getting close to them. All helicopters are capable of performing a visual search, and those that perform nighttime scene medevacs have searchlights. Some air medical programs utilize Forward Looking Infrared (FLIR) devices mounted to the nose of the aircraft that allow the detection of missing persons by sensing body heat. Effective integration of air medical programs in search-and-rescue operations requires preplanning and training. Some discussion of expenses also likely needs to occur, since often these calls do not result in the actual transport of a patient by air.

Aerial Lighting

Most medevac helicopters have a strong searchlight that can effectively illuminate an area the size of a football field. While use of a helicopter searchlight is not as cost-effective method of routinely providing illumination, it can provide rapid, mobile visualization in critical situations. Beyond initially locating patients, the aircraft can provide lighting while rescuers access and provide initial care to patients that are scattered across a large incident, or are located in the water or in a difficult-access area. It should be noted, however, that the aircraft will produce a significant amount of noise that may make communications among ground rescuers difficult.

Mass Casualty Incidents

In incidents with multiple injured patients, air medical transport can be utilized to distribute patients among appropriate trauma facilities to prevent any one center from becoming overwhelmed. Depending on the incident location, the strategy may be to fly the most seriously injured patients, or alternatively to drive the most critical to nearby trauma centers, while flying less critical but serious patients to more distant trauma facilities.

Mass Gatherings

Mass gatherings of people present EMS systems with unique problems. Normal traffic patterns throughout an entire city or region may be disrupted significantly. In addition to challenges in accessing and transporting patients associated with the event itself, access to healthcare facilities in the area may be obstructed. These facilities may also be overwhelmed with ambulatory patients from the event. Air medical transport may play roles in removing patients from the event itself, allowing non-event patients to continue to access healthcare facilities in the area, and distributing patients to more distant hospitals when local facilities are overwhelmed.

Go Teams

Air medical programs may be able to support local EMS by transporting hospital-based physician/nurse anesthetist teams who are specially trained and equipped for scene response. These responses typically involve incidents with protracted extrications in which there is concern that a field surgical procedure may be required. Such teams may also play a role in selected mass casualty incidents and disaster situations. Go team response requires much preplanning and coordination among local EMS, the sending hospital, and the local air provider.

High-Rise Emergency Aerial Teams (HEAT)

Local Fire Services and EMS may team with air medical providers to be able to insert firefighter caregivers onto the roofs of large burning buildings. In addition to being able to assist in firefighting and to initiate medical care, these personnel can be a significant calming influence to prevent building occupants from unnecessarily jumping. Firefighters and paramedics trained in this fashion can also be inserted to provide care and rescue in other challenging locations, such as on the decks of sinking ships, the tops of water towers, and the edges of cliffs. In order to be performed safely, such maneuvers require specialized equipment and regular training by all involved.

Summary

The successful integration of air medical transport into local EMS system is dependent upon effective preplanning and coordination at many different levels. With the proper degree of understanding and insight into air medical operations, the medical director can play a pivotal role in ensuring that air services are utilized efficiently and effectively.

Bibliography

Air Medical Physician Association. Rodenberg H and Blumen IJ, eds. *Air Medical Physician Handbook.* 1999.

Annual medical crew survey. *AirMed.* 1999;5(5):27–33.

Annual transport statistics and fees survey. *AirMed.* 1999;5(4): 20–23.

National Association of EMS Physicians. Air medical dispatch: guidelines for trauma scene response. *Prehosp Disaster Med.* 1992;7:75–78.

National Association of EMS Physicians. Criteria for prehospital air medical transport: non-trauma and pediatric considerations. *Prehosp Disaster Med.* 1994;9:2.

CHAPTER 51

Interfacility Transport

Ronald B. Low, MD

Introduction

Choosing the "closest" versus "most appropriate" receiving hospital has been and remains a source of controversy within EMS. However, those issues are resolved when the patient first goes to the hospital, there will be instances where a patient needs to be moved from one hospital to another. Frequently, these moves are to a center with special capabilities: burn centers, trauma centers, neonatal centers, and so on. As financing of medical care evolves, more patients will move for financial reasons: moving indigent patients to government-owned hospitals and insured patients to "in system" hospitals. As corporate planners continue to "remove excess bed capacity," patients will be moved from hospitals that are full to hospitals with open beds. Some patients will ask to be transferred for personal reasons, such as being closer to family.

Level of Care

Several types of vehicles can be used to move patients between hospitals. The patients will be cared for by a variety of caretakers. Family or friends can drive many relatively stable patients in their own car; an example would be the renal transplant patient going to a transplant center after a kidney becomes available. EMS planners realize that private transport is sometimes efficient and appropriate. The next level of care is the "invalid coach" or "ambulette." These vehicles may be the most efficient way to transport stable patients with mobility problems, such as amputees, the mentally impaired, and "old stroke" patients. Most states regulate these vehicles and their drivers as a special category of bus, taxi, or limousine. These patients do not need treatment skills. Operators of these services are not often required to train drivers and attendants with prehospital medical skills. Some states do require first-aid training; this seems prudent.

Standard ambulances are often used for critical-care transport between facilities. In some instances, this may represent the best available option. Usually, this type of transport is not what the vehicle, onboard equipment, and crew training were designed for. Overuse of field units for interfacility transport makes them unavailable for prehospital response. In some rural areas, the desire to keep scarce field units available locally is the main justification for calling an outside transportation service.

Dedicated interfacility transport services vary in their intent and design. Many are critical-care transport services; some are specialized to one type of patient. Generally, these services are designed to provide care that would be unavailable aboard an ambulance designed for prehospital work. Examples of such care include a much wider variety of intravenous medication infusions, more complex ventilators and respiratory care, multichannel monitoring, and invasive blood pressure measurements.

Some transport services are very focused. Examples include neonatal, cardiac, transplant, military casualty, and very long distance transport teams. When assessing the need for specialty services, it is necessary to match the anticipated needs of the patient with the training, experience, equipment, and capability of the available transport teams. Focused experience and niche-specific equipment are two important "up sides" of specialty transport teams. "Down sides" include higher costs, limited reduced efficiency and reduced transport experience for both the niche team and the general critical-care transport teams. Boundary areas between niches may also become problematic. Should an obstetrical (OB) unit or a neonate unit be sent when a referring hospital calls for help with a woman in premature labor?

Availability is usually an issue. The interhospital transport team is rarely standing by, near the patient, when the doctors decide to transport the patient. If a local ambulance is standing by, it is often the fastest way to get the patient to a tertiary care center. Under ideal circumstances, a helicopter might be able to make a round trip from the tertiary care center to the transferring hospital and back as quickly. Using that time as a "baseline," the only way to shorten the time is to summon a helicopter as soon as the need is evident but before the patient is "stable enough to transfer." This shortening of time requires forethought and coordination between referring hospital and transfer service. Any of the following may lengthen the time beyond "baseline":

1. Waiting for a niche team to assemble and reconfigure a vehicle.
2. Weather delays, particularly for air transport.
3. Waiting for a transport team that is already out with another call.
4. Using "three point transfers," where a transport team leaves its base, goes to the referring hospital, then to the receiving hospital, drops off the patient, then returns to its base.

Personnel

The composition of transport team has been and remains a significant source of controversy. People who market critical-care transport teams frequently tout the training and experience of the transport team as a selling point for their service. Intuitively, it seems that well trained, experienced, and procedurally competent team members are needed to care for critically ill patients. Realistically, many transported patients do not need en route interventions nor immediate complex decision making. While some of the transported patients have little chance of survival, most patients benefit from en route intensive care. For those patients, the benefit depends on: (1) the interventions which could potentially help the patient, (2) the total clinical experience of the team member, (3) the crewmember's experience with this type of patient, (4) the training level of the crewmember, (5) the equipment available, (6) the space available, and (7) the team member's transport experience and familiarity with the vehicle and equipment. The few research efforts to show the value of one type of team over another have been small and limited by design flaws. There have been no prospective randomized controlled trials where a patient was entered into a study, then randomized to be transported by one type of team or another.

Most transport teams do not carry physicians; those teams that do include physicians usually use resident physicians in training. These doctors are not considered ready for unsupervised practice in the hospital; yet they are often the best trained but inexperienced crewmembers. The teams that do not carry physicians typically assert that a direct medical oversight physician could make complex decisions. This doctor usually makes decisions based on relatively infrequent radio or telephone communication. Some studies show some minimal benefit of this type of medical oversight for prehospital care; however, there is no research demonstrating the effectiveness of this medical oversight for long interhospital transports.

Almost all hospital-based critical-care interhospital transport teams use nurses as team members. Usually, these nurses have years of relevant hospital-based experience before they join the transport teams. After joining the transport teams, the nurses typically have several weeks of special training and apprentice experience. The training includes endotracheal intubation, clinical protocols, radio operations, extrication techniques, scene safety, vehicle equipment use (including litter and lifting techniques) and vehicle emergency procedures.

Some transport teams include paramedics as a permanent crewmembers, who have usually been hired for their previous experience with scene safety, extrication techniques, litter use and lifting, and other prehospital skills. Typically in this mode, paramedics are taught how to manage the ventilators and monitoring equipment. Usually, the paramedics are taught more extensive pharmacology; however, choice of drug therapy is usually left to other team members or direct medical oversight.

Some transport programs use intermediate or basic level EMTs for dispatching, driving, or other ancillary support. Interhospital transport services rarely use basic or intermediate level EMTs as permanent patient-care crewmembers. Many teams will add other medical specialists on an ad hoc basis. Respiratory therapists or intra-aortic balloon pump technicians may join the team when use of their special skills is anticipated.

Vehicle

Any vehicle may perform transfers; ground ambulances, rotor, and fixed-wing aircraft are most commonly used. Special boats are sometimes used between islands and coastal areas. The vehicles needed by any given service will depend on the number and types of nearby hospitals and the availability of other transport services. Helicopters may reduce transport time; however liftoff and landing operations generally take a minimum of five minutes. This time can be considerably longer if the patient is very heavy or if multiple life support devices must be moved concomitantly. Helicopters usually have little advantage over ground transport for distances of 20 miles or less. All civilian helicopters are relatively noisy (around 100dB); some urban areas ban their use altogether or restrict their use during certain times. Ground ambulances are usually operational in weather that has grounded airplanes and helicopters. Ground ambulances offer advantages of cost and safety; time is rarely the most important issue. For example, neonatal teams are generally more concerned about providing an appropriate level of care than in reducing transport time.

Rotor wing services generally offer a dedicated team and ready availability. The maximum speed of EMS helicopters varies from 100 to 200 mph. Weather conditions may slow a mission down.

Available fixed-wing air ambulances have more than twice the speed of helicopters. For some missions of over 100 miles and most missions over 200 miles, airplane transfer is faster. Fixed-wing transfers usually involve the extra time and expense of ground ambulance trips from the referring hospital to a nearby airport, then again from an airport to the receiving hospital. Fixed-wing transfers can fly in worse weather than helicopters, but not in any weather. Most helicopter ambulances are prohibited from flying in poor visibility and no civilian helicopter is certified to fly when there is icing. Most fixed-wing ambulances can fly under instrument flight rules and in some icing. Since the quality, experience, and availability of air ambulance services vary greatly, it is prudent to make contact with the service, know its capabilities, and have a standing arrangement prior to the event.

Specific Transfers

Interhospital transfer involves a minimum of two hospitals and a transfer service. In some circumstances, this model may not be the fastest. There may not be a helicopter service nearby. Sometimes, particularly in densely populated cities, there may not by nearby sites to safely land helicopters. In sparsely populated areas, fixed-wing aircraft may be useful, and separate services may be needed to move the patient between hospital and airport. Often, more complex models can be anticipated. Planning and existing protocols

can smooth the process of exchanging the patient and information. Many aspects of interhospital transfer are generalizable; the model and protocols apply to all transfers of patients from a smaller hospital with limited resources to a larger, tertiary care center. Some transfers are integral to the system design. Trauma systems may be the most common systems in the country. Many other systems are also used: burn center systems, maternal-fetal systems, and so on. The EMS planner should develop standards for these transfers. The standards should minimize medical complications, reduce legal liability and improve system efficiency.

Trauma

The underlying theory of trauma system designation is a focus on expertise, experience, and commitment. Most trauma systems have three levels of trauma center, although at least one largely rural state has four levels. Densely populated New York City has only one level. Generally, Level III trauma centers commit to having one physician readily available to treat an injured patient, along with minimal amounts of blood available in a blood bank, basic lab and radiology support, and other basic needs. Level I trauma centers commit to having in-house emergency physician coverage, immediately available specialty surgeons, extensive laboratory support, radiology capability and research commitment.

All EMS systems put considerable design effort into ensuring that patients requiring a trauma center will be appropriately triaged to one from the scene of injury. Most of these systems provide for considerable overtriage, therefore there will be many more patients with minor injuries transported to a trauma center than badly injured patients sent to a hospital that is not a trauma center. Nonetheless, trauma patients are one of the largest groups of patients transfered. There are three main reasons for this: (1) even a sophisticated triage system will still "miss" some patients with subtle injuries; (2) some patients will find their way to the initial hospital outside of the EMS system; (3) in many rural areas the trauma system is designed with the expectation that many patients will be transported from a lower-level hospital to a higher-level hospital. In most of these systems, the Level III hospital performs initial stabilization and retriage. Most patients moved from a Level II to a Level I center are transfered for neurosurgical interventions.

Timeliness is usually the most important factor in the interhospital transport of trauma patients, since the major killers of trauma victims are shock and brain injury. The goal of the transport is to bring the patient to definitive intervention before shock or neurological injury becomes irreversible. Sometimes the transport team provides some procedure that local hospital personnel are unable to perform. The most commonly performed procedures are intubation and intravenous access. The ideal trauma system will designate the receiving hospital and transport system ahead of time. The system expectations should also be clear to the sending hospital, the receiving hospital, and the transport team, so that minimal time is lost while the transport team does maneuvers that were not done by the sending hospital.

Burns

Compared to other injuries, burns usually progress slowly. Burn centers give special expertise to wound healing and infection prevention. In the hours immediately following a burn, the main life threats are loss of intravascular volume and concomitant injury. Among the concomitant injuries are inhalation burn injuries to the airway, and poisonings. If inhalation burns seem likely, early intubation is prudent. A rare but dramatic complication is a sudden airway obstruction by swelling after seemingly normal breathing. A moving ambulance is a difficult place to monitor for stridor, then intubate through a swollen airway. Carbon monoxide and cyanide are the most common poisons. Cyanide works very quickly; it is unlikely to be an issue by the time a patient is ready for interhospital transfer. In the absence of hyperbaric oxygen, providing high concentrations of inhaled oxygen is the best available therapy, and can be easily provided at the local hospital and during transport. Significant increases in altitude during flight are problematic for patients suffering from carbon monoxide poisoning. Calculations of fluid requirements depend on careful estimation of time and burn size, measurement of urine volume and concentration, and, when available, hemodynamic monitoring. To the extent that the transport team can provide these services, they may offer significant benefit to the early resuscitation of burn patients. Burns certainly need to be kept clean during transport. Dressing the wounds helps keep them clean, provide early antimicrobial activity, and reduce pain. Dressing the wounds may make analysis of the burns more difficult to assess at the burn center.

Spinal Trauma

Spinal cord injuries are frequently associated with additional trauma, and these patients are initially managed with other trauma victims. Following stabilization, these patients may benefit from the experienced treatment and rehabilitative services available at spinal cord centers. Transfer is rarely time-critical. Transfer arrangements will usually be determined by safety, convenience, cost, and mechanical stability. Depending on the nature of the injury and the time since injury, the main consideration may be preventing movement and extending the injury. Although in cases of high cervical lesions, the team should be proficient in airway management, many spinal injured patients may be safely transported by basic EMT.

Obstetrical

Almost all OB transfers are for the fetus. Some anticipated transfers for scheduled procedures can be done by private vehicle. Many transfers are for unanticipated conditions, usually premature labor or pre-eclampsia. Federal COBRA/EMTALA laws define any woman in active labor as "unstable." These patients can be transferred only when the expected benefits are clear. Premature infants delivered at a neonatal center are more likely to survive than similar infants delivered at other hospitals; however few systems proceed with transfer unless en route delivery is unlikely. The most reliable indication that delivery may occur soon is cervical dilation of greater than 4cm. Fetal distress warrants C-section prior to transport. As en route time is usually critical, helicopter transport is often the preferred method. Helicopter transfer is very rarely associated with in-flight delivery. Long-distance airplane transfers have a higher incidence of in-flight delivery. Ideally, OB transfers are made in vehicles with enough space and personnel to deliver intensive care to a newly delivered infant and to attend to the mother. Prior to managing OB patients in a transfer setting, the crews should be trained to handle the relatively large number of possible problems or complications that can occur in rapid succession.

Pediatric and Neonatal

As outlined above, even under the best of circumstances, some mothers will deliver markedly premature infants at hospitals without the equipment or trained personnel to care for them. Neonates require a disproportionate number of interhospital transfers, but some older children will also need to be transferred. Many local hospitals can care for a child with uncomplicated dehydration or uncomplicated surgical conditions. A much smaller number of hospitals are prepared to care for children with sepsis or other severe forms of shock. A relatively small number of hospitals are prepared for operative repair of complex developmental abnormalities, or for workup of complex inherited metabolic derangements. Compared to other patients, young children are more susceptible to dehydration and hypothermia. Young children have airways that are relatively small, floppy, and easily occluded. The current standard of care is to bring critically sick children to specialty centers designed to care for them. Children being transferred between hospitals may need special equipment. Commonly needed items include pediatric endo-tracheal tubes, transport isolettes, low volume ventilators, and IV infusion pumps. Some medication is specific to pediatric illness, for example, prostaglandin. The American Academy of Pediatrics has published transport guidelines based upon expert consensus. These guidelines list specific equipment needs and recommend formal pediatric training and competence of the transport crew.

Poisoning

Some poisoned patients need complex management or specific antidotes. These patients frequently have multisystem compromise; they may need respiratory and hemodynamic support. Surgery may be needed for an envenomated extremity or chemical burns. Time may be critical. When a specific antidote is needed but not available at the referring hospital, flying the antidote to the patient may be of enormous benefit. Ideally, the transport team will have experience with the type of poisoning and its therapy.

Cardiac

A large and growing number of heart patients are transferred between hospitals. Heart disease is fairly common, the number of heart centers is relatively small, and new aggressive interventions are improving outcome for these patients. Following occlusion of a coronary artery, the ultimate extent of cardiac damage depends on how quickly the artery can be reopened. One therapy, intravenous thrombolytic agents, can be given at many hospitals. Prompt angio-plasty may be more effective than thrombolytic agents; and invasive therapy may be needed to "back up" thrombolysis. Intra-Aortic balloon pump support may stabilize patients awaiting a re-vascularization procedure. Angioplasty and bypass are usually done at centers committed to 24-hour availability of cardiac bypass capability. Many patients are transferred to designated heart centers early in the process of myocardial infarction. In the early phases of a myocardial infarction (MI), the main dangers to the patient are dysrhythmia, pump failure, and extension of the MI. Interhospital transfer can minimize these risks by: (1) speedy transfer; (2) in some cases, starting IV thrombolysis; (3) careful monitoring of rhythm and hemodynamics; (4) treating dysrhythmias with drugs, cardioversion, defibrillation or pacemakers; (5) and treating pump failure with IV infusions and intra-aortic balloon pumps (IABP). Treating pump failure with IV infusions may increase cardiac workload, extend the MI, and exacerbate dysrhythmias. Noninvasive arterial blood pressure measurement can be inaccurate, especially in the EMS setting. Titrating IV pressors requires invasive hemodynamic monitoring. IABP decreases cardiac workload, but requires significant equipment, space, and a two-person medical crew. Optimally a helicopter or ground vehicle used for these transports will be adequately large, powerful, and well equipped to provide all monitoring and IABP treatment options. If these teams and vehicles are not available, it may still be advisable to move the patient to a heart center in the less than ideal circumstances. There is no research enabling one to calculate the risks of transfer under certain conditions and compare that risk to the risk of staying at the smaller hospital.

Medical Oversight

Medical oversight is one of the more complicated and controversial issues surrounding interhospital transport. There are unresolved "turf" issues between medical specialties and between medical professionals of differing levels of training: EMTs, nurses, PAs, resident and attending physicians.

Most interfacility transports are routine and uncomplicated. Compared to pre-hospital transport, a disproportionate number require advanced procedures and complex decision making. These complex transports may involve multichannel monitors. Patients may receive multiple efficacious but potentially dangerous drugs. Some patients will need transport

INTERFACILITY TRANSPORT

ventilators, advanced airway devices, intra-aortic balloon pumps, tube thoracostomy or internal and external pacemakers. Many of these devices were designed for use in a hospital; most are not proven in the more varied circumstances of an ambulance. Interfacility transports are potential subjects to intense EMTALA scrutiny. Understanding the risk-benefit ratio for interventions, or whether to transport at all, requires an understanding of all of these issues, as well as a knowledge of the personnel and equipment at each referring facility and accepting facility.

Ideally, medical oversight physicians will have the training and experience needed to meet these challenges. Thorough knowledge of the capabilities of outlying hospital may require actually working there, or at least making several visits and spending time talking with several people on that hospital staff. Participating in actual transports will provide useful experience and insight. These measures require a substantial time commitment. Some services use multiple direct medical oversight physicians (DMOPs) and/or multiple medical directors. This has the advantage of spreading out the workload and concentrating specialty expertise: a traumatologist for trauma transports or a neonatologist for neonatal transports. The disadvantage of this system is that each of these physicians will have less experience with the crews, vehicles, referring facilities, receiving hospitals, and the progressively more complex rules and laws. In a real time scenario it is important to give the "benefit of the doubt" to the referring physician who has seen the patient and knows the local capabilities.

Most transports need only a modicum of direct medical oversight and more extensive audit and review by retrospective indirect medical oversight. When indirect medical oversight determines that policies and procedures were not followed; review should determine if: (1) that the circumstances were quite unusual (2) remedial education is needed or (3) the policies need improvement. There is little down side to having physicians from multiple specialties involved with indirect medical oversight. It may also be useful to have the participation of other EMS customers: other EMS services, nursing personnel from both sending and receiving hospitals, local hospital physicians, and those responsible for legal and administrative issues. Indirect medical oversight is often well suited to correct system problems associated with inappropriate transfers, "wallet biopsies," or inadequate stabilization by referring hospitals. Indirect medical oversight should offer in depth, deliberative

analysis and recommendations to all of the participants involved. This should be well integrated into a quality management (QM) process that is itself integrated into the hospital QM processes.

Ideally, medical oversight will be involved with research projects. Potential projects could: find the limits of hospital-based technology used on ambulances, discover new techniques or invent new technology when needed, improve direct medical oversight, and quantify the broader systems issues of who benefits from transport and who does not.

Legal Issues

Local and state legal issues, as the names suggest, vary from region to region. In general, many applicable laws were not written with complex inter-hospital transfers in mind which often "stretch" laws governing the equipment, training and scope of practice for an EMS vehicle. Generally, laws were written with scene pickup and delivery to a local hospital in mind. To the extent that some laws were written with interhospital transfers in mind, those laws may not keep up with dynamically changing medical science, medical economics, and federal law. Some specific questions have arisen: (1) If a patient is to be moved from a hospital in one state to a referral center in another state, what are the licensing requirements for the medical crew, medical control physicians, and vehicle? (2) When a transport team does not include a physician with an unrestricted license, when does "observation" and "protocol directed therapy" turn into "diagnosis" and "medical treatment"? (3) When has the transport team crossed the line and practiced medicine? (4) If a patient loses signs of life during a transport, can he be pronounced dead? (5) Does the pronouncement have to be made by a physician? (6) Can the direct medical oversight make the pronouncement without seeing the patient? (7) What is the time and location of death? (8) Does resuscitation need to be continued until the vehicle reaches its destination? Practically, many services find it more expedient to continue a fruitless resuscitation than to try to pronounce a patient dead while en route; however an unnecessary red lights and siren traffic accident death usually changes that practice.

Federal Law

EMTALA stands for Emergency Medical Transfer and Active Labor Act. COBRA stands for Consolidated Omnibus Budget Reconciliation Act which was part of that large budget bill. The "anti-dumping" parts of the law were meant to prevent hospitals from turning away indigent patients in immediate need of care. Successive versions of the laws have expanded the obligations of hospitals. The laws apply to hospitals that take federal money in virtually any form including Medicare, Medicaid, Champus, or grants. Almost all U.S. hospitals are included. Multiple other federal laws apply to specific situations; federal air regulations apply to air ambulances; federal rules about disaster management apply if a federal disaster is declared. These other laws are dealt with in other appropriate chapters of this book.

The following aspects of the laws particularly apply to transfers between hospitals:

(1) If a patient presents to an emergency department, then that hospital is obligated to see that the patient has an examination. Many independent observers conclude that federal officials enforce the law aggressively, perhaps beyond the letter of the law. As the law is interpreted and enforced, the examination of the patient should probably be done by a licensed independent practitioner (LIP). Usually, the LIP would be an attending physician.

(2) The examination should include any necessary laboratory tests or radiographs.

(3) After an adequate examination, the LIP would have to determine if the patient was "stable" or in "active labor." ("Active labor" does not seem to have a medical definition but represents an "unstable" patient)

(4) If the patient is "stable" and not "in active labor", then the hospital has no further COBRA/EMTALA federal obligation to the patient.

(5) If the patient is "unstable" or "in active labor," then the hospital has an obligation to care for the patient until he becomes "stable" or is no longer in "active labor." Whatever services the hospital normally offers, the hospital must offer to the covered patient. For example, if the hospital normally offers orthopedic coverage, then the hospital must offer that care to any "unstable" patient who needs emergent orthopedic treatment.

(6) The hospital can legally transfer an "unstable" or "laboring" patient to another hospital ONLY if one of the following conditions is met:

a. The patient requests the transfer. The patient has to be fully informed about the risks and benefits of the transfer. This informed consent and all other elements of the transfer must be clearly documented.

b. The hospital does not offer a service that the patient urgently needs. The accepting hospital must be contacted and must explicitly agree to accept the patient. When a patient is transferred for this reason, the referring hospital must clearly document what service is needed and an explicit statement that this service is not available at the referring hospital. Transfer documents must clearly state the reasons for transfer.

(7) If an on call physician refuses to respond to a patient in the ED, the patient can be transferred, but the referring and accepting hospitals are obligated to report the fact that the on call physician refused to respond.

(8) Under newer laws (as they are interpreted), the nearest appropriate hospital with special resources may be obligated to accept the transfer of patients needing that level of care. For example, a nearby trauma center may be obligated to accept the transfer of a badly injured patient from a non-trauma center.

(9) If the transfer vehicle is operated by a hospital, many observers believe that the operator of the vehicle becomes bound by COBRA laws once the patient boards the vehicle. For example, a helicopter ambulance would be considered a flying piece of the base hospital; once a patient boards the helicopter, then the sponsoring hospital has all of the COBRA obligations to care for the patient. Similar considerations apply to remote clinics or other facilities run by a hospital.

(10) Transfer documents that accompany the patient must include explicit statements about the reason for transfer and all relevant medical records, including radiographs and lab results.

Bibliography

Barquist E, Pizzutiello M, Tian L, et al. Effect of trauma system maturation on mortality rates in patients with blunt injuries in the Finger Lakes Region of New York State. *Journal of Trauma-Injury Infection & Critical Care.* 2000;49(1):63–70.

Castillo CY, Lyons TJ. The transoceanic air evacuation of unstable angina patients. *Aviation Space & Environmental Medicine.* 1999;70(2):103–106.

Clay M, Mullins RJ, Hedges JR, et al. Mortality among seriously injured patients treated in remote rural trauma centers before and after implementation of a statewide trauma system. *Medical Care.* 2001;39(7):643–653.

Conroy MB, Rodriguez SU, Kimmel SE, et al. Helicopter transfer offers a potential benefit to patients with acute stroke. *Stroke.* 1999;30(12):2580–2584.

Dardis R, Roberts G, Phillips J. A cost-benefit evaluation of helicopter transfers to the Beaumont neurosurgical unit. *Irish Medical Journal.* 2000;93(2):50–51.

Domeier RM, Hill JD, Simpson RD. The development and evaluation of a paramedic-staffed mobile intensive care unit for inter-facility patient transport. *Prehospital & Disaster Medicine.* 1996;11(1):37–43.

Gebremichael M, Borg U, Habashi NM, et al. Interhospital transport of the extremely ill patient: the mobile intensive care unit. *Critical Care Medicine.* 2000;28(1):79–85.

Holt J, Fagerli I. Air transport of the sick newborn infant: audit from a sparsely populated county in Norway. *Acta Paediatrica.* 1999;88(1):66–71.

Koury SI, Moorer L, Stone CK, et al. Air vs ground transport and outcome in trauma patients requiring urgent operative interventions. *Pre Emerg Care.* 1998;2(4):289–292.

Nathens AB, Jurkovich GJ, Cummings P, et al. The effect of organized systems of trauma care on motor vehicle crash mortality. *JAMA.* 2000;283(15):1990–1994.

Sampalis JS, Denis R, Lavoie A, et al. Trauma care regionalization: a process-outcome evaluation. *Journal of Trauma-Injury Infection & Critical Care.* 1997;46(4):565–579.

Wills VL, Eno L, Walker C, et al. Use of an ambulance-based helicopter retrieval service. *ANZ Journal of Surgery.* 2000;70(7):506–510.

Prehospital Providers in the Emergency Department

52

James M. Atkins, MD
Russell W. Hartung, MD

Introduction

EMS providers interact with emergency department (ED) personnel in three main arenas. The first is during training; the second is during transfer of patient care from the prehospital to the hospital environment; and the third occurs when the provider is actually employed in the EDs. Although the first two arenas are fairly well established, the appropriate clinical activities of EMS personnel who are employed as staff in the ED are areas of ongoing controversy.

As EMS has matured, questions have naturally arisen about the appropriate boundaries of practice. In recent years there has been an ongoing discussion about whether an expanded role might be found in the community. It has been postulated that certain patients could be treated in the field or referred directly to a primary care setting; that underserved patients could be cared for by mobile practitioners; and that providers could serve a public health role in injury prevention and screening.

Another discussion has taken place regarding the role of EMS providers in the ED itself. The fact that the ED is a useful training site for EMS students has not been challenged, and they are regularly found in EDs, learning about everything from diagnosing rhythm disturbances to interacting with patients and families during a crisis.

On the other hand, the role of EMS providers as hospital employees has been challenged by nursing groups and has become an ongoing legal controversy. Others have felt that incorporating EMS providers into the ED staff makes sense, in terms of both putting their skills to use and in allowing them to keep those skills honed for use in the field. Use of EMS providers in other areas of the hospital has not been challenged as vigorously as it has in the ED. They have, for example, been used to monitor cardiac rhythms on telemetry units and in cardiac rehabilitation units, since recognition of cardiac arrhythmias is an area in which EMS providers are well trained.

This chapter addresses the incorporation of students into the ED, the interaction which occurs when a patient is brought into the ED by ambulance, and the use of field providers as ED staff.

Students in the ED

Most educators agree that exposure to patient care in an ED is valuable in the training of an effective EMS provider. If properly supervised, the student can gain insight into the breadth of the emergency care of patients. In addition they can gain practice with skills such as interacting with patients during an emergency, reading rhythm strips, starting IVs, and setting clinical priorities.

Appropriate supervision of the student in the ED is an important consideration. Course directors and instructors must establish clearly defined goals and objectives, lists of procedures to be performed, and performance evaluations. It is important to orient the nurses or physicians who will be supervising the EMS providers to the educational needs, limitations, and performance expectations of the students. The clinical experience can be enhanced if a preceptor from the training program is present, although this is not always feasible because of lack of sufficient staff. Having nurses and physicians ride along with EMS units can provide understanding about their prehospital colleagues that is difficult to obtain in any other way. This experience will be helpful in both the education and subsequent professional interaction with EMS personnel.

Goals for the educational experience include patient assessment, obtaining vital signs, specific skill performance (IVs, reading rhythm strips, airway skills), taking reports from incoming EMS units, and general observation of patient care in the ED. In EDs that staff a hospital-based ambulance service, the student can also ride along with experienced EMS providers. The ability of students to follow the patient through their ED care after assisting on the prehospital run can be especially insightful. The ability to see the progression of an illness and response to therapy helps the student gain a better perspective on the care they will provide in the field.

It is helpful in setting up the educational goals to remember that nurses and prehospital personnel have different roles and different educational backgrounds. Field providers perform patient care using focused protocols. These protocols are important in gathering and transmitting patient information and in determining the treatment of the patient. On the other hand, nurses have a broader base of education and generally do not function in a protocol-driven fashion in the ED, except to triage and to facilitate initial treatment. ED training programs for prehospital students must recognize these differences. Similarly, nursing personnel need to understand the role and the educational needs of the EMS students with whom they interact.

Problems occasionally occur with education of EMS personnel in the ED, and these problems should be anticipated. These can arise from a lack of understanding of the educational objectives by students or proctors, from an ignorance by staff regarding the amount of training the student has already received, from disagreements regarding clinical freedoms in the ED, from an uneasiness with relatively untrained personnel being in the position of interacting with patients, and from a fear of legal consequences of actions taken by students. The more experienced the ED staff is with prehospital care, and the better the educational objectives and parameters are established, the less likely it is that problems will arise, and the better the educational experience will be.

The issue concerning continuing education of EMS personnel in the ED is a similar but slightly different issue as opposed to initial education. In 1980 it was demonstrated that EMT-Bs lost 50% of their basic skills and paramedics lost 61% of their basic skills within two years of training. Ongoing education and skills practice are crucial. This is especially true in rural areas, where low run volumes may result in an even faster deterioration in skill level. The ED is a natural resource for ongoing education. In addition, the side-by-side human interaction can often minimize the problems and misunderstandings that may arise between EMS personnel and ED personnel.

Clinical Interface: The Emergency Department

The interaction between EMS personnel and ED staff can vary significantly based on the size of the ED and on regional differences in protocol. For example, in some areas, the most common level of provider is the paramedic. At this level there are often extensive standing orders that allow a great deal of treatment in the field without consultation with direct medical oversight. In other areas, EMT-Bs are most commonly found. In these regions, very little advanced care is administered in the field, and the ED staff is more likely to need to intervene early for critically ill patients. In still other regions, the most common advanced EMT is the Critical Care or Intermediate level EMT. In this type of system, the EMT can provide many of the same treatments that can be provided by a paramedic, but they must first present the case over the radio to the direct medical oversight physician and receive an order to carry out these treatments. Thus the interaction between the physician and the EMT in this system is much more frequent. This is highly variable, however, since in some areas that have a preponderance of Intermediate or Critical Care level EMS providers, there is no radio system available.[1]

In most systems that depend heavily on mid-level EMTs, the radio interaction is probably the most significant interaction that takes place. The physician is ultimately responsible for the medication order, and thus depends on the accuracy of the radio presentation. A logical presentation that conveys the important information accurately is crucial. These communications go more smoothly when the providers and physicians are sufficiently familiar with each other. Since the physician on the radio is often not the same physician who interacts with EMS personnel during indirect medical oversight activities, it is helpful to create situations outside the ED environment where physicians and EMTs can interact. Setting up periodic sessions in which each of the emergency physicians must interact with and educate EMTs can allow the two groups to understand each other better, thus significantly improving the stressful interactions that occur over the radio.

Feedback regarding common mistakes or problems can also be discussed during teaching sessions, although immediate feedback at the time of patient presentation is often the most effective. This is frequently the best time to point out physical findings that may have been overlooked, or to have the EMT try one more attempt at the IV or intubation that was missed. For example, if a patient who was described as short of breath turns out to also have marked neck vein distension that was unrecognized, the best time for pointing it out and discussing how it relates to the patient's symptoms is immediately after the patient is delivered. This will not only target the educational point to the personnel who were involved but will deliver it at a time when they are most interested and ready to receive it. In doing so one must be sensitive to the way this information is delivered. Like anyone else, the EMT may feel publicly humiliated and demoralized if he is made to feel foolish in front of their colleagues. If the feedback is directed to one person specifically, it may be best to deliver it out of hearing range of the rest of the staff. If the feedback relates to more of a "team" issue, it is appropriate to speak with the crew as a whole. In any case, criticism or case review should be done out of the hearing range of the patient and the family.

If the crew had a hard time intubating a patient, starting an IV, or performing any other procedure, it can be particularly educational to have them make another attempt while they are in the ED with the patient on steady ground and under the direct supervision of the physician. This allows them a chance to "succeed" in the skill, and will help avoid the loss of confidence that can occur if they complete the run without having succeeded. It also allows the emergency physician to directly observe their technique and discover any errors that might otherwise result in continued failure in the future.

Providers in the ED

A significant percentage of EDs use prehospital providers for patient care.[1] EMTs are engaged in a wide variety of behaviors, many of which have been felt by nursing groups to be traditional nursing duties. In some settings they were functioning independently and had replaced nursing positions. As a result of this practice and of the scrutiny of this issue on a state-by-state basis by nursing organizations, a significant controversy has arisen. The central question is usually: What standing do EMTs have in the in-hospital setting and what nursing functions are delineated in law and require a license for their performance?

When exploring this issue, one must first understand why having EMS personnel work in the ED has been a developing trend. There are several reasons for

this, which include the availability of valuable skills and personnel cost considerations.

As EMS has developed, there have been increasing numbers of EMS providers who are available and looking for work in hospitals. In places where the availability of EMS providers is greater than the availability of nurses, this is an especially important factor. There is also the issue of the use and the maintenance of valuable skills. Not only does the experience the provider receives in the ED help them in the field, but their experience and training are valuable in the ED.

The issue is especially poignant when the hospital runs an ambulance service. If the EMS providers work in the ED when they are not out on a call, they get valuable experience, either through their own roles or through observing the staff. In addition, there is a financial incentive. Instead of having downtime while the providers wait for their next call, they can assist with patient-care activities in the ED. This is a more efficient use of staffing, and results in better trained EMTs. Problems arise because of the overlap between what the EMTs are trained to do and what nurses are trained to do. For example, both groups are trained in starting IVs, giving certain medications, and assessing patients. There is a tendency, then, for EMTs to be used as substitutes for nurses. This is attractive to hospital administrators, since EMTs are generally paid less than nurses, and since there is a shortage of nurses in many areas of the country. Nursing groups, however, have been concerned about the encroachment into nursing practice.

As a result of these concerns, nursing groups on all levels have been looking very closely at these developments. Various state nursing associations have developed position statements regarding the role of EMS providers in the ED. These statements have cited both patient-care concerns and the risk of losing nursing jobs to less expensive EMS providers. These statements have cited the difference in training, the licensure status, and the nature of the work as the basis of their concerns. In some cases, legislation has been sought which would further define and limit the scope of practice of field personnel in the in-hospital environment.

Nurses have much more training in the foundations of medical practice such as physiology and pharmacology, and are licensed to perform "nursing functions" independently. EMTs are trained in the use of specific protocols in a variety of situations, and are well trained in specific tasks. The nursing associations believe that EMS providers do not have the aggregate knowledge to assess body systems that nurses have. EMS providers, on the other hand, have pointed out that it makes little difference whether an IV is started in the field or in the ED; the task is the same. They point out that the claims that patient care suffers when EMTs are allowed to perform traditional nursing functions in the ED have no basis in proof. They also cite the shortage of nursing personnel available especially in rural and other underserved areas.

This controversy has led to high-profile conflicts in some states. For example, in Alabama, the state hospital association asked for assistance from the Alabama Committee of Public Health in defining acceptable practice for EMTs in the ED.[2] The Committee developed a document called Rules of Hospitals which, among other things, stated that "If emergency department paramedics (EDPs) are utilized in the support of emergency services, the EDPs shall be limited to performing tasks only in the hospital's emergency service area under direct supervision of the physician and/or registered nurse." They set a minimum of one RN or MD to supervise each two EDPs. They required that the medical staff and governing body approve the use of EDPs in the emergency service area and specify the scope of services they may render. Duties performed by the EDP included: assisting with the triage and initial assessment of patients; carrying out or assisting with the monitoring of patients, administration of medications, initiation and discontinuance of intravenous therapy; and assisting with procedures and treatments as directed. The Alabama State Nurses Association countered that the Board of Nursing alone had the authority to establish the boundaries of nursing practice, and that the Board of Public Health did not have the authority to promulgate such rules.

In 1988 an opinion was rendered by the General Counsel of the New York State Department of Health, which stated that Public Health Law only authorizes an EMT to staff a certified ambulance and is not intended as a means for authorizing individuals to provide healthcare services outside of the prehospital setting.[3] "An EMT, unless also licensed as a nurse, may not perform activities in a hospital if such activities constitute the practice of nursing. EMTs would not be prohibited from rendering assistance to the hospital's staff if such activities could be performed by individuals who did not require professional licensure."[3]

In New York State, a 1998 letter was sent from the State Education Department to hospitals stating that EMTs have no legal standing in the hospital setting.[4] "They may not perform any activity that cannot be performed by any unlicensed person." It specifically stated that EMTs may not remove sutures, may not initiate IVs, and may not insert or remove Foley catheters. "If they do perform such activities they are threatened with charges of practicing the profession of nursing without a license." The Public Health Law was amended by the legislature in 1992 to clarify that EMT authorization to perform medical or nursing procedures applies to the prehospital setting only. The Nurse Practice Act (Article 139 of State Education Law) states that "only a person licensed or otherwise authorized under this article shall practice nursing."

The New York State Nurses Association and the State Education Department of New York have specifically stated that performing sterile irrigations, performing sterile dressings or wound care, performing tracheostomy suctioning, performing tracheostomy care, ventilating with a bag valve mask unit for clients under 12 years of age, and connection of IV catheters to IV solutions (both medicated and non-medicated) are nursing functions. An exemption is granted that allows the performance of nursing tasks by unlicensed personnel to students who are enrolled in courses which are registered with the state, who are performing these duties as part of their clinical experience.[5]

Liability may be a consideration as well. In some cases, the uncertainty over the legal standing of EMS personnel in the ED has led both malpractice carriers and hospital attorneys to question the liability of the practice. Others have pointed out that the potential for liability always exists but that if the job descriptions, scope of practice, and supervisory requirements are spelled out in department policy and followed, liability from this type of arrangement should be minimal. The effect of applicable laws varies from state to state; however what is true in New York or Alabama may not be true in another state.[6]

In some places, EMTs function in a limited and mostly technical capacity in the ED. Their responsibilities include taking vital signs, performing CPR, applying sterile dressings, applying bandages, administering oxygen, applying physical restraints, assessing pupillary reaction, immobilizing suspected extremity fractures, performing oral suctioning, ventilating with the bag valve mask, cleaning equipment or rooms, setting up and stocking equipment, transporting patients and supplies, stocking rooms, teaching patients crutch walking, and assisting within the defined limits of the role.[7]

A separate issue is the use of the ED as a place where EMS personnel can perform prehospital skills for continuing education. In other words, allowing EMTs to start IVs, perform intubations, and so on, under the direct supervision of a nurse or physician is felt by many to be a distinct issue from hiring these same people as staff. This distinction has sometimes been lost in the ongoing debate but is being kept alive in the EMS community. The ED is one of the few places where physicians and nurses trained in emergency care can directly observe the EMS provider performing procedures on patients. Since EMS personnel are responsible for performing these same procedures in the field without supervision, periodic direct observation is very important.

The issue of ongoing education and maintenance of clinical skills has been a continuing controversy. Many state nursing associations have interpreted the laws to only allow performance of such skills as IV canulation and intubation by EMTs if they are enrolled in state-registered educational programs. This has been a source of frustration among some EMS medical directors, who realize that the best place for EMS providers to perform these skills under direct supervision, for the purpose of ensuring quality care in the field, is in the emergency department. There will always be EMS providers who have completed their "state-registered" educational programs, but whose skills have become rusty. It is argued that the medical director needs to be able to respond by setting up additional practice and observation as it becomes necessary. This is best accomplished in the ED under the direct observation of the physicians and nurses.

In some regions specific policies have been developed which allow EMS providers to start IVs in the ED but only under the direct supervision of a nurse. This allows the provider to gain the ongoing experience in a skill which will be needed in the field but ensures that the nurse remains at least in a supervisory role for the procedure. A similar situation is being tried in some EDs regarding intubation. In this case it is the ED physician who directly supervises the provider in intubating a patient.

Some regional EMS councils are formalizing this relationship between the EMT and the ED as an ongoing, continuing medical education "course." In other areas, the EDs have simply developed this rela-

tionship as an individual ED policy. Discussion about this issue needs to continue, and policy needs to be developed and negotiated at the state and regional level, so that EMS personnel can continue to receive effective continuing education without putting the hospitals at increased liability for providing this opportunity.

Even in cases where EMS providers are not allowed to actually practice their prehospital skills in the ED, the side-by-side working relationship that develops when they are employed in the ED helps foster a greater understanding and familiarity between the emergency physicians and the EMTs than would generally be seen in other departments. This is especially useful in a system where many of the field procedures carried out by the EMTs require direct medical oversight.

Running an ambulance service out of the ED staffing it with EMTs who are part of the ED staff is not without its internal problems. For example, if EMTs work in the ED when they are not out on a call, it means that they have to leave on a moment's notice when a call does come in. Making an ED function smoothly when a portion of the staff regularly "disappears" can be a challenge, and requires a significant amount of flexibility in roles in such a department. For example, EMTs might generally do the EKGs. When a 9-1-1 call comes in, and the EMTs leave, nursing must take up the slack. This can sometimes lead to frustration, especially if the staff member does not realize the provider has been called away and then wastes time looking for that person. The most formidable "Catch 22" inherent in this type of system is that when the ED is busy, it is frequently a result of the high volume of EMS calls. Thus the frequency with which the EMTs are gone is directly proportional to how badly they are needed.

Another problem when EMTs work under the restrictions imposed by nursing practice is the schizophrenia caused by the dual role the EMTs play. In the field they are credentialed to run codes, intubate, and decompress tension pneumothoraces; in the emergency department they are unable to even hang IVs, and often are assigned the less skilled functions which are nevertheless crucial to running an ED. Most of the time this is not a significant problem and the individuals work well together. In fact, in some EDs many of the nurses also work as volunteer EMTs and understand the dichotomy of field versus hospital privileges. But occasionally the providers joke that, in the ED, EMT really means "Every Menial Task."

When there is a regular EMS staff in the ED, students who come in for clinical time tend to get a better experience. Not only are there veteran EMS providers in the department from whom they can learn but they get the additional exposure of a ride with one of the busier departments in the region. Thus the experience derived from working in the ED gets disseminated through education of new providers.

Suggestions

ED functions can be productive but should not involve assumption of nursing roles which would violate individual state Nursing Practice acts. Administrators are advised to research the situation in their own state. There should be written policies delineating the duties of EMS personnel and specifying to whom they are responsible. In some EDs the EMS providers have been seen as supporting the nursing role; and generally function under nursing supervision. This may not be true in situations like application of splints, in which case the physicians will often supervise and will be the final arbiter of whether the splint is acceptable and properly applied.[8]

It is sometimes a problem keeping EMS and nursing activities separate, especially in a busy ED when an EMS provider is asked by a physician to perform a nursing function. Physicians not familiar with the dichotomy sometimes are confused by the fact that EMTs are allowed to do certain functions in the field and may ask the EMT to perform the same function in the ED. Tasks allowed by EMTs should be spelled out in detail, and the staff should be in-serviced on which tasks are allowed in the ED and which are not.

Identifying EMS providers as separate from nurses, with a name tag or a different uniform, can help in keeping staff and patients from becoming confused. This may prevent them from being asked to perform an inappropriate task.

The EMS director and ED director must research the legal standing of EMS providers in the ED, this can differ from state to state. Perceptions can also differ based on the historical and political relationship between nursing and EMS. When the use of EMS providers in the ED is something new, the staff should be involved in the process.

Summary

EMS personnel interface with EMS on many levels. This interaction starts when they are students and continues as they transfer a patient to ED staff during a call. In addition, in some areas EMS personnel are used as staff in the ED. This last area of interaction has caused some confusion and generated some controversy because of the overlap between nursing training and EMS training. The resolution of this issue may differ from state to state. Even within relatively strict guidelines, EMS personnel can be a great asset to the smooth and efficient functioning of an ED, and they can gain valuable experience through their ED work.

References

1. Allerman G, et al. Use of prehospital care providers in emergency department: a national survey. *J Emerg Nurs.* 1985;11(1):33–39.
2. Alabama Emergency Nurses Association takes a stand against proposed emergency department paramedics with broad emergency department functions. *J Emerg Nurs.* 1992;18(5):464–468.
3. Letter from Peter J. Millock, General Counsel, NY State Department of Health, February 8, 1988.
4. Letter from Susan Mekus, Professional Assistant to the Executive Secretary of the State Education Department, Office of the State Board of Nursing, March 10, 1988.
5. Letter from Milene A. Sower, Ph.D., R.N., Executive Secretary New York State Education Department Board of Nursing, March 10, 1988.
6. Ingalls J. Historical Review of Emergency Medical Services, EMT roles, and EMT utilization in Emergency Departments. *J Emerg Nurs.* 1985;11(1):27–32.
7. Pediatric Hospitals Use Paramedics to Free Nurses. *ED Management.* 1995;7(11):127–129.
8. Regulation of prehospital nursing practice: a national survey. *J Emerg Nurs.* 1993;19(5):437–440.

Inappropriate Use and Unmet Need

53

Mark Henry, MD

Introduction

Emergency Medical Service Systems have been promulgated throughout the country in an effort to afford the ill and injured access to effective emergency care.[1] For improved health outcomes, patients must appropriately access these services. Inappropriate use or misuse of EMS is a potential waste of resource and possible diversion of needed service from another in need. Under use of resources can result in poor health outcome, since effective resources either were not accessed or were not available to those in need.

Inappropriate use of emergency medical services and unmet need for EMS have been proposed as useful measures of appropriateness of ambulance utilization since the early 1970s, when federal leadership resulted in growth of EMSS across the country.[2,3] Following the rapid expansion of EMS over the past three decades, one might believe that the major question today is whether there is overuse of service. Yet there are major national campaigns to address unmet need for major illness and injury. It is useful to consider both parameters together, as they are closely interrelated. The relationship of inappropriate use and unmet need, findings from the literature, and a discussion of some of the multiple factors which affect the appropriate use of EMS service lead to reconsideration of the values of these measurements in EMS system analysis today.

Definitions

Unmet Need

Gibson defined "unmet need" as the proportion of patients with a clinical need for ambulance services who did not receive it. He proposed it was a crucial measure of the ambulance system effectiveness, measured by clinical evaluation of all arrivals (ambulance and non-ambulance) at hospital emergency departments taken as the sampling frame.[2] Reasons for unmet need might include: a patient did not request it, they did not know how to access the system, or their request was denied. The measure of unmet need could be used by health planners, to develop systems which coordinate hospital services with emergency medical services, and for effective means to educate the public on methods for effective use of these services. Not only would the measure be of interest to health planners, but to emergency physicians as a means to assess the adequacy of ambulance services in their hospitals and within their EMS system.[3]

Inappropriate Use

Inappropriate ambulance use is simply defined as the proportion of all ambulance patients who do not need such care, and, according to Gibson, it exists for only one reason; that is, the ambulance dispatcher inappropriately accepted the request for the service.

Relationships

These measures are interrelated, as seen from the two-by-two table from which they can both be derived (fig. 53.1). Within the construct of the two-by-two table, unmet need would be a "false negative error" as a measure of system performance. In contrast to unmet need, inappropriate use would constitute a false positive error within the EMS system.

As might be expected when EMS Systems were initially developing, unmet need was high. Looking at data from 3,000 ambulance runs and 5,000 emergency department (ED) patient surveys in Chicago in 1969, while 84% of ambulance cases were true emergencies, only 38% of ED cases who were in clinical need of ambulance transportation actually received it.[2] There was a low inappropriate use rate but signifi-

	Patient Needed Ambulance Service	
PATIENT USED AMBULANCE SERVICE	YES	NO
Yes	a	b
No	c	d
Unmet Ambulance Need Inappropriate Ambulance Use	c/a + c b/a + b	

FIGURE 53.1. *A 2x2 table defining inappropriate use and unmet need for ambulance service. After Gibson.*[3]

cant of unmet need. Three years later, a similar analysis in Erie County, New York showed unmet need of 55% and inappropriate use of 31%.[3]

Patient interviews, attending physician rating of acuity, and medical records were used in the Chicago study, whereas the criteria of need in Erie County were from retrospective chart review by a trained trauma nurse. While comparison of the data from these two studies is limited since different methodologies were used, what is striking and hardly unexpected are the high rates of unmet need—the very reason EMS systems were being promoted with federal dollars.

Sensitivity and Specificity

Using the same table (fig. 53.1) Gibson proposed for inappropriate use and unmet need, he coined terms for ambulance indices of sensitivity and specificity. An ambulance specificity index can be calculated as d/b + d, the proportion of all patients not needing an ambulance who didn't receive one. Likewise, the sensitivity index is the proportion needing ambulance service who actually received it, a/a + c. Ideally, the goal for both sensitivity and specificity would be 100%. But this is unrealistic, and if there were a trade-off, one would hope to err by providing ambulance service to a patient who didn't need it rather than denying service to one who had need.

Likewise, inappropriate use and unmet need targets ideally would be 0%, denoting maximum efficiency and effectiveness. But this again is unrealistic. And because of the interrelationship, as one strives to reduce unmet need, inappropriate use is bound to increase. And if one tries to reduce inappropriate use, unmet need will rise. Most importantly, one has to accept and be cognizant of the interrelationship of use and need.

For example, with prehospital trauma triage, a certain amount of unnecessary use of EMS service is bound to occur if one includes less specific criteria (such as mechanism of injury without anatomic or physiologic findings) in an effort to improve sensitivity. In this context, is planned overtriage of trauma victims (to increase sensitivity) accurately described as "inappropriate" transport?

Roles of Dispatch and Medical Oversight

Emergency medical dispatch decisions can have a major impact on inappropriate use rates but are less likely to reduce unmet need. If an ambulance is only dispatched to those in obvious need, then nearly all patients transported by ambulance will have need of it. The inappropriate use of ambulance service will approach 0%; and the "appropriate" use will approach 100%. One can't use an ambulance inappropriately if it is never dispatched. However, decreasing inappropriate use by overly strict criteria for dispatch will invariably increase the number of times an ambulance is denied to someone who did need the service, and increase the unmet need.

The overall rate of unmet need in a community is less likely to be influenced by the dispatch decision than by public education on when and how to call for ambulance service. While dispatch decisions can increase unmet need by not dispatching an ambulance when one was needed, it is more likely that unmet need exists because a request for ambulance transport was never made on the patient's behalf.

Medical oversight of dispatch is an essential element of a modern EMS system. The medical director should approve the policies and protocols which address the response of the system to a call to 9-1-1. Should an ambulance be dispatched on all calls? If not, what calls are screened out and receive no ambulance response? What is the prioritization among multiple calls? Is transport expected once an ambulance is dispatched? What about field triage by EMTs and paramedics? All these questions are medical issues and will directly or indirectly affect the appropriate use of ambulances.

Medical oversight also plays a key role in addressing unmet need for ambulance service within a community. The medical director can include measurements of unmet need within the EMS system quality improvement programs. Educational programs for patients, the public, and the medical community conducted to decrease unmet need of targeted populations of patients should be consistent with the regional EMS Systems programs and their effectiveness analyzed when assessing change in the system.

Contributing Factors

There are multiple factors that influence the call for EMS, and all contribute to the appropriate use of the EMS system. The patient or someone on behalf of the patient must first make the request for EMS assistance. The decision to seek help can be influenced in large part by public education on when and how to use an ambulance. The availability of centralized communications such as 9-1-1 and public education on when and how to access 9-1-1 will increase requests for assistance. A system's response and threshold for dispatch may be influenced by the availability of ambulances and other EMS resources. The emergency medical dispatch policies, protocols, and training are key to the EMS system, and require significant oversight by the EMS medical director. Quality management (QM) reviews of the EMS system that address both inappropriate use and unmet need are fundamental for feedback to the multiple stakeholders, and to make change. To assess unmet need, systematic reviews of all ED patients, whether transported by ambulance or arriving by other means, need to be conducted.

Current Research and Programs

There are multiple studies in the literature addressing inappropriate use of ambulances. Both cost consciousness and the era of managed competition have caused reexamination of both the need for ambulance transport as well as the need for ED care. Multiple articles look at related issues such as the accuracy of dispatch assessments and the EMT's ability to triage at the scene. Indeed, current jargon includes the "partnership" between traditional public services such as EMS and for profit health businesses such as managed care organizations (MCO). In this environment, labels such as "inappropriate" are often interpreted as not requiring service, not reimbursable, or causing burden to the system.

Rarely do inappropriate use publications simultaneously examine unmet need. Yet unmet need exists, and efforts to reduce it are promulgated for different types of emergency patients, such as chest pain, stroke, dissecting thoracic aortic aneurysm, and mo-

tor vehicle crash victims. For many patients, the benefit of accessing the health system via ambulance transport is a reduction in time to care within the hospital setting itself, with improved outcomes independent of other benefits resulting from therapeutic interventions given enroute.

Inappropriate Ambulance Use

The literature has frequently focused on inappropriate use rates, and usually excluded unmet need. Some of the reported inappropriate use rates are alarming high, but there is considerable variation and one must look closely at the methods before drawing conclusions from the rates alone. In one study of pediatric EMS use, inappropriate ambulance transport was reported to be 61%, but excluded trauma team activations and those in need of immediate resuscitation.[4] Other studies note inappropriate use rates of 11% (Billittier),[5] 28% (Kost),[6] 38% (Gardner),[7] 45% (Brown),[8] 52% (Morris).[9]

Problems in comparing one study to another and extrapolating findings are evident from the very fact that the methods used to define "inappropriate" vary widely. Methods and analysis are often subjective or retrospective, have different exclusion criteria, or are based on information and findings not available until after a patient has been fully evaluated in the emergency department. For example, compare the following two methods to determine inappropriate use. Kost conducted a retrospective chart analysis and deemed ambulance transportation unnecessary unless the medical record revealed any of the following criteria: requiring CPR, respiratory distress, altered mental status, seizure, immobilization, inability to walk, admission to intensive care, ambulance recommended by medical personnel, motor vehicle collision, or parents not on scene. Billittier used a prospective design and determined ambulance use to be medically necessary if the physician completing the study form (after observing or assessing the patient) agreed with any of the following: unable to ambulate, patient required/could have required out-of-hospital emergency care, patient required/could have required expedient transport to the ED, patient had imminent potential for harm to self or others, or transport medically appropriate for some other reason. The primary outcome in each study was the rate of inappropriate use.

It is not surprising that the results would vary widely when different criteria are used to define the outcome. Many investigators mention this lack of uniform definition as they adopt their own. A Delphi methodology to establish criteria for the study of appropriate ambulance transport is another attempt to address this problem.[10] Poverty, lack of transportation, and alcohol are frequently cited factors associated with increased rates of inappropriate ambulance use.

POOR OR PUBLIC INSURANCE

Poverty or having public assistance insurance (such as Medicaid) is frequently cited as a demographic factor linked with high rates of inappropriate ambulance use. Brown noted 85% inappropriate use for patients with Medicaid as compared to 22% with private insurance. Camasso-Richardson noted 82% of patients with Medicaid who were transported by ambulance were inappropriate. Billittier noted that of the inappropriate transports in his study, 59% were insured by Medicaid versus 13% insured by private insurance.

Multiple reasons for higher use rate among the poor have been offered: lack of alternate transportation, lack of access to other health care, perception that there was no charge for the service. Association of low income with high ambulance demand was predicted and has been substantiated by studies across the country. Early estimates of ambulance need expected the highest demand for ambulance service in low-income neighborhoods, since patients may not have a regular physician.[11] Analysis of ambulance use rates in 142 communities in Massachusetts bore out these predictions, showing higher demand for ambulance correlated with populations more than 65 years of age and living below the poverty line.[12]

NO ALTERNATIVE TRANSPORTATION

Among inappropriate transports, lack of alternative transportation has also been cited as a major reason noted by patients or their caregivers to access emergency department care by ambulance. The association with lack of transportation and poverty is obvious. Many indicated they would take an alternate method of transportation if available, leading to recommendations to offer other options for transport as a means to decrease ambulance use.[4]

ALCOHOL INTOXICATION

In America and Europe, alcohol intoxication has been noted as a factor affecting ambulance transport. In a study looking at urban and rural ambulance utilization in Sweden, the dominating symptom of alcohol intoxication accounted for 11% of urban missions versus 2% in the rural area. The difference in social structure between urban and rural areas was associated with this finding.[13]

In a study in suburban Connecticut, alcohol intoxication was deemed as a medically inappropriate but legally mandated ambulance run, accounting for 20% of their inappropriate ambulance transports.[8] A British study classified all ambulance transports of patients with alcoholic intoxication as unnecessary.[14] Alcohol intoxication is listed as a non-emergency in the Salt Lake City EMS Abuse Ordinance and classified as an unlawful request for service.

How should alcohol intoxication be labeled: an appropriate or inappropriate transport? There are different perspectives. Certainly every emergency physician has witnessed arrival of intoxicated patients transported by ambulance and may have questioned their need for EMS. But likewise, physicians have been cautioned, usually by experience, not to rush to judgment, since intoxication can mask significant underlying pathology. Zachariah begins a commentary on ambulance misuse with just such a case, where paramedics mistook a young man who was only responsive to pain as intoxicated and advised his girlfriend to have him sleep it off and call back if necessary. Still unresponsive in the morning, another crew returned and transported him to the trauma center where he underwent delayed evacuation of an epidural hematoma.[15]

The role of ambulance transports as part of our social safety net has been discussed for over 30 years. Consider this perspective from a community medicine administrator in Los Angeles in 1971.

"Just as emergency rooms throughout the country have been found to be substitute sources of primary care for disadvantaged populations, public emergency ambulances appear to be fulfilling much the same role. It may be that the mobile dimension brought to the health care by the ambulance is in some way proportional to the immobility of the population it serves. The unconscious, alcoholic skid-row habitué without friends, relatives, or funds would seem to represent an extreme case of immobility and a prime candidate for ambulance service. Unlike public emergency rooms which usually provide some service to anyone who presents himself, the services of emergency ambulances can be controlled by dispatch policies, thus confounding the influence of social factors in [ambulance] demand analysis."[16]

When using labels such as "inappropriate" it is important to remember that societal expectations regarding appropriate use of an ambulance service may differ from region to region, and the public's view of need may differ from the opinion of hospital-based physicians.

Unmet Need

One of the few studies to examine both inappropriate use and unmet need is a Canadian study examining all ED arrivals in four cities in Alberta in 1980 and 1981. Trained nurses observed 6,405 ED arrivals and classified them according to criteria previously published by Schuman showing overall rates of unmet need and inappropriate use of 58% and 42% respectively.[17,18] Lower rates of both inappropriate use and unmet need were found in cities with paramedic versus nonparamedic ambulance systems.

Analyzing ambulance needs for the general ED population is an ambitious undertaking, and perhaps this is why it has been reported so seldom in the literature. Studies and programs aimed at specific patient populations do address unmet need. Patients with heart attacks or strokes, and victims of motor vehicle crashes are three examples where there is acknowledged unmet need for ambulance transport and EMS system activation. Targeted educational programs to promote increased EMS utilization for these populations are widely promulgated.

CARDIAC

Attempts to influence cardiac patients to enter the EMS system have been longstanding and are aimed at reducing time to definitive care as well as providing therapeutic interventions at the scene and enroute to the hospital.

A program in Gotesburg, Sweden is an example of a regional educational program designed by doctors, a nurse, and a copywriter with a special interest in advertising, which was able to demonstrate a reduction in time to care. The aim was to reduce time delays to therapeutic intervention for patients with suspected myocardial infarction (MI). The program used the Swedish 9-1-1 equivalent: Heart-Pain-90 000 and resulted in a savings in 20 minutes in median time delay to the intensive care unit (ICU) for suspected MI and 40 minutes with confirmed MI. There was no increase in ambulance utilization and a minor increase in ED visits for chest pain (9%).[19]

STROKE

Time to care for stroke victims is a most important parameter for improved outcome, especially if patients are to benefit from fibrinolytic treatment with short therapeutic windows. Studies show that activation of EMS is the single most important factor in rapid hospital triage and treatment of stroke. Individuals calling 9-1-1 arrive earlier to the hospital and get evaluated sooner once they reach the hospital.[20]

In one study, patients arriving by EMS were found to have significantly shorter times to being seen by the emergency physician (0.33 vs. 0.50 hours) and shorter time to CT scan (0.5 hours) when compared to those arriving by other means.[21] These authors note that "the influence of EMS on delays associated with rapid medical care of stroke victims reaches beyond the out-of-hospital transport phase."[21]

As a result multiple agencies are targeting educational efforts to teach the public how to recognize stroke and to call 9-1-1. Since patients themselves rarely call, studies have looked to target populations most likely to call for help, such as family, caregivers, and coworkers, as well as populations that could call more often, such as large employers.[20]

MOTOR VEHICLE CRASH VICTIMS

Needless deaths from motor vehicle crashes were and remain one of the major reasons to establish EMS systems in the U.S. To reduce needless deaths from accidents on rural highways, the U.S. Department of Transportation, National Highway Traffic Safety Administration (NHTSA) helped develop and distributes the National Standard Curriculum for Bystander Care to encourage early action by bystanders who come upon a motor vehicle crash.[22] The curriculum addresses the bystander who is the vital link between the EMS system and the victim, encouraging lay people who recognize an event to call 9-1-1 for early mobilization of EMS and to stop and help until EMS arrives.

Contributors to EMS Utilization

In order to affect inappropriate use and unmet need, the EMS system has to acknowledge the multiple factors that influence the decision to call for help as well as the response to that call. The patient and other callers to 9-1-1 first make the request for help. Public education efforts on appropriate use of 9-1-1 influence this decision. The 9-1-1 centers and emergency medical dispatchers decide how to respond to this request. Hospitals, physicians, insurers all have opinions on the appropriateness of the call. Society at large, through legal decisions and laws and regulations, implicitly and explicitly define appropriate use of EMS. Medical oversight at each stage of the decision tree is vital.

The Call for Help

PATIENT

While the patient is the focus of ambulance response, it is usually not the patient who calls 9-1-1, but rather someone on the patient's behalf. Major impediments to the call for help are patient denial and choosing to ignore atypical symptoms.

CALLER

Most of the time it is not the patient making the call to 9-1-1 but rather a family member or significant other, friend, co-worker, or bystander. The implications are two-fold. First, a patient may be dependent on someone else making a call on his behalf if help is ever to arrive. Second, the dispatcher is getting information from someone other than the patient.

Clawson and Dernocoeur in *Principles of Emergency Medical Dispatch,* describe four types of callers. First-party callers are the persons with the problem. Second-party callers are directly involved with or near the patient, such as the wife of a man who has chest pain or someone who was in a motor vehicle crash who is calling for someone else. The third-party caller is neither directly involved with the patient nor in close proximity to the incident, but is reporting an event such as a car crash they just passed on the highway, or a man collapsed on the street that they see from their window. Or they may be relaying a request for an ambulance—as a security guard in a building who is told there is an emergency and to call for help. The fourth-party caller is a report of an emergency request relayed from another public service agency. In a breakdown by caller type in three locales, first-party callers account for 9–15% of calls, second-party for 63–80%, third-party for 0–9% and fourth-party for 2%. In a separate report of caller party in 157 randomly selected traffic accident cases, there was only 1 first-party caller, 26 (16.5%) second-party callers, 129 (82.1%) third-party callers, and 1 fourth-party.[23]

Some studies of inappropriate use and unmet need have looked at who called for help, and its effect on appropriateness. Morris and Cross note that of 1000 calls, only 39 were made by patients and the major caller parties were relatives (358), neighbors (177), police (99) and employers (51). Gardner looked at factors affecting the decision whether to call an ambulance. The patients themselves made very few calls. Most calls were made by relatives, friends, and passers-by. Gardner observed that calls by relatives were more likely to be justified as they knew the patient, whereas friends and passers-by were not good judges. Employers were more likely to make justified calls for help, perhaps due to the obligatory first-aid training for businesses employing more than 50 people. Gardner felt teachers were likely to make unnecessary ambulances calls either to "cover themselves" or because no one was free to transport the child. Gardner advocated more public teaching and education about first-aid treatment of minor trauma as a means to reduce unnecessary ambulance runs.

9-1-1

When a centralized and easy-to-remember number for emergencies such as 9-1-1 is introduced and promoted, one can expect to find an increase in the number of calls for ambulance, including a number where the need is questionable, if not unnecessary. In many parts of the country, there is no secondary number promoted for emergencies—so less than emergent calls are placed as 9-1-1 calls[2] Non-emergency use of 9-1-1 is not only an EMS issue but may be promoted for other public services as well. For example, in some regions the public is told to call 9-1-1 for all police requests, whether to report a robbery in progress or a loud group of teenagers who are "disturbing the peace." In the latter instance the caller may well feel it is not a true emergency and not want to bother the 9-1-1 number, but is instructed by the system to do so. By analogy, a range in requests for medical need can be expected if 9-1-1 is the only phone number promoted, and the medical dispatcher must be aware that every call is neither a true emergency nor is it the intention of the caller to request that an ambulance be dispatched.

EMERGENCY MEDICAL DISPATCH

Emergency medical dispatch (EMD) is a cornerstone of appropriate EMS response. Training and protocols for EMD have been developed addressing how to interrogate callers, prioritize calls, and provide pre-arrival initial treatment instructions. The role of medical oversight is essential to approve the training, protocols, and policies that are used. While the importance of this EMD seems obvious, most states have no legislation related to standards, training, certification, and medical oversight of EMD.[23]

Inappropriate ambulance transports cannot occur if an ambulance is not dispatched. What options are available to an EMD other than ambulance dispatch? If a call funneled through 9-1-1 of a medical nature reaches an EMD and common sense dictates that no ambulance is needed, one option is not to send one for every call. Other options include referring calls to a nurse advice line for screening or dispatching a first responder unit to do an evaluation at the scene. What is important is that any response other than ambulance dispatch be clearly articulated and easily understood, be in writing, and be approved by the medical director.

Clawsen categorizes non-ambulance dispatch as OMEGA-level response to cover situation such as: referral of calls for asymptomatic poisonings and overdoses to a regional Poison Control Center; dispatch of other agencies besides EMS to homes where an expected death occurred; and options to assist caregivers when physical assistance may be needed but not ambulance transport, as when a patient has fallen out of bed at home and need aid returning to their usual resting place.[23]

In one urban system, fire apparatus first responders with AEDs rather than ambulances were dispatched to automatic 9-1-1 alarms and motor vehicle incidents lacking definitive caller information. Results showed faster triage for paramedic/transport backup, faster basic care and AED use if needed, and greater availability of ambulances, since ambulances were freed from high volumes of calls (>60%) not needing immediate transport or any transport at all.[24]

The Role of Public Education

Why does a person call 9-1-1 to request emergency medical service? And likewise, why do they choose not to call? The answers to these questions are key determinants to reducing unmet need and inappropriate requests for help.

There are well known initiatives by organizations such as the American Heart Association (AHA), to reach the general population, which advocate use of 9-1-1 for patients who may be having a heart attack or a stroke. Educational efforts by the AHA aimed at the general public encourage recognizing when a fellow human is in trouble, coming to their aid, and accessing help. The National Standard Curriculum for Bystander Care likewise encourages recognition of

an emergency, coming to another's aid and making the call for help. Both these educational efforts advocate a call to 9-1-1 as an early step, often before detailed information is known.

Look at some of the instruction given to the lay public in *Heartsaver CPR: A Comprehensive Course for the Lay Responder* of when to call 9-1-1 for heart attack or stroke:[25]

"How to recognize a heart attack?" stresses pain as the most important and most common symptom, but it notes: "Not all warning symptoms occur in every heart attack. People who are having a heart attack may have vague signs. They may say they feel lightheaded, faint, short of breath, or nauseated, or they may describe their chest discomfort as an ache, heartburn, or indigestion. These vague signs of a heart attack are more common in women, people with diabetes, and the elderly."

After acknowledging the common reaction of denial, it stresses, "When a person with symptoms . . . tries to downplay . . . you must take responsibility and act at once. Phone 9-1-1 or send someone to phone 9-1-1—for 2 reasons—EMS can treat potential complications and alert hospitals to speed time of hospital treatment."[25]

The section "How to Recognize a Stroke" includes the following signs and symptoms. "A stroke is the rapid onset of neurologic problems, including weakness or paralysis of one or more limbs (particularly the arms), facial weakness, difficulty speaking, visual problems, intense dizziness, altered responsiveness, or severe headaches." Facial droop, arm weakness and speech difficulties are highlighted as red flags.

After emphasizing the importance of the system ability to alert hospitals to prepare for rapid evaluation and therapy, the section concludes with the following paragraph.

"Family members and bystanders often fail to phone 9-1-1 when a stroke occurs. Do not make the mistake of thinking that the stroke victim's symptoms are caused by alcohol or drug intoxication or medical conditions such as low blood sugar. *If you suspect that a person is having a stroke, do not delay; phone 9-1-1 or other emergency response number immediately.*"[25]

MOTOR VEHICLE CRASH VICTIMS

The National Standard Curriculum for Bystander Care, distributed by NHTSA, is a program to promote more effective bystander actions to reduce deaths from rural highway crashes.[24] Developed by an expert panel and with enthusiastic support from several states, this five-part report is a deliberate attempt to encourage bystander involvement and teaches the following steps:

1. Recognizing the emergency
2. Deciding to help
3. Contacting the EMS system and informing them of the location and nature of the emergency
4. Preventing further injuries
5. Assessing the victim(s), and
6. Providing life-sustaining care in order to ensure that the victim still has a chance of surviving when EMS arrives.[26]

The panel felt that existing first-aid materials avoided the very difficult process of how a bystander would recognize an emergency exists. The failure to recognize an emergency, along with reluctance to get involved or to contact EMS, were reasons which led to under-use of EMS services. For the program to succeed, "local EMS and law enforcement personnel need to support the program by having improved lines of communication with bystanders since their actions and attitudes may have an impact on whether or not the helper bystander ever stops to help again." Within the course content there are multiple objectives that encourage the bystander to call EMS even if they are unsure if there is a critical injury. Consider proposed content for two objectives aimed to get the bystander to act even when it is not clear if there is serious injury:

Objective 3.12:

Given a video of a crash scene where it is not immediately obvious that the victims are seriously hurt, demonstrate how to describe the situation to the dispatcher.

Discuss how to answer the dispatcher's question, "Is this an emergency?" or "What is your emergency?"

Helping in an emergency often involves acting in the face of uncertainty. The examples should be emotionally involving. They should show models of bystanders who are uncertain but are still able to take action to help.

And Objective 6.5:

Given a video of a crash scene, describe what you should do if no one appears to be seriously injured.

Call the police or EMS even if there are no obvious injuries.

Many people will say they are fine even when they are not. After a crash, people tend to be distracted and may not realize that they are injured. Many people don't realize that the following could be signals of serious injury: pain in the neck, back, chest, or abdomen, a headache, a blow to the head, or a brief period of unconsciousness.[26]

Impact of Education on Ambulance Utilization

The sections included above which address unmet need were selected to show the emphasis given to: (1) bolstering the confidence of bystanders to take action, even if there is uncertainty; (2) the fact that patients may deny the significance of their symptoms; and (3) the inclusion of multiple signs and symptoms which might indicate stroke, myocardial ischemia or significant injury meant to increasing the probability of not overlooking a serious event.

What are the implications of the above public education when evaluating inappropriate use and unmet need? By necessity, inclusion of mechanism of injury and acting in the face of uncertainty will lead to calls where there is no injury or minor injury and an ambulance was not needed, with the trade-off being earlier calls for the small number of cases where early intervention prevents death and/or serious disability. Likewise the inclusion of vague or less specific symptoms of myocardial ischemia and stroke will decrease unmet need but with a progressive increase in ambulance requests for patients who do not know these diseases.

Equally important are educational programs used by regional EMS programs on appropriate use of emergency services in general. It is harder to construct guidance for all types of emergencies than for specific conditions. Likewise, the balance has to be struck between promoting advice sensitive enough to address unmet need while limiting requests for conditions where there is no added value. This same issue has been discussed in many EMS circles in recent years as systems "strive to identify criteria that will allow us to make decisions about the proper use of EMS resources . . . without the risk of jeopardizing the system and its resources, without risk of medical legal consequences, and without risk to the patient."[27]

Questions of why a bystander called and their prior education about when to call 9-1-1 (if any) should be of great interest to medical directors and administrators of an EMS System. Especially lacking in the literature are queries of the third-party callers and second-party callers who do not accompany the patient to the emergency department, the very people who make the majority of calls for help. Yet this information is important feedback to educators about the effectiveness of their programs, to physicians studying correlation of symptoms at the scene with hospital diagnosis, and to the EMS system and all its components, which are set in motion by the caller's request for help.

Response to the Call

Once a response is dispatched to a call for help there are still other options To reduce inappropriate ambulance transports, a patient might be left at the scene, treated and released, offered alternative transportation, and/or transported to a facility other than an ED.

DISPATCHER ACCURACY WITH FIELD FINDINGS
Neely looked at the agreement between dispatch nature and severity codes and paramedic field findings in part to see if callers at dispatch could safely be referred to a nurse advice telephone line or alternative EMS service.[28] The patient was the caller 11% of the time. Overall agreement failed to meet the predetermined threshold of 75%. Four nature/severity code combinations did reach agreement: urgent breathing, urgent diabetic, urgent falls, and urgent overdoses. The greatest disparity was in motor vehicle crashes. Paramedics using the same protocols as the dispatchers downgraded severity 29% of the time and upgraded severity 5.4% of the time.

It is not surprising that there is disparity between dispatch and scene findings in the Neely study. Only 11% of the time can the dispatcher speak directly to the patient. Nor is it surprising that there is greatest disparity with motor vehicle crashes, when it is even more likely that the 9-1-1 notification is by a third-party caller. The results substantiate the belief in many systems that except for some discrete and clearly defined situations, field evaluation is prudent. On-scene medical evaluation is a valuable service.

EMT FIELD TRIAGE
Multiple studies have looked at the provider's ability at the scene to determine whether ambulance transport is warranted. Hauswald noted that only 11% of patients were judged as able to be triaged for alternate transport, and over half of these were mistriaged.[29] Hunt noted that emergency physicians judged 30% of transports unnecessary and paramedics agreed 76% of the time.[30] The paramedic undertriaged 92 (11%) of 825 patients. Schmidt reported that EMTs categorized 79% of patients as needing ambulance transport and only 1% as treat and release while 3–11% of patients determined not to need ambulance transport had a predetermined critical event needing ambulance transport.[31] All advocated further study.

The various criteria used to determine whether ambulance transport was required included: whether the ED differential diagnosis indicated the potential need for an intervention en route (Hauswald); need for prehospital intervention, expedient transport, pain, potential for self harm, other (Hunt); needs ambulance, alternate transportation, own physician, treat and release (Schmidt).

Strategies employing field triage are formally in place in some systems. Different strategies may be used.[32] In one system, if the public-service first responder does not feel the agency's paramedic ambulance is required, a private ambulance is contacted for transport, which in turn bills the patient. In other systems, protocols exist which allow providers to deny transport after evaluation at the scene, but as of this writing, they are seldom used.

On-scene paramedics should be wary of patient denial when gathering the history, especially if an ambulance has been requested for a specific and serious complaint. Most patients arriving at the ED don't want to have an emergency. Even less likely do they want to be transported by ambulance. More often than not, anxious recognition and acknowledgement of symptoms and signs result in a call for EMS, since the caller believes a serious medical problem exists. Patients are hoping that a medical professional will tell them they don't have a problem, and will play down or minimize symptoms if encouraged to do so.

As Zachariah points out, defining ambulance transport as misuse is missing the point and classifying EMS as a transportation business. "Patients call seeking medical care and transportation, not just transportation. Thus they may not see the Chevy in the drive-way as a viable alternative to calling 9-1-1."

INAPPROPRIATE USE AND UNMET NEED

Moreover, since many EMS services depend on transport of a patient for reimbursement and most of the cost has already been borne in sending out a crew and assessing the patient, there is questionable value and probable economic loss in putting so much energy into denying transport at the scene.

ALTERNATE TRIAGE AND TRANSPORTATION BASED ON INSURANCE

Managed care organizations (MCOs) have been strong advocates of alternative and parallel systems so "their" patients are screened by their dispatchers and brought to "their" urgent care centers or network hospitals. Since they only want their patients culled from the mix, the biggest obstacle is the request for a public emergency medical service to perform financial triage and offer different standards of care based on insurance classification. In addition, while the potential for research via long-term follow-up of patients undergoing triage by dispatchers and field providers would seem optimal in a managed care environment, there has been a reluctance if not outright refusal from MCOs to share their triage protocols and the results of their experience. But pertinent to every triage protocol is the predicted mistriage rate. Both the protocols and the follow-up data are needed for medical direction to analyze the risk/benefit profile before implementing triage protocols to screen out any calls to 9-1-1, be it at dispatch or in the field.

EMS INITIATED NON-TRANSPORTS DISGUISED AS A REFUSAL OF MEDICAL ASSISTANCE (RMA)

It is far better to acknowledge and to have a written policy addressing those clear and evident cases (such as when a bystander calls for a motor vehicle passenger who has no injury), when both the provider and "patient" agree no intervention (including transport) is requested and/or needed than to use an RMA as a "legal" release. Unfortunately, in some systems, RMAs are used to avoid transport when in fact it is the EMS personnel who initiate this decision. This is a dangerous practice since the intent undermines the value of any RMA, and the provider is being untruthful with the patient. One can't really say "I don't believe you need EMS care—now I want you to sign a statement saying you are refusing my care and releasing me from liability." In addition to being unprofessional, such a practice perpetuates the system problem of not having a straightforward and more truthful description for these cases, such as "unfounded." In some cases it is outright absurd. A good

example is a QM review on a chart because there were no vital signs on a "patient" who left at the scene but had been called in as a "man down." This patient had refused any medical evaluation since he was sunbathing in a park when a neighbor looking out the window across the street called 9-1-1 on his behalf.

What Is Appropriate?

There are many ways that appropriate use is defined, and it is useful to remember that the different players involved in requesting, providing, evaluating, regulating, and paying for emergency services may have different operational definitions of what constitutes appropriate emergency care. Consider the following perspectives.

Healthcare administrators and an economist analyzed demand for emergency ambulance service in Los Angeles in 1971 and sought to predict volume of "medical emergencies and emergency-like incidents" which would be handled by a public emergency ambulance system. Here is their working understanding of the EMS system role: "The bulk of a community's true, life-threatening medical emergencies are generally handled by this system, since real emergencies are usually of such a catastrophic nature as to leave few alternatives. Many of the demands on such a system are, of course, far less medically threatening conditions. Most calls do, however, involve cases whose associated anxiety or pain is sufficient to warrant immediate response."[11]

Criteria to judge appropriateness constructed by hospital-based physicians seem to vary with the eye of the beholder. For example, in some studies, admission to an ICU was a criterion for appropriate use of the ambulance, but admission to a non-ICU bed was not. In others, the physicians had the benefit of laboratory tests and final diagnosis before they made their determination. They may or may not consider the presenting symptoms or the education of the caller that influenced the decision to call (or not call) 9-1-1. This variance results in a wide range of findings. What is important is to remember what criteria were used before interpreting the results and comparing to other studies. Otherwise the published findings of inappropriate use and unmet need rates are less than helpful, and can be confusing. A reported 62% inappropriate use rate is worse than a coin flip. On the other hand, with a rate of 11%, it may be questionable if there is a real problem.

Arguments with insurance companies over what qualifies for ED reimbursement are well known. Insurance companies have refused to reimburse for emergency evaluation and treatment based on the discharge diagnosis rather than the presenting symptoms, a position that has led to prudent layperson legislation in many states and for federal government insurers. Ambulance agencies believe that the prudent layperson standard should apply to them as well, since they have experienced denial of payment.

What is the impact of prudent layperson legislation on access to emergency care for those insured by a managed care plan? Consider the weight that one state gives to public education campaigns in defining emergency conditions which would be reasons to seek emergency care. In this excerpt from an article in an emergency physicians' newsletter, an Assistant Attorney General discusses New York State's 1997 Managed Care Bill of Rights, and in particular one of the limits on Plan "second guessing:"

> There are a number of limitations on Plan denials under the prudent layperson standard. First is the increasing popularity of layperson health information provided by the mass media. This information, often advising consumers that an urgent or emergent medical condition could underlie seemingly benign symptoms, will lead the prudent layperson to seek emergency treatment.

> As an example, the *Reader's Digest*, read by millions of laypeople, alerted readers in a recent article that the symptoms of a heart attack include "pressure, fullness, discomfort and squeezing in the chest, pain spreading to shoulders, neck or arms; sweating; lightheadedness; fainting; nausea and shortness of breath." Under the prudent layperson standard, a Plan should be required to pay benefits if a patient presents at the ED with any one or more of these symptoms.[33]

Goals

The goals of an EMS system will help define how inappropriate use and unmet needs are defined and addressed. Societal and legal definitions will of course need to be considered as they may directly impact on the EMS system's role. At times social and legal definitions may be congruent with the medical opinion; at other times they may diverge. For example, if a town hall directive states the homeless will be gathered off the street in subfreezing temperatures and the police are to call EMS for transport of those who will not or cannot walk, then that is an appropriate EMS call. In locals where a call to 9-1-1 for a person with alcohol intoxication is legally defined as misuse of the system, a particular transport may be medically appropriate but legally inappropriate.

There may be strong advocacy for certain patient populations, be it from the medical community or patient advocate groups, which argue for ambulance transport of all patients who may possibly have a particular illness. And there will always be the vulnerable populations, the poor, the addicted, the intoxicated, who are least able to advocate for themselves and find themselves with medical need but few options for care. The entire population is the EMS system constituency, and the public ultimately expects medical oversight to determine what is in the medical best interest of the population, regardless of the current political climate or prevailing attitudes in society.

When it comes to day-by-day operations, it is ultimately medical oversight that approves the dispatch protocols and field triage directives, and selects the indicators to evaluate system performance and achievement of its goals.

Future Directions

Measuring inappropriate use and unmet need are useful measures to judge the efficiency and effectiveness of an EMS system. Both should be included in regular quality improvement programs. Prospective studies of interest could look simultaneously at (1) the rates of inappropriate use of EMS, (2) the unmet need for EMS services, and (3) the reasons for calling or not calling 9-1-1 to access EMS. Once measurements are made and analyzed, achievement of goals can be evaluated and efforts made to realize improvement.

Include All Stakeholders

To measure either inappropriate use or unmet needs requires all components of the system to participate, from communication center through hospital discharge. To set criteria for either parameter—inappropriate use or unmet need—which will represent the community standard and have face value, multiple players need be included, such as dispatch centers, community health educators, physicians, system administrators, community advocates, and hospitals. State and local laws and ordinances which address use of emergency ambulance service, prudent layperson laws, and advice from local health plans regarding when to call 9-1-1 and options for alternative access, are helpful to review. What is the public expectation? Is EMS viewed as part of the health safety net? What about intoxicated patients? Does the EMS system care them for? If not, what are the alternatives? Widespread community consultation is helpful to gather broad-based support, since these analyses require sustained effort, cooperation among multiple agencies, and commitment to detail to obtain the essential data elements.

Start with Unmet Need

A fundamental question in assessing appropriate use of 9-1-1 is who do we want to come by ambulance? Which patients are we designing the system for and are we meeting their needs. For example, one can start with the obvious cases such as trauma and myocardial ischemia. Then look at the criteria currently used to educate people when to call and protocols used by dispatchers for these types of calls. Unmet need is studied by evaluating all patients in the ED regardless of mode of arrival. This allows evaluation of why patients with the target illness did not call 9-1-1 as well.

Once there is agreement on some targeted populations, one can define the complaints they might make at the scene that would warrant a call to 9-1-1. For example with education about signs of stroke, asymmetric weakness would be expected to be both sensitive and specific. But what about dizziness or severe headache? They may improve sensitivity but at what expense to specificity? What is the position of the EMS and general medical community on signs and symptoms for public education for stroke in the region?

Studies Objectives

The first step is to construct a method to analyze factors affecting the decision to call for help. This will include both who made the call as well as prior or current advice on why and when to call 9-1-1. For example, did the parents call the doctor who then advised them to call an ambulance? (The consulted physician's recommendation on calling 9-1-1 has usually been found to be inappropriate, unless they initiated the call directly.) Or had a bystander read a recent *Reader's Digest* article on access to 9-1-1? Current materials on when to call 9-1-1 should be reviewed,

such as instructions to school nurses, advice in first-aid textbooks, prudent layperson laws, education efforts by the Red Cross or AHA, and state EMS and EMSC educational materials, so that the criteria used to judge appropriateness can be compared to current educational curricula and medical recommendations.

A method to contact the persons who called for help can be developed to assess their rationale and whether prior instructions influenced their decision. In cases where EMS was not accessed, assess the rationale for the patient or guardian seeking other transportation to the ED. Ideally, a questionnaire can be completed when the decision maker is still available. For example, following ambulance dispatch, the call-back number of the person calling for help might be used to later elicit the rationale for the call. The ED personnel or research assistants can use the same questionnaire to assess factors influencing the patients' decision on whether to call 9-1-1. True system study requires integration of dispatch center records, EMS records, and ED records and offers opportunities to assess performance of the multiple decision points within the system.

Measurements and Criteria

The criteria selected to define appropriate use may be selected from other studies or developed locally. Criteria should be carefully selected and consideration given to: information from the caller to dispatcher, the patients' chief complaints, vital signs and physical findings, therapeutic interventions, ability to ambulate, admission to a hospital, differential diagnosis. Information available to the dispatcher and provider on the scene versus information only known after ED evaluation should be separated, since they define two different data points of decision making.

When deciding whether ambulance transport was needed, consider the value of the medical evaluation itself, whether or not the patient received prehospital treatments. Consider for example, victims of motor vehicle crashes. Only a small percentage of motor vehicle crash victims require any operative intervention, and the number requiring life-saving surgery is smaller yet. The most common trauma triage criteria for motor accidents are vehicle deformity and high speed. A bystander who calls 9-1-1 may have little other information, especially if the victim is conscious and breathing. But a finding of hypotension itself predicts a high likelihood of a need for major operative intervention and/or mortal injury, and warrants mobilization of a trauma team on an emergent basis.[34] This medical evaluation is a direct benefit of the EMS system. Similar arguments can be made for patients with myocardial ischemia and stroke.

Feedback to All Players

Stakeholders to whom the findings will have interest include medical directors of dispatch agencies, EMTs, paramedics, emergency nurses, physicians, and the public at large. Authors of educational materials promoting EMS use might be contacted, whether the findings suggest a need for change or affirm the utility of the current approach.

Summary

Inappropriate use and unmet need are indicators of efficiency and effectiveness of an EMS system, and have been recommended as parameters to gauge system performance since the inception of modern EMS. Both indicators should be routinely measured as part of system evaluation and quality improvement. It should be clear that these indicators are interrelated, and an effort to impact unmet need could influence the inappropriate use rate and vice versa.

Since inappropriate use and unmet need are medical measures, their evaluation is appropriately the responsibility of the medical director or the medical oversight committee.

Nearly every component of an EMS system contributes to appropriate use. The cooperation and participation of all players, from the 9-1-1 operator through the hospital, will be required in order to obtain the information needed to analyze the system and to make change. The 9-1-1 center, the bystander who calls for help, educators who teach the public how to recognize an emergency and call 9-1-1, the dispatcher, the paramedics, and the hospitals caring for emergency patients must all be included in this effort.

Measuring these parameters is no easy task, but assuring that one meets the needs of patients is the fundamental goal; and doing it efficiently allows for the best use of one's resources. An accurate measurement of these indices, like the actual response to a call for help, requires the cooperation of all parties. An unwillingness to participate will identify weak links in the system.

Much of the difficulty in influencing inappropriate use and unmet need is the work required upstream, long before the call for help arrives. Understanding the reasons behind a call for help and interceding before the next call is made, as with other upstream efforts, may be hard to do but promises a payoff well worth the effort expended.

References

1. EMS System Act of 1973, Public Law 93-154. Washington, DC, 1973.
2. Gibson G. Evaluative criteria for emergency ambulance systems. *Soc Sci Med*. 1973;425–454.
3. Gibson G. Measures of emergency ambulance effectiveness: unmet need and inappropriate use. *JACEP*. 1977;6:389–392.
4. Camasso-Richardson K, Wilde JA, Petrack EM. Medically unnecessary pediatric ambulance transports: a medical taxi service? *Acad Emerg Med*. 1997;4:1137–1141.
5. Billittier AJ, Moscate R, Janicke D. A multisite survey of factors contributing to medically unnecessary ambulance transports. *Acad Emerg Med*. 1996;3:1046–1050.
6. Kost S, Arruda J. Appropriateness of ambulance transportation to a suburban pediatric emergency department. *Prehosp Emerg Care*. 1999;3:187–190.
7. Gardner GJ. The use and abuse of the emergency ambulance service: some of the factors affecting the decision whether to call an emergency ambulance. *Arch Emerg Med*. 1990;7:81–89.
8. Brown E, Sindelar J. The emergent problem of ambulance misuse. *Ann Emerg Med*. 1993;22:646-650.
9. Morris DL, Cross AB. Is the emergency ambulance service abused? *Br Med J*. 1980;121–123.
10. Chu KH, Gregor MA, Maio RF, et al. Derivation and validation of criteria for determining the appropriateness of nonemergency ambulance transports. *Prehosp Emerg Care*. 1997;1(4):219–226.
11. Aldrich CA, Hisserich JC, Lave LB. An analysis of the demand for emergency ambulance service in an urban area. *Am J Public Health*. 1971;61:1156–1169.
12. Cadigan RT, Bugarin CE. Predicting demand for emergency ambulance service. *Ann Emerg Med*. 1989;18:618–621.
13. Brismar B, Dahlgren B, Larsson J. Ambulance utilization in Sweden: analysis of emergency ambulance missions in urban and rural areas. *Ann Emerg Med*. 1984;13:1037–1039.
14. Morris DL, Cross AB. Is the emergency ambulance service abused? *British Medical Journal*. 1980;3:121–123.
15. Zachariah BS. The problem of ambulance misuse; whose problem is it, anyway? *Acad Emerg Med*. 1999;6:2.
16. Hisserich JC. Reply to Dr. Gibson (letter). *Am J Public Health*. 1971;61(11):2160–2061.
17. Schuman LJ, Wolfe H, Sepulveda J. Estimating demand for emergency transportation. *Med Care*. 1977;15:738–749.
18. Rademaker AW, Powell DG, Read JH. Inappropriate use and unmet need in paramedic and nonparamedic ambulance systems. *Ann Emerg Med*. 1987;16:553–556.

19. Herlitz J, Blohm M, Hartford M, et al. Follow-up of a 1-year media campaign on delay times and ambulance use in suspected acute myocardial infarction. *European Heart Journal.* 1992;13:171–177.

20. Wein TH, Staub L, Felberg R, et al. Activation of emergency medical services for acute stroke in a nonurban population. *Stroke.* 2000;31:1925.

21. Morris DL, Rosamond WD, Hinn AR, et al. Time delays in accessing stroke care in the emergency department. *Acad Emerg Med.* 1999;6:218–223.

22. National Standard Curriculum for Bystander Care. DOT HS 807 872; October 1992.

23. Clawson JJ, Dernocoeur KB. *Principles of Emergency Medical Dispatch.* 3rd ed. Salt Lake City: Priority Press; 2001.

24. Key CB, Calderon D, Persse DE, et al. Prospective evaluation of the effects of only dispatching fire apparatus first responders to automatic 9-1-1 alarms and motor vehicle incidents lacking definitive caller information. *Acad Emerg Med.* 2000;7:476 (abstract).

25. Heartsaver CPR: A Comprehensive Course for the Lay Responder. American Heart Association. 1999.

26. *National Standard Curriculum for Bystander Care.* U.S. Department of Transportation. National Highway Traffic Safety Administration. DOT HS 807 872, October 1992.

27. Krohmer JR. Appropriate emergency medical services transport. *Acad Emerg Med.* 1999;6:5–7.

28. Neely KW, Eldurkar JA, Drake MER. Do emergency medical services dispatch nature and severity codes agree with paramedic field findings? *Acad Emerg Med.* 2000; 7:174–180.

29. Hauswald M, Brillman J, Raynovich W, et al. Training paramedics to determine who does not need ambulance transport. *Acad Emerg Med.* 1999;6:474-a(abstract).

30. Hunt JD, Gratton MC, Campbell JP. Prospective determination of medical necessity for ambulance transport by on-scene paramedics. *Acad Emerg Med.* 1999;6:447.

31. Schmidt T, Atcheson R, Federiuk C, et al. Evaluation of protocols allowing emergency medical technicians to determine need for treatment and transport. *Acad Emerg Med.* 2000;7:663–669.

32. Otto LA. Inappropriate use. In: Kuehl AE. *Prehospital Systems and Medical Oversight.* 2nd ed. St Louis: Mosby-Year Book; 1994.

33. McArdle EF. A guide to understanding the prudent layperson standard for managed care payment of emergency services. *Empire State EPIC.* 1998;Nov:1–4.

34. Henry MC, Hollander JE, Alicandro JM, et al. Incremental benefit of individual American College of Surgeons Trauma Triage Criteria. *Acad Emerg Med.* 1996;3: 992–1000.

Introduction

An important aspect of medical oversight is the creation and implementation of medical treatment protocols for the out-of-hospital care provider. Developed by the medical director, often with input from the regional medical community, protocols serve as the guidelines or the standards of care for the EMS system.

The following chapters review clinical conditions commonly encountered in the practice of out-of-hospital care. In general, the chapters are symptom-based as opposed to diagnosis-based, since often the exact diagnosis cannot be identified in the field. Each chapter provides an overview of the clinical condition, along with considerations for protocol development and for potential pitfalls.

The use of protocols calls on both the physician and the field provider to possess a good working knowledge of the various protocols. Protocols are only helpful when they are invoked for the proper patient clinical conditions. Field providers or physicians choosing the wrong protocol may cause harm to patients.

Clinical conditions can overlap; for example, the hypotensive patient might also complain of shortness of breath. The role of the direct medical oversight physician is to help the out-of-hospital care provider identify the primary problem and to direct treatment toward improving the patient's condition.

Procedures

David P. Thomson, MD

Introduction

Among the most controversial issues in EMS are those related to which procedures provider should be authorized to perform, and the situations in which those procedures are indicated. Although many municipalities provide a paramedic response for their community, several authors have questioned the value of the procedures that are performed.[1–7] However, other authors have shown that paramedic procedures have definite advantages.[8–15]

One of the major problems in trying to define appropriate procedures to be done in the field is that there are over two dozen levels of prehospital providers defined by state laws in this country. The Department of Transportation (DOT) EMT-Basic (EMT-B) curriculum authorizes EMT-Bs to perform some advanced skills, such as endotracheal intubation and assisting patients in the administration of epinephrine for allergic reactions or with inhalation treatments for bronchospasm.[16] In addition, although states may allow a wide range of procedures, most medical directors significantly limit the procedures available to the providers.

Some medical directors seem reluctant to authorize even a simple IV, while others encourage an aggressive approach, including paralysis for intubation. What skills should an EMS system use? This question has never been well studied. With more direct physician supervision, the opportunity exists to tailor the system to the local needs, without regard to artificially described levels. The medical director should consider the needs of the patients, the skills of the paramedics, the cost of training and equipment, and the likelihood of success within the individual system. This chapter provides some guidance and background regarding the selection of procedures currently available.

The procedures a medical director authorizes must be related to the individual region.[17] Considerations here include the patient mix, travel times, and the availability of backup services. A service that treats a high volume of urban trauma might place greater emphasis on immobilization and airway control and minimize time spent on the scene. Rural systems may require procedures that would be precluded by the short transport times of a municipal system. The availability of backup is another consideration. In a rural setting the nearest hospital may not be equipped, either in staffing or facilities, to care for a severely injured patient.[18] Although air medical services have alleviated some of this problem, they are not always available. The rural provider will need the training and authorization to perform highly "advanced" procedures if he is to have any hope of keeping certain patients alive until he can transport the patient to an appropriate facility.[19]

The difference between providers is primarily in the procedures they are allowed to perform. Each state has developed its own terminology corresponding to advanced-level, intermediate-level, and basic-level providers. Within each of these categories are often several subgroups of providers. Even region there may be little uniformity in which procedures are authorized. A basic unit in one region may be authorized to perform some procedure that advanced units in another area are prohibited from using. There is frequently little correlation between the needs of the local region and the level of training of the providers serving there.

The decision to determine the level of service is a difficult one. For many medical directors, the fiscal state of the community seems to be the guiding principal. Two axioms seem to guide this decision: (1) ALS is more expensive, and (2) a high call volume is necessary to maintain ALS skills. The idea that more advanced procedures should cost significantly more appeals to intuition, but investigation proves this incorrect. Ornato performed a brief analysis of the cost differential between a mixed BLS/ALS system and an all-paramedic system; there was a difference of only $2.88 per run.[20] This analysis did not factor in any increased risk of litigation in a mixed or BLS-only system, nor did it evaluate the potential savings in hospital costs that early intervention may provide.

In the West German EMS system, which uses physicians to provide prehospital care, it was estimated that early intervention with trauma patients in one region alone saved $28 million yearly due to prevention of death, $15.5 million due to preventing disability, and $800,000 yearly in ICU costs.[15] For this last figure it is important to note an ICU charge of $160 per day. This is ten to twenty times less than the cost of an ICU bed in most U.S. hospitals. While it is possible that providing ALS in the field is cost-effective, the cost-effectiveness of the individual procedures must be addressed.

Garrison has done an excellent job of looking at the cost-effectiveness of pediatric intraosseous infusion, providing a solid model for systems to use when assessing cost-benefit ratios.[21] As healthcare funds become tighter and the number of prehospital modalities expands, medical directors will need to show that the therapies chosen are cost-effective. Certainly among the costs one must consider the initial cost difference involved in training and skill maintenance. The recent addition of Amiodarone to the Advanced Cardiac Life Support (ACLS) protocols has added another concern, because of the cost of this medication. In some jurisdictions such medications have been replenished from hospital stocks. Rulings regarding "anti-kickback" laws have ended this practice for many services, placing them in the position of having to purchase the replacement medications with their own funds. Some volunteer services will no doubt have to downgrade their service level to remain solvent.

Skill retention has been cited as a reason for not permitting rural and suburban paramedics to perform some procedures. In 1977, Skelton and McSwain looked at skill degradation among Kansas City paramedics.[22] Their results indicated that the basic skills of short-board immobilization and Hare traction splint application degraded at a faster rate than the skills of intubation and IV access. They suggested that this was an effect of a continuing education program that placed an increased emphasis on the advanced skills.

An investigation of English ambulance staff concluded that, regardless of the effectiveness of the training, skill retention can only be ensured by providing an adequate monitoring system.[23] The skills taught in the Basic Trauma Life Support (BTLS) course degrade with time, in spite of frequent field experience with trauma patients.[24] Regardless of the technical difficulty of the procedure or the setting in which it is performed, skill maintenance among prehospital care providers requires careful education and ongoing quality assurance. If these are provided, the overall frequency of performance of a procedure for the individual provider becomes largely irrelevant.

The comments of McSwain and Pepe regarding endotracheal intubation provide some insight into the role of the medical director regarding procedures: "prehospital personnel with *inadequate training and inadequate supervision* should not use the ET tube."[25] "Key to predictable success in the performance of endotracheal tube placement is the *quality of initial training, the frequency of performance, and the close scrutiny by supervisors expert in emergency* endotracheal intubation techniques."[26]

Patient Assessment Procedures

The most fundamental procedures a prehospital care provider performs are those related to patient assessment. These skills are often afforded relatively little time in the initial training of healthcare providers, and it is a rare system that reviews these skills in a rigorous fashion. Yet these procedures are the cornerstone of any treatment.

HISTORY AND PHYSICAL ASSESSMENT

The prehospital provider must be able to gather a concise and accurate history and physical in a minimal amount of time. This provides the basis for any treatment rendered in the field and may help guide the treatment in the emergency department. The need to rapidly assess and treat trauma victims has been the impetus for the creation of the BTLS and Pre-Hospital Trauma Life Support (PHTLS) courses, but the assessment principles taught in these courses may be applied to any patient, regardless of the illness. When used for all patients, these assessment procedures ensure that the information needed to provide good patient care is gathered. BTLS and PHTLS help direct the provider to the critical problems, which are frequently overlooked in a less systematic evaluation. Providers should be encouraged to use these tools as part of their assessment of every patient they see.

VITAL SIGNS

Field personnel are expected to take vital signs on every patient. As with every procedure, though, vital sign assessment should have an indication and a proper sequence. BTLS has placed the vital sign assessment in the secondary survey, where it will not interfere with the identification and treatment of life-threatening problems. In patients without obvious life-threatening problems, vital signs are thought to help unmask a previously hidden injury.

Although vital signs are expected to be taken with each patient encounter, often they are not obtained. Spaite prospectively studied the frequency with which vital signs were omitted.[27] Even with an observer present, blood pressure or pulse were not taken in 37% of patients. This was an urban study, and it could be argued that short transport times precluded vital sign assessment in some cases. Moss has reviewed the data for nonurban areas of Arizona.[28] He found that optically scanned charts were missing either systolic blood pressure, diastolic blood pressure, pulse rate, or respiratory rate 15% to 18% of the time. Many of these transports involved long distances, which should have provided the providers adequate time. A study of the Los Angeles County system showed that as patient age decreased, so did the frequency of vital sign assessment.[29] Vital signs were rarely obtained on patients less than 2 years old. The providers surveyed felt significantly less confident in their ability to assess vital signs in the pediatric age group than in their ability with adults.

In 1978, Cayten attempted to look at the ability of basic EMTs, paramedics, and emergency department nurses to correctly assess a variety of physical parameters.[30] His research showed that there was consistent error by all groups, with systolic blood pressures being most accurately assessed. Diastolic blood pressure readings taken by the EMTs and paramedics were accurate only 54% of the time. He noted that there was significant error among the nursing personnel and that the level of training of both the nurses (which included registered, graduate, and licensed practical nurses) and the EMTs did not affect the performance. Although he tried to set tolerance limits for errors that would reflect clinical significance, perhaps the accuracy he demanded is not necessary in emergency care.

Another source of error may be related to the tools one uses. One paper has noted that a significant number of ambulance sphygmomanometers are inaccurate.[31] Medical directors must provide methods to ensure the accuracy of these measurements as part of their quality management plan. These plans must address both the equipment and the skills involved.

A 1994 study using a standardized blood pressure model showed a very large difference in the accuracy of blood pressures obtained in a quiet environment versus a moving ambulance.[32] In a convenience sample of ambulance sphygmomanometers in the Milwaukee area, 73% of the devices tested were either inaccurate or unreliable.[33] Thus it must always be remembered that in treating patients there may be a significant error in the vital signs as relayed by the provider, particularly in a moving ambulance.

No one has ever looked at the specific utility of the various measures that are obtained in the field. Until this research is performed, medical directors should insist that providers attempt to obtain the pulse, blood pressure, and respiration of every patient and repeat these readings as frequently as the clinical situation warrants or allows. Although the individual reading may in itself be less than perfectly accurate, development of a trend may help guide the course of treatment.

Most systems also use some rating scales to rank the case severity. These rating scales can take on major importance for an EMS system because they often form the basis for decisions about destination hospitals and the mode of transport. Because these measures have subjective components, medical directors must clearly define the terms and ensure that their personnel understand the parameter being assessed. In Cayten's study, he noted better than 95% agreement in assessing level of consciousness.[30] Menegazzi has found excellent agreement between paramedics and emergency physicians in assessing patients with the Glasgow Coma Scale,[34] a commonly used rating tool. Similar studies have been conducted on global case severity rating systems.[35] Although the nature of these overall ratings requires more subjective judgment, the authors found excellent reliability. Although some may view these types of numerical ratings as research tools, the ability to support a triage decision with a concise number may help the medical director in both the political and medico-legal arenas if questions arise.

Airway Management

Effective management of the patient's airway is the most essential skill in the care for critically ill and injured patients. Many devices are available for field airway care; however, few were thoroughly investigated before use in prehospital care.

Supplemental Oxygen Administration

The nasal cannula and oxygen mask have long been accepted as part of the repertoire of the EMT-B. Oxygen administration is frequently considered a benign procedure, and many services provide some form of supplemental oxygen to all of their patients. The standard teaching for EMTs was expressed by Caroline: "When in doubt, give oxygen."[36]

Although oxygen is a very safe agent, it must still be treated as a drug. As with any drug it is important to realize the indications, contraindications, dosages, and routes of administration. Because of its frequency of use (in some systems every patient receives oxygen) medical directors should pay special attention to the education of providers and assurance of the appropriateness of this treatment.

Finally the cost of administering a medication unnecessarily should be factored into this decision. This needs to include both the cost of the drug (oxygen) and the materials to administer it (cannula or mask). Written protocols and medical command help eliminate unnecessary oxygen use.

As a practical matter the determination of hypoxia in the field historically has been difficult, prompting Caroline's statement. In spite of all the hazards listed above, unless the service has access to pulse oximetry, oxygen administration for most patients is still the safest practice. In patients with a history of COPD, the protocol should encourage incremental increases in oxygen supplementation, rather than immediate high flow oxygen. If the paramedic finds that the patient loses respiratory drive, he or she should be prepared to assist ventilation. Protocols may be devised that restrict oxygen use in otherwise healthy individuals without systemic involvement, but medical directors should err on the side of supplemental oxygen whenever there is any question, particularly if pulse oximetry is not available.

Ventilation

Classically, prehospital care providers have been taught to use the bag-valve-mask (BVM), which was felt to provide an improvement over mouth-to-mouth ventilation by allowing supplemental oxygenation. This technique was borrowed from the operating room, where it had met with great success. The primary problem that anesthesiologists found was gastric insufflation, which they solved in the operating room by the use of cricoid pressure (Sellick maneuver). Unfortunately, the application of the BVM in the moving ambulance has brought less satisfactory results.[37,38] In the operating room the most common use of the BVM is preoxygenation before intubation. It is not routinely used for more than a few minutes in this setting.

For many "basic" systems, the BVM is the only device available for assisting ventilation. As such, it is often used for long periods. When used by a single rescuer in the back of a moving ambulance, the actual volume delivered to the patient may be small. This is because the BVM requires the provider to perform an airway maneuver and mask seal with one hand, while squeezing the bag with the other hand. Significant volumes may be lost from around the mask. When a resuscitation bag is squeezed with one hand, the volume may be as small as 500 cc.[39] Several authors have suggested that two providers be used whenever BVM ventilation is attempted, one to provide the airway maneuver and mask seal and another to squeeze the bag.[34,40]

The EMT-B curriculum recommends that this is ideally a two-person procedure and, with only one person managing the airway, that the order of priority of airway management is (1) mouth-to-mask, (2) two-person BVM, (3) flow-restricted oxygen powered ventilation device, and finally (4) one-person BVM ventilation.[41] When combined with an additional crew member to perform chest compressions, this can lead to a very tight fit in an ambulance. Unfortunately, many EMS systems budget for only one patient caregiver in the back of the ambulance, with that person frequently feeling like a "one-armed paperhanger."

Mask design and size may have a significant impact on the ability to ventilate the patient.[42,43,44] Facial trauma, dentition, and congenital anomalies may all present problems for the prehospital rescuer who attempts to ventilate a patient with a bag-valve-mask. Some systems have abandoned the BVM in favor of using a bag with the Esophageal Obturator Airway (EOA), but studies do not support this practice.[45] An investigation by Rhee demonstrated that the BVM, combined with aggressive management of secretions, can provide an adequate airway for patients whose mental status is slightly depressed but not sufficiently so as to allow direct endotracheal intubation.[46] This suggests that the EOA provides no advantage over the BVM in the management of airway secretions.

Oxygen content of the BVM may vary, depending on the ventilatory frequency and the reservoir used. To ensure an FiO2 level of 1.0, the bag must have a reservoir consisting of either a demand valve or a 2.5 liter reservoir (for a 1500 cc adult bag).[47] Other reservoirs, such as tubes, may provide significant lower FiO2 levels.

THE DEMAND VALVE

Some systems allow the use of a demand valve, or oxygen powered resuscitator. This device connects directly to the oxygen tank and allows the paramedic to deliver a breath by pressing a trigger. Since it is actuated by a finger, it allows the paramedic to use both hands to provide the airway maneuver and seal, while delivering the breath with only one finger. This solves the problem of ensuring volume delivery but deprives the rescuer of any sense of lung compliance. Many of these devices have a pressure relief valve, which may provide some protection against barotrauma, although studies proving this are lacking.

MOUTH-TO-MASK VENTILATION

In an effort to devise a simple compromise between mouth-to-mouth and BVM ventilation, mouth-to-mask ventilation was invented. This procedure allows the use of supplemental oxygen by connecting a tube to the mask. It prevents direct rescuer-to-patient contact, which can be important for both aesthetic[48] and infection control reasons.[49] Because no additional hands are needed to squeeze the resuscitation bag, both hands can be used to effect the airway maneuver and mask seal. The use of the rescuer's lungs to power the device allows larger tidal volumes to be delivered,[37] and the rescuer may be able to overcome decreases in compliance by exerting greater force with his or her breathing.

Unfortunately, greater gastric insufflation occurs with increases in airway pressures,[50] potentially increasing the risk of regurgitation and aspiration. Because expired air is used to drive the ventilation, it is impossible to achieve 100% oxygen concentrations, but concentrations up to 50% may be possible.[51]

In a study using infant mannequins, Terndrup and Warner demonstrated that use of mouth-to-mask ventilation in this age group has significant advantages over the mouth-to-mouth or BVM methods.[52] They found that there were higher peak airway pressures using pediatric bags. When they used a pediatric bag, the FiO2 level was 0.8 at a flow rate of 10 liters per minute. With the mouth-to-mask technique they achieved an FiO2 of 0.9.

Concerns regarding infections, especially with HIV and hepatitis, have led to increased awareness of these devices as a substitute for mouth-to-mouth ventilation. Melanson and O'Gara surveyed providers on their willingness to perform mouth-to-mouth resuscitation in four different scenarios.[53] While the responses varied given the case scenario, the availability of a barrier device dramatically improved the likelihood that a responder would provide mouth-to-mouth ventilation. Unfortunately, of their respondents, 44% rarely or never carried one of these devices. A variety of devices are available, including both masks and foil sheets. The former have the advantage of distancing the patient from the rescuer, while the latter have been made small enough to attach to a key chain. In spite of their small size, the foils appear to provide good protection, so long as care is taken to avoid cutting them with the patient's or rescuer's teeth.[54] Medical directors may wish to recommend these devices for those individuals who may respond while off duty.

Procedures for Active Airway Management

The gold standard for airway management has long been the endotracheal tube. Because this device has traditionally been reserved for physicians, alternative airways, most notably the EOA, Pharyngeal Tracheal Lumen (PTL) airway, and the Esophageal Tracheal Combitube™ (ETC) have been advocated by some for prehospital airway management (table 54.1). In addition to these devices, the laryngeal mask is being seen more often in the emergency and prehospital setting.

ENDOTRACHEAL INTUBATION

Endotracheal intubation (ET) is the optimal method of managing the unstable airway. Its use in prehospital care has been controversial, with proponents citing its efficacy and critics claiming that it is a difficult technical skill that should be reserved for highly trained physicians.

The ET has many advantages. It isolates the airway from secretions or gastric contents. When connected to a bag-valve-mask, a prehospital care provider can supplement both the oxygenation and ventilation of a patient without having to worry about airway maneuvers. Gastric insufflation, a major problem in the patient who is being mask ventilated, is eliminated. If

TABLE 54.1

Comparison of Airway Management Devices

DEVISE	DIFFICULTY OF USE	LIKELIHOOD OF COMPLICATIONS	COST	DEFINITIVE TREATMENT?	MEDICATION ADMINISTRATION	PEDIATRIC USE
BVM	++++	++	+	No	No	Yes
ET	+++	++	++	Yes	Yes	Yes
EOA	++	++++	+++	No	No	No
PTL	+	+++	++++	No	No	No
LMA	+	++	+	Possibly	No	Yes
ETC	+	+++	++++	No	No	No

Difficulty of use: How difficult it would be for a single paramedic to initiate and maintain the airway.

Likelihood of complications: The possibility of hypoxia, airway trauma, aspiration, or unrecognized esophageal ventilation.

Cost: All these assume a resuscitation bag will be used.

Note: These ratings are subjective judgements of the author based on the information in the text.

the patient has significant pulmonary pathology, positive end-expiratory pressure (PEEP) can be applied by way of the ET, improving oxygenation in patients who might otherwise remain hypoxic. Medications can be administered through the ET, providing a route when IV access is not possible. ET is inexpensive, usually costing less than five dollars. The tube may be placed using several different techniques, which adds to its versatility in the prehospital setting.

When compared to the EOA and oropharyngeal airways, patients who received an ET during prehospital cardiac arrest had an improved survival rate.[55] These patients also appeared to have good neurological recovery, and experienced a quality of life similar to patients with coronary artery disease.

Criticism of ET intubation by non-physicians in the out-of-hospital setting has focused on the concern that it is a very difficult procedure, potentially fraught with complications. Stewart looked at methods to train paramedics in ET intubation.[56] Their study found that paramedics could be trained to intubate using a variety of methods, including operating room, mannequin, and animal laboratory experience. The success rates for field intubation ranged from 76% to 92%, depending upon the seniority of the operator. This suggests that even if mannequins alone are used for training, paramedics can be taught to correctly intubate more than 75% of the time. Stratton performed a similar study with like results.[57]

In their study comparing ET intubation to esophageal airways, Shea found that training paramedics to perform ET intubation took approximately 7 hours, while training with the EOA took 4 hours,[58] an insignificant difference given the clear superiority of the endotracheal tube. In a study of skill retention by medical students who were trained in intubation as part of an ACLS course, 70% of students were able to successfully intubate 2 to 3 months after initial training, despite the lack of any reinforcement in the interim.[59] With minimal training, paramedics have been trained to provide nasotracheal intubation.[60] Finally, paramedics have been shown to be superior to physicians in performance of selected motor skills.[61] Clearly, the difficulty of this manual procedure has been greatly exaggerated.

Complications, primarily unrecognized esophageal intubation, have led some systems away from allowing their paramedics to intubate. The complication rate appears to vary greatly from system to system and is probably related to the protocol used for patient selection. In the Alameda County system, Pointer had a relatively high rate of unrecognized esophageal intubation, 5 in 383 attempts (1.3%).[62] Stewart demonstrated a rate of 0.4% for this complication,[63] while Jacobs in Boston and Guss in San Diego had no complications.[64,65] In Stewart's study, he concluded that all of the unrecognized esophageal intubations resulted from protocol violations (inadequate auscultation of the lung fields and epigastrium). Pointer reached this same conclusion. An alarming observational study was conducted in Orlando, Florida in 1997.[66] In this study the authors, Katz and Falk, found a 25% rate of misplaced endotracheal tubes in patients arriving in their emergency department. Because they did not question the paramedics regarding their placement verification procedures, it is not possible to know how these error occurred. The authors point out that most of the studies have been performed in systems where academic emergency physicians provide close supervision of the system; this was not present in this system. While some might read this to condemn all ET intubation programs, it appears that the problem is not with the procedure, but with the training and supervision. This article, and the accompanying editorial by Delbridge and Yealy[67] dramatically point out that if medical directors are going to permit their providers to perform any invasive procedure that they must provide close supervision and follow-up.

A review of methods for detecting esophageal intubation among anesthesia patients suggests that auscultation may be insufficient.[68] Birmingham indicated that even with careful chest and epigastric auscultation, presumably performed in a quiet operating room, a significant rate of unrecognized esophageal intubations could occur. He noted that this has been a significant cause for malpractice actions against anesthesia personnel. His conclusion was that prevention of esophageal intubation requires capnometry.

Endobronchial tube placement, primarily in the right mainstem bronchus, is another potential hazard. Bissinger noted a 7% rate of endobronchial tube placement, with another 13% of emergency patients having endotracheal tubes positioned near the carina.[69] He recommended that tubes be placed to 21 cm in women and 23 cm in men and that tubes be shortened before placement. His series did not describe any actual harm that occurred from endobronchial tube placement, but several theoretical concerns were addressed.

Intubation of the pediatric population has been another area of concern. This was addressed by a study of the Fresno system, where a 64% success rate was seen.[70] The authors found that intubation was attempted on only 67% of eligible patients. This may have been secondary to the providers lack of experience with intubation in general (it had only recently been authorized in this system) and with pediatric intubation in particular. Given that the BVM and endotracheal tubes are the only available pediatric airways, and that most pediatric arrests have respiratory causes, clearly providers need to possess the skills and equipment to expertly manage children's airways. Gausche and her colleagues in Los Angeles looked at this problem.[71] Using an every other day system of randomization, they assigned patients to either BVM only or to BVM followed by ET intubation. Using survival and neurological status as outcome markers, they could find no difference between the two types of airway management. Until this study is replicated in several different systems, medical directors should target pediatric airway management as a high-priority area for quality management.

Cervical spine movement during ET intubation has always been a significant concern because many of the patients who require intubation are at high risk for cervical spine injuries. A 1991 study indicated intubation, regardless of technique, results in less cervical spine displacement than BVM ventilation.[72]

ET intubation may mean the difference between adequate and inadequate care in the back of an ambulance. No other method of airway management will permit a single attendant to control ventilation, monitor lung compliance, remove secretions, prevent aspiration, and perform the myriad other tasks often asked of the lone provider. In air-medical transport, endotracheal intubation is critical, because the patient care crew is unable to monitor many of the signs that signal airway compromise, and it is not always possible to land to re-check breath sounds or assess stridor. In addition, in some rotorcraft adequate space is not available to optimally perform ET intubation while the patient is in flight.

METHODS OF ENDOTRACHEAL INTUBATION

Several methods of ET intubation are available; these include direct oral intubation, nasotracheal intubation, digital intubation, and lighted stylet intubation. The gum bougie, a well known adjunct in Europe, has recently been seen in the U.S. as well.

DIRECT ORAL INTUBATION (LARYNGOSCOPIC INTUBATION)

Direct oral intubation is the most common method of intubation. There are several advantages to this method of intubation: Because the operator sees the pathway of the ET tube, placement is felt to be more sure, although some have questioned this reasoning.[57] Direct laryngoscopy allows the removal of any foreign bodies that may be obstructing the airway. This method also appears more efficient because the route is visualized and the tube placed without searching for the airway.

Disadvantages of this technique include the need for the patient to be able to tolerate the laryngoscope, which requires either sufficient depression of the mental status or pharmacological adjuncts. Trismus, not uncommon in the head-injured patient, also prevents this route of intubation. Although paralytic agents, such as succinylcholine, have been used by prehospital care providers, this practice is not common.[48,73] Generally, the patient must be supine, which places significant limitations on the paramedic whose patients are not always conveniently positioned.

Several authors have raised concerns regarding this intubation route in the patient with potential cervical spine injuries. The ATLS manual advocates oral endotracheal intubation with "inline manual cervical immobilization" as the means to intubate apneic trauma patients, but only if they do not have maxillofacial injuries.[74] Bivins indicates that patients with potential cervical spine injuries should have their airway managed by either nasotracheal intubation or cricothyrotomy because of the risk of worsening an injury with manual traction and direct laryngoscopy.[75] Other authors have produced conflicting studies.[76,77] Walls encourages the use of oral ET intubation in the trauma patient, but only if the technique can be performed in a "gentle . . . manner."[78] He suggests that the best method is probably rapid sequence intubation using succinylcholine or rapid tranquilization.

For those medical directors who feel uncomfortable having their paramedics use succinylcholine, sedation with an opioid (reversible with naloxone) or with a benzodiazepine (reversible with flumazenil) could be considered. Etomidate is a nonopioid nonbarbiturate that is capable of inducing the rapid onset of hypnosis, allowing for intubation to be facilitated. Its major advantage is its lack of cardiovascular depression.[79,80] It also has the advantage that it does not completely depress respirations, so patients are not completely dependent on the caregiver's ability to maintain the airway. Regardless of the pharmacological adjunct used, the objective has to be a gentle procedure. Patients who are fighting the intubation attempt and gagging on the laryngoscope blade are at much higher risk of injury. Probably the most realistic statement regarding this question was by Joyce, who warns that any airway maneuver may affect the cervical spine, no matter what modality is used.[81] Therefore in any patient with a potential cervical spine injury rescuers must aggressively manage the ABCs while paying as much attention as possible to minimizing cervical spine motion.

NASOTRACHEAL INTUBATION

Another commonly used route for tracheal intubation is by way of the nasal passages. This generally requires that the person have some respiratory effort to guide the tube into the trachea, although adjuncts, such as the flexible lighted stylet, may facilitate this route in the apneic patient.[82] It is ideal for the patient who cannot be placed recumbent, either because of

entrapment or because of their clinical condition (e.g., congestive heart failure). Nasotracheal intubation is well tolerated by the awake patient. Since it does not require jaw opening, the patient with trismus may by intubated without pharmacological adjuncts. Although there are no good models for teaching the technique, still has been applied with a low complication rate.[58]

In the Louisville EMS system, paramedics who had been trained in endotracheal intubation were authorized to perform nasotracheal intubation.[58] They achieved a 71% success rate with this intubation modality without receiving any hands-on training in humans before performing the procedure. This success rate compares favorably with the 75% to 98% success rates for direct oral intubation. Another study showed no difference in success rates between the orotracheal and nasotracheal routes.[83] Some authors feel the nasotracheal technique may involve less manipulation of the cervical spine than laryngoscopic intubation, concluding that nasotracheal intubation is the only non-surgical airway maneuver to use in blunt trauma victims.[61]

Concerns regarding this method of intubation have come from several areas. Passage of a tube through the nose tends to make the very friable mucosa bleed. Even if the nares are prepared with a vasoconstrictor and lubricant, bleeding may become a problem. Most adults can tolerate a tube larger than 4mm, the minimum tube size required for ventilation. Sinusitis has also been cited as a complication, but this is related to the duration of intubation. Should tube size or sinusitis become concerns, the tube can be replaced when the patient is stable in the hospital. There is considerable concern over perforation of the cribriform plate with subsequent intracranial placement, although the incidence of this appears to be exceedingly rare.[84] Many caregivers have difficulty in locating the trachea, but use of the Endotrol™ directable tube or flexible lighted stylet may aid in this problem.

In the noise of the prehospital environment, it may be difficult to hear the breathing of the patient to help guide the tube. The bell of the stethoscope can be placed over the open tube to facilitate this. Commercial devices, such as the Beck Airway Airflow Monitor (BAAM™) can also be used to amplify the breath sound.[85] Because this technique is used only on spontaneously breathing patients, concerns regarding esophageal intubation should be minimal. End-tidal CO_2 detectors can be used to eliminate any shred of doubt.

PROCEDURES

DIGITAL INTUBATION

Digital intubation is the original method of ET intubation. It is an excellent way to orally intubate the unresponsive patient who is entrapped or is otherwise in an awkward position for laryngoscopy.[86] When batteries fail, digital intubation may be the only method available. Like direct oral intubation the tube is placed under guidance, but unlike the laryngoscopic method, the landmarks are palpated, not seen. Because visualization is not necessary, this modality is useful when there are secretions or bleeding. The primary disadvantage of the digital technique involves the risk one incurs when one places the fingers into another person's mouth. Of course, gloves should always be worn. A dental prod or mouth gag is used to keep the mouth open during the procedure. The prod should be used regardless of mental status in case the patient awakens during the procedure.

LIGHTED STYLET INTUBATION

A rigid stylet, tipped with a light, can be used to intubate a patient without laryngoscopy.[87] It has many of the advantages of the digital technique but is safer in that the operator need not reach into the patient's mouth. The paramedic holds the tip of the patient's tongue with a gauze square, thus opening the airway and raising the epiglottis. The ET tube, with the stylet in place, is formed into a hockey-stick shape. It is inserted into the mouth and trachea while watching the passage of the light in the end of the stylet. This technique is best performed in a partially darkened room or ambulance, because bright sunlight may limit the ability of the operator to visualize the glow the stylet produces. This method offers the additional advantage that tube placement can be easily verified simply by reinserting the stylet.[88] The lighted stylet technique has also been described to assist nasotracheal intubation.[89,90] There are several manufacturers of lighted stylets, some of which are small enough for infant use.

GUM BOUGIE

This device is essentially a semi-rigid stylet. Although available in Europe for a number of years, it has only recently come to the U.S. Used with a laryngoscope, the gum bougie is placed in the trachea much like an ET tube. Because of its smaller diameter and stiffness, it can often be placed more easily than an ET tube. Experienced users of this device say that they can feel the tracheal rings, helping verify the ET placement. Once the bougie is in place, the ET tube is slid over the bougie and into the trachea, using a Seldinger-like technique.

ESOPHAGEAL OBTURATOR AIRWAY (EOA)/ ESOPHAGEAL GASTRIC TUBE AIRWAY (EGTA)

The EOA was first described by Michael in 1968.[91] The original design was invented for use in the coronary care unit. It was later refined and promoted primarily as a tool to allow prehospital personnel to control the airway when they are unable to provide ET intubation.[92] It gained amazingly widespread use despite a dearth of clinical studies.

The American Heart Association classifies this technique as II b, which they define as "A therapeutic option that is not well established by evidence but may be helpful and probably not harmful."[93] The primary advantage of this device is that it allows the provider to ventilate the patient without being concerned over gastric distention or regurgitation. An improvement, the EGTA, features a lumen in the esophageal tube through which a nasogastric tube can be placed to evacuate the stomach. Advocates report blood gas results equivalent to those obtained with ET intubation.[94-96] Several other authors agree that EOA are useful when the patient cannot be endotracheally intubated or if the patient has such copious gastric contents that aspiration is a hazard.[54,97,98]

Esophageal airways essentially are a BVM with an obturator; as such, they suffer from some of the same problems as the bag-valve-mask. The operator must still provide both a mask seal and an airway maneuver, so ideally the device should be used with two paramedics to perform ventilation. It is difficult to effect a seal on edentulous patients,[42] and its use is contraindicated in patients who are less than 15 years of age. Caustic ingestion or esophageal pathology are also contraindications to the use of this device. Esophageal perforation has been described,[99] as has unrecognized tracheal intubation[100] and gastric rupture due to cuff failure.[101] Esophageal tube placement with an EOA has been suggested to help aid in ET intubation, but Gatrell cites two instances where both the esophageal obturator and ET tubes were placed in the esophagus, and this error was not recognized.[102]

Most of the studies mentioned thus far were performed in the hospital setting. In an early prehospital study, Schofferman found adequate blood gas levels in a series of 18 patients ventilated with the EOA by paramedics.[103] Twelve of these patients had a spontaneous supraventricular rhythm; six were undergoing

CPR. The mean $PaCO_2$ level in the arrested patients was 62 mmHg, while those with a rhythm had a $PaCO_2$ level of 40 mmHg. The patients all underwent ET intubation in the emergency department, and subsequent blood gas levels were obtained, but no comparisons were made. This is the only prehospital study in which the EOA was seen in a favorable light. Auerbach and Geehr looked at the prehospital setting in two prospective studies.[104,105] In the first of these they obtained blood gas levels from patients who had undergone EGTA intubation in the field. The patients were then endotracheally intubated, and the gas levels were redrawn 5 minutes after the new airway was established. Their results demonstrated a significant improvement in both oxygenation and ventilation following ET intubation in the emergency department. The follow-up study was performed after paramedics were trained in ET intubation. They compared a group of patients who were treated using an ET tube with a group of patients treated in the field with the EGTA. There was a substantial difference in age between the two groups, the EGTA group being younger. No difference was detected in downtime or field times. Oxygenation, ventilation, and pH level were all significantly better among those patients who had received ET intubation. Similar results were reported by Smith.[106] They found the EOA could not be passed in 18% of patients, which is worse than the rates quoted for ET intubation failures in many systems. Bass concluded that the complication rate of the EGTA, when compared with the reported successes with ET intubation, made the EGTA an airway of last resort for use only when ET intubation could not be achieved.[107] Smith and Bodai reviewed the literature in 1983 and concluded that the EOA was a poor substitute for ET intubation in the prehospital setting.[108] This conclusion was reaffirmed in a somewhat more recent paper by Hankins.[109] Although it appears that the sun has set on esophageal airways, they are still commercially available; medical directors should be aware of the past as they evaluate devices in the future.

THE PHARYNGO-TRACHEAL LUMEN AIRWAY (PTL) AND THE ESOPHAGEAL TRACHEAL COMBITUBE (ETC)

The tracheoesophageal airway, a precursor of the PTL and the ETC, was developed because of the incidence of ET placement of the esophageal obturator. This device allowed the patient to be ventilated through the mask if the tube passed into the esophagus or by way of the tube should it enter the trachea.[110,111] Difficulties with mask ventilation prompted the creation of two other devices, the Pharyngo-Tracheal Lumen Airway (PTL) and the Esophageal Tracheal Combitube™ (ETC). These devices are similar in design, both essentially being a double lumen tube with a distal and a proximal balloon. The distal balloon is inflated once the device is in place and is designed to occupy the trachea or esophagus. The proximal balloon is larger, designed to occupy the oropharynx when inflated. The inner lumen is similar to an ET tube, while the outer lumen is truncated PTL or perforated ETC to allow ventilation if the long tube is placed in the esophagus. Both of these devices are placed blindly. The operator then uses breath sounds and chest movement to determine whether the distal lumen is in the esophagus or trachea.

Niemann at Harbor-UCLA initially tested the PTL in an animal study, with the device deliberately placed in the esophagus.[112] They were able to demonstrate ventilatory efficiencies and blood gas levels equivalent to those seen with ET tubes. Included in their report was a pilot study on six patients in cardiac arrest. They drew blood gas levels on patients who were endotracheally intubated, then replaced this device with the PTL™. After a stabilization period, gas levels were again collected. No difference in blood gas values was seen between the two devices. In a study of the ETC in patients undergoing anesthesia, it appeared to provide better oxygenation than conventional endotracheal airway management.[113] Frass then used the ETC on patients who suffered cardiac arrest in the hospital and noted that the ETC provided adequate oxygenation and ventilation in all of these patients. He concluded that the ETC was a useful device for airway management. Bartlett's group has demonstrated that the PTL can provide significant protection for the airway in the setting of upper airway hemorrhage.[114] Atherton looked at the use of the ETC in the field.[115] In this study the device was compared with the endotracheal tube using an alternate day design. The ETC was used as a backup airway on days when the endotracheal tube was primary. When the ETC was used as the primary airway, it was successfully placed 72% of the time. When used as a backup for failed endotracheal tube placement, successful placement occurred in 64% of patients. The endotracheal tube, as the primary airway, was placed 84% of the time. McMahan compared the PTL with the endotracheal tube and found no difference in the rate of successful intubation.[116] In a study comparing these two devices along with the laryngeal mask and the oral airway, Rumball and MacDonald found little difference between these two devices, and they felt that both were superior to the use of an oral airway and BVM.[117]

The major concern regarding the use of these airways has been the need for the paramedic to discriminate between esophageal and endotracheal placement. The difficulty in making this determination has been one of the major stumbling blocks preventing paramedics from using the endotracheal tube. As noted previously, the use of breath sounds or chest rise to determine the placement of a tube is not foolproof, even in a quiet operating theater.[62] When providers were trained in the use of the PTL and then retested 6 weeks after training, they were unable to correctly determine the site of placement in over 40% of cases.[118] The authors concluded that paramedics using this device need extensive training in assessment of tube placement.

When these devices are placed in the esophagus (the most likely location) the trachea cannot be suctioned without deflating the oropharyngeal balloon. While resuscitation medications could potentially be administered, it is unlikely that any significant amount would reach the bronchial tree. Like the EOA, the ETC has a long list of contraindications. It should not be used in pediatric patients, patients with a gag reflex, or patients who have ingested caustic substances.[119]

Both the PTL and the ETC have been touted as airways that can be placed when ET tubes cannot be inserted. Multiple attempts at ET intubation without success might be an indication to use these devices. They have also been authorized for use in some states by paramedics who are not permitted to perform ET intubation, although it appears they may be at least as difficult to use correctly as an ET tube. While it is considered more difficult to train personnel in the use of the ET tube, both Hunt[101] and Atherton[99] showed that the PTL and the ETC both require significant ongoing training and supervision. Neither is superior to a correctly placed ET tube. Paramedics should be trained in all the methods of ET tube insertion, and significant amounts of ongoing education should be devoted to intubation skills. If the medical director elects to use other devices as backup, he needs to realize that their use will also require substantial training and supervision. Confirmation of placement with an end-tidal CO_2 detector or other method should still be performed. The Self-Inflating Bulb (SIB) has been used successfully to confirm proper placement of the ETC.[120] While these devices appear to be suitable backups for ET intubation, they still require training. Medical directors electing to use these devices should spend considerable time training their providers in the correct indications, methods of use, and verification needed to safely perform these skills.

LARYNGEAL MASK AIRWAY (LMA)

The laryngeal mask airway (LMA) was first used as an alternative to ET tube ventilation in operating rooms in Great Britain in 1983.[121] Because of its purported ease of use and efficacy, this device has appeal as a useful field airway adjunct.[122] A study comparing the LMA to ET intubation in 19 patients undergoing elective surgery showed that paramedics and respiratory therapists were able to successfully ventilate the patients in less time and with less attempts at placement when using the LMA. There has been some suggestion that the LMA may also have the advantage of minimizing cervical spine motion when being placed.[123] Cases have been described of the use of the LMA where patients are trapped with limited access preventing ET intubation.[124] One of the major disadvantages to this airway is that it does not protect against aspiration.[125] Although paramedics found it more difficult to place than either the PTL or the Combitube, one Canadian study demonstrated that with a short course of training the LMA could provide an acceptable alternative airway.[114]

Tools for Confirming Airway Placement

END-TIDAL CO_2 DETECTORS/MONITORS

Medical directors should insist on the use of a CO_2 detection technique in any patient who has been intubated. This has been shown to be the most reliable method of determining ET placement in a perfusing patient.[62] At the present time, both electronic and chemical devices are available for detection of exhaled CO_2. Studies have demonstrated the utility of these devices in the prehospital[126,127] and emergency department settings.[128] These devices should be used for all intubated patients, especially when the patient was intubated by a blind technique, such as digital intubation.

Electronic devices are also being marketed. In the prehospital market, most of these provide only a yes or no indication of the detection of CO_2. Quantitative monitoring of end-tidal CO_2 has been available in the hospital for several years. There is increasing miniaturization of these devices, making them more useful in the prehospital environment. Some monitors designed for the prehospital and interfacility transport environment contain integral end-tidal CO_2 modules. Use of these devices will allow the provider to accurately titrate the degree of ventilation to the patient's needs, preventing the severe hyperventilation that occasionally occurs.

OTHER TECHNIQUES

Aside from the devices described above, two other ways of confirming ET tube placement deserve mention. Lighted stylets, both of the rigid and flexible type, can be used to confirm placement of a tube inserted by another method. The use of a large syringe to aspirate the airway has also been advocated. This device is commercially available as the Esophageal Intubation Detector (EID). In this situation the syringe is attached to the endotracheal tube and the plunger is rapidly withdrawn. If the tube is in the esophagus, it will collapse from the vacuum and the operator will not be able to withdraw air. In the trachea, because it will not collapse, the syringe will aspirate air. Several studies have demonstrated the utility of this device in the operating room, where all researchers noted it to be 100% accurate at detecting esophageal intubation in adults.[129-133] A study by Jenkins demonstrated the utility of this device in the prehospital and emergency department setting.[134] Although there were only two esophageal intubations in their series of 90 patients, they were both detected. The authors noted that there were no false negatives, despite the presence of a large hemothorax in one patient and pulmonary edema in nine patients.

It is absolutely essential that medical directors choose a method for auxiliary confirmation of tube placement and insist on its use. The risk of an undetected esophageal intubation is minimized when one (or more) of these auxiliary techniques is used. Not using these tools or having protocols not properly performed risks not only the patient's life, but it also jeopardizes the paramedic, the medical director, and the EMS system.

INVASIVE AIRWAY PROCEDURES

When ET intubation has failed or when the anatomy of the face has been so distorted so as to prevent placement of an ET tube, a surgical airway may be lifesaving. Cricothyrotomy has usually been the route used in emergencies and by non-surgeons. Tracheotomy has been considered too difficult and too complicated to perform in the emergency situation. Alternatives to formal cricothyrotomy have included "minicricothyrotomy" and translaryngeal needle ventilation.

CRICOTHYROTOMY

This procedure has a long history, but it fell into disfavor after Jackson implicated it as a cause of airway stenosis in 1921.[135] Like so many techniques, it was later resurrected as a method of emergency airway management. Some authors feel it is the method of choice for management of apneic patients with suspected cervical spine injuries.[61] McGill reviewed 3 years of data at Hennepin County Medical Center.[136] During this period, 38 cricothyrotomies were performed in their department, primarily for failure of other airway management techniques. Twelve patients were long-term survivors. There was a 39% complication rate, which included placement of the tube through the thyrohyoid membrane, prolonged procedure times, and hemorrhage from the incision. Only one survivor had permanent dysphonia. He stated that the complication rate is much higher than others have quoted, but this was due to the emergency nature of the procedures in the series.

A series of 69 patients who underwent cricothyrotomy by flight nurse/paramedics in the field was reviewed by Boyle.[137] He reported a complication rate of 8.7%, all of which occurred in patients who were in traumatic cardiac arrest at the time of the procedure. In another series of air-medical service patients, no complications were seen among 20 patients on whom the procedure was performed.[138] Their indications included maxillofacial or cervical trauma or the failure of other methods of airway management when patients were in arrest. None of the arrested patients survived, but seven of the maxillofacial trauma patients survived.

Spaite and Joseph reviewed the records of 20 patients who presented to a Level 1 trauma center after undergoing prehospital cricothyrotomy.[139] Their results were not encouraging in that only one patient survived without neurological complications. They concluded that many of the massively injured or arrested patients probably did not benefit from this procedure and that the indications for this procedure in the prehospital setting should be very narrowly defined. Other investigators have had better success. Nugent found that when flight nurses performed cricothyrotomy, 27% of their patients survived to hospital discharge.[140] Their retrospective study also noted that during the first year the procedure was performed primarily on victims in cardiac arrest. In subsequent years, this population made up a minority of the patients. This suggests that as the flight nurses became more comfortable with the procedure, they began to use it earlier, which may explain their good results. The lesson here is that if paramedics are authorized to perform this procedure, they need to perform it as soon as the indications arise, rather than using it only on patients in cardiac arrest.

MINICRICOTHYROTOMY

Several studies have looked at minimizing the amount of surgical expertise and the size of the device placed through the cricothyroid membrane. Yealy has shown that adequate tidal volumes can be delivered using a 4 mm catheter.[122,123] Campbell has used an 8.5 French (2.8 mm) central venous catheter to ventilate dogs with conventional BVM techniques.[141] The Seldinger technique has been used to percutaneously place larger diameter devices.[142] These studies suggest that it may be possible to cannulate the trachea percutaneously with larger diameter devices, eliminating the need for a special high-pressure connection, without requiring a formal cricothyrotomy.

Commercial devices are available for performing minicricothyrotomy. One of these, the Pertrach, consists of a needle, wire, dilator, and cannula. This procedure is performed by making a small skin incision, through which the needle is introduced into the cricothyroid membrane. Air is aspirated to confirm position, then a dilator is passed through the breakaway needle to spread the tissues. The tube is then placed into the airway. When compared to conventional cricothyrotomy, paramedics found this technique to be just as successful as the conventional method but felt it was more difficult to perform.[143]

TRANSTRACHEAL JET VENTILATION

Transtracheal jet ventilation, occasionally called needle cricothyrotomy, is one of the simplest methods of invasive airway access, but unfortunately it is also one of the most underutilized. This is probably because of the perception that it can only be used for a very short time. The ATLS manual states that this technique can provide adequate oxygenation for only 30 to 45 minutes.[144] However, the technique they describe is not jet ventilation, but apneic oxygenation. Frame has been able to demonstrate adequate oxygenation when using 14 and 16 gauge catheters in cats with total airway obstruction, applying the ATLS technique. Use of an 18 gauge catheter did result in hypoventilation.[145] Ventilation requires that a 50 psi source, such as is available directly from a wall connection or oxygen tank regulator sidearm, be used in conjunction with a 14 or 16 gauge catheter. It can be performed indefinitely, since a 16 gauge catheter will allow flow rates in excess of 50 liters per minute.[146] If extrapolated to 20 breaths per minute, this is equivalent to a tidal volume of 950cc,[147] which is more than adequate to ventilate most adult patients.

Aspiration has also been a concern with this method, because it, like the surgical cricothyrotomy, is often used in patients with massive upper airway injury or hemorrhage. When Yealy looked at this problem using Gastrograffin as the marker, he found no evidence of aspiration when the head of the bed was at a 30-degree angle, noting mild aspiration only in two of six animals who were set at a 45-degree angle.[148] He concluded that at 30 degrees or less the jet ventilator provided sufficient airway protection. As most patients in critical condition are transported in the supine position, this should not be a problem. In patients with a totally obstructed airway there may be an increased risk of barotrauma. Stothert has shown that in these patients inspiration times greater than 1 second or expiration times of less than four times the inspiration time have a greatly increased risk of barotrauma or hemodynamic compromise.[149]

When assembled, the device consists of a connection for a high pressure (50 psi) source, a connecting line, a spring loaded trigger valve, and a tube with a Luer lock connection. This connects to the catheter. This is a high pressure system and will not work if it is fed from a 125-liter flow meter. The tubing must be the same as that used to connect a ventilator to a wall connection. Oxygen tubing, like that used for a mask or cannula, will not work. Supplies to make this device are usually available locally from the respiratory supply company or respiratory therapy departments of local hospitals. The medical director must ensure that the supplies are available and assembled well ahead of the time they are needed.

VENTILATORS

Some systems, especially air-medical systems and ground systems specializing in interhospital transfers, use portable mechanical ventilators. These devices are usually battery or oxygen powered, and they are produced by a variety of manufacturers.[150] Some are designed for transport only, while others can be used during CPR. Some of these devices are designed as simple resuscitators, while others have many of the features of hospital ventilators, such as oxygen mixers, pressure gauges, and PEEP. They have the advantage of freeing the attendant from the task of manually ventilating the patient with a resuscitation bag. They also tend to produce a consistent volume, preventing the variation in ventilation that occurs with manual bagging. Costs vary.

Like any medical device, ventilators require some care to perform properly. Some have specialized cleaning requirements. The volume produced by the ventilator should be checked with a spirometer at the beginning of use and on a regular basis during transport. If the ventilator is pressure cycled, the volume may change as lung compliance changes. Paramedics using this type of ventilator should be aware of this effect. Some ventilators will continue to cycle even when their oxygen supply is cut off; the paramedic must be vigilant in this regard. Medical directors who permit their EMS service to use ventilators must be sure that there is a clear protocol governing their use. Frequent continuing education is also mandatory when using these devices.

Adjuncts for Airway Management

Oxygen is routinely given to most ambulance patients in the United States today. The public considers it to be life-giving and without side effects. Paramedics are often of a similar mind. As mentioned before, oxygen is a drug with both benefits and side effects. In addition, increasing emphasis on cost-effective medical care discourages the use of a drug that may have no effect on the patient. Often, in spite of oxygen administration, unrecognized hypoxia may occur. However, until the advent of pulse oximetry, there was no method of assessing adequate oxygenation in the prehospital setting.

The arrival of pulse oximeters and their miniaturization in the 1980s provided medical caregivers with another parameter for assessing patients. One article described pulse oximetry as the "fifth vital sign."[151] Studies have demonstrated that pulse oximetry can be performed reliably in the prehospital setting. Aughey compared the pulse oximeter reading obtained in the field with the saturation of a simultaneously obtained blood gas level.[152] Her group demonstrated excellent correlation between the reading of the pulse oximeter and the co-oximeter. McGuire and Pointer found that paramedics were able to follow the patient's response to respiratory interventions more closely by use of oximetry.[153] Silverston found

that pulse oximetry was able to provide an early clue for finding developing pneumothorax, as well as helping to guide the caregivers in selection of appropriate airways.[154] When used during endotracheal intubation the pulse oximeter can help prevent unrecognized hypoxia from occurring.[155] Cydulka demonstrated that when a relatively conservative saturation of 97% was used, pulse oximetry could substantially decrease the unnecessary oxygen use.[156] This decrease in oxygen use was shown to produce substantial cost savings, without an apparent decrement in patient care.

In the air-medical setting, pulse oximetry has been proven valuable.[157,158] In helicopter transport the flight crew may be relatively isolated from the patient due to noise and packaging, making detection of hypoxemia difficult. The altitude changes associated with fixed wing transport may rapidly produce hypoxemia. These changes are often detected by the pulse oximeter before there is clinical evidence.

As with any monitoring device, some control and education are necessary to guide the paramedic. Although both of the above authors demonstrated the device was reliable, it may give erroneous numbers due to local hypoperfusion, hypotension, movement of the probe, fingernail polish, bright lights, carboxyhemoglobinemia, anemia, or other patient or equipment problems.[159,160] Special probes may be needed for small children, adding to the expense of the device. As with all types of monitoring devices, providers must be cautioned to treat the patient, not the monitor.

There is a wide range of monitor types and prices, ranging from several hundred to several thousand dollars. Prices for these units have been rapidly dropping. The less expensive versions usually have a single digit probe and an LED readout. As one moves up in price the units display waveforms and may have interchangeable probes for digits, ears, noses, or other areas. Most pulse oximeters look at the oxygenation at the time of the arterial pulse and depend upon plethysmography for timing. Some of the high-end monitors are able to synchronize with the EKG, allowing more accurate monitoring of the patient, who may have peripheral hypoperfusion or is on vasopressors. When added to the signs commonly assessed, pulse oximetry can be a valuable adjunct, but only if its use is audited and the medical director provides ongoing guidance.

NASOGASTRIC TUBES

Nasogastric (NG) tubes may be useful in selected adults at risk for vomiting and aspiration, and in in-

PROCEDURES

fants where gastric distention may cause respiratory compromise. In systems with short transport times NG tube placement is probably not useful, but in long-distance transports it may decrease the chance of airway compromise. These tubes may be placed through the mouth or the nose in adults. Children tolerate the oral route better because of concern over adenoidal bleeding with nasal passage. When used for aspiration only and not for fluid or medication administration, they should enjoy a low complication rate. Even an endotracheal placement would be unlikely to cause much harm. Take care to avoid aspiration, and suction should be available during the procedure. Providers must be cautioned against placing NG tubes in patients with craniofacial injuries because of the risk of cribriform plate disruption and intracranial placement.

NEEDLE THORACOSTOMY

The placement of a needle to relieve tension pneumothorax is often used in ground EMS systems. Some air-medical services have also authorized the placement of a formal tube thoracostomy by their crews.

The placement of a needle in the midclavicular line, second intercostal space can produce dramatic results in a patient suffering from a tension pneumothorax. This procedure should be considered in any patient who suffers from rapid cardiopulmonary decompensation. Although tracheal deviation or decreased breath sounds are commonly accepted as signs of a tension pneumothorax, they may not always be accurate.[161] Providers should be encouraged to perform this procedure in any patient who has a precipitous course, especially if there is a history of COPD, asthma, or chest trauma. Trauma patients with obvious subcutaneous emphysema can benefit from the early application of this technique. The procedure appears to be safe and simple. Eckstein and Suyehara reviewed their experience in a series of over 6000 trauma patients.[162] Their conclusion, based on the 108 patients in this series who received needle decompression, was that this was a potentially life-saving intervention, with a low complication rate. If the catheter is placed into the lung parenchyma, the puncture will be small and should heal rapidly. The resultant pneumothorax is an open one, and therefore the patient should suffer little further compromise. Although inappropriate placement generally results in the considerable morbidity of a tube thoracostomy, patients who are candidates for this procedure usually have other injuries that will require a hospital stay.

If the patient is intubated, the catheter may be placed and left open to the air. If the patient is spontaneously breathing, a one-way valve must be created to prevent reentry of air during inspiration. One way valves, such as the Heimlich valve, are available. Condoms may be used by puncturing the condom with the catheter and then unrolling it after it has been placed in the patient. Surgical gloves have been used, but when compared to condoms, they produce unacceptable air leakage.

TUBE THORACOSTOMY

This common surgical procedure is used to evacuate air or blood from the pleural space. Its use in the field has commonly been limited to air-medical services or military situations. The primary advantage of this technique is that it can rapidly evacuate a large amount of blood from the trauma patient's pleural space, converting a tension hemothorax into an open hemothorax. In some cases this may be life-saving, but in others the patient can exsanguinate from the tube, depending upon the source of the bleeding. If this occurs in the field, however, it is unlikely that the tube would have contributed to the patient's demise.

If the transport time is sufficiently long, tube thoracostomy may be a useful procedure. The tube must be placed under sterile conditions, and it is difficult to provide even a modicum of sterility at many scenes. This may lead to empyema, should the patient survive. The technique has several areas where the operator must be careful, placement in the wrong interspace can result in injury to the abdominal organs, the heart or great vessels. Use of trocars or Kelly clamps to place the tube may cause injury to the lung parenchyma or other thoracic structures.

Once the tube has been secured, one must decide what to do with the free end of the tube. If the patient is intubated the tube may be left open, creating an open pneumothorax. For a patient who is not intubated, a one-way valve must be created to prevent entry of air into the thorax during inspiration. Historically water seals were used, but these are highly impractical outside the hospital. More recently, commercially manufactured chest tube drainage bottles have been manufactured, many of which do not require instillation of water to seal the system. Because of their bulk, they are difficult to use in the prehospital setting. The Heimlich valve, essentially a rubber flapper valve in a tube, is the most practical device for the paramedic. It may be connected to suction is required, and if there is a large amount of drainage, a urinary catheter bag may be attached to collect the drainage.

Other devices, such as the McSwain Dart, have also been used for chest decompression, but they confer no advantage over a venous catheter and are mentioned here only to discourage their use. In addition, catheters are usually carried by prehospital care providers, so they are readily available if the patient suddenly decompensates. For most EMS systems, needle thoracostomy is the safest, most rapid, and most effective way of providing pleural decompression.

Venous Access

When the primary purpose of ALS in prehospital care was cardiac care, it was obvious that IVs were needed for medication administration. Indeed, when combined with airway management and defibrillation skills, IV access has allowed the paramedic to provide care equivalent to that given in many emergency departments. However, when trauma patients became part of the paramedic's practice, considerably less agreement could be found regarding the benefits of IV fluids.

In an often quoted article, McSwain state that prehospital IV starts added 12.2 minutes to the on-scene time.[163] He questioned whether this delay was beneficial to the patient in cardiac arrest. Similar times were found in a study of the Sacramento EMS system.[6] Given that the delay resulted in an average of less than 1 liter of fluid administered, Smith concluded that IVs were unwarranted in trauma victims, who would benefit more from earlier surgical intervention. The times these authors quote were not directly measured, so there may have been other activities that contributed to the times.

Similar times for IV starts have also been reported in the South Carolina EMS system.[164] Blaisdell quoted these data in his 1984 address to the American Association for the Surgery of Trauma.[1] He concluded that in an urban system with short transport times, scoop-and-run techniques were preferable to IV access being obtained at the scene. The volume of fluid administered has also come into question. Kaweski's review of fluid administration in San Diego found there was no effect on survival with prehospital fluids.[4] However, computer modeling of prehospital hemorrhage suggests that fluid administration in the field provides an advantage in both blood pressure and survival.[165] As noted below, it is unclear whether raising blood pressure confers a survival advantage in

the clinical setting. Aprahamian has noted an improvement in survival for abdominal trauma patients when provided IV fluids.[166] The setting in which the prehospital IV is placed may engender a higher complication rate, and this also must be accounted for when evaluating the utility of IV therapy. Lawrence has noted a significantly higher rate of phlebitis and febrile illness when patients had IVs started in the field versus the ED.[167]

Numerous studies have been published that dispute the claim that paramedic-started IVs significantly delay transport. In one of the few studies to directly measure the time for procedures, Pons found that IV access required less than 3 minutes in all patients. This included time to draw blood, which prolonged the procedure. When a second IV line was required, it took only 1.25 minutes for placement.[168] Another study measuring IV start times found an average time of 2.8 minutes, with a 91% success rate. They also found a high success rate for lines placed while en route.[169] A 95% success rate for en-route IV starts in trauma patients was seen by Slovis, who also noted an 80% en-route IV success rate in medical patients.[170] O'Gorman found that IV lines could be initiated while en route with as much success as at the scene, leading him to suggest that prehospital IVs could be performed in "zero-time."[171] In a study of penetrating cardiac wounds the Denver group found that their paramedics could perform several procedures on these patients and still have an average on-scene time of less than 11 minutes.[172] For major trauma patients in Tucson, the average on-scene time was 8.1 minutes, with the sicker patients receiving more procedures and having a shorter scene time.[173] A 1994 study was done in both urban and non-urban settings measuring IV success rate and time.[174] In both, the success rate was greater than 97% at establishing an IV. More than 94% of lines in both settings were established in less than 4 minutes.

There is considerable debate regarding the appropriate amounts and types of fluid for trauma resuscitation.[175] While it may turn out that vigorous fluid resuscitation in the field produces no improvement or is even harmful, at present the clinical data are controversial. Many authorities believe that in uncontrolled hemorrhage, vigorous fluid resuscitation increases blood pressure, resulting in an increase in blood loss. Accelerating the blood loss is the dilution of coagulation factors and oxygen-carrying capacity. Some patients, however, are so hypotensive as to need at least enough resuscitation to maintain a modicum of blood flow to vital organs to prevent cardiac arrest. It has been suggested that maintaining the minimum blood pressure to provide cerebral perfusion may be the answer. While mental status has been suggested as the vital sign of significance here, it is likely that this will be applicable only to young victims of penetrating trauma. In the study done in Houston of almost 600 patients who were hypotensive secondary to penetrating torso injuries, the group that had a delay in aggressive fluid resuscitation until operative intervention had improved outcomes.[176] Clinical trials in this area are difficult to perform and to interpret, because there is no uniformity in the site and mechanism of the wounds. Animal studies of hemorrhage suggest that some level of hypotension may be beneficial.[177] Medical directors should follow this controversy closely, as it is fundamental to the way in which trauma victims are optimally resuscitated.

While speed is of paramount importance for the trauma patient, the effectiveness of field therapy may be more critical to the medical patient. In Australia, Potter noted a decrease in early mortality among patients treated by ALS units, which included IV therapy.[13] No difference in overall mortality was seen, however. In contrast, a study of North Carolina intermediate EMTs, who were authorized to start IVs but not administer drugs, showed no advantage to prehospital IV placement.[178] In reality there was a significant delay in medication administration for patients with EMT-I started IVs. In medical patients, the only reason for IV access is immediate drug therapy. Systems where blood is obtained for laboratory studies should be cautioned about the risk of mislabeled tubes. Some hospitals will not process blood which has not been drawn by one of their own staff. If the provider is prohibited from medication administration, medical patients do not benefit from a prehospital IV.

Peripheral Lines

Traditionally paramedics have started IVs in the veins of the upper limbs. Some systems have also authorized the use of the external jugular vein as a "peripheral" site. The immediate complications appear to be limited to unsuccessful attempts and local infiltration. There is some risk of infection, so many hospitals require that "field" lines be changed soon after the patient arrives.[142] One of the major difficulties is finding a "good vein" in some patients, such as the chronically debilitated or intravenous drug abuser.

Many paramedics have a low comfort level in obtaining vascular access in pediatric patients.

In adult patients, most systems use 14 gauge to 20 gauge catheters, depending upon the nature of the patient's complaint and the caliber of the veins. For medical patients, catheter size makes little difference because flow rates for all of these are sufficient for drug administration. Most of these will also allow the administration of blood, although it may be rather slow when given through a 20 gauge tube. For patients requiring high volumes, short (3.2 cm/1.25 inch) 14 gauge catheters can provide high flow rates. Flow is directly proportional to the pressure gradient, inversely proportional to the length, and proportional to the diameter of the tube to the fourth power (Poiseuille's Law). Guisto has demonstrated that 12 gauge catheters can be used, with paramedics having an 84% success rate with this large IV.[179] This allows fluid rates as high as many 8.5 French central lines. When used with wide-bore tubing and a pressure bag, this catheter achieved a flow of nearly 900 cc per minute. Kits are available using the Seldinger wire technique to convert peripheral 14 gauge to 18 gauge IVs to an 8.5 French diameter IV. No studies are available to assess the utility of this technique in the prehospital setting.

For infants and pediatric patients, providers should be encouraged to look for access in the lower limbs. The dorsal veins of the foot and the greater saphenous vein can be cannulated by percutaneous means, and this area is often less "pudgy" than the upper limbs.

Central Venous Access

Many flight programs, but few ground ambulances, allow providers to place central venous catheters. In systems with short transport times this prohibition may be warranted, but if transport times are prolonged and peripheral access cannot be obtained, central venous cannulation may be life-saving. Central administration of medications in cardiac arrest may increase the likelihood that drugs will reach their target organs. Several sites are described: subclavian, internal jugular, and femoral veins. No studies are available to assess the utility or morbidity of those in the prehospital environment. Studies of in-hospital use of these techniques suggest that even subclavian catheterization, which many feel has the highest morbidity, can be performed successfully in over 90% of cases and has few complications.[180,181] Excellent reviews of the subclavian route, internal jugular, and femoral techniques can be referred to for details regarding the technique.[182,183]

One of the most exciting rediscoveries of the past several years has been intraosseous (IO) infusion. This technique was originally used early in the twentieth century to administer fluids and medications, but advances in IV technology caused IO infusions to fall into disuse. IO access today is primarily used in young children, where peripheral vascular access is unobtainable. IO techniques are easily taught, using readily available chicken and turkey legs as the model.[184] In the hands of paramedics and flight nurses this method enjoys a good success rate and is much easier to perform than percutaneous IV cannulation in small children.[185] Although most individuals rarely use the technique, the skill does not seem to deteriorate substantially over time.[186] It appears that any fluid or drug that can be administered intravenously can be given by the IO route.

The only absolute contraindication appears to be the presence of a fracture of the selected bone proximal to the site, and relative contraindications include congenital bone disease and penetrating through an area of burned tissue. Complications include fractures at the site of the infusion, which is most likely due to selection of too large of a needle in a small child, and bone marrow emboli. The latter problem was studied by Orlowski, who concluded that although there were notable amounts of emboli in the lung after IO infusion, they did not appear to affect the resuscitation and should be of no concern to rescuers considering this route.[187]

Because of the difficulty with vascular access in many pediatric patients, all paramedics should be familiar with IO infusion. One excellent way to acquire this training is through the Pediatric Advanced Life Support (PALS) course offered by the American Heart Association.

IV Summary

For trauma patients, IVs should be started while en route unless the patient has a prolonged extrication, in which case the IV may be started before transport. Medical patients should receive an IV line in the field only if they are to receive medications. "Prophylactic" lines should be discouraged. Strong medical oversight is essential to evaluate the use and success rates and provide guidance for this procedure. This applies to all IV procedures, but is especially important for services that place central lines or perform intraosseous infusion. Without proper supervision, IV access can change from a life-saving to a life-taking intervention.

Cardiac Procedures

Monitoring and Defibrillation

The original prehospital ALS service, Pantridge's Mobile Intensive Care Unit, was established to decrease the morbidity and mortality associated with cardiac events occurring outside the hospital.[188] Monitoring was performed by physicians from the coronary unit. Because of this there was no question about their ability to interpret arrhythmias. His success led to the establishment of other mobile coronary care units, eventually evolving into our present EMS systems. In North America, most of these systems have employed physician-surrogates rather than doctors. The ability to train these providers to accurately determine and treat rhythms has been the subject of numerous studies.

Training paramedics to assess arrhythmias and defibrillate has been done in courses ranging from 4 to over 40 hours. Some systems have decreased their arrhythmia teaching to only that needed to treat ventricular fibrillation and ventricular tachycardia. Such a program was used in Stockholm.[189] In an 8-hour session, paramedics were trained to recognize ventricular fibrillation and tachycardia and to use a defibrillator. The initial testing found an 88% pass rate, with 58 of 59 applicants eventually passing the test. When applied in the field, this group demonstrated a 98% accuracy in their ability to diagnose and treat these rhythms. Follow-up studies have confirmed the efficacy of this system.[190–192]

Members of a volunteer EMS unit in Connecticut were trained to recognize ventricular fibrillation in a 4-hour course, with a 10-hour "standard" course being given as a control.[193] No differences in the ability of these providers to recognize and treat fibrillation were seen.

Early defibrillation is clearly the key to treatment of out-of-hospital cardiac arrest. A study in Wisconsin demonstrated a clear improvement in survival after implementation of the EMT-Defibrillation program when compared to historical controls.[194] This study emphasized the importance of rapid defibrillation, since there were no survivors when the response was greater than 8 minutes. As Eisenberg demonstrated in 1980, time to definitive care is the critical determinant in cardiac arrest survival,[10] and defibrillation is definitive care for most cardiac arrests.

The advance of microcomputing technology has provided an alternative to manual defibrillation in the form of the semi-automated and automated external defibrillators (AED). These devices are placed on the patient with self-adhesive electrodes and are designed to recognize ventricular fibrillation and deliver an electrical countershock. The semi-automated defibrillator requires the operator to press a button on the device to deliver the energy, while the automatic model requires only that the operator attach the leads, then stand away from the patient. These have the advantage of requiring no training in arrhythmia recognition and less than 4 hours of training in their use. The designs of AEDs attempt to be 100% specific for ventricular fibrillation and rapid ventricular tachycardia; they are not supposed to deliver a shock to patients with other rhythms. Their sensitivity is therefore somewhat diminished, and very fine ventricular fibrillation may not be treated because the unit may consider it to be asystole. This is probably not of great importance, because both patients with fine fibrillation and asystole have extremely poor chances of survival. The AHA has endorsed the use of these devices.[195]

When Seattle firefighters were trained to use automatic defibrillators, survival to discharge increased from 19% with CPR alone to 30% with the defibrillator.[196] The fully automated versions are simple enough that laypersons with only CPR training have been taught their use.[197] A one-year follow-up study demonstrated that these skills are easily retained.[198] Indeed, their application is so easy that some authors feel that correct assessment of vital signs may be the limiting factor in their use.[199]

No studies have been performed to assess the use of these devices in pediatric patients. It seems likely though that a device could be developed that would allow the paramedic to enter the patient's age or weight, and the machine would then calculate the correct dose. Because the incidence of primary fibrillatory arrest in children is low, the low demand for such a defibrillator might make it prohibitively expensive.

Paramedic training programs require several hundred hours beyond basic EMT training, and much of this time is involved with rhythm analysis and treatment. Cardiac rhythm determination is a difficult skill to teach and learn. Its application in the rear of a moving ambulance, with a 4-square-inch display, motion artifact, and the other demands of caring for a critical patient makes it an even more difficult skill to apply. It is likely that if full spectrum arrhythmia detection is desired, paramedics need extensive initial training and frequent continuing education. The direct medical oversight physician should ask specific questions regarding rate, regularity, QRS duration, and relationship of the P wave to the QRS complex.

External Cardiac Pacing

The idea of cardiac pacing dates from 200 years ago, but it was not until the 1950s that the first transcutaneous pacemakers were developed. In the intervening years the technology of transvenous pacemakers overtook that of the transcutaneous pacemaker, which fell into disuse. During the past decade, transcutaneous pacemakers for use in the emergency setting have been rediscovered and greatly improved.

When used promptly in patients suffering from hemodynamically significant bradycardias, transcutaneous pacing appears effective in the prehospital setting. Vukov showed that transcutaneous pacing was an important procedure among patients transferred by helicopter for acute cardiac problems.[200] Eitel found transcutaneous pacing was easy for prehospital providers to learn and apply.[201] O'Toole demonstrated survival in all patients who had pacing initiated immediately on bradyasystolic arrest.[202] Emphasis here is placed on early initiation of pacing, since pacing is increasingly ineffective when delayed.[203] In the Eitel study there were no differences in outcome, regardless of whether the patient was paced.[201] The author felt that this reflected the long down-time of the patients. Hedges alternate-day control trial of prehospital transcutaneous pacing also reached a similar conclusion.[204]

Despite his enthusiasm for transcutaneous pacing in the interhospital transfer environment, Vukov was not able to extend this endorsement to the use of this procedure in the treatment of prehospital bradyasystolic cardiac arrest.[205] The benefits clearly outweigh the complications, and the current AHA guidelines advocate early transcutaneous pacing in conjunction with medications. The most prevalent problem with transcutaneous pacing currently is the tendency to delay initiation of pacing, and in sometimes spending too long a period of time using an ineffective energy setting.

Although not currently commercially available, transcutaneous burst pacing at high pulse rates (200–280 bpm), has been shown to be effective in terminating supraventricular tachycardias.[206] This may prove to be an attractive modality for unstable patients with PSVT who might otherwise require cardioversion.

Transcutaneous cardiac pacing is an important modality in those patients suffering from symptomatic bradycardia unresponsive to pharmacological intervention. When the patient suffers from a bradyasystolic arrest, transcutaneous pacing must be initiated immediately to be effective. The use of combination pacing/defibrillation pads should be standard in any patient who appears to be suffering from a cardiac event. Having these pads in place early will allow the paramedic to either defibrillate or pace without delay, should the need arise. The lack of significant side effects and the safety of this treatment indicate that this modality should be available to all paramedics.[207]

Pericardiocentesis

Pericardiocentesis is described in ACLS as the procedure of choice for treating cardiac tamponade.[208] It may be a life-saving intervention when an effusion results in hemodynamic compromise. Its use in the prehospital setting has not been investigated, and ACLS reserves its use for physicians because of concern regarding complications, such as myocardial or coronary artery injury. In the patient suffering from pulseless electrical activity (PEA) due to cardiac tamponade, pericardiocentesis may theoretically produce a perfusing rhythm. Given the poor prognosis of PEA, it seems unlikely that these patients could come to much more harm from this procedure. Although Callaham discourages the use of this technique in the patient with a traumatic tamponade, this is because it may delay the implementation of thoracotomy, which is not available in the prehospital setting.[209]

Medical directors may wish to include pericardiocentesis as part of the protocol for PEA. However, its use is strictly reserved for patients in whom fluid challenge and needle thoracostomy have not produced pulses. The prehospital care provider should use the subxyphoid approach, placing the needle to the left of the xyphoid and aiming at the left shoulder at a shallow angle. This technique minimizes the likelihood of injuring other important structures. It must be emphasized that this procedure should only be used as a final resort, when all other therapies have failed.

Patient Packaging

Before the appearance of organized EMS services and paramedic training, motor vehicle crash victims were often extricated without the use of any form of spinal immobilization. Patients often presented to the hospital with completed spinal cord injuries.[210] Immobilization has since become one of the most fundamental interventions provided by prehospital providers. It is not, however, without its problems.

Spinal Immobilization

Immobilization has been considered important not only for victims of motor vehicle crashes, but also in patients who suffer falls and gunshot wounds. Even falls from the standing position, especially in the elderly, may result in spinal injuries. In some areas, gunshot wounds are the leading cause of spinal cord injuries, while nationwide they are the third most common source of spinal injury.[211] Although occult spinal injuries may be difficult to reliably detect in the field, studies have noted the discomfort caused by the use of backboards and collars, and have questioned whether immobilization should be performed in the absence of signs and symptoms.[212] Domeier and his colleagues in Michigan reviewed a large group of patients with spinal fractures.[213] They concluded that patients with altered mental status, neurologic deficit, spinal pain, evidence of intoxication, and suspected extremity fracture were more likely to have significant spinal injuries.

Muhr, Seabrook, and Wittwer were able to demonstrate that the use of a clearance algorithm had the potential to decrease immobilization by one third.[214] Spinal immobilization is not practiced throughout the world. In a unique comparative study Hauswald and his colleagues in New Mexico and Malaysia compared neurologic outcomes between immobilized and unimmobilized blunt trauma victims.[215] In the Malaysian system none of the patients received any form of prehospital spinal immobilization. The New Mexican series immobilized all studied patients. Their results indicated that there was less neurologic injury in the Malaysian population than in the New Mexican group. This study has significant limitations, which are described in an accompanying editorial by Orledge and Pepe.[216] Taken together, these studies point out the need for research in even the most "basic" areas of prehospital care.

Hankins describes some clinical criteria indicating which patients might be eligible for clinical clearance.[217] They recommend that none of the following be present: No extremes of age (<12, >65yo), no altered mental status, including language barriers, no neurologic deficits, no distracting injuries, and no midline or paraspinal pain or tenderness. They recognize that this is somewhat of a high-risk area, and recommend that medical directors look closely at their system to see which, if any, criteria for spinal clearance can be safely applied within their individual systems. While his group did not come to a conclusion as to the details of how these patients should be tracked, they were clear that any system implementing clearance criteria must have a solid quality management (QM) program in place to provide ongoing evaluation of these criteria.

Apart from its primary purpose, spinal immobilization permits the patient to be easily log-rolled, should vomiting occur. When properly immobilized, the patient is secured in the ambulance, an important consideration should the ambulance be involved in an crash. For unruly patients, spinal immobilization may decrease the security risk, making the journey safer for both patient and provider.

Cervical Collars

The first step in immobilizing the blunt trauma victim is manual stabilization of the head, followed by placement of a rigid cervical collar. Numerous collars are available on the market, ranging from cloth covered foam rubber to stiff plastics of various designs. The soft collar provides no immobilization and has no place in prehospital care.[218] Perhaps the most commonly used collar is the Philadelphia collar, a two-piece device made of rigid foam. McCabe compared cervical spine motion on radiographs with volunteers immobilized in Philadelphia, hard extraction, and two versions of the Stifneck Collar.[219] The Stifneck collars were better than either the Philadelphia or hard extraction collars in immobilizing the patient in all directions except extension. Dick, in a review of all spinal immobilization devices, was also enthusiastic about the Stifneck collar, stating that it provided the best immobilization among all collars tested.[220] A number of similar plastic collars are currently available, but limited data are available regarding their effectiveness. Regardless of the collar used, the medical director must emphasize that this is only one part of complete cervical immobilization.

Spine Boards

The spine board is the most common method of cervical immobilization in the U.S. Minimal amounts of motion were seen by Podolsky when the board was combined with tape and sandbags.[192] Graziano and Cline state that the lack of movement associated with short-board stabilization of the cervical spine makes this the standard of comparison for all other devices.[221,222] Howell has demonstrated that the use of a collar does make a difference in immobilization when combined with the short board or Kendrick Extrication Device.[223] The ideal method is to have the patient placed in a cervical collar, then have the short board placed behind the patient. The head of the board should be padded to prevent pulling the patient into extension.[224] Once the patient is secured to the short board, the patient is then extricated to a long spine board and strapped down. If the patient must be extricated rapidly, however, the patient is placed in a collar and removed directly to a long board. This procedure provides an adequate compromise between spinal protection and other considerations, such as cardiopulmonary status and scene safety. Care must be taken to manually support the spine when this technique is used. Since no studies have demonstrated the safety of the latter technique, providers should be instructed to use this only when rapid extrication is indicated.

For immobilization of children there are several commercially available devices. For smaller children a short board, well padded under the torso, can be used. Markenson described using the Kendrick Extrication Device for pediatric immobilization.[225] Because of its versatility with both adult and pediatric patients, he suggests that this is "an ideal device" for pediatric immobilization.

Although immobilization protects the spine from further injury, it may compromise ventilation. Even in children, who would be unlikely to suffer from COPD, spinal immobilization produced a significant decrease in forced vital capacity.[226] Providers must be ready to assist with ventilation, should immobilization result in compromise.

Cervical Immobilizers

Just as there are many different collars, so too are there many different devices to immobilize the head to the board. The only study that looked at these devices found that the two commercially available immobilizers tested did not control the pediatric patients well in flexion and extension when used without a collar. When a collar was used, the immobilization was as effective as that of a short board with tape, but not as good as a long board with sandbags and tape.[227] Sandbags are no longer routinely recommended. The mass of the sandbag in a moving ambulance, especially with pediatric patients, would seem to pose a danger if the taping is less than optimal. Log-rolling a vomiting patient can also be a difficult proposition when heavy sandbags are used. For these reasons, as well as because of the unaesthetic nature of tape residue, Dick advocates the use of commercially available head immobilizers.[228]

When an immobilizer is added to the Philadelphia collar (Philadelphia Red E.M. Collar with Head Immobilizer/Stabilizer), the stability of the cervical spine was as good as or better than found with a short spine board.[229] The spine board was used without a collar, which is not the usual method of immobilization. These results once again point out the importance of a cervical immobilizer and collar combination.

Extremity Splints

Splinting of limbs in the prehospital setting today is primarily performed to control pain and to protect neurovascular structures. It is often forgotten that the major impetus for splinting of limbs came from the significant decrease in mortality that occurred with the use of the Thomas traction splint during the First World War.[230] Today several types of splints are available to paramedics. The Thomas splint and its variations are commonly used for fractures of the femur. Patients with these injuries can be afforded significant relief when traction is properly applied. Although these are simple devices, it is just as important to review their indications and use on a regular basis, as Skelton demonstrated in Kansas City.[21] Providers must be cautioned not to focus on splint placement while ignoring other aspects of care, such as spinal immobilization or cardiopulmonary status.

The development of vacuum and pneumatic splints devices in the past 20 years has changed the management of fractures in the prehospital setting. Much of the original teaching regarding fractures was to "splint it where it lies." Usually board splints were used and served well. The appearance of pneumatic splints in the early 1970s required the paramedic to reposition the limb to conform to the splint. The extent to which a paramedic repositions limbs in the field must be delineated in the system procedure manual. One popular EMT text suggests that angulated long-bone fractures be splinted in anatomic position, unless resistance is encountered.[231] It

recommends any dislocation be splinted without reduction.

Both pneumatic and vacuum splints work well, barring leaks. Most are radiolucent to a sufficient extent to allow radiological assessment. Pneumatic splints are usually made of clear plastics, which allow some visual inspection of wounds and skin color. Vacuum splints are made of a rubberized cloth bladder filled with beads. Both types of devices will provide some degree of tamponade if there is an open wound. The major drawback with this type of splinting device is the possibility of failure if the splint is damaged. Just as with traction splints, providers must be warned against caring so much for the limb that they lose sight of the patient.

The out-of-hospital care provider should be encouraged to use extremity splints only when the mechanism involves only one or two limbs and is not likely to involve multiple organ systems. For most patients the long board will provide adequate limb immobilization and is much quicker to apply. On occasion, providers become involved in placing traction splints for femur fractures, while the pelvic or abdominal injuries are relatively neglected. Medical directors must be vigilant in both their education and QM programs to prevent this from occurring. With multiple trauma, time is of the essence and life threats take precedence over limb threats.

Pneumatic Anti-Shock Garments (PASG or MAST Suits)

McSwain called the pneumatic anti-shock garment (PASG) ". . . the most controversial device in prehospital care of the 1980s."[232] Originally developed as a device to control hemorrhage, the pneumatic garment evolved into the G-suit of military aviators and astronauts. This device was then returned to its original use during the Vietnam War, where it was felt to dramatically improve survival from wounds. This experience was brought back from Vietnam by the combat medics, many of whom became paramedics. In a report from 1976, Civetta described PASG use with the Miami Fire Rescue service. He felt the PASG was a significant device and advocated its incorporation into civilian EMS service.[233] By 1983, however, questions had arisen about its efficacy in the urban environment.[234] A 1985 study from Houston found there to be no difference in the trauma score on presentation to the emergency department with or without the PASG.[235] When this group looked only at penetrating abdominal trauma, their results again showed no improvement over controls.[236] Despite these investigations, McSwain argues in favor of the use of the PASG.[230] He cites laboratory investigations indicating that the PASG has an effect on blood pressure and that it controls hemorrhage in the area beneath it. He goes on to state that the complication rate is low and that clinical trials have demonstrated no harm.

When ventilatory compromise was investigated in healthy volunteers, no compromise was seen.[237] These authors caution that this might not be the case with patients in a shock state. Cayten has shown a higher-than-predicted survival rate among profoundly hypotensive (BP ≤ 50 mmHg) patients when the PASG was used.[238] Lloyd has proposed a multicenter trial of PASG, but no one has developed this study.[239] Domeier and his colleagues, writing for the NAEMSP, critically evaluated the literature and classified uses for the PASG in a manner similar to the AHA.[240] The only class I (usually indicated, useful, and effective) recommendation was that the PASG be used in the case of hypotension due to ruptured abdominal aortic aneurysm. Class IIa indications include hypotension due to pelvic fracture, anaphylactic shock that is otherwise unresponsive, lower extremity hemorrhage, and severe traumatic hypotension where there is no palpable pulse. They also have a long list of class IIb recommendations. More important are the class III uses, which they define as inappropriate therapy which may be harmful. These class III uses include: adjunct to CPR, diaphragmatic rupture, penetrating thoracic injury, pulmonary edema, lower limb splint, abdominal evisceration, acute cardiac disease, including cardiogenic shock, and in the presence of a gravid uterus.

If they are going to use the garment, providers should be encouraged to place the PASG on the long board or stretcher before extricating the patient, rather than attempting to place it while en route. Rural systems need to take a different look at PASG, since prolonged transport time studies have not been conducted.

Summary

What should be the basic repertoire for EMS? Aside from rendering basic first-aid for minor injuries, the system should be able to rapidly assess the patient for life-threatening problems and have the tools to begin the patient resuscitation. Suggested procedures are listed in table 54.2.

The procedures a medical director will authorize determines the system ability to respond to its patients. Procedures should be based on the needs of the population the system serves, not on arbitrary distinctions among provider levels. The repertoire may be limited by the amount of time available to the medical director and providers for continuing education and skills practice. Safe and effective prehospital procedures require an effective QM program. The medical director must provide the oversight, guidance, and discipline to ensure the procedures meet the needs of the patients and the system.

References

1. Blaisdell FW. Trauma myths and magic: 1984 Fitts lecture. *J Trauma.* 1985;25(9):856–863.
2. Cales RH. Advanced life support in prehospital trauma care: an intervention in search of an indication? (editorial). *Ann Emerg Med.* 1988;17(6):651–653.
3. Gold CR. Prehospital advanced life support vs. "scoop and run" in trauma management. *Ann Emerg Med.* 1987;16(7):797–801.
4. Kaweski SM, Sise MJ, Virgilio RW. The effect of prehospital fluids on survival in trauma patients. *J Trauma.* 1990;30(10):1215–1219.
5. Reines HD, Bartlett RL, Chudy NE, et al. Is advanced life support appropriate for victims of motor vehicle accidents?: the South Carolina highway trauma project. *J Trauma.* 1988;28(5):563–570.
6. Smith JP, Bodai BI, Hill AS, et al. Prehospital stabilization of critically injured patients: a failed concept. *J Trauma.* 1985;25(1):65–70.
7. Trunkey DD. Is ALS necessary for pre-hospital trauma care? (editorial). *J Trauma.* 1984;24(1):86–87.
8. Aprahamian C, Thompson BM, Towne JB, et al. The effect of a paramedic system on mortality of major open intra-abdominal vascular trauma. *J Trauma.* 1983;23(8):687–690.
9. Baxt WG, Moody P. The impact of advanced prehospital emergency care on the mortality of severely brain-injured patients. *J Trauma.* 1987;27(4):365–369.
10. Eisenberg MS, Copass MK, Hallstrom A, et al. Management of out-of-hospital cardiac arrest: failure of basic emergency medical technician services. *JAMA.* 1980;243(10):1049–1051.
11. Hearne TR, Cummins RO. Improved survival from cardiac arrest in the community. *PACE.* 1988;11(2):1968–1973.
12. Honigman B, Rohweder K, Moore EE, et al. Prehospital advanced trauma life support for penetrating cardiac wounds. *Ann Emerg Med.* 1990;19(2):145–150.
13. Potter D, Goldstein G, Fung SC, et al. A controlled trial of prehospital advanced life support in trauma. *Ann Emerg Med.* 1988;17(6):582–588.

TABLE 54.2

ALS Procedures

PROCEDURE	INDICATION	TEACHING	DIFFICULTY OF USE	COMMENTS
History and physical	Patient encounter	2	3	Basic to all other procedures; requires training to be accurate and fast
Vital signs	Patient encounter—no other more important procedures pending	3	3	Should be attempted with each patient, but should not interfere with life-saving procedures
Supplemental oxygen	Hypoxia; all patients when pulse oximetry is not available or not functioning	1	1	Not a benign drug, but should be applied liberally in the absence of pulse oximetry
Bag-valve-mask	Hypoventilation; preoxygenation prior to intubation	2	5	Most difficult skill to perform properly under prehospital conditions; should be viewed as precursor to intubation
Demand valve	Hypoventilation; preoxygenation prior to intubation	2	4	Alternative to BVM; may allow a better mask seal than the BVM; no sense of compliance changes
Mouth-to-mask	Hypoventilation; preoxygenation prior to intubation	1	3	Underutilized technique
Endotracheal intubation				
Direct oral intubation	No trismus; tolerates laryngoscope	4	4	Most common; requires patient to be supine; alternatives should be taught
Nasotracheal intubation	Breathing; unable to lie supine	3	4	Safe; easy to teach
Digital intubation	Unresponsive	4	4	Use a mouth gag or bite block
Lighted stylet	Unresponsive	3	3	Requires a dark area
EOA/EGTA	Excessive vomitus (obturator only); no indication as a primary airway management tool	2	3	Obsolete for ventilation; may be useful for controlling vomitus during intubation
PTL/ETC	Legal restrictions barring use of ET intubation	4	4	Poor substitutes for ET intubation
Cricothyrotomy	Need for airway management but unable to place ET tube	5	5	Should be performed rarely if intubation skills are good; should be practiced frequently
Transtracheal jet ventilation	Need for airway management but unable to place ET tube	3	4	Relatively easy alternate airway; requires special equipment; Misplacement can cause massive subcutaneous emphysema
Minicricothyrotomy	Need for airway management but unable to place ET tube	4	4	Several manufacturers and devices
End-tidal CO_2 detection	Intubation	1	1	Mandatory after any intubation or cricothyrotomy
Pulse oximetry	Assessment for hypoxia	2	3	May be useful in titrating oxygen therapy; benefits for COPD patients, multiple casualty incidents (where oxygen is limited)

TABLE 54.2 (CONTINUED)

PROCEDURE	INDICATION	TEACHING	DIFFICULTY OF USE	COMMENTS
Endotracheal intubation (cont.)				
NG tubes	Vomiting with risk of aspiration; gastric decompression	3	4	Useful for long transport; use only for aspiration of gastric contents; not recommended for medication administration in the field
Needle thoracostomy	Tension pneumothorax; EMD	2	2	Should be performed promptly for tension pneumothorax
Tube thoracostomy	Pneumothorax; hemothorax	5	5	Limited use in long transports, hemothorax
Medication administration				
Peripheral intravenous access	Fluid or medication administration prior to arrival at hospital	3	2	Most common; should have clear access indications; overused for "prophylactic access"
Central intravenous access	High volume fluid or critical medication administration; lack of peripheral access	4	4	Not as difficult or risky as some believe; may be lifesaving in severe trauma patients with long transports
Intraosseous access	Fluid or medication administration in a critical pediatric patient	3	3	Line of choice in critical pediatric patients
Cardiac monitoring	Patients at risk for dysrhythmias	5	4	Requires continual education to maintain dysrhythmia recognition skills
Other Procedures				
Defibrillation	Ventricular tachycardia or fibrillation	2	2	Automated defibrillators decrease the amount of training required
External cardiac pacing	Symptomatic bradycardia	2	2	Only successful if initiated early
Pericardiocentesis	EMD after failure of fluid resuscitation and bilateral needle thoracostomy	3	4	Should be available as a last resort
Spinal immobilization	All patients at risk for spinal injury (significant blunt force; penetrating injuries of the trunk)	2	3	Basic skill, but high risk; should receive more continuing education
Traction splints	Isolated femur fractures and hemodynamic stability	3	4	Few indications except long distance transports; other techniques more efficient for urban/suburban setting
Vacuum-pneumatic splints	Isolated limb fractures and hemodynamic stability	2	2	Use in preference to traction splints
Pneumatic shock garments	Penetrating wounds under area of device; pelvic or lower limb fractures	2	3	Use much more limited than in past

1 = easy, 5 = very difficult.

14. Pressley JC, Severance HW, Raney MP, et al. A comparison of paramedic versus basic emergency medical care of patients at high and low risk during acute myocardial infarction. *J Am Coll Cardiol.* 1988;12(6): 1555–1561.

15. Riediger G, Fleischmann-Sperber T. Efficiency and cost-effectiveness of advanced EMS in West Germany. *Am J Emerg Med.* 1990;8:76–80.

16. EMT: B National Standard Curriculum. Washington, D.C., U.S. Department of Transportation, National Highway Traffic Safety Administration, 1995.

17. Smith JP, Bodai BI. The urban paramedic's scope of practice. *JAMA.* 1985;253(4):544–548.

18. Waller JA. Urban-oriented methods: Failure to solve rural emergency care problems. *JAMA.* 1973;226(12): 1441–1446.

19. Hedges JR. Load and go—where?: the non-urban perspective of scoop and run. Unpublished paper, 1989.

20. Ornato JP, Racht EM, Fitch JJ, et al. The need for ALS in urban and suburban EMS systems (editorial). *Ann Emerg Med.* 1990;19(12):1469–1470.

21. Garrison HG, Downs SM, McNutt RA, et al. A cost-effectiveness analysis of pediatric intraosseous infusion as a prehospital skill. *Prehosp Disaster Med.* 1992;7(3): 221–227.

22. Skelton MB, McSwain NE. A study of cognitive and technical skill deterioration among trained paramedics, *JACEP.* 1977;6(10):436–438.

23. Walters G, Blucksman E. Retention of skills by advanced trained ambulance staff: implications for monitoring and retraining. *BMJ.* 1989;298:649–650.

24. Werman HA, Keseg DR, Glimcher M, et al. Retention of basic trauma life support skills. *Prehosp Disaster Med.* 1990;5(2):137–144.

25. McSwain NE. Editorial comment on: Hankins DG, Carruthers N, Frascone RJ, et al. Complication rates for the esophageal obturator airway and endotracheal tube in the prehospital setting. *Prehosp Disaster Med.* 1993; 8(2):117–121.

26. Pepe P, Zachariah BS, Chandra NC. Invasive airway techniques in resuscitation. *Ann Emerg Med.* 1993;22(2 pt 2):393–403.

27. Spaite DW, Criss EA, Valenzuela TD, et al. A prospective evaluation of prehospital patient assessment by direct in-field observation: failure of ALS personnel to measure vital signs. *Prehosp Disaster Med.* 1990;5(4): 325–334.

28. Moss RL. Vital signs records omissions on prehospital patient encounter forms. *Prehosp Disaster Med.* 1993; 8(1):21–27.

29. Gausche M, Henderson DP, Seidel JS. Vital signs as part of the prehospital assessment of the pediatric patient: a survey of paramedics. *Ann Emerg Med.* 1990; 19(2):173–178.

30. Cayten CG, Herrmann N, Cole LW, et al. Assessing the validity of EMS data, *JACEP.* 1978;7(11):390–396.

31. Jones JS, Ramsey W, Hetrick T. Accuracy of prehospital sphygmomanometers. *J Emerg Med.* 1987;5:23–27.

32. Prasad NH, Brown LH, Ausband SC, et al. Prehospital blood pressures: inaccuracies caused by ambulance noise? *Am J Emerg Med.* 1994;12:617–620.

33. Cady CE, Pirrallo RG, Grim CE. Ambulance sphygmomanometers are frequently inaccurate. *Prehosp Emerg Care.* 1997;1:136–139.

34. Menegazzi JJ, Davis EA, Sucov AN, et al. Reliability of the Glasgow coma scale when used by emergency physicians and paramedics. *J Trauma.* 1993;34(1):46–48.

35. Keeler JL, Shuster M, Rowe BH. Reliability of prehospital rating scales for case severity and status change. *Am J Emerg Med.* 1993;11(2):115–121.

36. Caroline N. *Emergency medical treatment: a text for EMT-As and EMT-Intermediates.* Boston: Little, Brown; 1987:133.

37. Elling R, Politis J. An evaluation of emergency medical technicians' ability to use manual ventilation devices. *Ann Emerg Med.* 1983;12(12):765–768.

38. Lande S. EMT ventilation skills (letter). *Ann Emerg Med.* 1988;17(1):107.

39. Harrison RR, Maull KI, Kennan RL, et al. Mouth-to-mask ventilation: a superior method of rescue breathing. *Ann Emerg Med.* 1982;11(2):74–76.

40. Jesudian MCS, Harrison RR, Keenan RL, et al. Bag-valve-mask ventilation; two rescuers are better than one: preliminary report. *Crit Care Med.* 1985;13(2):122–123.

41. Samuels DJ, Maull KI, Bock HC, et al. *Emergency Medical Technician: Basic, National Standard Curriculum, U.S. Department of Transportation, DOT HS 808 149, August 1994.

42. Stewart RD, Kaplan RM, Pennock B, et al. Influence of mask design on bag-mask ventilation. *Ann Emerg Med.* 1985;14(5):403–406.

43. Palme C, Nystrom B, Tunnell R. An evaluation of the efficiency of face masks in the resuscitation of newborn infants. *Lancet.* 1985;1:207–210.

44. Terndrup TE, Canter RK, Cherry RA. A comparison of infant ventilation methods performed by prehospital personnel. *Ann Emerg Med.* 1989;18(6):607–611.

45. Bryson TK, Benumof JL, Ward CF, The esophageal obturator airway: a clinical comparison to ventilation with a mask and oropharyngeal airway. *Chest.* 1978; 74(5):537–539.

46. Rhee KJ, O'Malley RJ, Turner JE, et al. Field airway management of the trauma patient: the efficacy of bag mask ventilation. *Am J Emerg Med.* 1988;6(4):333–336.

47. Campbell TP, Stewart RD, Kaplan RM, et al. Oxygen enrichment of bag-valve-mask units during positive-pressure ventilation: a comparison of various techniques. *Ann Emerg Med.* 1988;17(3):232–235.

48. McCormack AP, Damon SK, Eisenberg MS. Disagreeable physical characteristics affecting bystander CPR. *Ann Emerg Med.* 1989;18(3):283–285.

49. Cydulka RK, Connor PJ, Myers TF, et al. Prevention of oral bacterial flora transmission by using mouth-to-mask ventilation during CPR. *J Emerg Med.* 1991;9: 317–321.

50. Johannigman JA, Branson RD, Davis K, et al. Techniques of emergency ventilation: a model to evaluate tidal volume, airway pressure, and gastric insufflation. *J Trauma.* 1991;31(1):93–98.

51. Caroline N. *Emergency medical treatment: a text for EMT-As and EMT-Intermediates.* Boston: Little, Brown; 1987:140.

52. Terndrup TE, Warner DA. Infant ventilation and oxygenation by basic life support providers: comparison of methods. *Prehosp Disaster Med.* 1992;7(1):35–40.

53. Melanson SW, O'Gara K. EMS Provider reluctance to perform mouth-to-mouth resuscitation. *Prehosp Emerg Care.* 2000;4:48–52.

54. Rossi R, Linder KH, Ahnefeld FW. Devices for expired air resuscitation. *Prehosp Disaster Med.* 1993;8(2):123–126.

55. Hillis M, Sinclair D, Butler G, et al. Prehospital cardiac arrest survival and neurologic recovery. *J Emerg Med.* 1993;11:245–252.

56. Stewart RD, Paris PM, Pelton GH, et al. Effect of varied training techniques on field endotracheal intubation success rates. *Ann Emerg Med.* 1984;13(11):1032–1054.

57. Stratton SJ, Kane G, Wheeler NC, et al. Prospective study of manikin-only versus manikin and human subject endotracheal intubation training of paramedics. *Ann Emerg Med.* 1991;20(12):1314–1318.

58. Shea SR, MacDonald JR, Gruzinski G. Prehospital endotracheal tube airway or esophageal gastric tube airway: a critical comparison. *Ann Emerg Med.* 1985;14(2):102–112.

59. Nelson MS. Medical student retention of intubation skills. *Ann Emerg Med.* 1989;18(10):1059–1061.

60. O'Brien DJ, Danzl DF, Hooker EA, et al. Prehospital blind nasotracheal intubation by paramedics. *Ann Emerg Med.* 1989;18(6):612–617.

61. Pepe PE, Copass MK, Joyce TH. Prehospital endotracheal intubation: rationale for training emergency medical personnel. *Ann Emerg Med.* 1985;14(11):1085–1092.

62. Pointer JE. Clinical characteristics of paramedics' performance of endotracheal intubation. *J Emerg Med.* 1988;6:505–509.

63. Stewart RD, Paris PM, Winter PM, et al. Field endotracheal intubation by paramedical personnel. *Chest.* 1984;85(3):341–345.

64. Jacobs LM, Berrizbeitia LD, Bennett B, et al. Endotracheal intubation in the prehospital phase of emergency medical care. *JAMA.* 1983;250(16):2175–2177.

65. Guss DA, Posluszny M. Paramedic orotracheal intubation: a feasibility study. *Am J Emerg Med.* 1984;2:399–401.

66. Katz SH, Falk JL. Misplaced endotracheal tubes by paramedics in an urban emergency medical services system. *Ann Emerg Med.* 2001;37:32–37.

67. Delbridge TR, Yealy DM. "A" is for airway . . . also for action. *Ann Emerg Med.* 2001;37:62–64.

68. Birmingham PK, Chesney FW, Ward RJ. Esophageal intubation: a review of detection techniques. *Anesth Analg.* 1986;65:886–891.

69. Bissinger U, Lenz G, Kuhn W. Unrecognized endobronchial intubation of emergency patients. *Ann Emerg Med.* 1989;18(8):853–855.

70. Aijan P, Tsai A, Knopp R, et al. Endotracheal intubation of pediatric patients by paramedics. *Ann Emerg Med.* 1989;18(5):489–494.

71. Gausche M, Lewis RJ, Stratton SJ, et al. Effect of out-of-hospital pediatric endotracheal intubation on survival and neurological outcome: a controlled clinical trial. *JAMA.* 2000;283(6):783–90.

72. Hauswald M, Sklar DP, Tandberg D, et al. Cervical spine movement during airway management: cinefluoroscopic appraisal in human cadavers. *Am J Emerg Med.* 1991;9(6):535–538.

73. Dronen SC, Merigian KS, Hedges JR, et al. A comparison of blind nasotracheal and succinylcholine-assisted intubation in the poisoned patient. *Ann Emerg Med.* 1987;16(6):650–652.

74. *Advanced Trauma Life Support Program for Physicians.* 5th ed. Chicago: American College of Surgeons; 1993.

75. Bivins HG, Ford S, Bezmalinovic Z, et al. The effect of axial traction during orotracheal intubation of the trauma victim with an unstable cervical spine. *Ann Emerg Med.* 1988;17(1):25–29.

76. Rhee KJ, Green W, Holcroft JW, et al. Oral intubation in the multiply injured patient: the risk of exacerbating spinal cord damage. *Ann Emerg Med.* 1990;19(5):511–514.

77. Holley J, Jorden R. Airway management in patients with unstable cervical spine fractures. *Ann Emerg Med.* 1989;18(11):1237–1239.

78. Walls RM. Airway management. *Emerg Med Clin NA.* 1993;11(1):53–60.

79. Levine RL. Pharmacology of intravenous sedatives and opioids in critically ill patients. *Crit Care Clinics.* 1994;10:709–731.

80. Mendel PR, White PF. Sedation of the critically ill patient. *Int Anesthesiol Clinics.* 1993;10:185–200.

81. Joyce SM. Cervical immobilization during orotracheal intubation in trauma victims (editorial). *Ann Emerg Med.* 1988;17(1):88.

82. Verdile VP, Chiang J-L, Bedger R, et al. Nasotracheal intubation using a flexible lighted stylet. *Ann Emerg Med.* 1990;19(5):506–510.

83. Krisanda TJ, Eitel DR, Hess D, et al. An analysis of invasive airway management in a suburban emergency medical services system. *Prehosp Disaster Med.* 1992;7(2):121–126.

84. Kastendieck JG. Airway management. In: Rosen P, Baker FJ, Barkin RM, et al. *Emergency Medicine: Concepts and Clinical Practice,* 2nd ed. St Louis: Mosby; 1988:41–68.

85. Krishel S, Jackimczyk, Balazs K. Endotracheal tube whistle: an adjunct to blind nasotracheal intubation. *Ann Emerg Med.* 1992;21:33–36.

86. Stewart RD. Tactile orotracheal intubation. *Ann Emerg Med.* 1984;13:175–178.

87. Ellis DG, Jakymec A, Kaplan RM, et al. Guided orotracheal intubation in the operating room using a lighted stylet: a comparison with direct laryngoscopic technique. *Anesthesiology.* 1986;64:823–826.

88. Stewart RD, LaRosee A, Kaplan RM, et al. Correct positioning of an endotracheal tube using a flexible lighted stylet. *Crit Care Med.* 1990;18:97–99.

89. Verdile VP, Heller MB, Paris PM, et al. Nasotracheal intubation in traumatic craniofacial dislocation: use of the lighted stylet. *Ann J Emerg Med.* 1988;6:39–41.

90. Hung OR, Lung KE, Multari J, et al. *Clinical Trial of a New Light-Wand Device for Nasotracheal Intubation in Surgical Patients.* Presented at the Canadian Anesthesiologists Society, 1993.

91. Don Michael TA, Lambert EH, Mehran A. "Mouth-to-lung" airway for cardiac resuscitation. *Lancet.* 1968;2:1329.

92. Don Micheal TA, Gordon AS. The oesophageal obturator airway: a new device in emergency cardiopulmonary resuscitation. *BMJ.* 1980;281:1531–1534.

93. Cummins RO, ed. *Advanced Cardiac Life Support.* AHA; 1994:1–17.

94. Don Michael TA. The esophageal obturator airway: a critique. *JAMA.* 1981;246(10):1098–1101.

95. Hammargren Y, Clinton JE, Ruiz E. A standard comparison of esophageal obturator airway and endotracheal tube ventilation in cardiac arrest. *Ann Emerg Med.* 1985;14(10):953–958.

96. Meislin HW. The esophageal obturator airway: a study of respiratory effectiveness. *Ann Emerg Med.* 1980;9(2):54–59.

97. Johnson KR, Genovesi MG, Lassar KH. Esophageal obturator airway: use and complications. *JACEP.* 1976;5(1):36–39.

98. Smock SN. Esophageal obturator airway: preferred CPR technique. *JACEP.* 1975;4(3):232–233.

99. Harrison EE, Nord HJ, Beeman RW. Esophageal perforation following use of the esophageal obturator airway. *Ann Emerg Med.* 1980;9(1):21–25.

100. Yancey W, Wears R, Kamajian G, et al. Unrecognized tracheal intubation: a complication of the esophageal obturator airway. *Ann Emerg Med.* 1980;9(1):18–20.

101. Crippen D, Olvey S, Graffis R. Gastric rupture: an esophageal obturator airway complication. *Ann Emerg Med.* 1981;10(7):370–373.

102. Gatrell CB. Unrecognized esophageal intubation with both esophageal obturator airway and endotracheal tube. *Ann Emerg Med.* 1984;13(8):624–626.

103. Schofferman J, Oill P, Lewis AJ. The esophageal obturator airway: a clinical evaluation. *Chest.* 1976;69(1):67–71.

104. Auerbach PS, Geehr EC. Inadequate oxygenation and ventilation using the esophageal gastric tube airway in the prehospital setting. *JAMA.* 1983;250(22):3067–3071.

105. Geehr EC, Bogetz MS, Auerbach PS. Prehospital tracheal intubation versus esophageal gastric tube airway use: a prospective study. *Am J Emerg Med.* 1985;3:381–385.

106. Smith JP, Bodai BI, Aubourg R, et al. A field evaluation of the esophageal obturator airway. *J Trauma.* 1983;23(4):317–321.

107. Bass RR, Allison EJ, Hunt RC. The esophageal obturator airway: a reassessment of use by paramedics. *Ann Emerg Med.* 1982;11(7):358–360.

108. Smith JP, Bodai BJ, Seifkin A, et al. The esophageal obturator airway: a review. *JAMA.* 1983;250(8):1081–1084.

109. Hankins DG, Carruthers N, Frascone RJ, et al. Complication rates for the esophageal obturator airway and endotracheal tube in the prehospital setting. *Prehosp Disaster Med.* 1993;8(2):117–121.

110. Berdeeh TN. One-year experience with the tracheoesophageal airway. *Ann Emerg Med.* 1981;10(1):25–27.

111. Eisenberg RS. A new airway for tracheal or esophageal insertion: description and field experience. *Ann Emerg Med.* 1980;9(5):270–272.

112. Niemann JT, Rosborough JP, Myers R, et al. The pharyngo-tracheal lumen airway: preliminary investigation of a new adjunct. *Ann Emerg Med.* 1984;13(8):591–596.

113. Frass M, Franzer R, Zhrahal F, et al. The esophageal tracheal combitube: preliminary results with a new airway for CPR. *Ann Emerg Med.* 1987;16(7):768–772.

114. Bartlett RL, Martin SD, Perina D, et al. The pharyngeo-tracheal lumen airway: an assessment of airway control in the setting of upper airway hemorrhage. *Ann Emerg Med.* 1987;16(3):343–346.

115. Atherton GL, Johnson JC. Ability of paramedics to use the Combitube™ in prehospital cardiac arrest. *Ann Emerg Med.* 1993;22(8):1263–1268.

116. McMahan S, Ornato JP, Racht EM, et al. Multi-agency, prehospital evaluation of the pharyngeo-tracheal lumen (PTL) airway. *Prehosp Disaster Med.* 1992;7(1):13–18.

117. Rumball CJ, MacDonald D. The PTL, Combitube, laryngeal mask, and oral airway: A randomized prehospital comparative study of ventilatory device effectiveness and cost-effectiveness in 470 cases of cardiorespiratory arrest. *Prehosp Emerg Care.* 1997;1:1–10.

118. Hunt RC, Sheets CA, Whitley TW. Pharyngeal tracheal lumen airway training: failure to discriminate between esophageal and endotracheal modes and failure to confirm ventilation. *Ann Emerg Med.* 1989;18(9):947–952.

119. Johnson JC, Atherton GL. The esophageal tracheal combitube: an alternate route to airway management. *JEMS.* 1991;16(5):29–35.

120. Wafai Y, Salem MR, Baraka A, et al. Effectiveness of the self-inflating bulb for verification of proper placement of the Esophageal Tracheal Combitube™. *Anesth Analg.* 1995;80:122–126.

121. Brain ALJ. The laryngeal mask airway: a new concept in airway management. *Br J Anaesth.* 1983;55:801–805.

122. Davies PRF, Tighe SQM, Greenslade GL, et al. Laryngeal mask airway tube insertion by unskilled personnel. *Lancet.* 1990;336:977–979.

123. Pennant JH, Pace NA, Gajraj NM. Role of the laryngeal mask airway in the immobile cervical spine. *J Clin Anesth.* 1993;5:226–230.

124. Greene MK, Roden R, Hinchley G. The laryngeal mask airway: two cases of prehospital trauma care. *Anaesthesia.* 1992;47:688–689.

125. Reinhart DJ, Simmons G. Comparison of placement of the laryngeal mask airway with endotracheal tube by paramedics and respiratory therapists. *Ann Emerg Med.* 1994;24:260–263.

PROCEDURES

126. MacLeod BA, Heller MB, Gerard J, et al. Verification of endotracheal tube placement with calorimetric end-tidal CO_2 detection. *Ann Emerg Med.* 1991;20(3):267–270.

127. Ornato JP, Shipley JB, Racht EM, et al. Multicenter study of a portable, hand size, colorimetric end-tidal carbon dioxide detection device. *Ann Emerg Med.* 1992;21(5):518–523.

128. Anton WR, Gordon RW, Jordan TM, et al. A disposable end-tidal CO_2 detector to verify endotracheal intubation. *Ann Emerg Med.* 1991;20(3):271–275.

129. Wee MYK. The oesophageal detector device: assessment of a new method to distinguish oesophageal from tracheal intubation. *Anaesthesia.* 1988;43:27–29.

130. O'Leary JJ, Pollard BJ, Ryan MJ. A method of detecting oesophageal intubation or confirming tracheal intubation. *Anaesth Intens Care.* 1988;16:299–301.

131. Anderson KH, Hald A. Assessing the position of the tracheal tube: the reliability of different methods. *Anaesthesia.* 1989;44:984–985.

132. Williams KN, Nunn JF. The oesophageal detector device: a prospective trial on 100 patients. *Anaesthesia.* 1989;44:412.

133. Zaleski L, Abello D, Gold MI. The esophageal detector device: does it work? *Anesthesiology.* 1993;79(2):244–247.

134. Jenkins WA, Verdile VP, Paris PM. The syringe aspiration technique to verify endotracheal tube position. *Am J Emerg Med.* 1994;12:413–416.

135. Jackson C. High tracheostomy and other errors: the chief causes of chronic laryngeal stenosis. *Surg Gynecol Obstet.* 1921;32:392–395.

136. McGill J, Clinton JE, Ruiz E. Cricothyroidotomy in the emergency department. *Ann Emerg Med.* 1982;11(7):361–364.

137. Boyle MF, Hatton D, Sheets C. Surgical cricothyroidotomy performed by air ambulance flight nurses: a 5-year experience. *Am J Emerg Med.* 1993;11:41–45.

138. Miklus RM, Elliott C, Snow N. Surgical cricothyroidotomy in the field: experience of a helicopter transport team. *J Trauma.* 1989;29(4):506–508.

139. Spaite DW, Joseph M. Prehospital cricothyroidotomy: an investigation of indications, technique, complications, and patient outcome. *Ann Emerg Med.* 1990;19(3):279–285.

140. Nugent WL, Rhee KJ, Wisner DH. Can nurses perform surgical cricothyroidotomy with acceptable success and complication rates? *Ann Emerg Med.* 1991;20(4):367–370.

141. Campbell CT, Harris RC, Cook MH, et al. A new device for emergency percutaneous transtracheal ventilation in partial and complete airway obstruction. *Ann Emerg Med.* 1988;17(9):927–931.

142. Corke C, Cranswick P. A Seldinger technique for minitracheostomy insertion. *Anaesth Intens Care.* 1988;16:206–207.

143. Johnson DR, Dunlap A, McFeeley P, et al. Cricothyroidotomy performed by prehospital personnel: a comparison of two techniques in a human cadaver model. *Am J Emerg Med.* 1993;11(3):207–209.

144. *Advanced Trauma Life Support Program for Physicians.* 5th ed. Chicago: American College of Surgeons; 1993:54.

145. Frame SB, Timberlake GA, Kerstein MD, et al. Transtracheal needle catheter ventilation in complete airway obstruction: an animal model. *Ann Emerg Med.* 1989;18(2):127–133.

146. Yealy DM, Stewart RD, Kaplan RM. Myths and pitfalls in emergency translaryngeal ventilation: correcting misimpressions. *Ann Emerg Med.* 1988;17(7):690–692.

147. Yealy DM, Stewart RD, Kaplan MS. Clarifications on translaryngeal ventilation (letter). *Ann Emerg Med.* 1988;17(10):1130.

148. Yealy DM, Plewa MC, Reed JJ, et al. Manual translaryngeal jet ventilation and the risk of aspiration in a canine model. *Ann Emerg Med.* 1990;19(11):1238–1241.

149. Stothert JC, Stout MJ, Lewis LM, et al. High pressure percutaneous transtracheal ventilation: the use of large gauge intravenous-type catheters in the totally obstructed airway. *Am J Emerg Med.* 1990;8(3):184–189.

150. Nolan JP, Baskett PJF. Gas-powered and portable ventilators: an evaluation of six models. *Prehosp Disaster Med.* 1992;7(1):25–34.

151. Porter RS, Merlin MA, Heller MB. The fifth vital sign. *Emergency.* 1990;22(3):37–41.

152. Aughey K, Hess D, Eitel D, et al. An evaluation of pulse oximetry in prehospital care. *Ann Emerg Med.* 1991;20(8):887–891.

153. McGuire TJ, Pointer JE. Evaluation of a pulse oximeter in the prehospital setting. *Ann Emerg Med.* 1988;17(10):1058–1062.

154. Silverston P. Pulse oximetry at the roadside: a study of pulse oximetry in immediate care. *BMJ.* 1989;298:711–713.

155. Mateer JR, Olson DW, Stueven HA, et al. Continuous pulse oximetry during emergency endotracheal intubation. *Ann Emerg Med.* 1993;22(4):675–679.

156. Cydulka RK, Shade B, Emerman CL, et al. Prehospital pulse oximetry: useful or misused? *Ann Emerg Med.* 1992;21(6):675–679.

157. Melton JD, Heller MB, Kaplan R, et al. Occult hypoxemia during aeromedical transport: detection by pulse oximetry. *Prehosp Disaster Med.* 1989;4(2):115–121.

158. Valko PC, Campbell JP, McCarty DL, et al. Prehospital use of pulse oximetry in rotary wing aircraft. *Prehosp Disaster Med.* 1991;6(4):421–428.

159. Craft TM, Blogg CE. Pulse oximetry at the roadside (letter). *BMJ.* 1989;298:1096.

160. Cockcroft S, Dodd P. Pulse oximetry at the roadside (letter). *BMJ.* 1989;298:1096.

161. Ross DS. Thoracentesis. In: Roberts JR, Hedges JR, eds. *Clinical Procedures in Emergency Medicine.* Philadelphia: WB Saunders; 1985:85.

162. Eckstein M, Suyehara D. Needle thoracostomy in the prehospital setting. *Prehosp Emerg Care.* 1998;2(2):132–135.

163. McSwain GR, Garrison WB, Artz CP. Evaluation of resuscitation from cardiopulmonary arrest by paramedics. *Ann Emerg Med.* 1980;9:341–345.

164. Border JR, Lewis FR, Aprahamian C, et al. Panel: prehospital trauma care—stabilize or scoop and run. *J Trauma*. 1983;23(8):708–711.

165. Wears RL, Winton CN. Load and go versus stay and play: analysis of prehospital IV fluid therapy by computer simulation. *Ann Emerg Med*. 1990;19(2):163–168.

166. Aprahamian C, Thompson BM, Towne JB, et al. The effect of a paramedic system on mortality of major open intra-abdominal vascular trauma. *J Trauma*. 1983;23(8):687–690.

167. Lawrence DW, Lauro AJ. Complications from IV therapy: results from field-started and emergency department-started IVs compared. *Ann Emerg Med*. 1988;17(4):314–317.

168. Pons PT, Moore EE, Cusick JM, et al. Prehospital venous access in an urban paramedic system—a prospective on-scene analysis. *J Trauma*. 1988;28(10):1460–1463.

169. Jones SE, Nesper TP, Alcouloumre E. Prehospital intravenous line placement: a prospective study. *Ann Emerg Med*. 1989;18:244–246.

170. Slovis CM, Herr EW, Londorf D, et al. Success rates for initiation of intravenous therapy en route by prehospital care providers. *Am J Emerg Med*. 1990;8:305–307.

171. O'Gorman M, Trabulsy P, Pilcher DB. Zero-time prehospital IV. *J Trauma*. 1989;29(1):84–86.

172. Honigman B, Rohweder K, Moore EE, et al. Prehospital advanced trauma life support for penetrating cardiac wounds. *Ann Emerg Med*. 1990;19(2):145–150.

173. Spaite DW, Tse DJ, Valenzuela TD, et al. The impact of injury severity and prehospital procedures on scene time in victims of major trauma. *Ann Emerg Med*. 1991;20(12):1299–1305.

174. Spaite DW, Valenzuela TD, Criss EA, et al. A prospective in-field comparison of intravenous line placement by urban and nonurban emergency medical services personnel. *Ann Emerg Med*. 1994;24:209–214.

175. Pollack CV. Prehospital fluid resuscitation of the trauma patient: an update on the controversies. *Emerg Med Clin NA*. 1993;11(1):61–70.

176. Bickell WH, Wall MJ, Pepe PE, et al. Immediate versus delayed resuscitation for hypotensive patients with penetrating torso injuries. *N Engl J Med*. 1994;331:1105–1109.

177. Silbergleit R, Satz W, McNamara RM, et al. Effect of permissive hypotension in continuous uncontrolled intra-abdominal hemorrhage. *Acad Emerg Med*. 1996;3(10):922–926.

178. Donovan PJ, Cline DM, Whitley TW, et al. Prehospital care by EMT's and EMT-I's in a rural setting: prolongation of scene times by ALS procedures. *Ann Emerg Med*. 1989;18(5):495–500.

179. Guisto JA, Iserson KV. The feasibility of 12-gauge intravenous catheter use in the prehospital setting. *J Emerg Med*. 1990;8:173–176.

180. Emerman CL, Bellon EM, Lukens TW, et al. A prospective study of femoral versus subclavian vein catheterization during cardiac arrest. *Ann Emerg Med*. 1990;19(1):26–30.

181. Arrighi DA, Farnell MB, Mucha P, et al. Prospective, randomized trial of rapid venous access for patients in hypovolemic shock. *Ann Emerg Med*. 1989;18(9):927–930.

182. Dronen SC. Subclavian venipuncture. In: Roberts JR, Hedges JR, eds. *Clinical Procedures in Emergency Medicine*. Philadelphia: WB Saunders; 1985:304–321.

183. Wyte SR, Barker WJ. Central venous catheterization: internal jugular approach and alternatives. In: Roberts JR, Hedges JR, eds. *Clinical Procedures in Emergency Medicine*, Philadelphia: WB Saunders; 1985:321–332.

184. Fuchs S, LaCovey D, Paris P. A prehospital model of intraosseous infusion. *Ann Emerg Med*. 1991;20(4):371–374.

185. Smith RJ, Keseg DP, Maney LK, et al. Intraosseous infusions by prehospital personnel in critically ill pediatric patients. *Ann Emerg Med*. 1988;17(5):491–495.

186. Glaeser PW, Hellmich TR, Szewczuga D, et al. Five-year experience in prehospital intraosseous infusions in children and adults. *Ann Emerg Med*. 1993;22(7):1119–1124.

187. Orlowski JP, Julius CJ, Petras RE, et al. The safety of intraosseous infusions: risks of fat and bone marrow emboli to the lungs. *Ann Emerg Med*. 1989;18(10):1062–1067.

188. Pantridge JF, Geddes JS. A mobile intensive-care unit in the management of myocardial infarction. *Lancet*. 1967;2:271–273.

189. Jakobsson J, Nyquist O, Rehnqvist N. Concise education of ambulance personnel in CG interpretation and out of hospital defibrillation. *Eur Heart J*. 1987;8:229–233.

190. Jakobsson J, Nyquist O, Rehnqvist N, et al. Prognosis and clinical follow-up of patients resuscitated from out-of-hospital cardiac arrest. *Acta Med Scand*. 1987;222:123–132.

191. Jakobsson J, Nyquist O, Rehnqvist N. Cardiac arrest in Stockholm with special reference to the ambulance organization. *Acta Med Scand*. 1987;222:117–122.

192. Jakobsson J, Nyquist O, Rehnqvist N. Effects of early defibrillation of out-of-hospital cardiac arrest patients by ambulance personnel. *Eur Heart J*. 1987;8:1189–1194.

193. Bradley K, Sokolow AE, Wright KJ, McCullough WJ. A comparison of an innovative four-hour EMT-D course with a 'standard' ten-hour course. *Ann Emerg Med*. 1988;17(6):613–619.

194. Olson DW, LaRochelle J, Fark D, et al. EMT-Defibrillation: the Wisconsin experience. *Ann Emerg Med*. 1989;18(8):806–811.

195. Cummins RO, Thies W. Encouraging early defibrillation: the American Heart Association and automated external defibrillators. *Ann Emerg Med*. 1990;19(11):1245–1248.

196. Weaver WD, Hill D, Fahrenbruch CE, et al. Use of the automatic external defibrillator in the management of out-of-hospital cardiac arrest. *N Engl J Med*. 1988;319(11):661–666.

197. Moore JE, Eisenberg MS, Cummins RO, et al. Lay person use of automatic external defibrillation. *Ann Emerg Med*. 1987;16(6):669–672.

198. Cummins RO, Schubach JA, Litwin PE, et al. Training lay persons to use automatic external defibrillators: success of initial training and one year retention of skills. *Am J Emerg Med.* 1989;7:143–149.

199. Hunt RC, McCabe JB, Hamilton GC, et al. Influence of emergency medical systems and prehospital defibrillation on survival of sudden cardiac death victims. *Am J Emerg Med.* 1989;7(1):68–82.

200. Vukov LF, Johnson DQ. External transcutaneous pacemakers in interhospital transport of cardiac patients. *Ann Emerg Med.* 1989;18(7):738–740.

201. Eitel DR, Guzzardi LJ, Stein SE, et al. Noninvasive transcutaneous cardiac pacing in prehospital cardiac arrest. *Ann Emerg Med.* 1987;16(50):531–534.

202. O'Toole KS, Paris PM, Heller MB. Emergency transcutaneous pacing in the management of patients with bradyasystolic rhythms. *J Emerg Med.* 1987;5:267–273.

203. Syverud SA, Dalsey WC, Hedges JR. Transcutaneous and transvenous cardiac pacing for early bradyasystole cardiac arrest. *Ann Emerg Med.* 1986;15:121–124.

204. Hedges JR, Syverud SA, Dalsey WC, et al. Prehospital trial of emergency transcutaneous cardiac pacing. *Circulation.* 1987;76(6):1337–1343.

205. Vukov LF, White RD. External transcutaneous pacemakers in prehospital cardiac arrest (letter). *Ann Emerg Med.* 1988;17(5):554–555.

206. Grubb BP, Samoil D, Temesy-Armos P, et al. The use of external noninvasive pacing for the termination of supraventricular tachycardia in the emergency department setting. *Ann Emerg Med.* 1993;22(4):714–717.

207. Vukmir RB. Emergency cardiac pacing. *Am J Emerg Med.* 1993;11(2):166–176.

208. Cummins RO, ed. *Advanced Cardiac Life Support Textbook.* Dallas: American Heart Association; 1994:Ch.13.

209. Calliham M. Pericardiocentesis. In: Roberts JR, Hedges JR, eds. *Clinical Procedures in Emergency Medicine.* Philadelphia: WB Saunders; 1985:208–225.

210. Green BA, Eismont FJ, O'Heir JT. Pre-hospital management of spinal cord injuries. *Paraplegia.* 1987;25:229–238.

211. Kihtir T, Ivatury RR, Simon R, et al. Management of transperitoneal gunshot wounds of the spine. *J Trauma.* 1991;31(12):1579–1583.

212. Lerner EB, Billittier AJ IV, Moscati RM. The effects of neutral positioning with and without padding on spinal immobilization of healthy subjects. *Prehosp Emerg Care.* 1998;2(2): 112–116.

213. Domeier RM, Evans RW, Swor RA, et al. Prehospital clinical findings associated with spinal injury. *Prehosp Emerg Care.* 1997;1:11–15.

214. Muhr MD, Seabrook DL, Wittwer LK. Paramedic use of a spinal injury clearance algorithm reduces spinal immobilization in the out-of-hospital setting. *Prehosp Emerg Care.* 1999;3:1–6.

215. Hauswald M, Ong G, Tandberg D, Omar Z. Out of hospital spinal immobilization: its effect on neurologic injury. *Acad Emerg Med.* 1998;5(3):214–219.

216. Orledge JD, Pepe PE. Out-of-hospital spinal immobilization: is it really necessary. *Acad Emerg Med.* 1998; 5(3):203–204.

217. Hankins DG, Rivera-Rivera EJ, Ornato JP, et al. Spinal immobilization in the field: clinical clearance criteria and implementation. *Prehosp Emerg Care.* 2001;5:88–93.

218. Podolsky S, Baraff LJ, Simon RR, et al. Efficacy of cervical spine immobilization methods. *J Trauma.* 1983; 23(6):461–465.

219. McCabe JB, Nolan DJ. Comparison of the effectiveness of different cervical immobilization collars. *Ann Emerg Med.* 1986;15(1):50–53.

220. Dick T, Land R. Spinal immobilization devices. Part 1: cervical extrication collars. *J Emerg Med Serv.* 1982;12: 26–32.

221. Graziano AF, Scheidel EA, Cline JR, et al. A radiographic comparison of prehospital cervical immobilization devices. *Ann Emerg Med.* 1987;16(10):1127–1131.

222. Cline JR, Scheidel E, Bigsby EF. A comparison of methods of cervical immobilization used in patient extrication and transport. *J Trauma.* 1985;25(7):649–653.

223. Howell JM, Burrow R, Dumontier C, et al. A practical radiographic comparison of short board technique and Kendrick Extrication Device. *Ann Emerg Med.* 1989; 18(9):943–946.

224. Schriger DL, Larmon B, LeGassick T, et al. Spinal immobilization on a flat backboard: does it result in neutral position of the cervical spine? *Ann Emerg Med.* 1991;20(8):878–881.

225. Markenson D, Foltin G, Tunik M, et al. The Kendrick Extrication Device used for pediatric spinal immobilization. *Prehosp Emerg Care.* 1999;3:66–69.

226. Schafermeyer RW, Ribbeck BM, Gaskins J, et al. Respiratory effects of spinal immobilization in children. *Ann Emerg Med.* 1991;20(9):1017–1019.

227. Huerta C, Griffith R, Joyce SM. Cervical spine stabilization in pediatric patients: evaluation of current techniques. *Ann Emerg Med.* 1987;169(10):1121–1126.

228. Dick T, Land R. Spinal immobilization devices. Part 3: full spinal immobilizers. *J Emerg Med. Serv.* 1983;2:34–43.

229. Joyce SM, Moser CS. Evaluation of a new cervical immobilization/extrication device. *Prehosp Disaster Med.* 1992;7(1):61–64.

230. Dick T. Prehospital splinting. In: Roberts JR, Hedges JR, eds. *Clinical Procedures in Emergency Medicine.* Philadelphia: WB Saunders; 1985:576–597.

231. Grant HD, Murray RH, Bergeron JD. *Emergency Care.* 5th ed. Englewood Cliffs, NJ: Prentice Hall; 1990: 251–253.

232. McSwain NE. Pneumatic anti-shock garment: state of the art. *Ann Emerg Med.* 1988;17(5):506–525.

233. Civetta JM, Nussenfeld SR, Rowe TR, et al. Prehospital use of the military anti-shock trouser (MAST). *JACEP.* 1976;5(8):581–587.

234. Mackersie RC, Christensen JM, Lewis FR. The prehospital use of external counterpressure: does MAST make a difference? *J Trauma.* 1984;24(10):882–888.

235. Bickell WH, Pepe PE, Wyatt CH, et al. Effect of anti-shock trousers on the trauma score: a prospective analysis in the urban setting. *Ann Emerg Med*. 1985;14(30):218–222.

236. Bickell WH, Pepe PE, Bailey ML, et al. Randomized trial of pneumatic antishock garments in the prehospital management of penetrating abdominal injuries. *Ann Emerg Med*. 1987;16(6):653–658.

237. Riou B, Pansard J, Lazard T, et al. Ventilatory effects of medical antishock trousers in healthy volunteers. *J Trauma*. 1991;31(11):1495–1502.

238. Cayten CG, Berendt BM, Byrne DW, et al. A study of pneumatic antishock garments in severely hypotensive trauma patients. *J Trauma*. 1993;34(5):728–735.

239. Lloyd S. MAST and IV infusion: do they help in prehospital trauma and management? *Ann Emerg Med*. 1987;16(50):565–567.

240. Domeier RM, O'Connor RE, Delbridge TR, Hunt RC. Use of the pneumatic anti-shock garment (PASG): a position paper of the National Association of EMS Physicians. *Prehosp Emerg Care*. 1997;1(1):32–35.

CHAPTER 55

Pharmacotherapy

Adrian D'Amico, MD

Out-of-hospital medical oversight requires prudent and expeditious use of pharmacological agents. Over the past several years, numerous drugs have appeared that have significant implications for the out-of-hospital provider. The EMS medical director must sift carefully through the list of available medications and incorporate those that are clearly indispensable and review those medications that have promise but require further scrutiny. This chapter provides an overview of the common principles regarding out-of-hospital pharmacotherapy. In addition, common medications currently available to the out-of-hospital care provider are reviewed. Pitfalls in pharmacotherapy will be discussed. Newer agents that may become integral to future out-of-hospital systems will be discussed.

All recommendations made in this chapter are simply guidelines for the medical director to use in his development of out-of-hospital protocols, and are not to be construed as standards of practice.[1] Each new medication that will appear in the future must undergo careful study for relevant use within the system for which the medical director is responsible.

Early hospital clinicians recognized that many pharmacological agents garnered greater success when administered earlier in the evolution of certain acute illnesses. The logical consequence of improved survival with early administration of medications was the addition of many pharmacological maneuvers to the out-of-hospital environment. Table 55.1 lists medications currently in use in the state of Pennsylvania.[2]

The medications available within a typical EMS system demands strict medical oversight. The medical director is charged with the choice of drugs for out-of-hospital use, based on ACLS guidelines, local standards, and state-approved drug lists. Jurisdictions vary as to the type and number of drugs carried by field providers.[3]

While it is desirable to carry a broad range of medications to meet a variety of patient requirements, the medical oversight physician must understand the real cost of stocking medications, developing protocols, providing initial training, and continuing education. Adding succinylcholine, for example, to a field drug list might require extensive provider training, protocol revision, and the development of procedures for dealing with the short shelf life. Amiodarone, which recently attained Class II status in the revised American Heart Association (AHA) treatment guidelines,[4] is costly and cumbersome to administer; therefore, it's out-of-hospital status must be carefully evaluated. Drugs should not be added to the armamentarium simply because they are available and offer promise. The medical oversight physician must consider potential risks and benefits over existing therapies. For example, although diltiazem is a useful drug for supraventricular tachycardia (SVT) in the hospital, the cost of adding this agent to the out-of-hospital drug list may not be justified in a service that treats few cases of SVT.

Scant outcome data are available for the use of pharmacological agents in the out-of-hospital setting.[5] A 1992 national conference adopted a system of classifying cardiac interventions based on supporting scientific evidence, later revised in the *Guidelines 2000 for Cardiovascular Resuscitation and Emergency Cardiac Care*.[4] All out-of-hospital interventions should be classified in a similar manner based on available scientific evidence. This classification system permits reliable assessment of medications based on research evidence, and should serve to guide the medical oversight physician in evaluation of new out-of-hospital medications. See Table 55.2.

TABLE 55.1

Medications Currently in Use in the State of Pennsylvania

Adenosine	Glucagon	Sodium Bicarbonate
Albuterol	Heparin lock flush	Sterile water for injection
Amiodarone	Hydrocortisone Na Succinate	Terbutaline
Aminophylline	Lidocaine HCL	Verapamil
Aspirin	Isoproterenol HCL	Benzocaine/Tetracaine (topical
Atropine Sulfate	Magnesium Sulfate	only)
Bretylium	Meperidine	Heparin IV drip (interfacility
Calcium Chloride	Metaproterenol	transport only)
Dexamethasone Na Phosphate	Midazolam	IIb/IIIa inhibitors (interfacility
Diazepam	Morphine Sulfate	transport only)
Diltiazem	Naloxone HCL	Nitroglycerin IV drip (interfacility
Diphenhydramine	Nitroglycerin ointment	transport only)
Dobutamine	Nitroglycerin spray	IV electrolyte solutions
Dopamine	Nitroglycerin sublingual tablets	Dextrose
Droperidol	Nitrous oxide	Lactated Ringer's
Epinephrine	Oxytocin	Sodium Chloride
Furosemide	Procainamide	Normosol

Routes of Administration

The out-of-hospital care provider must understand the available routes of administration of indicated drugs, as well as their proper doses. Providers must realize that numerous drugs have beneficial effects through a particular route of administration but might be detrimental if administered via an inappropriate route.[6]

In the out-of-hospital environment, often the optimal route of administration is the parenteral route. The advantages include a rapid onset of action and clearly predictable effects. Parenteral drugs can be administered to treat the patient who is unable to orally ingest a necessary drug, as well as to deliver the medications into the patient's system more quickly and efficiently.

Oral

Medications administered via the oral (PO) route have limited utility because of the slow rate of absorption via the gastrointestinal tract. Patients with altered mental status are at risk for choking and aspiration and should not receive PO medications.

Aspirin is the only medication available in a PO form which, because of its value in the initial management of the acute coronary syndrome, should be available to out-of-hospital providers. Numerous studies have demonstrated the value of aspirin in the reduction of post myocardial infarction mortality.[7] Aspirin is now included in out-of-hospital protocols

for the management of chest pain. Exclusion to the use of aspirin include allergy or a history of gastrointestinal bleed related to prior use of aspirin or nonsteroidal antiinflammatories.

Subcutaneous

Certain medications can be administered into the subcutaneous layer of the skin where vascular networks promote efficient absorption of a drug. Epinephrine is the prototypical drug in this class administered for the treatment of allergic disorders. Because subcutaneous absorption is dependent on local blood flow, there may be a significant reduction in absorption in conditions that decrease local perfusion in skin, such as hypotension or shock-like states.

Sublingual

The sublingual route permits absorption of a drug into the systemic circulation via the vascular network of the mucous membranes in the floor of the mouth. Nitroglycerin is the prototypical drug in this class, exhibiting rapid and predictable absorption.

Intramuscular

The intramuscular (IM) route is a common route of drug administration but generally exhibits slow absorption in comparison to the intravenous (IV) route. The absorption of an IM medication is dependent upon the regional vascular supply; physiological states

TABLE 55.2

Classification of Therapeutic Interventions in CPR and ECC

- **Class I** Therapeutic option that is definitely recommended, is supported by excellent evidence, and has proven efficacy and effectiveness.
- **Class IIa** Therapeutic option for which the weight of evidence is in favor of its usefulness and efficacy.
- **Class IIb** Therapeutic option that is acceptable and useful, and has fair to good supporting evidence.
- **Class III** Therapeutic option that is inappropriate, is without scientific supporting data, and may be harmful.
- **Class Indeterminate** Therapeutic option with insufficient evidence to support a final class status, but can still be recommended.

that diminish blood flow either acutely or chronically can have a dramatic impact on the absorption of an IM medication. For example, shock-like states can adversely affect IM absorption; therefore, it is not the recommended route of administration for patients with decreased blood flow to the skin or muscle regions. In a patient with unstable VT, the use of IM lidocaine would result in delayed absorption of the drug and therefore delayed onset of drug action.

Intraosseous

In children of any age, the intraosseous route (IO) can be used for many medications when IV access is not readily available.[8-11] Most medications that are administered parenterally can be administered via the IO route, including the common cardiac drugs given during advanced resuscitation, with the exception of sodium bicarbonate. The IO route of administration requires specific training of personnel, since the technique requires specialized equipment and expertise not normally found in most out-of-hospital training programs. The costs of initiating this training and continuing education are significant, and must be considered in the context of other programs that may be more cost-effective.[12] Potential complications of the procedure include tibial fracture, injury of the epiphyseal plate, and infection at the access site.[8-11] These complications, albeit rare, require the medical director to closely monitor the performance of this type of invasive procedure in the pediatric patient.

Inhalational

Some medications, such as metaproterenol, albuterol, and atropine, can be aerosolized and administered into the tracheobronchial tree in the awake patient. This is especially true for patients with reversible airway obstruction, such as asthma or chronic obstructive pulmonary disease (COPD). These inhalational medications, commonly used in the field, have simplified the treatment of spontaneously breathing patients with bronchospasm, and have eliminated the dangerous practice in the past of administration of aminophylline, which is fraught with many complications.

Intravenous

Most drugs used in the field are intended to be administered via the IV route. The rate of absorption of an IV administered drug is generally immediate and predictable. Unfortunately, the IV route is also fraught with risks inherent in the rapid delivery of a drug directly into the peripheral or central circulation.

The rate of drug administration varies dependent upon the drug type, class, and patient condition. Drugs may be administered via rapid IV push (adenosine), slow IV push (furosemide), repeated boluses (lidocaine), or drip infusion titrated to effect (dopamine). To be effective, adenosine must be administered via rapid IV push, due to its short half-life in the peripheral circulation. Likewise, epinephrine during cardiac arrest is ideally administered via rapid IV push, since the desired effect generally is immediate. To enhance delivery of drugs to the central circulation during cardiac arrest, the dose of epinephrine should be followed by a 20–30 ml fluid bolus, and the extremity should be elevated.[1]

Certain drugs are to be given by slow IV push, such as furosemide or morphine sulfate, whose anticipated effects are slower in onset. Several medications are to be given by slow infusion, such as dopamine or dobutamine. Medications given by slow infusion generally have potent hemodynamic effects and must be titrated slowly to achieve the desired effect. Drug infusions are often difficult to maintain in a moving ambulance, since administration pumps are not universally available in the field.

Recently, more providers are being called upon to provide interfacility transport of patients; the medical director must review and recommend the drugs which will be maintained during transport via intravenous infusion. Also, the type and variability of infusion pumps must be reviewed so as to provide proper instruction and medical oversight of providers involved in interfacility transports.

Endotracheal

When IV access is delayed or unavailable, certain drugs can be given directly into the tracheobronchial tree via an endotracheal tube. The rate of absorption is essentially equal to the IV route. The dose of endotracheal drugs is typically 2 to 2.5 times the IV dose.[1] The specific drugs administered endotracheally include lidocaine, epinephrine, atropine, and naloxone.[1] Common mnemonics for these agents are LEAN and NALE.

Rectal

The rectal route has been studied as a route of administration for certain drugs readily absorbed from the rectal mucosa.[13] This is of special benefit in the pediatric patient. Clinical studies have demonstrated the reliable results and ease of administration of diazepam in the control of seizures in the pediatric population.[14] Rectal administration usually results in a slower onset of action than the IV route but is of specific benefit in children, such as when IV access is technically difficult in an actively seizing child.

The efficacy of rectally administered diazepam to a pediatric population has been reliably studied.[14] Diazepam has been shown to be effective when administered rectally by a syringe containing 0.5 mg/kg as the initial dose in a seizing child to a 14G plastic IV catheter (with needle removed) and advancing the catheter assembly 4–6 cm into the rectum. Diazepam administered in this manner should be flushed with 5 cc of saline fluid. Rectally administered diazepam may cause respiratory depression, and appropriate precautions should be undertaken.

Cardiac Medications

Vasopressin

Vasopressin is an endogenous neuropeptide hormone produced by the posterior pituitary gland. When used in pharmacologic doses in resuscitation, it promotes intense vasoconstriction by stimulating receptors on vascular smooth muscle cells.[15] In experimental models of ventricular fibrillation in cardiac arrest, vasopressin given intravenously in doses of 0.4 to 0.8 units/kg promoted greater myocardial blood flows than low-dose (0.045 mg/kg) or high-dose (0.2 mg/kg) epinephrine. Although vasopressin had a more gradual onset of action than epinephrine, the effect appeared to be more sustained. Vasopressin also appeared to be more effective after prolonged intervals of cardiac arrest without losing its vasoconstrictive effects.[15]

Vasopressin has been shown to improve myocardial blood flow and cerebral perfusion in the porcine model of cardiac arrest.[16,17] In 1996, eight adult cases of in-hospital cardiac arrest resuscitated with vasopressin after unsuccessful defibrillation and epinephrine were reported.[18] Three patients lived to hospital discharge with no reported neurologic deficits. Lindner then designed a randomized, double-blind trial using 40 units of vasopressin compared to standard doses of epinephrine in 40 out-of-hospital patients with VF resistant to defibrillation.[19] There was a statistically significant improvement in restoration of spontaneous circulation and 24-hour survival in the vasopressin group, but only an observed trend toward improved hospital discharge survival. Although these results appear promising, no large trials have to date been completed. Vasopressin has received class IIb status in the *Guidelines 2000* and is recommended as an alternative to epinephrine in the treatment of shock refractory VF.[4] It is Class Indeterminate in situations such as asystole and/or pulseless electrical activity as well as vasodilatory shock such as the sepsis syndrome.[4]

Vasopressin is not without risk, and the potentially detrimental effects of vasopressin must be considered. First, vasopressin has a relatively long half-life (~18 minutes) and may cause persistent vasoconstriction early after resuscitation. Reductions in blood flow to the coronary, renal, and adrenal circulation[20,21] have been documented. Peripheral vasoconstriction may increase mean aortic pressure and potentially affect the postischemic left ventricle. Vasopressin also exerts a hypercoagulable action that has been associated with increased risk of thrombotic events.[22] The potential consequences of these unwanted effects on cardiac arrest victims who have widespread atherosclerotic vascular disease are unknown. Despite these considerations, vasopressin is an important agent in the treatment of cardiac arrest, and is well recognized by the AHA. It is probable that epinephrine as currently recommended is not the ideal vasopressor for prolonged cardiac arrest. Optimal vasopressor therapy in the future will include vasopressin with or without other medications.

Epinephrine

Epinephrine is of benefit in the cardiac arrest patient because of its alpha-adrenergic receptor properties. These effects increase blood flow to the heart and brain during CPR.[23] The beta adrenergic effects of epinephrine may actually be harmful and have been implicated in increased myocardial work during ischemia.[24] In the past, epinephrine has been the catecholamine of choice in cardiac arrest. Despite its universal use, there appears to be little evidence demonstrating improvement of outcome in the cardiac arrest patient. Epinephrine was carefully reviewed in the *Guidelines 2000* curricula and new recommendations have surfaced.

The standard dose of epinephrine (1 mg) in common use is not based on body mass but stems from the anecdotal use of intracardiac epinephrine in the operating room.[25] The dose became 1 mg without clinical research to determine an effective dosing regimen based on mass.

Several studies have been performed to determine the dose-response curve of epinephrine and suggested that the optimal dosing range was 0.045–0.20 mg/kg.[26] A review of these trials did not demonstrate statistically significant improvement in survival rates to hospital discharge when compared with standard dose epinephrine.[27] The clinical trials that investigated the utility of high-dose epinephrine in cardiac arrest were not sufficiently convincing to modify the AHA recommendations in 1992 regarding epinephrine dosing.[28]

However, most of the high-dose epinephrine trials administered the higher dose late in the cardiac arrest. The recommended adult dose of epinephrine remains 1 mg IV of the 1:10,000 concentration repeated every 3 to 5 minutes followed by a 20 cc flush of IV fluid to deliver the dose into the central circulation. The *Guidelines 2000* curriculum reviewed a number of clinical trials comparing high dose and standard dose epinephrine, and it appears that higher epinephrine doses may increase coronary perfusion pressure with beneficial effects, but likewise may worsen myocardial function after resuscitation. Because of the potentially conflicting results in the studies, high-dose epinephrine is not recommended in routine use, but can be considered if 1 mg. doses are unsuccessful.[4] This is classified as Class Indeterminate use of epinephrine.

Epinephrine exhibits excellent bioavailability after endotracheal administration, and therefore the endotracheal route of administration should be used promptly in the absence of venous access. A dose of 2–2.5 mg is required.[1]

Epinephrine can also be given by continuous infusion, although the utility of such infusions must be tailored to the particular system. An infusion can be prepared by placing epinephrine hydrochloride into 250 cc of NS and titrating to a specific hemodynamic endpoint.[1]

Acute anaphylaxis may also require epinephrine administration. Epinephrine 1:1000 is administered in a subcutaneous manner at a dose of 0.01 mg/kg (0.01 cc/kg) to a maximum 0.5 mg in adults.[29] For adult patients refractory to subcutaneous epinephrine or into acute cardiovascular collapse, 0.3–0.5 mg (3–5 ml) epinephrine 1:10,000 is administered slowly, over 3 to 5 minutes via the IV route.[29]

Epinephrine is a potent vasoactive catecholamine and can cause severe hypertension, tachycardia, and increased myocardial oxygen consumption. The direct medical oversight physician (DMOP) must be confident that the field provider has sufficiently established the "arrest" state before epinephrine is administered. Low-flow states with subsequent profound hypotension may mimic the "arrested" state in the noisy environment of a field resuscitation, and the use of epinephrine may be deleterious. Personnel must carefully assess and monitor vital signs.

Dopamine

Dopamine is a chemical precursor of norepinephrine, exerts its effects by stimulating adrenergic receptors in a dose-dependent fashion.[30] At dosage ranges from 1–2 mcg/kg/min, there is stimulation of dopaminergic receptors to produce renal and mesenteric vasodilatation. At this dosage range, there is also stimulation of alpha-adrenergic receptors, which produces an increase in venous tone. At a dosage range of 2–10 mcg/kg/min, dopamine stimulates both beta-1 adrenergic receptors, which causes increased cardiac output, as well as alpha-adrenergic receptors, which also affects cardiac output and results in a modest increase in systemic vascular resistance. At doses greater than 20 mcg/kg/min, dopamine exerts primarily prominent alpha-adrenergic effects, such as vasoconstriction, which results in an increase in systemic and peripheral vascular resistance, as well as preload.

Dopamine is indicated for hemodynamically significant hypotension without hypovolemia with a systolic blood pressure less than 90 mmHg with evidence of clinical shock.[1]

Dopamine should not be used in doses greater than 20 mcg/kg/min, because of the profound generalized vasoconstriction from the stimulation of alpha-adrenergic receptors. Dopamine can also induce a tachycardia and can result in various ventricular and supraventricular arrhythmias. By increasing peripheral resistance, dopamine can worsen pulmonary congestion and increase myocardial lactate production.

Nausea and vomiting are frequent side effects. Extravasation of dopamine may cause tissue necrosis and sloughing of skin. Patients using monoamine oxidase inhibitors should receive a much lower dose of dopamine because of the direct drug interaction.

Dobutamine

Dobutamine is a synthetic sympathomimetic amine that is a potent inotropic agent. It stimulates beta-1 and alpha-1 adrenergic receptors in the heart. Its effect on peripheral adrenergic receptors leads to a mild vasodilatory response, which leads to a direct rise in cardiac output. Dobutamine results in less tachycardia than dopamine at conventional doses, and produces a beneficial rise in cardiac output without a concomitant rise in myocardial oxygen demand.[1]

Dobutamine is generally administered at a dosage range of 2–20 mcg/kg/min and is indicated in those patients with pulmonary congestion but a low cardiac output manifested clinically by hypotension.[1] Dobutamine may be superior to dopamine in those patients with mild-to-moderate hypotension and evidence of congestive heart failure (CHF) where it is desirable to promote primarily inotropic effects in the heart without the undesirable effects of tachycardia and peripheral vasoconstriction.[30] Studies of out-of-hospital dobutamine use show that this agent may be useful in selected cases of CHF.[31] Dobutamine may be combined with dopamine for additive effects to maintain arterial pressure in patients with pulmonary congestion and low cardiac output.

Dobutamine can cause tachycardia and arrhythmias at higher doses, and frequently results in headache, nausea, and tremor. Out-of-hospital care providers may not be familiar with dobutamine because of the traditional use of dopamine, but the benefits and pitfalls of dobutamine cannot be overstated. The medical director should carefully consider the addition of dobutamine to protocols.

Nitroglycerin

Nitroglycerin is a valuable drug, and familiarity with its drug profile is critical for the out-of-hospital care provider. It is the cornerstone agent in the treatment of patients with suspected ischemic chest pain and signs and symptoms of CHF who present to the field provider.[32]

Nitroglycerin causes relaxation of vascular smooth muscle and relieves angina pectoris in part by producing peripheral venodilatation with reduction in preload volume to the heart. Nitroglycerin also dilates large coronary arteries and can antagonize coronary vasospasm.[1] It is available for out-of-hospital use both in a tablet form and an aerosol spray for sublingual administration.[33]

Nitroglycerin is the drug of choice in the field for the treatment of chest pain of suspected ischemic origin and for CHF. It offers significant benefits in the management of CHF, including ease of administration and rapid titratability. Tablets have been traditionally used, but the aerosol spray offers greater convenience of administration. The use of IV nitroglycerin is generally impractical in the field but may be used during interfacility transports, familiarity with infusion devices and potential complications of intravenous nitroglycerin should be reviewed.

The recommended sublingual dosage of nitroglycerin is 0.3–0.4 mg in either the tablet or aerosol form. Oral administration results in some deactivation of the drug in the liver, and patients with potential or real liver failure may require dosage adjustment. The use of rapid multiple doses of sublingual nitroglycerin is highly effective in the out-of-hospital treatment of CHF when compared with treatment protocols using morphine and furosemide.[34]

Typically, nitroglycerin can cause transient hypotension, especially in patients who are hypovolemic, and fluids should be cautiously administered to counteract changes in blood pressure. This is secondary to its potent hemodynamic effects primarily on the venous system, causing a drop in venous return to the heart. Headache is common after nitroglycerin administration, and patients receiving nitroglycerin in the field should be warned of this unpleasant side effect. Patients who are using sildenafil (Viagra) should not receive nitroglycerin because of the potential harmful interaction with nitroglycerin and resulting severe hypotension.[35]

Not all chest pain encountered in the out-of-hospital setting is cardiac in origin. Nitroglycerin administration should be limited to patients with chest pain suspected to be cardiac in origin. Administration of nitroglycerin to a patient with chest pain secondary to aortic dissection or pulmonary embolism may adversely impact the patient's hemodynamics.

Atropine

Atropine, which stimulates sinus node discharge and enhances atrioventricular node conduction, is the parasympatholytic agent of choice for symptomatic bradycardia.[1] While there are no randomized, controlled out-of-hospital trials, atropine may be beneficial in nodal bradycardia. The data concerning the utility of atropine in pulseless idioventricular rhythm and asystole are inconclusive. A clinical trial of 21 patients was performed without improvement in mortality with the use of atropine in these specific dysrhythmias.[36]

The recommended initial dose is 0.5–1.0 mg IV in the adult patient.[1] The dose may be repeated at 5-minute intervals until the desired response is achieved. The total dose should be restricted to 2–3 mg if possible to avoid the adverse effects of an atropine-induced tachycardia.

Atropine may also be useful in patients with cholinesterase poisoning. The dose of atropine in this condition is larger and is titrated to effect.

The administration of atropine should never delay the initiation of transcutaneous pacing (TCP). If the patient's condition is severe, the DMOP should instruct the out-of-hospital care providers to immediately begin TCP.

In less acute situations the DMOP must query the out-of-hospital care provider regarding progressive bradycardic rhythms that exhibit ventricular escape activity. The request for lidocaine in these circumstances must be rejected due to the potential suppressive effects on the ventricular myocardium that is manifesting a desirable physiological response. Atropine instead should be used to provide the desired chronotropic effect.

Atropine should also be used cautiously in patients exhibiting asymptomatic bradycardias, since an increase in heart rate may be deleterious in patients with underlying coronary artery disease, especially during myocardial ischemia. Atropine has been reported harmful in some patients with cardiac block at the His-Purkinje level (type II AV block) and third degree heart block.

Antiarrythmic Medications

Adenosine

Adenosine is the out-of-hospital drug of choice for the treatment of paroxysmal SVT of the reentrant type. Its half-life of 5 seconds makes this drug ideal for rapid conversion of supraventricular rhythms with minimal hemodynamic consequences.[37] Adenosine transiently interrupts cardiac impulse propagation through the AV node, thereby terminating AV nodal reentrant rhythms.[1]

Adenosine has earned a place in the ACLS treatment algorithms and is part of many standard out-of-hospital protocols for the treatment of SVT.[38,39] Generally, the attempted conversion of atrial flutter or atrial fibrillation will not be successful with adenosine, but the short-lived AV block that occurs may unmask the underlying mechanism of the tachycardia. The dosage of adenosine is 6 mg rapid IV bolus over 1 to 3 seconds. This should be accompanied by a 20 cc NS flush.[1] A 12 mg IV bolus should be given if termination of the SVT does not occur within 12 minutes. Although more expensive than verapamil,[39] adenosine is a safer antiarrythmic. The consequences of administering adenosine for a misinterpreted ventricular tachycardia are less than those of inappropriate verapamil administration.[1]

The most frequent side effects of IV adenosine administration are flushing and chest pain.[40] These effects usually abate promptly, but the patient should be warned before adenosine administration. Adenosine has minimal lasting hemodynamic effects, because of its ultra-short half-life, and rarely produces hypotension. Transient AV block may occur and may unmask underlying atrial arrhythmias such as atrial fibrillation or atrial flutter.

Several drugs interact with the action of adenosine. Theophylline and other methylxanthines block the receptor responsible for adenosine action. Dipyridamole, on the other hand, blocks adenosine uptake and potentiates the drug.

Amiodarone

Intravenous amiodarone is effective and safe in the treatment of patients with hemodynamically destabilizing ventricular arrhythmias refractory to conventional antiarrythmic therapy.[41,42] Amiodarone has been well studied in patients with life-threatening ventricular arrhythmias.[43] A meta-analysis was performed to determine the impact of amiodarone on mortality and sudden death in patients with acute myocardial infarction (MI) or congestive heart failure.[43] There appeared to be a clear mortality reduction in arrhythmic-induced sudden death alone.

Amiodarone does appear to improve the likelihood of successful out-of-hospital cardiac resuscitation to hospital admission but not necessarily to hospital discharge.[44] Amiodarone has been reported to be effective in refractory VF even in low-dose administration. Petrovic observed that doses as low as 150 mg IV were effective in the conversion of refractory VF in two instances.[1]

Is amiodarone the preferred antiarrythmic agent? The AHA recommends that amiodarone be used in patients with "impaired heart function" for both atrial and ventricular arrhythmias.[4] Amiodarone appears to have a lower incidence of proarrhythmic effects when compared to other agents in similar circumstances.

Amiodarone is available currently in an intravenous form which must be diluted in saline or dextrose in water and administered intravenously through a filtered needle. This makes the drug cumbersome for out-of-hospital use; hopefully the manufacturers will provide a form of amiodarone that is easily administered in the field. Amiodarone may cause hypotension and bradycardia, which can be avoided by slow drug infusion.

Verapamil and Diltiazem

Verapamil and diltiazem are calcium antagonists that have great utility for the treatment of supraventricular tachycardias, and in the control of ventricular response in rapid atrial flutter and fibrillation.[45] Both drugs exert negative chronotropic effects on the heart, while verapamil also exerts a strong negative inotropic effect. As a result, diltiazem produces less unwanted hemodynamic side effects, such as hypotension and decreased cardiac output. Both drugs slow conduction and prolong the refractoriness of the AV node. Diltiazem may play a greater role for the treatment of hemodynamically significant atrial flutter or fibrillation.

Since diltiazem produces dose-dependent depression of AV nodal conduction, it is effective in the treatment of paroxysmal SVT by interrupting reciprocation at the AV node. It also may be considered for patients in CHF because of its minimal depressant effects on the left ventricle.

The provider, faced with a patient in an obvious atrial fibrillation with a rapid ventricular response and subsequent hemodynamic compromise, should probably choose diltiazem before electrical cardioversion.

The dosage of IV diltiazem is 0.25 mg/kg in a bolus fashion, typically 20 mg in an adult. A repeat bolus dose of 0.35 mg/kg may be given 15 minutes after the initial bolus if there is no observed effect. These dosages are recommended for both paroxysmal SVT and the slowing of a rapid atrial flutter and fibrillation.[1]

Verapamil remains a useful drug when used with caution. The dosage of verapamil is 2.5–5.0 mg IV over 1–2 minutes.[1] The dose should be administered over a longer period of time (3 minutes) in older patients. A repeat dose of 5–10 mg may be given in 15–30 minutes. The out-of-hospital care provider should monitor the patient for rhythm change, hypotension, and worsening CHF.

Both of these drugs (verapamil to a greater extent than diltiazem) may produce transient hypotension, especially in patients with left ventricular dysfunction. Intravenous beta-blocking agents should not be used concomitantly with diltiazem because of the synergism of their hemodynamic effects and the risk of hypotension and depressed IV dysfunction. Patients on oral beta-blocking agents should receive diltiazem cautiously although this situation does not contraindicate the use of diltiazem. Patients exhibiting severe CHF should not receive diltiazem unless the underlying etiology is AF, in which case slowing of the ventricular rate may have immediate beneficial effects.

A major pitfall in the out-of-hospital treatment of SVT is the variable ability of practitioners to interpret arrhythmias. One study found misinterpretation of the arrhythmias of 30 out of 73 patients.[46] Inadvertent administration of either drug to a patient in ventricular tachycardia (VT) may produce severe hemodynamic compromise.[1]

Lidocaine

Lidocaine has been the traditional choice for the treatment of ventricular arrhythmias including ventricular ectopy, VT and VF. Lidocaine does possess a narrow therapeutic range, and toxicity can easily occur. According to the AHA *Guidelines 2000*, lidocaine is recommended for persistent VF and pulseless VT after defibrillation and epinephrine (Class Indeterminate), control of severe PVCs (Class Indeterminate) and hemodynamically stable VT (Class IIb).[4] Lidocaine has clearly lost its preeminent status in treatment of ventricular arrhythmias secondary to amiodarone and procainamide. Lidocaine should be given to patients who are at risk for significant malignant ventricular dysrhythmias to prevent recurrence. Lidocaine is the drug of choice for the suppression of ventricular ectopy, but it should be reserved for patients with symptomatic ectopy in the acute setting, such as myocardial ischemia or after conversion of VF or VT.

For refractory VF and pulseless VT, an initial dose of 1.0–1.5 mg/kg is recommended.[1] In addition to the initial dose, a subsequent dose of 1.0–1.5 mg/kg can be given for refractory ventricular rhythms to a total dose of 3 mg/kg.[1]

It is of paramount importance to stress the need to administer lidocaine by the multiple bolus technique instead of continuous infusion. The pharmacokinetics of lidocaine are more predictable and reliable in the field when given by multiple boluses. Due to the altered pharmacokinetics in the arrested heart, only the multiple bolus technique is recommended. Since the clearance of lidocaine is decreased in the arrested heart, a single dose of lidocaine should produce therapeutic levels. After spontaneous circulation is restored, additional lidocaine should be administered. Lidocaine can also be given via the endotracheal route, and dosing should be 2–2.5 times the IV dose to obtain therapeutic levels.

Lidocaine is metabolized in the liver, and maintenance doses should be decreased in the setting of reduced hepatic blood flow, such as during acute myocardial infarction, CHF, or shock states. The initial loading dose of lidocaine remains the same in these conditions (1.0–1.5 mg/kg); however, additional boluses should be reduced by 50% (0.25 mg/kg). The maintenance dose should also be reduced in patients over 70 years old.

Once the most aggressively used out-of-hospital cardiac medication, lidocaine is fraught with potential toxicities of which the DMOP must be aware and vigilant. The DMOP may be confronted with an out-of-hospital report of "frequent PVCs" and a request for the administration of lidocaine. The DMOP must query the field provider regarding the "clinical" significance and setting of the reported ectopy, because that will predict the need for pharmacological treatment. Ventricular ectopy in the absence of significant risk factors or active symptomatology warrants only ongoing cardiac monitoring.

Lidocaine should not be given to patients who exhibit high-degree AV block, since these patients may be entirely dependent upon the spontaneous automa-ticity of the myocardium when the conduction system is failing. Currently, none of the above drugs are recommended for prophylactic use in the setting of chest pain, since no clinical study has demonstrated clear benefit. In the non-arrest state, the rate of administration and total dosage of lidocaine must be monitored to prevent side effects and dysrhythmias.

Bretylium

Bretylium is an agent recommended in the past for patients with refractory ventricular fibrillation. Bretylium is complex drug; a recent review of the evidence by the AHA prompted its removal from the ACLS algorithms due to a high occurrence of side effects. At the time of this publication, Bretylium is not available from the manufacturer and is not recommended for use.

Procainamide

Procainamide, which has ventricular and atrial stabilizing effects, is used in some out-of-hospital systems for the treatment of arrhythmias. The clear advantage of procainamide is its combined antiarrythmic effects for both atrial and ventricular arrhythmias. Procainamide is particularly useful in patients with arrhythmias secondary to Wolf-Parkinson-White syndrome (WPW).

However, the usefulness of procainamide is tempered by its potential hypotensive effects during its administration. The use of procainamide warrants close monitoring and careful titration, both of which are difficult to maintain during out-of-hospital evaluation and treatment. In refractory VT or VF, the recommended IV dose is a total of 17 mg/kg administered at a rate of 30 mg/min by infusion.[1] Typically, the infusion rate is much faster, but there are no substantiating clinical studies to support a higher rate of infusion. The bolus technique of administration can result in toxicity such as hypotension, which must be tempered against the potential benefits.

Procainamide can cause hypotension and prolongation of the QRS interval; infusions must be very closely monitored. This drug should also be avoided in instances of QT prolongation and Torsades de Pointes. The difficulty of administering procainamide also limits its use.

Sodium Bicarbonate

Traditionally, sodium bicarbonate therapy had been used to buffer the acidemia that occurs in low-flow states, such as cardiac arrest, in the field. Sodium bicarbonate is only indicated in unique situations. These unique clinical circumstances include preexisting metabolic acidoses, hyperkalemia, or tricyclic antidepressant overdose where the benefit of bicarbonate therapy has been demonstrated. The IV dosing recommendation of sodium bicarbonate is 1 mEq/kg.[1]

There is evidence in animal models that the administration of sodium bicarbonate results in the generation of CO_2, which has been shown to produce intracellular acidosis and subsequently worsen central venous acidosis during CPR.[47] The administration of sodium bicarbonate can also result in hypernatremia and hyperosmolality.

Other Medications

Aspirin

Aspirin has become a mainstay of acute therapy in the setting of myocardial ischemia. Its effect on improved mortality was clearly demonstrated in the ISIS-2 trial; where a clear reduction in mortality was shown in 30 days following acute infarction.[48] The initial dose is 162–325 mg orally, usually given via chewable tablet form for convenience. Aspirin has been widely accepted and most chest pain protocols now include aspirin.

Aspirin use is widespread and out-of-hospital providers need to be wary of patients with a history of allergy, particularly anaphylaxis, in response to aspirin. Aspirin should be withheld if allergy is suspected; currently there are no alternatives for out-of-hospital use such as ticlodipine, which is used in hospital management for suspected intolerance of aspirin.

Inhaled Bronchodilators

The prompt recognition and treatment of bronchospasm in the field is of paramount importance in the prevention of severe morbidity from unrecognized respiratory failure. Acute respiratory distress in whole or in part secondary to acute bronchospasm is one of the most common complaints presenting in the field.

Once the diagnosis of acute bronchospasm is confirmed, the initial management includes supplemental oxygen and beta-agonist aerosolized agents. Beta-adrenergic agonists produce bronchodilation in airways by stimulation of beta-2 receptors and, in addition, inhibit mediator release and promote mucociliary clearance.

Aerosol therapy has become the preferred route of administration of beta-adrenergic agonists. The aerosol route results in optimal local absorption of a relatively small dose of drug with minimal systemic absorption and few side effects. Beta-adrenergic drugs are analogs of naturally occurring sympathomimetic catecholamines. The most commonly used bronchodilator agents are metaproterenol and albuterol. These drugs possess greater beta-receptor specificity than older agents such as isoproterenol or isoetharine.

The ability to administer aerosolized medications in the field has dramatically improved the acute management of bronchospasm. In the past, epinephrine and aminophylline were used primarily for acute bronchospasm with obvious adverse effects. These medications are still useful for bronchodilation but pose risks in the field, especially in patients susceptible to toxicity from increased sympathomimetic activity, such as the very old or very young and those with co-morbid illnesses. A study comparing metaproterenol alone with subcutaneous epinephrine and a combination of metaproterenol and epinephrine in the asthmatic out-of-hospital patient suggested that metaproterenol alone was as effective in achieving bronchodilation.[49] This lent support to the notion that use of aerosolized medications alone is effective in the treatment of the bronchospastic patient. The use of multiple doses of aerosolized beta-agonists in the field is efficacious, and demonstrates a safety profile well within acceptable limits.

The potential pitfalls of aerosolized beta-adrenergic agonists in the field are minimal. There is little systemic absorption of aerosolized medications, and therefore systemic toxicity rarely occurs. To obtain maximum efficacy from the aerosolized route, the patient must be cooperative and understand the nature of the treatment that requires deep inspiratory efforts to promote efficient delivery of microscopic droplets. Out-of-hospital care providers must be adequately trained in the delivery process of aerosolized medications, and must be able to coach patients in the proper breathing techniques during the administration process.

Anticonvulsant Medications

The appropriate out-of-hospital pharmacological management of a seizure depends on the prompt recognition of tonic or clonic activity and a possible underlying etiology. A seizure may be a primary or idiopathic event, or it may be secondary to multiple etiologies, such as metabolic derangements, inflammatory or infectious states, structural injury to the CNS, or generalized illness.

Before any pharmacological considerations, the field provider must address the airway and provide lifesaving measures to maintain ventilatory support, supply oxygen, and prevent aspiration. A seizure in and of itself is not typically life-threatening and the first priority remains respiratory status. The care provider must not be so distracted by a seizure to fail to search for a treatable etiology in the field. For example, a seizure in a child may be secondary to hyperpyrexia and therefore reassurance to the family and direct medical oversight communication may be sufficient, although transport is probably warranted in most cases.

One etiology of seizures is hypoglycemia; the providers must search for evidence of hypoglycemia and treat the patient accordingly. Head injury with structural damage to the CNS may result in a seizure, and the treatment priorities are directed to the primary injury. It is imperative to treat a seizure in the field when failure to do so might result in acute respiratory, insufficiency, cardiac compromise, or place the patient in grave danger.

The most commonly used anticonvulsant is diazepam, a short-acting benzodiazepine with well-recognized and reliable properties. IV diazepam is administered 5 mg over 2 minutes, typically up to 10 mg in adults, watching for respiratory depression.[1] Diazepam has a rapid onset of action, achieving maximal CNS concentrations 1–2 minutes after IV administration.[1] The half-life of diazepam is 15–90 minutes. The rectal route of diazepam administration (0.2–0.5 mg/kg) has been shown to be very effective in the pediatric population when IV access is difficult and prolonged seizure activity warrants ablation of the event.[13,14] Lorazepam may also be used to control seizures (1–4 mg over 2–10 min).[1] Phenytoin and phenobarbital, two other commonly used anticonvulsants, are generally reserved for hospital administration. Midazolam is a short-acting benzodiazepine which likely will have an increased field role.

Fosphenytoin (Cerebryx®) is a new anticonvulsant whose active metabolite is phenytoin. It is soluble in aqueous solutions and readily absorbed via the intramuscular route, an advantage over phenytoin. It also has fewer cardiovascular effects in comparison to phenytoin, and may supplant phenytoin.

The greatest pitfall in the pharmacological management of seizures is the potential to compromise respiratory and hemodynamic status. Since many idiopathic seizures stop spontaneously, aggressive treatment usually is not warranted; prolonged seizures and status epilepticus must be aggressively treated.[50]

A seizure is a dramatic event and the out-of-hospital care providers may not search for underlying causes, such as hypoglycemia, which is easily treated. Failure to recognize a significant head injury manifesting a secondary seizure will delay the appropriate treatment for CNS injury.

Neuromuscular Blocking Agents

The use of intubation adjuncts, such as neuromuscular blocking agents, is a cornerstone in the management of the difficult airway. The medical director must evaluate the potential benefits of these agents in light of the risks associated with their use. These agents, if used in the field, require close scrutiny of the provider and rigid adherence to protocols.[51,52]

Neuromuscular blocking agents are classified either as depolarizing or non-depolarizing agents, depending on their interaction with the neuromuscular junction.[53] They are used for supplemental muscle relaxation and can be of tremendous advantage in the uncooperative patient, especially when associated with a head injury. The potential risk of increased intracranial pressure with the stimulation of the airway reflex can be blunted by using these drugs.

The primary hazard in the use of a neuromuscular blocking agent is the inability to manage the airway when paralysis and subsequent apnea occur. The out-of-hospital use of these agents must be tempered by the medical director's confidence in the airway skills of the field providers. The prototypical agent in this class is succinylcholine, which depolarizes the postsynaptic junction and competitively inhibits the affects of acetylcholine. The duration of a single dose is 3–5 minutes. Potential vagal stimulation may require the concomitant use of atropine in the child or in adults receiving multiple doses. The recommended IV dose is 1.0–1.5 mg/kg.[53]

Non-depolarizing agents competitively block the effects of acetylcholine at the neuromuscular junction. In theory, this does not produce the fasciculations as seen with depolarizing agents. The two agents in this class in common use and of potential field use are pancuronium and vecuronium. Rocuronium, a newer non-depolarizing agent, offers promise as a safer alternative to succinylcholine. It has a comparable speed of onset in the range of 65 to 80 seconds when used in doses of 0.9 to 1.2 mg/kg, but it concomitantly has prolonged action, similar to vecuronium and atracurium.[54]

Pancuronium is a long-acting neuromuscular blocking agent with an onset of action of 2–5 minutes and a duration of action of approximately 60 minutes. The recommended IV dose is 0.1 mg/kg with repeated doses exhibiting a cumulative effect.[56] Reversal can be achieved with cholinesterase inhibitors, such as neostigmine, with concomitant use of atropine to minimize the cholinergic effects of neostigmine. Vecuronium has few pitfalls in comparison with pancuronium, which is why it has been recommended as the ideal longer-acting neuromuscular blocking agent for out-of-hospital use. The use of priming doses, that is, the administration of a subparalytic dose before a smaller than usual "intubating" dose, has been shown to have a more rapid onset of paralysis than a single dose of vecuronium. Unfortunately, the long interval between the priming and intubating dose, generally 4–6 minutes, has made this impractical for the emergent intubation in the field. Vecuronium has a shorter onset and duration of action than pancuronium and does not exhibit cumulative effects with repeated doses, as does pancuronium. Vecuronium has an onset of action of approximately 3 minutes and a duration of action of 30–35 minutes. Its recommended IV dose is 0.1 mg/kg.[53]

Succinylcholine may produce profound muscle fasciculations with resulting hyperkalemia, hyperthermia, or histamine release. In certain pathological states the hyperkalemic response may be profound, such as severe nonacute burns or severe muscle trauma.[55] Fasciculations may be prevented by pre-administration of a subparalytic dose (0.01 mg/kg) of pancuronium. Pancuronium may cause a rise in heart rate or blood pressure because of its vagolytic effects. Pancuronium may also cause release of histamine, with subsequent end organ effects.

Glucose

Hypoglycemia is a common cause of altered consciousness in the out-of-hospital setting. In one series, 8.5% of patients with altered level of consciousness were found to be hypoglycemic.[13] Symptomatic hypoglycemia has been demonstrated in both diabetic and non-diabetic patients.[13] As a result, many out-of-hospital care protocols recommend the routine administration of 50% dextrose (D50) as part of a "coma cocktail" to patients presenting with altered

level of consciousness. The drug of choice for the parenteral treatment of hypoglycemia in patients with IV access is 50% dextrose, supplied in 50 ml prefilled syringes. In a study of 51 patients documented a mean increase of serum glucose concentration from baseline of 166 mg/dl with a range of 37 to 379 mg/dl following the injection of 50 ml of D50 in hypoglycemic patients.[56] This study suggested that the magnitude of change of serum glucose level cannot be predicted from a single ampule of D50.

Recent literature has questioned the practice of routinely administering D50 in the patient with altered level of consciousness. Multiple studies in animals and humans have demonstrated increased neurological impairment and mortality in subjects with hyperglycemia after a neurological insult.[56] Hyperglycemia may produce its detrimental cerebral effect in the setting of hypoxia or ischemia due to an increase in the amount of substrate for anaerobic glycolysis and an accelerated accumulation of brain lactic acid.[57] This suggests that D50 and glucose containing IV solutions should be avoided in patients at risk for cerebral ischemia (i.e., acute stroke, cardiac arrest). Ideally, the administration of D50 should be limited to patients with documented hypoglycemia.

Conveniently, the use of rapid glucose reagent strips in the out-of-hospital setting provides an easy and reliable method for documenting hypoglycemia. Rapid glucose reagent strips require a drop of blood (via venipuncture or finger stick) applied to the strip. Estimation of serum glucose level can then be read via strip in approximately 1–2 minutes. Hogya found the Chemstrip BG® to be 100% sensitive and 88% specific for the out-of-hospital detection of hypoglycemia.[58] Reagent strips provide a rational means of detecting hypoglycemia in the field in patients with altered level of consciousness, and provide a rational basis for D50 administration.[59] In addition, Hogya noted that the cost of a single Chemstrip BG® to be less than 1/10 the cost of an ampule of D50. Glucometer analysis of serum glucose is now also commonly performed, due to competitive cost of the devices and the reliability of the readings.

Some systems include thiamine (vitamin B_1) as part of the series of drugs administered to the unconscious patient. Thiamine administration initiates the treatment of Wernicke's encephalopathy, a rare cause of unconsciousness. Although common wisdom suggests that a single bolus of hypertonic dextrose can precipitate such an event, the scientific evidence for this is lacking.[59] There is no evidence to support delaying the administration of dextrose until thiamine can be administered.

Glucagon

Unfortunately, D50 can only be administered via the IV route. Therefore D50 cannot be administered to the patient with altered level of consciousness without IV access. Glucagon, a naturally occurring polypeptide administered via the IM or subcutaneous route, is useful in reversing hypoglycemia in patients without IV access. Glucagon acts on liver glycogen, converting it to glucose. Therefore patients must have liver glycogen stores for glucagon to work. Patients with hepatic glycogen depletion (starvation, chronic alcoholism, chronic illness, or impaired liver function) may not respond to glucagon.

Glucagon is packaged as a lyophilized powder and must be mixed with a diluent provided in the packaging. Glucagon administered in a dose of 1–5 mg has a slower onset of action than D50 (8–10 minutes for a 1 mg dose) with a duration of action of 10–30 minutes.[65,66] Side effects of glucagon include nausea and vomiting. Glucagon may cause extreme hypertension in pheochromocytoma, and is therefore contraindicated in patients with this disorder. Glucagon produces a positive inotropic effect on the heart and may be useful in the reversal of hypotension associated with beta blocker overdose, calcium channel overdose, and anaphylactic shock.[60–65] For these indications, glucagon should be given IV in a dose titrated to effect.

Antihypertensives Medications

Although it is rare for patients to engage EMS for the chief complaint of asymptomatic hypertension, out-of-hospital care providers often encounter patients with hypertension. Hypertension may be part of the patient's primary problem (i.e., chest pain or CHF), secondary to pain or anxiety, or found unexpectedly during assessment of routine vital signs.

Hypertension is often treated in the field with nontraditional agents, such as morphine and nitroglycerin. Both agents will decrease blood pressure and may be appropriate for treatment of significant hypertension associated with chest pain of suspected cardiac origin or CHF.

Nifedipine, a calcium channel blocker, had been used in the hospital and out-of-hospital settings to decrease blood pressure.[66–70] A 10 mg nifedipine capsule chewed and then swallowed by the patient has been effective in reducing blood pressure.[71] However, nifedipine administration has also been associated with symptomatic hypotension and heart block.[74] In addition, the single oral dose cannot be accurately titrated or reversed. Hypovolemia and the concomitant use of other antihypertensive agents may predispose patients to complications. The use of chewed nifedipine is not recommended.

Hypertension can be identified, and options exist for its treatment in the out-of-hospital setting. However, the rationale for treating hypertension in this setting has been questioned. There is probably no benefit to the short-term treatment of hypertension in the asymptomatic patient. To be effective, antihypertensive therapy must occur over the long term and must be monitored.

The treatment of hypertension associated with pain or anxiety should be corrected at the cause (i.e., administration of analgesics to control pain resulting from a fracture). The treatment of hypertension associated with an acute neurovascular or cardiovascular process is controversial and must be individualized. Patients probably benefit from mild blood pressure reductions in hypertensive emergencies, such as CHF, aortic dissection, subarachnoid hemorrhage, and hypertensive encephalopathy. These diagnoses can be suggested by patient presentation, but definitive diagnosis cannot be made in the out-of-hospital setting.

Likewise, hypertension may be seen in the setting of an acute stroke. In the past, elevated blood pressure in the face of an acute neurological event was aggressively decreased to normal ranges. This practice is fraught with danger. Several authors have demonstrated that in patients with acute stroke and moderate hypertension (systolic blood pressures 170–220 or diastolic blood pressures from 90–120 mmHg), cerebral blood flow was negatively correlated with decreases in blood pressure.[72,73] In the setting of an acute cerebrovascular insult, reduction of hypertension may reduce cerebral perfusion pressure and decrease cerebral blood flow in areas of viable tissue surrounding the ischemic cerebral brain. Therefore, lowering the blood pressure may exacerbate ischemic brain injury. The known risk (i.e., hypotension, heart block, exacerbation of ischemic brain injury) should be balanced with the unclear benefit of reducing blood pressure in the asymptomatic patient. Should the DMOP elect to initiate antihypertensive therapy, adequate monitoring must be ensured.

Opioid and Benzodiazepine Antagonists

The unconscious overdose patient provides a clinical and therapeutic challenge to the out-of-hospital care provider and medical command physician. Ideally the etiology of the overdose can be rapidly identified and its toxidrome reversed. Naloxone is commonly used in the "coma cocktail" administered to patients with decreased level of consciousness.[59,74] Naloxone, an opioid antagonist, reverses the effects of opioids including respiratory depression, sedation, and hypotension. Naloxone works faster when administered IV but also works when administered IM or subcutaneously. This is helpful in the out-of-hospital setting, especially when dealing with chronic IV drug abusers who may lack venous access. The IM dose provides a more prolonged effect.

Basic resuscitative measures, including establishing the airway, breathing, circulation, and suctioning, should not be ignored while waiting for naloxone to take effect. Although providers should prepare for intubation of patients with profound respiratory depression, they might want to delay the procedure until the naloxone takes effect. There is a danger of narcotized patients traumatically self-extubating once the profound respiratory depression is reversed.

The initial dose of naloxone is 0.4–2 mg administered IM, IV, or subcutaneously. This dose may be repeated every 3–5 minutes. In the controlled, hospital setting, naloxone is often titrated to effect; however, rapid opioid reversal is often desired in the out-of-hospital setting. Although this may be appropriate in the patient unable to protect the airway, precipitation of acute opioid withdrawal and violent behavior has been demonstrated after rapid reversal.[75]

Several opioids, including pentazocine, propoxyphene, and some synthetic "designer" opioids, may require high doses of naloxone for reversal (6–8 mg).[76] Therefore, higher requirements of naloxone should be considered in selected patients with these overdoses.

Abrupt reversal of opioid intoxication, as mentioned above, may lead to acute opioid withdrawal, including nausea, vomiting, tachycardia, seizures, and violent behavior.[75,77] Hoffman has suggested the selective use of naloxone for patients with clinical evidence of opioid intoxication (i.e., decreased level of consciousness, myosis, and decreased respiratory rate).[59] Some have recommended that naloxone be administered only in patients with suspected opioid overdose and significant respiratory depression.

The mean serum half-life of naloxone administered intravenously is 1 hour, with a duration of action of 2–3 hours.[76] Many opioids, including methadone, propoxyphene, and heroin, have a longer half-life than naloxone. This suggests, but has not been thoroughly demonstrated, that patients given naloxone and released by providers could lapse back into altered level of consciousness and respiratory depression.[78] Another pitfall with the administration of naloxone is that the opioid overdose may be associated with the concomitant use of alcohol or other depressives. Naloxone may not adequately reverse the respiratory or cardiovascular depression in these patients.

Nalmefene, a relatively new opiate antagonist, is more potent than naloxone, has a longer serum half-life (greater than 10 hours), and in the ED setting has been reported to be well tolerated.[78,79] Using a titrated dose 0.5–1 mg IV, nalmefene may be useful in the out-of-hospital setting, especially in the opioid overdose patient who may refuse or not otherwise require hospital transport. Onset of action begins within 2 minutes and peaks within 5 minutes.[80] Nalmefene's higher cost, slower onset of action, and limited clinical studies in the field setting limit its usefulness at this time. In addition, nalmefene may cause a prolonged period of withdrawal in opioid-dependent patients.

Activated Charcoal

Activated charcoal has proven to be beneficial in a variety of poisonings. It is not absorbed from the gastrointestinal tract and has the property of adsorbing to many toxins, thus allowing them to pass through the gut and out of the body. The adsorption occurs within 1–2 minutes of contact with the toxin. Activated charcoal can adsorb to substances that have passed through the pylorus into the small bowel. Activated charcoal is equal to or more effective than syrup of ipecac for decontamination in awake overdose patients.[81] In patients with a decreased level of consciousness who present more than 1 hour after overdose, activated charcoal was more effective than gastric lavage followed by activated charcoal.[81]

Activated charcoal does not effectively bind to the following substances: acids, alkalis, arsenic, bromide, DDT, ethanol, ethylene glycol, heavy metals, iodide, iron, lithium, methanol, potassium, or tobramycin. Activated charcoal is indicated for nearly all significant poisons except those listed above. Activated charcoal is contraindicated in caustic ingestions and in the presence of an ileus or bowel obstruction.

The typical adult dose is 30–100 gm mixed with water as a slurry. Children up to 12 years old may receive 15–30 gm. Use 1–2 gm activated charcoal/kg in infants. Activated charcoal may be mixed with sorbitol to provide a more palatable flavor and to serve as a cathartic, speeding elimination from the body. Activated charcoal premixed with water or sorbitol is definitely easier for out-of-hospital use.

Potential complications of activated charcoal administration include vomiting, aspiration pneumonitis, constipation, and charcoal empyema when given through a lavage tube that has perforated the esophagus. Activated charcoal use in patients who have ingested caustic agents may limit the endoscopic evaluation of injury to the gastrointestinal tract.

Out-of-hospital care providers may find patients to be reluctant to drink the black and gritty charcoal. The providers can be instructed to place a lid on the cup of charcoal and encourage the patient to drink without looking at the mixture. Activated charcoal tends to be very messy, especially when administered in the back of a moving ambulance. In summary, activated charcoal is a rapidly effective agent with few or no serious side effects, and is useful for administration in the out-of-hospital setting, especially if transport times are prolonged.

Magnesium

Over the past few years, magnesium has gained recognition as a clinically important electrolyte and effective therapeutic agent.[82] Some of the conditions in which magnesium has been successfully used include asthma, cardiac arrhythmias, acute myocardial infarction, and eclampsia. These conditions are frequently seen in the out-of-hospital environment, so it would be reasonable to include magnesium as another tool for EMS. One survey of state-approved drugs for EMS systems showed that five states suggested magnesium sulfate should be carried.[3] The specifics of different clinical settings in which magnesium could be helpful in the out-of-hospital environment follow.

Magnesium has been successful in the treatment of VT and VF in cases where standard therapy (e.g., lidocaine and bretylium) have failed.[83,84] It is also considered to be the drug of choice for the treatment of Torsades de Pointes.[85,86] Hypomagnesaemia can exacerbate digitalis-related arrhythmias even with therapeutic digitalis levels. In patients with suspected digitalis toxicity and cardiac arrhythmias, magnesium therapy should be considered.[87]

For cardiac arrhythmias in the out-of-hospital environment, magnesium can be given as a slow IV bolus of 2 gm of magnesium sulfate diluted in 10 cc of NS or D5W.[85] The DMOP should consider magnesium in the patient with refractory ventricular arrhythmias and history of risk factors for common causes of hypomagnesaemia, such as alcoholism, malabsorption, and diuretics.

Several studies have suggested that magnesium may be useful in severe bronchospasm associated with asthma.[84,88,89] Although inhaled bronchodilator (beta-agonists) remain the mainstay of out-of-hospital treatment for bronchospasm, magnesium may be administered in severe refractory cases. Magnesium has a bronchodilator effect and may improve ventilation in spontaneously breathing and intubated patients.[90,91] For severe bronchospasm, magnesium can be given as a slow IV bolus of 2 gm of magnesium sulfate diluted in 10 cc of NS or D5W.

Some authors have noted that serum magnesium levels fall transiently in the immediate post myocardial infarction period.[92] This finding has prompted investigation into whether magnesium therapy may be beneficial in this setting. Studies have provided evidence suggesting that magnesium may be of value in reducing arrhythmias and mortality following acute myocardial infarction.[93,94] A loading dose of magnesium can be considered for patients with suspected acute myocardial infarction as a slow IV bolus of 2 gm of magnesium sulfate diluted in 10 cc of NS or D5W.

In spite of some controversies, for decades IV magnesium has been considered the treatment of choice for the management of eclamptic seizures.[95] The recommended loading dose in the out-of-hospital setting is 4–6 gm of IV.

Magnesium is relatively contraindicated in patients with renal failure. In addition, patients may experience a burning sensation with IV administration. Toxic levels or rapid IV administration of magnesium may cause hypotension, weakness, decreased deep tendon reflexes, and respiratory depression. Providers should monitor the patient for possibility of toxicity. However, toxicity is very rare with the doses to be used in the field, with the exception of the larger doses administered for preeclampsia/eclampsia.

Calcium

The therapeutic use of calcium in the out-of-hospital environment is limited. Although calcium ions play a critical role in myocardial contractility and impulse formation, several studies in the cardiac arrest setting failed to show any benefit from calcium administration.[85] Calcium salts are available in two different preparations for IV administration: (1) calcium chloride 10%, which contains 13.4 mEq of calcium; and (2) calcium gluconate 10%, which contains 4.6 mEq of calcium. This difference should be considered when specific doses of calcium need to be administered. The most common clinical situations in which calcium can be of benefit in the field are life-threatening arrhythmias associated with hyperkalemia and hemodynamic instability secondary to calcium channel blocker toxicity.

Patients with a history of renal failure who present with sudden onset cardiac arrest or life-threatening arrhythmias should be considered at high risk for hyperkalemia. Calcium chloride is usually given for severe hyperkalemia with level above 7.0 mEq/L. Calcium chloride is administered in a 10–20 cc IV dose in a slow infusion over 10 minutes.[96] Calcium antagonizes the toxic effects of hyperkalemia for approximately 30 minutes but does not alter the serum potassium levels.[97] Of course, other standard therapy to reduce the hyperkalemia and for life support should be used.

The cardiovascular manifestations of calcium channel blocker toxicity can be treated with IV calcium. Calcium salts increase the concentration of extra-cellular calcium, helping to overcome the blockade.[98] Initial calcium therapy is 10 ml of calcium chloride 10% IV. Its effect is transient, and higher doses may be necessary in cases of refractory life-threatening toxicity. Unfortunately, treatment failure is not uncommon, and other life-supporting therapies should be initiated.

Cases

Case 1

Paramedics are on-scene with a 63-year-old male with a history of atherosclerotic heart disease and CHF who presents a profound respiratory distress and signs and symptoms of CHF. Paramedics note that he is complaining of chest pain similar to his typical angina, which was unrelieved by one of his nitroglycerin tablets before medics arrived. They found the patient's medications include digoxin and furosemide 40 mg per days and potassium. He has not taken his meds today. Vital signs are pulse-96, respirations-32, BP-210/110, pulse ox-89%.

The physical exam reveals positive JVD, rales three quarters of the way up both lung fields, and marked peripheral edema. EKG is a sinus rhythm with a rate of 96. The paramedics have initiated a precautionary IV and placed the patient on oxygen. Under protocol the paramedics have administered one sublingual nitroglycerin spray and administered 40 mg of furosemide IV.

WHAT ADDITIONAL ORDERS SHOULD THE DMOP PROVIDE?

Aggressive use of nitroglycerin is required in this case to both decrease preload and provide relief for chest pain. Even in the absence of chest pain, nitroglycerin could be administered as a out-of-hospital treatment for CHF as long as the patient's systolic blood pressure was maintained. The patient could be aggressively treated by the crew with sublingual nitroglycerin sprays 2–3 sprays every 3–5 minutes.

Case 2

Paramedics are on-scene with a 75-year-old female with a history of atherosclerotic heart disease, status post-coronary artery bypass, who called EMS for generalized weakness. Upon arrival, they find an elderly female in no acute distress. Her meds include nitroglycerin patch and an anti-hypertensive Tenormin®. The patient shows no other symptoms other than weakness at this time.

Her pulse is 50, respirations-12, blood pressure-130/84, pulse ox-98%. The patient's lungs are clear. The rest of her physical exam is unremarkable. The cardiac monitor reveals a sinus bradycardia rate of 50 without ectopy. The paramedics have initiated a precautionary line of saline at KVO. They are requesting to administer 1 mg of atropine to increase the heart rate.

HOW SHOULD THE DMOP PROCEED?

This patient is in a stable bradycardic rhythm possibly secondary to the beta blocker that she is taking on a regular basis. In addition, this patient is stable and asymptomatic and therefore does not require atropine at this time. An increase in this patient's heart rate may be deleterious secondary to her underlying coronary artery disease. An external pacemaker could be applied but not turned on as a precautionary measure.

Case 3

The paramedics are on the scene with an 84-year-old male with signs and symptoms consistent of CVA. The patient has a past history of hypertension and TIAs and now presents with right-sided upper and lower extremity weakness. The onset of the symptoms was gradual, beginning approximately 2 hours prior to calling the field crew. The patient's medications include multiple unknown antihypertensives. On physical exam the patient's pulse is 70, respirations 14, blood pressure 220/108. Physical exam is remarkable for an awake, alert elderly male with obvious right, upper, and lower extremity weakness. The paramedics are requesting to administer several nitroglycerin sprays to lower the patient's blood pressure.

HOW SHOULD THE DMOP PROCEED?

Although this patient is hypertensive and appears to be having a stroke, the risk of acutely treating this patient's probable chronic hypertension probably outweigh the unclear benefits. This patient is stable and does not appear to be having a hypertensive emergency. The paramedics should place the patient on oxygen, an EKG monitor, and initiate IV access. If available, the paramedics could measure the patient's serum glucose level via Chemstrip and treat it appropriately.

Case 4

The paramedics are on-scene with a 25-year-old male found unresponsive in an alley way. Drug paraphernalia were found at the patient's side, although bystanders are not helpful in providing additional information about the patient's collapse. Upon examination, the medics find the following vital signs: pulse-90, respirations-6, BP-140/90, pulse ox-92%. The patient's pupils are pinpoint and minimally reactive. His lungs are clear and the patient has obvious track marks on both arms and in the neck. The medics note that they are assisting the patient's ventilations via bag-valve-mask and are unable to obtain IV access.

WHAT ORDERS SHOULD BE GIVEN BY DIRECT MEDICAL OVERSIGHT?

Should the patient not respond, the out-of-hospital care provider should be prepared to intubate the patient, having all the necessary equipment ready, including suction. The crew should be aware that oc-casionally patients under the influence of opioids become violent when reversed with naloxone.

Summary

The selection and implementation of drugs for out-of-hospital use requires careful oversight by the responsible medical director. Adherence to evidence-based indications and careful attention to the requirements of the out-of-hospital providers will help to insure patient safety and appropriate use of medications.

The AHA guidelines provide a critical framework for the use of cardiac and other resuscitative medications. The use of other additional protocols must be tempered by the weight of evidence and the anticipated safety profile in the individual command system.

The skills of the field providers will provide guidance for the medical director in the choice of safe medications and protocols. Every system and its providers have unique requirements; it is incumbent upon the medical director to be acutely aware of these individual needs, and to provide medical oversight accordingly.

References

1. Cummins RO, ed. Cardiovascular pharmacology 1. In: *Textbook of Cardiac Life Support*. Dallas: American Heart Association; 1994.
2. Pennsylvania EMS formulary. 1994.
3. Delbridge TR, Verdile VP, Platt TE. Variability of state-approved emergency medical services drug formularies. *Prehosp Dis Med*. 1994;9:S55.
4. Cummins RO, ed. *Circulation*.(supp). 2000;102:8.
5. Shuster M, Chong J. Pharmacologic interventions in prehospital care: a critical appraisal. *Ann Emerg Med*. 1989;18:192–196.
6. Shuster M, Chong J. Pharmacologic intervention in prehospital care: a critical appraisal. *Ann Emerg Med*. 1989;18:201–207.
7. ISIS-2 (Second International Study of Infarct Survival) Collaborative Group. Randomized trial of intravenous streptokinase, oral aspirin, both or neither among 17,187 cases of suspected acute myocardial infarction. *Lancet*. 1988;2:349–360.
8. Chameides L, ed. Vascular access. In: *Textbook of Pediatric Life Support*. Dallas: American Heart Association; 1990:37–46.
9. Glaeser PW, Losek JD. Emergency intraosseous infusion in children. *Am J Emerg Med*. 1986;4:34.
10. Iserson KV, Criss E. Intraosseous infusions: a usable technique. *Am J Emerg Med*. 1986;4:540.
11. Fiser DH. Intraosseous infusion. *N Engl J Med*. 1990; 322:1579.

12. Garrison HG, Downs SM, McNutt RA, et al. A cost-effective analysis of pediatric intraosseous infusion as a prehospital skill. *Prehosp Dis Med*. 1992;7:221–227.

13. Fuchs S. Managing seizures in children. *Emerg Ped*. 1990;47–52.

14. Dieckmann RA. Rectal diazepam for prehospital pediatric status epilepticus. *Ann Emerg Med*. 1994;23:216–219.

15. Gazmuri RJ. *Crit Care Med*. 2000;28(4):1236–1238.

16. Lindner KH, Prengel AW, Pfenninger EG, et al. Vasopressin improves vital organ blood flow during closed-chest cardiopulmonary resuscitation in pigs. *Circulation*. 1995;91:215.

17. Lawrence ME, Price L, Riggs M. Inpatient cardiopulmonary resuscitation: Is survival prediction possible? *South Med J*. 1991;84:1462.

18. Lindner KH, Prengel AW, Brinkmann A, et al. Vasopressin administration in refractory cardiac arrest. *Ann Intern Med*. 1996;124:1061.

19. Lindner KH, Dirks B, Strohmenger HU, et al. Randomized comparison of epinephrine and vasopressin in patients with out-of-hospital ventricular fibrillation. *Lancet*. 1997;349:535.

20. Tang W, Weil MH, Sun S, et al. Epinephrine increases the severity of post resuscitation myocardial dysfunction. *Circulation*. 1995;92:3089–3093.

21. Prengel AW, Lindner KH, Wenzel V, et al. Splanchnic and renal blood flow after cardiopulmonary resuscitation with epinephrine and vasopressin in pigs. *Resuscitation*. 1998;38:19–24.

22. Grant PJ, Tate GM, Davies JA, et al. Intra-operative activation of coagulation: a stimulus to thrombosis mediated by vasopressin? *Thromb Haemost*. 1986;55:104–107.

23. Michael JR, et al. Mechanisms by which epinephrine augments cerebral and myocardial perfusion during cardiopulmonary resuscitation in dogs. *Circulation*. 1984;69:822–835.

24. Ditchey RV, Lindenfeld J. Failure of epinephrine to improve the balance between myocardial oxygen supply and demand during closed-chest resuscitation in dogs. *Circulation*. 1988;78:382–389.

25. Beck C, Leighninger D. Reversal of death in good hearts. *J Cardiovas Surg*. 1962:3:27–30.

26. Brown CG, Taylor RB, Werman HA, et al. Effect of standard doses of epinephrine on myocardial oxygen delivery and utilization during CPR. *Crit Care Med*. 1988;16:536–539.

27. Brown CG, Werman HA, Davis EA, et al. The effects of graded doses of epinephrine on regional myocardial blood flow during CPR in swine. *Circulation*. 1987;75:491–497.

28. Brown CG, Werman HA, et al. Comparative effects of graded doses of epinephrine on regional brain blood flow during CPR in a swine model. *Ann Emerg Med*. 1986;15:1138–1141.

29. Bochner BS, Lichtenstein LM. Anaphylaxis. *N Eng J Med*. 1986;324:1785–1790.

30. Levy D, Lyons E. Pharmacology of antiarrythmic and vasoactive medications. In: Tintinalli JE, ed. *Emergency Medicine: A Comprehensive Study Guide*. 4th ed. New York: McGraw Hill; 1986:183.

31. Oberg B, Sorenson MB. Out-of-hospital treatment with dobutamine. *Prehosp Dis Med*. 1992;8:247–249.

32. Bledsoe BE. *Out-of-Hospital Emergency Pharmacology*. 3rd ed. Englewood Cliffs, NJ: Simon and Schuster; 1992:127–130.

33. Rottmann SJ, et al. Nitroglycerin lingual aerosol in prehospital emergency care. *Prehosp Dis Med*. 1989;4:11.

34. Hoffman JR, Reynolds S. Comparison of nitroglycerin, morphine and furosemide treatment of presumed pulmonary edema. *Chest*. 1987;92:586–593.

35. Conti C. Viagra, the latest cardiovascular drug. *Clin Cardiol*. 1998;21:616.

36. Coon GA, Clinton JE. Use of atropine for bradyasystolic out-of-hospital arrest. *Ann Emerg Med*. 1981;10:462–467.

37. Bertolet BD. Adenosine: diagnostic and therapeutic uses in cardiovascular medicine. *Chest*. 1993;104:1860–1871.

38. Gausche M. Persse DE, Sugarman T, et al. Adenosine for the prehospital treatment of paroxysmal SVT. *Ann Emerg Med*. 1994;24:183.

39. Belhassen B, Viskin S. What is the drug of choice for the acute termination of paroxysmal supraventricular tachycardia: verapamil, adenosine triphosphate or adenosine? *PACE*. 1993;16:1735.

40. CammHelmy I, Herre JM, Gee G, et al. Use of intravenous amiodarone for emergency treatment of life-threatening ventricular arrhythmias. *J Am Coll Cardiol*. 1988;12:1015–1022.

41. Levine JH, Massumi A, Scheinman MM, et al. Intravenous amiodarone for recurrent sustained hypotensive ventricular tachyarrhythmias. *J Am Coll Cardiol*. 1996;27:67–75.

42. Leak D. Intravenous amiodarone in the treatment of refractory life-threatening cardiac arrhythmias in critically ill patients. *Am Heart J*. 1986;111:456–462.

43. Amiodarone Trials Meta-Analysis Investigators. Effect of prophylactic amiodarone on mortality after acute myocardial infarction and in congestive heart failure: meta-analysis of individual data from 6500 patients in randomized trials. *Lancet*. 1997;350:1417–1424.

44. Kudenchuk PJ, Cobb LA, Copass MK, et al. Amiodarone for resuscitation after out-of-hospital cardiac arrest due to ventricular fibrillation. *N Engl J Med*. 1999;341:871–878.

45. Dougherty AH, Jackman WM, et al. Acute conversion of paroxysmal supraventricular tachycardia with intravenous diltiazem. *Am J Card*. 1992;70:587–592.

46. Madsen CD, Pointer JE, Lynch TG. A comparison of adenosine and Verapamil for the treatment of supraventricular tachycardia in the prehospital setting. *Ann Emerg Med*. 1955;25:649–655.

47. Weil MH, Rackow EC, Trevino R, et al. Difference in acid base state between venous and arterial blood during cardiopulmonary resuscitation. *N Eng J Med*. 1986;315:153–156.

48. ISIS-2 (Second International Study of Infarct Survival) Collaborative Group. Randomized trial of intravenous streptokinase, oral aspirin, both or neither among 17,187 cases of suspected acute myocardial infarction. *Lancet.* 1988;2:349–360.

49. Quadrel M, Lavery RF, Jaker M, et al. A prospective, randomized trial of epinephrine, metaproterenol and epinephrine and metaproterenol in the prehospital treatment of adult asthma. *Prehosp Dis Med.* 1995;26(4):469–473.

50. Pellegrino TR. Seizures and status epilepticus in adults. In: Tintinalli JE, ed. *Emergency Medicine: A Comprehensive Study Guide.* 4th ed. New York: McGraw Hill; 1996: 1032.

51. Hedges JR, Dronen SC, et al. Succinylcholine assisted intubations in prehospital care. *Ann Emerg Med.* 1988; 17:469–472.

52. Rhee KJ, O'Malley RJ. Neuromuscular blockade: assisted oral intubations versus nasotracheal intubation in the prehospital care of injured patients. *Ann Emerg Med.* 1994;23:37–42.

53. Savares JJ. Pharmacology of muscle relaxants and their antagonists. In: Miler RD, ed. *Anesthesia.* 4th ed. New York: Churchill Livingston; 1994:417–487.

54. Magorian T, Flannery KB, Miller RD. Comparison of rocuronium, succinylcholine an vecuronium for rapid sequence induction of anesthesia in adult patients. *Anesthesiology.* 1993;79:913–918.

55. Roberts JR, Hedges JR. *Clinical Procedures in Emergency Medicine.* 2nd ed. Philadelphia: W.B. Saunders; 1991: 34–35.

56. Adler PM. Serum glucose changes after the administration of 50% dextrose solution. *Am J Emerg Med.* 1986; 4:504–506.

57. DeCourten-Meyers G, et al. Hyperglycemia enlarges infarct size in cerebrovascular occlusion in cats. *Stroke.* 1988;19:623.

58. Hogya P, Yealy DM, Paris PM, et al. The rapid prehospital estimations of blood glucose using chemstrip bG. *Prehosp Dis Med.* 1989;4:109–113.

59. Hoffmann RS, Goldfrank LR. The poisoned patient with altered level of consciousness: controversies in the use of a coma cocktail. *JAMA.* 1995;274:562–569.

60. Hall-Boyer K, Zaloga GP, Chernow B. Glucagon: hormone or therapeutic agent? *Crit Care Med.* 1984;12: 584.

61. Vukmir RB, Yealy DM. Glucagon: prehospital therapy for hypoglycemia (abstract). *Ann Emerg Med.* 1989;18: 479.

62. Salzberg MR, Gallagher EJ. Propanolol overdose. *Ann Emerg Med.* 1980;9:26.

63. Weinstein RS. Recognition and management of poisoning with beta-adrenergic blocking agents. *Ann Emerg Med.* 1984;13:1123.

64. Ramoska EA, Spiller HA, et al. A one year evaluation of calcium channel blocker overdose: toxicity and treatment. *Ann Emerg Med.* 1993;22:196.

65. Zaloga GP, Delacy W, Holmboe E, et al. Glucagon reversal of hypotension in a case of anaphylactic shock. *Ann Int Med.* 1986;105:65.

66. Ellrodt AG, Ault MJ, Riedinger MS. Efficacy and safety of sublingual nifedipine in hypertensive emergencies. *Am J Med.* 1985;79:19–25.

67. Ellrodt AG, Ault MJ. Calcium channel blockers in acute hypertension. *Am J Emerg Med.* 1985;3:16–24.

68. Davidson RC, Bursten SC, Keeley PA. Oral nifedipine for the treatment of patients with severe hypertension. *Am J Med.* 1985;79:26–30.

69. Wachter RM. Symptomatic hypotension induced by nifedipine in the acute treatment of severe hypertension. *Arch Intern Med.* 1987;147:556.

70. Davidson RC, Bursten SL, Keeley PA. Oral nifedipine for the treatment of patients with severe hypertension. *Am J Med.* 1985;79:26.

71. Heller MB, Duda JR, Maha RJ, et al. Use of nifedipine for field management of severe hypertension (abstract). *Ann Emerg Med.* 1987;16:520.

72. Lisk DR, Grottaj C, Lamki LM. Should hypertension be treated after stroke? *Arch Neurol.* 1993;50:855.

73. Powers WJ. Acute hypertension after stroke: the scientific basis for treatment decisions. *Neurology.* 1993;43: 461.

74. Yealy DM, Paris PM, Kaplan RM. The safety of prehospital naloxone administration by paramedics. *Ann Emerg Med.* 1990;19:902–905.

75. Gaddis GM, Watson WA. Naloxone associated patient violence: an overlooked toxicity. *Ann Pharmaco.* 1992; 26:196.

76. Smith JA, Stenbach GL. Narcotics. In: Tintinalli JE, ed. *Emergency Medicine: A Comprehensive Study Guide.* 4th ed. New York: McGraw Hill; 1996:772–773.

77. Yealy DM, Paris PM, Kaplan RM. The safety of prehospital naloxone administration by paramedics, *Ann Emerg Med.* 1990;19:902–905.

78. Kaplan JL, Marx JA. Effectiveness and safety of intravenous nalmefene for emergency department patients with suspected narcotic overdose: a pilot study. *Ann Emerg Med.* 1993;22:187–190.

79. Barsan WG, Seger D, Danzi DF. Duration of antagonist effects of nalmefene and naloxone in opiate induced sedation for emergency department patients. *Am J Emerg Med.* 1989;7:155–161.

80. Nalmefene: a long acting injectable opioid antagonist. *Medical Letter.* 1995;27:97–98.

81. Merigian KS, Woodard M, Hedges JR. Prospective evaluation of gastric emptying in the self poisoned patient. *Am J Emerg Med.* 1990;6:479–483.

82. Tso EL, Barish RA. Magnesium: clinical considerations. *J Emerg Med.* 1992;10:735–745.

83. Iseri LT. Magnesium and cardiac arrhythmias. *Magnesium.* 1986;5:111–126.

84. Iseri LT, Chung P, Tobias J. Magnesium therapy for intractable ventricular tachyarrhythmias in normomagnesemic patients. *West J Med.* 1983;138:823–828.

85. American Heart Association: Guidelines for cardiopulmonary resuscitation and emergency cardiac care. *JAMA.* 1992;268:2135–2302.

86. Tzivoni D, Banai 5, Schuger C, et al. Treatment of Torsades de Pointes with magnesium sulfate. *Circulation.* 1988;77:392–397.

87. Seller RH, Cangiano J, Kim KE, et al. Digitalis toxicity and hypomagnesaemia. *Am Heart J.* 1970;79:57–68.

88. Tso EL, Barish RA. Magnesium: clinical considerations. *J Emerg Med.* 1992;10:735–745.

89. Iseri LT. Magnesium and cardiac arrhythmias. *Magnesium.* 1986;5:111–126.

90. Don MR, Wrenn KD, Slovis CM, et al. When asthma attack turns deadly: principles of aggressive effective interventions. *Emerg Med Rep.* 1991;12:179–186.

91. Rolla G, Bucca C, Bugiana M, et al. Reduction of histamine induced bronchoconstriction by magnesium in asthmatic subjects. *Allergy.* 1987;42:186–188.

92. Rasmussen HS, Norregard P, Lindeneg O. Intravenous magnesium in acute myocardial infarction. *Lancet.* 1986; 1:234–235.

93. Teo KK, Yusuf S, Collins R, et al. Effects of intravenous magnesium in suspected acute myocardial infarction: overview of randomized trials. *Br Med J.* 1991;303: 1499–1503.

94. Ceremuzynski L, Jurgiel R, Kulakowski P, et al. Threatening arrhythmias in acute myocardial infarction are prevented by intravenous magnesium sulfate. *Am Heart J.* 1989;118:1333–1334.

95. Sibai BM. Magnesium sulfate is the ideal anticonvulsant in preeclampsia-eclampsia. *Am J Obst Gynecol.* 1990; 162:1141.

96. Wilson HF, Barton C. Fluids and electrolyte problems. In: Tintinalli JE, ed. *Emergency Medicine: A Comprehensive Study Guide.* 4th ed. New York: McGraw Hill; 1996.

97. Janson CL, Marx JA. Fluid and electrolyte balance. In: Rosen P, et al., eds. *Emergency Medicine: Concepts and Clinical Practice.* 3rd ed. St. Louis: Mosby; 1992:113.

98. Smilkstein S. Common cardiac medications. In: Rosen P, et al., eds. *Emergency Medicine: Concepts and Clinical Practice.* 3rd ed. St. Louis: Mosby; 1992:131.

CHAPTER
56

Analgesia

Paul M. Paris, MD, FACEP, LLD (Hon.)

Introduction

Pain and suffering are not confined within hospital boundaries. While prehospital personnel are usually focused on the ABCs, the treatment of pain should also be considered an important priority in the care of ill and injured patients.[1,2] The National Association of EMS Physicians (NAEMSP) currently supports every EMS system having a policy to address prehospital pain management.[3] "NAEMSP believes that the relief of pain and suffering of our patients must be a priority for every EMS system. NAEMSP recommends that prehospital pain protocols should address the following issues:

a. Mandate for pain assessment.

b. Tools for pain measurement.

c. Indications and contraindications for prehospital pain management.

d. Non-pharmacologic interventions for pain management.

e. Pharmacologic interventions for pain management.

f. Patient monitoring and documentation before and after analgesia.

g. Transferring information to receiving medical facility.[3]

The challenge of treating pain in the prehospital setting is to use agents and techniques that are not only effective but safe, and do not lead to physiological compromise or a delay in diagnosis upon arrival in the emergency department.[4,5] Because of inordinate fears of "masking the diagnosis" and the desire to prevent side effects, many EMS systems have opted for little or no use of pharmacological analgesics. Providing analgesia has been largely ignored in prehospital care education.[1] Few EMS texts devote any significant attention to this topic. Most systems do not even have protocols to treat pain and suffering other than ischemic chest pain. Prehospital providers are frustrated by not being able to offer patients more than the "bite the bullet" approach to providing relief from acute pain.

Few clinical studies have examined the safety and efficacy of analgesics in the field.[6–14] All healthcare providers must make the provision of relief of pain and suffering one of their most important responsibilities in both the hospital and prehospital settings. This philosophy recognizes that all clinicians must be guided by the principle of "First, do no harm" and that some patients seen in the field may be so physiologically compromised that analgesia may need to be delayed. However, this group of patients is the minority of those seen in the field with moderate-to-severe pain. It should be stressed that there are many pathological consequences of untreated acute pain.[2] This philosophy was well summarized by Evans when he said "To allow a patient to suffer unnecessary pain does harm to the patient—a violation of the first ethical principle of medicine."[15] In a recent editorial Baskett states "The blame for 'oligoanalgesias' must be laid at the door of physicians in authority who have, through ignorance, underplayed the physiologic and psychological benefits of analgesia and overplayed the potential of deleterious side effects of agents that are commonly available."[16]

Unfortunately, no ideal analgesic exists; however, to simply delay the administration of any agents until arrival at the hospital is inhumane in many cases. The agents to be discussed are nitrous oxide, opioids, ketamine, and nonsteroidal anti-inflammatories. Another vital aspect of patient care for pain is the use of proper communication techniques.

Nitrous Oxide

Nitrous oxide-oxygen mixtures fulfill many of the properties desired for a prehospital analgesic.[17–19] Sev-

In choosing an analgesic for the field, desirable properties should be—

1. Safety.
2. Efficacy.
3. Ease of administration.
4. Rapid onset.
5. Short duration.
6. Low abuse potential for patient and staff.
7. Reversible.

FIGURE 56.1. *Desired characteristics.*

eral field studies have demonstrated the safety and efficacy of self-administered 50% nitrous oxide in prehospital care.[20–22] All studies have confirmed that the majority of patients with moderate-to-severe pain from a variety of sources will achieve significant pain relief. In a 16-year study of over 2,700 patients in the city of Pittsburgh, significant analgesia was achieved in over 80% of patients.[23] One of the major advantages of the use of nitrous oxide is that it is relatively devoid of serious side effects. In 1994, an alert entitled "Controlling exposure of nitrous oxide during anesthetic administration" provided guidelines to prevent environmental levels from exceeding their recommended standards. In a moving vehicle, or one with a fan, short-term administration should be safe for the providers; although well designed protocols must be written and followed in using this gas mixture. A prototype of a nitrous oxide protocol concludes this chapter; it includes the absolute and relative contraindications to nitrous oxide administration.[24]

Opioids

Opioid analgesics have been used in many systems for over two decades. In most, morphine sulfate is the analgesic of choice for ischemic chest pain that is not relieved with administration of nitrates.[25] For noncardiac pain, most physicians have been reluctant to use opioids such as morphine because of exaggerated fears of producing side effects. For many types of pain, opioids can be titrated by the IV route to produce safe and effective analgesia.[13,26] One of the major benefits of opioids is that most side effects can be rapidly reversed with an opioid antagonist, such as naloxone, which is carried by most EMS systems.

Fentanyl is an opioid that is rarely available on ground ambulances, but it has been well described for helicopter use. A study done in air-transported patients with fractures showed that fentanyl could be administered safely and effectively in the prehospital environment.[27] The same authors also demonstrated that fentanyl could be safely used in the air transport of pediatric trauma patients.[27] It has many potential advantages for the prehospital environment. Fentanyl is much more potent than morphine due to its lipid solubility, ability to cross the blood-brain barrier, and ability to bind to opiate receptors. The desirable characteristics of fentanyl include short half-life and duration of action of 60 minutes or less; lack of histamine release is important since release of histamine results in vasodilation. Opioid-induced hypotension is rare with fentanyl, but in patients who are only able to maintain normal systemic pressure due to extreme sympathetic drive, fentanyl can blunt the sympathetic response and theoretically lower blood pressure. Should this occur, fluid administration or alpha-adrenergic agents are used to restore blood pressure.

One of the newer opioids which may have some future use in the prehospital environment is remifentanil.[28] The advantage of this agent is that it is a potent, quick-acting opioid with a very short half-life. Due to the fact that this drug is metabolized in the plasma by hydrolysis, it has a half-life of less than ten minutes. There are no descriptions in the literature of the use of this agent, but for brief procedures such as splinting or other acutely painful states, there may be some benefit to its use in the field environment.

Opioid Agonist-Antagonists

Some characteristics of the opioid agonist-antagonist class of analgesics make them ideally suited for prehospital use. Drugs in this group include nalbuphine and butorphanol. The primary benefits of this class are the ceiling on respiratory depression, minimal euphoria and limited abuse potential, lack of biliary spasm, and minimal hemodynamic effects. Stene described the prehospital use of nalbuphine in 46 patients with moderate-to-severe pain due to multiple trauma, burns, fractures, and intraabdominal conditions.[29] The agent was partially to completely effective in 89% of patients and was without any major untoward effects. Nalbuphine also causes very minimal, if any, hemodynamic changes. Since that early study, others have confirmed the value of intravenous nalbuphine in the field.[30,31] One of the other advantages of this drug is that it is not a controlled substance, easing some of the paperwork required when using morphine. Butorphanol is now available as a nasal spray.[32,33] This agent and route of administration have many theoretical benefits in the prehospital environment, but studies have yet to be reported on the field use of nasal butorphanol. The use of the agonist/antagonist class of analgesics in the field may result in patients in the ED requiring somewhat higher doses of pure opiate agonists to achieve adequate analgesia.[34]

Ketamine

Ketamine is a dissociative anesthetic that is structurally related to phencyclidine, and it has some unique properties. The dissociative state produced by ketamine is characterized by analgesia and amnesia, while preserving airway protective reflexes.[35–37] Since ketamine is a bronchodilator, it can be used to treat severe asthma.[38,39] While this agent has little indication for routine prehospital care, it can be used as a field anesthetic for unusual situations, such as field amputations.[40] Ketamine has also been described as a useful agent for field surgical procedures during disasters, especially among children.[41]

Non-Steroidal Anti-Inflammatory Agents

Currently few EMS systems routinely use aspirin, acetaminophen, or other non-steroidal anti-inflammatory (NSAID) drugs or specific COX-2 inhibitors. Aspirin is now the standard of care as an antiplatelet drug in the treatment of acute myocardial infarction. Now that parenteral NSAIDs and COX-2 inhibitors are available, this class may have an expanded prehospital role as an analgesic. NSAIDs are particularly well suited for treatment of urethral and biliary colic.[42] These drugs may also potentiate the analgesic action of opiates.[43] While these agents do not work as quickly as opiates, if given at the scene they will frequently have beneficial effect before the patient arrives at the hospital. These agents should not be considered as a substitute for opiates and nitrous oxide but as another helpful adjunct with selected indications. The major side effects to consider with a single-dose use in the field would be allergic reactions and platelet inhibition. They should therefore be withheld in the field if the patient has known allergies to NSAIDs or if the antiplatelet effect may exacerbate an underlying problem.

Communication Techniques

The most ignored aspect of providing prehospital relief to those with pain and suffering is the powerful effects that can result from therapeutic communication techniques.[44] These techniques can be mastered by all providers and can bring a significant degree of comfort to patients without use of pharmacological agents. Jacobs points out that many patient responses to an injury or illness are occurring at an unconscious level and that "every word, phrase, sentence, pause, voice inflection, and gesture can initiate automatic psycho-physiologic effect."[45] An example of a suggested dialogue for a patient with burns is as follows:

"I'll bet you can imagine some place you'd rather be than here. As a matter of fact, go ahead and do that now while we get you bandaged up. Think of your favorite place. When you are there in your mind's eye, look around and notice all the things there are to notice. Listen to the sounds. Feel the good feelings. There might even be a special aroma you can smell. When you are really experiencing that place, let me know by raising your index finger. Good."

While many prehospital providers may feel uncomfortable with guided imagery techniques such as this, they all should recognize the powerful implications of their verbal and nonverbal communication. Providers should be capable of engaging patients in a way that distracts them from their injury or illness.

Distraction can also be very helpful while prehospital providers are performing potentially painful interventions, such as starting an IV line or splinting a fracture. Music has been shown to be effective in decreasing pain of laceration repair in emergency departments, and could be adapted for use on an ambulance.

Words should be chosen carefully when communicating, "mild discomfort," is more useful than terms such as "bee sting," "prick," or "shot."

Pitfalls

The major pitfall regarding analgesia is the attitude that it should not be provided in the field, but should wait for hospital evaluation. Safe and effective prehospital pharmacological and non-pharmacological techniques are appropriate for the majority of patients. These techniques will not "mask" the diagnosis or worsen the patient's condition. Pain is subjective and should be measured by the patient's words and not

The following protocol for the non-cardiac analgesia use of nitrous oxide stresses the psychological support that can be provided by prehospital caregivers.

1. Develop a rapport with the patient with appropriate reassurance and encouragement.
2. Properly prepare the equipment necessary to administer the gas.
3. Offer nitrous oxide to the patient if there are no contraindications to its use. The patient should self-administer the gas via a mask or mouthpiece.

   NOTE: When using nitrous oxide-oxygen mixtures, remember that it induces a trancelike state in patients, thereby making them particularly sensitive to suggestion. This can be used to increase the therapeutic effect of the gas, but caution must be taken since idle conversation may be misinterpreted by the patient and have detrimental effects. Sample instructions would be "We're going to give you some oxygen with pain relieving medicine in it to help relieve your discomfort. To get the medicine, you have to hold the mask (or mouthpiece) firmly to your face and breathe normally. In a minute or two, you will feel calm and relaxed and you may feel a little drowsy. Your arms and legs may feel a little heavy as you begin to feel more comfortable. Just relax and let the medicine work for you."

4. Immobilization and splinting if necessary.
5. Gentle handling and movement.
6. Monitor the patient's vital signs every 5–10 minutes.

Contraindications

1. Obvious intoxication
2. Altered level of consciousness
3. Pregnancy (except during labor)*
4. Suspected pneumothorax
5. Decompression sickness
6. Suspected bowel obstruction
7. Patients with blood pressure <90 mmHg or respirations <8
8. Chronic obstructive pulmonary disease (COPD)*

*This is a relative contraindication

Notes

1. All inflow ventilating fans must be operating in the patient compartment during administration of this agent.
2. Studies have shown that female dental assistants have a higher rate of spontaneous abortions if they work around nitrous oxide than a control group. The exact risk is not clear but it would seem to be a reasonable policy to have female prehospital providers who are considering pregnancy or may possibly be pregnant to limit their total time in the patient-care compartment of the ambulance when nitrous oxide is being used. Finally, it is also desirable for EMS systems to monitor the use of the agent with a log and consider using a locking system to limit the temptation of providers to abuse the agent.

Cases

Case 1

The paramedics are called to see a 25-year-old male complaining of severe lumbar pain that started while lifting a refrigerator. The vital signs are blood pressure of 130/86, pulse 88, and respiration of 14. The neurological examination and remainder of examination are unremarkable.

How would you direct the care of this patient?
The paramedics' appropriate treatment of this patient's pain should involve a kind, compassionate, caring approach combined with the use of nitrous oxide if available. The nitrous oxide should be started before any attempt is made to move the patient. The efficacy of the nitrous oxide will be improved if the paramedics present the benefits and efficacy of inhalational analgesia to the patient in a positive light. It also cannot be overemphasized how important gentle handling is in cases such as this. Patients are very quick to gauge how caring the providers are in terms of language, nonverbal communication, and patient handling.

Case 2

The paramedics call to direct medical oversight to report that they are seeing a 70-year-old male complaining of severe abdominal pain radiating to his groin. The vital signs are a blood pressure of 70 by palpation with a pulse of 120 and a respiratory rate of 20. The patient has a past history of hypertension and coronary artery disease.

How would you direct the care of this patient?
This is one of the few times where the axiom "First do no harm" precludes the initial use of a pharmacological analgesic. This presentation is very compatible with a ruptured abdominal aortic aneurysm. Because of the major hemodynamic instability that is occurring in this patient, the primary consideration should be very rapid transport to the hospital, with communication with the receiving facility to allow the hospital to begin preparation for the staff and resources that may be necessary to save this patient's life. Patient communication techniques may actually be very calming. Even the presentation of oxygen in a positive reassuring way can allay some anxiety.

Case 3

You are asked to give orders on a 22-year-old female who was working in a restaurant and had hot oil spilled over both lower extremities with resultant 10% body surface second- and possibly third-degree burns.

How would you direct the care of this patient?
This patient would be a candidate for use of 50% nitrous oxide or an IV opioid. If nitrous oxide was not available or was ineffective, there should be no reluctance to slowly titrate IV opioids such as morphine. The goal would not be total elimination of all pain but achieving the state where the patient is relatively comfortable and able to tolerate the pain.

FIGURE 56.2. *Nitrous Oxide/Non-Cardiac Pain Protocol.*

expectations of how much a patient should be suffering for a given condition.

Another pitfall is to believe that there is a "uniform" dose of analgesic that will bring elimination of pain when using pharmacological therapy. Particularly with the use of opioids, there is tremendous interpatient variability. The best way to approach is to slowly titrate, monitoring for side effects and efficacy, until the desired result is reached.

A particularly common pitfall is the belief that the degree of pain can be gauged by vital signs or facial expressions. The pain literature repeatedly documents the unreliability of either vital signs or facial expression in assessing the severity of pain. The only scale that should be used is verbal expression. A helpful technique to use is a 1–10 verbal analogue scale, with 10 representing the worst pain the patient has ever experienced.

Another pitfall is to fail to distract the patient while performing painful procedures. Just the opposite usually occurs where the provider calls attention to every step of the procedure, using terms that are intended to soften the insult but usually actually magnify it.

Summary

Treating acute pain and relieving suffering should be a primary missions of all healthcare providers. Unfortunately, EMS providers have not been given the tools or training to satisfactorily accomplish this worthy mission. While patient "safety" and "doing no harm" must always be considered, these should not be used as excuses for "doing no good" for patients with acute pain treated in the field.

References

1. Stewart RD. Pain control in prehospital care. In: Paris PM, Stewart RD, eds. *Pain management in emergency medicine*. Norwalk, CT: Appleton & Lange; 1987:19:313–321.
2. Clinical Practice Guideline. Acute pain management: Operative or medical procedures and trauma. Agency for Health Care Policy and Research, U.S. Department of Health and Human Services, AHCPR Pub. No. 92-0032. Rockville, MD, 1992.
3. Alonso-Serra H. National Association of EMS Physicians: Standards and Clinical Practice Committee, 2001. (to be published)
4. Verdile VP, Stewart RD. The prehospital management of pain. In: May HL, ed. *Emergency medicine*. 2nd ed. Boston: Little, Brown; 1992:626–630.
5. Stewart RD. Analgesia in the field. *Prehosp Disaster Med.* 1989;4:31–35.
6. DeVellis P, Thomas SH, Wedel SK. Prehospital and emergency department analgesia for air-transported patients with fractures. *Prehosp Emerg Care.* 1998;2:293–296.
7. Thomas SH, Benevelli W, Brown DF, Wedel SK. Safety of Fentanyl for analgesia in adults undergoing air medical transport from trauma scenes. *Air Med J.* 1996;15:57–59.
8. Kozak FJ, Chapman C, Hart MM. Utilization of pain medication in the out-of-hospital setting [abstract]. *Prehosp Emerg Care.* 1997;1:180.
9. Chambers JA, Guly HR. The need for better prehospital analgesia. *Arch Emerg Med.* 1993;10:187–192.
10. Ricard-Hibon A, Leroy N, Magn M, et al. [Evaluation of acute pain in prehospital medicine]. *Ann Fr Anesth Reanim.* 1997;16:945–949.
11. Stene JK, Stofberg L, MacDonald G, et al. Nalbuphine analgesia in the prehospital setting. *Am J Emerg.* 1988;6:634–639.
12. White LJ, Cooper JD, Chambers RM, Gradisek RD. Prehospital use of analgesia for suspected extremity fractures. *Prehosp Emerg Care.* 2000;4:205–208.
13. Gray A, Johnson G, Goodacre S. Paramedic use of nalbuphine in major injury. *Eur J of Emerg Med.* 1997;4:136–139.
14. Ricard-Hibon A, Chollet C, Saada S, et al. A quality control program for acute pain management in out-of-hospital critical care medicine. *Ann Emerg Med.* 1999;34:738–744.
15. Evans WO. The undertreatment of pain. *Indiana Med.* 1988;81:848–850.
16. Baskett PJ. Acute pain management in the field. *Ann Emerg Med.* 1999;34:784–785.
17. Stewart RD. Nitrous oxide. In: Paris PM, Stewart RD, eds. *Pain management in Emergency Medicine*. Norwalk, CT: Appleton & Lange; 1988:221–239.
18. Burton JH, Stewart RD. Nitrous oxide. In: Paris PM, Grass JA, eds. *Textbook of Acute Pain Management*. W.B. Saunders. (in preparation)
19. Paris PM, Yealy DM. Pain management. In: Rosen P, et al, eds. *Emergency Medicine*. 5th ed. St Louis: Mosby Year Book.
20. Johnson JC, Atherton GL. Effectiveness of nitrous oxide in rural EMS system. *J Emerg Med.* 1991;9:45–53.
21. Yealy DM, Paris PM, Kaplan RM, et al. The safety of prehospital naloxone administration by paramedics. *Ann Emerg Med.* 1990;19:902–905.
22. Donen N, Tweed WA, White D, et al. Prehospital analgesia with Entonox. *Can Anaesth Soc J.* 1982;29:275–279.
23. Personal conversation between Paul M. Paris, MD and Richard Kaplan, MD.
24. Mosesso V, Stewart RD, Paris PM, et al. *City of Pittsburgh ALS Protocols* (adaptation); 1994.
25. Bruns BM, Dieckmann R, Shagoury C, et al. Safety of prehospital therapy with morphine sulfate. *Am J Emerg Med.* 1992;10:53–57.
26. Paris PM, Weiss LD. Narcotic analgesics: the pure agonists. In: Paris PM, Stewart RD, eds. *Pain Management in Emergency Medicine*. Norwalk, CT: Appleton & Lange; 1988:125–156.

27. DeVellis P, Thomas SH, Wedel SK, et al. Prehospital Fentanyl analgesia in air-transported pediatric trauma patients. *Ped Emerg Care*. 1998;14:321–323.

28. Glass PS, Gan TJ, Howell S. A review of the pharmacokinetics and pharmacodynamics of remifentanil. *Anes Analg*. 1999;84:S7–14.

29. Stene JK, Stofberg L, MacDonald G, et al. Nalbuphine analgesic in the prehospital setting. *Am J Emerg Med*. 1988;6:634–639.

30. Hyland-McGuire P, Guly HR. Effects on patient care of introducing prehospital intravenous nalbuphine hydrochloride. *J Accid Emerg Med*. 1998;15:99–101.

31. Chambers JA, Guly HR. Prehospital intravenous nalbuphine administered by paramedics. *Resuscitation*. 1994;27:153–158.

32. Joyce TH, Kubicek MF, Skjonsby BS, et al. Efficacy of transnasal butorphanol titrate in postepisiotomy pain: a model to assess analgesia. *Clin Ther*. 1993;15:160–167.

33. Diamond S, Freitag FG, Diamond ML, et al. Transnasal butorphanol in the treatment of migraine headache pain. *Headache Quarterly, Cut Ther and Res*. 1992;3:164-170.

34. Houlihan KP, Mitchell RG, Flapan AD, Steedman DJ. Excessive morphine requirements after prehospital nalbuphine analgesia. *J Accid Emerg Med*. 1999;16:29–31.

35. Bennett CR, Stewart RD. Ketamine. In: Paris PM, Stewart RD, eds. *Pain Management in Emergency Medicine*. Norwalk, CT: Appleton & Lange; 1988:295–310.

36. Green SM, Rothrock SG, Lynch EL, et al. Intramuscular ketamine for pediatric sedation in the emergency department: safety profile in 1,022 cases. *Ann Emerg Med*. 1998;31:688–697.

37. Green SM, Clem KJ, Rothrock SG. Ketamine safety profile in the developing world—survey of practitioners. *Acad Emerg Med*. 1996;3:598–604.

38. Sarma VJ. Use of ketamine in acute severe asthma. *Acta Anaesthesiol Scand*. 1992;36:106–107.

39. Jahangir WM, Islam L. Ketamine infusion for post-operative analgesia in asthmatics: a comparison with intermittent meperidine. *Anesth Analg*. 1993;76:45–49.

40. Bioin JF. Infusion analgesia for acute war injuries: a comparison of pentazocine and ketamine. *Anaesthesia*. 1984;39:560–564.

41. Dick W, Hirlinger WK, Mehrkens HH. Intramuscular ketamine: an alternative pain treatment for use in disasters? In: Manni C, Magnalini SI, eds. *Emergency and Disaster Medicine: Proceedings of the Third World Congress in Rome, 1983*. Berlin: Springer-Verlag, 1985:167–172.

42. Goldman G. Biliary colic treatment and acute cholecystitis prevention by prostaglandin inhibitor. *Dig Dis Sci*. 1989;34:809–811.

43. ParisPM, Stewart RD. Analgesia and sedation. In: Rosen P, ed. *Emergency Medicine: Concepts and Clinical Practice*. 3rd ed. St Louis: Mosby-Year Book; 1992:201–229.

44. Goldfarb B. Prehospital pain management: providing physical and psychological care. *Prehosp Care Reports*. 1992;2:73–80.

45. Jacobs TJ. *Patient communications*, Englewoods Cliffs, NJ: Brady; 1991.

Shortness of Breath

Thomas D. Fowlkes, MD

Introduction

Shortness of breath (SOB) is one of the most frequently encountered complaints in the out-of-hospital setting. The patient with dyspnea presents one of the most challenging management problems for both the out-of-hospital care provider and the direct medical oversight physician. Early interventions can frequently lead to dramatic patient improvement prior to arrival at the hospital. Unfortunately, there has been little research on the out-of-hospital management of patients with dyspnea.

In the emergency department (ED), the assessment of the patient with respiratory distress can be difficult even for an experienced physician with assistance of tests not available to the out-of-hospital care provider, such as radiography and EKG. The challenge for the direct medical oversight physician is to rely entirely on the history and physical findings as relayed by the provider to form a working diagnosis and initiate out-of-hospital therapy. The physician must be cognizant that the perceptions of the out-of-hospital provider may be influenced by commonly disseminated misperceptions regarding the relationship of selected signs and symptoms and ultimate diagnosis. Until very recently, there have been almost no objective measures of the severity of respiratory distress in the field.

The risk-to-benefit ratio must be weighed for each intervention contemplated for use in the out-of-hospital setting. Treatments that are indicated for certain conditions are contraindicated in other conditions. Some of the treatments for specific illnesses may harm the patient if the out-of-hospital diagnosis is incorrect. The interventions that may be used in a given out-of-hospital setting depend on the level of training and skill of the providers, as well as the extent of direct medical oversight.

Evaluation

When presented with a case of respiratory distress, the direct medical oversight physician must form an initial differential diagnosis of possible etiologies. Of these, life-threatening conditions must be rapidly identified and appropriately treated. For most paramedics, the major differential diagnosis of a patient with SOB is bronchospasm versus congestive heart failure (CHF). They often have protocols that are broken down into these two entities, but they tend not to think of other common, potentially life-threatening illnesses, such as pulmonary embolus or pneumonia. Table 57.1 is a partial list of the differential diagnosis of the patient with dyspnea. Given the unreliability of physical findings in patients with dyspnea and the variability in paramedics' skill in interpreting these subjective findings, objective measurements may greatly enhance our ability to focus our evaluation and treatment.

In the future, objective measures of airway obstruction, oxygenation, and ventilation will be used to assess the severity of respiratory distress and help

TABLE 57.1
Non-Traumatic Etiologies of Dyspnea
■ Bronchospasm: Asthma, Emphysema, Bronchitis, COPD
■ Cardiogenic pulmonary edema—CHF
■ Non-cardiogenic pulmonary edema—ARDS
■ Spontaneous pneumothorax
■ Pneumonia
■ Pulmonary embolus
■ Physiological hyperventilation (e.g., metabolic acidosis)
■ Psychogenic
■ Upper airway obstruction
■ Pleural effusion
■ Neuromuscular disease
■ Anaphylaxis

differentiate the etiology. Pulse oximetry is rapidly becoming the standard of care. It provides an easily used and non-invasive means of reliably detecting hypoxemia in the field.[1,2] Field studies have shown that a significant number of cases of hypoxemia detected by pulse oximetry were not suspected on clinical grounds.[3] At present, cost is the primary impediment to its widespread use in the field. However, the cost savings to systems from reduced oxygen usage for non-hypoxemic patients may offset the cost of the pulse oximeters.[4] Capnography is already established as a reliable means of confirming endotracheal tube placement, and in the future may be useful in the field to assess the adequacy of ventilation. Measurements of peak expiratory flow rates (PEFR) provide an objective measurement of airflow obstruction. An ED study suggested that the PEFR could be used to differentiate CHF from COPD, but a field study done to confirm this initial report failed to show benefit of this modality to make a diagnostic differentiation.[5,6] Although theoretically PEFR could be used to objectively measure the degree of airway obstruction, one small field study showed that it was difficult to obtain accurate readings.[7] In the ED, use of the PEFR has become the standard of care to grade the severity of airway obstruction in asthma, and to guide therapy.[8]

Without the use of technology as such, the direct medical oversight physician should be very attuned to asking "how many word" dyspnea a patient has. When a patient has less than 5 word dyspnea the condition should be considered severe, requiring aggressive interventions.

Treatment

As with all fields of medicine, the basic premise of out-of-hospital care must be: "First, do no harm." The goal of the medical director should be to treat those life-threatening conditions that are treatable in the field without worsening other potentially serious medical conditions if the out-of-hospital diagnosis is incorrect.

There has been very little research on the out-of-hospital treatment of patients with respiratory distress. MacLeod evaluated 118 patients presenting with SOB in an urban EMS system with direct medical oversight, and found that when the ED diagnosis was bronchospasm or CHF, the out-of-hospital diagnosis was correct 86% and 82% of the time respectively.[9] For these two conditions, appropriate treat-

ment was given in 98% and 92% respectively. In 24 patients with other ED diagnoses, out-of-hospital diagnosis matched ED diagnosis in only 33% of cases, but acceptable treatment was given in 79%. This study shows that paramedics are able to evaluate and treat appropriately the common conditions of bronchospasm and CHF with direct medical oversight. For other diseases, paramedics are less accurate in their assessment but appropriate treatment (primarily supportive) is usually given. It must be emphasized that these findings cannot be generalized to other EMS systems or other levels of providers without analysing the direct medical oversight component.

Bronchospasm (COPD/Asthma)

Often the diagnosis of bronchospasm is strongly suggested by the past history and the patient's medications, and confirmed by typical findings on physical examination. It is helpful to ascertain the severity of prior episodes, especially the need for previous intubation, steroids, and/or oxygen dependence.

Prehospital provider training has traditionally overemphasized the possible precipitation of respiratory arrest by use of high-flow oxygen in COPD patients who retain carbon dioxide. Clearly one of the most lethal problems in COPD patients is hypoxia, and an important goal of out-of-hospital treatment should be to correct hypoxemia. Providers are sometimes reluctant to use more than nasal cannulas for the bronchospastic patient. Venturi masks provide precise oxygen concentrations between 24% and 50%, and it is not unreasonable to begin oxygen therapy with these or low-flow oxygen via nasal cannula. However, if the patient shows signs of hypoxemia or is even suspected of being hypoxemic, higher-flow oxygen should be used as necessary to correct the hypoxemia. The likelihood of precipitating respiratory arrest is very small and can be dealt with by providers trained in advanced airway management. Even if unable to intubate, the provider can usually adequately ventilate the patient with a bag-valve-mask. In the future, more widespread use of pulse oximetry in the field should greatly enhance the ability to recognize and treat hypoxemia.

Inhaled beta$_2$-agonists have emerged as the first-line treatment of bronchospasm both in the ED and in the field. Inhaled beta$_2$-agonists have been shown to be a safe and effective treatment for reactive airway disease in the field. Providers can be trained to reliably distinguish patients who will benefit from beta$_2$-

agonists by the history, physical examination, and medications. In addition, few side effects from inhaled selective beta$_2$-agonists are seen.[10]

Beta$_2$-agonists may be given parenterally or inhaled via metered dose inhaler (MDI) or nebulized aerosol. Previously, subcutaneous epinephrine or terbutaline have been used extensively for bronchospasm; however, the inhaled route has replaced this procedure as the first choice because fewer side effects are seen and the drug is directly delivered to the site of action. Subcutaneous beta-agonists may still be used as adjunctive treatment in severe bronchospasm in the young asthmatic or as treatment of anaphylaxis; they should be used as last resorts in the older COPD/asthma patient with possible coronary artery disease.

Nebulized aerosol and MDI delivery of beta$_2$-agonists have been shown to be equally effective when used appropriately; however, good hand-breath coordination is required.[11] This may not be possible for patients in severe respiratory distress.[12] Therefore, nebulized aerosol is recommended for out-of-hospital use. The recommended dose for aerosol treatments is albuterol 2.5 mg or metaproterenol 5% solution 0.3 cc in 2.5 cc saline. For severe bronchospasm, this dose may be repeated or may be used continuously during the transport. For small children, one-half the adult dose is appropriate. Nebulized aerosols can also be successfully used when applied to a tracheostomy site. For out-of-hospital use, the nebulized aerosol treatment should be powered by oxygen from a portable oxygen supply.

Intravenous aminophylline, once a common out-of-hospital modality, now has few field indications. It has largely been replaced by the more efficacious beta$_2$-agonists. In addition, the low therapeutic index and the need for drug-level monitoring, along with serious doubts about its beneficial effects in the acute management of bronchospasm, have resulted in much less use of aminophylline in out-of-hospital settings.

One of the most difficult situations a provider can face is a patient who has bronchospasm and severe hypoxia, who is combative and agitated, and who is not allowing therapeutic interventions to be initiated. One agent that may offer theoretical benefit in this difficult situation is ketamine. Ketamine is a dissociative anesthetic that also causes bronchodilation. Despite a report of five cases in the emergency department setting, and anecdotal evidence of field benefit, there are no published field trials of this agent.[13]

Dyspnea in a patient with COPD may be secondary to CHF, pneumonia, pneumothorax, pulmonary embolus, or arrhythmias. Treatment must keep those possible disorders in mind. Bronchospasm may play a role in CHF; thus, patients with CHF may benefit from, as well as not be harmed by, beta$_2$-agonists. The direct medical oversight physician (DMOP) should err in favor of beta$_2$-agonists when the exact diagnosis is in doubt.

Congestive Heart Failure (CHF)

The working diagnosis of acute pulmonary edema is clearest when there is no previous history of COPD/asthma and there is a prior history of CHF, coronary artery disease, or hypertension. A recent retrospective study shows a reduction in mortality for those patients with a discharge diagnosis of CHF who received out-of-hospital treatment with nitroglycerin, furosemide, or morphine compared with those patients who received only oxygen. However, there was also an apparent increase in mortality in those patients who were "mistreated" with the above medications but who ultimately had a diagnosis other than CHF.[14]

There is some evidence to suggest that nitrates are the preferred first-line treatment in the out-of-hospital treatment of pulmonary edema. In a out-of-hospital study by Hoffman of presumed pulmonary edema, patients who received nitroglycerin and furosemide fared better than patients who received morphine and furosemide.[15] These results should be interpreted cautiously, however, since there were several methodological problems with the study. Another important finding of this study was that 23% of the patients were ultimately given a diagnosis other than pulmonary edema.

The beneficial effects of nitroglycerin in pulmonary edema are well described.[16] The primary side effect of nitroglycerin is hypotension, which can be a problem in the patient who is already relatively hypotensive or dehydrated.[17] Often the hypotension, which may be accompanied by bradycardia, is transient and resolves spontaneously or with symptomatic therapy.[18] Hypertensive patients with pulmonary edema should be treated aggressively. Initially two sublingual 0.4 mg nitroglycerin should be administered and then 1 to 2 every 3 to 5 minutes as long as the systolic blood pressure is maintained above 120. Although certainly not widely used at present, Bertini found in a retrospective study that the out-of-hospital use of intravenous nitrates improved the short-term prognosis in acute pulmonary edema.[19]

Morphine can be used as a second-line treatment, but one must keep in mind the risks and benefits. Although all of the actions of morphine in CHF are not well understood, it clearly reduces myocardial oxygen consumption by decreasing both preload and afterload. There is some research to suggest that it also may increase coronary blood flow.[20] Another advantage is the decrease in anxiety of the patient that may facilitate increased cooperation. Morphine, however, can decrease the respiratory drive, especially if the underlying condition is not CHF, although this concern is probably overstated. It may also cause hypotension, which may not respond to opioid antagonists, but frequently responds to fluid administration.

Another second-line agent in the out-of-hospital treatment of CHF is furosemide. There has been much debate regarding furosemide as a venodilator, but clearly it has a role in the treatment of CHF as a diuretic. Therefore, in patients with severe CHF, especially if already on furosemide, out-of-hospital treatment with approximately twice the oral dose will at the very least minimize the delay in diuretic therapy, and may improve outcome.

The newest modality being studied for field treatment of pulmonary edema is CPAP (continuous positive airway pressure). In the ED, this modality is gaining support as a means to quickly improve pulmonary edema, decreasing the need for endotracheal intubation.[21] A prospective study is testing the feasibility of administering CPAP to patients with presumed cardiogenic pulmonary edema in the field.[22]

Upper Airway Obstruction

While upper airway obstruction in adults is uncommon, it is a life-threatening emergency and must be considered in patients with acute respiratory distress. Foreign-body aspiration is the most frequent cause in children. The diagnosis may be suggested by a history of onset while eating and the presence of inspiratory distress or stridor, as opposed to expiratory distress with bronchospasm. Recently, there has been more recognition of retropharyngeal infections, including epiglottitis, as a cause of airway obstruction in adults. In addition, angioedema secondary to ACE inhibitors is increasing.

It is critical to rapidly identify the choking victim and to relieve the obstruction with the Heimlich maneuver or with direct laryngoscopy and Magill forceps. If these maneuvers are not successful and the patient cannot be ventilated, field cricothyrotomy or jet ventilation may be lifesaving. Jet ventilation can be taught to paramedics but is usually not included in the standard paramedic curriculum. Special equipment, including a direct connection to a 50-psi O_2 source, is required. It must be remembered that standard 15-lpm O_2 or a BVM connected to a trans-tracheal catheter will not provide adequate ventilation.[23]

Pneumonia

Pneumonia is especially common in patients with COPD, alcoholism, or immunosuppression, and in elderly or institutionalized patients. The diagnosis may be suggested by cough, sputum production, fever/chills, or a friction rub. Pneumonia is infrequently considered by providers in the field. Rales commonly are heard with pneumonia and often equated with CHF by paramedics. The presence of rales alone often prompts a request for furosemide, nitroglycerine, and morphine. Field treatment is primarily supportive with oxygen to treat hypoxemia, although bronchodilators may help alleviate dyspnea caused by reactive airways. If the patient has a fever and is clinically dehydrated, fluid resuscitation would be indicated.

Pulmonary Embolus

Pulmonary (PE) embolus is a relatively common life-threatening condition that is under-considered in the field. Out-of-hospital treatment is primarily supportive, but the advent of thrombolytic treatment requires the DMOP to consider this diagnosis and ensure expeditious transport. The most common symptoms of a pulmonary embolus are chest pain and shortness of breath, but atypical presentations are as much the rule as the exception. Treatment for CHF, especially furosemide and nitroglycerin, can potentially have adverse effects for the hemodynamically unstable patient with a pulmonary embolus.

Pneumothorax

Spontaneous pneumothorax is an uncommon cause of dyspnea. Pleuritic chest pain is often a prominent component, but the history and physical findings are notoriously unreliable. Fortunately, only 1% to 2% of spontaneous pneumothoraces progress to tension pneumothoraces. Tension pneumothorax is a clinical, not a radiographic, diagnosis. Provider curricula include the signs of tension pneumothorax, but some providers are not trained in needle decompression. Protocols should include specific indications for needle decompression (i.e., unilateral diminished breath sounds with tracheal deviation and hypotension or cyanosis). This intervention is dangerous if the diagnosis is incorrect, but lifesaving if there is a tension pneumothorax.

Protocols

The development of protocols for treating the adult non-trauma patient with respiratory distress is difficult. It is impractical to have one protocol for all cases of respiratory distress so it is necessary to construct protocols for the different problems that require different treatments in the field (upper airway obstruction, bronchospasm, acute pulmonary edema, and anaphylaxis). Integral to these protocols is an outline of the relevant history and physical findings that guide the provider to the appropriate protocol. Each protocol should include specific indications and exclusions for its use.

In addition, guidelines for determining the severity of respiratory distress should be included. Early direct medical oversight contact should be mandated for cases of severe dyspnea. Cases of severe respiratory distress will benefit from early intubation.

Controversies

Perhaps the most common pitfall is that providers place too much reliance on a given physical finding to diagnose the etiology of dyspnea. Physical findings are often unreliable despite the experience of the examiner, and do not necessarily correlate with the severity of respiratory distress.

This problem is compounded, since the differential diagnosis for SOB is often CHF versus COPD. There is a common misunderstanding that rales equal CHF and wheezing equals asthma/COPD. Field providers are most often not accurate in their assessment of venous distention and pedal edema. Table 57.2 shows the large overlap in the physical findings that occurs in conditions causing dyspnea, particularly CHF and COPD.

The field team may draw a conclusion about what the underlying diagnosis is and then allow that bias to slant the report given to the DMOP. For example, it would not be unusual for a paramedic to examine a patient and find wheezing and attribute it to COPD as opposed to recognizing the possibility of "cardiac asthma." On the other hand, wheezing may be absent with severe airflow obstruction. The risks and

TABLE 57.2				
COPD vs. CHF				
	RALES	**WHEEZE**	**JVD**	**PEDAL EDEMA**
COPD	+	+++	++	+
CHF	+++	+	+++	++

Key:
+   May be present
++ Often present
+++ Usually present and prominent

benefits must be weighed before ordering treatment. There are risks if the working diagnosis is incorrect. The safety of various interventions for those two respiratory conditions are compared in table 57.3.

The DMOP should take into account the skills of the providers, the transport time, and the severity of the respiratory distress in determining which interventions will be performed in the field. In general, on-scene time for the severely dyspneic patient should be limited to approximately 10 minutes, unless endotracheal intubation is performed.

Psychogenic hyperventilation is a dangerous diagnosis to make over the radio. Many serious conditions such as pulmonary emboli, hypoxia, sepsis, and metabolic acidosis can be indistinguishable from psychogenic hyperventilation. Reassurance and oxygen are acceptable initial treatment for each of these conditions. Pulse oximetry is helpful in ruling out hypoxemia as a cause of hyperventilation. Having patients re-breathe into a paper bag should not be done, since it is clearly inappropriate treatment for the other, more serious possibilities.

One of the pitfalls that occurs regularly in asthma is for the provider to underestimate the severity of an asthma attack. The patient may not look severe, may have few wheezes, and may be thought to be improv-

TABLE 57.3					
Treatment of CHF vs. COPD					
	OXYGEN	**DIURETICS**	**BETA-AGONIST**	**NTG**	**MS**
COPD	+++	–	+++	+–	–
CHF	+++	++	+	+++	++

–   Potentially harmful
+– Risks exist, limited if any benefit
+   Limited risk, uncertain if any benefit
++ Useful but not without some side effects or risk
+++ Safe, minimal risk

ing, only to have the sudden onset of extremely severe dyspnea, agitation, and respiratory arrest.

Summary

Dyspnea is a common but unfortunately difficult complaint to diagnose and treat in the field. Providers are limited in their ability to accurately identify physical findings. Often the understanding of dyspnea is simply to equate rales with CHF and wheezing with COPD/asthma. The DMOP should rely on the patient's history, past medical history, and home medications to formulate a working diagnosis and to guide safe field treatment.

Supportive treatment (e.g., oxygen, airway management, prophylactic IV, monitor) and expeditious transport to the emergency department are always indicated. If the etiology is clear, aggressive treatment should be begun in the field, to attempt to avoid further deterioration and to improve outcome. However, the DMOP should keep foremost in his mind: "First, do no harm!"

Cases

Case 1

A 74-year-old male with a history of 4 previous MI's and "an enlarged heart" is seen by the paramedics after worsening SOB for the last 2 days. The patient has been unable to lie down to sleep at night and is unable to walk to the bathroom without severe dyspnea. He denies chest pain. Medications include digoxin, furosemide, and nitroglycerin, but his wife states he has been out of his meds for 4 days. Paramedics report patient sitting upright on couch in severe respiratory distress, able to speak only one to two words at a time. P-110 RR-32 BP-196/110, heart regular, sinus tach on monitor; lungs-rales throughout; abdomen-unremarkable; skin-diaphoretic; 2+ pedal edema.

HOW WOULD YOU DIRECT THE MANAGEMENT OF THIS PATIENT?

This case depicts classic CHF and will likely be recognized as such by both the paramedics and the DMOP. The challenge in this case is to provide aggressive enough treatment to turn this patient around and hopefully avoid intubation. Since the diagnosis is relatively certain and the blood pressure is elevated, aggressive use of sublingual nitroglycerin will provide

the most benefit. Also, since the patient has previously been on furosemide and has not had any for several days, IV furosemide would be appropriate. The severity of this case also warrants the judicious use of small, frequent doses of IV morphine sulfate, keeping in mind the caveats discussed above.

If the patient does not respond to initial treatments or his mental status deteriorates, the patient may require intubation and assisted ventilation. This is a potential candidate for awake, sitting nasal intubation if the paramedics are appropriately trained. The success of nasotracheal intubation by paramedics depends on adequate training and opportunity for practicing this skill. In addition, the availability of a CO_2 detection technique or some other reliable method to confirm endotracheal tube placement is highly desirable. This patient would also be an excellent candidate for CPAP or BiPAP.

Case 2

Paramedics are at a local nursing home where they were called for a 76-year-old female with SOB for approximately the last 4 hours. The patient also complains of right-sided chest pain that is worse with inspiration. Patient has a history of two prior CVAs and is completely bedridden due to left hemiparesis. No other significant past history. Vital signs include a pulse-116, respirations-28 and BP-104/68. The patient is alert and oriented in moderate respiratory distress. Her skin is warm/dry, without cyanosis; heart —regular, tachycardia; monitor-sinus tachycardia; lungs-rales in the bases; abdomen-soft, non-tender.

HOW WOULD YOU PROCEED?

In this scenario the diagnosis is unclear and the patient does not fit nicely into any of the specific protocols. The most likely diagnoses are pneumonia and pulmonary embolus, although certainly CHF and metabolic acidosis are possible. Given the patient's mental status and degree of respiratory distress, immediate intubation is not indicated. To avoid further complicating the picture or precipitating hemodynamic compromise, basic supportive measures (high-flow oxygen, IV of NS or LR, monitor) and expeditious transport should be adequate for this patient. Since this patient may have a pulmonary embolus and the blood pressure is only 104/68, a fluid challenge would be reasonable. Diuretics are potentially dangerous since the patient's volume status is not known.

Case 3

You are consulted by paramedics who are at the home of a 60-year-old female who has had worsening SOB and intermittent chest pain for the last 3 days. The patient currently does not have pain but is sitting upright in a dining room chair wearing home oxygen at 2 lpm and is only able to speak short phrases. She has a past history of "emphysema," requiring several hospitalizations and home oxygen. The patient also had a myocardial infarction 6 months ago. Her medications include Albuterol and Atrovent inhalers, Theodur, Lasix, Isordil, and Captopril. She is awake but slightly drowsy in moderate-to-severe respiratory distress. P-80 RR-36 BP-144/96; skin-slight cyanosis of nailbeds; heart-irregular, monitor-atrial fibrillation at 80; lungs-breath sounds decreased at bases, wheezes in upper fields bilaterally; abdomen-soft, non-tender.

HOW WOULD YOU PROCEED?

Directing field treatment in such cases is particularly difficult for the DMOP. Without actually examining the patient yourself and getting a chest x-ray, it is very difficult to determine whether this exacerbation is primarily due to COPD, CHF, or, as is more likely, a combination of the two. In such cases, supportive measures are paramount, with intubation as required by the clinical condition. Beyond this, specific treatments should only be used if they are unlikely to cause deterioration in the patient's condition if the working diagnosis is incorrect, and if they are likely to have a beneficial effect. (table 57.3.) Beta-agonist treatment would likely be useful in this case, since there is at least some degree of bronchospasm, and if the etiology is found to be primarily cardiac there would be limited risk.

References

1. McGuire TJ, Pointer JE. Evaluation of a pulse oximeter in the out-of-hospital setting. *Ann Emerg Med.* 1989;17:1058–1062.
2. Sughey K, Hess D, Eitel D, et al. An evaluation of pulse oximetry in out-of-hospital care. *Ann Emerg Med.* 1991;20:887–891.
3. Bota GW, Rowe BH. Continuous monitoring of oxygen saturation in out-of-hospital patients with severe illness: the problem of unrecognized hypoxemia. *J Emerg Med.* 1995;13:305–311.
4. Howes DW, et al. Justification of pulse oximeter costs for paramedic out-of-hospital providers. *Prehosp Emerg Care.* 2000;4:151–155.
5. McNamara RM, Cionni DJ. Utility of peak expiratory flow rate in the differentiation of acute dyspnea. *Chest.* 1992;101:129–132.
6. Kelly JM, Delbridge TR, Sullivan MP, et al. Assessment of the usefulness of peak expiratory flow rate to differentiate out-of-hospital CHF and COPD patients. *Prehosp Dis Med.* 1994;9(supp 3):S56.
7. Heller MB, Melton JB, Paris PM, et al. Data collection by paramedics for out of hospital research (abstract). *Ann Emerg Med.* 1988;17:414.
8. Rubsamen DS. The doctor, the asthmatic patient, and the law (editorial). *Ann Allergy.* 1993;71:493–494.
9. MacLeod BA, et al. The accuracy of out-of-hospital diagnosis in patients with dyspnea (abstract). *Ann Emerg Med.* 1990;19:459.
10. Eitel DR, et al. Out of hospital administration of inhaled metaproterenol. *Ann Emerg Med.* 1990;19:1412–1417.
11. Hawkins J, et al. Metered-dose aerosolized bronchodilators in out-of-hospital care: a feasibility study. *J Emerg Med.* 1986;4:273–277.
12. Cabanes LR, et al. Bronchial hyperresponsiveness to methacholine in patients with impaired left ventricular function. *N Engl J Med.* 1989;320:1317–1322.
13. L'Hommedieu CS, Arens JJ. The use of ketamine for the emergency intubation of patients with status asthmaticus. *Ann Emerg Med.* 1987;16:568–571.
14. Wuerz RC, Meador SA. Effect of out-of-hospital medications on mortality and length of stay in congestive heart failure. *Ann Emerg Med.* 1992;21:669–674.
15. Hoffman JR, Reynolds S. Comparison of nitroglycerin, morphine, and furosemide in treatment of presumed out-of-hospital pulmonary edema. *Chest.* 1987;92:586–593.
16. Bussman WD, Schapp D. Effects of sub-lingual nitroglycerin in emergency treatment of severe pulmonary edema. *Am J Cardiol.* 1978;41:931–934.
17. Wasserberger J, Balasubramaniam S. Complications in out-of-hospital use of nitroglycerin. *Ann Emerg Med.* 1982;11:116.
18. Wuerz R, Swope G, Meador S, et al. Safety of out-of-hospital nitroglycerin. *Ann Emerg Med.* 1994;23:31–36.
19. Bertini G, et al. Intravenous nitrates in the out of hospital management of acute pulmonary edema. *Ann Emerg Med.* 1997;30:493–499.
20. Leaman DM, Nellis SH, Zelis F, et al. Effects of morphine sulfate on human coronary blood flow. *Am J Cardiol.* 1978;41:324–326.
21. Bernsten AD, Holt AW, Vedig AE, et al. Treatment of severe cardiogenic pulmonary edema with continuous positive airway pressure delivered by face mask. *N Engl J Med.* 1991;325:1825–1830.
22. Kosowsky JM, Gasaway MD, et al. EMS transports for difficulty breathing: is there a potential role for CPAP in the out of hospital setting? *Acad Emerg Med.* 2000;7:1165.
23. Yealy DM, Plewa MC, Stewart RD. An evaluation of cannulae and oxygen sources for pediatric jet ventilation. *Amer J Emerg Med.* 1991;9:20–23.

Chest Pain

Sandra M. Schneider, MD
James I. Syrett, MD

Introduction

In the early 1960s out-of-hospital care of chest pain patients focused on rapid transport and in-hospital care. In 1967 Pantridge and Geddes reported successful resuscitation of 100% of 10 out-of-hospital cardiac arrest victims with 50% long-term survivors.[1] This led to modern advanced life support with increased capabilities in the field. In the case of cardiac ischemia nearly all techniques available for resuscitation (airway management, arrhythmia control, etc.) were introduced in the out-of-hospital practice. Field times increased. Although this was often misunderstood by non-emergency personnel, it allowed paramedics to assess patients, and provided stabilization at the scene before transport.

The goal of cardiac care has always been preservation of myocardial tissue. Rest, oxygenation, and prevention of hypotension in the field prevent further damage to the myocardium. However, this approach did little to reperfuse damaged tissue. Today ischemia can be reversed and myocardial tissue preserved if circulation is restored rapidly, through either thrombolysis or acute angioplasty within 6 hours. Rapid transport has again become the goal of acute out-of-hospital cardiac care. Time means myocardium.

Evaluation and Treatment

Chest pain is a common out-of-hospital complaint. In 1995 there were approximately 4.6 million ED visits for non-traumatic chest pain or 27.7 visits/ 1000 people.[2] But only 12% to 30% of patients presenting to an emergency department with chest pain are found to have an acute myocardial infarction.[3–5] Applying standard cardiac protocols for all patients with chest pain is not only expensive and time-consuming but at times may have detrimental results. Nitroglycerin, for example, can compromise patients whose chest pain results from a pulmonary embolism.

Thrombolytics may be deadly to a patient with aortic dissection.

A careful history can lead the out-of-hospital provider to a correct "category" of diagnosis most of the time. Since 100% accuracy in the diagnosis of chest pain is not possible, even with the advanced measures in the hospital utilizing technology and expertise, the out-of-hospital provider cannot be expected to accurately diagnose a patient. However, the out-of-hospital provider may be able to place the patient in a risk category based on the symptoms and modifying risk factors. At all times, however, the patient should be treated as if they have the most serious likely illness.

Cardiac Ischemia

Cardiac pain is usually, but not always, substernal, heavy, crushing discomfort that may radiate to the neck or arms. Radiation to the neck is particularly sensitive for cardiac disease.[6] Accompanying diaphoresis is a suggestive sign. Although cardiac disease is generally seen in middle-age men and older women, patients who use amphetamines or cocaine or those with insulin-dependent diabetes may have ischemic disease at a much younger age. Significant risk factors are listed in table 58.1.

TABLE 58.1
Risk Factors for Cardiac Ischemia
Smoking
Hypertension
Cocaine/Amphetamine Use
Male Gender
Hyperlipidemia
Women Post-menopausal
Family History
Congenital Heart Disease

Subtle details of the history can be extremely helpful to create an accurate suspicion of the correct diagnosis. Providers should be taught to obtain and report the important descriptors of chest pain that are sometimes remembered by use of the mnemonic PQRST (table 58.2).

Elderly patients and those with diabetes are more prone to have "silent" ischemia. These patients present with sudden onset of shortness of breath (flash pulmonary edema), diaphoresis, general weakness, or syncope.[7] Other patients may have an atypical presentation with isolated arm or jaw pain, epigastric discomfort, or (in some cases) back pain. Some patients experience typical symptoms but denial may lead to a history that is ambiguous or misleading. Repeated questioning and a healthy degree of suspicion can help identify these patients.

Although only a few patients with chest pain will actually have an acute myocardial infarction or even an ischemic cardiac pain, all patients with suggestive symptoms, especially those with risk factors, should be treated as if they have acute cardiac disease.

Patients should be monitored, have an IV established with fluids at a slow rate, and receive oxygen. All patients should receive aspirin unless contraindicated by allergy. Aspirin is a cheap and readily available treatment that has been shown to benefit patients with myocardial infarction. ISIS-2 established the beneficial effects of administering aspirin immediately during suspected acute myocardial infarction and its continuation for one month after the event. It was found that the absolute improvement from aspirin administration alone was 26 fewer deaths per 1000 patients treated. Administration of aspirin within the first four hours of the onset of symptoms was found to be most beneficial.[8] While the benefit of aspirin administration has long been established, the actual administration rates are disappointedly low. Studies have shown that actual administration of aspirin occurs in only 45% to 69% of eligible patients.[9-10]

The protocol-driven nature of prehospital care lends itself to improve on these administration rates. The possibility exists that if aspirin is not given by out-of-hospital care providers, it may never be given. In one study the institution of protocol-driven aspirin administration lead to 85% of eligible patients receiving aspirin with no increase in adverse events from its administration.[11] This rate was significantly higher than previously published rates.

Standing protocols for the management of chest pain should now include the use of aspirin. While varying doses and forms of aspirin have been proposed, the most widely used is four 81 mg "baby aspirin" tablets in all patients with a presentation suggestive of myocardial ischemia or infarction. These dissolving tablets are well tolerated, easier to swallow, and more rapidly absorbed than other preparations. Acceptable contraindications to administration are definite allergy to aspirin or a history of active gastrointestinal bleeding. Rectal preparations can be utilized in patients unable to protect their airway, or to swallow, or with severe nausea or vomiting.

The 12-lead electrocardiogram (EKG) remains the quickest method of diagnosing cardiac ischemia or infarction. Rapid diagnosis and treatment of patients with acute myocardial infarction has been shown to improve patient mortality and morbidity.[12] Studies have shown that while there is an increased on-scene time to perform an out-of-hospital EKG (2–3 minutes), the time to thrombolysis is significantly reduced, leading to an overall time saving and 4% reduction in mortality.[13-15] This has prompted the American Heart Association Guidelines 2000 to make the institution of a prehospital EKG program a Class 1 recommendation.[16]

While the principles of electrocardiography have been known since 1842, its clinical use to diagnose coronary artery occlusion began is 1932 and its lead arrangement is unchanged since 1942. Technology has advanced to a point that out-of-hospital providers have portable, robust, and accurate EKG machines available for them to use.[17-19]

With the development of appropriate EKG machines, it has become clear that precise interpretations are important because they dictate immediate management strategies on arrival at hospital, and may also dictate the diversion of the patient to a more appropriate but more distant facility. It has been found

---

TABLE 58.2

Historical Aspects of Chest Pain

P—What **provoked** the pain or what was the patient doing when the pain started?

Q—What is the **quality** of pain; is it burning, aching, squeezing, stabbing?

R—Is there any **radiation** of the pain; does it go to neck, jaw, back, or arms?

S—How **severe** is the pain? On a scale of 1–10, with 10 being the worst pain of one's life, what is the pain currently and what was it earlier?

T—What are the **temporal** aspects of the pain? How long has it been present? Has it occurred before, and when?

that the EKG interpretation is far more accurate in diagnosing acute myocardial infarction than any history taken or examination done by the on-scene personnel.[13]

Currently three methods of out-of-hospital EKG interpretation exist: computer algorithms integrated into the EKG machine, direct paramedic interpretation, or transmission of the EKG to a base-hospital physician for interpretation. In one study computer algorithm interpretation of tracings taken in a pre-hospital setting were comparable to interpretation by a cardiologist significantly better than paramedic interpretation, and could reliably be used to determine if a patient was having a myocardial infarction.[20] Additional benefits of computer interpretation is that it is significantly cheaper than having a dedicated physician on call, and it is a consistent method that does not depend on the relative experience of the personnel.

Early identification of possible transmural involvement should lead to diversion of the patient to a site where acute angioplasty can be performed within 3 hours. Ideally the door to angioplasty time should be less than 1 hour. If no such site is within reasonable transport time, then the patient should be transferred to a site where thrombolytics can be administered rapidly. In cases where transport time is excessive, thrombolytics may be given in the field. In addition, notification of the hospital by the out-of-hospital team can decrease time to thrombolytics by allowing the hospital to be prepared and the thrombolytics mixed and awaiting the patient.[18]

"Safe" Transport

Despite the availability of sophisticated prehospital care systems, many patients with chest pain continue to delay coming to the ED. Massive public education efforts designed to heighten awareness of cardiac symptoms and their importance have had little impact on patients' denial of potential danger and delays in seeking prompt treatment. Even when patients decide to seek treatment, they may use their own automobile, often on the advice of their physicians. Continued public education, often through popular television shows and national access to 9-1-1 will hopefully improve this situation. Clearly more education is needed, beginning with healthcare professionals.

All patients should receive supplemental oxygen that theoretically improves oxygen delivery to the myocardium. Oxygen therapy may be titrated with the use of pulse oximetry to monitor the arterial content of oxygen non-invasively. It is a rapid, inexpensive, and non-invasive clue to oxygen needs, but its results must be interpreted with caution. There is a tendency to think that any result greater than 90% is good, when results in the low 90s may correlate with a PO_2 level in the 50s. Pulse oximetry may not be accurate in patients with severe hypotension, peripheral vasoconstriction, dark nail polish, or dyshemoglobinopathies.

Patients should receive increased amounts of oxygen until their O_2 saturation is > 95% (unless the patient also has significant lung disease). The patient with severe COPD should be watched for the development of confusion or somnolence, an indication of CO_2 retention. Any patient with continued low saturations that are believed to be accurate despite maximal supplemental oxygen should be considered for possible intubation or rapid transport.

Pain Relief

Regardless of the etiology of chest pain, pain relief should be attempted, provided it does not endanger the patient's hemodynamic status. The relief of pain reduces anxiety and decreases the catecholamine effect, decreasing myocardial oxygen consumption. This is particularly beneficial in preserving the myocardium, but it also improves overall patient comfort.

There are three major analgesics used to provide acute pain relief in the field: opioids, nitroglycerin, and nitrous oxide.

Opioids are very helpful since they provide both analgesia and anxiolysis. Morphine, the most commonly used opioid for chest pain, decreases systemic and peripheral vascular resistance and decreases the cardiovascular response to stress. Morphine is also believed to have the potentially beneficial action of decreasing coronary artery resistance. Hypotension is an idiosyncratic reaction to morphine that may occur more often when the rate of administration exceeds 5 mg morphine per minute or when given to elderly or vasoconstricted patients. This hypotension is often associated with a slowing of the pulse. The hypotension is almost always self-limited and responds to administration of fluids.

Nitroglycerin decreases myocardial oxygen demand and may also increase collateral blood flow. It may also be effective in patients with esophageal spasm. When using nitroglycerin, it is desirable to have an IV initiated as soon as possible to treat hypotension or bradycardia that may occasionally occur as a result of the nitroglycerin.

Nitrous oxide has less hemodynamic effects but does relieve apprehension and some pain. It may be used in the field when opioids and nitroglycerin are contraindicated by hypotension or drug allergy. Nitrous oxide should not be combined with opioids, since the combination may result in a significant decrease in cardiac output.

Perhaps the most commonly ignored form of providing comfort to patients in pain is proper use of communication techniques. These can be particularly helpful in patients having ischemic chest pain, since the patients may have many fears associated with the pain.

Other Causes of Substernal Chest Pain

Despite all the attention cardiac disease receives, most chest pain patients will have another, non-cardiac cause for their discomfort. Some of the most serious causes include dissecting aortic aneurysm, pulmonary embolism, pericarditis, and tension pneumothorax. In addition, some patients will have chest trauma which is not covered in this chapter.

There are many other causes of chest pain that may cause a patient to call 9-1-1 to go to the hospital. In some cases, these are minor. In other cases out-of-hospital treatment for presumed myocardial infarction could interfere with, or worsen, the underlying condition. This section will be a brief outline of those entities that may produce chest pain. Some are very rare and difficult to detect even with advanced technology. Concern for these causes should *not* prevent appropriate treatment of acute myocardial infarction.

DISSECTION OF THE THORACIC AORTA

This rare disorder causes sudden onset of severe central pain in the chest, often radiating to the back and neck, and at times into the abdomen. The pain begins suddenly and may be accompanied by nausea, vomiting, and diaphoresis. The dissection is caused by a tear in the intimal lining of the aorta, thought to be due to cystic medial necrosis. Once that tear occurs, it may propagate into the ascending aorta to involve the pericardium, coronary arteries, and other cardiac structures. If the dissection progresses in the opposite direction, it may involve the arch of the aorta down to and including the abdominal aorta. It may interfere with the blood supply to one or more peripheral vessels, leading to loss of a peripheral pulse, or neurologic finding such as a hemiparesis or blindness of one eye, or may involve the renal arteries.

The pain is severe; however, the patient may otherwise appear to be having a myocardial infarction. When the coronary arteries are involved, EKG changes may be noted. The diagnosis is often missed even during hospital care. The diagnosis is most often suggested by a chest radiograph but it can be normal. Definitive diagnosis often can only be made by CT or angiogram, which in some cases may be normal as well. An aortic dissection most commonly occurs in a middle age to elderly patient with long-standing hypertension (table 58.3).

Iatrogenic dissections can occur after aortography. Familial cases have been described. It would be nearly impossible to imagine that an out-of-hospital provider could make this diagnosis outside the hospital. Treatment with thrombolytics, while life-saving and tissue-sparing for a myocardial infarction, would, in this case, be potentially lethal. Nitroglycerin and aspirin should have no effect on outcome.

PERICARDITIS

Pericarditis causes sudden or gradual onset of chest pain similar to a myocardial infarction. It is felt in the central area of the chest often with radiation to the left shoulder, epigastrium, neck, or back. Fever, dyspnea, and dysphagia may be present. In many patients, pericarditis causes only minor pain, while in others the pain is severe, stabbing, or knife-like. Moving or breathing can often aggravate the pain. The classic finding in pericarditis is pain relieved by sitting, worse when recumbent. The classic physical finding of a friction rub is difficult enough to hear in an emergency department, and would be almost impossible to distinguish out-of-hospital. However, if heard, pericarditis should be considered. The EKG

TABLE 58.3
Risk Factors for Aortic Dissection
Long-standing hypertension
Congenital valve disease
Chest trauma
Marfan's syndrome
Pregnancy
Connective tissue disorders
Familial
Atherosclerosis
Aortic coarctation
Turner's Syndrome

may show diffuse ST-T wave changes suggestive of an extensive myocardial infarction.

Pericarditis is most often caused by viral infection (Coxsackie virus, Echovirus, HIV) but can also be seen as a result of other infections (bacterial, fungal), connective tissue disorders, Dressler's syndrome, uremia, or malignancies (particularly those involving the chest) (table 58.4).

Administration of thrombolytics to patients with pericarditis may be potentially harmful. Hemorrhage into the pericardium may result in tamponade. Aspirin should cause no major problem; anti-inflammatory drugs are part of the recommended treatment. Nitroglycerin should have no effect.

PERFORATION OF THE ESOPHAGUS

Perforation of the esophagus may occur as a result of instrumentation of the esophagus. Rarely it occurs from vomiting, referred to as Boerhaave's syndrome. Boerhaave's is classically described to follow a large meal often with copious amounts of alcohol, followed by vomiting against a dysfunctional lower esophageal sphincter. Perforation generally occurs at the lower end of the esophagus, with spillage of gastric contents into the left chest. Pain begins shortly after the vomiting episode and is accompanied by constant pain radiating into the shoulders, back, and neck, accompanied by shortness of breath, and diaphoresis. Physical exam may reveal subcutaneous air or Hamman's sign, a loud crunching sound in the chest from mediastinal emphysema. The abdomen may be tender, and at times rigid. Hypotension and signs of shock may develop rapidly (table 58.5).

While esophageal perforation is not associated with significant hemorrhage, the use of thrombolytics is

---

TABLE 58.5

Risk Factors for Esophageal Perforation

Recent instrumentation of the esophagus
Recent forceful vomiting
Recent significant abdominal blunt trauma
Heimlich Maneuver
Accidental insufflation of compressed air
Malignancy
Foreign body/caustic ingestion
Alcoholism

---

contraindicated, since immediate surgery is necessary for this highly fatal condition. Out-of-hospital administration of thrombolytics would be contraindicated if esophageal perforation is considered. Aspirin administration should be of little consequence; however, the vasodilation associated with nitroglycerin administration could produce profound hypotension.

PULMONARY EMBOLISM

Pulmonary embolism (PE) is the great masquerader. It can present with relatively mild symptoms of dyspnea to severe dyspnea, syncope, and shock. The chest pain is classically described as pleuritic but can be crushing, heavy, sharp, or even absent. Small pulmonary emboli may be asymptomatic. The presentation can be easily confused with myocardial infarction or anxiety. Because of the anxiety that often is associated with PE, the dyspnea may be misinterpreted to be hyperventilation.

Most patients have at least one risk factor for a PE; however, these may be unknown to the out-of-hospital provider. These risk factors are listed in table 58.6.

An EKG may show changes of an acute infarction with ST-T changes and T wave inversions. Other EKG changes include right axis deviation and clockwise rotation of the anterior forces in the limb leads. However, the most common EKG finding in a patient with pulmonary embolism remains sinus tachycardia without acute changes.

Out-of-hospital treatment of a patient with suspected PE should include administration of oxygen to keep the O_2 saturation above 95%. Many providers may be tempted to treat the "hyperventilation" with a paper bag. Such treatment can be dangerous in the patient with a PE, increasing the arterial CO_2 and further compromising the pulmonary physiology of the victim. Therefore, paper bags and other similar rebreathing devices should not be used in the field. A

TABLE 58.4

Patients At Risk for Pericarditis

Connective tissue disease (Scleroderma, Rheumatoid arthritis, SLE)
Taking procainamide, hydralazine, methyldopa
Recent chest trauma
Recent viral syndrome
Chronic renal failure—uremia
Malignancy
Post radiation
Recent cardiac surgery
Recent myocardial infarction
Known tuberculosis
HIV

CHEST PAIN

TABLE 58.6
Risk Factors for Pulmonary Embolism
Congestive heart failure
Myocardial infarction
COPD
Pregnancy
Oral contraceptives/estrogen replacement
DVT (current or previous history)
Previous PE
Prolonged immobilization (recent travel)
Obesity
Malignancy
Hypercoagulable states
Recent surgery
Extremity trauma
Burns
Post Partum

patient with a PE can be easily assumed to have an acute MI. Aspirin treatment should have no detrimental effect, but nitroglycerin can cause hypotension. Use of thrombolytics would be potentially beneficial in these patients. However, it would be preferable to wait until further in-hospital diagnostic procedures, provide a definitive diagnosis.

PNEUMOTHORAX

Most commonly the pain of a pneumothorax is pleuritic and of acute onset. However, it can be confused with acute myocardial infarction, especially when the accompanying dyspnea is severe. Dyspnea and tachycardia are present in most patients with a significant pneumothorax. The patient with a tension pneumothorax may present with shock (secondary to decreased filling of the heart) and rapid deterioration. Bilateral tension pneumothoraces may occur in patients with airway disease (COPD/asthma) or with trauma, and can lead to rapid death. Decreased breath sounds and hyperresonance are classical physical signs of a pneumothorax and may be appreciated in the field; however, in noisy environments, they may be missed. Other signs suggestive of a pneumothorax include subcutaneous emphysema, tracheal deviation (with a tension pneumothorax), jugulovenous distention, and hypotension. Some conditions that predispose to a pneumothorax are listed in table 58.7.

Treatment of a suspected pneumothorax begins with administration of oxygen to assure oxygenation.

If a tension pneumothorax is suspected, a needle thoracostomy should be performed as soon as possible, followed by tube thoracostomy once the patient arrives in the emergency department. Patients who require air transport are of particular concern. Air pressure changes can increase the size of a pneumothorax. Tube thoracostomy should be considered prior to air transport of any patient with suspected pneumothorax.

Patients with pneumothorax rarely have EKG changes that would suggest acute transmural myocardial infarction. However, administration of thrombolytics could cause hemorrhage during the tube thoracostomy. Administration of aspirin or nitroglycerin should have no beneficial or adverse effects.

Treatment Challenges
Atypical Chest Pain

Perhaps the most confusing patients are those with some components of cardiac pain and some symptoms of gastrointestinal pain (e.g., the patient with a little burning, a little belching, or a mild dyspnea). These individuals are difficult to diagnose even in the emergency department. Patients at risk of cardiac disease—previous history of MI, over age 40 (50 in women), heavy smokers, hypertensives—should be presumed to have cardiac disease even if the story is atypical. These patients should receive oxygen, an IV line, and monitoring until their symptoms are better analyzed in the ED. Avoid labeling these high-risk patients as "crocks," since very often they will later develop true cardiac disease.

Silent Myocardial Infarction

One should beware of patients, particularly the elderly or those with diabetes or hypertension, who present with acute dyspnea, fatigue, or acute pulmonary

TABLE 58.7
Risk Factors for Pneumothorax
COPD
Previous pneumothorax
Asthma
Other chronic lung conditions
Recent instrumentation of the chest (central line, bronchoscopy)
Recent chest trauma
Tobacco

edema. These symptoms may indicate a silent MI. Patients with a silent MI are five times as likely to have life-threatening complications and three times as likely to die than patients with atypical chest pain.

Chest Pain in Elderly Patients

Less than 40% of patients over the age of 85 describe chest discomfort or pain with acute MI. Common presenting symptoms in this group include acute confusion, weakness, dyspnea, and acute pulmonary edema.

The elderly often have liver dysfunction, which may interfere with lidocaine metabolism; infusion rates need to be reduced by approximately 50%. The elderly are also more susceptible to the sedative, hypotensive, and respiratory suppression effects of opioids.

Hypotension

The acute cardiac ischemia patient with hypotension (including those precipitated by opioid or nitroglycerin therapy) is a difficult management problem. Though analgesics seem indicated for pain relief, they may cause hemodynamic compromise. In some patients the decrease in preload or afterload may actually cause the cardiac output to increase. Patients with a borderline low blood pressure, such as 90 to 100 mmHg systolic, may be treated with very small doses of morphine sulfate (1–2 mg IV) titrated to the desired effect. Patients who become hypotensive (excluding those in CHF) may respond to a fluid challenge. Patients with significant hypotension in the field should be rapidly transported. Nitrous oxide can provide anxiety relief generally without hypotension, although pain relief may be variable. Nitrous oxide should not be combined with opioid use, since the combination may decrease cardiac output.

Hyperventilation

Patients hyperventilate for a variety of reasons, including anxiety, pain, pulmonary embolism, and aspirin toxicity. In the past, it was popular to treat many of these patients with a paper bag to elevate their PCO_2 level. The hypoxemia caused by rebreathing expired air can cause disaster if the "hysterical" patient really has a pulmonary embolism. Rebreathing masks should be used with extreme caution and only if a pulse oximeter is available. Paper bags should be totally avoided in the field.

Women

The chest pain of cardiac ischemia is more likely to be atypical in women. Women are more likely to be under-diagnosed than men. Functional testing such as exercise EKGs (treadmill) are poorer diagnostic tests in women. Finally, even when the history is controlled (same history scripted for men and women) women are more likely to be dismissed as having non-cardiac pain. A heightened suspicion is necessary for women with cardiac type chest pain.

Controversies

The use of thrombolytic therapy and acute angioplasty has revolutionized the care of the acute cardiac patients. The public is increasingly aware of the phrase "time is muscle." Many out-of-hospital providers are eager to add thrombolytic therapy to their patients even earlier than upon arrival. While the time element suggests improved outcome, if clot is lysed earlier, there are drawbacks to this approach. While chest pain patients are commonly seen by the out-of-hospital provider, patients with acute MI are encountered rarely. Each provider is likely to see only a few MI patients in a year. Thrombolytic therapy is not straightforward. Serious refractory dysrhythymias occur frequently, a situation difficult to handle in a moving vehicle. The rare patient with a contraindication or other condition (such as aortic dissection) is a disaster. A recent meta-analysis of 9 studies (extracted from an initial pool of 145 studies) showed that there was a 58-minute reduction in time to thrombolytic if it was given prehospital; and there was a significant decrease in mortality.[21] This result was not dependent on the quality of training nor the experience of the provider. The GREAT report shows prehospital administration of thrombolytics saved 130 minutes and led to a 50% decrease in mortality at one year.[22] The five-year mortality rate was 25% in those who received prehospital thrombolytics and 36% in those receiving drugs in the hospital.[23] A delay in thrombolytics of 30 minutes shortens average life expectancy by one year, according to this data. Based on this evidence, the European Society of Cardiology and the European Resuscitation Council suggest the use of prehospital thrombolytics whenever transport time is expected to be greater than 30 minutes or the door-to-needle time is greater than 60 minutes.[24]

However, the American Heart Association Committee on Emergency Cardiovascular Care is more conservative. It recommended prehospital thrombolytic therapy when a physician is present or when transport is greater than 60 minutes.[25] It urged EMS to concentrate on rapid transport and early diagnosis.

EMS routinely brings acutely ill patients to the ED. However, in a system where small amounts of time are crucial to survival, this protocol may need to be reconsidered. European studies have considered direct EMS to CCU transfers with a decrease in time to thrombolytics.[26] Most US centers now administer thrombolytics in the ED, negating the advantage of direct admission to the CCU. However, there may be a role for direct admission to a cardiac catheterization lab in certain facilities.

The biggest time delay in cardiac care is not EMS or door-to-needle, but is delay by the public to initiate care. Public service education has had limited effectiveness, and for only brief periods of time. EMS providers have tremendous interface with the public. EMS providers as a group should adopt the role of public educators with organized groups, and informally with friends and family.

Despite years of advertising 9-1-1, patients persist in using a private vehicle when coming to the hospital with chest pain. Advertisements and public service announcements have little impact. With the advent of managed care and gatekeeper functions, more patients call their physician prior to coming to the ED, even when potentially seriously ill. Although 54% of patients with chest pain, in one study, called their physicians, only 3.5% were told to call 9-1-1.[5] Of those who were told to call 9-1-1, 86% did so; of those who were not told to call 9-1-1, only 2% did so. Gatekeepers could enhance the use of 9-1-1, which has been proven to be the most appropriate form of transport for cardiac patients. Yet, even today, many managed care companies and physicians continue to send their chest pain patients, and themselves, to the ED by private vehicle.

Protocols

The BLS protocols for patients with chest pain should be directed towards the evaluation and treatment of airway and breathing problems. The application of oxygen should be relatively universal for all patients with chest pain. Additional treatments, including patient assisted medication administration (i.e., nitroglycerin), should be addressed in BLS protocols.

Protocols for advanced providers must recognize that all chest pain is not cardiac in nature. In addition, treating all chest pain patients with nitroglycerin may be detrimental. Unfortunately the diagnosis of myocardial ischemia is difficult in the out-of-hospital setting. However, out-of-hospital providers can often stratify patients based on their symptoms and risk factors. Some medical directors will include the EKG as part of their chest pain protocol, to increase diagnostic accuracy.

Chest pain protocols addressing cardiac ischemia must insure adequate oxygenation, mitigation of symptoms (chest pain, anxiety, arrhythmias), and prevention of hypotension. In addition, urgent transport to a center capable of restoring myocardial circulation through either thrombolysis or acute angioplasty should be part of a cardiac ischemia protocol.

Protocols dealing with non-cardiac chest pain should seek to identify causes that may lead to rapid death (i.e., dissecting aortic aneurysm). For the most part, these causes are difficult to diagnose in the field, and treatment options are limited. However, the provider's field assessment may raise suspicions.

Summary

Of patients over the age of 40 years presenting with chest pain to a hospital, only about 80% will have symptoms and signs that suggest acute coronary disease. Of these, only 12% will have proven acute MI.[5] The majority of patients with chest pain will have an alternate diagnosis; often one listed in table 58.8.

Many will never be definitely diagnosed. However, the out-of-hospital treatment of these patients is exactly the same as those with acute coronary syndromes. Any patient who has a history suggestive of myocardial disease should be treated as such (with IV, oxygen, and monitor). Where there is strong suspicion of PE, thoracic dissection, pneumothorax, pericarditis, or esophageal perforation, protocols may need to be adjusted. Aspirin and nitroglycerin (for pain) should be given.

The use of thrombolytics in the field at this time cannot be considered routine. Use of thrombolytics can be considered where distances are great, there is tight control of out-of-hospital providers, and EKGs are available. Thrombolytics should be withheld whenever an alternative diagnosis such as thoracic dissection or esophageal rupture is possible.

TABLE 58.8

Chest Pain Considerations

Causes of concern to out-of-hospital provider
  Acute myocardial infarction
  Acute coronary syndrome
  Dissection of the thoracic aorta
  Pericarditis
  Esophageal perforation
  Pleuritic chest pain
  Pulmonary embolism
  Pneumothorax

Other causes of chest pain
  Constant substernal chest pain
  Idiopathic hypertrophic subaortic stenosis
  Esophageal spasm
  Peptic ulcer disease
  Biliary colic
  Pancreatitis
  Intestinal gas entrapment
  Valvular heart disease (AS, MVP, IHSS)
  Pneumonia
  Pulmonary hypertension
  Pleuritis
  Bronchitis
  Muscular strain
  Costochondritis
  Rib fracture
  Thoracic outlet obstruction
  Spinal disc compression
  Spinal degenerative joint disease
  Herpes/Zoster
  Anxiety
  Hyperventilation
  Malingering

Cases

Case 1

"Medic command, this is medic one. We are currently at a local bank seeing the vice president, who is 50 years old. The patient states there is nothing wrong with him; his co-workers overreacted. He states he began having indigestion about an hour after eating. The indigestion was partially relieved by belching, although some chest discomfort continues. The patient has some mild nausea and SOB. He has never had similar pain before. The patient is on an anti-hypertensive, brand unknown, and he smokes two packs a day. No allergies, took two aspirin last evening for a headache. On physical examination, his blood pressure is 140/100, pulse 110 and regular, respirations are 28 and unlabored. The patient is cool, clammy and his clothes are soaked with sweat. His chest is clear to auscultation. The monitor shows a normal sinus rhythm. There appears to be ST elevation on the 12-lead. We have an ETA of 10–15 minutes."

HOW WOULD YOU PROCEED?

This is a typical patient at high risk for an acute MI. The patient has many risk factors and relatively classic pain, although he may be subjectively denying his symptoms. Short field time is appropriate, since he may be a candidate for thrombolysis. Transmission of an EKG may mobilize personnel for rapid administration of thrombolysis. The paramedics may be able to screen for contraindications to thrombolytics. Transfer to a facility with emergency angioplasty capabilities is appropriate. Aspirin should be given.

SAMPLE ORDERS

1. Oxygen 2 L/min by nasal canula.
2. IV NS at KVO rate.
3. Apply a cardiac monitor.
4. Administer one nitroglycerin tablet or buccal spray every 5 minutes, as long as blood pressure remains above 100 systolic or until chest discomfort is eliminated.
5. Aspirin 325 mg po.
6. Expeditious transport to a hospital with angioplasty capabilities.
7. Frequent check of vital signs.

Case 2

"We are at the home of an 85-year-old female who called with a complaint of being sick. The patient is extremely vague about her history. When she got up this morning, she was feeling well. Shortly after eating breakfast, she began to feel weak and lightheaded. She broke out in a sweat, and it was more difficult for her to breathe while she walked around. She denies any pain. The patient has a past medical history of cardiac disease. She had a myocardial infarction approximately 1 year ago with similar symptoms. The patient is currently on Lasix, Digoxin, Ecotrin, Synthroid, Procardia, Peri-Colace, Halcion, Periactin, Timoptic, and Allopurinol. The patient is lying in bed, somewhat diaphoretic. Vital signs—blood pressure 90/60, respirations are 28 and mildly labored, pulse is 80. Chest has rales at the bases. There is 2+

pitting edema of the ankles. Monitor is showing a normal sinus rhythm. ETA is 5 minutes."

HOW WOULD YOU PROCEED?

This elderly patient poses several problems. She does not present with chest pain, but rather a variety of vague symptoms, which together should suggest ischemic cardiac disease (particularly since the same symptoms occurred with the previous myocardial infarction). The patient is hypotensive and requires a reduced dose of analgesics. If her respiratory distress were severe, diuretics could be given but might worsen her hypotension.

SAMPLE ORDERS

1. Oxygen.
2. IV NS KVO.
3. Cardiac monitor.
4. Small doses of morphine (1–2 mg) IV.
5. Aspirin 325 mg po.

Case 3

"We are seeing a 28-year-old female complaining of severe substernal chest pain and SOB. Her symptoms began approximately one hour ago while she was playing tennis and the pain is still present despite rest. She describes it as a heavy pressure radiating into her jaw and down her arm. She also complains of SOB.

"The patient has previously been well. She is on no medications. She admits to using cocaine regularly and did some crack this morning just before getting the pain. Also, be advised, she may be pregnant.

"On physical exam, she is cold and clammy, BP 150/100, pulse 120, regular respiration 25. Chest is clear. Monitor shows a sinus tachycardia with occasional PVCs. ETZ is 10 minutes."

HOW WOULD YOU PROCEED?

This menstruating female would normally be in a low-risk group but her use of cocaine puts her at high risk for cardiac damage. She should be treated as a possible myocardial infarction.

SAMPLE ORDERS

1. Cardiac monitor.
2. IV KVO.
3. Oxygen, 10 L by face mask.
4. Pain relief (morphine or nitrates) en-route to hospital.
5. Aspirin 325 mg po.

References

1. Pantridge JF, Geddes JS. A mobile intensive care unit in the management of myocardial infarction. *Lancet.* 1967;2:271–273.
2. Burt CW. Summary statistics for acute cardiac ischemia and chest pain visits to United States EDs, 1995–1996. *Am J Emerg Med.* 1999;17:552–559.
3. Eppler E, Eisenberg MS, Schaeffler S, et al. 9-1-1 and emergency department use for chest pain: result of a media campaign. *Ann Emerg Med.* 1994;24:202–208.
4. Herletz J, Karlson BW, Liljeqvist J, et al. Early identification of acute myocardial infarction and prognosis in relation to mode of transport. *Am J Emerg Med.* 1992; 10:406–412.
5. Schneider SM, Cobaugh DJ, Leahey NF. Gatekeepers: a missed opportunity for safe transport. *Acad Emerg Med.* 1998;5:587–592.
6. Jonsbu J, Rollag A, Aase O, et al. Rapid and correct diagnosis of myocardial infarction: standardized case history and clinical examination provide important information for correct referral to monitored beds. *J Intern Med.* 1991;229:143–149.
7. Bayer AJ, Chandra JS, Farag RR, Pathy MSJ. Changing presentation of myocardial infarction with increasing age. *J Am Geri Soc.* 1986;34:263–266.
8. ISIS-2 Collaborative Group. Randomized trial of intravenous streptokinase, oral aspirin, both or neither among 17187 suspected acute myocardial infarction: ISIS-2. *Lancet.* 1988;2:349–360.
9. Sakethou BB, Conte FJ, Noris M, et al. Emergency Department use of aspirin in patients with possible acute myocardial infarction. *Ann Intern Med.* 1997;127:126–129.
10. Krumholz HM, Radford MJ, Ellerbeck EF, et al. Aspirin in the treatment of acute myocardial infarction in elderly medicare beneficiaries. *Circulation.* 1995;92:2841–2847.
11. Davis EA, Syrett JI. Improving aspirin administration in ischemic chest pain. *Ann Emerg Med.* 2000;36(4): Suppl 38 (abstract).
12. Weaver WD, Cerqueira M, Hallstrom AP, et al. Prehospital-initiated vs hospital-initiated thrombolytic therapy: the myocardial infarction triage and intervention trial. *JAMA.* 1993;270(10):1211–1216.
13. Davis EA, Syrett JI, Breneman SM. Clinical indicators of myocardial infarction in an out-of-hospital setting. *Ann Emerg Med.* 2000;36(4):Suppl 32 (abstract).
14. Foster DB, Dufendach JH, Barkdoll CM, et al. Prehospital recognition of AMI using independent nurse/paramedic 12-lead ECG evaluation: impact on in-hospital times to thrombolysis in a rural community hospital. *Am J Emerg Med.* 1994;12:22–31.
15. Canto JG, Rogers WJ, Bowlby LJ, et al. The prehospital electrocardiogram in acute myocardial infarction: is its full potential being realized? *J Am Coll Cardiology.* 1997;29:498–505.
16. International Consensus on Science. Guidelines 2000 for cardiopulmonary resuscitation and emergency cardiovascular care. *Circulation.* 2000;102 (Suppl): I172–I203.

17. Matteucci C. Sur in phenome physiologique product par les muscles en contraction. *Ann Chim Phys*. 1842;6:339–341.
18. Wolferth CC, Wood FC. The electrocardiographic diagnosis of coronary occlusion by the use of chest leads. *Am J Med Sci*. 1932;183:30–35.
19. Fye WB. A history of the origin, evolution and impact of electrocardiography. *Am J Cardiol*. 1994;73:937–949.
20. Syrett JI, Daher AF, Davis EA, et al. ECG interpretation: man vs machine. *Acad Emer Med*. 2000;7; 5 Suppl: 478 (abstract).
21. Morrison IJ, Verbeek PR, McDonald AC, et al. Mortality & pre-hospital thrombolysis for acute myocardial infarction: a meta-analysis. *JAMA*. 2000;283:2686–2692.
22. Rawles J. Halving mortality at one year by domiciliary thrombolysis in the Grampian Region Early Anistreplase Trial (GREAT). *J Am Coll Cardiol*. 1994;23:1–5.
23. Rawles JM. Quantification of the benefit of early thrombolytic therapy: five year results of Grampian Region Early Anistreplase Trial (GREAT). *J Am Coll Cardiol*. 1997;30:1181–1186.
24. The pre-hospital management of acute heart attacks: recommendations of a task force of the European Society of Cardiology and the European Resuscitation Council. *Eur Heart J*. 1998;19:1140–1164.
25. ACLS. Era of Reperfusion *Circulation*. 2000;102 (Suppl): I172–I203).
26. Ljosland M, Weydahl PG, Stumberg S. Pre-Hospital ECG reduces the delay of thrombolysis in acute myocardial infarction. *Tidsskrift for Den Norske Laegeforenig*. 2000;120:2247–2249.

Dysrhythmias

Donald M. Yealy, MD

Introduction

E MS physicians often use the same approach in the field and the hospital to provide or guide patient care, even though the goals in each area differ. The care of patients with dysrhythmias before hospital arrival focuses on treating all life-threatening or imminently life-threatening rhythm changes within minutes. In the ED and in the hospital, a longer period is available to achieve these goals, plus identify other non-lethal rhythms and deliver definitive long-term treatment. It is this confusion over the basic goals of dysrhythmia management in these two settings that complicate medical oversight.

This chapter discusses a pragmatic method of providing medical oversight for non-arrest dysrhythmias. The most important field observations and actions will be highlighted to help simplify the approach when giving direct medical oversight or creating written protocols. A decidedly "low tech" approach to the problems will be used, emphasizing simple tools including a brief history, physical exam, and standard 3-lead field EKG monitor. Similarly, the interventions suggested will be limited to those that are effective and easily given in the out-of-hospital setting. In general, the approach offered is consistent with the 2000 American Heart Association Advanced Cardiac Life Support Guidelines, although areas where simplification or an alternative approach are offered will be highlighted.

Evaluation

Three basic sources of information are available during the assessment of field dysrhythmias: patient history, physical examination, and the EKG. Rarely will any one of these suffice in choosing a treatment option; rather, the combination of these three data sources can help streamline care.[1,2]

Four steps can be used to manage patients with dysrhythmias in the field. Often, treatment decisions can be started before completing all steps, allowing an economy of effort.

Step One: Identify Symptoms and How They Relate to the Rhythm?

Two groups of patients present with dysrhythmias: asymptomatic patients or those with incidental rhythm changes, and patients with symptomatic rhythm changes. Incidental dysrhythmias may relate to the symptoms but are the result (not the cause) of another problem and do not worsen immediate outcome. Patients with an incidental dysrhythmia or who are asymptomatic rarely require field rhythm-directed treatment.

Those with incidental dysrhythmias require treatment of any underlying acute condition (e.g., analgesia for pain, or fluids for hypovolemia). A 67-year-old male patient with a history of "extra heart beats" transported for an isolated ankle injury displays a sinus tachycardia (from pain) and occasional premature ventricular complexes but no other symptoms or abnormalities on physical exam. He requires splinting and analgesia, not antidysrhythmics. This should not be confused with dysrhythmias with symptoms, such as frequent or complex ventricular extrasystoles associated with ischemic chest pain.

Step Two: Identify Stable and Unstable Patients

Since asymptomatic or incidental dysrhythmias usually require no direct treatment, the prehospital focus is shifted to those dysrhythmias associated with symptoms. Although many patients display symptoms attributable to the change from a "normal" rhythm, most tolerate these well. Two broad categories can be created to classify patients based on the severity of symptoms: stable and unstable. Unstable patients are likely to suffer harm or deteriorate; the providers and EMS physician must identify these patients and rapidly intervene. The best method of identifying unstable patients is to seek signs of inadequate end-organ perfusion that are a result of the rhythm disturbance.[2] A few short historical questions and physical exam steps can accomplish this in minutes.

The following must be sought in the initial phases of patient evaluation:

- Hypotension—often arbitrarily defined as a systolic blood pressure below 90 mm Hg.
- Chest pain, shortness of breath, or rales (signifying inadequate myocardial perfusion)
- Altered consciousness, from mild agitation or somnolence to obtundation or coma (signifying CNS hypoperfusion)

Delayed capillary refill and lowered skin temperature can identify poor perfusion; however, the subjective nature of these observations and multiple other causes limit their utility in the field.

Assessing instability is not an "all or none" phenomenon but a continuum. The presence of either a severe sign/symptom or >one sign/symptom of hypoperfusion is diagnostic of an unstable rhythm; a single mildly abnormal finding suggests "borderline" stability. The blood pressure is the simplest method of assessing circulatory adequacy, but it alone may be insufficient in accurately classifying patients. A patient with a blood pressure of 90 mm Hg systolic, rales, and a depressed sensorium is clearly unstable; if awake and with no rales, chest pain or other symptoms, he occupies a "borderline" position due to the singular mild finding. Similarly, agitation suggests mild CNS hypoperfusion and "borderline" stability, while coma is associated with more profound derangement and instability.

In the absence of clear evidence of instability, each patient can receive a more complete evaluation, although the total prehospital time interval should not be unduly prolonged. Stable and borderline patients are usually treated with pharmacologic agents. Unstable patients need rapid therapy, usually with electrical interventions such as external countershock or pacing. Symptomatic but stable or borderline unstable patients can be initially treated with pharmacologic agents, with other electrical devices nearby in the case of deterioration. The more extreme, the sign

or symptom of instability (e.g., coma versus mild anxiety), the more the provider should move toward aggressive treatment.

Step Three: Classify the EKG Findings

After assessing stability, the field providers need to categorize the EKG. Again, it is tempting to use a traditional approach, separating dysrhythmias into dozens of categories. In the field evaluation, a simpler scheme can be used based on the assessment of stability and three EKG features: QRS complex rate, regularity, and duration.

EKG interpretation is performed in two ways: by command physicians receiving transmitted tracings, or by the field teams. Transmitted tracings are hampered primarily by technical problems (which occasionally can cloud salient features) or limitations in the reader's skills (which are best addressed by ongoing education when needed). Field providers can learn the basics of EKG interpretation, and most can classify the common and lethal rhythms with accuracy. However, misclassification of QRS duration and rate occurs in up to 20% to 30% of tachycardias.[3] Protocols and direct medical oversight decisions must assume that the potential for misclassification exists and take actions to minimize the adverse outcomes that can result. Our strategies outlined below apply to both field and transmitted interpretation. In all steps, EKG interpretation must be done from a printed strip and not "guess-timated" from the monitor to lessen the risk of misclassification.

Rate

Initially, the rate should be classified as fast (>120/minute), slow (<60/minute), or normal/near normal (60–120/minute) based on the frequency of QRS complexes over six seconds multiplied by ten. After the estimation of rate, sinus P waves should be sought in those patients with normal or fast rates. These sinus P waves always precede the QRS complexes and have a consistent appearance and relationship (i.e., distance) to the QRS complexes.

As a simple rule, all **unstable** patients with non-sinus fast (no discernible P waves and QRS rate >120/min) rhythms deserve immediate countershock with 100 Joules. Often, lower energy levels can convert specific rhythms (SVT or atrial flutter), but little benefit is gained by attempting to make fine distinctions in these unstable patients. Although changes in heart rate that fall into the "normal" range can cause symptoms, these are usually of little importance in the field management.

Slow dysrhythmias require no further classification after assessing stability. All other details (e.g., P wave characteristics, Type I or II second degree block, junctional versus ventricular escape) are of little value in the prehospital management of patients. Slow stable dysrhythmias need no intervention besides monitoring for deterioration. Slow unstable dysrhythmias require external pacing (preferred) or atropine (0.5–1.0 mg IV in adults up to 2–3 mg total). Transcutaneous pacing is best done as early as possible to maximize clinical capture and restoration of perfusion.[4–5]

Previously, isoproterenol (2 mg in 250–500 cc of crystalloid titrated to heart rate and symptoms) was suggested for atropine-resistant bradycardias. With the availability of external pacemakers in the field and the poor clinical effectiveness of isoproterenol, this treatment is not currently recommended. In adults, epinephrine and dopamine infusion should be employed only when heart rate has been normalized but hypotension persists.

Direct medical oversight may request field providers to measure the QRS duration in symptomatic bradycardia. Theoretically, a QRS of >0.12 seconds (three small boxes on the EKG strip) may represent ventricular escape and worsen with atropine. In practice, clinical harm is rarely seen and is easily treated with transcutaneous pacing, allowing this step to be omitted.

Regularity and Duration

In contrast to bradycardias, if the ventricular rate is fast, the regularity and duration of the QRS complexes should be assessed. Regularity is divided into two categories: mostly or completely regular, and chaotic (or "irregularly irregular" without any pattern). Chaotic rhythms are usually due to atrial fibrillation, irrespective of the appearance of the baseline or QRS duration. Other less common causes include multifocal atrial tachycardia and frequent extrasystoles (either atrial, ventricular, or junctional).

To ease the process of measuring duration and assessing regularity, the field teams should be asked to run an EKG strip. From this, they or direct medical oversight (if transmitted) can measure in "small boxes" how wide the QRS duration is and look for irregularity. Each small box represents 0.04 seconds

at normal paper speed. Asking or training providers to seek out "How many small boxes wide is the QRS complex?" will limit mathematic or conversion errors. Similarly, evaluating printed strips helps with detecting irregularity, which may be difficult to appreciate on a monitor if the ventricular rate is > 150/minute. In these cases, close tracking on a six-second EKG strip may help detect chaos and identify atrial fibrillation.

Those rhythms with a QRS duration of less than 3 "small boxes" (0.12 seconds) are termed narrow complex dysrhythmias. Conversely, any rhythm with a QRS duration of greater than 3 "small boxes" is considered a wide complex dysrhythmia. Nearly all narrow complex rhythms originate from atrial or nodal (i.e., supraventricular) sources. Wide complex rhythms can originate from a ventricular source or a supraventricular source. In the latter situation, some abnormality in ventricular conduction is responsible for the prolonged QRS duration. In the field, attempts to separate the myriad causes of wide complex tachydysrhythmias rarely alter therapy, which is based on the clinical stability of the patient, basic history, and the simple EKG characteristics defined above.

UNSTABLE TACHYDYSRHYTHMIAS

Aside from sinus tachycardia, all other unstable patients with a wide complex tachydysrhythmia (WCT) or a narrow complex tachydysrhythmia (NCT) deserve countershock(s), irrespective of the exact source (ventricular or supraventricular). The QRS duration will help dictate care after countershock (successful or unsuccessful) but does not fundamentally drive the initial care in unstable patients with a tachydysrhythmia.

The initial energy level used to treat tachycardias is based on the QRS pattern. If the QRS pattern is regular (or nearly regular) in any **unstable** patient with a tachydysrhythmia, 100 Joules should be used, followed by increasing energy up to 360 Joules if unsuccessful. As noted previously, some rhythms may require less energy but attempts to carefully titrate this life-saving therapy in unstable patients is of little pragmatic benefit. Also, although some experts recommend synchronized countershock so as to avoid post-countershock ventricular fibrillation (VF), this step is not mandatory and often not possible due to sensing problems.

In those subjects with an unstable non-sinus WCT (no P waves seen, QRS greater than 3 "small boxes"), lidocaine should be given after successful countershock. The initial dose of lidocaine is 1–1.5 mg/kg, followed by 0.5–0.75 mg/kg every 5–10 minutes (up to 3 mg/kg). A continuous drip (2–4 mg/min[1,2]) after initial bolus dosing will maintain steady serum levels and effects, but is not practical in most EMS systems unless prolonged transport times are anticipated and pumps are available. Alternatives include procainamide (15–18 mg/kg IV over 20 mins unless side effects occur) and amiodarone (5 mg/kg over 10 mins), though lidocaine remains an excellent post-WCT prophylactic drug. Conversely, no follow-up drugs are needed in the field after cardioverting an NCT.

If countershock fails in an unstable patient with a WCT, give either amiodarone (5 mg/kg) or lidocaine (1–2 mg/kg) as a bolus and repeat the countershock. The recent AHA guidelines suggest amiodarone be the "first line agent" in unstable—especially pulseless WCT (presumed ventricular tachycardia), although direct comparisons to lidocaine are lacking; either seems to be a reasonable choice until further data are available.[1,2]

If the QRS complexes are chaotic, the most common diagnosis is atrial fibrillation. When chaos and a QRS duration of >3 "small boxes" appear together, atrial fibrillation with altered conduction is the diagnosis. All unstable fast chaotic rhythms should be cardioverted with 50–100 Joules unsynchronized initially and titrated up as needed. No post-countershock medications are needed.

One practical point: If regularity versus irregularity cannot be established during assessment of a patient with an unstable WCT or NCT, 100 Joules is a good starting energy level for countershock. Similarly, if simplicity of treatment protocols is sought, 100 Joules is reasonable for all unstable non-sinus tachycardias, since the extra energy delivered to the rapid atrial fibrillation patient is unlikely to cause harm or worsen discomfort compared to 50 Joules.

Step Four: Focus Actions to Evaluate Stable But Symptomatic and "Borderline" Patients

Up to this point, little specific history and only a few basic physical exam and EKG reading skills have been required. This is intentional, so as not to "clutter" the field evaluation of those who need it the most (the unstable patient) or don't need it at all (the asymptomatic patient). The remaining patients are those with symptoms, albeit none clearly identifying instability. Here, a few questions and actions can help to deliver the appropriate prehospital care.

History

An abridged past medical history alone can influence field therapy; the field teams should focus on cardiac-related problems in stable patients. For example, patients who present with a new onset WCT with a history of previous myocardial infarction are much more likely to have ventricular tachycardia than a supraventricular rhythm with abnormal conduction. Similarly, those with a history of a previous dysrhythmia who present with similar symptoms again are likely to have recurrence rather than a new dysrhythmia. Neither of these clinical rules is infallible, but these data can help guide therapy. Other points are also helpful; for instance, a patient with a history of poorly controlled hypertension presenting with a low blood pressure suggests a dramatic change, prompting more aggressive treatment.

History can influence the dosing of field agents. Subjects with liver or heart failure, and those age 65 and older, should receive lower lidocaine infusion rates. Those patients with renal failure are at risk for hyperkalemia and rhythm changes. The current medications can provide a clue to any previous conditions or guide field drug therapy. A patient treated with digoxin or a beta blocker plus coumadin for "palpitations" may have atrial fibrillation present. Finally, although rare, a brief search for drug allergies may help avert a complication later. The key is to ask the field team to do a focused history, looking for information regarding heart disease and other specific conditions.

Physical Exam

In addition to a search for signs of instability, some manipulations can help when assessing and managing tachycardias. Specifically, actions that alter AV node conduction ("vagal maneuvers") can help terminate or uncover a specific dysrhythmia.[2,6] In the patient under 50 years old, carotid body massage can be attempted; this procedure is often restricted or prohibited in the field because of poorly documented concerns about embolization. The Valsalva action can be used with massage in young patients or as the sole maneuver in those over 50 years old. Other maneuvers, including ocular and rectal massage, ice packs or cold-water dunking, and rapid inflation of pneumatic anti-shock garments, are of dubious value and are not recommended.

Stable Narrow Complex Tachydysrhythmias

In patients who are symptomatic but stable, or with one "borderline" symptom of instability (e.g., dizzy or anxious with a low blood pressure) certain actions are indicated. Patients with a regular NCT between 120 and 140/minute are likely to have a sinus tachycardia and require no antidysrhythmic treatment. Stable patients with a regular NCT at a rate of 140/minute or greater should have vagal maneuvers performed in an attempt to terminate the rhythm. Sometimes, this maneuver uncovers sinus P waves, clarifying the sinus or atrial etiology. When P waves are seen, treatment is directed at the cause, not the rhythm.

Those with minor symptoms (e.g., isolated subjective dizziness or "palpitations") do not require field treatment beyond vagal maneuvers. For those with more prominent symptoms during a regular NCT at 140/minute or greater, give adenosine (6–12 mg as a rapid IV bolus followed with a flush).[1-3,6] The smaller initial dose (6 mg) is effective about 60% of the time, and it should be repeated within two minutes at the higher dose if no effect is seen. If adenosine causes slowing followed by a return to tachycardia, repeat or larger doses will not help—the cause is a non-reentrant source, often an atrial rhythm, either atrial tachycardia, fibrillation, or flutter.

Adenosine is effective in 85% to 90% of patients with a regular NCT. Even in those who "fail," adenosine may uncover hidden sinus or flutter waves, clarifying the diagnosis. The drug has a duration of effect of 20 seconds or less, and recurrence of an NCT may occur in 10% to 58% of cases. It is common for patients to complain of transient chest pain, flushing, or dyspnea during adenosine treatment. Some patients may experience bradycardia or asystole after adenosine; usually, this lasts seconds but may require temporary external pacing if prolonged. Contrary to popular belief, adenosine can occasionally terminate ventricular tachycardia, although the majority of patients are unaffected.[7]

Verapamil (2.5–5 mg IV initially followed by 5–10 mg in 15 minutes if unsuccessful) and diltiazem (0.15 mg initially, followed by 0.20–0.25 mg in 15 minutes if unsuccessful) will terminate 85% to 90% regular NCT.[8,9] However, both can cause hypotension and congestive heart failure (though diltiazem is alleged to have slightly lower rates of this in equipotent doses); because of these disadvantages, many prefer adenosine in the field. Whenever giving adenosine, verapamil, or diltiazem in the field, it must be absolutely clear that the QRS duration is less than 3 "small boxes" (0.12 seconds). This will help avoid the hemodynamic collapse that can occur with these drugs in VT or atrial fibrillation with an accessory pathway. Most patients tolerate the transient effects of adenosine, often "fooling" providers into thinking no harm is possible if given in error (the potential harm is real, albeit less frequently than with calcium channel blockers). If hypotension occurs after IV verapamil or diltiazem in the absence of bradycardia, it is treated with saline infusions, intravenous calcium salts (5–10 cc of a 10% $CaCl_2$ solution), or catecholamines (dopamine or epinephrine).

Current research suggests that even with close monitoring WCT are erroneously classified as narrow in up to 20% of cases; therefore, many medical oversight physicians prefer to avoid verapamil or diltiazem and use adenosine to treat all regular and symptomatic NCT.

For those patients with a chaotic NCT, atrial fibrillation is the likely rhythm; if mildly symptomatic and stable, no field treatment is required. An example is an elderly patient with an irregular NCT at a rate of 130/minute complaining of weakness; although rapid atrial fibrillation can contribute to the symptoms, no field treatment is needed in the absence of other clear signs or symptoms of decompensation. Those with instability deserve immediate countershock with 50 to 100 Joules. If transport is prolonged and either borderline symptoms or a rate of 140–180/min, verapamil (2.5–5 mg IV) or diltiazem (0.15–0.25 mg/kg IV) will control the ventricular rate in 85% to 90% cases of rapid atrial fibrillation, with diltiazem display a slightly lower incidence of hypotension compared to verapamil.[8,9]

One pitfall in the treatment of stable NCT must be highlighted: When the rate is >220/minute, the risk of decompensation rises and the ability to detect irregularity is limited.[2] Therefore, all adults with a very fast NCT—heart rate > 220/minute—should be either cardioverted with 100 Joules or treated with adenosine plus prepared for cardioversion; as the rate rises > 250/minute, cardioversion is the best choice given the risk of deterioration.

Stable Wide Complex Tachydysrhythmias

As noted earlier, WCT can be due to VT or SVT with abnormal conduction. Until proven, field providers should assume all new WCT are due to VT. Hospital data recently suggests that about two-thirds of patients with a new WCT have VT; with a history of previous myocardial infarction, this frequency of VT increases to 90%. Although it is possible to assemble evidence to detect supraventricular rhythms from a detailed exam and 12-lead EKG these data are not easily obtainable in the field. Thus, actions in managing WCT should either treat or cause no harm in VT.

All unstable patients with a WCT should be cardioverted with 100 Joules, with escalating energy doses if needed. When stable or borderline, a few simple measures can help stratify patients. It is always an option to observe this group, intervening only if conditions worsen.

If P waves precede each QRS complex during a stable WCT a rate of 140/minute or less, a supraventricular source (especially sinus or atrial tachycardia) is likely, although VT is a remote possibility. Treatment focuses on correcting any potential causes (e.g., pain, hypovolemia, hypoxemia) and observation. Irregular QRS complexes suggest atrial fibrillation or multifocal atrial tachycardia; neither requires field rhythm directed therapy in stable patients, although other actions (e.g., oxygen, bronchodilators) may be needed.

When no clear P-QRS relationship exists, differentiating between SVT and VT is difficult during a WCT. These key features help decide a clinical course of action:

- Patients with new onset WCT and a history of previous myocardial infarction or VT very likely will have VT.

- VT will not often slow during vagal maneuvers; therefore, slowing of a WCT during these efforts suggest SVT. The absence of change does *not* diagnose VT.

- Most VT does not respond to adenosine, where SVT slows or terminates. Conversely, lidocaine has little effect on most SVT and will terminate 75% to 85% of VT.

- VT is usually regular and rarely seen at a rate of >220/minute. Any chaotic WCT should be considered atrial fibrillation with abnormal conduction. When a chaotic WCT at a rate of >220/minute occurs, atrial fibrillation with the Wolff-Parkinson-White syndrome is present; this rhythm is prone to deterioration.

From these clinical observations, the following scheme can be used in approaching stable or borderline (one minor sign or symptom of instability alone) patient with a WCT:

- All stable patients with a regular WCT at a rate of 120–220/minute should receive vagal maneuvers. Those who slow should receive adenosine (6–12 mg IV). If no slowing with vagal maneuvers occurs, one of three paths should be taken:

- *Young (age <50 years) previously healthy patients with a stable (or borderline) regular WCT that slows with vagal maneuvers should receive adenosine. If this fails or non-response to vagal maneuvers exists, assume VT and give lidocaine (1.0–1.5 mg/kg up to 3 mg/kg) or amiodarone (5 mg/kg over 5 minutes).* The AHA has emphasized the role of amiodarone over lidocaine[1] in spite of limited direct comparisons. If lidocaine converts the rhythm, repeat boluses at 5–10 minutes of 0.5 mg/kg should be given during transport to prevent recurrence. Many continuous infusions after lidocaine loading are impractical in the field unless prolonged transport times are likely and pumps are available.

- Patients with a history of a previous myocardial infarction or VT, or over the age of 50 years presenting with a stable regular WCT should be treated with lidocaine or amiodarone as outlined above.

- Because of the risk of deterioration, any patient with a WCT at a rate of > 220/minute deserves countershock with 100 Joules, irrespective of symptoms.

- Patients with a chaotic WCT usually have atrial fibrillation with altered conduction; if stable with a heart rate of <200/minute, they deserve close observation and rapid transport. If the rate elevates to 220/minute or higher, immediate countershock with 100 Joules is indicated.

Other agents are available but have a limited role in the field. Procainamide (50–100 mg IV every 1–2 minutes up to a maximum of 15–18 mg/kg or until side effects occur) treats both VT and SVT but is difficult to give in the field.

Controversies

Rhythms Strips versus Monitor Interpretation

Besides clearly abnormal rhythms (e.g., obvious VT or severe bradycardia), EKG interpretation should be taken from a tracing and not from the monitor screen. It is tempting to avoid obtaining strips, but misclassifications may result from a "screen look." Strips are valuable in the ED evaluation, documenting conditions prior to and after field treatment, which helps unravel the causes in certain dysrhythmias. At least two leads should be sampled.

Synchronization and Sedation During Countershock

When possible, it is preferable to deliver any countershock synchronized with the intrinsic QRS complexes. Synchronization helps avoid depolarization during the vulnerable phases of repolarization, theoretically decreasing the risk of post-countershock ventricular fibrillation. During most dysrhythmias, this is not a problem; the defibrillator unit senses the underlying QRS pattern and delivers the shock at the appropriate time. When the rhythm is extremely fast or irregular, or the QRS complexes are markedly abnormal (i.e., very wide or small), sensing is difficult. In these cases, an unsynchronized countershock is appropriate. Electrophysiologic data do not support the notion that this will increase the likelihood of VF. If post-countershock VF occurs, repeat countershock is usually successful in restoring an organized rhythm.

The usual controversy surrounding field countershock is other than the arrest in unstable but awake patients. Medical oversight must clearly communicate the need for this unpleasant but life-saving intervention in those patients near death to improve outcomes. Sedation with a benzodiazepine prior to countershock may improve patient comfort; however, countershock should not be delayed in unstable patients while awaiting clinical sedation.

Prophylactic Lidocaine for PVCs

In the past, lidocaine was given for all patients with suspected acute coronary ischemia and any evidence of ventricular ectopy. Newer data suggest that most patients do not benefit from this medication, and some may be harmed. If the PVCs are asymptomatic or trivial, there is no proven benefit from treatment.

PVCs associated with more pronounced symptoms should receive an antidysrhythmic, usually lidocaine. Although oft-cited lists of ominous EKG "warning" signs exist (e.g., multiform, >6 minute, couplets, R-on-T, or runs of PVCs), treatment of these and other asymptomatic PVCs does not confer any benefit.

Do not use prophylactic lidocaine for all patients with chest pain—lidocaine may reduce the risk of VF but will increase the risk of asystole. Instead, base the therapy on the effect of the PVCs on symptoms or if the aforementioned higher risk patterns are seen.

Pediatric Dysrhythmias

When evaluating pediatric tachycardias, a crucial difference compared to adults must be stressed. Children under the age of 5 years can sustain a sinus tachycardia at much higher rates (up to 225/minute) in response to physiologic stresses. Therefore, a search for hypovolemia, hypercarbia, and hypoxemia is mandatory in stable children with NCT before drug therapy is used. A volume challenge with 10–20 cc/kg of saline is useful prior to other therapies.

Although some guidelines make a distinction between energy levels when performing synchronized versus unsynchronized countershock, the utility of this distinction is dubious. To keep treatments simple but effective, unstable children deserve countershock with 2 Joules/kg. Otherwise, antidysrhythmic principles are similar to those outlined earlier, with agents given in the appropriate mg/kg doses.

Pediatric non-arrest bradycardias are also usually secondary to another cause, often respiratory distress. When symptomatic, these rhythms are treated primarily with epinephrine and airway maneuvers, and rarely need transcutaneous pacing or atropine (0.02 mg/kg/dose).

Torsades de Pointes

This rare dysrhythmia classically presents with paroxysms of syncope and polymorphic ("twisting") wide QRS complexes, each lasting 20 to 30 seconds (fig. 59.1). Torsades de Pointes (TdP) in adults is usually "pause dependent," flourishing when the intrinsic heart rate drops below 80–100/minute. A variety of antidysrhythmics (essentially all aside from lidocaine, and calcium channel or beta adrenergic blocking agents), antihistamines, antimicrobials, and psychoactive drugs, along with metabolic disorders, can precipitate TdP. Field treatment consists of countershock

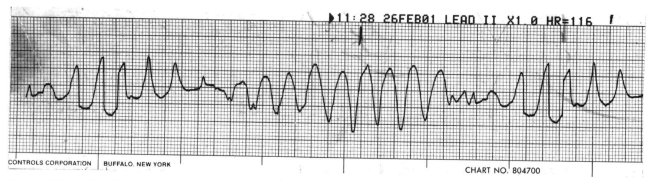

FIGURE 59.1. *The classic one-lead EKG appearance (lead II here) of Torsades de Pointes. Note the shifting of the QRS complex axis and appearance.*

when unstable and transcutaneous pacing or isoproterenol (titrated to a heart rate >120/minute). Magnesium sulfate, 2 grams as a rapid intravenous bolus, is also suggested for those who fail countershock.

A more practical problem with TdP is the search for it; specifically, patients with VT or VF often display some changes in QRS complex appearance. Field providers may mistake these variations for the classic (but rare) QRS twisting. If recurrent polymorphic VT occurs in a patient with one or more of the above risks, treatment should be started. Otherwise, orders and protocols should focus on the treatment of common VT.

Rhythm Disturbances in Renal Failure Patients

This group often falls prey to metabolic derangements that alter rhythms, in addition to having high rates of underlying heart disease. Hyperkalemia is a common complication of renal failure that can cause a bradycardia or a wide complex rhythm, although the latter is usually not above a rate of 100–120/min and often much slower. Treatment should include IV calcium (10cc of 10% of $CaCl_2$), bicarbonate (1–2 ampules IV), albuterol nebulizer treatments, and insulin plus glucose. The first three interventions rapidly shift potassium; these should be part of protocols for any renal failure patient with new onset symptomatic bradycardia or a wide complex rhythm. Because of the risk of hypoglycemia, insulin and glucose infusions in the field are best done under direct medical oversight supervision rather than by protocol.

Lidocaine can cause asystole in the presence of hyperkalemia, and the role of other agents, including amiodarone, is unknown in the rare event of hyperkalemia and new onset WCT.[10] If a rhythm-specific

intervention is needed in unstable patients with suspected hyperkalemia, electricity—pacing for slow, countershock for fast rates—is a safe choice.

Protocols

When creating protocols, focus on the simple data points and steps. For example, both the bradycardia and tachycardia protocols should start with a division between "Stable/No symptoms" and "Symptomatic and unstable or borderline"; those in the "Stable/No symptoms" category should be observed, rapidly transported, and monitored, with prophylactic IV and oxygen. As a corollary, unstable patients with bradycardia or tachycardia should receive prompt electrical therapy (pacing or countershock), airway support, monitoring, and IV insertion occurring either in tandem with or after electrical therapy. Remind the providers to save rhythm strips and to give sedation if possible, but not to withhold life-saving treatment trying to "get a good strip" or titrating sedation. Unless the signs of instability are subtle direct medical oversight contact should follow the initial treatment of unstable patients.

For patients symptomatic without signs of instability, ask the field teams to assess a rhythm strip first. In the tachycardia protocols, these three things should be asked: rate, QRS duration in "small boxes," and regularity. If direct medical oversight is part of the protocol then is the time to seek advice. Narrow complex tachycardias that are regular deserve either vagal maneuvers (Valsalva with carotid massage if no history of stroke) or adenosine by protocol. Those patients with irregular narrow complex rhythms deserve calcium channel blocker therapy if symptomatic but stable. Patients with wide complex regular rhythms who are stable or "borderline"

DYSRHYTHMIAS

should receive lidocaine or amiodarone, and counter-shock if this fails or deterioration occurs. Finally, those with irregular WCTs should be transported without therapy unless unstable; in which case, they should be treated with countershock.

Summary

Prehospital dysrhythmia evaluation must be tailored to the time restraints, physical limitations, and out-come needs that are specific to the field setting. Decision trees should be simple and effective, focusing on treating patients, not rhythms. Protocols must identify and treat all unstable patients; those subjects without symptoms or with trivial symptoms do not require rhythm-directed therapies. For symptomatic but stable patients, a few key steps should be taken to help manage each case.

Cases

Case 1

A 52-year-old male presents with weakness and dys-pnea. He is somnolent with rales in all lung fields. His blood pressure is 60 mm Hg palpable, and his heart rate is 40/minute, confirmed on the EKG monitor.

HOW WOULD YOU PROCEED?

This is an unstable patient with bradycardia. A rhythm strip should be obtained and either atropine or immediate transcutaneous pacing (latter preferred) administered to elevate the heart rate to >60/minute and resolve symptoms.

Case 2

A 22-year-old female with a history of "a rapid heart beat" complains of palpitations. She is not taking any medications currently, and she denies any other symptoms. Her blood pressure is 102/66 mm Hg with a heart rate of 180/minute and regular; the lung exam is clear.

HOW WOULD YOU PROCEED?

This is a stable tachycardia; further evaluation should include an EKG strip to determine QRS regularity and duration. Figure 59.2 identifies her rhythm to be a regular NCT (less than "3 boxes" wide). Vagal maneu-vers should be performed. If these fail, either close observation and transport or adenosine 6–12 mg IV can be chosen. Verapamil (5 mg IV) or diltiazem (0.15–0.25 mg/kg—often 15 mg initially) would also be reasonable for this stable patient. If she was clearly unstable (hypotension, altered sensorium, or difficult breathing), immediate cardioversion with 100 Joules (after sedation, if possible) would be indicated.

Case 3

A 72-year-old 85 kg male with a previous myocardial infarction and "skipped heart beats" presents with dizziness. His medications include procainamide, diltiazem, and nitroglycerin. His initial vital signs are: blood pressure-92/40 mm Hg; heart rate-160/minute and regular; respirations-18/minute. His lung fields are clear; he denies chest pain; and he is awake and oriented.

HOW WOULD YOU PROCEED?

This is a "borderline" unstable patient, with one find-ing (mild hypotension) suggesting poor perfusion; an EKG strip must be obtained. In this case, a regular WCT (QRS > 3 boxes wide, fig. 59.3) at a rate of 175/minute is seen. From his history and EKG, VT is likely. The best course is to give lidocaine (1.0–1.5 mg/kg IV—100–150 mg in this patient; and repeat up to 3 mg/kg total **or** amiodarone (5 mg/kg, or 350–500 mg IV). "Rounding up" slightly is the best course in these cases (though giving multiples of the

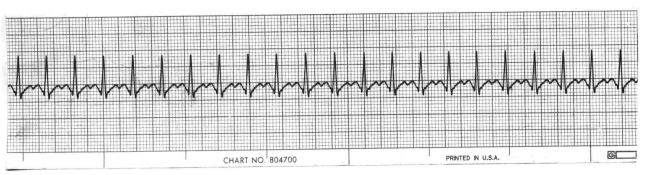

FIGURE 59.2. *A regular NCT (QRS < "3 boxes" wide).*

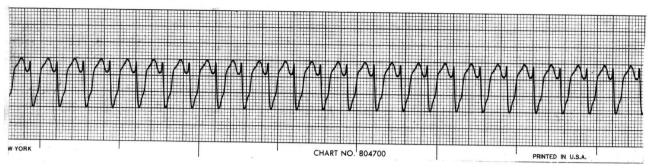

FIGURE 59.3. *In this case, a regular WCT (QRS > "3 boxes" wide).*

recommended dose is not prudent). If treatment fails or deterioration is noted, cardioversion with 100 Joules is indicated. If lidocaine is successful, a continuous drip and follow bolus should be given. If worsening hypotension or any other sign of hypoperfusion develops, immediate countershock is indicated.

References

1. Advanced Cardiovascular Life Support, Section 5: Pharmacology I: Agents for arrhythmias. *Resuscitation.* 2000; 46(1–3):135.
2. Yealy DM, Delbridge TR. Dysrhythmias. In: Rosen P, et al, eds. *Emergency Medicine: Concepts and Clinical Practice.* 5th ed. St. Louis: CV Mosby Co.; 2001.
3. McCabe J, Menegazzi JJ, Adhar G, Paris PM. Intravenous adenosine in the prehospital treatment of supraventricular tachycardia. *Ann Emerg Med.* 1992;21:358–361.
4. Hedges JR, Syverud SA, Dalsey WC, et al. Prehospital trial of emergency transcutaneous pacing. *Circulation.* 1987;76:1337–1340.
5. Paris PM, Stewart RD, Kaplan RM, et al. Transcutaneous pacing for bradyasystolic cardiac arrest in prehospital care. *Ann Emerg Med.* 1985;14:320–323.
6. Wrenn K. Management strategies in wide QRS complex tachycardia. *Am J Emerg Med.* 1991;9:592–597.
7. Wilber DJ, Baerman J, Olshansky B, et al. Adenosine-sensitive ventricular tachycardia: clinical characteristics and response to catheter ablation. *Circulation.* 1993;87: 126–134.
8. O'Toole KS, Heller MB, Menegazzi JJ, Paris PM. Intravenous verapamil in the treatment of paroxysmal supraventricular tachycardia. *Ann Emerg Med.* 1990;19: 279–285.
9. Wang HE, O'Connor RE, Megargel RE, et al. The use of diltiazem for treating rapid atrial fibrillation in the out-of-hospital setting. *Ann Emerg Med.* 2001;37:38–45.
10. McLean SA, Paul ID, Spector PS. Lidocaine-induced conduction disturbance in patients with systemic hyperkalemia. *Ann Emerg Med.* 2000;36:615–618.

Cardiac Arrest

Vince Mosesso, MD

Introduction

For those involved in EMS, cardiac arrest represents the pinnacle of challenges. The cardiac arrest brings to bear the very essence of what EMS providers are. The cardiac arrest thrusts upon the system the challenge of life and death. While cardiac arrest is a straightforward diagnosis and its treatment delineated by well-defined protocols, this condition symbolizes the struggle for life which medicine is all about. These cases not only test medical knowledge and clinical skills in an unforgiving time-pressured manner, but they invoke strong physiological and emotional forces both in caregivers and in bystanders as well. Newer field personnel experience an unmatched surge of adrenaline, while old-timers may view such calls as hopeless and routine. Both responses may hinder the out-of-hospital care provider from functioning as efficiently and expeditiously as possible.

The annual incidence of sudden cardiac arrest in the United States is estimated at 220,000.[1] Most cardiac arrests are due to the uniformly fatal rhythm of ventricular fibrillation (VF), but the percentage of victims found in VF varies based on the time interval from collapse to initial assessment. Reports based on patients being monitored note VF in about 75% of cases, whereas prehospital studies vary from 40% to 60%.[2-6]

Although no reliable nationwide data exist, the survival rate from out-of-hospital cardiac arrest (OOHCA) is generally considered to be a dismal 5% to 10%. About two-thirds of these survivors are intact or minimally impaired neurologically. This is based on published studies, over time, of cardiac arrest in specific areas, which report a range of survival from 0% in Houston to 50% in Rochester, MN, after introducing a police automated external defibrillator (AED) program.[4,7-11] Similar success has been described in demonstration projects in Chicago airports and in a group of casinos with on-site responders trained and equipped with AEDs.[12,13] These marked improvements in survival seem to confirm that time to defibrillation is the most important determinant of survival. While use of AEDs by on-site personnel may be shown to significantly decrease mortality and morbidity, about three-fourths of all OOHCAs occur at the victim's residence.[14] This limits the potential effectiveness of public access defibrillation unless the home situation is also addressed.

The provision of the highest quality care to victims of sudden cardiac arrest requires that a dedicated system, often referred to symbolically as The Chain of Survival, be in place and in a constant state of readiness. Call takers at the Public Safety Answering Point (PSAP) must be trained to recognize potential cardiac arrest calls and promptly dispatch appropriate units, including the closest emergency responder with defibrillation capability. Equipment must be properly stocked and in working condition. Personnel must be well trained, equipped with appropriate resources, and empowered with the authority to immediately initiate life-saving interventions. Finally, a direct medical oversight physician who understands the out-of-hospital cardiac arrest scenario, knows the providers' capabilities and resources, and is able to provide expert and levelheaded guidance, must be continuously available.

It is the medical director's responsibility to ensure that all of these components of the system are in place. Stewart has described the importance of strong and authoritative medical oversight and writes that "without dedicated medical leadership, the EMS system of a community flirts with mediocrity."[15] He developed a partnership between EMS administration and medical oversight in Pittsburgh that has yielded a model of collaboration to assure high-quality care. Another example of the importance of strong medical oversight can be found in the city of Houston, where the annual survival rate from ventricular fibrillation improved from 0% to 21% over a five-year period. This was attributed to the hiring of a medical director who became actively involved in training personnel in cardiac arrest management and implemented immediate defibrillation on standing orders.[10]

System Evaluation and Management

To be effective at reducing mortality from out-of-hospital cardiac arrest, the EMS system must be well prepared and in a constant state of readiness. However, excellent EMS is only one component of what must be a community-wide public safety system, which has become known as a Chain of Survival. This includes a computerized emergency call center with 9-1-1 access, prioritized dispatching, and pre-arrival instruction; rapid response by first responders who are able to defibrillate; and a well-informed public which is willing to act. Attention to these areas is necessary to enable medical oversight physicians and field personnel to provide the highest possible care to the patient in cardiac arrest.

Rapid Response and Early Defibrillation

The most important determinant of survival from sudden cardiac death is the rapidity with which treatment is provided.[4,16] Current research indicates that the most important intervention to affect survival rates is defibrillation. While it is estimated that 70% to 80% of patients in VF can be successfully converted to a perfusing rhythm if countershocked within three minutes of the onset of VF, this success rate deteriorates rapidly with every passing moment.[17] Studies in the 1980s demonstrated a significant benefit from CPR if initiated within five minutes of collapse and if followed by advanced life support (defibrillation) within twelve minutes.[18,19] Larsen reported in 1993 on the survival effect of time to initiation of various interventions and developed the following equation: Survival rate = 67%—(2.3% per minute to CPR)–(1.1% per minute to defibrillation)—(2.1% per minute to ACLS).[20] Whether early CPR and early ACLS are more important for survival, from early defibrillation remains controversial.

Valenzuela combined data from several systems to develop a model of the impact of time to both defibrillation and onset of CPR; the analysis reveal a decrease in survival of 7% to 10% for each minute that passes before defibrillation; however initiation of CPR within five minutes of collapse approximately doubles survival—if defibrillation is delivered within ten minutes.[21] This ten minute window of opportunity is often squandered.

A series of events must all occur in swift succession for EMS providers to have a chance at a successful resuscitation. These events include:

- recognition of arrest by the public
- notification of public safety answering point (PSAP)
- dispatch of response unit
- initiation of response
- arrival at scene
- arrival at bedside
- delivery of therapy

Since delay in achieving any of the above tasks correlates directly with increased mortality, it is the medical director's and administration's responsibility to work together to improve all these components of the system. For example, the medical director should be aware of exactly what are the dispatch interval, response interval for first and advanced responders, and the interval from call receipt to first shock.

It is incumbent upon the medical director to determine if the public can be better served by involvement of other public safety agencies, such as police and fire. If these agencies are able to respond to a significant number of calls more quickly than EMS, then strong consideration should be given to their use as first responders (FRs) to provide CPR, airway management and early defibrillation. Successful use of AEDs by fire-first responders has been reported in King County, WA[22] and of police-first responders in Rochester, MN[10,23] and Pittsburgh.[6,24] These programs have shown benefit even if FRs arrive only two minutes earlier than EMS. The best utilization of resources and the best way to achieve early defibrillation must be determined on the local level, taking care to avoid undue influence of political factors.

Public Awareness and Involvement

Local EMS, led by medical oversight should strive to increase the public's awareness of how to recognize sudden cardiac arrest and of what they should do to help. Resuscitation rates will not improve without increased bystander involvement, including rapid call to 9-1-1, prompt initiation of CPR, and use of an AED. There should be continual effort to increase the proportion of the general population with CPR training. While EMS resources for the above efforts may be limited, this does not preclude advocating for appropriation of local, regional, state, and even federal funds to achieve these goals.

Training and Equipment

Cardiac arrest is a condition that demands timeliness and accuracy of proper interventions. It is ruthlessly unforgiving to delays in administering proper therapy. Therefore, all field personnel must be extremely well versed in recognizing and instituting initial treatment for this condition. Field crews must be able to work synchronously with each other so that multiple critical interventions can be performed as rapidly as possible. Field providers should run through practice scenarios so that system-wide protocols that reflect the most efficient utilization of personnel can be instituted, and so that crews become proficient at working together. These practical scenarios also allow medical oversight to evaluate current protocols, policies, and equipment, and to implement modifications that facilitate a more rapid and efficient provision of care.

Personnel must be able to utilize various specialty pieces of equipment with the utmost proficiency in this setting. Therefore, it may be beneficial for periodic review of the use of equipment such as monitor-defibrillators, external pacers, pulse oximetry, CO_2 detectors, and mechanical CPR devices; and of skills such as endotracheal intubation and intraosseous infusion. Even in busy systems there are often a significant proportion of personnel who do not perform these various skills or use specific equipment for months at a time.

Policies Specific to Cardiac Arrest

ADVANCE DIRECTIVES

System policies should provide field personnel with guidance on recognition and application of a patient's advance directives, based on state law and regulations. While this is often a tedious and unpleasant task, there is an increasing awareness of the importance for all healthcare providers to search for and abide by advance directives even in the emergency setting. Personnel should receive education in the ethical principle of patient autonomy and the local regulations regarding patient directives. The specific operational details must be put in place prospectively to avoid confusion and misunderstanding at the patient bedside.

DETERMINATION OF DEAD-ON-ARRIVAL STATUS

Policies elaborating specific criteria for when field crews can and cannot declare a person dead on arrival (DOA) must be implemented to avoid both treatment delays and inappropriate resuscitative efforts. These should address special circumstances such as hypothermia and trauma in addition to "routine" medical arrests. The policy should include specific steps that personnel must take after making the DOA declaration; these may include notification of police, the coroner or the medical examiner. EMS providers should also be trained to provide support and guidance to family and bystanders.

CESSATION OF RESUSCITATION EFFORTS

An important decision to be made in treating out-of-hospital cardiac arrest is whether to cease resuscitative efforts in the field or to transport to the local emergency department. This is a complex issue with social and ethical implications beyond pure medical decision-making. A growing body of evidence in the medical literature has found that patients who receive appropriate advanced cardiac life support, remain in asystole for greater than 20 to 30 minutes and are then transported to a hospital are unlikely to be resuscitated.[25] The American Heart Association (AHA) have endorsed the concept that, after an adequate trial of advanced cardiac life support, resuscitation should be ceased and there is no medical reason to transport these patients to the hospital.[26–29] This principle is applicable only to the patient with sustained pulselessness from a suspected cardiac etiology and does *not* apply to patients with drug overdose, hypothermia, and other special conditions.

There has been some concern that ceasing resuscitative efforts at the scene would be poorly accepted by family and friends, but this was found to be false in at least two studies.[30,31] These reports suggest that non-transport is well accepted and often preferred if proper counseling and explanation are given to family members at the scene. Nonetheless, circumstances at the scene may suggest that transport to the hospital should be done for purely social concerns, such as arrests occurring in public locations, unexpected death in the very young, and in the case of extremely distraught and unaccepting family. The direct medical oversight physician should rely on information relayed by the field crew to make this determination. Field crews should be trained in dealing with survivors of deceased loved ones prior to implementing such a policy.

Quality Management

While a comprehensive and effective quality management (QM) program is in essence a continual reappraisal of the entire system, in this section we will point out only a few items that deal specifically with cardiac arrest. Perhaps the most important issue is timeliness of service. In the treatment of cardiac arrest, time reduces directly to survival. The faster a system can access a patient, provide defibrillation, and manage the airway correlates directly with success rate. Therefore, a high priority should be given to evaluating these important time intervals, including call received to unit dispatched, dispatch to unit arrival, patient access time after unit arrival on scene (although often not measurable directly), and call received to first defibrillation. The QM program should also review proper protocol implementation, skills performance such as intubation, EKG interpretation and IV initiation; and the timeliness of these procedures as well.

The Utstein style for reporting of cardiac arrest data attempts to provide some common denominators for comparing resuscitation rates among various systems.[32] Systems should utilize this format in order to compare their performance with that of other systems.

Patient Evaluation and Treatment

Direct Medical Oversight

While it is critical that field personnel provide initial care through standing orders so that interventions are performed as rapidly as possible, it is just as important that direct medical oversight be involved after this initial period. The use of intermediaries who relay information between the physician and the field crew causes unnecessary delay and promotes miscommunication. These problems become magnified in critical conditions such as cardiac arrest.

The direct medical oversight physician (DMOP) must know the system intimately. This includes a thorough understanding of patient-care protocols, a working knowledge of the medications that field personnel have available and how they are supplied, and what equipment potentially needed for treatment of cardiac arrest is available—such as external pacemakers, CO_2 detectors, esophageal detector devices, pulse oximeters, automatic ventilators, mechanical CPR devices, and intraosseous infusion devices. It is also helpful if the DMOP and provider are familiar with each other and have worked together previously.

Perhaps the most important attribute that the physician can bring to the situation is a calm demeanor and clear thinking. Field personnel are caught in an uncontrolled setting which is often quite raucous and complicated by anxiety-ridden bystanders and family members. Field personnel also have many psychomotor skills to perform and can become thoroughly occupied by practical necessities at the scene. The following case provides an illustration of this point.

The patient, who collapsed at a family gathering, was wedged between the bathtub and the commode, covered with stool, and being tugged at by numerous panicked relatives. Simply taking care of the logistics of maneuvering the patient into a position so that defibrillation and airway management could be properly performed, getting bystanders out of the way, and paying some attention to becoming unnecessarily soiled was itself quite a challenge for the EMS crew. The DMOP's ability to elicit a past medical history of renal failure, a missed dialysis session, and the recognition of a wide QRS bradycardia suggested the presence of severe hyperkalemia. The administration of sodium bicarbonate and calcium chloride led to the patient's subsequent resuscitation.

The DMOP should take advantage of his distance from the scene and should use the resultant solitude to gather all the important data available and evaluate the situation as a whole. He should ensure that basics of care are done, including prompt defibrillation of VF, proper airway management, absolute confirmation of endotracheal tube placement, and the basic steps of the appropriate protocol. He should then determine if special interventions are indicated and decide when transport to the hospital should be initiated versus cessation of resuscitative efforts at the scene.

A significant challenge is to accomplish all of this with conservative use of the radio. This is perhaps the biggest trap for the novice or inexperienced DMOPs. Directives must be as brief and concise as possible while still being very precise and understandable. Avoid soliciting information that will not change your instructions to the field team or the preparation of the receiving facility. Much data of interest or even of use in the ED will not influence out-of-hospital treatment. Extreme diligence in use of radio time will avoid unnecessary distraction of field personnel.

Differential Diagnosis

While a majority of cardiac arrests are due to myocardial ischemia or primary VF, and require standard ACLS care, the DMOP must be the watchdog for those situations when a specific intervention may be appropriate and could lead to the successful resuscitation of a patient who otherwise would die. The most common and important of these situations are listed in the AHA algorithms for pulseless electrical activity and asystole and are elaborated further in the new course "ACLS for Experienced Providers."[33,34] The astute physician will pick up clues to these conditions and prompt out-of-hospital providers to investigate further and treat accordingly, or if the situation is obvious, be able to provide guidance for these uncommon cases. These interventions are often outside the scope of protocols or are rarely performed. A few specific examples follow.

TRAUMA

Perhaps the most obvious atypical cardiac arrest is that associated with major trauma, which in some cases may be occult. Patients found in cardiac arrest with no signs of life, especially if in asystole, are unsalvageable and should be pronounced at the scene.[35] Patients who arrest after EMS arrival, particularly those with penetrating trauma, have a very low survival rate.[36] Of all patients in cardiac arrest due to trauma, victims of penetrating trauma to the heart have the highest likelihood to survive. This is due to containment of hemorrhage in the pericardial sac, which is potentially treatable

Direct medical oversight physicians should insure that field personnel initiate rapid transport of potentially salvageable patients; initial defibrillation and airway management are the only two interventions that should be done on the scene. If crews are properly trained, needle decompression of suspected tension pneumothorax should be done immediately as well; venous access and volume infusion should be accomplished en route to the hospital.

HYPERKALEMIA

Another condition providers may not think of is the presence of hyperkalemia, as in the example discussed earlier. While this is probably a fairly unusual cause of cardiac arrest, it is an entity that the DMOP should know to consider, since it can be treated in the field with intravenous calcium chloride and bicarbonate boluses. In 1994 a case of severe hyperkalemia was reported leading to cardiac arrest, including 26 continuous minutes of asystole, with subsequent complete recovery.[37]

ASTHMA

Asthmatic patients present a particularly challenging scenario. These patients are often severely hypoxic and hypercapnic when they arrest. Therefore, the initial management should be to assure adequate oxygenation and ventilation. Field personnel may be particularly distraught in these cases, as often the patient is young and arrests after their arrival. The DMOP must confidently guide field personnel to achieve adequate airway patency and ventilation, either by intubation or other airway adjuncts, in a patient who may have trismus and/or laryngeal spasm. Use of bag-mask device may allow successful ventilation when placement of an invasive airway is not possible. Direct medical oversight should recall the high incidence of tension pneumothorax in these patients and should consider ordering empiric bilateral chest decompression.[38]

Positive pressure ventilation does not alleviate bronchospasm and therefore appropriate pharmacological therapy should be intensely administered. This includes inhaled and parenteral bronchodilators (including consideration of intravenous epinephrine), intravenous magnesium, and intravenous corticosteroids (not essential out of hospital). Another good alternative is ketamine, a dissociative anesthetic with bronchodilator activity. These drugs are in addition to standard cardiac arrest management.

HYPOTHERMIA

Another difficult situation is the severely hypothermic patient. Field personnel will usually be alert for this condition in patients with acute exposures in cold weather and cold-water immersions. The astute DMOP will consider this diagnosis in patients predisposed to chronic or secondary hypothermia when it may not be so obvious, and should be alert to hypothermia in patients apparently DOA. Field personnel should be reminded that these patients require prompt transport for rewarming and that the usual ACLS protocols, other than initial defibrillation and airway management, usually are not effective.

HYPOVOLEMIA

Occult hypovolemia is another etiology that direct medical oversight may assist in detecting. An example is the case of a middle-aged male who collapsed and was found to be in a tachycardic rhythm at a rate of 160 without pulses or other signs of life. Paramedics obtained a history of diabetes and checked blood sugar with a chemical reagent strip; the glucose level was markedly elevated. The physician's questioning elicited a history from the patient's wife of increasing urinary frequency and thirst over the past week; therefore, the presence of diabetic ketoacidosis with severe hypovolemia was entertained and the patient was given a large volume of crystalloid fluid with subsequent resuscitation. Other conditions where the DMOP may be able to elicit clues would be previous diagnosis of abdominal aortic aneurysm or GI bleeding.

DRUG OVERDOSE AND TOXIC AGENTS

Many drugs in overdose and chemical agents used in terrorism may induce cardiac arrest. Direct medical oversight should be alert to clues that such a condition exists based on available historical and examination findings, and should have ready access to specific intervention regimens for identified agents. Tricyclic antidepressant overdose, while declining in frequency, is still a relatively common overdose that can lead to wide-complex tachycardia, severe hypotension, seizure, and arrest. Sodium bicarbonate may be life-saving early rather than late in the arrest. Nerve agents such as sarin produce cholinergic toxicity and should be treated in the field with atropine in much higher doses than usual. Consideration of the patient's medications and potential exposures may help guide therapy. The point, however, is that experienced DMOP must be vigilant for such situations and must avoid assuming that every "cardiac arrest" is secondary to cardiac ischemia.

Care After Resuscitation

Provider training currently places heavy emphasis on initial resuscitative interventions, stressing ACLS protocols. There is much less training in caring for patients after the return of spontaneous circulation. These critical patients, whose life is now in the hands of the field crew and their direct medical oversight, require specifically tailored care. The role of the physician is to assess each patient individually and to determine the appropriate post-resuscitative therapy for each patient. This, of course, includes ensuring adequacy of ventilation and oxygenation, maintenance of blood pressure either with fluids or vasopressors or both, and any specific therapeutics which may seem appropriate. Use of anti-arrhythmic agents for ventricular arrhythmias must be carefully considered, especially in the face of AV block or bradycardia; there may be a role for external pacing in these patients as well. Direct medical oversight should insist on frequent updates on patient condition and watch for any trends in deterioration. This should include vital signs, EKG monitoring, pulse oximetry, and reassessment of lung sounds and neurologic status.

The DMOP should also be prepared to deal with a wide variety of arrhythmias, as these are common in the post-arrest setting. While many paramedics are very adept at EKG interpretation, their training usually encompasses common or lethal arrhythmias. Post-arrest rhythms often are complex and do not fit neatly into textbook categories. Direct medical oversight may need to elicit descriptions of these rhythms in systems that do not use telemetry in order to make appropriate therapeutic decisions. Paramedics should be guided to provide specific critical information, such as correlation of P waves to the QRS and the width of the QRS complex, when precise rhythm diagnosis would alter management.

Finally, consideration should be given for prompt transport in special situations based on resources available at the receiving facility. For example, immediate cardiopulmonary bypass is being studied at one center for patients with witnessed arrest and short down times.[39]

Controversies

Airway Management

Recent research has highlighted the risks associated with out-of-hospital intubation, leading to a reconsideration of whether endotracheal intubation should be the preferred and routine method of airway management for all advanced out-of-hospital care providers. High rates of unrecognized misplaced tubes were found in two recent studies.[40,41] Further, one of these, a study of pediatric patients in the Los Angeles County EMS system, did not find any benefit to intubation over ventilation with bag-valve-mask.[41] These findings mandate that medical oversight carefully assess and evaluate system performance and determine if individual providers maintain sufficient experience with this skill to adequately eliminate the associated risks. Systems solutions, including use of secondary confirmation methods (e.g., end-tidal CO_2

detection and use of esophageal-detector devices) and other airway adjuncts (e.g., esophageal-tracheal Combitube or laryngeal mask airway), and a strong QM program should be implemented. Consideration should be given to limiting the number of personnel permitted to perform intubation or assuring that all providers maintain adequate levels of experience.

Defibrillation or CPR First?

While the gospel of contemporary resuscitation preaches defibrillation as soon as a defibrillator is available, recent animal and human studies suggest that for prolonged arrest there may be benefit in providing CPR and medications prior to initial defibrillation. Menegazzi found improved resuscitation rates in swine which had been in VF for 8 minutes if CPR and a drug cocktail consisting of epinephrine, lidocaine, bretylium, propranolol, and a free radical scavenger were administered prior to shock.[42] This concept has gained increased interest after Cobb found improved survival in Seattle if first responders performed CPR for 90 seconds before defibrillating.[43]

Also relevant to this concept is preliminary research that uses mathematics based on chaos theory to quantify the VF waveform.[44] This research has yielded a tool, the scaling exponent, which is highly correlated with duration of VF and predictive of defibrillation outcome.[45,46] This finding may lead to technology that will allow caregivers to more accurately treat VF—whether to first shock or provide other life support care.

Defibrillation Waveform: Biphasic or Monophasic?

Increasingly, AEDs and manual defibrillators are utilizing biphasic rather than the traditional monophasic waveforms. The biphasic waveform, now uniformly used in implanted defibrillators, affords some economy in device cost, size, and energy expenditure. Studies have demonstrated that lower-energy biphasic waveform (about 150 Joules) is at least equivalent to monophasic in efficacy of converting VF, and may cause less myocardial injury.[47–49] Further research is needed to determine the optimal energy level and type of biphasic waveform, and whether there is benefit to increasing energy levels if initial shocks are unsuccessful. However, there is currently insufficient evidence to warrant discarding current monophasic devices simply to obtain biphasic technology.

Anti-arrhythmic Medications

The AHA Guidelines 2000 make a number of recommendations regarding anti-arrhythmic medications that will require consideration of revisions in protocols and medication inventory. It is important to appreciate that the purpose of the guidelines is to present the best overall treatment options for various conditions under ideal circumstances; they have been developed from an international perspective and to cover all care settings. Implementation of specific treatment protocols must consider system and personnel factors that may make certain recommendations more or less applicable to an individual setting. The most obvious example would be that certain drugs listed in the guidelines are not FDA approved for use in the United States.

Both lidocaine and amiodarone are listed as acceptable options for treatment of shock-refractory VF. Lidocaine is Class Indeterminate, whereas amiodarone is a Class IIb recommendation.[50] This reflects the level of evidence, not efficacy. One randomized trial compared outcomes in patients who remained in VF after three countershocks; 246 patients received amiodarone and 258 a placebo. Survival to hospital admission was improved in the amiodarone group (44% vs. 34%, P=0.03) but there was no difference in survival to hospital discharge (13%).[47] This presents a dilemma for medical oversight. Amiodarone is expensive and logistically more difficult to administer than lidocaine, and there is no evidence of survival benefit beyond hospital admission. Yet, the AHA guidelines indicate amiodarone to have stronger supporting evidence than lidocaine, and marketing efforts have touted it as state-of-the-art therapy. Further, amiodarone may be useful for other tachyarrhythmias, ventricular and supraventricular, particularly in patients with impaired heart function. Medical oversight must consider this issue carefully and continually review new research findings. Whatever decision is made, field personnel should be thoroughly educated as regards the rationale for the decision. Lidocaine retains a Class IIb recommendation for stable ventricular tachycardia.

Bretylium is no longer listed in the AHA Guidelines 2000 algorithms.[52]

Protocols

Protocols provide a system-wide standard so that field personnel and direct medical oversight understand and are facile in the system's approach to various conditions. Standing orders are those steps of individual protocols which field personnel are permitted to perform without direct medical oversight. Cardiac arrest is one of the indisputable conditions when out-of-hospital personnel should operate initially with standing orders and not delay critical interventions in order to contact the physician. The extent of these standing orders will be system specific, but should at a minimum include EKG rhythm determination, immediate defibrillation for VF and pulseless ventricular tachycardia, definitive airway management, and intravenous access. Additional reasonable standing orders include administration of first-line ACLS drugs, such as epinephrine.

Protocols for cardiac arrest should address step-by-step treatment for the various cardiac arrest rhythms and acceptable treatment options, generally from which the on-line command physician can guide patient-specific therapy. Many systems use the emergency cardiac care guidelines developed and promulgated by the AHA as the basis for their cardiac arrest protocols.[53] References for medication dosages, drip mixtures, administration rates, and other data useful in the arrest situation should be readily available to both field providers and direct medical oversight. Criteria for determination of DOA status, recognition of advance directives, and cessation of resuscitation in the field, as discussed earlier, should also be included. Local considerations should include level of training and experience of personnel, transport times, and unique or high-frequency patient populations.

Summary

Caring for the patient in cardiac arrest is the final struggle in the war between life and death for medical personnel. While certain actions may be routine, this condition is clearly the ultimate challenge for the EMS system. Medical oversight must provide leadership and guidance to field personnel. While initial care may be provided through standing orders, the challenge to the DMOP as well as the providers, is to effectively battle against the constraints of time and to astutely discover the special circumstances for which specific therapy may lead to the saving of a life.

Cases

Case 1

Medics are dispatched to a 54-year-old male who is "going in and out of consciousness." Upon arrival, the patient is pulseless, apneic, and in ventricular tachycardia. Medics defibrillate three times in rapid succession without rhythm conversion. They intubate, initiate an IV, and administer epinephrine 1 mg IV. While contacting direct medical oversight, they defibrillate again and note temporary conversion to sinus tachycardia without pulses. The patient reverts to ventricular tachycardia.

DIRECT MEDICAL OVERSIGHT: SCENARIO A

The physician orders lidocaine 1.5 mg per kg IV push and defibrillation one minute after drug administration. These orders are carried out and there is brief conversion to sinus rhythm, but degeneration into ventricular tachycardia quickly recurs. The physician orders epinephrine 1 mg IV every 5 minutes and orders an additional dose of lidocaine 1.5 mg per kg IV push followed by defibrillation. Defibrillation is unsuccessful and the physician orders procainamide 100mg over 1 minute repeated every 5 minutes up to 1 gm. The arrest is worked for about 45 minutes and the patient is in asystole and is finally pronounced.

SCENARIO B

The DMOP orders lidocaine 1.5 mg per kg IV push followed by defibrillation. Again, the patient converts briefly to a sinus rhythm, which then degenerates into ventricular tachycardia. The physician asks for any available history and the paramedics respond that the patient has a past history of hypertension and was recently discharged from the hospital after admission for new onset atrial fibrillation. They also report that he was started on a new but unknown medication. The physician then asks for a description of the rhythm. The paramedics review the EKG, and describe the rhythm as a wide complex tachycardia, fairly regular, and with a regularly alternating amplitude. After looking more carefully at the rhythm, medics recognize that it may be Torsades de Pointes (multi-focal ventricular tachycardia). The physician orders magnesium sulfate 2 g IV push followed by defibrillation. The rhythm converts to sinus, but again degenerates into ventricular tachycardia. The physician orders an additional 2 g of magnesium sulfate IV followed by defibrillation. This time the patient converts to and remains in sinus tachycardia. He regains pulses and a blood pressure and is transported to the ED where his condition stabilizes. At the hospital, it is confirmed that the patient had been started on quinidine for medical therapy of new atrial fibrillation.

- elicit more complete history;
- obtain description, not just name, of EKG rhythm;
- treat identified specific conditions aggressively.

Case 2

The air medical crew responds to the scene of a motor vehicle accident with multiple casualties. Ground EMS initially direct one crewmember to the ambulance for a middle-aged female in cardiac arrest. As the crewmember begins to evaluate the patient, his partner calls him to assist with another patient, who is still entrapped. Direct medical oversight is contacted to give preliminary notification of multiple patients with major trauma. The flight crew reports they have two patients: a middle-aged female in cardiac arrest from blunt trauma whom ground EMS is attempting to resuscitate without success, and a potentially critical middle-aged male entrapped for over 20 minutes to whom they are just now gaining access. They report that they will not fly the patient in traumatic arrest per protocol and will provide further information on the male patient as soon as possible.

DIRECT MEDICAL OVERSIGHT: SCENARIO A

The physician concurs with this decision and awaits further reports.

SCENARIO B

The DMOP asks that one member of the crew perform a quick assessment of the patient in traumatic arrest assuring that:

a. there have been no signs of life since ground EMS arrival;
b. there are no signs of life by flight crew examinations;
c. there is no evidence of an acutely reversible condition such as tension pneumothorax, airway obstruction or ventricular fibrillation.

The flight crew agrees to perform this assessment and notes that the patient has markedly poor lung compliance upon ventilation. Breath sounds on the left are totally absent. After checking depth of tube insertion, the flight medic performs needle thoracostomy on the left chest that results in a rush of air and improved ventilatory compliance. The patient develops weak carotid and femoral pulses. Meanwhile, the

other flight crewmember reports that the entrapped patient is alert and oriented, is in no significant respiratory distress, and has a pulse of 100 and a blood pressure of 110 systolic. Thus, the decision is made to fly the patient who was initially in traumatic arrest to a trauma center, while the patient initially entrapped is transported by ground.

KEYS TO THE CASE:

- directing crew to check critical criteria for pronouncing death at the scene, which may be overlooked due to on-scene distractions;
- actively listening and interacting with providers even on a "preliminary report."

Case 3

Paramedics are called to the home of a 44-year-old female who collapsed in front of her family. Family members state that the patient, who is now pulseless and apneic, had been feeling very weak and lethargic since awakening a few hours earlier and was recently discharged from the hospital after a heart operation. Paramedics quickly apply the quick-look paddles, note VF, and defibrillate. The EKG rhythm converts to a supraventricular tachycardia with weak pulses. While contacting direct medical oversight, pulses are lost and paramedics intubate the patient.

DIRECT MEDICAL OVERSIGHT: SCENARIO A

The DMOP orders epinephrine 2 mg through the endotracheal tube and administration of IV fluid wide open as soon as venous access is obtained. The medics quickly initiate a large-bore IV and begin fluid administration. The patient's rhythm degenerates into VF and the physician orders defibrillation. The rhythm does not convert and the physician orders lidocaine 1.5 mg per kg IV. There is a brief conversion to a supraventricular tachycardia with questionable pulses. The physician orders continuation of IV fluid as well as initiation of a dopamine drip. Upon loss of pulse, the physician orders epinephrine 1 mg IV push. The patient subsequently goes into VF and is unable to be resuscitated.

SCENARIO B

The DMOP orders epinephrine 2 mg down the endotracheal tube and administration of IV fluid wide open as soon as venous access is achieved. As IV fluids are begun, the patient again goes into VF and is defibrillated into a supraventricular rhythm without pulses. The physician asks for further information concerning the cardiac surgery and medics learn from family that the patient was discharged several days ago after open heart surgery for valve replacement. The physician orders the paramedics to perform pericardiocentesis; they are able to aspirate 60 cc of blood. The patient develops weak carotid pulses but no peripheral pulses. The DMOP orders a two-liter bolus of crystalloid IV fluid and dopamine drip run wide open. After a few additional minutes of CPR, the patient develops weak antecubital pulses and a systolic blood pressure of 80. Dopamine is titrated to maintain a blood pressure of 90 systolic and the patient is transported to the ED.

KEYS TO THE CASE:

■ eliciting more complete history of present illness;

■ recognizing potentially reversible cause of pulseless electrical activity;

■ directing medics to perform specific, aggressive interventions for identified conditions.

References

1. American Heart Association. *2001 Heart and Stroke Statistical Update.* Dallas, TX: American Heart Association, 2000.

2. Yusuf S, Venkatesh G, Teo KK. Critical review of the approaches to the prevention of sudden death. *Am J Cardiol.* 1993;72:51F–58F.

3. Schaffer WA, Cobb LA. Recurrent ventricular fibrillation and modes of death in survivors of out-of-hospital ventricular fibrillation. *N Eng J Med.* 1975:293:259–262.

4. Eisenberg MS, Horwood BT, Cummins RO, et al. Cardiac arrest and resuscitation: a tale of 29 cities. *Ann Emerg Med.* 1990:19(2):179–186.

5. Mitchell RG, Guly UM, Roberson CE. Paramedic activities, drug administration and survival from out-of-hospital cardiac arrest. *Resuscitation.* 2000:43:95–100.

6. Mosesso VN, Davis EA, Auble TE, et al. Use of automated external defibrillators by police officers for treatment of out-of-hospital cardiac arrest. *Ann Emerg Med.* 1998;32:200–207.

7. Becker LB, Ostrander MP, Barrett J, et al. Outcome of CPR in a large metropolitan area—Where are the survivors? *Ann Emerg Med.* 1991;20:355–361.

8. Westfal RE, Reissman S, Doering G. Out-of-hospital cardiac arrests: an 8-year New York City experience. *Am J of Emerg Med.* 1996;14(4):364–368.

9. Cobb LA, Weaver WD, Fahrenbruch CE, et al. Community-based interventions for sudden cardiac death: impact, limitations, and changes. *Circulation.* 1992;85(1 Suppl):98–102.

10. Pepe PE, Mattox KL, Duke JH, et al. Effect of full-time, specialized physician supervision on the success of a large, urban emergency medical services system. *Clin Care Med.* 1993;21:1279–1286.

11. White RD, Hankins DG, Bugliosi TF. Seven years' experience with early defibrillation by police and paramedics in an emergency medical services system. *Resuscitation.* 1998;39:145–151.

12. Page RL, Joglar JA, Kowal RC, et al. Use of automated external defibrillators by a U.S. airline. *N Eng J Med.* 2000;343:1210–1216.

13. Valenzuela TD, Roe DJ, Nichol G, et al. Outcomes of rapid defibrillation by security officers after cardiac arrest in casinos. *N Eng J Med.* 2000;343:1206–1209.

14. Becker L, Eisenberg M, Fahrenbruch C, et al. Public locations of cardiac arrest: implications for public access defibrillation. *Circulation.* 1998;97:2106–2109.

15. Stewart RD. Medical direction in emergency medical services: the role of the physician. *Emerg Med Clinics of NA.* 1987;1:119–132.

16. Roth R, Stewart RD, Rogers K, et al. Out-of-hospital cardiac arrest: factors associated with survival. *Ann Emerg Med.* 1984;13:237–244.

17. Weaver WD, Cobb LA, Hallstrom AP, et al. Factors influencing survival after out-of-hospital cardiac arrest. *J Am Coll Cardio.* 1986;7:752–757.

18. Cummins RO, Eisenberg MS, Hallstrom AP, et al. Survival of out-of-hospital cardiac arrest with early initiation of cardiopulmonary resuscitation. *Am J Emerg Med.* 1985;3:114–119.

19. Eisenberg MS, Copass MK, Hallstrom AP, et al. Treatment of out of hospital cardiac arrest with rapid defibrillation by emergency medical technicians. *N Eng J Med.* 1980;301:1379–1383.

20. Larsen MP, Eisenberg MS, Cummins RO, et al. Predicting survival from out-of-hospital cardiac arrest: a graphic model. *Ann Emerg Med.* 1993;22:1652–1658.

21. Valenzuela TD, Roe DJ, Cretin S, et al. Estimating effectiveness of cardiac arrest interventions: a logistic regression survival model. *Circulation.* 1997;96:3308–3313.

22. Weaver WD, Hill D, Fahrenbruch CE, et al. Use of the automatic external defibrillator in the management of out-of-hospital cardiac arrest. *N Eng J Med.* 1988;319: 661–666.

23. White RD, Asplin BR, Bugliosi TF, et al. High discharge survival rate after out-of-hospital ventricular fibrillation with rapid defibrillation by police and paramedics. *Ann Emerg Med.* 1996;28(5):480–485.

24. Davis EA, Mosesso VN. Performance of police first responders in utilizing automated external defibrillation on victims of sudden cardiac arrest. *Prehosp Emerg Care.* 1998;2:101–107.

25. Kellerman AL, Hackman BB, Somes G. Predicting the outcome of unsuccessful prehospital advanced cardiac life support. *JAMA.* 1993;270:1433–1436.

26. Bonin MJ, Pepe PE, Kimball KT, et al. Distinct criteria for termination of resuscitation in the out-of-hospital setting. *JAMA.* 1993;270:1457–1462.

27. Kellerman AL. Criteria for dead-on-arrivals, prehospital termination of CPR, and do-not-resuscitate orders. *Ann Emerg Med.* 1993;22:47–51.

28. Gray WA, Capone RJ, Most AS. Unsuccessful emergency medical resuscitation—are continued efforts in the emergency department justified? *N Eng J Med.* 1991;325:1393–1398.

29. American Heart Association. Guidelines 2000 for cardiopulmonary resuscitation and emergency cardiovascular care: international consensus on science. *Circulation.* 2000;102(suppl I):I-12–21.

30. Delbridge TR, Fosnocht DE, et al. Field termination of unsuccessful out-of-hospital cardiac arrest resuscitation: acceptance by family members. *Ann Emerg Med.* 1996;27(5):649–654.

31. Schmidt TA, Harrahill MA. Family response to death in the field. *Ann Emerg Med.* 1993;22:918.

32. American Heart Association. Recommended guidelines for uniform reporting of data from out-of-hospital cardiac arrest: the "Utstein style." *Resuscitation* 1991;22(1):1–26.

33. American Heart Association. Guidelines 2000 for cardiopulmonary resuscitation and emergency cardiovascular care: international consensus on science. *Circulation.* 2000;102(suppl I):I-142–152.

34. American Heart Association. *Instructor's Manual: Advanced Cardiac Life Support for Experienced Providers.* Dallas, TX: American Heart Association; 1999.

35. Priest ML, Campbell JE. The trauma cardiopulmonary arrest. In: Campbell JE, ed. Basic trauma life support for paramedics and advanced EMS providers. 3rd ed. Englewood Cliffs, NJ: Brady; 1995;292–300.

36. Rosemurgy AS, Norris PA, Olson SM, et al. Prehospital traumatic cardiac arrest: the cost of futility. *J Trauma.* 1993;35(3):468–474.

37. Quick G, Bastani B. Prolonged asystolic hyperkalemic cardiac arrest with no neurologic sequelae. *Ann Emerg Med.* 1994;24:305–311.

38. Josephson EB, Goetting MG. Bilateral tube thoracostomies (abstract). *Ann Emerg Med.* 1989;18:457.

39. Tisherman SA, Safar P, Abramson NS, et al. Feasibility of emergency cardiopulmonary bypass for resuscitation from CPR-resistant cardiac arrest: a preliminary report. *Ann Emerg Med.* 1991;20:491.

40. Katz SH, Falk JL. Misplaced endotracheal tubes by paramedics in an urban emergency medical services system. *Ann Emerg Med.* 2001;37:32–37.

41. Gausche M, Lewis RJ, Stratton SJ, et al. Effect of out-of-hospital pediatric endotracheal intubation on survival and neurological outcome: a controlled clinical trial. *JAMA.* 2000;283(6):783–790.

42. Menegazzi JJ, Seaberg DC, Yealy DM, et al. Combination pharmacotherapy with delayed countershock vs standard advanced cardiac life support after prolonged ventricular fibrillation. *Prehosp Emerg Care.* 2000;4(1):31–37.

43. Cobb LA, Fahrenbruch CE, Walsh TR, et al. Influence of cardiopulmonary resuscitation prior to defibrillation in patients with out-of-hospital ventricular fibrillation. *JAMA.* 1999;281(13):1182–1188.

44. Sherman L, Callaway C, Menegazzi J. Ventricular fibrillation exhibits dynamical properties and self-similarity. *Resuscitation.* 2000;47:163–173.

45. Callaway C, Sherman L, Scheatzle M, et al. Scaling structure of the electrocardiographic waveform during prolonged ventricular fibrillation in swine. *Pacing Clin Electrophysiol.* 2000;23:180–191.

46. Callaway C, Sherman L, Mosesso VN, et al. Scaling exponent predicts defibrillation success for out-of-hospital ventricular fibrillation cardiac arrest. *Circulation.* 2001;103.

47. Cummins RO, Hazinski MF, Kerber RE, et al. Low-energy biphasic waveform defibrillation: evidence-based review applied to emergency cardiovascular care guidelines: a statement for healthcare professionals for the American Heart Association Committee on Emergency Cardiovascular Care and the Subcommittees on Basic Life Support, Advanced Cardiac Life Support, and Pediatric Resuscitation. *Circulation.* 1998;97:1654–1667.

48. Bardy GY, Marchlinski FE, Sharma AD, et al. Transthoracic Investigators: multicenter comparison of truncated biphasic shocks and standard damped sine wave monophasic shocks for transthoracic ventricular defibrillation. *Circulation.* 1996;94:2507–2514.

49. Poole JE, White RD, Kanz KG, et al. Low-energy impedance-compensating biphasic waveforms terminate ventricular fibrillation at high rates in victims of out-of-hospital cardiac arrest. *J Cardiovasc Electrophysiol.* 1997;8:1373–1385.

50. American Heart Association. Guidelines 2000 for cardiopulmonary resuscitation and emergency cardiovascular care: international consensus on science. *Circulation.* 2000;102(suppl I):I-147–149,I-116–117.

51. Kudenchuk PJ, Cobb LA, Copass MK, et al. Amiodarone for resuscitation after out-of-hospital cardiac arrest due to ventricular fibrillation. *N Eng J Med.* 1999;341:871–878.

52. American Heart Association. Guidelines 2000 for cardiopulmonary resuscitation and emergency cardiovascular care: international consensus on science. *Circulation.* 2000;102(suppl I):I-122.

53. American Heart Association. Guidelines 2000 for cardiopulmonary resuscitation and emergency cardiovascular care: international consensus on science. *Circulation.* 2000;102(suppl I).

Hypotension and Shock

Ron Roth, MD

Introduction

Shock is the ultimate life-threatening emergency that must be recognized and treated early to prevent progression and subsequent morbidity and mortality. Unfortunately, the identification and treatment of shock in the out-of-hospital setting is fraught with many difficulties and potential pitfalls. Patient assessment is often limited by the challenging out-of-hospital environment and lack of diagnostic and therapeutic options. In addition, the early stages of compensated shock with subtle alterations in mental status and vital signs are easily overlooked or misinterpreted by out-of-hospital care providers.

Shock is a complex physiologic process that can be defined as the widespread reduction in tissue perfusion, which if prolonged, can lead to cellular and organ dysfunction and death. In the early stages of shock, a series of complex compensatory mechanisms act to preserve critical organ perfusion.[1] As a result, the patient with a potentially lethal injury or medical condition may have vital signs (pulse, blood pressure and respirations) within normal limits.

Out-of-hospital care providers often equate "normal" vital signs with normal cardiovascular status. The field team may be lulled into a false sense of security if the early signs of shock are overlooked, only to be caught off guard when the patient "crashes" during transport. Early recognition and aggressive treatment of shock may prevent progression to the profound stages of shock and death in potentially salvageable patients. Compounding the problem, the tools available for the diagnosis of shock in the field are very limited. Primarily, the direct medical oversight physician must rely on the observations of the field team, along with the clinical history. Likewise, the tools for treating shock in the field are restricted to fluid infusion, intravenous inotropes/pressors, the application of the pneumatic anti-shock garment (PASG), or a combination of these.

Time is a critical factor in the out-of-hospital treatment of shock. This chapter will identify several pitfalls associated with the diagnosis and treatment of shock, and will help establish an overall thought process for dealing with shock in the out-of-hospital arena.

Evaluation

The initial problem with the evaluation of shock in the field is the accuracy of the providers assessment. Cayten found an error rate of over 20% for basic EMTs obtaining vital signs in a non-emergent setting.[2] While the tolerance limits set by the researchers were relatively strict and many of the "errors" would have no clinical significance, several errors were noted to be quite large. The researchers suggest that when critical medical decisions will be based on the data gathered in the field, multiple measures should be obtained.

In the noisy field environment, providers often measure blood pressure by palpation rather than auscultation. Blood pressure by palpation provides only an estimate of systolic pressure. Without an auscultated diastolic pressure, the pulse pressure (difference between systolic and diastolic pressure) cannot be calculated. A decrease in the pulse pressure may provide an early clue to the presence of hypovolemic shock.[1]

As previously mentioned, "normal" vital signs do not necessarily correlate with the presence or absence of shock. For children, the norm of 120/80 mmHg is not applicable. In addition, an adult with previous hypertension may actually be relatively hypotensive with a blood pressure of 120/80 mmHg and may require emergent treatment. Therefore, the patient's age, size, and present and past medical history must be taken into consideration, along with the blood pressure.

Abnormal vital signs must be correlated with the overall clinical presentation provided by the field crew. A petite 45 kg 16-year-old female with lower abdominal pain and a reported blood pressure of 88/palpation may have a ruptured ectopic pregnancy or may normally run a blood pressure of 88 systolic. An elderly patient with significant epistaxis may be hypertensive due to catecholamine release and vasoconstriction despite being relatively volume depleted. Therefore, in the diagnosis and treatment of shock, the out-of-hospital care provider must look for the signs and symptoms of system-wide reduction in tissue perfusion, such as tachycardia, tachypnea, mental status changes, and cool, clammy skin (table 61.1). Overall the clinical presentation of shock depends on the patient's degree of compensation and the etiology of the shock state.

Previously healthy victims of acute hypovolemic shock may maintain relatively normal vital signs with up to 25% blood volume loss.[1] Sympathetic nervous system stimulation with vasoconstriction and increased cardiac contractility can maintain blood pressure in the face of decreasing vascular volume. In some patients with intra-abdominal bleeding (e.g. abdominal aneurysm, ectopic pregnancy) the pulse may be relatively bradycardic despite significant blood loss. Obviously it is beneficial to recognize hypovolemia early before significant alterations in vital signs and organ damage occur.

Despite their limited efficacy, orthostatic vital signs are often evaluated in the emergency department. The most sensitive test is lying to standing with a pulse increase of 30 bpm after one minute of standing.[3] Symptoms of lightheadedness or dizziness would also be considered a positive test. Orthostatic blood pressure checks are rarely done in the field.

Occasionally they are performed serendipitously by the patient who refuses treatment while lying down, then stands up to leave the scene and suffers a syncopal episode. This demonstration of orthostatic hypotension is often helpful in convincing the patient to allow treatment and transport.

In the past, testing capillary refill was recommended as a clinical test for hypovolemia. However, in a study of patients with evidence of hypovolemia, Schringer and Baraff found capillary refill not to be a useful test for mild to moderate hypovolemia.[4] For a 450 ml blood loss the sensitivity of capillary refill in detecting hypovolemia was 11%, with a specificity of 89%, thus suggesting that capillary refill is not a useful test for evaluating shock.

Out-of-hospital providers often provide estimates of blood loss on-scene for trauma victims. These estimates may influence therapeutic interventions, including fluid administration. A recent study suggests that they are not accurate at estimating spilled blood volumes.[5]

Hypoxia is a common theme for many shock states. Therefore it is important for the out-of-hospital provider to recognize patients with inadequate oxygenation; however, a study by Brown suggests that the detection of hypoxia in the prehospital setting without a pulse oximeter may be difficult.[6]

In summary, while technology may be the future solution, the current evaluation of the potential shock victim in the out-of-hospital setting is challenging due to limited assessment skills and diagnostic tools. Both the provider and the direct medical oversight physician must be cautioned on placing too much emphasis on a single set of vital signs or a limited assessment.

Treatment

All treatment approaches to shock must include the following basic principles:

1. Establish and maintain the A B Cs (Airway, Breathing, Circulation).
2. Administer oxygen to maintain adequate oxygen saturation (SaO_2 >94%) and ensure adequate ventilation.
3. Control blood/fluid losses.
4. Monitor the patients vital signs, EKG monitor and oxygen saturation.
5. Prevent additional injury or exacerbation of existing medical conditions.

TABLE 61.1
Signs and Symptoms of Shock

Cardiovascular
- hypotension, tachycardia, arrhythmias

Central Nervous System
- confusion, agitation
- alterations in level of consciousness

Respiratory
- tachypnea, dyspnea

Skin
- pallor, diaphoresis
- cyanosis, mottling

6. Protect the patient from the environment.
7. Determine need for early definitive care.

Once these basic principles are addressed, the field team should attempt to identify the etiology of the shock state. Often the etiology is obvious and the initial management options are very straightforward. For example, the out-of-hospital treatment of a young previously healthy college student with hypotension secondary to severe vomiting and diarrhea includes intravenous fluids. The treatment of cardiogenic shock in an unresponsive elderly patient with ventricular tachycardia obviously requires prompt defibrillation by the field crew. The patient suffering from severe anaphylaxis after an insect sting may require both fluids and vasopressors (epinephrine) to optimally reverse hypotension.

Occasionally, the primary problem may be strongly suspected but not readily treatable in the field (e.g., pulmonary embolism). Less often, but most difficult to manage, is the patient in shock without an obvious cause. The hypotensive cardiac patient and the hypotensive trauma victim without obvious injuries are challenging conditions to manage.

To aid in the evaluation and treatment of shock it is often useful for the physician and the out-of-hospital care provider to categorize etiologies of shock. Most providers are familiar with the pump—fluid—pipes model of the cardiovascular system, with the pump representing the heart; pipe, the vascular system; and fluid, the blood. Using that analogy figure 61.1 divides the causes of shock into four general categories:

The etiologies of shock by the categories are listed in table 61.2. Categorizing shock into these four categories helps the prehospital care provider and the direct medical oversight physician (DMOP) organize their thoughts and develop treatment modalities.

Knowing the limited treatment options for the management of hypotension in the out-of-hospital setting (fluids, inotropes/pressors, PASG) and

having the etiologies of shock and hypotension placed in four categories, a treatment scheme can be developed.

The treatment of hypotension and shock caused by hypovolemia is relatively straightforward. Treatment includes replacement of fluid volume and possibly the use of PASG. In the United States, crystalloids are the fluid of choice for the initial field resuscitation of the hypovolemic patient.[7] The amount of fluids that should be provided, however, remains controversial.[7–14]

Treating distributive shock involves the combination of vasoactive medications, to constrict the dilated vasculature, and fluids, to fill the expanded vascular tree. Commonly used vasoactive medications used in the out-of-hospital setting for distributive shock include epinephrine and dopamine. While epinephrine is easily administered via several routes (subcutaneous, intramuscular, endotracheal, or intravenous—bolus or drip), the drug has significant side effects. Dopamine has side effects similar to epinephrine and must be administered via drip infusion. Drips are difficult to maintain without infusion pumps in the field. The PASG may also be useful in distributive shock because of its ability to increase peripheral vascular resistance.[15]

Obstructive causes of shock are often difficult to diagnose and treat. If possible, the obstruction should be removed (i.e., the pneumothorax decompressed). However, when the primary problem cannot be treated successfully in the field (i.e., pulmonary embolus), fluids may be helpful in increasing preload and temporarily overcoming the obstruction.

As in obstructive shock, treatment of cardiogenic shock requires individualization. Cardiogenic shock secondary to arrhythmias including bradycardia and tachycardia will most likely be obvious and should be treated appropriately. Pump failure is as difficult to diagnosis and treat in the field as it is in the emergency department without invasive monitoring. Adult patients without obvious pulmonary edema may benefit

FIGURE 61.1		
Pump—Fluid—Pipe Model of Shock		
TYPE OF SHOCK	**DISORDER**	**EXAMPLE**
Hypovolemic	decreased fluids	hemorrhage, GI loss, burns
Distributive	increased pipe size	spinal cord injury, anaphylaxis, sepsis
Obstruction	pipe obstruction	pulmonary embolus, tension pneumothorax, cardiac tamponade
Cardiogenic	pump problems	MI, arrhythmia, cardiomyopathy

TABLE 61.2
Etiologies of Shock

Hypovolemia
  A. External fluid loss
    1. Hemorrhage
    2. Gastrointestinal losses
    3. Renal losses
    4. Cutaneous loss
  B. Internal fluid loss
    1. Fractures
    2. Intestinal obstruction
    3. Hemothorax
    4. Hemoperitoneum

Cardiogenic Shock
  A. Myocardial infarction
  B. Arrhythmias
  C. Cardiomyopathy
  D. Acute valvular incompetence
  E. Myocardial contusion

Obstructive Shock
  A. Pulmonary embolism
  B. Tension pneumothorax
  C. Cardiac tamponade
  D. Severe aortic stenosis
  E. Venacaval obstruction

Distributive Shock
  A. Drug induced
  B. Spinal cord injury
  C. Sepsis
  D. Anaphylaxis
  E. Anoxia

from fluid challenges of approximately 150cc–300cc of crystalloid with reevaluation of vital signs after each fluid challenge. An improvement in the patient's condition with fluid suggests that improving preload would be beneficial to the cardiovascular status of the patient. A worsening of the patient's condition with a fluid challenge or obvious pulmonary edema on initial evaluation would make additional fluid challenges inappropriate. Therefore, treatment with inotropes/pressors such as dopamine or dobutamine would be more appropriate. Ideally, these medications should be initiated at low doses in the field and then titrated to effect. The provider and direct medical oversight physician must realize that drips are often difficult to manage in the field and must be watched very closely.

In a few disconcerting situations the primary etiology for shock is not obvious and may not be identifiable by the field team. Looking at the individual etiologies of shock, (1) hypovolemic, (2) distributive,

(3) cardiogenic, and (4) obstructive, the bottom line in the treatment of shock in the out-of-hospital setting is whether or not to give fluids. In hypovolemic, distributive, and obstructive shock, fluids are an appropriate initial treatment for hypotension. Some cases of cardiogenic shock will respond to fluids. However, fluids should not be given to patients in cardiogenic shock with florid pulmonary edema. Fluids are also not appropriate when cardiogenic shock has been precipitated by a treatable arrhythmia. In other cases, response to fluid challenges should dictate whether additional fluid challenges should be given or trial of inotropes or pressors should be used.

The treatment of shock must be somewhat service/location-specific. In the urban setting with short transport times, the victim of a penetrating cardiac wound might benefit most from airway maintenance and rapid transport to the hospital without intravenous access being attempted in the field.[16] On the other hand, with longer transport times such as in the rural setting, a similar patient might benefit from carefully titrated crystalloid volume infusion during the transport time. Fluids could be initiated while the patient is enroute to the hospital, thereby prolonging neither scene time nor time until definitive care.[17]

Unfortunately, the ideal quantity of fluids to administer in the out-of-hospital setting is not known, especially in the trauma victim with uncontrolled hemorrhage. However, when rapid fluid infusion is required, fluids should be infused with either pressure bags or manual pressure on the IV bag.[18]

Isotonic crystalloids are currently the fluid of choice for out-of-hospital resuscitation in the United States.[7] However, several centers have initiated studies to examine alternate fluids. Hypertonic saline, colloids, and artificial blood substitutes have been proposed to replace isotonic saline.[19,20] Problems with these alternate fluids include cost, allergic reactions, coagulopathy, and lack of studies demonstrating clinical benefit versus isotonic crystalloids.[20] As a result, none of the alternative fluids has gained wide acceptance.

Occasionally shock will be refractory to initial attempts at resuscitation. This may be a reflection of the need for definitive care in the hospital (i.e., thoracotomy, laparotomy). If after vigorous field treatment the patient remains hypotensive, other etiologies for the hypotension must be considered. Refractory hypotension may be the result of inadequate volume replacement, inadequate oxygenation, cardiac tamponade, tension pneumothorax, acidemia, myocardial infarction, or medications.

Controversies

Unfortunately, the literature lacks definitive studies on the treatment shock in the out-of-hospital setting. In fact there are very few randomized controlled studies supporting most of the interventions that are performed in the field.[21] Out-of-hospital treatment is largely based on anecdotal reports, limited scientific studies, personal experience, and the extension of hospital treatment regimens.[21-23] As a result, there is considerable controversy with respect to the treatment of shock, especially trauma, in the out-of-hospital setting. Logic would suggest that if an intervention works in the ED that it would likely work in the field, so long as time to definitive treatment was not delayed.

The benefit of any prehospital procedure must be weighed against any potential risk. A major pitfall associated with the performance of out-of-hospital procedures for the shock victim, is that they may delay definitive care.[12] It is clear from the work of Pantridge in Belfast that, for victims of myocardial infarction, some aspects of definitive care can be delivered in the field (defibrillation and arrhythmia management).[24] However, for trauma victims with internal hemorrhage, definitive care can only be provided in the hospital. Therefore, any procedure that significantly delays delivery of definitive care must be critically proven before implementation.

Hemorrhage is a common cause of shock in the trauma victim. Treatment schemes for hemorrhagic shock in the past have included aggressive fluid resuscitation and the use of PASG to restore normal vital signs.[7] This rational was based on animal studies using controlled hemorrhage models; however, over the past ten years, studies and clinical trials have challenged the time-honored practice of attempting to restore a normal blood pressure in a patient with uncontrolled hemorrhage.[7-13] These studies suggest that volume resuscitation prior to controlling hemorrhage may be detrimental. Possible mechanisms for worse outcomes include dislodgement of clot, dilution of clotting factors, decreased oxygen carrying capacity of the blood, and exacerbation bleeding from injured vessels in the thorax or abdomen.[7,9,10] The optimal level of hypotension in patients with uncontrolled hemorrhage states in the field has yet to be determined.

Studies by Martin in Houston and Kaweski in San Diego, suggest that mortality following trauma is not influenced by prehospital administration of fluid.[8,11] Survival to hospital discharge rates were not significantly different for patients receiving fluids versus patients not receiving fluids in the field. Both studies were performed in systems with relatively short scene and transport times. In addition, the Houston study only evaluated victims of penetrating trauma.

Excess fluid administration can cause problems in the out-of-hospital setting. Trauma victims with isolated head injuries who receive excess fluids can develop worsened cerebral swelling. In addition, excess fluids may precipitate congestive heart failure in susceptible individuals.

Several investigators have looked at the time it takes to initiate interventions in the field, primarily in trauma victims. Unfortunately their findings provide a mixed picture. Smith analyzed 52 cases of prehospital stabilization for multiple trauma victims and found that the time for IV insertion exceeded the transport time in all cases. In addition, over one-fourth of the IV attempts were unsuccessful and only one liter of fluid was infused on average in the most critical patients.[16]

However, in separate studies Honigman, Jacobs and Eckstein, on the other hand, found that on-scene time did not correlate with the number of various prehospital procedures performed, including intubation, PASG application, or IV insertion.[25-27] In the study by Jacobs evaluating the impact of Advanced Life Support (ALS) compared to Basic Life Support (BLS) in trauma, investigators reported that ALS-resuscitated patients had higher Champion trauma scores upon arrival to the hospital.[26] In addition, ALS interventions did not delay transport time to the hospital as compared to BLS units. Eckstein described a 3.9 times higher adjusted survival rate for patients receiving IV fluids in the field versus patients not receiving fluids; however, this difference did not achieve statistical significance in their study.[27]

Other investigators have described the feasibility of starting IV access while actually en route to the hospital. They have coined the term "Zero-time Prehospital IV."[17] While several studies suggest that advanced procedures can be performed on-scene or during transport without increasing scene time, strong medical oversight and adequate provider training are essential.

In the early 1960s PASG were touted as a non-invasive, life-saving device that would raise systemic blood pressure, make vascular access easier, tamponade internal bleeding, and splint fractures.[28-31] By the 1980s the PASG were widely accepted and included in the American College of Surgeons Committee on

Trauma recommendations for hypotensive trauma patients. More recently, detractors of the PASG suggest that time spent on applying the device delays the time until definitive care, and the device has questionable benefits.[15,32–36] In addition, they suggest a harmful effect of PASG, especially in patients with penetrating thoracic trauma.[15,32–37] Transport delays to apply the PASG and exacerbation of uncontrolled hemorrhage are proposed mechanisms for the harmful effect of PASG. Adding to the controversy, two studies have shown a trend to improved survival for a subset of trauma victims with a systolic blood pressure less than 50 mmHg.[36–38] Despite the controversy, some systems continue to use the device while medical oversight in others have removed PSAG from the ambulances.

The National Association of EMS Physicians has authored a position paper based on a review of 375 clinical reports addressing the use of PSAG for various clinical conditions.[37] In summary, the position paper lists the application of PSAG as class I (usually indicated, acceptable, effective) for hypotension due to ruptured abdominal aneurysm. Class II indications (acceptable, uncertain efficacy) include hypotension due to pelvic fracture, anaphylactic shock, otherwise uncontrollable lower extremity bleeding, and severe traumatic hypotension. Class III indications (application may be harmful) include diaphragmatic rupture, penetrating thoracic injury, cardiac tamponade, and cardiogenic shock. The authors of the position paper admit that many of their recommendations are not as a result of data from adequate clinical trials.[37]

The true controversy about the use of any procedure done in the field is whether the procedure truly makes a difference in patient outcome.[27] With regards to the PASG and IV fluid therapy, the questions have yet to be answered. The difficulty for both the fluid issue and PSAG is that trauma is a heterogenous "disease." Treatment of shock due to a given penetrating thoracic trauma may require a different treatment strategy from another. The role of "normalizing" blood pressure for multiple trauma victims with serious head injuries remains unclear. Since the majority of studies for both IV fluids and PASG were performed in urban settings with primarily penetrating trauma victims and rapid transport times, their application in the rural/wilderness setting is untested.

Protocols

A treatment protocol for treating shock in the field should keep the following factors in mind:

1. Need to establish and maintain the ABCs.
2. Need for definitive care.
3. Transport time to the hospital.
4. Resources in the field.
5. Skills of the prehospital care provider in the field.

Protocols developed for the out-of-hospital treatment of shock must take into consideration the heterogenicity of the disease state, the limited assessment and treatment options, and the environment in which the protocols will be applied. Protocols for the inner city may not be appropriate for the rural setting. The level of training of providers must also be taken into consideration. Ideally, medical oversight would use evidence-based medical decision-making when developing treatment protocols. Sadly, the literature is scant for randomly controlled studies that support much of what is done or recommended in the out-of-hospital setting.[39]

Summary

In summary, hypotension is a relative term for patients in the field and must be correlated with the patient's clinical condition including age, size, and present and past medical history. Ideally, the provider must identify signs of systemic decreased tissue perfusion and the presence of shock. Treatment modalities for shock and hypotension are limited to fluids, inotropes/pressors, and PASG trousers. Often the primary problem causing hypotension in the field is obvious and can be treated. Occasionally the primary problem precipitating the hypotension is obvious but not readily treated in the field.

The most difficult to manage are those hypotensive patients without an obvious cause for their hypotension. The ultimate question in the treatment of shock is whether to give or withhold fluids. Fluids are the traditional initial treatment for hypotension caused by hypovolemic shock, distributive shock, and obstruction. Some cases of cardiogenic shock will respond to fluids. However, fluids should not be given to patients in cardiogenic shock with florid pulmonary edema. The response to fluid challenges should dictate the use of additional fluid challenges, or the use of inotropes/pressors. Ultimately, the potential benefit of performing any procedure in the field must be weighed against the potential risk of delaying definitive care.

Cases

Case 1

Paramedics report that they are seeing a 65-year-old male with a history of an abdominal aortic aneurysm, coronary artery disease, and recent prostate surgery with an indwelling urinary bladder catheter, who was complaining of abdominal pain and dizziness on standing. The patient is alert and oriented with a BP of 60/palp, pulse of 95, respirations of 16. Medics note that he is pale and diaphoretic. Their evaluation is remarkable for clear lungs and no evidence of JVD or peripheral edema. The abdomen is slightly distended and tender. Monitor shows sinus rhythm at a rate of 95. The medics are 25 minutes from the nearest hospital and are requesting orders from direct medical oversight. The patient is taking oral antibiotics and has no allergies.

HOW WOULD YOU DIRECT THE MANAGEMENT OF THIS PATIENT?

Although the parties involved in this case were rightly concerned about a leaking abdominal aortic aneurysm, other etiologies of hypotension and shock in this patient may include a perforated abdominal viscus, myocardial infarction, gastrointestinal bleeding, or sepsis.

Fluid therapy would be appropriate for hypovolemic, cardiogenic, distributive, or obstructive shock with no signs of fluid overload. Suspecting an abdominal catastrophe, the DMOP should instruct the field personnel to expedite transport. IV access should be established en route. A fluid challenge of 300–500cc of crystalloid should be rapidly infused under pressure. PASG could be applied and inflated en route in an attempt to raise systolic blood pressure and to tamponade possible internal bleeding. The patient should be reevaluated frequently and the operating room and surgical team should be notified.

Case 2

A 65-year-old man with a history of hypertension, coronary artery disease, and myocardial infarction was working on his roof on a hot, sunny day. He struck a beehive with his hammer and suffered a fall approximately six feet from the roof.

Upon arrival of the two-person paramedic crew, the patient was found unresponsive, lying on the ground. A primary survey was performed and the airway was secured by endotracheal intubation. During their report to direct medical oversight the paramedics noted that the patient was relatively bradycardic, heart rate 65, blood pressure of 60/systolic, and had clear and equal lung sounds. Secondary survey revealed no signs of external or obvious sources of internal bleeding, urticaria, facial swelling, internal or external trauma, or arrhythmias. The paramedics estimate a 20-minute transport time to the nearest trauma center.

HOW WOULD YOU DIRECT THE MANAGEMENT OF THIS PATIENT?

The etiologies of hypotension in this patient are possibly endless (table 61.3). However, the initial evaluation and treatment would be independent of the etiology. The patient showed no signs of fluid overload; therefore, interventions to be performed by the paramedics en route to the hospital should include large-bore intravenous access and a fluid challenge of at least 150cc of an isotonic crystalloid. The PASG trousers could also be inflated during transport. Response to these interventions should dictate further therapy.

The actual patient in this case scenario remained hypotensive despite inflation of the PASG and repeated fluid challenges (200 cc trial infused rapidly under pressure for a total of one liter). A dopamine drip was initiated with moderate improvement of the patient's blood pressure and perfusion. However, the patient remained unresponsive and without spontaneous movement.

Evaluation at the trauma center revealed a cervical spine fracture and EKG changes suggestive of an inferior wall myocardial infarction.

Case 3

Paramedics have initiated hospital transport of a 25-year-old female who cut both of her wrists in an apparent suicide attempt. Upon arrival of the paramedics at the scene, the patient was awake, but drowsy,

TABLE 61.3
Possible Etiologies of Hypotension in Case 2

1. Internal bleeding	7. Myocardial infarction
2. Spinal cord injury	8. Drugs
3. Dehydration	9. Tension pneumothorax
4. Cardiac contusion	10. Anaphylaxis
5. Sunburn	11. Cardiac arrhythmias
6. Cardiac tamponade	

with active bleeding from both wrists. The field team estimates a 900 cc blood loss on scene. The bleeding is now controlled with direct pressure, and two large-bore IV catheters have been established. The patient's present blood pressure is 60 mmHg systolic. Normal saline IV are running wide open.

How would you direct the management of the IV fluids for this patient?

Clearly, this patient is suffering from hypovolemic shock and requires fluid resuscitation. In this case, the hemorrhage is controlled and fluids should be administered at a wide open rate with pressure applied to the IV fluid bag to increase the flow. Unlike the uncontrolled hemorrhage model, where aggressive fluid administration may lead to increased bleeding, the bleeding is controlled. Therefore, fluid volume should be rapidly replaced.

References

1. American College of Surgeons, Committee on Trauma. *Advanced Trauma Life Support Program for Doctors: Instructors Manual.* Chicago: American College of Surgeons; 1997.
2. Cayten CG, Herrmann N, Cole LW, Walsh S. Assessing the validity of EMS data. *JACEP.* 1978;7:390–396.
3. Knopp R, Claypool R, Leonard D. Use of the tilt test in measuring acute blood loss. *Ann Emerg Med.* 1980;9:72–75.
4. Schriger DL, Barraff LJ. Capillary refill—Is it a useful predictor of hypovolemic states? *Ann Emerg Med.* 1991;20:601–605.
5. Moscati R, Billittier AJ, Marshall B, et al. Blood loss estimation by out-of-hospital emergency care providers. *Prehosp Emerg Care.* 1999;3:239–242.
6. Brown LH, Manring EA, Kornegay HB, et al. Can prehospital personnel detect hypoxia without the aid of pulse oximeters? *Am J Emerg Med.* 1996;14:43–44.
7. Pepe PE, Eckstein M. Reappraising the prehospital care of the patient with major trauma. *Emerg Med Clin NA.* 1998;16:1–15.
8. Kaweski SM, Sise MJ, Virgilio RW. The effect of prehospital fluids on survival in trauma patients. *J Trauma.* 1990;30:1215–1219.
9. Kowalenko T, Stern S, Dronen S, et al. Improved outcome with hypotensive resuscitation of uncontrolled hemorrhagic shock in a swine model. *J Trauma.* 1992;33:349–353.
10. Stern S, Dronen S, Birrer P, et al. Effect of blood pressure on hemorrhagic volume and survival in a near fatal hemorrhage model incorporating a vascular injury. *Ann Emerg Med.* 1993;22:155–163.
11. Martin R, Bickell W, Pepe P, et al. Prospective evaluation of preoperative fluid resuscitation in hypotensive patients with penetrating truncal injury: a preliminary report. *J Trauma.* 1992;33:354–362.
12. Bickell WH. Are victims of injury sometimes victimized by attempts at fluid resuscitation? (editorial). *Ann Emerg Med.* 1993;22:225–226.
13. Bickell WH, Wall MJ, Pepe PE, et al. Immediate versus delayed resuscitation for hypotensive patients with penetrating torso injuries. *N Engl J Med.* 1994;331:1105–1109.
14. Silbergleit R, Satz W, McNamara RM, et al. Effect of permissive hypotension in continuous uncontrolled intra-abdominal hemorrhage. *Acad Emerg Med.* 1996;3:922–926.
15. O'Connor RE, Domeier RM. An evaluation of the pneumatic anti-shock garment (PASG) in various clinical settings. *Prehosp Emerg Care.* 1997;1:36–44.
16. Smith P, Bodai BI, Hill AS, Frey CF. Prehospital stabilization of critically injured patients: a failed concept. *J Trauma.* 1985;25:65–70.
17. O'Gorman M, Trabulsy P, Pilcher DB. Zero-time Prehospital IV. *J Trauma.* 1989;29:84–86.
18. White SJ, Hamilton WA, Veronesi JF. A comparison of field techniques used to pressure-infuse intravenous fluids. *Prehosp Disaster Med.* 1991;6:129–134.
19. Vasser MJ, Fisher RP, O'Brien PE, et al. A multicenter trial for resuscitation of injured patients with 7.5% sodium chloride. The effect of added dextran 70. The multicenter group for the study of hypertonic saline in trauma patients. *Arch Surg.* 1993;128:1003–1011.
20. Bickell WH, Bruttig SP, Millnamow GA, et al. The use of hypertonic saline/dextran versus lactated Ringer's solution as a resuscitation fluid after uncontrolled aortic hemorrhage in anesthetized swine. *Ann Emerg Med.* 1992;21:1077–1085.
21. Callaham M. Quantifying the scanty science of prehospital emergency care. *Ann Emerg Med.* 1997;30:785–790.
22. Garrison HG, Benson NH, Whitley TW, et al. Paramedic skills and medications: practice options utilized by local advanced life support medical directors. *Prehosp Disaster Med.* 1991;6:29–33.
23. Brown LH, Collins K, Gough JE, et al. An evidence-based evaluation of EMS protocols. *Prehosp Emerg Care.* 1999;3:31–36.
24. Pantridge JF, Geddes JS. A mobile intensive care unit in the management of myocardial infarction. *Lancet.* 1967;2:271–273.
25. Honigman B, Rohweda K, Moov EE, et al. Prehospital advanced trauma life support for penetrating cardiac wounds. *Ann Emerg Med.* 1990;19:145–150.
26. Jacobs LM, Sinclair A, Beiser A, D'Agostino RB. Prehospital advanced life support: benefits in trauma. *J Trauma.* 1984;24:8–13.
27. Eckstein M, Chan L, Schneir A, et al. Effect of prehospital advanced life support on outcomes of major trauma patients. *J Trauma.* 2000;48:643–648.
28. Gaffney FA, Thal ER, et al. Hemodynamic effects of medical antishock trousers. *J Trauma.* 1981;21:931–937.
29. Flint LM, Brown A, Richardson JD, Polk HC. Definitive control of bleeding for severe pelvic fractures. *Ann Surg.* 1979;189:709–716.

30. Cutler BS, Daggett WM. Application of the "G-Suit" to the control of hemorrhage in massive trauma. *Ann Surg.* 1971;173:511–514.

31. McSwain NE Jr. Pneumatic antishock garment: state of the art 1988. *Ann Emerg Med.* 1988;17:506–525.

32. Bickell WH, Pepe PE, et al. Effect of antishock trousers on the trauma score: A prospective analysis in the urban setting. *Ann Emerg Med.* 1985;14:218–222.

33. Mattox KL, Bickell WH, Pepe PE, et al. Prospective randomized evaluation of antishock MAST in post-traumatic hypotension. *J Trauma.* 1986;26:779–786.

34. Mackenzie RC, Christensen BS, Lewis FR. The prehospital use of external counterpressure: does MAST make a difference? *J Trauma.* 1984;24:882–888.

35. Gold CR. Prehospital advanced life support vs. "scoop and run" in trauma management. *Ann Emer Med.* 1987;16:797–801.

36. Mattox KL, Bickell WH, Pepe PE, et al. Prospective MAST study in 9-1-1 patients. *J Trauma.* 1989;29:1104–1112.

37. Domeier RM, O'Connor RE, Delbridge TR, et al. Use of the pneumaticanti-shock garment. *Prehosp Emerg Care.* 1997;1:32–35.

38. Cayten CG, Berendt BM, Byrne DW, et al. A study of pneumatic antishock garments in severely hypotensive trauma patients. *J Trauma.* 1993;34:728–735.

39. Callaham M. Quantifying the scanty science of prehospital emergency care. *Ann Emerg Med.* 1997;30:785–790.

Trauma

Susan M. Dunmire, MD

Introduction

Appropriate out-of-hospital management of the trauma patient can have a major impact on overall patient morbidity and mortality. While controversy exists as to how much out-of-hospital intervention is indicated in the trauma patient, recent studies have been elucidating which interventions may benefit the patient and which may be harmful. In past discussions on the treatment of the trauma patient, guidelines may have been oversimplified, not accounting for the mechanism of injury, injury severity, and location of the EMS provider in relation to the nearest hospital. Experience and scientific studies indicate that simplified philosophies such as "scoop and run" and "stay and play," while applicable in certain situations, no longer should be universally applied to all trauma patients.

Evaluation and Treatment

Penetrating Trauma

The management of the patient with penetrating injuries, particularly to the head, neck, chest, or abdomen, is usually straightforward. These patients should undergo a rapid survey followed by immobilization and rapid transport to the nearest regional trauma center.

Depending on the distance to this trauma center, decisions regarding airway management may differ. If transport is short (less than 20 minutes) and the out-of-hospital team is able to achieve adequate oxygenation and ventilation with a facemask or with a bag-valve-mask (BVM), time should not be taken at the scene for attempts at intubation. Not only is intubation time-consuming, but it is particularly challenging in the trauma victim due to secretions or blood in the airway, inadequate suction, and often lack of neuromuscular blockade for the semi-responsive, combative patient.

Should active airway intervention become necessary due to inability to oxygenate or ventilate with the BVM or a prolonged distance to the trauma center, attempts at intubation may be made while the patient is en route to the hospital. Orotracheal intubation is the preferred route for the trauma patient. Techniques such as digital intubation are particularly helpful in the setting of the unresponsive patient with large amounts of blood or secretions in the airway. Training out-of-hospital personnel in alternate airway techniques such as digital and lighted stylet intubation and use of the Combitube may be extremely useful in the trauma setting.

Most studies indicate that patients suffering penetrating trauma do not benefit from massive fluid resuscitation in the out-of-hospital setting. Intravenous access should be attempted if there is time during transport, but should not delay scene time in the patient with penetrating trauma. If IV access is established, crystalloid may be infused judiciously. If transport to the nearest regional trauma center is prolonged, it is recommended that fluid be infused to keep the patient's mean blood pressure above 40 mm Hg, but not with the goal of normalizing the blood pressure.

Blunt Trauma

The management of the patient suffering from blunt trauma often requires a longer "scene time" due to extrication and immobilization. There is a paucity of literature on airway management in the victim of blunt trauma, but the studies that have been done suggest there is improved survival if a patient with a Glasgow Coma Score of < 8 undergoes endotracheal intubation in the field.[1–3] In one study, field intubation decreased mortality from 57% to 36% in patients with severe head injury, and from 50% to 23% in patients with isolated head injury.[1]

Intubation is particularly challenging in the patient with facial and head trauma; orotracheal intubation is the preferred route. The out-of-hospital provider must use his judgment based on the difficulty of the airway and the distance to the hospital as to whether to take the time for endotracheal intubation at the scene. If two attempts are unsuccessful, rapid transport to the hospital while assisting ventilation with a BVM is advised.

The role of fluid resuscitation in the blunt trauma patient is unclear, and requires further study. Current recommendations are that IV access be attempted en route to the hospital and crystalloid be infused at a moderate rate if the patient is hypotensive. The goal is not to normalize the blood pressure, but to elevate and maintain enough systolic pressure to sustain cerebral perfusion and oxygenation.

Controversies

Intravenous Fluid Resuscitation

Recent clinical research indicates that out-of-hospital fluid resuscitation may be detrimental in the patient with penetrating trauma to the torso.[4] A large prospective study in which victims of penetrating trauma were randomized to receive out-of-hospital fluid resuscitation versus delaying fluid resuscitation until they reached the operating room, indicates that patients undergoing out-of-hospital resuscitation had a higher mortality and more postoperative complications than the group with delayed fluid resuscitation. There is speculation that an increase in hydraulic pressure in the vessels increases bleeding and potentially dislodges any clots that had formed at the site of bleeding. Massive fluid resuscitation with crystalloid undoubtedly dilutes the body's clotting factors.

Scoop and Run vs. Stay and Play

As stated earlier, this age-old controversy over-simplifies the treatment of trauma. The appropriate treatment of a victim of trauma must take into consideration the mechanism of injury, patient stability, availability of resources, and distance to the regional trauma center. Clearly this is less of an issue in patients with penetrating trauma where the benefit of the "scoop and run" philosophy has been supported by studies. Some experts postulate that there is no benefit to EMS transport of trauma patients if they are within 15 to 20 minutes from a trauma center. One recent study comparing trauma victims who were transported by paramedics versus private vehicle demonstrated a mortality rate of 28.8% for the EMS transport group versus 14.1% for those arriving in private vehicles.[8] With the exception of securing an airway in a blunt trauma victim, there is no indication for prolonging scene time in any trauma victim. Clearly all studies support the importance of rapid transport to a regional trauma center where definitive care can be rendered.

Does the Patient Need a Trauma Center?

It is crucial that the out-of-hospital provider be able to rapidly and accurately identify those patients who may benefit from the resources available at a trauma center. The correct triage of trauma victims is challenging in that it must be completed rapidly, and frequently much important data is missing. Although trauma scoring systems are useful in predicting who will die from trauma, they cannot be used alone to predict who will benefit from a trauma center. Most out-of-hospital systems base the trauma triage decision on a combination of the revised trauma score, the mechanism of injury, and the judgment of the provider. It is recommended that trauma victims with a revised trauma score of <11 should be transported to a regional trauma center. Some of the more common mechanisms of injury used as indicators for transport to a regional trauma center include:

- Major damage to the vehicle
- Falls > 15 feet
- Rollover of vehicle
- Extrication > 20 minutes
- Fatality within the same vehicle
- Pedestrians struck by a vehicle

An under-appreciated and under-emphasized factors in trauma triage decision-making are the judgments of the provider and the direct medical oversight physician. Although such judgment is useful in triaging a patient to a regional trauma center who otherwise would not have met criteria, the reverse is not true. Judgment should never override trauma scoring and mechanism of injury in diverting a patient away from a trauma center.

Protocols

In developing protocols for the triage and treatment of the trauma patient, multiple factors must be considered. The provider must take into consideration mechanism of injury, clinical markers of injury, and physiologic signs of instability. In theory, considering the mechanism of injury should improve the accuracy of trauma triage; however, Henry found that considering some mechanism criteria actually worsened triage specificity.[9,10] The American College of Surgeons and the American College of Emergency Physicians (ACEP) have published trauma triage guidelines to assist out-of-hospital providers.[11,12] It is estimated that these guidelines result in over-triage by approximately 30%. Figure 62.1 is a triage algorithm developed by ACEP to assist systems with the development of trauma triage protocols.

Protocols for treatment of the trauma patient should be straightforward and allow the provider maximum autonomy. Scene time should not be delayed while the provider waits for direct medical oversight. All protocols should be focused on providing the necessary interventions with rapid transport to a trauma center.

Trauma Scoring

Trauma scoring systems were first developed over twenty years ago in an attempt to determine the severity of injury and guide the out-of-hospital provider to the appropriate triage of certain patients to a regional trauma center. A variety of scoring systems exist today; however, the major scoring systems used in the out-of-hospital setting are the Revised Trauma Score (RTS) and the Out-of-Hospital Index (PI).

The PI scores four variables (systolic blood pressure, pulse, respiratory status, and level of consciousness) and each variable can be rated 0–5 with 0 being a normal value. In one study which incorporated a fifth variable of penetrating torso trauma worth 4 points, patients with a score <4 had a 0.6% incidence of requiring surgery and no deaths.[13] For patients with a score > 3, 47% required emergent surgery and 23% died. The study authors recommended triage of patients with a score >3 to a regional trauma center. A Canadian study found a PI of > 3 to be 98% sensitive in identifying mortality due to trauma, but only 59% sensitive in predicting which patients will require surgery within 24 hours.[14]

The RTS is one of the most common out-of-hospital scoring systems. (fig. 62.2) It combines the Glasgow Coma Score with respiratory rate and systolic blood pressure. It is recommended that any patient with an RTS<11 be transported to a trauma center.[12]

Most literature suggests that provider judgment is almost as good as trauma scoring in predicting the need for triage to a trauma center.[15–17] Training in the use of a trauma scoring system to be used in conjunction with judgment is recommended. Factors such as the provider's level of training, distance to the trauma center, and availability of rotorcraft may all play a role in the decision as well. Each trauma system must determine acceptable levels of over- and under-triage and how to best achieve these goals.

Summary

Management of trauma in an efficient, well organized fashion by out-of-hospital providers can have a major effect on patient morbidity and mortality. Rapid transport of the severely injured trauma patient to a regional trauma center, and airway management, are the only factors that have ever been shown to make a significant difference in patient survival. While airway interventions and fluid resuscitation may be necessary and life-sustaining en route to the trauma center, they are rarely a priority at the scene. All out-of-hospital systems should work toward the common goal of the "golden ten minutes" of out-of-hospital time for the trauma patient in order to optimize patient survival. This can only be accomplished through concise protocols, continued training and cumulative experience.

Cases

Case 1

A 54-year-old male sustains a gunshot wound to the neck. Upon arrival of the out-of-hospital team (1 paramedic, 1 EMT), the patient is lying supine, unresponsive. A large wound is noted over the left lateral neck and a smaller wound in the right posterior neck. On primary survey, respirations are shallow at a rate of 24 per minute and there are equal breath sounds bilaterally. A large amount of blood is exiting the left neck wound. Although the patient moans occasionally, there is no localizing response to verbal or painful stimuli. A carotid pulse is present, but there is no palpable brachial pulse. Transport time to the nearest trauma center is 10 minutes.

The patient is placed supine on a stretcher. The EMT assists ventilations with a BVM and applies in line stabilization to the neck while the paramedic finishes the secondary survey. The paramedic then attempts to intubate the patient, but is unsuccessful

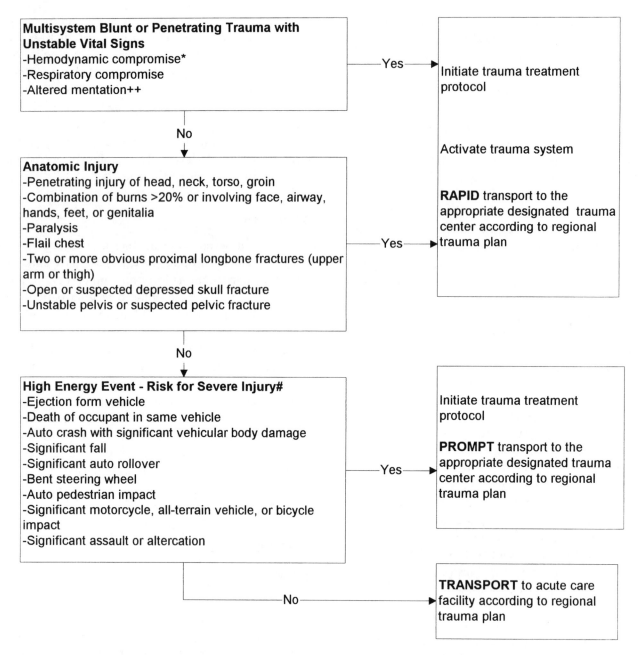

Multisystem Blunt or Penetrating Trauma with Unstable Vital Signs
-Hemodynamic compromise*
-Respiratory compromise
-Altered mentation++

—Yes—→ Initiate trauma treatment protocol

Activate trauma system

RAPID transport to the appropriate designated trauma center according to regional trauma plan

No ↓

Anatomic Injury
-Penetrating injury of head, neck, torso, groin
-Combination of burns >20% or involving face, airway, hands, feet, or genitalia
-Paralysis
-Flail chest
-Two or more obvious proximal longbone fractures (upper arm or thigh)
-Open or suspected depressed skull fracture
-Unstable pelvis or suspected pelvic fracture

—Yes—→

No ↓

High Energy Event - Risk for Severe Injury#
-Ejection form vehicle
-Death of occupant in same vehicle
-Auto crash with significant vehicular body damage
-Significant fall
-Significant auto rollover
-Bent steering wheel
-Auto pedestrian impact
-Significant motorcycle, all-terrain vehicle, or bicycle impact
-Significant assault or altercation

—Yes—→ Initiate trauma treatment protocol

PROMPT transport to the appropriate designated trauma center according to regional trauma plan

—No—→ **TRANSPORT** to acute care facility according to regional trauma plan

*In addition to hypotension: pallor, tachycardia or diaphoresis my be early signs of hypovolemia.

+Tachypnea (hyperventilation) alone will not necessarily initiate this level of response.

++Altered sensorium secondary to sedative-hypnotics will not necessarily initiate this level of response.

#High energy event signifies a large release of uncontrolled energy. Patient is assumed injured until proven otherwise, and multisystem injuries might exist.

Determinants to be considered by medical professionals are direction and velocity of impact, patient kinematics and physical size, and the residual signature of energy release (e.g., major vehicle damage). Clinical judgment must be exercised and may upgrade to a high level of response and activation. Age and comorbid conditions should be considered in the decision.

FIGURE 62.1. *Prehospital—Model triage algorithm. From: ACEP: Guidelines for trauma care systems. Ann Emerg Med 22:1088, 1993.*

		Score
A. Respiratory Rate	10–24	4
	25–35	3
	>36	2
	1–9	1
	0	0
B. Systolic Blood Pressure	>89	4
	70–89	3
	50–69	2
	1–49	1
	0	0
C. Glasgow Coma Score	13–15	4
	9–12	3
	6–8	2
	4–5	1
	<4	0

FIGURE 62.2. *Revised Trauma Score.*

due to the amount of blood in the airway. The paramedic attempts an IV and is successful in placing one 16-gauge IV in the antecubital fossa. IV fluids are initiated at a rapid rate. The patient is rolled onto a long board and loaded into the ambulance. The paramedic continues to assist ventilations while the EMT drives to the regional trauma center.

Time at the scene: 23 minutes
Transport time: 8 minutes

DISCUSSION

There were some major mistakes made in the management of this patient. This patient is in hemorrhagic shock after sustaining a penetrating wound to the neck. The primary survey identified a spontaneously breathing patient with an unprotected airway as well as frank shock with a systolic blood pressure of < 80 mm Hg (no palpable brachial pulse). His RTS is approximately 9 with an obvious need for a trauma center. Cervical spine immobilization was an appropriate decision due to the blast injury to the neck. If it is impossible to place a cervical collar due to limitation in the ability to apply direct pressure to the wound, then in-line stabilization is the next best alternative.

With a trauma center less than 10 minutes away, the team should have immobilized the patient, applied a face mask of oxygen or assisted ventilation with a bag valve mask and applied direct pressure to the bleeding wound. Time should not have been taken for IV placement or active airway inter-

vention in what would be anticipated to be a difficult intubation.

Case 2

A 23-year-old female is the unrestrained driver in a single-vehicle, high-speed MVA in which her vehicle struck a utility pole. A rescue unit consisting of one paramedic and one EMT arrives on scene to find the patient entrapped on the driver's side. Her head is slumped back against the headrest and she is moaning. She does respond to questioning, but her answers are slurred. She complains of her chest hurting. Transport time to nearest trauma center is 25 minutes.

While the EMT works to free the patient's legs, the paramedic enters the passenger door and performs a primary survey. The patient has decreased breath sounds on the right with crepitance of the right chest wall. Her BP is 86/P, pulse of 140 and respiratory rate of 30. While extrication is in progress, the paramedic applies oxygen by facemask and initiates a 14-gauge IV of lactated Ringer's infusing at a rapid rate. Once extrication is complete, the patient is immobilized. Her respiratory distress markedly worsens and the paramedic prepares to intubate. She is orotracheally intubated and tube placement is confirmed; however, she has absent breath sounds on the right. The patient now has no palpable brachial pulse, but does still have a weakly palpable carotid pulse.

The patient is loaded into the ambulance. With a 25-minute time to the nearest trauma center, the paramedic asks direct medical oversight for permission to decompress her presumed tension pneumothorax. A 14-gauge IV catheter is inserted into the second intercostal space and the patient's brachial pulse returns. The remaining transport is without incident.

Time at the scene: 25 minutes
Transport time: 26 minutes

DISCUSSION

This case of blunt trauma was managed appropriately by the crew and the DMOP. On primary survey, the patient is found to be in respiratory distress and hypotensive. Her RTS is 10 (GCS of 14, respiratory rate of 30 and systolic blood pressure of 86) indicating that she will require a trauma center. The paramedic made good use of the extrication time to initiate oxygen and an IV. As soon as the patient was extricated it was clear that she would not maintain her airway for a 25-minute transport time and the decision was made to intubate her.

With further deterioration of her vital signs, the paramedic realized the necessity of decompression of the pneumothorax and direct medical oversight appropriately agreed. Although the scene time was 25 minutes, 15 minutes of this time was used for extrication. Identification and rapid treatment of these life-threatening airway problems resulted in a good outcome.

References

1. Winchell RJ, Hoyt DB. Endotracheal intubation in the field improves survival in patients with severe head injury. *Arch Surg.* 1997;132:592–597.
2. Durham LA, Richardson RJ, Wall MJ, et al. Emergency center thoracotomy: impact of out-of-hospital resuscitation. *J Trauma.* 1992;32:775–779.
3. Copass MK, Oreskovich MR, Bladergroen MR. Out-of-hospital cardiopulmonary resuscitation of the critically injured patient. *Am J Surg.* 1984;148:20–26.
4. Bickell WH, Wall MJ, Pepe PE, et al. Immediate versus delayed fluid resuscitation for hypotensive patients with penetrating torso injuries. *N Engl J Med.* 1994;331: 1105–1109.
5. Gervin AS, Fischer RP. The importance of prompt transport in salvage of patients with penetrating heart wounds. *J Trauma.* 1982;22:443–448.
6. Smith JP, Bodai BI, Hill AS, et al. Out-of-hospital stabilization of critically injured patients: a failed concept. *J Trauma.* 1985;25:65–70.
7. Pons PT, Moore EE, Cusick JM, et al. Out-of-hospital venous access in an urban paramedic system—a prospective on-scene analysis. *J Trauma.* 1988;28:1460–1463.
8. Demetriades D, Chan L, Cornwell E, et al. Paramedic versus private transportation of trauma patients. *Arch Surg.* 1996;131:133–138.
9. Henry MC. Evaluation of American College of Surgeons trauma criteria in a suburban and rural setting. *Am J Emerg Med.* 1996;14:124–129.
10. Henry MC, et al. Incremental benefit of individual American College of Surgeons trauma triage criteria. *Acad Emerg Med.* 1996;3:992–1000.
11. American College of Emergency Physicians. Guidelines for trauma care systems. *Ann Emerg Med.* 1993;22: 1079–1100.
12. American College of Surgeons Committee on Trauma. Out-of-hospital Resources for Optimal Care of the Injured Patient. Chicago: American College of Surgeons; 1993.
13. Koehler J, et al. A multi-center validation of the out-of-hospital index. *Ann Emerg Med.* 1987;16:380–385.
14. Plant JR, MacLeod DB, Kortbeek J. Limitation of the out-of-hospital index in identifying patients in need of a major trauma center. *Ann Emerg Med.* 1995;26:133–137.
15. Simmons E, et al. Paramedic injury severity perception can aid trauma triage. *Ann Emerg Med.* 1995;26:461–468.
16. Ornato J, et al. Ineffectiveness of the Trauma Score and the CRAMS Scale for accurately triaging patients to trauma centers. *Ann Emerg Med.* 1985;14:1061–1064.
17. Fries GR, et al. A prospective comparison of paramedic judgment and trauma triage in the out-of-hospital setting. *Ann Emerg Med.* 1994;24:885–889.

CHAPTER 63

Obstetric and Gynecologic

William J. Angelos, MD

Introduction

It is important for the direct medical oversight physician (DMOP) to have a well established knowledge of obstetrics and gynecology to appropriately guide treatment and management of these patients in the field. Most out-of-hospital obstetric cases will be unremarkable, with minimal interventions such as oxygen and an intravenous line. Some cases, however, such as imminent delivery or severe vaginal bleeding, can be a very challenging clinical encounter. Out-of-hospital deliveries are not uncommon and can have the potential for significant complication with associated morbidity and mortality.[1] Training of most out-of-hospital care providers is minimal for obstetric emergencies, and their field experience is variable, especially for complicated cases. Taking care of an obstetric or gynecologic emergency can be stressful and demanding on the prehospital personnel. The amount of stress and anxiety that a situation produces will be dependent on the prehospital care provider's previous experiences, level of training, and the type of equipment they carry with them.

The tone of the out-of-hospital care provider's voice over the radio can be the first indicator that a difficult situation is in progress. A knowledgeable DMOP can alleviate some of the anxieties of the care provider as well as provide needed medical guidance for these patients. Understanding these extreme situations can help to improve the patient's outcome and help prehospital personnel deal with the stressful and sometimes overwhelming situation.

Evaluation

Important historical and physical information should be obtained by the out-of-hospital personnel. If the patient is pregnant, information such as number of previous pregnancies and deliveries; due date; previous perinatal complications; membrane rupture; contraction onset, duration and interval; and vaginal bleeding should be sought. Physical findings such as vital signs and fetal movement should also be part of the report that the prehospital personnel obtains. If there is a history of precipitous delivery or the patient has the urge to push or is pushing, examination of the introitus should be performed. If there is a presenting part and the patient is pushing, an imminent delivery is inevitable, and the prehospital care-giver should prepare to deliver the baby.

It is important for the out-of-hospital care provider to recognize and treat problems that arise during pregnancy, labor, and delivery. Bleeding and abdominal pain are common complaints during pregnancy and can be from a variety of etiologies. Knowing what trimester the patient is in will help narrow the differential diagnosis (table 63.1).[2] The DMOP should aggressively treat bleeding in pregnancy (all trimesters) and consider the potential for hypovolemia.

Women in child-bearing age who present with abdominal pain can have a wide spectrum of etiologies (table 63.2).[3] The DMOP should develop a working diagnosis and supportive plan from the information that is supplied by the out-of-hospital care provider. This plan should be explained to the prehospital provider caring for the patient, especially if subtle etiologies are being considered.

TABLE 63.1	
Differential Diagnosis of Vaginal Bleeding	
	CONSIDERATIONS
PREGNANT PATIENT	Ectopic pregnancy, threatened AB, placenta previa, abruptio placenta, bloody show
NON-PREGNANT PATIENT	Ectopic pregnancy, dysfunctional uterine bleeding, degenerating fibroid, menses, trauma, cancer, hyperplasia

TABLE 63.2	
Differential Diagnosis of Abdominal Pain	
	CONSIDERATIONS
OB/GYN RELATED	Ectopic pregnancy, PID, torsion of the ovary, degenerating fibroid, threatened AB, ruptured ovarian cyst, endometriosis
OB/GYN NON-RELATED	Gastroenteritis, appendicitis, cholecystitis, SBO, PUD, gastritis, diverticulitis, perforation, peritonitis

TABLE 63.3
Signs and Symptoms of Preeclampsia
Systolic Blood Pressure greater than 160
Diastolic Blood Pressure greater than 110
Increasing Pedal Edema
Headache
Epigastric/RUQ Abdominal Pain

Treatment

Pregnant Patient— Preeclampsia/Eclampsia

The out-of-hospital care provider has limited resources in the field to treat a preeclamptic or eclamptic patient. An IV line should be established, as well as oxygen by a non-rebreather mask. If the patient is seizing, 5 to 10 mg of diazepam should be ordered IV at a rate of 2mg/min. If there is no IV access, diazepam can be given rectally with a syringe and angiocath (5mg–10mg). If the unit carries magnesium it should be given to all preeclamptic patients with a diastolic pressure of greater than 100 with symptoms (headache, visual complaints, RUQ pain), and all eclamptic patients (table 63.3). Four grams of 10% magnesium sulfate in 250 cc of D_5W IV can be given safely over 15 minutes.[4] Special attention should be made to maintaining an airway and for rapid transport to the hospital. If no intravenous access can be established, 5 grams of magnesium can be given intramuscular in each buttock.[5]

Pregnant Trauma Patient

The pregnant trauma patient should be treated with special consideration. Basic trauma life support should be carried out accordingly with high flow oxygen, immobilization, and large bore IVs. The pregnant patient's physiology is different from a non-pregnant patient and these differences should be known to the physician giving medical command. In the last trimester the blood volume has increased 50% above baseline, the heart and respiratory rate have also increased by at least 10%, blood pressure is lower, and cardiac output is increased (table 63.4).[6] Because of the increase in blood volume, signs of shock may

occur later than normal or be absent with considerable amount of blood loss.[7,8] Gastric motility is also decreased, which increases the risk of aspiration.

It is important that all pregnant trauma patients in the second and third trimester should be transported in the left lateral decubitus position. This can be accomplished after the patient is immobilized on a long board by lifting the right side of the board approximately 15 degrees with blankets or sand bags. This position allows for the uterus to be moved off the inferior vena cava and facilitates blood return to the heart to maintain uterine flow.[8,9] If at all possible, fetal heart tones should be assessed by the medics without delaying transport. Usually the heart tones can be heard with a stethoscope after 20 weeks of gestation. Variation of normal fetal heart tones (normal-120–160) may be the first sign that maternal circulation is compromised as well as indicate fetal hypoxia. If vaginal bleeding is present, the possibility for uterine rupture or placental separation is likely.[7,9] In this situation the prehospital provider should not perform a digital vaginal exam because of the potential to aggravate the condition.

Pneumatic anti-shock garments (PASG) have a limited role in the trauma pregnant patient. If there are signs or symptoms of hypovolemia, the PASG suit can be inflated on the legs only. The PASG suit can also be used to splint lower extremity fractures as needed.[7,9]

TABLE 63.4
Physiology Changes in Pregnancy
Blood volume increases greater than 50% of baseline
Heart rate increased 10% to 15%
Respirations increased 10% to 15%
Cardiac output increased
Blood Pressure is lower or normal

Pregnant Patient in Cardiac Arrest

Resuscitation methods for the pregnant arrested pregnant patient are different for the non-pregnant patient. The out-of-hospital care provider should "load and go" with interventions and resuscitation measures en route, as the success of emergent caesarean section in the emergency department correlates directly with the length of time the patient has been in arrest.

Communication with the obstetrician and a neonatal resuscitation team should be made regarding the possibility of a C-section. If available, subspecialty team members should be prepared to meet the patient in the emergency department. Being prepared and ready in the emergency department will give the neonate every possible chance of survival. There are reported cases of good neurologic outcome of the neonate if the C-section is done within the first 15 minutes of the arrest.[10–12]

Imminent Delivery

All women who are in active labor should have oxygen by face mask applied and a large bore intravenous line of a crystalloid solution established, which usually can be done en route to the hospital. Every effort should be made to insure delivery in the hospital. When the provider calls for direct medical oversight it is important for the DMOP to get the appropriate information as well as to remind the field team to expedite transport if at all possible.

Understandably, not all patients will be amenable to being moved to the back of the ambulance as the delivery is advancing; however, it should be explained to the patient that if there is a problem with the delivery, help is only a drive away. Only truly imminent deliveries justify out-of-hospital deliveries. All too often the prehospital care provider will state that they have an imminent delivery and call back to command 45 minutes later when the infant is born! Paramedics should not wait around for delivery, but should be reminded what constitutes a true imminent delivery (table 63.5). The occasional practice of waiting for the delivery should be discouraged; however in some instances inhospital delivery cannot occur if a true imminent delivery is present. The field teams must be encouraged to begin transporting the patient in labor to the hospital.

If a delivery is about to take place, it is important for the prehospital care providers to be prepared emotionally and technically. Most experienced providers will have been involved in some aspect of a delivery in the past. Even though they may have

TABLE 63.5
Signs and Symptoms of Imminent Delivery
Presenting part is visible at the introitus
Patient has urge to push
Increasing bloody show
Bulging perineum

previous knowledge and experience, a delivery can be stressful, and the DMOP must help alleviate these problems as well as give technical information. An area should be designated for resuscitation of the neonate, and appropriate airway equipment should be ready.

The delivery in most cases will progress with little intervention. Once the head is delivered, the nares and mouth should be suctioned out with a bulb syringe unless there is meconium. The umbilical cord should be double clamped and divided after the remaining body is delivered. The baby should be immediately dried and evaluated.

Prolapse of the Umbilical Cord

There are several potential complications associated with vaginal deliveries. One such complication is the prolapse of the umbilical cord. If the provider reports the umbilical cord is prolapsed while the patient is in labor, the provider should be instructed not to push the cord back into the vagina. The provider should wrap the cord in sterile gauze, which should be moistened with sterile saline or water. It is recommended to keep the presenting part off the pelvic brim.[13] The provider should be instructed to insert two fingers of a sterile gloved hand into the vagina and lift the presenting part off the bony pelvis. The patient is then placed in a knee-chest position to allow gravity to help take pressure off the cord. This will improve umbilical blood follow and reduce the chance of hypoxia to the neonate. This maneuver should be done while in transit to the hospital and should by no means delay transportation. It is important to remind the prehospital crew to stabilize the patient on the stretcher when in the knee-chest position. If the delivery is imminent, then the providers should proceed as discussed earlier.

Nuchal Cord

Another complication of vaginal delivery is a nuchal cord. If there is an umbilical cord wrapped around the fetus' neck, the provider should be instructed to attempt to gently lift the cord over the head. If the cord is tight and cannot be lifted over the neonate's head, the prehospital care provider should suction out the oral pharynx and nares before double clamping and cutting the cord. This maneuver will clear the airway and allowed the neonate to breath.

Meconium

If thick meconium is present, the care provider should be instructed to suction out the hypopharynx with a bulb syringe. The provider should be told not to stimulate the neonate so that respirations are not initiated. Once the delivery is complete, the prehospital provider should intubate the neonate and suction through the endotracheal tube as it is being withdrawn from the airway. This procedure should be continued until the majority of the meconium has cleared or the newborn becomes bradycardic (<80 bpm). The provider should not bag the neonate or stimulate it until the meconium is cleared. In some cases, the provider will be in a situation where meconium is not totally clear and the neonate has become bradycardic. In this case, the provider will need to ventilate and oxygenate the infant. Endotracheal intubation is not required if watery or thin meconium is present. The provider's skill and the equipment available will determine how much airway control will be achieved. The DMOP should know what the prehospital system is capable of and make medically sound decisions based on this information.

Breech

The problem that arises with a breech presentation is that the presenting part does not adequately dilate the cervix, making spontaneous delivery difficult. Morbidity and mortality is significantly higher even if delivery occurs in the labor and delivery room of a hospital.[14] It is almost impossible to give proper instructions over the radio for a breech delivery. The best approach is to have the providers support the presenting part, letting the delivery occur spontaneously. When the head presents, the paramedics can place two fingers forming a V into the vagina to allow the neonate to breathe. Simultaneously, the providers should move the patient into the back of the ambulance for expeditious transport. Oxygen should be administered to the mother and an intra-venous line should be established en route to the hospital. They should not push the presenting part back into the vagina, but allow the delivery to proceed spontaneously.

Shoulder Dystocia

In most deliveries the shoulders will be delivered easily. If the shoulders by chance become impeded, the prehospital care providers can have an assistant hyperflex the mother's hips against her abdomen and apply mild suprapubic pressure (not fundal pressure). Gentle posterior traction of the head will relieve the dystocia.[15] If this maneuver by itself does not work, the DMOP should instruct the provider to rotate the shoulders while suprapubic pressure is being applied. This can be accomplished by having the provider apply two fingers on the front part of the top shoulder (anterior) and rotate the neonate toward the back into an oblique position.[16,17] The success of freeing of the shoulders will depend primarily on the experience of the care provider and the ability of the DMOP to provide precise instruction.

If at all possible, have the provider get the patient into the ambulance early before delivery problems arise. This will allow them to drive for help while managing the complication.

Post Delivery—Care of the Neonate

Once the umbilical cord is divided, the neonate should be placed in a supine, head down position with head turned to the side. Normally, the newborn begins to breathe and cry almost immediately after birth. If respirations do not occur or are infrequent, suctioning of the mouth and pharynx should be performed. Also, stimulating the feet or back may initiate breathing. The neonate should be dried and kept warm. If the neonate is stable, the infant can be held close to the mother's chest to decrease heat loss.

A helpful method in evaluating the newborn's condition is using the one and five minute Apgar scores (table 63.6). Scores between 4 and 6 at one minute may indicate a mildly to moderately depressed infant, whereas scores below 3 represent a severely depressed infant.[18] If warming and stimulating the neonate do not initiate the infant's respirations, the prehospital provider will need to resuscitate the infant. First, the prehospital care provider should place the infant on oxygen and assess the patient's color and respiratory status. If respiratory status does not

TABLE 63.6			
APGAR Scoring System			
SIGN	**0**	**1**	**2**
Heart Rate	Absent	Below 100	Over 100
Respiratory Effort	Absent	Slow, irregular	Good, crying
Muscle Tone	Flaccid	Some flexion of extremities	Active motion
Reflex Irritability	No response	Grimace	Vigorous cry
Color	Blue, pale	Body pink, extremities blue	Pink

improve, it may be necessary to start bag/mask ventilation of the neonate until spontaneous respirations occur. If bag/mask ventilation does not improve symptoms, chest compression should be initiated. Chest compressions can be performed by having the provider place both thumbs on the lower one-third of the sternum with fingers wrapped around the torso in support of the back.[19] The thumbs should be positioned side by side on the sternum just below the line of the two nipples. The sternum is compressed, 1/2 to 3/4 of an inch downward and at a rate of approximately 120 times per minute. If the neonate's respiratory, heart rate and color do not improve with chest compression, the neonate will require intubation. If this does not correct the situation, medications may be warranted. Epinephrine is indicated if spontaneous heart rate is less than 80 beats per minute despite adequate ventilation with 100% O_2 and chest compressions. The dose is 0.01 to 0.03 mg/kg of 1/10,000 solution. This can be given down the endotracheal tube.

Intravenous access is difficult in the prehospital setting on a neonate and time should not be delayed trying to establish IV access. An alternative is to establish an intraosseous line if drugs and fluid are needed to resuscitate. The provider should be instructed that if they are having difficulties with the infant and/or mother, he should get the patient into the back of the ambulance and transport to the closest appropriate facility.

Postpartum Hemorrhage

Blood loss greater than 500 cc after the third stage of labor is considered abnormal. Even after delivery, bleeding can occur anywhere along the reproductive tract. Bleeding at the placenta is usually controlled by uterine contractions. Usually, early postpartum bleeding is either from uterine atony or lacerations to the genital tract (table 63.7).[20] If bleeding is significant, the providers should establish a line of crystalloid and give a large bolus of fluid with reassessments of the patient's vitals.

A quick abdominal exam should be performed to evaluate the uterus. If the uterus is soft and boggy, this suggests uterine atony. If the uterus is firm and contracted, the source of bleeding is most likely a laceration of the genital tract. Unfortunately, these findings are often difficult to discern in the field. Out-of-hospital treatment is mainly IV crystalloids and oxygen. The provider should expedite transportation of the patient to the hospital.

Delivery of the Placenta

In most cases, the placenta will deliver spontaneously. The prehospital care provider should not wait for delivery of the placenta, but transport the mother and neonate to the hospital. Physical signs that the placenta is about to be delivered are that the uterus becomes globular in shape, the umbilical cord lengthens and there may be a gush of blood just prior to the delivery. If the placenta is delivered prior to arrival to the hospital, the placenta should be saved for pathologic evaluation.

TABLE 63.7
Differential Diagnosis Early Postpartum Hemorrhage
Uterine Atony
Laceration
Retained placenta
Uterine Rupture
Uterine Inversion

Vaginal Bleeding—The Pregnant Patient

As mentioned earlier, all pregnant patients should be placed on high flow oxygen and have an intravenous line of a crystalloid solution. The amount of bleeding and the change in vital signs will determine how much fluid will be required. If the vital signs are stable (appropriate for pregnancy) and minimal blood loss has occurred, a 300–400 cc bolus should be ordered. If there are unstable vitals, moderate to severe bleeding, or even subjective complaints (i.e. light-headed, dizzy), a larger bolus, preferably using a pressure bag, should be given until the vital signs are corrected or symptoms improved. Instruct the provider to recheck vitals after the fluid bolus and report the results. It is important to err on the side of too much volume than not enough in these patients. Supportive care is the major prehospital concern and transport to an appropriate hospital should be expedited for the unstable patient.

Abdominal Pain with Vaginal Bleeding

All patients of child-bearing years with abdominal pain and vaginal bleeding should be treated as possible ectopic pregnancies until proven otherwise.[21-23] The provider should be instructed to establish two large bore intravenous lines with an isotonic crystalloid solution and to administer oxygen by mask. A fluid bolus of 500 cc during transport is prudent if there is no underlying cardiac or renal disease. Evidence of hypotension in the setting of a "normal" heart rate may be a sign of intraperitoneal blood and would warrant more aggressive fluid resuscitation.[24] If there are signs of hypovolemia, the PASG suit would be another alternative to increase blood pressure and possibly reduce the amount of intraperitoneal bleeding.

Vaginal Bleeding without Pain

The lack of abdominal pain with vaginal bleeding does not mean that the patient has a less urgent condition. Vaginal bleeding alone can be life-threatening. All patients should be placed on oxygen and an intravenous line established with a crystalloid solution. A fluid bolus of 500 cc should be given en route depending on the estimated blood loss and the vital signs. For every 1 cc of blood loss, 3 cc of crystalloid is needed to replace intravascular volume. Obviously if vitals are unstable or there are symptoms of hypovolemia, a larger fluid bolus should be given.

Pitfalls

Allowing out-of-hospital deliveries to take place when an imminent delivery is not present is a common pitfall. It is important to ask specific questions to the prehospital providers to determine if the delivery is truly imminent. If the patient is pushing and there is a presenting part that can be seen at the introitus, then it is justified to proceed with the delivery in the field. Even if this scenario were present, it is recommended to at least have the patient in the back of the ambulance. If there is a problem with the delivery, the providers can initiate transport to the hospital expeditiously.

An unprepared or poorly equipped provider is another potential pitfall. If a delivery is to take place in the field, the out-of-hospital provider must be prepared and equipped for airway management and resuscitation. The airway kit should be open with the appropriate blades and endotracheal tubes available. Suction should also be readied. A card or tape with pediatric doses of medication should be available both for the provider and for the DMOP.

Failure to consider ectopic pregnancy in women of child-bearing years with abdominal pain with or without vaginal bleeding can be a serious oversight. Consider initiating intravenous access in all women of child-bearing age. Not all ectopic pregnancies will initially have vaginal bleeding. Also, the blood pressure and pulse can be normal initially and signs of shock delayed. Giving a modest fluid bolus to a young healthy woman will not be harmful.

Failure to transport a pregnant third trimester trauma patient in the left lateral decubitus position is another pitfall. There will be a time when a prehospital provider consults the DMOP with a trauma patient who is pregnant and a blood pressure of 70/40. While there is the potential for hypovolemia, the simple maneuver of turning the patient may be all that is needed.

Failure to communicate early with the obstetrician or the neonatal personnel can also be problematic. In certain situations (i.e., abnormal presentation) it is important that the obstetrician as well as the neonatologist be contacted immediately so that they are ready for the patient when the ambulance arrives.

Summary

Most obstetrical and gynecological problems in the field will be uneventful, but they have potential for complications. It should be routine that oxygen is administered and an intravenous line established on all women of child-bearing age who have symptoms of gynecologic or obstetric origin. The DMOP can reduce the prehospital complication with good judgment and direction. Also, the DMOP can be involved with continuing education for the prehospital care provider, with reviewing obstetric and gynecologic emergencies as well as neonatal resuscitation, with both formal and informal lectures.

Cases

Case 1

Paramedics state that they are on scene with a 23-year-old female Gl P0 who is in labor. She is 38 weeks pregnant with no prenatal complications. Contractions began three hours ago that are now three minutes apart. The paramedic states that there is no presenting part and the membranes haven't ruptured. The DMOP responds: Establish an intravenous line of lactated ringers at KVO en route, administer high flow oxygen by mask and expedite transport.

DISCUSSION

This case is an example of uncomplicated, early labor. The patient is a primigravida with only contractions and no sign of impending delivery. The paramedics should expedite transport and can perform their interventions on the way to the hospital.

Case 2

EMT-B providers report that they are seeing a 27-year-old female G5P4 who is 39 weeks pregnant and has a history of precipitous deliveries. The patient now has the urge to push. The infant's head can be seen at the introitus. The membranes ruptured 30 minutes ago with the onset of contractions. The DMOP instructs the provider to set up for an imminent delivery. High flow oxygen by mask should be administered and, if possible, an IV of crystalloid solution. Also, the providers should be instructed to have an area set up for neonate resuscitation. After delivery, the cord should be double clamped and cut, and the neonate should be wrapped in a blanket and given to the mother. If the infant is stable, the mother should be instructed to hold it close to her chest to diminish heat loss. The providers should expedite transport after delivery. The placenta can be delivered en route or at the hospital.

DISCUSSION

It is obvious that this delivery is going to occur within minutes; the prehospital providers should be prepared. If possible, the providers should get the patient into the back of the ambulance so that if any problems arise, they can easily begin transport to the hospital.

Case 3

Paramedics report that they are evaluating a 25-year-old female G0P0 who developed abdominal pain and slight vaginal bleeding. This pain and bleeding is not typical for her menses and her last period was 7 weeks ago. All vital signs are stable. The DMOP requests them to establish a large bore intravenous line of crystalloid and run in 500 cc en route, also to administer oxygen by mask and reconsult if there is a change in vitals or new symptoms.

DISCUSSION

All women of child-bearing years with abdominal pain with or without vaginal bleeding should be considered to have an ectopic pregnancy. Most ectopic pregnancies present with normal blood pressure and heart rate. The providers should start a large bore IV and give a bolus of fluid. If the vital signs are unstable, the PASG suit would be appropriate.

Case 4

EMT-Bs are on the scene of a motor vehicle crash. The driver is a 35-year-old female who is 35 weeks pregnant. She is complaining of lower extremity pain and neck pain after hitting a telephone pole. Vitals: BP-70/P, HR-100, RR-24. The DMOP has them immobilize the patient with a cervical collar, long board, high flow oxygen by mask and expedite transport. He instructs the providers to place the patient in the left lateral decubitus while transporting and to reassess the vitals. Also a bolus of fluid would be appropriate and the amount would depend on whether or not the BP corrected with moving the patient in the left lateral decubitus position.

DISCUSSION

All pregnant trauma patients in the second and third trimester should be transported in the left lateral decubitus. Also, the pregnant patient's physiology is different, which can confuse the picture; their blood volume is increased, and signs of shock may appear late.

Case 5

A 23-year-old, 36-weeks-pregnant female calls paramedics because her legs have become more swollen over the past few days. She is also complaining of a headache. Paramedics report that the blood pressure is 160/100, pulse is 100 and respirations are 24. She has no previous history of hypertension. Paramedics would like to not transport her to the hospital; hoping she could follow up with her obstetrician within a week. The DMOP indicates that this is a serious condition and transport should be done expeditiously with seizure precautions. Place the patient on high flow oxygen by face mask and establish an IV of crystalloid. Caution should be made not to overload the patient with fluids.

DISCUSSION

It is difficult to make the diagnosis of preeclampsia in the field. There are no medications that the prehospital care provider carries that are approved for lowering the BP in a pregnant patient. If the diastolic blood pressure is above 100 and the patient has no prior history of hypertension, the prehospital care provider can give magnesium if their unit carries it and the transport time is long (> 30 mins). For the most part, the prehospital care is rapid transport with interventions en route.

Case 6

A 27-year-old female G1P0 is found seizing at home. The seizures have been going on for 15 minutes. The blood pressure is 220/110. Paramedics are requesting orders. The DMOP directs the paramedics to maintain an airway and to administer high flow oxygen by mask. An intravenous line should be rapidly started and 5 mg of diazepam should be given IV line over 2½ minutes. If the seizures do not stop after 2 minutes, another 5 mg should be given. Special attention should be given for maintenance of the airway as well as rapid transport to the hospital.

DISCUSSION

The life-saving interventions for the mother and fetus are to control the seizure and to reduce the blood pressure. Diazepam and magnesium are temporizing measures. The patient should be transported to the hospital as rapidly as possible, since definitive treatment for eclampsia is delivery of the baby. Communication should be made with the obstetrician and neonatal team, while the patient is being transported.

References

1. Verdile VP, Tutsock G, Paris PM, Kennedy R. Out-of-hospital deliveries: a five-year experience. *Prehosp Disaster Med.* 1995;10:10–13.
2. Green-Thompson RW. Antepartum hemorrhage. *Clin Obstet Gynecol.* 1982;9:479–515.
3. Staniland JR, Ditchburn J, DeDombal FT. Clinical presentation of acute abdomen: study of 600 patients. *Br J Med.* 1972;3:393–398.
4. Pritchard JA. Management of preeclampsia and eclampsia. *Kidney Int.* 1980;18:259–266.
5. Sibai BM, Graham JM, McCubbin JH. A comparison of intravenous and intramuscular magnesium sulfate regimens in preeclampsia. *Am J Obstet Gynecol.* 1984;150:728.
6. Cruikshank DP. Anatomic and physiologic alterations of pregnancy that modify the response to trauma. In: Buchsbaum HJ, ed. *Trauma in Pregnancy.* Philadelphia: WB Saunders; 1979.
7. Pearlman MD, Tintinalli JE. Evaluation and treatment of the gravida and fetus following trauma during pregnancy. *Obstet Gynecol Clin North Am.* 1991;18:371.
8. Lavery JP, Staten-McCormick M. Management of moderate to severe trauma in pregnancy. *Obstet Gynecol Clin North Am.* 1995;22:69.
9. Neufield JD, Moore EE, Marx JA, et al. Trauma in pregnancy. *Emerg Med Clin North Am.* 1987;5:623.
10. Weber CE. Postmortem ceasarean section: review of the literature and case reports. *Am J Obstet Gynecol.* 1971;110:158.
11. Katz VL, Dotters DJ, Droegemueller W. Perimortem ceasarean delivery. *Obstet Gynecol.* 1986;68:571.
12. Lopez-Zeno JA, Carlo WA, O'Grady JP, et al. Infant survival following delayed postmortem ceasarean delivery. *Obstet Gynecol.* 1990;76:991.
13. Barnett WM. Umbilical cord prolapse: a true obstetrical emergency. *J Emerg Med.* 1989;7:149–152.
14. DeGrespigny LJC, Pepperell RJ. Perinatal mortality and morbidity in breech presentation. *Obstet Gynecol.* 1979;53:141.
15. Gherman RB, Goodwin TM, Souter I, et al. The McRoberts' maneuver for the alleviation of shoulder dystocia: how successful is it? *Am J Obstet Gynecol.* 1997;176:656–661.
16. Resnik R. Management of shoulder girdle dystocia. *Clin Obstet Gynecol.* 1980;23:559–564.
17. Woods, CE, A principle of physics as applicable to shoulder delivery. *Am J Obstet Gynecol.* 1943;45:796.
18. Drage JS, Berendes H. Apgar scores and outcome of the newborn. *Pediatr Clin North Am.* 1966;13:635–642.
19. Todres ID, Rogers MC. Methods of external cardiac massage in the newborn infant. *J Pediatr.* 1975;86:781–782.
20. Watson P. Postpartum hemorrhage and shock. *Clin Obstet Gynecol.* 1980;23:985–1001.
21. Jones EE. Ectopic pregnancy: common and some uncommon misdiagnoses. *Obstet Gynecol Clin North Am.* 1991;15:55.

22. Abbott JT, Emmans L, Lowenstein SR. Ectopic pregnancy: ten common pitfalls in diagnosis. *Am J Emerg Med*. 1990;8:515.

23. Gonzales FA, Waxman M. Ectopic pregnancy: a prospective study on differential diagnosis. *Diag Gynecol Obstet*. 1981;3:101–109.

24. Snyder HS. Lack of a tachycardic response to hypotension with ruptured ectopic pregnancy. *Am J Emerg Med*. 1990;8:23–26.

Pediatric

Susan Fuchs, MD

Introduction

Despite the fact that pediatric calls account for only 10% of ambulance runs, they provoke a disproportionate degree of concern and anxiety for prehospital care providers, and in turn, the medical oversight. Approximately one half of pediatric ambulance runs are trauma-related, such as motor vehicle crashes and falls, with the other half for medical complaints, especially respiratory distress and seizures.[1–3] There is also a bimodal age distribution of the calls: 0–3 years and 13–18 yrs.[1] The majority of calls for children under 3 years are medical, whereas the majority of adolescent calls are trauma-related.[1,2]

Prehospital care providers may be uncomfortable with pediatric patients. This can be due to limited knowledge and skills obtained during initial training, infrequent field experience, or a lack of continuing education. It can also be due to weight-based drug doses and equipment size variations in children (table 64.1). Although in a recent survey, 70% of nationally registered EMS providers answered that they were comfortable to some degree handling a critical pediatric call, 76% also wanted a national mandate on pediatric continuing education.[4] In fact, this survey identified infants and toddlers (age birth to 3 years) as the pediatric age group causing the most concern.[4] In addition, empathy in treating ill and injured children plays a large role. Therefore their anxiety is often expressed during radio communications, making it difficult to obtain a clear picture of the severity of the patient's condition. The direct medical oversight physician (DMOP) can hopefully provide guidance, improve patient outcome, and ultimately alleviate some of these anxieties.

A DMOP should recognize that there is an underutilization of medical oversight for prehospital pediatric calls. Some of the reasons include: lower acuity level of many younger patients, poor recognition of distress, and no specialized call-in requirements for children.[5]

A knowledgeable DMOP should realize the problematic areas in prehospital care provider training that lead to these problems. Although the new national standard curricula for all levels of providers have shifted focus from problem-based to assessment-based protocols, some older responders were trained under the problem-based system. Decisions about whether rapid transport versus field treatment and intervention, as well as triage or bypass decisions, are often in a constant state of flux.[5] The DMOP should know the system's patient illness/injury algorithms, triage, and bypass rules, so cases are managed properly and on a consistent basis.[6]

The Problem

Due to the federal Emergency Medical Services for Children (EMSC) program, there has been an enormous growth in the number of protocols and algorithms for pediatric patients.[7] In addition, the NAEMSP model algorithms were developed to try to solve some of the differences across systems.[8] The particular protocol or algorithm chosen in a system should be based upon several factors including the structure of the system (one-tiered vs two-tiered; EMT-B vs paramedics), scope of practice decisions, transport times, continuing education requirements, skills retention, system QM, and of course, resources.

Rather than concentrating on specific protocols, this chapter highlights some important issues regarding pediatric patients including: patient assessment, respiratory distress respiratory arrest, shock, trauma, and seizures.[9]

Evaluation

This is the area where children are truly different. An accurate assessment of a pediatric patient is the key to proper field evaluation and treatment and, in turn, appropriate direct medical oversight. It is important

TABLE 64.1

Weight-based Drug Doses and Equipment

MEDICATION	DOSE	MAXIMUM SINGLE DOSE	ROUTE/ COMMENT
Activated charcoal	< 1 Year 1–2 gm/kg > 1 Year 25–50 gm	n/a	PO, NG tube
Adenosine	0.1 mg/kg if not effective, 0.2 mg/kg	12 mg	IV, IO rapidly
Albuterol	unit dose vial (2.5 mg)	n/a	aerosol inhalation

Amiodarone
  For pulseless VF/VT
 	
  For perfusing tachycardia
	5 mg/kg
	
	Loading dose: 5 mg/kg
		15 mg/kg/day	IV, IO rapid bolus
			
			IV over 20–60 minutes

Atropine	0.02 mg/kg	0.5 mg child, 1.0 mg adolescent 0.1 mg minimum	IV, ET, IO
Calcium chloride (10%)	20 mg/kg	500 mg	IV, IO slowly
Dextrose (25%) Newborn (10%)	2–4 ml/kg 1–2 ml/kg		IV, IO IV, IO
Diazepam	IV, IO 0.1–0.3 mg/kg PR 0.5 mg/kg initial 0.25 mg/kg subsequent	10 mg 10 mg	IV, IO slowly rectal
Diphenhydramine	1 mg/kg	50 mg	IV, IO, IM

Epinephrine
  For symptomatic bradycardia
 	
  For pulseless arrest
 	
  For anaphylaxis
	IV, IO 0.01 mg/kg (1:10,000)
	
	ET: 0.1 mg/kg (1:1000)
	
	First dose:
	IV, IO: 0.01 mg/kg (1:10,000)
	ET: 0.1 mg/kg (1:1000)
	Subsequent doses: repeat initial dose or increase up to 10 times (0.1 mg/kg 1:1000)
	
	0.01 mg/kg (1:1000) SQ
		0.5 mg
		
		0.35 mg
			For newborn resuscitations dose is:
			IV, IO, ET 0.01–0.03 mg/kg 1:10,000
			
			Repeat every 3–5 minutes
			
			SQ

Furosemide	1 mg/kg	40 mg	IV, IO
Lidocaine (1%)	1 mg/kg	100 mg	IV, IO, ET
Magnesium sulfate	25–50 mg/kg	2 gm	IV, IO Rapid infusion for Torsades or suspected hypo-magnesemia 10–20 minute infusion for asthma
Naloxone	0.1 mg/kg	n/a	IV, IO, ET
Procainamide	Loading dose: 15 mg/kg		IV, IO over 30–60 minutes
Sodium bicarbonate (8.4%) Newborn (4.2%)	1 mEq/kg 2 mEq/kg	n/a n/a	IV, IO slowly IV, IO slowly

to remember that assessments and interventions should be tailored to each child in terms of their age, size, and developmental level.

A new useful learning tool that may be beneficial for providers is the "Assessment Triangle," which looks at Appearance, work of Breathing, and Cir-culation. This tool was developed by the Pediatric Education for Paramedics Task Force and has been incorporated into the new Pediatric Education for Prehospital Professionals (PEPP) program, as well as Advanced Pediatric Life Support (APLS).[10,11]

A brief overview of the Pediatric Assessment Triangle (PAT) will demonstrate how well it fits into overall patient assessment. The PAT allows the prehospital provider to develop a general impression of the child as well as determine if life support is needed urgently. The three parts of the triangle are done by watching and listening to the patient, and do not require equipment. They can be accomplished from across the room and can be completed in 30 to 60 seconds.[11]

Appearance—This is the most important component as it determines the severity of injury or illness. It consists of five characteristics, the "TICKLES" mnemonic: Tone, Interactiveness, Consolability, Look/gaze and Speech/cry. Assessment of tone includes: Is the child moving vigorously or is he limp? Interactiveness reflects how alert the child is; does he react to a voice, or an object? Does the child reach for a toy, or are they uninterested? Is the child Consolable; can they be comforted? Look/gaze: Does the child look at the EMS provider or care-giver or does the child have a blank expressionless face? Speech/cry: Is the cry or voice strong or weak?[11]

Work of Breathing: This portion can give the provider a quick indication of oxygenation and ventilation, and can be done without a stethoscope. The characteristics to note include: (1) abnormal airway sounds such as grunting, wheezing, muffled sounds; (2) abnormal positioning such as the tripod position, sniffing position, or refusing to lie down; (3) retractions: are they present, and if so where; and (4) the presence of nasal flaring.[11]

Circulation to the skin: This helps determine the adequacy of perfusion to vital organs. It can be determined by three characteristics: (1) pallor, which reflects inadequate blood flow; (2) mottling, which is due to vasoconstriction; and (3) cyanosis, which is blue coloration of the skin and mucous membranes.[11]

If there is an abnormality in one or more aspects of the triangle, this can help the provider decide how severely ill or injured the child is, and the most likely physiologic abnormality. For example, abnormal appearance and breathing point to a respiratory problem, while abnormal appearance and circulation point to a circulatory disorder. Abnormalities in all three areas point to a critically ill child who requires rapid scene interventions.[11]

The next step in patient assessment is the ABCDEs:

A—Airway: Assessment of the patient's airway should include: Is it patent? Is the child maintaining his/her own airway, or is assistance needed in the form of airway positioning: jaw thrust, chin-lift, oral airway, nasal airway, bag-valve-mask, or endotracheal tube?[11,12]

B—Breathing: This involves obtaining a respiratory rate, which varies with age (it decreases with increasing age), and can be very difficult in a crying child. A child in respiratory distress will usually breathe fast, but as they tire, it will decrease, which is an ominous sign. When one listens to the chest, are there any adventitous sounds: grunting, stridor, wheezing, rales, rhonchi, or no sounds (no air movement)? Depending upon available equipment, the use of a pulse oximeter can help determine oxygen saturation and the need for supplemental oxygen and/or assisted ventilation.[11,12]

C—Circulation: Determining heart rate and strength of peripheral pulses (radial) can be accomplished together. Heart rate varies with age (it decreases as children get older), and can also increase with fever and anxiety, but a heart rate below the normal range is worrisome, and can imply pending arrest. If peripheral pulses are weak, central pulses should be checked as a means of assessing circulation. Capillary refill, which should be less than 2 seconds, can be assessed with the evaluation of the temperature and color of the extremity. Cold, blue, pale, or mottled extremities indicate poor circulation and shock. Although obtaining a blood pressure is part of the vital signs, in children it is often inaccurate because of a wrong size cuff or a fighting child. A normal blood pressure in the face of some of the above abnormalities should not make a prehospital care provider comfortable. In fact, hypotension in a child is a late finding of shock.[11,12]

D—Disability: This is a brief assessment of level of consciousness (mental status). The key is a quick assessment done initially as general appearance, so this is a recheck. It is not necessary to memorize a pediatric Glasgow Coma Scale, as a rapid assessment uses the mnemonic AVPU: alert and playful, crying but consolable, crying and unconsolable, responsive to painful stimuli, alternating level of consciousness.[12,13]

E—Exposure: While parts of the ABCDs require that parts of the body be exposed for a complete assessment, it is necessary to assure that all of the child's body has been examined to fully evaluate any abnormalities. At the same time, it is also important to prevent heat loss and hypothermia.[11]

Treatment

Based on the above assessment, it should be possible for field providers to relay useful information to the DMOP. From this information it may be possible to group the child into one of several assessment-based categories which can guide appropriate field therapy and transport guidelines.

Caveats

1. Basic life support alone is all that is required for the majority of prehospital pediatric care. In fact, one study demonstrated that only 12% of pediatric calls need ALS care.[14]
2. There should be frequent updates of prehospital pediatric protocols based on recent advances in pediatric emergency care.[15]
3. Often the best field treatment decision is no treatment at all. When patient assessment is confusing, rapid transport with basic interventions to a facility that can manage the patient may be the best idea.[15]

Pitfalls

1. Vital signs must be interpreted carefully in the field. Inasmuch as they are stressed, as mentioned above they can vary widely, so an overall patient assessment (respiratory effort, breath sounds, pulse quality, skin color and temperature, level of consciousness) are more sensitive and useful. If vital signs are available, they should be compared with age-related norms. (table 64.2).[15]
2. The treatment should be no worse than the disease, and advanced treatment should avoid causing unnecessary distress or patient anxiety.[15] While all children in respiratory distress or shock require oxygen, an IV is not required in most patients with respiratory complaints.

Respiratory Distress

In the majority of infants and children, the cause of cardiopulmonary arrest is usually respiratory in origin. Therefore, if one can learn to recognize a child in respiratory distress, it is hoped that respiratory, and therefore cardiac, arrest can be prevented. There are many respiratory diseases unique to children; however, the underlying treatment is the same: maintenance of the airway with oxygenation and ventilation.

If a child is not breathing, basic procedures should be performed following current American Heart Association (AHA) guidelines for pediatrics: Stimulate and check responsiveness, position child ("sniffing

				TABLE 64.2				
				Pediatric Vital Signs				
Age	**Weight (kg)**	**Respiration Min-Max**	**Heart Rate Min-Max**	**Systolic Blood Pressure Min-Max**	**Distance (cm) Mid-Trachea to Teeth**	**Endo-tracheal Tube Uncuffed**	**Laryngo-scope Blade**	**Suction Cath.**
Premie	1–2	30–60	90–190	50–70	7–8	2.5–3.0	0 straight	5–6 F
Newborn	3–5	30–60	90–190	50–70	10	3.5	1 straight	6 F
6 MO	7	24–40	85–180	65–106	12	4.0	1 straight	8 F
1 YR	10	20–40	80–150	72–110	12	4.0–4.5	1–2 straight	8 F
3 YR	15	20–30	80–140	78–114	13–15	4.5–5.0	2 straight	8 F
6 YR	20	18–25	70–120	80–116	16	5.5	2–3 straight	10 F
8 YR	25	18–25	70–110	84–122	18	6.0 (cuffed)	2–3 straight/ curved	10 F
12 YR	40	14–20	60–110	94–136	20–22	7.0 (cuffed)	3 straight/ curved	12 F
15 YR	50	12–20	55–100	100–142	22–24	7.0 (cuffed)	3 straight/ curved	12 F
18 YR	65	12–18	50–90	104–148	24	7.0–8.0 (cuffed)	3 straight/ curved	12 F

position"), open airway (chin-lift, jaw thrust), check breathing, give 2 breaths. If there is no chest movement, reposition the airway, give 2 more breaths: if there is no chest rise and fall, suspect foreign body obstruction: give 5 back blows then 5 chest thrusts in infants < 1 yr or 5 abdominal thrusts (Heimlich manuever) in children >1 yr, remove the foreign body if visualized, open the airway, and resume rescue breathing.[16]

Evaluation of the respiratory rate and effort are the first keys to determining respiratory distress. Tachypnea is often an early sign of respiratory distress; however, the normal respiratory rate varies with age, but it can also increase due to fever or fear.[12] Therefore, assessment of respiratory mechanics and effort is also important. A child with nasal flaring and/or retractions (intercostal, subcostal, supraclavicular) is in distress, as is an infant (or any child) with grunting respirations. Auscultation of the chest may reveal wheezing, rales, rhonchi, or prolonged expirations (lower airway disease), and the presence of stridor is a clue to upper airway problems. Even if these children are not cyanotic, they all require supplemental high-flow oxygen such as a face mask at 12–15L/min. If the child is cyanotic, oxygen with assisted ventilation may be required. The use of a pulse oximeter is useful to determine if the child is receiving adequate oxygen en route. A low saturation (<94%) should prompt an increase in oxygen flow or an alternate delivery method such as a non-rebreather mask. Frequent reassessment is required en route, with decisions for additional therapy based upon provider reports.

Evaluation, the infant and young child in respiratory distress should be in the parent's/guardian's arms if possible. Another important factor is mental status, as a child who is becoming tired will not be able to breathe as fast or as hard as needed, and a decreasing respiratory rate is an ominous sign. On the other hand, an anxious child may resist therapy and become more distressed, so any interventions should be non-anxiety producing and may be accomplished easily with the parent's assistance.

The key is not to worry if the child has asthma, bronchiolitis, croup, or epiglottitis, but to assure an open airway and provide supplemental oxygen. The "Blow-by O_2" method vs. face mask includes the administration of oxygen by "blow-by"—holding the face mask 1–2 inches in front of the child's face, but slightly above the nose and mouth. Another option is to place the oxygen tubing through the bottom of a paper or plastic (not styrofoam) cup and hold it in a similar location; if aerosol nebulization set-ups are available, 3 cc of saline can be placed in the nebulizer (instead of medication), and administered by the parent if possible.

Caveats

1. The primary cause of cardiac arrests in children is an underlying respiratory problem. Failure to recognize that an infant or child is in respiratory distress can lead to hypoxia, bradycardia, and ultimately cardiac arrest.
2. Recognition that a child is in respiratory distress is more important than making a specific diagnosis.
3. Evaluation of respiratory rate and effort can be performed from a distance, with the child in a parent's arms.
4. High-flow oxygen should be provided to all children in respiratory distress, by a means that does not agitate the child.
5. Assisted ventilation is required in children who are apneic, those who are cyanotic despite oxygen, or when the respirations are too slow and/or shallow to provide adequate air exchange.

Pitfalls

1. Oxygen should be given to any child with tachypnea, retractions, or grunting respirations; cyanosis is a later finding.
2. Do not force a child to lie supine if they prefer to sit upright, as infants and children in respiratory distress will often assume a position of comfort to help them maintain their own airway.
3. A specific diagnosis is not necessary (e.g., croup vs. epiglottitis or asthma vs bronchiolitis), as the basic prehospital management is no different.
4. Intravenous access is not required in most cases of respiratory distress and may actually lead to worsening distress secondary to agitation and crying.

Shock

In simple medical terminology "shock" means failure to perfuse vital organs.[12] Shock is also a continuum ranging from compensated (normal blood pressure) to decompensated (hypotension).[17] Many prehospital care providers equilibrate shock with hypotension or low blood pressure, which may be useful for adults, but provides many problems when caring for a child. It would be hard to argue with a systolic pressure below 70 mmHg in anyone, but the normal systolic blood pressure of a 2-year-old can be 90 mmHg, which is low for most adults. The recent Pediatric Advanced Life Support (PALS) guidelines characterize hypotension as: term neonates (0–28 days) SBP <60 mmHg, infants (1–12 months) SBP < 70 mm Hg, children (1–10 yrs) SBP <70 +(2× age in years), beyond 10 yrs SBP <90 mm Hg.[17] The next problem is obtaining an accurate blood pressure in a child, which requires the proper-sized cuff, a cooperative child, a quiet environment, and knowledge of the various age-based norms. Obviously, there are easier and more accurate methods to assess a child's circulatory status available to prehospital care providers.

Heart rate is the key parameter, initially and upon repeated assessments. A child who is in shock has an elevated heart rate long before their blood pressure begins to drop. Therefore, tachycardia mandates further investigation for some of the underlying causes such as: fever, anxiety, hypovolemia, or hypoxia.[12] Heart rate, like respiratory rate and blood pressure, varies with age, so knowledge of the norms are needed to know if tachycardia is present in the first place (see table 64.2). Clinical assessment of stroke volume is easily performed by assessing pulse quality (strength), and comparing peripheral and central pulses. The presence of a strong radial pulse means that a child probably is not in shock. On the other hand, a weak, thready radial pulse should mandate a comparison with a brachial or carotid pulse. A discrepancy can be due to peripheral vasoconstriction, as in hypothermia, but it can also be a sign of diminished stroke volume.[12] Since decreased skin perfusion is another early sign of shock, another reliable sign is the assessment of peripheral vascular resistance. This can be done in several ways: by determining capillary refill, skin color, and skin temperature. Delayed capillary refill (> 2 seconds), and mottled skin (uneven or marbled appearance) indicate low cardiac output and shock.[12]

The effects of shock on the brain are demonstrated by a change in the level of consciousness. While this may be subtle, it is often useful in children as a child over 2 months should be able to recognize and respond to his parents' faces. Therefore, failure to recognize one's parents is an early sign of inadequate blood flow to the brain.[12] A decreasing level of consciousness—from awake, to responsive to voice (sleepy), to responsive to pain, and finally to unre-

sponsive—is an ominous sign. Other parameters to assess should include muscle tone and pupillary responses. While blood pressure is often difficult to obtain, it can be used as a baseline and to identify trends along with the other parameters.

While identification of shock is the prime goal, it is usually beneficial to determine the cause of shock to focus the prehospital treatment. Shock in children tends to result from hypovolemia; which most commonly occurs in gastroenteritis/dehydration and trauma. Another form of shock is distributive, due to a maldistribution of blood as occurs in sepsis or anaphylaxsis. The least common form in children is the most common in adults—cardiogenic shock resulting from an arrhythmia, congestive heart failure, or congenital heart disease.[12] After a cardiopulmonary arrest in a child, the heart often appears to be in cardiogenic shock.

The goal of the therapy of shock is the restoration of adequate blood volume, which is done in the field by the intravenous (IV) or intraosseous (IO) administration of 20 cc/kg of a crystalloid such as Ringer's lactate or normal saline as fast as possible. If a child's weight is unknown, a length-based resuscitation tape can be utilized for fluids, drug dosing as well as equipment size.[18] After initial fluid resuscitation, patient reassessment should be performed, focusing on the parameters mentioned above. This fluid bolus should be repeated if there is not an adequate response such as decreased heart rate or improved capillary refill. After the next bolus and patient reassessment, further management should be based upon the child's status, etiology of shock (if known or suspected), and transport time. High-flow oxygen should be given to all children in shock.

Obviously, the major difficulty in these situations may be the ability of the provider to establish IV access. It has been demonstrated that it is very difficult and time-consuming to establish IV access in young ill children.[19] In some situations, rather than waste precious moments of transport time, it may be useful to "load and go" and search for access en route. Another method is to limit the number of attempts or time allowed for IV access before IO cannulation is attempted in the appropriate patient.[20]

Due to limited pediatric research, there is currently no indication to support the use of the pneumatic antishock garment (PASG) to improve blood pressure or obtain IV access.[21]

The decisions of the DMOP regarding initial and subsequent interventions and treatment should be based upon the reports received from the field, provider skills and training, accepted protocols for the region, and repeated patient assessment once therapy is initiated.

Caveats

1. The assessment of shock in a child is not based solely upon blood pressure, as hypotension is a late finding.
2. Evaluation of heart rate, capillary refill, and peripheral pulses are more reliable and easier to assess, than blood pressure.
3. Basic treatment is no different from adults, and involves the administration of crystalloid at 20 cc/kg as fast as possible.
4. As IV access may be difficult, IO infusion is a viable alternative for children, even those above 6 years of age.[17]
5. High-flow oxygen should be provided to all children in shock.

Pitfalls

1. If the report reveals an ill or injured child with tachycardia and a normal blood pressure, the child may nevertheless be in shock.
2. While IV access and fluids are the first line treatment for children in shock, if transport time is short, scene time should not be delayed to obtain IV access. The prehospital care providers should "load and go," and attempt IV or IO access en route. On the other hand, if there is prolonged extrication time, IV access or IO access should be attempted prior to transport, so therapy can be given en route.[21]
3. If rapid fluid infusions are needed, do not assume that a "wide open" rate will do the job. It may be necessary to infuse the fluid under pressure (pressure bag or squeezing).
4. Do not be afraid to give an infant or child too much fluid, as very few conditions will put them into pulmonary edema. What fluid they do not need will be excreted as urine.

Trauma and Trauma Triage

Some of the differences between pediatric and adult trauma are related to the mechanism of injury. Most pediatric trauma is blunt injury, as occurs in a motor vehicle crash, rather than penetrating. Head trauma is the most common area of the body injured by chil-

dren.[22] In addition, children often have occult injuries, especially involving the liver and spleen, which can result in significant blood loss. The basic approach and treatment of a pediatric trauma patient vary little from that of an adult. The keys remain airway control with cervical spine stabilization, breathing, circulation, disability, and exposure.

All trauma patients should receive supplemental high flow oxygen and immobilization. If an appropriate sized cervical collar is not available, suggest towels and tape, neither sandbags nor IV fluid bags. The most important factor is to assure that the airway is open and the child is breathing. Suctioning the airway, and positioning (jaw thrust) may accomplish this task. High-flow supplemental oxygen is best given by a pediatric face mask. If BVM ventilation is required assure the rise and fall of the chest, in addition to improvement in the patient's color. Circulatory assessment should include heart rate, capillary refill, peripheral pulse strength, color and temperature of extremities, and level of consciousness. IV fluids should be administered to victims of multiple trauma with decompensated shock (hypotension) or significant blood loss.[22] The decision whether to start an IV at the scene should be based upon patient severity and the anticipated transport time. The sooner IV access can be obtained, the sooner 20 cc/kg of crystalloid (lactated Ringer's or .9 normal saline) can be infused. It can be very difficult to start an IV in a child, so if valuable time is being wasted at the scene, it is often beneficial to transport and attempt IV access while en route. Once the initial fluid bolus has been administered, the child should be reassessed, and an additional bolus (20 cc/kg) given as warranted. While concerns have been raised in adult patients that aggressive fluid resuscitation for uncontrolled bleeding will result in normalization of the blood pressure and increased bleeding, these studies involved adults with penetrating injury, and similar studies have not been performed in children.

There is no indication for the use of a PASG in children. While it is still included in the current ATLS curriculum for adults, its only use may be for hypotension with a clinically unstable pelvic fracture.[22,23] Disability assessment should include level of consciousness, and a check of the pupils. Exposure refers to a complete rapid secondary survey examination. It should be stressed that if a life-threatening injury is found during the initial assessment, the injury should be stabilized and then "load and go." If no such injury is found and time permits (scene times on trauma patients should be less than 10 minutes), the child can be fully examined (this can also be done en route). A child should be kept warm during transport, as their large body surface area allows them easily to become hypothermic, which can complicate their resuscitation.

When a prehospital provider calls for direct medical oversight regarding a pediatric trauma patient, a trauma score would be helpful to direct the patient to the appropriate facility, such as a pediatric trauma center. An ideal trauma score should be reliable, reproducible, simple, and able to predict patient outcome. It should be able to categorize patients so that severe injuries are not missed, and the score obtained by one observer should be the same as another observer using the same information.[24] This information can then be used by a prehospital care provider to communicate to the DMOP the severity of injury, which should then indicate to which hospital a patient should be transported (based on previously existing trauma triage criteria).

Several adult scores are in existence (trauma score, revised trauma score, injury severity score, CRAMS score), but it is difficult to apply these scores to pediatric patients. The Pediatric Trauma Score (PTS) was developed to overcome this problem, as this score combines anatomic variables and physiologic variables.[24] The components include: size, airway, systolic blood pressure, central nervous system (level of consciousness), skeletal injury, and cutaneous injury. Each is scored from −1 to +2, with a range of scores from −6 to +12 (see table 64.3).[24] Research has demonstrated that a PTS of +8 or less will identify those patients in whom mortality is likely to occur (inverse relationship between decreasing PTS and increasing mortality).[24] From this information, prehospital decisions about pediatric trauma patient transport can be made for the region and reinforced by the DMOP.

In many regions of the country, rather than use a specific trauma score, trauma center criteria have been developed. These criteria allow prehospital care providers to bypass local hospitals in favor of a designated trauma center. Some of these criteria are based upon vital signs (e.g., hypotension), airway difficulties, injuries (gun shot wound to chest), or mechanisms of injury.

Caveats

1. The initial approach to a pediatric trauma patient is the same as that of an adult: airway with cervical spine stabilization, breathing, circulation, disability and exposure.
2. As the majority of childhood trauma is blunt injury, there may be multi-system injury, as well as occult abdominal injury.
3. Head injury is the most common site of injury. Airway control, breathing, and administration of high-flow oxygen, possibly with hyperventilation, are the most important therapeutic maneuvers.
4. Children can easily become hypothermic.
5. There is no indication for the use of a PASG in children.
6. A car seat, if intact, can be used to immobilize an infant or child. A cervical collar should still be applied, and towels can be used as padding along the head. Tape should then be used across the forehead to secure the infant.

TABLE 63.3			
Pediatric Trauma Score (PTS)			
COMPONENT	**+2**	**+1**	**−1**
Size	> 20 kg	10–20 kg	< 10 kg
Airway	Normal	Maintainable	Unmaintainable
CNS	Awake	Obtunded	Comatose
Systolic BP	> 90 mmHg	50–90 mmHg	< 50 mmHg
Open Wounds	None	Minor	Major or penetrating
Skeletal	None	Closed fracture	Open/multiple fractures
Range −6 to +14; <9 identifies high mortality			

If proper sized BP cuff is not available, BP can be assessed by assigning:
+2 pulse palpable at radial or brachial artery
+1 pulse palpable at groin
−1 no pulse palpable.

7. Transport of a pediatric trauma patient should be to a facility that is able to handle the patient.

Pitfalls

1. Infants and children can have serious internal injuries without evidence of external trauma.
2. If the appropriate size cervical collar/immobilization equipment is not available, towels and tape can be used to secure the head; do not use IV bags or sandbags.
3. If there is evidence of severe head injury (unequal pupils, seizures, unresponsive patient), assist ventilation with bag-valve-mask and 100% oxygen, at an age-appropriate rate (30 per min <12 months and 20 per min >1 yr), do not hyperventilate unless there is equipment to insure that the PCO_2 is no less than 30 mmHg (table 64.2).[21]
4. After a full evaluation, the child should be covered, and the transporting vehicle warmed to avoid hypothermia.
5. IV access and the administration of crystalloid (20 cc/kg) should be done quickly, but should not prolong scene time.

Seizures

Due to the 5% incidence of febrile seizures in children under 7 years of age, it is not surprising that seizures account for many prehospital transports.[25,26] Prehospital care providers are often anxious about the call for several reasons: Will the child still be seizing when they arrive? What interventions will be needed? The DMOP should be concerned about the cause of the seizure as well as field treatment; however, providers should not have to diagnose the cause of the seizure before appropriate therapy and transport.

Although there are many causes of seizures the basic prehospital management remains the same: assessment of airway, breathing, and circulation. If a child is still seizing, the first priorities are assuring a patent airway and breathing, procedures such as chin-lift, or jaw thrust may be required. Suction should be available, and the crew should be ready to assist ventilation with a BVM if the respiratory rate is slow, or absent, or the child is cyanotic, even just around the lips. All patients should also have supplemental oxygen administered during a seizure. The use of anticonvulsants should be based upon several factors; the length of the seizure, patient history (e.g., known seizure disorder), patient medications, possible etiology (e.g., low blood sugar), transport time, and ability and comfort level of the providers to provide adequate or additional airway support (intubation if needed). There are several medications and routes available to administer anticonvulsants, including IV or rectal diazepam or IM midazolam. It is important for medical oversight to decide which medication and route are preferred, so the proper techniques and dosages can be taught to the providers.[25] A finger-stick glucose level (Dextrostix®, Chemstrip®) should be performed prior to the initiation of anticonvulsants. If a high fever is suspected as the cause, the child can be cooled with towels en route, not with ice or cold packs. The providers should reassess the patient frequently en route, even if the seizure stops. They should also be made aware that the seizure may recur en route.

If upon the providers' arrival the child has stopped seizing, additional time can be spent obtaining information from the parents or caretakers after the child has been assessed and found to be in stable condition. The possibility of a fall during or after the seizure should be determined quickly so appropriate immobilization can be performed if necessary. Information regarding the presence of fever prior to the seizure, recent illness, type of movements (jerking, rigid, flaccid), extremities involved (legs and/or arms, both sides or one side), eye movements (staring, rolling back), loss of continence (urine and/or stool), underlying medical problems, medications, allergies, and family history (of seizures) will provide help in establishing the etiology once the child is seen and evaluated at the hospital.[27] During transport it will be necessary to perform repeated evaluations of the child with regard to airway and breathing, reporting any changes while en route.

If the seizure is prolonged (>15 minutes) or persistent, the use of an anticonvulsant is warranted. Diazepam can be administered by several routes: IV or IO (0.1–0.3 mg/kg IV at a rate no greater than 1 mg/min) with maximum single dose of 10 mg; this can be repeated up to 3 times, with doses spaced 10 minutes apart. Rectal administration (0.5 mg/kg for the first dose, 0.25 mg/kg for any subsequent dose), can be done by attaching a syringe of the IV formulation of the drug to a 14G or 16G plastic intravenous catheter or a 10Fr suction catheter, and advancing it 4-6 cm into the rectum. The catheter should be flushed with air (keep the catheter in place and fill the syringe with air), or 5cc of saline. Since the major side effect of diazepam is respiratory depression, it is mandatory to have a BVM ready prior to administration, and to reassess the patient frequently.

Midazolam is another medication that can be used for seizure control. Although it is not considered a first-line drug, it can be used via the intramuscular route. The dose is 0.1 mg/kg IM and is given into the lateral thigh, the buttocks or the upper arm (if the child is >18 months and only a small volume of medication is used). It takes effect in approximately 15 minutes.[28]

Caveats

1. Assessments of airway, breathing, and circulation remain key.
2. All children should receive supplemental oxygen during a seizure; however, since respirations can be slow, shallow, or irregular, the child may need assisted ventilation as well.
3. Not all seizures require anticonvulsant therapy.
4. Transport of a child after a seizure is mandatory, as the etiology cannot be determined from the field.

Pitfalls

1. During a seizure, control of the airway with proper head position, suctioning, oxygen, and assessment and/or assistance of breathing are more important than stopping the seizure.
2. After a seizure, if a child is post-ictal, airway positioning and oxygen remain a priority.
3. If a decision is made to use anticonvulsants (especially benzodiazepines), the DMOP should assure that the crew is aware of the side effect of respiratory depression, and has the necessary equipment and training to manage the patient.

Recent Changes

The recent PALS guidelines have a few changes that are worth noting. The first is the extension of the age for IO infusion to those >6 years of age.[17] The locations to gain IO access remain the same (anterior tibia, medial malleolus, and distal femur), but a provider will need to realize that in some cases a larger-gauge needle may be necessary. An 18G needle is likely to bend during insertion when placement is attempted into the femur of a 7 year old; a 13G needle is more appropriate).

The initial dose of epinephrine for cardiac arrest remains 0.01 mg/kg (0.1 mL/kg of 1:10,000 solution) via the IV or IO route and 0.1 mg/kg (0.1 mL/kg of 1:1000 solution) via the endotracheal route. The same dose is recommended for subsequent doses, given every 3–5 minutes. The use of high dose epinephrine 0.1 to 0.2 mg/kg (0.1 to 0.2 mL/kg of 1:1000) by IV or IO may be considered.[17]

Amiodarone has been introduced as an option for the treatment of pulseless ventricular tachycardia (VT) or fibrillation (VF), similar to the new adult algorithms. The dose for pediatrics is 5 mg/kg bolus via IV or IO. The other alternative drugs include lidocaine (1 mg/kg bolus IV/IO/ET) or magnesium 25–50 mg/kg IV/IO for Torsades de Pointes of hypomagnesemia).[17] Amiodarone has also been added as an option to the treatment algorithm for VT (5 mg/kg IV over 20–60 minutes). Other options for VT/VF include procainamide 15 mg/kg IV over 30–60 minutes or lidocaine 1 mg/kg IV bolus (for wide complex VT only). Bretylium has been deleted.[17] An addition is that automatic external defibrillators may be used in children >8 years of age (>25 kg weight) in cardiac arrest in the prehospital setting.[17]

Controversies

A National Task Force on education for EMS providers identified several areas in the education of providers that are controversial.[21] While some of these areas have been mentioned previously (the need for vascular access, provision of hyperventilation, lack of use of pneumatic antishock garment), the main controversy remains the scope of practice in pediatric airway management. A wide range of options exist, from BVM ventilation to endotracheal (ET) intubation, rapid sequence induction, use of laryngeal mask airways, surgical cricothyrotomy, and retrograde intubation.[17,21] The method of airway support used in the system should be based upon the skill level of the providers, equipment and medications available, on-going training and experience, transport times, and medical oversight.

One key fact remains: proficiency in BVM ventilation is mandatory for all prehospital care providers.[17] A recent study demonstrated, that there was no increase in survival or neurologic outcome in those children who received ET intubation compared to BVM ventilation.[29] While the results of this study may not apply to all EMS systems, several areas deserve highlighting. ET intubation, while the "gold standard," is often an infrequently performed skill, and not without its complications. Therefore, ongoing experience, training, the use of techniques for evaluating ET tube placement, and quality management of complication rates are required. In some systems, rapid transport times may not justify ET intubation.[17,30] Although some systems have effectively used paralytics to facilitate pediatric ET intubation, the use of rapid-sequence induction requires close medical oversight.[21,31,32] Additional techniques such as needle cricothyrotomy and retrograde intubation, while taught in courses for physicians, should not be included in the pediatric essential airway skills for prehospital providers.[21]

Summary

While pediatric calls account for only a small percent of runs, they cause an inordinate amount of anxiety. Some of the factors, such as training and appropriate equipment, can be addressed beforehand; other aspects cannot. The level of comfort when giving direct medical oversight on pediatric calls will be discerned by the prehospital care providers.

Patient assessment skills are the cornerstone of therapy, as treatment and triage decisions are based on this information. At a minimum, all ill or injured infants and children should be transported on oxygen, but further decisions regarding IV access and/ or medications should be based upon the age of the child, transport time, and the information related by the prehospital care providers. Frequent reassessment should be performed en route, in many cases, a child will have "turned around" by the time he arrives at the emergency department due prehospital care and expertise.

Cases

Case 1

The prehospital care providers report that a 9-month-old male has had a cold for 3 days, that he is breathing 60 times a minute, that the pulse is 160, and that he feels a bit warm. They are unable to get an accurate blood pressure, as the cuff is too big.

How would you proceed?
The DMOP should ask a few more questions. Is the child grunting or wheezing? Are there retractions? What is the child's level of consciousness? As long as

the child's level of conscious is adequate (awake, even if irritable), high-flow oxygen should be provided. This can be done by blow-by or mask; if the child is very sleepy, difficult to arouse, or the respiratory rate is abnormal, the providers may have to provide assisted ventilation en route, using a BVM device. This infant is in respiratory distress; the cause is not important. Providing high-flow oxygen is the key. An IV is not necessary and may agitate the infant, causing increased respiratory distress.

Case 2

A 6-year-old has had vomiting and diarrhea for 2 days. Her pulse is 130, respiratory rate 24, and blood pressure 110/70 mm Hg. She is sleepy but easily arousable; her radial pulse is strong. Depending upon the transport time, all that may be needed is expeditious transport. On the other hand, if transport time is long (>20 minutes), if the providers can establish an IV, they can start a crystalloid fluid bolus (20 cc/kg) of Ringer's lactate or normal saline. In any case, repeated assessment of the patient en route is required, and if the heart rate increases, or blood pressure drops, rapid fluid replacement is required.

Discussion
This child is not in shock, but is dehydrated (note the elevated heart rate). An IV is not needed, and may waste time if transport time is short. For prolonged transport time, an IV would be beneficial, but should not delay scene time, and an IO is inappropriate, due to the level of consciousness.

Case 3

A 14-year-old was riding his bike when he was struck by a car travelling about 35 mph. He was thrown across the road, and witnesses say he lost consciousness for 1 minute. He is now able to say his name, but is confused. He has a deformity of his right thigh and right forearm. He has abrasions to his abdomen and a large laceration of his scalp. His pulse is 140; respiratory rate is 20; blood pressure is 84/60. He is currently immobilized on a backboard and CID, and a cervical collar has been applied. The scalp laceration stopped bleeding with direct pressure, and is covered with a dressing. The right forearm is immobilized, and there is a strong radial pulse, but the pulse at the right ankle is weak, and the foot is cool. The providers are asking if they can apply and inflate the PASG.

HOW WOULD YOU PROCEED?

Splinting the leg as it currently lies in a PASG will not correct the circulation problem in the leg, or for the youngster in general. Slight manipulation and straightening of the thigh, and rechecking the pulses are indicated. This child requires a rapid infusion of IV fluids, as well as high flow oxygen, as he is in shock. Rapid transport to an appropriate trauma facility should not be delayed. The crew should be instructed to keep the DMOP posted of any changes in the patient's condition while en route.

This child has multisystem injuries: head, abdomen (possibly liver or spleen), and extremity trauma. His pulse is elevated, and his blood pressure low, which indicate shock due to blood loss. The scalp laceration alone probably is not causing this; he could lose a large amount of blood into his thigh, but another hidden area is a liver or spleen injury. Key points are immobilization with cervical spine stabilization, and assessment of the airway and breathing. Circulatory status of his leg is questionable without some manipulation. Assessment of disability (level of consciousness) reveals that he is awake but confused, so it is abnormal. IV fluids, oxygen, rapid transport with repeated assessments should be stressed. Based upon this youngster's injury and PTS (+1), transport should be to a pediatric trauma facility, if available in a reasonable timeframe.

Case 4

A 3-year-old has had a seizure, which lasted 5 minutes. She has never done this before, and was well earlier. Now she is sleepy, but arousable, and recognizes mom. She feels very warm, her heart rate is 120, respiratory rate is 22 (unlabored), and blood pressure is 96/60.

DISCUSSION

As long as she didn't fall and strike her head or neck, the child can be transported without immobilization. No specific therapy is required, such as an IV, but oxygen and suction equipment should be readily available in case the child has another seizure en route. This child is probably post-ictal, which can explain her sleepiness. Although this was probably a febrile seizure, that diagnosis cannot be made in the field. A thorough examination in the ED is required to make this diagnosis and exclude other causes.

References

1. Tsai A, Kallsen G. Epidemiology of pediatric prehospital care. *Ann Emerg Med.* 1987;16:284–292.

2. Kallsen GW. Epidemiology of pediatric prehospital emergencies. In: Dieckmann RA, ed. *Pediatric Emergency Care Systems: Planning and Management.* Baltimore: Williams and Wilkins; 1992.

3. Institute of Medicine. Risking our children's health: a need for emergency care. In: Durch JS, Lohr KN, eds. *Emergency Medical Services for Children.* Washington, DC: Academy Press; 1993.

4. Glaeser PW, Linzer J, Tunik MG, et al. Survey of nationally registered emergency medical service providers: pediatric education. *Ann Emerg Med.* 2000;36:33–38.

5. Dieckmann RA. Medical direction. In: Dieckmann RA, ed. *Pediatric Emergency Care Systems: Planning and Management.* Baltimore: Williams and Wilkins; 1992.

6. Luten RC, Stenklyft PH. Early recognition of illness. In: Dieckmann RA, ed. *Pediatric Emergency Care Systems: Planning and Management.* Baltimore: Williams and Wilkins; 1992.

7. American Academy of Pediatrics, Committee on Pediatric Emergency Medicine. Available on-line resources. In: Seidel JS, Knapp JF, eds. *Childhood Emergencies in the Office, Hospital and Community: Organizing Systems of Care.* Elk Grove Village, IL: American Academy of Pediatrics; 2000.

8. Mulligan-Smith D, O'Connor RE, Markenson D. NAEMSP Model Pediatric Protocols. Health Resources and Services Administration, Maternal and Child Health Bureau, National Highway Traffic Safety Administration. Washington, DC: EMSC National Resource Center; 2000. (http://www.ems-c.org)

9. Fuchs S, Paris PM. EMS physicians. In: Dieckmann RA, ed. *Pediatric Emergency Care Systems: Planning and Management.* Baltimore: Williams and Wilkins; 1992.

10. Dieckmann RD, Gausche M, Brownstein D. *Pediatric Education for Paramedics Student Manual.* Sacramento, CA: EMS Authority; 1996.

11. American Academy of Pediatrics. Pediatric assessment. In: Dieckmann RA, Brownstein DR, Gausche-Hill M, eds. *Pediatric Education for Prehospital Professionals Textbook.* Sudbury, MA: Jones and Bartlett Publishers; 2000.

12. Chameides L, Hazinski MF, eds. Recognition of respiratory failure and shock. In: *Textbook of Pediatric Advanced Life Support.* Dallas: American Heart Association; 1997.

13. Illinois Medical Services for Children. Pediatric Initial Assessment ALS/ILS/BLS Guideline. In: Illinois EMSC Pediatric Resource Manual. Springfield, IL: Dept. of Public Health; 1997.

14. Seidel JS, Henderson DP, Ward P, et al. Pediatric prehospital care in urban and rural areas. *Pediatrics.* 1991;88:681–690.

15. Hoffman SH, Dieckman RA. Prehospital illness treatment. In: Dieckmann RA, ed. *Pediatric Emergency Care Systems: Planning and Management.* Baltimore: Williams and Wilkins; 1992.

16. American Heart Association. Guidelines 2000 for cardiopulmonary resuscitation and emergency cardiovascular care. Part 9: Pediatric basic life support. *Circulation.* 2000;102(suppl I): I 253–I 290.

17. American Heart Association. Guidelines 2000 for cardiopulmonary resuscitation and emergency cardiovascular care. Part 10: Pediatric advanced life support. *Circulation.* 2000;102(suppl I): I 291–I 342.

18. American Academy of Pediatrics. Resuscitation tape. In: Dieckmann RA, Brownstein DR, Gausche-Hill M, eds. *Pediatric Education for Prehospital Professionals Textbook.* Sudbury, MA: Jones and Bartlett Publishers; 2000.

19. Rossetti VA, Thompson BM, Aprahamian C, et al. Difficulty and delay in intravascular access in pediatric arrests. *Ann Emerg Med.* 1984;13:406.

20. Chameides L, Hazinski MF, eds. Vascular access. In: *Textbook of Pediatric Advanced Life Support.* Dallas: American Heart Association; 1997.

21. Gausche M, Henderson DB, Brownstein D, et al. Education of out-of-hospital emergency medical personnel in pediatrics: report of a national task force. *Ann Emerg Med.* 1998;31:58–64.

22. American Academy of Pediatrics. Trauma. In: Dieckmann RA, Brownstein DR, Gausche-Hill M, eds. *Pediatric Education for Prehospital Professionals Textbook.* Sudbury, MA: Jones and Bartlett Publishers; 2000.

23. American College of Surgeons, Committee on Trauma. Musculoskeletal trauma. In: *Advanced Trauma Life Support Program for Doctors.* Chicago: American College of Surgeons; 1997.

24. Tepas JJ. Prehospital trauma scoring and triage. In: Dieckmann RA, ed: *Pediatric Emergency Care Systems: Planning and Management.* Baltimore: Williams and Wilkins; 1992.

25. American Academy of Pediatrics. Medical emergencies. In: Dieckmann RA, Brownstein DR, Gausche-Hill M, eds. *Pediatric Education for Prehospital Professionals Textbook.* Sudbury, MA: Jones and Bartlett Publishers; 2000.

26. Gonzalez del Rey JA. Febrile seizures. In: Barkin EM, ed. *Pediatric Emergency Medicine: Concepts and Clinical Practice.* St Louis, MO: Mosby; 1997.

27. Fuchs, S. Managing seizures in children. *Emergency.* 1990;47–52.

28. American Academy of Pediatrics. Intramuscular and subcutaneous injections. In: Dieckmann RA, Brownstein DR, Gausche-Hill M, eds. *Pediatric Education for Prehospital Professionals Textbook.* Sudbury, MA: Jones and Bartlett Publishers; 2000.

29. Gausche M, Lewis RJ, Stratton SJ, et al. Effect of out-of-hospital pediatric endotracheal intubation on survival and neurologic outcome: a controlled clinical trial. *JAMA.* 2000;283:783–790.

30. Glaeser P. Out-of-hospital intubation in children (editorial). *JAMA.* 2000;283:797–798.

31. Brownstein DR, Shugerman R, Cummins P, et al. Prehospital endotracheal intubation of children by paramedics. *Ann Emerg Med.* 1996;28:34–39.

32. Sing RF, Reilly PM, Rotondo MF. Evaluation of out-of-hospital rapid sequence intubation of the pediatric patient. *Acad Emerg Med.* 1996;3:41–45.

CHAPTER 65

Poisoning and Overdose

Daniel J. Cobaugh, PharmD
Sandra M. Schneider, MD

Introduction

Between 1995 and 1999, the American Association of Poison Control Centers (AAPCC) reported over 8.6 million poisonings in the United States.[1-5] Over 91% of these cases were prehospital exposures that occurred in the home. Of the 3,884 poisoning fatalities reported during this time frame, 37% involved an out-of-hospital respiratory or cardiac arrest. Between 1995 and 1999, over 5.6 million accidental poisonings in children less than 6 years of age were reported. Although the majority of unintentional poisoning exposures involve children, major morbidity and mortality have become relatively rare in pediatric poisoning victims. The incidence of pediatric poisoning mortality has changed over the last four decades. In 1964, over 600 pediatric poisoning deaths were reported by poison centers.[6] From 1995 through 1999, there were 104 pediatric poisoning deaths reported by U.S. poison centers. Prevention efforts, along with enhanced patient care, research, and regulatory efforts, have been effective in reducing this number. The role of more sophisticated approaches to out-of-hospital care should not be minimized when considering this trend.

Fumes/gases/vapors, hydrocarbons, and analgesics were the substances most often implicated in the reported fatalities described in table 65.1. Carbon monoxide (CO) was responsible for all of the pediatric deaths from fumes/gases/vapors in the 1995 through 1999 data. Thirty-five of the pediatric poisoning fatalities between 1995 and 1999 were due to medications. Although analgesics are most prevalent, iron supplements, antidepressants, cardiovascular medications, and oral hypoglycemics are also represented.

A number of toxicity risks begin to present with the onset of adolescence. Suicide attempts begin to rise in adolescence. Also, toxicity and sudden death secondary to inhalant abuse is a significant problem in this age group. Toxicity from illicit substances, including newer agents such as gamma hydroxybutyrate (GHB) and methylenedioxymethamphetamine (MDMA), is now seen frequently in adolescents. Recently news reports have described dance clubs in large cities that have begun to utilize private ambulance services, given the large number of exposures, to transport MDMA and GHB abusers to emergency departments. In many respects, poisoning and overdose in older adolescents and adults are more complex. Most often, toxic exposures in adults are the result of a suicide attempt. This often involves exposure to a wide variety of substances including prescription, non-prescription, and illicit drugs. These "polypharmacy" overdoses can have very complicated clinical presentations, given the multitude of pharmacologic and toxicologic effects of the agents involved. Substances found in the workplace, such as hydrofluoric acid and methylene chloride, pose a significant risk for adults. Children and adults are equally at risk for exposure to environmental poisons such as carbon monoxide. Toxic exposures in pregnant women present unique challenges. Risk to the fetus must be assessed in each situation, based on the degree of transplacental distribution of the involved substance and the toxicity profile of the involved substance in the fetus.

Out-of-hospital management of victims of poisoning and overdose presents challenges for emergency medical technicians, paramedics, and direct medical oversight physicians (DMOP). It would be impossible to review the entire spectrum of poisoning in a brief chapter. Therefore, substances with significant risk for out-of-hospital morbidity and mortality which have known out-of-hospital interventions will be the focus of this chapter.

General Approach

Out-of-hospital personnel and medical command physicians have several responsibilities in the manage-

TABLE 65.1			
Pediatric Poisoning Deaths, 1995–1999			
SUBSTANCES—NON-PHARMACEUTICALS	**NUMBER OF FATALITIES**	**SUBSTANCES—PHARMACEUTICALS**	**NUMBER OF FATALITIES**
Alcohols	2	**Analgesics**	13
Ethanol	1	Acetaminophen	3
Isopropanol	1	Aspirin	1
Bites and Envenomations	1	Codeine	1
Rattlesnake	1	Ibuprofen	1
Chemicals	1	Methadone	4
Diethylene glycol vehicle for acetaminophen	1	Morphine	1
		Phenylbutazone	1
		Potassium	1
Cleaning Substances	8	**Anesthetics**	1
Cleaner	2	Ketamine	1
Condenser coil cleaner	1	**Anticonvulsants**	3
Degreaser	1	Carbamazepine	1
Drain opener	1	Fosphenytoin	1
Rust remover	1	Valproic acid	1
Tire cleaner	1	**Antidepressants**	5
Wheel cleaner	1	Amitriptyline	1
Cosmetics/Personal Care	4	Desipramine	3
Baby oil	1	Doxepin	1
Hair oil	1	**Antihistamines**	1
Mouthwash (ethanol)	1	Promethazine	1
Nail polish remover (acetone)	1	**Antimicrobials**	1
Essential Oils	1	Ceftriaxone	1
Citronella oil	1	**Cardiovascular Drugs**	3
Foreign Body	2	Digoxin	1
Activated charcoal	2	Nifedipine	1
Fumes/Gases/Vapors	22	Propranolol	1
Carbon monoxide	22	**Cough and Cold Products**	1
Heavy Metals	1	Phenylpropanolamine	1
Mercury	1	**Electrolytes and Minerals**	5
Hydrocarbons	11	Iron	5
Chlorodifluoromethane	1	**Gastrointestinal Preparations**	1
Lamp oil	2	Bismuth sub-salicylate	1
Lighter fluid	5	**Hormones and Hormone Antagonists**	1
Gasoline	1	Glipizide	1
Motor oil	1		
Paint thinner	1	**Sedatives/Hypnotics/Antipsychotics**	1
Insecticides/Pesticides	5	Chloral hydrate	1
Aluminum phosphate	1	**Stimulants and Street Drugs**	4
Carbamate	1	Cocaine	1
Organophosphate	3	Heroin	2
Plants	2	Methamphetamine	1
Cayenne pepper	1	**Unknown**	1
Pennyroyal tea	1	Unknown poison	1
Sporting Equipment	1	**Vitamins**	1
Gun bluing	1	Prenatal vitamins with iron	1
Tobacco	1		
Cigarette butts	1		

ment of poisoning. First and foremost, the scene must be assessed for safety. Then the potential for poisoning must be recognized. An assessment of the physical environment in which a comatose patient is found may lead the out-of-hospital provider to suspect that a toxic exposure has occurred. In other environments out-of-hospital providers need to be cognizant of the potential for toxicity. Second, the out-of-hospital provider needs to provide initial treatment in the management of the poisoned patient. This may include, but is not limited to, administration of ipecac syrup to induce emesis, administration of naloxone to reverse the effects of opiates/opioids, or dermal decontamination of the hazardous materials exposure. Out-of-hospital providers must also be prepared to manage the life-threatening sequelae of poisonings such as respiratory depression, hypotension, dysrhythmias, and cardiac arrest. It is impossible for any physician to have a working knowledge of all environmental and pharmacologic poisons.

Poison Center Resources

Poison centers across the United States can be accessed via a single nationwide toll-free number: **1-800-222-1222.** The regional poison center can provide a wealth of information to prehospital providers and medical command physicians managing patients with a toxic exposure. The centers are staffed 24 hours per day by specialists in poison information (SPIs), pharmacists, and nurses, with extensive clinical toxicology training. These SPIs are supported at all times by board-certified medical toxicologists who are available to consult directly with the medical command physician. The poison center can assist in identification of substances, assessment of toxicity potential, and provision of treatment recommendations. They also monitor the incidence of exposures/ poisonings, providing important epidemiologic information.

Out-of-Hospital Evaluation

In many patients the diagnosis of poisoning or overdose may be obvious. In children there is often a good history of the exposure. Adults are sometimes found with suicide notes, empty medication containers, or in suspicious circumstances that allow out-of-hospital providers to conclude that an overdose or poisoning has occurred. It is important for out-of-hospital personnel to determine if such evidence ex-

ists. Often the patient may have attempted to dispose of medication containers immediately following the ingestion, or family members may try to disguise an overdose scenario.

Once an overdose or poisoning is suspected, the degree of toxicity should be established rapidly. The toxicity risk can be estimated from the patient's symptoms and physical condition, as well as the poisons involved, the amount or concentration, the time since exposure, and in some cases the length of exposure. Sustained release formulations, commonly used for calcium channel blockers and theophylline products, may cause delayed onset of symptoms for several hours after ingestion. Patients may then deteriorate rapidly. Toxic effects of acetaminophen, cyclopeptide mushrooms, carbon tetrachloride, or chloroform may take days to become apparent. In some patients there is suspicion of overdose, but the substance involved is unknown. In others, symptoms do not correlate with the identified substance. Patients with immediate outward symptoms probably have a significant overdose, but it may not have reached full effect. If the patient is having symptoms that are not consistent with the identified poisons, believe the symptoms. Tables 65.2 and 65.3 describe toxidromes that may be helpful in determining the substance type in these cases.

At times an overdose or poisoning may be totally unsuspected, particularly in the trauma patient. In one study, nearly 50% of fatal motor vehicle accidents involved alcohol or drugs.[2] Overdose should be considered in trauma patients with unexplained hypotension, respiratory depression, seizures, or agitation. A widened QRS, bradycardia, hypotension, and severe agitation, unexplained by the patient's trauma, should lead to treatment of possible toxicity (such as tricyclic antidepressant toxicity). A decreased level of consciousness in adolescent and adult patients is often assumed to be drug-induced. In the absence of other physical evidence of overdose, other causes should be considered; hypoglycemia, infectious causes such as meningitis, and cerebral vascular accidents should also be considered. A useful mnemonic when considering the differential diagnosis of decreased level of consciousness is **(AEIOU TIPS).**

A—alcohol, acidosis
E—epilepsy
I—insulin (too much or too little)
O—overdose, opiates
U—uremia/hepatic

TABLE 65.2		
Toxidromes		
SYNDROME	**SIGNS AND SYMPTOMS**	**AGENTS**
Cholinergic Muscarinic	Salivation lacrimation, urination, defecation (diarrhea), GI pain, emesis, bradycardia, miosis	Organophosphates, carbamates, some wild mushrooms
Nicotinic	Tachycardia, hypotension, hypertension, seizures	Tobacco, organophosphates, carbamates
Anticholinergic	Dry mucus membranes, flushing, mydriasis, tachycardia, hyperthermia, delirium, coma	Cyclic antidepressants, diphenhydramine, antihistamines, some plants (Jimson weed)
Sympathomimetic	Seizures, tachycardia, hypertension, hyperthermia	Cocaine, theophylline, caffeine, phenylpropanolamine (diet pills)
Opioid	Coma, respiratory suppression, miosis	Heroin, morphine, fentanyl, diphenoxylate, propoxyphene, dextromethorphan
Late Hepatotoxicity	Mild initial symptoms, late onset jaundice, hepatic coma	Acetaminophen, some wild mushrooms, carbon tetrachloride, chloroform

T—trauma
I—infection
P—poisoning, psychiatric
S—shock

Age Considerations

With the exception of iron-containing vitamins, toddlers generally take small amounts of medications. However, pediatric patients exposed to even small doses of calcium channel blockers, diphenoxylate, or clonidine may have a precipitous decline in CNS and hemodynamic function. Histories are often more accurate following pediatric ingestions. Young adults may make suicidal gestures or attempts and experiment with mind-altering drugs. In suicide attempts, teenagers often ingest over-the-counter medications such as acetaminophen and iron; they may not manifest severe toxicity for 48 to 72 hours. Experimentation with some mind-altering agents such as GHB and MDMA may result in immediate severe, life-threatening sequelae. Abuse of readily available inhalants, such as cooking spray, can have catastrophic effects in adolescents, including sudden cardiac arrest. Often friends of the victim will try to conceal the fact that abuse preceded the event. The out-of-hospital provider is then faced with ruling out all causes of sudden cardiac arrest in an adolescent patient.

Older adults or elderly patients may have toxicity from a therapeutic misadventure (i.e., taking too many drugs, double-dosing through the day, taking drugs with interactions), or a change in their physiologic status (e.g., hepatic failure, renal failure, dehydration), resulting in toxicity. Changes in neurologic function secondary to toxicity in older adults may be missed and attributed to worsening dementia, and the like. They also take overdoses in suicide attempts. Often they are reluctant to discuss their intoxication.

Cardiac Arrest

Cardiac arrest is an ominous event in the poisoned patient. However, some patients have been resuscitated despite very prolonged CPR.[7] Unlike patients with coronary artery disease, victims of poisoning often have normal coronary arteries, normal myocardial function, and normal pulmonary function prior to their ingestion. In many of these patients, normal function can be restored if the patient survives the toxicity and arrest. Therefore, prolonged resuscitation may be indicated, particularly in young overdose patients. In some situations, such as tricyclic antidepressant or digoxin poisoning, standard measures need to be altered to include administration of a known antidote. Cardiopulmonary bypass (CPB) has been successfully used in a small number of arrested overdose patients,[7–9] particularly patients who have taken lethal amounts of calcium channel or beta blocker medications. Patients with serious calcium channel blocker, beta blocker overdoses, and overdose patients in cardiac arrest should be taken to institutions with emergency CPB capabilities, where available.

TABLE 65.3

Common Poisons and Clinical Effects

Clinical Effect	Agent Involved	Clinical Effect	Agent Involved
Decreased LOC	Alcohol Antipsychotics Barbiturates Benzodiazepines Beta Blockers Calcium Blockers Carbon Monoxide Clonidine Cyanide Cyclic Antidepressants GHB and analogs Ketamine Lithium Opioids	Sinus Tachycardia/ SVT	Amphetamines Antidepressants Antihistamines Antipsychotics Caffeine Cocaine Decongestants Theophylline
Agitation	Amphetamines Anticholinergics Antihistamines Caffeine Cocaine Cyclic Antidepressants Hallucinogenic amphetamines (MDMA) LSD PCP Theophylline	QRS and QT Prolongation	Beta Blockers Lithium Non-sedating antihistamines Phenothiazines Procainamide Quinidine Tricyclic Antidepressants
Seizures	Amphetamines Camphor Cocaine Cyclic Antidepressants Decongestants GHB and analogs Hallucinogenic amphetamines (MDMA) Isoniazid LSD Organophosphates	Ventricular Tachycardia	Amphetamines Caffeine Digitalis Glycosides Phenothiazines Tricyclic Antidepressants
Hypotension	Barbiturates Beta Blockers Calcium Blockers Clonidine Cyanide Cyclic Antidepressants Iron MAOIs Narcotics Organophosphates Phenothiazines	Mydriasis	Amphetamines Anticholinergics Caffeine Cocaine LSD MAOIs Nicotine PCP
Hypertension	Amphetamines Cocaine Ephedrine/Pseudoephedrine LSD MAOIs Phencyclidine	Miosis	Barbiturates Benzodiazepines Clonidine Opiates
Bradycardia/ Heart Block	Barbiturates Beta Blockers Calcium Blockers Carbamazepine Cyclic Antidepressants Digitalis Organophosphates Phencyclidine Phenytoin		

Decontamination

The standard of care for poisoned patient includes stabilizing the patient, limiting absorption, increasing elimination, and providing specific antidotes. Early attempts at gastric decontamination are helpful in decreasing systemic poison absorption. Some decontamination measures can be instituted in the out-of-hospital setting such as emesis (with syrup of ipecac) or administration of activated charcoal, dermal decontamination, and ocular irrigation. Activated charcoal can be given to limit absorption of retained drugs. Aggressive gastric decontamination is not indicated in asymptomatic patients with known nontoxic ingestions.

The primary purpose of gastric decontamination is to prevent further absorption of the poison and to decrease the risk for toxicity. Currently, four methods of gastrointestinal decontamination are employed —ipecac syrup-induced emesis, activated charcoal administration, gastric lavage, and whole bowel irrigation. Of these, ipecac syrup and activated charcoal play a role in out-of-hospital management of the poisoned patient; out-of-hospital initiation of whole bowel irrigation decontamination may be of benefit. This is based on the belief that gastrointestinal decontamination methods are most effective when initiated soon after ingestion. This is especially true in those situations in which transport to the emergency department may be prolonged. Despite the potential benefit, one study showed that out-of-hospital gastrointestinal decontamination was initiated in only 6 of 361 (2%) poisoned patients.[10] In all of these patients, ipecac syrup-induced emesis was the decontamination method of choice. In the emergency department, activated charcoal was administered to 70% of the patients who might have been suitable candidates for out-of-hospital activated charcoal. The median time to activated charcoal administration after arrival in the ED was 82 minutes.

Ipecac Syrup

Use of ipecac syrup to induce emesis has decreased dramatically over the last two decades and many emergency physicians have completely abandoned its use. In 1999 the AAPCC reported that ipecac was used to induce emesis on over 21,000 occasions as compared to use in over 104,000 poisoning cases in 1990.[5,11] Despite these trends, there may still be a limited role for the use of ipecac syrup in the out-of-hospital management of poisoned patients. Although utilization of ipecac has decreased over the last 10 years, many poison centers still recommend home and ambulance storage of ipecac syrup. One of the greatest challenges to the DMOPs is determining those selected situations in which ipecac syrup use can be beneficial and safe. In 1997 the American Academy of Clinical Toxicology (AACT) published a position statement on syrup of ipecac administration.[12] The AACT has determined that there is insufficient data to provide support for or against the use of syrup of ipecac after ingestion of a poison. They advise that ipecac should only be administered in patients who are awake and alert and who have ingested a potentially toxic amount of a substance.

Ipecac should not be administered beyond 60 minutes after ingestion, since its clinical effects diminish with time. Recommended syrup of ipecac doses can be found in table 65.4. All syrup of ipecac doses should be preceded or followed by 120–240 ml of water. In young children, their favorite beverage can be substituted for water. Expired ipecac can be used without loss of efficacy.[13] If vomiting does not occur by 20–30 minutes after administration, an additional dose can be administered. Additional doses of ipecac should be avoided and alternative approaches to the prevention of poison absorption should be considered. Syrup of ipecac is contraindicated in patients with a compromised airway or in patients who have ingested a substance that could rapidly compromise airway function. Syrup of ipecac is also contraindicated in patients who have ingested hydrocarbons and caustic substances. Table 65.5 provides a list of some substances for which indirect emesis is contraindicated.

Activated Charcoal

Activated charcoal (AC) plays an important role in the management of many poisoned patients. However, lithium, iron, ethanol, methanol, and ethylene

TABLE 65.4	
Ipecac Syrup Dosage Guidelines	
Age	**Dose**
6 months and less	Administer only under supervision of a physician
6–12 months	5–10 ml
1–12 years	15 ml
12 years and older	15–30 ml

TABLE 65.5
Contraindications to Induced Emesis
Cyclic Antidepressants
Calcium Channel Blockers
Beta Blockers
Theophylline
Strychnine
Camphor
Isoniazid
Ammonia
Sedative hypnotics including benzodiazepines, barbiturates, all sleeping medications
Batteries, battery acid
Corrosives—including drain openers, automatic dish washing detergent, oven cleaners
Hydrocarbons—especially mineral seal oil (furniture polish), gasoline, kerosene

glycol are not effectively adsorbed to activated charcoal due to their low molecular weights. Adsorption is thought to occur within one minute of exposure of the activated charcoal to the poison.[14] In adults, doses range from 25 to 50 grams. Some reference texts recommend a pediatric dose of 1 gram/kg. A commonly accepted pediatric dosage range is between 15 and 25 grams. The gritty texture of traditional AC slurries, along with the black color, decreases the palatability of these products. Along with problems associated with palatability, emesis has been shown to occur following the administration of AC. The incidence of vomiting may increase when AC-sorbitol slurries are administered as compared to AC-water slurries. Minocha reported a 12.5% incidence of emesis following administration of AC-water and a 15.5% incidence with AC-sorbitol.[15] Problems with palatability and vomiting represent pitfalls in the out-of-hospital administration of AC, but they should not preclude its use. Given AC's ability to cause vomiting, appropriate measures must be taken to protect the airway in patients with a decreased level of consciousness in order to decrease the risk of pulmonary aspiration of charcoal.

A cathartic such as sorbitol is often co-administered with AC to enhance movement of the charcoal-toxin complex out of the gastrointestinal tract. Co-administration of a cathartic is not absolutely necessary. Combination AC-sorbitol products should not be used in children, since they will provide an excessive amount of sorbitol to the child. Adverse effects of cathartics include diarrhea, fluid loss, dehydration, electrolyte loss, and subsequent acid-base disorders.

Dermal Decontamination

Following topical exposure to hazardous materials such as organophosphate pesticides, hydrofluoric acid, and hydrocarbons, early dermal decontamination is indicated. The provider should first protect herself with gloves, gown, and protective face mask, when indicated, to prevent self-exposure. Contaminated clothing should be removed, and all exposed skin irrigated with copious amounts of tepid water for at least 15 minutes. If solid or powdered toxins are present on the patient's skin, these should be removed prior to irrigation, since dilution with water may hasten absorption and potential for toxicity. The drainage water should be handled as contaminated waste. If ocular exposure occurs, the affected eye(s) should be irrigated with a gentle stream of lukewarm water for at least 15 minutes.

Specific Poisons

Benzodiazepines

Benzodiazepines are frequently ingested in intentional drug overdoses. In 1999, the AAPCC reported over 40,000 intentional ingestions of benzodiazepines.[5] Only seven of these fatalities involved a benzodiazepine alone. Most often, death from benzodiazepine poisoning involves co-ingestion of a benzodiazepine and at least one other agent.

The clinical features observed following exposure to a benzodiazepine vary based on the dose ingested, the route of exposure, and co-ingestion of other agents that affect the central nervous system. Following ingestion of a benzodiazepine alone, toxicity is usually limited. Parenteral overdose of a benzodiazepine or co-ingestion of other substances may result in more profound toxicities. Central nervous system and respiratory depression are the most common clinical features observed after toxic exposure to a benzodiazepine.

When toxicities occur secondary to a benzodiazepine exposure, airway management is the primary type of supportive care that needs to be provided. In significant recent ingestions, a single dose of AC may be administered to prevent benzodiazepine absorption. Induction of emesis with syrup of ipecac is not recommended due to the central nervous system effects of these agents. Flumazenil (Romazicon®) is available as an antidote for benzodiazepines. Flumazenil competes for benzodiazepine receptor sites in the central nervous system. The product information for flumazenil states that flumazenil is indicated for complete or partial reversal of the sedative effects of benzodiazepines.

Although the manufacturer states that flumazenil is indicated in benzodiazepine overdose, most clinical toxicologists have concluded that it has limited use in these situations.[16] This is due to the benefit versus risk ratio associated with this medication. Given the limited clinical effects that occur in isolated benzodiazepine poisonings, there is little need to use an antidote for management of the patient. The use of flumazenil in poly-pharmacy exposures that include a benzodiazepine can cause adverse effects. Specifically, use of flumazenil in mixed ingestions involving a tricyclic antidepressant and a benzodiazepine has resulted in development of seizures. Therefore, most clinicians are reluctant to use flumazenil in any poly-pharmacy ingestion involving agents that are known to cause seizures. Since the history of the ingestion is often inaccurate, flumazenil use should be avoided in poly-pharmacy ingestions. Additionally, administration of flumazenil to patients who are benzodiazepine-dependent can result in precipitation of benzodiazepine withdrawal. The most concerning manifestation of benzodiazepine withdrawal is seizures.

Calcium Channel Blocking Agents

Over the past years, prescribing of calcium channel blockers, such as diltiazem, nifedipine, and verapamil, has increased dramatically. Along with the increase in the use of these agents, there has been a dramatic increase in the number of accidental and intentional ingestions involving them. These agents may cause profound life-threatening hypotension, bradycardia, and asystole. Calcium channel blockers interfere with conduction through sinoatrial and atrioventricular nodes resulting in bradyarrhythmias, conduction disturbances, and a decrease in cardiac output. Hypotension occurs secondary to vasodilation and decreases in cardiac output.[17]

Even small quantities of calcium channel blockers (1–2 tablets) may cause significant morbidity or mortality in a pediatric patient. Asymptomatic patients who claim to have ingested these agents should be treated seriously. These drugs are commonly prescribed in sustained release preparations, which will have delayed onset (several hours) of symptoms, such as an extremely precipitous decrease in blood pressure to severe hypotension. Blood pressure monitoring, continuous cardiac monitoring, and pulse oximetry should be initiated immediately by out-of-hospital providers. As mentioned earlier, these patients may have a precipitous change in cardiovascular function with subsequent airway compromise.

Ipecac syrup should not be used to induce emesis due to the potential for rapid decreases in level of consciousness. AC is effective, and can be administered in the out-of-hospital setting as long as the patient is conscious. Symptomatic bradycardia may be treated with atropine, and when necessary a transcutaneous pacemaker. Calcium chloride may be of some benefit in calcium blocker toxicity. One gram of calcium chloride (the preferred calcium salt) should be administered as a 10% solution. Doses should be repeated 2–3 times until symptoms subside. Very large doses may be necessary (> 10 amps).[18] Calcium should not be administered in the setting of a combined ingestion of a calcium channel blocker and a digitalis glycoside until digoxin Fab fragments have been administered. Administration of calcium to the digoxin toxic patient can result in disturbances in cardiac contractility. Glucagon (1–10 mg) IV has also been beneficial in some patients and should be included in the standard approach to the patient with calcium channel blocker poisoning.[19] Hypotension should be treated with fluids challenges and vasopressors such as dopamine.

Carbon Monoxide

Sources of CO include fires, automobile exhaust, malfunctioning furnaces, indoor use of charcoal and propane grills, inadequately vented fireplaces, and cigarettes. Smokers often have carboxyhemoglobin levels of 5%.[20] CO poisoning is probably the number one cause of death from poisoning each year. Unfortunately, it is difficult to determine exactly how many people die each year because there is not mandatory reporting of CO poisoning in every state.

There are multiple mechanisms for CO poisoning. Classically, CO is known to displace oxygen from hemoglobin and increase the hemoglobin binding affinity of the remaining oxygen molecules.[21] This results in decreased oxygen delivery to tissue and many of the clinical effects of CO poisoning. This mechanism does not completely explain many of the effects of CO poisoning, including the delayed neurologic sequelae, that are sometimes observed. Additional research has shown that CO also binds to cytochrome oxidase and inhibits cellular respiration.[22] Additionally, it has been shown to cause the formation of oxygen-free radicals that cause lipid peroxidation and it is known to bind to myoglobin. This binding to myoglobin may explain many of the cardiac effects that are observed in CO poisoning.

The presentation of CO poisoning may differ depending on the source. For example, patients who are exposed due to a malfunctioning furnace may present with complaints of several days of nausea, vomiting, and headache. Often, they may not seek medical attention until something significant, such as loss of consciousness, has occurred in one or more of the victims. On the other hand, the patient who connects a hose to their automobile exhaust pipe in a closed garage may have a rapid change in level of conscious, hemodynamic instability, cardiac dysrhythmias, and seizures. Table 65.6 lists classic acute signs and symptoms of CO poisoning.

A number of delayed neurologic effects of CO have also been described.[23] These include dementia, amnesia, psychosis, parkinsonism, and peripheral neuropathy. The severity of signs and symptoms will depend on the duration of exposure and the concentration of CO that they are exposed to. In pregnancy, the fetus may be at greater risk than the mother, as the fetal carboxyhemoglobin may be higher than the maternal carboxyhemoglobin.[24]

As soon as CO poisoning is suspected, the patient should be moved to an area with fresh air, and high flow oxygen should be administered via a tight-fitting face mask. In these patients, the pulse oximeter reading may be normal as the device will measure carboxyhemoglobin as oxygenated hemoglobin. Due to out-of-hospital interventions, movement to fresh air and supplemental oxygen administration, the carboxyhemoglobin measurement in the ED will not reflect the peak carboxyhemoglobin. Table 65.7 shows the effects of fresh air, high flow oxygen, and hyperbaric oxygen on carboxyhemoglobin half-lives.

Victims of CO poisoning may also be treated with hyperbaric oxygen, which provides oxygen at 2.5 atmospheres and increases the amount of oxygen dissolved in the blood. The decision to use hyperbaric oxygen is dependent on the clinical presentation, the carboxyhemoglobin level, age, and medical history. The DMOP may want to consider diverting some patients to a facility with hyperbaric oxygen capabilities. Such patients include those who are initially unresponsive, experiencing chest pain, or pregnant. An absolute carboxyhemoglobin level that indicates a need for hyperbaric oxygen has not been determined. In some settings, a level of 25% is used, while 40% is used in other settings. The threshold for treating children and pregnant women with hyperbaric oxygen is lower. Depending on regional practices, the DMOP and out-of-hospital providers may consider diverting CO-poisoned patients to a hyperbaric facility. Guidelines should be prospectively developed if such facilities are available.

TABLE 65.6	
Clinical Manifestations in Carbon Monoxide Poisoning	
SYSTEM	**SIGNS AND SYMPTOMS**
Neurologic	Headache Dizziness Difficulty thinking Blurred vision Cognitive deficits Seizures Coma
Respiratory	Dyspnea Tachypnea Respiratory arrest
Gastrointestinal	Nausea Vomiting
Cardiovascular	Tachycardia Palpitations Chest pain Ventricular dysrhythmias Myocardial ischemia Hypotension Cardiac arrest
Skin	Erythema (Note—this is usually a post-mortem finding.)

TABLE 65.7	
Effects of Oxygen on Carboxyhemoglobin	
OXYGEN SOURCE	**AVERAGE CARBOXYHEMOGLOBIN HALF-LIVES (MINUTES)**
Ambient air	300–360
High flow oxygen	40–90
Hyperbaric oxygen	<30

Cocaine

The recreational use and abuse of cocaine continues to be common in the United States. Typical effects observed in cocaine toxicity are the result of the sympathetic storm from cocaine's potentiation of the neurotransmitters, epinephrine, and norepinephrine. In the early stimulation phase, neurologic effects observed include hyperexcitability, euphoria, muscle twitching, irritability, headache, and hallucinations.[25] Cardiovascular effects include bradycardia, tachycardia, chest pain, and hypertension.[26] Seizure activity may advance to status epilepticus. Agitation and seizures in the cocaine-toxic patient can be treated with benzodiazepines such as lorazepam or diazepam.

Since cocaine is most often abused by inhalation and intravenous injection, gastric decontamination is often not necessary. The exception to this is the case of the individual who is a body-packer or body-stuffer. The body-packer ingests bags of cocaine (containing huge amounts of drugs) as a means of transporting the drugs. These bags are usually of high quality and difficult to break. The body-stuffer is a person who swallows bags of cocaine to rid himself of evidence. These bags or balloons are often thin and prone to breakage, and may contain enough cocaine to cause serious toxicity. Activated charcoal should be administered in the field to either a body-packer or a body-stuffer. In the case of bag breakage, the AC will adsorb cocaine in the gastrointestinal track. Administration of AC can be followed later by irrigation and cleansing of the gastrointestinal tract to eliminate the bags of cocaine. The patient should be monitored, as ventricular arrhythmias are common.

Ethanol

The ethanol-intoxicated patient is most often an adolescent or adult who drank excessively in a social situation, but children are also potential victims of ethanol toxicity. Most commonly, this involves the child who accidentally ingests an ethanol-containing product, such as perfume or cologne, in the home setting.

Several mechanisms for ethanol toxic effects have been suggested. Unfortunately, there is a great deal of controversy regarding these mechanisms and their specific role in ethanol toxicity. Some literature has suggested that ethanol toxicity is due to the dissolution of ethanol in the lipid membrane of the cell. Other researchers have concluded that ethanol, like the benzodiazepines, may enhance the effects of GABA. Recently, the effects of ethanol on the inhibitory neurotransmitter N-methyl-d-aspartate were described. Most likely the ethanol mechanism of toxicity is complex and cannot be attributed to one single neurotransmitter or pathway. Ethanol-induced hypoglycemia is due to inhibition of gluconeogenesis and depletion of glycogen stores.[27]

Peak ethanol serum concentrations have been reported to occur between 30 and 100 minutes after an oral dose.[28] Based on studies in emergency department populations, the mean ethanol clearance rate ranges from 15 to 20 mg/dL/hr.[29] This will vary depending on the patient's experience with ethanol. For example, alcoholic patients may clear ethanol at a rate as high as 40 mg/dL/hr.

Ethanol toxicity is frequently the primary reason for a presentation to EMS. However, ethanol toxicity is often combined with other medical conditions, including trauma. The effects of ethanol will vary from patient to patient. Table 65.8 lists the most common clinical effects observed in acute ethanol toxicity. Co-ingestion of CNS depressant substances, such as benzodiazepines and GHB, can further complicate the picture of ethanol toxicity. Children are thought to be at greater risk for hypoglycemia than adults. Nonetheless, blood glucose monitoring should be done in all ethanol intoxicated patients.

Management of the ethanol-poisoned patient is primarily supportive. These patients are at increased risk for mental status changes that may impair airway control. In the out-of-hospital setting, dextrose should be administered to mitigate any ethanol-induced hypoglycemia. In adults, 50 ml of dextrose 50% should be administered followed by a dextrose infusion. The dextrose dose in children will vary based on age. There is limited role for out-of-hospital gastric decontamination in the patient with ethanol toxicity. Syrup of ipecac should never be used and ethanol is not well adsorbed by AC. In the setting of hypothermia, these patients should be warmed until their core body temperature returns to normal. In those patients with environmental hyperthermia and concomitant ethanol toxicity, aggressive external cooling should be utilized. Given the risk for co-existing morbidity in many ethanol-poisoned patients, specific attention must be focused on treating these other symptoms.

Foreign Body Ingestion

Foreign body ingestion is common, particularly in small children. The child is usually seen playing with a coin, only later to have the coin disappear. Because

TABLE 65.8	
Toxic Effects of Ethanol	
SYSTEM	**CLINICAL EFFECTS**
Central Nervous System	Euphoria Disinhibition Slurred speech Altered perception Impaired judgment Ataxia Hyperreflexia Combativeness Seizures Coma
Cardiovascular	Hypotension Tachycardia
Respiratory	Respiratory depression
Gastrointestinal	Abdominal pain Nausea Vomiting Hematemesis
Metabolic	Hypoglycemia Hypothermia Hyperthermia

they are frequently asymptomatic, there is an inclination to leave the child at home and allow nature to take its course ("this too shall pass"). However, esophageal erosion can occur, particularly with button batteries. Therefore, all children should be brought to the hospital for x-ray localization. Once the foreign body is in the stomach, it will generally pass into the feces without further difficulties.

Gamma Hydroxybutyrate

In 1960, gamma-hydroxybutyrate (GHB) was synthesized as an analog of the inhibitory neurotransmitter gamma-amino butyric acid.[30] Beginning in the late 1980s, GHB was sold in health food stores as a dietary supplement that enhanced bodybuilding, hastened weight loss, and induced sleep. In the 1990s, it became popular as a recreational drug due to its intoxicating and euphoria-inducing properties. Along with health food store sales, GHB has been listed as a "party drug" on web sites and advertised in bodybuilding magazines. GHB, which is popular with high school and college students, can be found at dance clubs and rave parties. A typical intoxicating dose ranges from 1 to 5 grams of the powder. Often, GHB is sold already mixed in liquid and dispensed by the water-bottle cap to the user.

Since 1992, the Drug Abuse Warning Network (DAWN) has reported over 3000 ED visits related to GHB. Between 1995 and 1998, the AAPCC reported 1 to 2 deaths per year from GHB and its analogs. In 1999 alone, 10 GHB deaths were reported by poison centers.

In humans, the largest GHB concentrations are in the basal ganglia. The sleep-inducing properties seem to be due to conversion of the gamma butyrolactone to GHB. GHB is considered to be an inhibitory neurotransmitter that induces central nervous system depression through regulation of dopaminergic neurons.[31] Although promotional information claimed that GHB had anabolic effects, through stimulation of growth hormone release, this is probably untrue. GHB is rapidly absorbed from the gastrointestinal tract, and exhibits clinical effects within 15 minutes. Peak serum concentrations have been observed at 1.5 to 2 hours after ingestion.

The primary effects of GHB and its analogs result from their ability to cause dose-related central nervous system depression. GHB doses of 10 mg/kg have resulted in mild CNS effects, including amnesia and hypotonia.[32] Drowsiness, dizziness, and euphoria have been observed in the 20 to 30mg/kg range and profound CNS depression and respiratory depression have occurred with doses above 50 mg/kg.[32] A unique characteristic of GHB exposure is that coma may last for a short period of time. The duration of coma is very short, and ranges from 1 to 2 hours in many patients. Often, these patients require intubation in the field or on presentation to the ED and are completely awake within 4 to 6 hours of presentation. The effects of these substances can be enhanced by co-ingestion of other CNS depressants, including ethanol and benzodiazepines.

GHB-related bradycardia is often associated with deterioration in mental status. Patients with bradycardia had a median initial GCS score of 4, compared to a median initial score of 9.5 for patients without bradycardia. In these patients, hypotension is usually accompanied by bradycardia and involves co-ingestion of other substances. Seizure-like activity has been reported. Vomiting is often associated with emergence from coma, but it can be seen at any time after ingestion of GHB. Esophageal burns are an interesting potential clinical effect associated with GHB.[33] Sodium hydroxide is used in the manufacture of GHB; if all of the sodium hydroxide is not consumed, the liquid could be strongly alkaline.

Along with acute toxicity, a GHB withdrawal syndrome has been described. This withdrawal syndrome consists of anxiety, agitation, tremors, insomnia, disorientation, paranoia, auditory and visual hallucinations, tachycardia, elevated blood pressure, and ocular-motor changes.[34]

These patients should be closely observed for changes in neurologic, respiratory, and cardiovascular status. Initial out-of-hospital management patients should include establishment of intravenous access as well as placement on a cardiac monitor and a pulse oximeter. Given the incidence of vomiting accompanied by CNS depression, aspiration precautions should be taken. Due to the potential for CNS depression, out-of-hospital intubation may be necessary. The need for intubation may be heightened with co-ingestion of other CNS depressant substances. There is limited role for gastric decontamination following ingestion of GHB. Ipecac syrup-induced emesis is contraindicated due to the CNS depression associated with these substances. Since absorption of GHB is rapid, AC may be of limited benefit. Symptomatic bradycardia can be treated with atropine. Hypotension can be treated with fluids and vasopressors. Seizures should be treated with benzodiazepines such as diazepam or lorazepam. Antagonists, such as naloxone and flumazenil, have limited effect in reversing the sedating effects of these substances. Given the relatively rapid reversal of mental status changes, these patients should be monitored closely so that they do not risk self-extubation.

Hazardous Materials

Hazardous materials are a potential threat not only to workers, but to out-of-hospital care providers and the population at large. Large communities can afford to have specialized Hazmat teams, but smaller communities rely on their EMS services. Some basic principles for handling hazardous materials are discussed in this section.

A hazardous material incident is any situation which may cause harmful contamination to the environment (air, water, or soil) or to personnel. In many cases the substance involved is unknown. Extreme caution should be used when approaching a scene. Realize that contamination flows downstream and by air currents. Areas where the chances of contamination are high are considered hot. Hot zones should be entered only by a limited number of personnel equipped with protective gear. A secondary area around the hot zone, a contamination reduction zone should be established for basic decontamina-

tion. Basic decontamination facilities need not be fancy—a water supply, an inflatable pool to collect run off, and plastic bags to double-bag exposed clothing and jewelry are often all that is necessary. Either treatment should take place beyond the contamination reduction zone unless a critical condition exists.

Identification of toxic substance may be aided by labels, placards and shipping papers. The U.S. Department of Transportation uses a 4-digit identification code.[35] A similar code by the National Fire Protection Association is described in table 65.9.[36] A patient decontaminated at the scene may still have the potential to contaminate an ambulance or hospital. Vomit and urine may add to the contamination risk. Additional decontamination on arrival to the ED is appropriate. The out-of-hospital providers should have protective gear and the ambulance itself may require decontamination.

Opioids

Out-of-hospital exposure to the opiates and opioids can occur in a variety of settings, such as abuse of heroin and fentanyl derivatives, or opioids used for

TABLE 65.9
National Fire Protection Association Classification of Hazardous Materials
BLUE = Health Hazard
4—Short exposure can be critical.
3—Short exposure can be serious—temporary or residual impairment.
2—Prolonged exposure can be serious—temporary or residual impairment.
1—Minor injury.
0—No injury.
RED = Combustible
4—Vaporizes in atmosphere conditions—burns easily.
3—Can be ignited at high temperatures.
2—Can be ignited at normal temperatures.
1—Must preheat before ignited.
0—Will not burn.
YELLOW = Explosive Hazard
4—Readily detonates.
3—Requires strong initiating source to explode or will explode with water.
2—Violent chemical reaction, but no explosion. May form explosive with water.
1—Becomes unstable at high temperature.
0—Stable.

pain control. Agents such as diphenoxylate, clonidine, and dextromethorphan may have opiate-like effects. Physicians and providers may not consider opiate toxicity in a patient taking over-the-counter cough preparations. In meperidine overdose, pupils may be dilated rather than constricted. Anticholinergic effects will predominate in diphenoxylate ingestions.

Treatment of exposure to these substances includes supportive care, consideration of gastric decontamination, and the use of specific narcotic antagonists. Administration of naloxone will result in rapid reversal of opiate/opioid toxicity, often precipitating opiate withdrawal. Usual initial adult dose of naloxone is 2 mg, although massive doses (10–20 mg) have been required to manage exposure to the fentanyl derivatives, diphenoxylate, and clonidine. Repeat doses of naloxone may be necessary to manage recurrence of toxic effects due to the short half-life of naloxone. Patients who respond to naloxone should be transported to the hospital for an observation period.

Salicylates

Although the incidence of pediatric salicylate poisoning has decreased over the last two decades, salicylates continue to present challenges to the prehospital providers who initially are responsible for care of these patients. Salicylate poisoning is usually categorized as acute, acute on chronic, or chronic. Acute exposures usually involve accidental exposures in children and intentional overdoses in adults as in the case described above. Acute-on-chronic exposures involve acute ingestion in an individual who is chronically using therapeutic doses of salicylates. Chronic salicylate toxicity often occurs following prolonged administration of large doses of aspirin and other salicylate-containing products for the treatment of pain.

Although the majority of salicylate exposures involve aspirin, other salicylates may be involved. These other salts provide different amounts of salicylate than aspirin and therefore an aspirin conversion factor is useful in determining the potential for toxicity. For example, a young child may ingest a topical medication that contains methyl salicylate. Methyl salicylate contains larger amounts of salicylate than aspirin and can be very toxic soon after exposure.

The clinical presentation of salicylate toxicity can be very complex and is dependent on the amount ingested, the time since the exposure, and the type of exposure (acute or chronic), as well as the presence of co-ingestants. Following acute exposure, salicylate

doses of greater than 150 mg/kg have the ability to cause toxicity. Doses between 150–300 mg/kg usually cause mild toxicity and doses between 300–500 mg/kg can cause moderate toxicity. The risk for severe toxicity is associated with doses above 500 mg/kg. Table 65.10 lists the common clinical effects associated with salicylate toxicity. In chronic salicylate toxicity, neurologic changes and laboratory changes may be present immediately upon presentation of the patient. In the out-of-hospital setting, salicylate toxicity may be overlooked and stroke, infection, or progression of dementia may be considered responsible for the patient's presentation.

Gastric decontamination may include syrup of ipecac-induced emesis, gastric lavage, and/or AC administration, depending on the clinical scenario. In children who have ingested a toxic amount of aspirin,

TABLE 65.10	
Clinical Manifestations in Salicylate Poisoning	
SYSTEM	**CLINICAL EFFECTS**
Gastrointestinal	Nausea Vomiting Gastrointestinal bleeding Pylorospasm with decreased gastric emptying
Neurologic	Tinnitus Decreased auditory acuity Hearing loss Vertigo Agitation Delirium Lethargy and coma Seizures Central nervous system hypoglycemia Cerebral edema
Respiratory	Tachypnea Hyperpnea Non-cardiogenic pulmonary edema
Acid/Base and Electrolytes	Large anion gap metabolic acidosis Respiratory alkalosis Hyponatremia Hypernatremia Hypokalemia
Metabolic	Hypoglycemia Hyperglycemia Hyperthermia
Coagulation	Hypoprothrombinemia Platelet dysfunction

syrup of ipecac can be used within 60 minutes of the ingestion. On the other hand, ipecac should not be used for a potentially toxic methyl salicylate ingestion, since methyl salicylate can have more rapid neurologic effects than aspirin. AC effectively adsorbs salicylates and should be a primary component of gastric decontamination in these patients.

Since salicylates are acids, they are found in an un-ionized form in a more acidic environment such as the urine. In their un-ionized form, salicylates are readily reabsorbed into the systemic circulation. In more alkaline environments, salicylates become ionized and they are less readily reabsorbed. Therefore, alkalinization of the urine to a pH of 8 is an effective method of enhancing elimination of ionized salicylate if normal urine output is maintained. This can be achieved by administering 1–2 mEq/kg of sodium bicarbonate.

Out-of-hospital providers need to be very careful in treatment of agitation in these patients. Administration of sedatives, such as benzodiazepines, can depress respiratory drive, worsen the acidosis, and increase salicylate absorption into tissue. Salicylate-poisoned patients must be adequately ventilated when sedative drugs are administered. Salicylate-induced seizures should be treated initially with benzodiazepines.

Serotonin Syndrome

Studies involving the induction of serotonin syndrome in animals were first published in the early 1960s.[37] Early reports in humans, due to monoamine oxidase inhibitors, date back to the 1950s. Although many medications have the ability to cause the serotonin syndrome, it was the emergence of the selective serotonin reuptake inhibitors (SSRIs) such as fluoxetine that increased awareness of this condition. Table 65.11 list medications implicated in the serotonin syndrome.

Although a number of mechanisms for the serotonin syndrome have been discussed in the literature, it is most likely due to excessive stimulation of the 5HT-1A receptor.[38] Stimulation of this receptor can be due to drug-drug interactions that result in excess serotonin, overdose with one or more serotonergic agents, and abuse of agents known to increase serotonin, such as MDMA.

Sternbach described a classic triad of symptoms associated with the serotonin syndrome.[39] This triad includes mental status changes, autonomic dysfunction, and neuromuscular abnormalities. Table 65.12

TABLE 65.11
Agents Implicated in the Serotonin Syndrome[2]

Increase Serotonin Synthesis
  L-tryptophan
Decrease Serotonin Metabolism
  Meclobemide
  Monoamine oxidase inhibitors
Increase Serotonin Release
  Amphetamine
  Cocaine
  Fenfluramine
  Methylenedioxymethamphetamine (MDMA)
  Reserpine
Inhibit Serotonin Reuptake
  SSRIs
  Tricyclic antidepressants
Other Serotonin Reuptake Inhibitors
  Amphetamine
  Cocaine
  Dextromethorphan
  Meperidine
  Methylenedioxymethamphetamine (MDMA)
  Venlafaxine
Direct Receptor Antagonists
  Buspirone
  Lysergic acid diethylamide
  Sumatriptan
Dopamine Agonists
  Amantadine
  Bromocriptine
  Bupropion
  Levodopa
Other Drugs
  Carbamazepine
  Dihydroergotamine
  Fentanyl
  Lithium
  Nefazodone
  Pentazocine
  Sumatriptan
  Tramadol
  Trazodone

describes specific clinical effects that are included in this triad.

These patients should be closely monitored for vital sign changes along with changes in mental status and neuromuscular function. Frequently, they only require supportive care until their symptoms resolve. In more critically ill patients, intubation and mechanical ventilation may be required. Depending on the history of the exposure, gastric decontamination may or may not be warranted. Ipecac syrup-induced emesis is contraindicated due to the potential for mental status changes. Activated charcoal is effective in adsorbing all of the agents listed on table 65.11 and should also be considered in recent ingestions. Benzodiazepines, such as lorazepam and diazepam, play a crucial role in the management of the patient with serotonin syndrome. If the patient is agitated or experiencing muscular rigidity, they are at significant risk for developing hyperthermia. Administration of a benzodiazepine to decrease agitation and/or

rigidity can also help to decrease temperature. Aggressive external cooling should also be used to treat hyperthermia.

Toxic Inhalants

Inhalant abuse has been a significant problem in society for many centuries. Inhalation of substances for illicit purposes can be traced back to ancient Greek culture. These substances are abused because they are described as causing feelings of euphoria and exhilaration. Inhalant abuse is most prevalent from 13 to 15 years of age. It has been described in children as young as 6 to 8 years of age. Inhalants are often abused by teenagers because they are relatively inexpensive and readily available. Many of these substances are commonly found in the home, so children do not need to make purchases. Also, these containers can be easily concealed and do not raise suspicion of drug abuse (such as other drug paraphernalia like needles and syringes) and are not regulated as controlled substances. Inhalants are sometimes described as gateway substances because their use is followed by use of other illicit substances including cocaine, hallucinogens, and opiates. Some inhalant abusers become chronic users and develop emotional dependency and physical complications from long-term exposure to these substances.

The organic solvents most often implicated in inhalant abuse are aliphatic, aromatic, and halogenated hydrocarbons. Nitrites, including isobutyl nitrite and amyl nitrate, are also abused through inhalation. Table 65.13 lists some commonly abused solvents. Most often solvents are inhaled by sniffing directly from the container or huffing from a cloth that has been moistened with the liquid chemical. In some cases, the so called "bagger" will pour the solvent into a bag and inhale from the opening in the bag or place their head inside of the bag in order to inhale as much of the solvent as possible. Occasionally, inhalant abusers will boil the solvent on a stove to enhance vaporization and subsequent inhalation.

Due to their ready absorption into fat, solvents are rapidly transported to the brain. Immediate absorption of the solvent from the lungs followed by distribution to the brain results in a rapid onset of effects. Once the organic solvent enters the CNS, it exhibits its depressant effect. Both myelin and the neuronal membrane have very high fat concentrations. The solvents also have defatting effects that result in the associated long-term neurologic effects.

TABLE 65.12

Clinical Manifestations of the Serotonin Syndrome

Mental Staus Changes
- Agitation
- Coma
- Confusion
- Delirium
- Disorientation
- Hallucinations
- Insomnia
- Mania
- Mutism

Autonomic Dysfunction
- Abdominal pain
- Blood pressure increases/decreases
- Diaphoresis
- Diarrhea
- Flushing
- Hyperthermia
- Lacrimation
- Mydriasis
- Salivation
- Shivering
- Tachycardia

Neuromuscular Abnormalities
- Akathisia
- Clonus
- Hyperactivity
- Hyperreflexia
- Incoordination
- Myoclonus
- Nystagmus
- Ocular oscillation
- Oculogyric crisis
- Opisthotonos
- Rhabdomyolysis
- Rigidity
- Seizures
- Tremor
- Trismus

Secondary Complications
- Acidosis
- ARDS
- Disseminated intravascular coagulation
- Renal failure
- Respiratory failure

TABLE 65.13

Products Implicated In Inhalant Abuse

Aerosol Propellants (Air Fresheners, Deodorant Sprays, Hair Sprays)
  Dimethyl Ether
  Butane
  Halogenated Fluorocarbons
    Carbon Tetrachloride
    Ethylene Chloride
    Perchloroethylene
    Trichloroethylene

Gas Fuels (Disposable Cigarette Lighters)
  Propane
  Butane
  Liquid Petroleum Gas

Chlorinated Solvents (Commercial Dry Cleaning/Degreasing Agents)
  Carbon Tetrachloride
  Dichloromethane
  Methanol
  Tetrachloroethylene
  Toluene

Solvents From Adhesives (Also includes paints, nail polish, varnish remover)
  Acetone
  Butane
  Cyclohexanone
  Toluene
  Xylene

The clinical presentation of organic solvent abuse may involve acute toxicity, chronic toxicity, and a withdrawal syndrome. Often these patients will present with an odor of the substance on their breath or clothes. Abusers may also have signs of paint or other products on their face or hands. Abusers may be observed frequently sniffing their clothes (which are soaked with the substance), or sniffing a pen, marker, correction fluid, or other substance. Abusers often hide the rags or clothes used to sniff the substance.

Most individuals who abuse inhalants are seeking the known behavioral effects of these substances. These include euphoria, excitation, and disinhibition. As these patients become disinhibited, they are less fearful and may participate in activities they would otherwise not participate in. Disinhibition may lead the individual to participate in behaviors that may result in traumatic injuries. Falls, motor vehicle crashes, and burns have all been reported after inhalant abuse. The risk for burn trauma is increased with these agents given their high flammability. Sexual assault has also been reported following inhalant abuse.

The neurologic toxicities of the organic solvents include slurred speech, ataxia, disorientation, decreased reflexes, and central nervous system depression. Other neurologic symptoms include headache, diplopia, mydriasis, and tinnitus. Eventually these patients can become stuporous. These agents can also have an anesthetic effect, making the patient less able to feel pain. At large doses, these agents may cause both visual and auditory hallucinations. None of these signs or symptoms is exclusive to inhalant abuse, so out-of-hospital care providers should be alert to other indicators of inhalant abuse as listed above.

On respiratory examination, wheezing, rales, and rhonchi may be noted. Gastrointestinal mucous membrane irritation with subsequent nausea and vomiting may occur. Coughing, sneezing, hypersalivation, and conjunctival irritation have also been associated with these agents. A "glue-sniffer's rash" around the mouth and nose has also been described.

These agents have the ability to cause vasodilation and the halogenated hydrocarbons can sensitize the myocardium to the effects of endogenous catecholamines. Myocardial catecholamine sensitization has the potential to cause ventricular dysrhythmias. This has been referred to as the "sudden sniffing death syndrome." Descriptions of this syndrome include a scenario in which the inhalant abuser is startled or discovered during the inhalation process. Being startled causes a catecholamine release that, combined with the myocardial catecholamine sensitization, causes the dysrhythmias.

Death following inhalation of organic solvents can occur via several mechanisms. These include asphyxia, suffocation, traumatic injury, aspiration, and the sudden sniffing death syndrome. Death from asphyxiation is possible given that these solvents have the ability to displace oxygen. Suffocation is an especial risk with baggers who physically place their heads inside of a paper or plastic bag to inhale the solvent.

Individuals who develop symptoms following inhalation of an organic solvent should be removed from the source of the exposure. Place the patient on high flow oxygen via a non-rebreather mask. Given the nature of the organic solvents, airway management, including intubation and assisted ventilation, may be required.

If the solvent has been spilled on the patient's clothes, in order to minimize dermal absorption, the clothes should be removed and the skin should be thoroughly washed. Although these agents are primarily abused through some form of inhalation, accidental ingestion may occur. Administration of ipecac syrup is contraindicated in these patients. Activated charcoal is minimally effective in adsorbing hydrocarbons and should be withheld unless there is evidence of co-ingestion. If the solvent has been splashed in the patient's eye, the eye should be irrigated for 15 minutes with copious amounts of tepid tap water. If contact lenses are in place, they should be removed to prevent trapping of the substance under or in the lenses.

These patients should be monitored for ventricular dysrhythmias. Ventricular dysrhythmias should be treated with antiarrhythmics and defibrillation. Caution should be exercised in using epinephrine in these patients, since the dysrhythmia may be due to myocardial catecholamine sensitization. In these cases, the use of epinephrine could exacerbate dysrhythmias.

Tricyclic Antidepressants

The tricyclic antidepressants (TCAs), such as amitriptyline and nortriptyline, are a group of medications that have significant potential to cause death following accidental and intentional ingestion. Although the introduction of the selective serotonin reuptake inhibitors has resulted in decreased prescribing of the TCAs, poisoning due to the TCAs still occurs.

Patients with TCA toxicity have the potential to become critically ill in a very short time frame. These patients can become comatose and experience cardiovascular toxicities within 30–60 minutes after exposure. The clinical manifestations of TCAs are listed in Table 65.14.

Close attention must be paid to the provision of aggressive out-of-hospital care including airway management, treatment of dysrhythmias, circulatory support, and treatment of seizures. Management of these patients can be very complex. Treatment with sodium bicarbonate is a key component in the treatment of TCA toxicity. Sodium bicarbonate is more effective in reversing TCA-induced dysrhythmias than traditional anti-arrhythmic medications such as lidocaine and phenytoin. Most toxicologists recommend use of bolus doses of sodium bicarbonate to reverse the effects of TCAs. Sodium bicarbonate doses of 1–2 mEq/kg are used to reach a target pH of 7.5. Procainamide should not be administered, since it can worsen TCA-induced dysrhythmias. Also, bretylium should be avoided due to its ability to cause hypotension. TCA-induced hypotension is often resistant to dopamine and requires treatment with norepinephrine. In the out-of-hospital setting, dopamine

is often the only available vasopressor. Paramedics should be directed to administer dopamine to patients with hypotension secondary to TCA toxicity. If dopamine is ineffective in increasing the patient's blood pressure, therapy with norepinephrine can be initiated.

Gastric decontamination plays a very important role in management of the patient with TCA toxicity. Due to the rapid changes in level of consciousness that occur, induction of emesis with syrup of ipecac is absolutely contraindicated. Activated charcoal effectively adsorbs TCAs and prevents their systemic absorption. The benzodiazepine antagonist flumazenil should not be administered in the setting of TCA toxicity. Seizures have occurred following administration of flumazenil to patients who have co-ingested TCAs and benzodiazepines.

Triage Criteria

There is a growing trend to develop specialized centers for handling Hazmat victims and victims of poisoning and overdose. Adequate treatment and decontamination facilities are essential, as well as immediate access to antidotes and laboratory support. Guidelines for facilities wishing to become regional toxicol-

TABLE 65.14	
Clinical Manifestations of Tricyclic Antidepressant Poisoning	
ORGAN SYSTEM	**COMMON CLINICAL EFFECTS**
Cardiovascular	Sinus tachycardia, QRS widening, QT prolongation, bundle branch block, atrioventricular block, premature ventricular contractions, ventricular tachycardia, ventricular fibrillation, bradycardia, asystole
	Hypotension
Neurologic	Lethargy, agitation, hallucinations, coma, seizures
Respiratory	Respiratory depression, aspiration, ARDS
Other	Increases in temperature, mydriasis, decreases in bowel sounds and urine output, dry flushed skin
	Rhabdomyolysis and renal failure may occur due to prolonged seizures or immobility

ogy treatment centers have been established and endorsed by several organizations including AACT.[15] Few facilities specializing in the care of poisoning victims currently exist, but as these facilities become more common, appropriate triage in the field will become necessary. Unstable patients (hemodynamically unstable or respiratory distress) may be more appropriately handled in a regional center, should one be close. In addition, patients who ingest unusual materials, victims of major industrial exposures, and patients ingesting drugs with high lethal potential (table 65.6) may be triaged to centers with special abilities when and where these exist. Local capabilities will determine local triage criteria.

Pitfalls/Controversies

One of the primary pitfalls in the out-of-hospital management of overdose patients is the inability to obtain an accurate history of the exposure. Patients who are truly suicidal are notoriously unreliable historians. In addition, the medications or drug of abuse cannot be identified, or the time of the ingestion cannot be estimated. Also, in situations where multiple medications are involved, it is difficult to determine which medication(s) was taken in a quantity significant enough to contribute to toxicity.

In many circumstances, the out-of-hospital personnel may be at risk for physical harm due to the combative and/or violent behaviors exhibited by overdose patients. One example of this would be the patient who becomes violent following exposure to cocaine or LSD. Two providers may not be capable of restraining this patient long enough to sedate prior to transport. Another example would be the patient who has experienced a decrease in LOC and respiratory depression secondary to an opioid exposure. If naloxone is administered in doses capable of completely reversing the effects of the narcotics, the patient typically becomes either violent upon arousal or experiences opiate withdrawal.

Another pitfall that should be considered is the situation in which toxicity is masked or forgotten due to the presence of trauma. Examples include the burn trauma patient who may have been exposed to both CO and cyanide in a fire. These life-threatening toxicities may be overlooked when providing initial stabilization and burn care. Often in cases of blunt and penetrating trauma, toxins such as ethanol, opiates, and cocaine may cause confusing symptoms (unexplained tachycardia or coma) and complicate care.

A growing number of adults mix several medications in their suicide attempts, often as many as four different medications plus alcohol. The field team may gather huge bags of medications and recite long lists of potential toxins. DMOPs may waste precious minutes researching all potential toxicities. Some simple rules are helpful. If it is several hours since ingestion and there is no evidence of a calcium channel blocker, beta blocker, tricyclic antidepressant, theophylline, or sustained release medication, then the patient can usually be treated according to presenting symptoms. If it has been less than 1 hour since ingestion, the patient should be treated with an IV and airway/hemodynamic monitoring, regardless of the suspected ingestant. Drug-drug interactions and significance of the ingestion can await discovery in the ED.

Refusals

There is considerable liability in not transporting potentially suicidal patients. Patients may take an overdose as a gesture, or they may have had earlier suicidal ideation, which they and the family now deny. On occasion, not only does the patient display dysfunction behavior, but also the patient's family and friends can be more dysfunctional than the patient. Patients who cry "wolf" should be believed and brought to the facility for toxicologic analysis and medical observation. Such patients may need psychiatric referral. No potentially suicidal overdose patient should be allowed to refuse transport to the hospital. When appropriate, an involuntary commitment should be obtained through normal procedures.

Summary

The overdose or poisoned patient can provide many challenges to the prehospital care provider and DMOP. Sometimes the exposure is obvious; however, often the offending substance is unknown, occult, or masked by other trauma or exposures. Once an exposure has occurred, the role of the out-of-hospital provider and DMOP is to establish the potential for toxicity. The toxicity can be estimated from the patient's symptoms, the toxins involved, and facts surrounding the exposure. The DMOP must keep in mind that some patients may deteriorate rapidly (i.e., tricyclic overdoses, calcium channel blocker overdoses) while others may have delayed onset of symptoms (i.e., acetaminophen, mushroom poisoning).

The treatment of the overdose patient must include the evaluation and initial treatment by the care provider. This treatment must include insuring the ABCs as well as limiting toxin absorption, increasing elimination, and providing specific antidotes. The DMOP must keep in mind several pitfalls associated with the care of the overdose patient, including the inability to obtain an accurate history, the potential masking of overdose symptoms due to the presence of trauma, and/or poly drug overdose. In addition, the care providers are at risk when treating the overdose patient, due to violent patients or due to exposure to hazardous materials. There is considerable liability in not transporting potentially suicidal overdose patients and care providers should be instructed to transport certain patients against their will. Since it is impossible for a DMOP to have a working knowledge of all potential toxins, the local poison center can be a valuable resource for toxin identification, assessment of potential toxicity, and treatment guidelines.

Cases

Case 1

Paramedics are on scene with a 24-year-old female who recently ingested "a bottle of pills" in a suicide attempt. They note that the patient has a history of depression, and was recently discharged from a psychiatric facility. The patient is somewhat confused, and complains of a dry mouth. Her vital signs include a blood pressure of 90/60, pulse of 140, and respirations of 18. Her pupils are dilated, and her lungs are clear. Her skin is warm and dry, and there is no evidence of trauma or needle marks. The paramedics on scene are unable to find a pill bottle. They have initiated an IV of normal saline, and are requesting further orders.

WHAT ORDERS WOULD YOU PROVIDE?

The identity of the drug ingested is not known. The patient has a toxidrome consistent with that of a tricyclic antidepressant, including the anti-cholinergic symptoms of dilated pupils, blurred vision, dry mouth, and tachycardia. The medics should be instructed to place the patient on a cardiac monitor, and to provide the width of the QRS complex. (In this case, the QRS width was 0.18 cm).

The widened QRS complex and hypotension suggest that this is a serious and potentially life-threatening overdose. The provider should contain the ABCs, (airway, breathing, and circulation), and watch closely for precipitous change in the patient's level of consciousness, seizures, arrythmias, or hypotension. A fluid challenge of 300 to 500 cc normal saline would be appropriate. In addition, sodium bicarbonate should be administered in a dose of 1 miliequivalent per kilogram. Sodium bicarbonate and fluid challenge could be repeated if the patient fails to respond. Urgent transport to an appropriate facility should be initiated. Police or other public safety officials could search the patient's home, looking for pill bottles, or other evidence of drug ingestion.

Case 2

Paramedics are called to the home of a 45-year-old male with a suspected narcotic overdose. A friend states that the patient ingested multiple narcotic pain pills in an attempt to get "high," approximately an hour ago. The friend became concerned when the patient was difficult to arouse. The patient is a chronic, daily user of narcotic tablets. Paramedics report that the patient is awake and alert, but somewhat drowsy. His airway is patent, and there is no respiratory distress. His blood pressure is 130/90, pulse of 70, respiratory rate is 12. Pupils are markedly constricted, and minimally reactive to light. Medics are requesting to administer 2 ml. of Naloxone IV.

WHAT ORDERS WOULD YOU PROVIDE?

Naloxone is frequently used to reverse opioid toxicity. In this case, naloxone is not indicated. This patient is awake and maintaining his own airway. Administering naloxone in this patient with chronic narcotic overdose will most likely precipitate an opioid withdrawal syndrome. This may convert this currently cooperative patient to a very uncomfortable, anxious, unmanageable patient. This is especially true if a large dose (2 mg. of naloxone) is administered.

Another consideration is the possibility of acetaminophen toxicity in this patient. Many opioids are combined with acetaminophen, and this patient may have self-administered a toxic dose of acetaminophen.

Case 3

A 25-year-old college student has, reportedly, ingested a large quantity of alcohol, along with multiple "other tablets." He is apparently distraught over the recent breakup with his girlfriend. He is currently awake, alert, and oriented, but somewhat drowsy. At this time he agrees to a paramedic evaluation, but refuses transport to the hospital.

HOW SHOULD YOU PROCEED?

If the patient allows, the paramedics should complete a physical exam, and initiate an IV access. The patient should be placed on oxygen, and a cardiac monitor. If available, the patient's blood glucose should be measured. The paramedics should also quickly initiate the appropriate legal proceedings for transporting the patient against his will. Although the exact procedure may vary by jurisdiction, often this includes a telephone call to the local mental health bureau, and/or assistance by the police. This patient must not be allowed to refuse transport. If the patient's level of consciousness decreases, he should be treated and transported immediately, without his verbal consent.

References

1. Litovitz TL, Felberg L, White S, et al. 1995 Annual report of the American Association of Poison Control Centers Toxic Exposure Surveillance System. *Am J Emerg Med.* 1996;14:487–537.
2. Litovitz TL, Smilkstein M, Felberg L, et al. 1996 Annual report of the American Association of Poison Control Centers Toxic Exposure Surveillance System. *Am J Emerg Med.* 1997;15:447–500.
3. Litovitz TL, Klein-Schwartz W, Dyer KS, et al. 1997 Annual report of the American Association of Poison Control Centers Toxic Exposure Surveillance System. *Am J Emerg Med.* 1998;16:443–497.
4. Litovitz TL, Klein-Schwartz W, Caravati EM, et al. 1998 Annual report of the American Association of Poison Control Centers Toxic Exposure Surveillance System. *Am J Emerg Med.* 1999;17:435–487.
5. Litovitz TL, Klein-Schwartz W, White S, et al. 1999 Annual report of the American Association of Poison Control Centers Toxic Exposure Surveillance System. *Am J Emerg Med.* 2000;18:517–574.
6. Baltimore CL, Meyer RJ. A study of storage, child behavioral traits, and mother's knowledge of toxicology in 52 poisoned families and 52 comparison families. *Pediatrics.* 1968;42:312–317.
7. Hendren WG, Schiever RS, Garrettson LK. Extracorporeal bypass for the treatment of verapamil poisoning. *Ann Emerg Med.* 1989;18:984–987.
8. McVey FK, Corke CF. Extracorporeal circulation in the management of massive propranolol overdose. *Anaesthesia.* 1991;46:744–746.
9. Larkin GL, Graeber GM, Hollingsed MJ. Experimental amitriptyline poisoning: treatment of severe cardiovascular toxicity with cardiopulmonary bypass. *Ann Emerg Med.* 1994;22:480–486.
10. Wax PM, Cobaugh DJ. Prehospital gastrointestinal decontamination of toxic ingestions: a missed opportunity. *Am J Emerg Med.* 1998;16:114–116.
11. Litovitz TL, Bailey KM, Schmitz BF, et al. 1990 Annual report of the American Association of Poison Control Centers Toxic Exposure Surveillance System. *Am J Emerg Med.* 1991;9:461–509.
12. American Academy of Clinical Toxicology and European Association of Poisons Centres and Clinical Toxicologists. Position statement: ipecac syrup. *J Tox Clin Tox.* 1997;35:699–709.
13. Grbcich PA, Lacouture PG, Kresel JJ, et al. Expired ipecac syrup efficacy. *Pediatrics.* 1986;78:1085–1089.
14. Chyka PA, Seger D. Position statement: single-dose activated charcoal. American Academy of Clinical Toxicology; European Association of Poisons Centres and Clinical Toxicologists. *J Tox Clin Tox.* 1997;35:721–741.
15. Minocha A, Krenzelok EP, Spyker DA. Dosage recommendations for activated charcoal-sorbitol treatment. *J Tox Clin Tox.* 1985;23:579–587.
16. Mathieu-Nolf M, Babe MA, Coquelle-Couplet V, et al. Flumazenil use in an emergency department: a survey. *J Tox Clin Tox.* 2001;39:15–20.
17. Kerns W 2nd, Kline J, Ford MD. Beta-blocker and calcium channel blocker toxicity. *Emerg Med Clin North Am.* 1994;12:365–390.
18. Henry M, Kay MM, Viccellio P. Cardiogenic shock associated with calcium-channel and beta blockers: reversal with intravenous calcium chloride. *Am J Emerg Med.* 1985;3:334–336.
19. Doyon S, Roberts JR. The use of glucagon in a case of calcium channel blocker overdose. *Ann Emerg Med.* 1993;22:1229–1233.
20. Wald N, Howard S, Smith PG, et al. Use of carboxyhaemoglobin levels to predict the development of diseases associated with cigarette smoking. *Thorax.* 1975;30:133–140.
21. Turner M, Hamilton-Farrell MR, Clark RJ. Carbon monoxide poisoning: an update. *J Accid Emerg Med.* 1999;16:92–96.
22. Hardy KR, Thom SR. Pathophysiology and treatment of carbon monoxide poisoning. *J Tox Clin Tox.* 1994;32:613–629.
23. Thom SR, Taber RL, Mendiguren II, et al. Delayed neuropsychologic sequelae after carbon monoxide poisoning: prevention by treatment with hyperbaric oxygen. *Ann Emerg Med.* 1995;25:474–480.
24. Caravati EM, Adams CJ, Joyce SM, Schafer NC. Fetal toxicity associated with maternal carbon monoxide poisoning. *Ann Emerg Med.* 1988;17:714–717.
25. Mueller PD, Benowitz NL, Olson KR. Cocaine. *Emerg Med Clin North Am.* 1990;8:481–493.
26. Goldfrank LR, Hoffman RS. The cardiovascular effects of cocaine. *Ann Emerg Med.* 1991;20:165–175.
27. Ernst AA, Jones K, Nick TG, et al. Ethanol ingestion and related hypoglycemia in a pediatric and adolescent emergency department population. *Acad Emerg Med.* 1996;3:46–49.
28. Cobaugh DJ, Gibbs M, Shapiro DE, et al. A comparison of the bioavailabilities of oral and intravenous ethanol in healthy male volunteers. *Acad Emerg Med.* 1999;6:984–988.
29. Brennan DF, Betzelos S, Reed R, et al. Ethanol elimination rates in an ED population. *Am J Emerg Med.* 1995;13:276–280.
30. Laborit H. Sodium 4-hydroxybutyrate. *Int J Neuropharmacol.* 1964;3:433–452.

31. Tunnicliff G. Sites of action of gamma-hydroxybutyrate (GHB)—a neuroactive drug with abuse potential. *J Tox Clin Tox.* 1997;35:581–590.

32. Chin RL, Sporer KA, Cullison B, et al. Clinical course of γ-hydroxybutyrate overdose. *Ann Emerg Med.* 1998;31: 716–722.

33. Dyer JE, Reed JH. Alkali burns from illicit manufacture of GHB. *J Tox Clin Tox.* 1997;35:553. (Abstract)

34. Craig K, Gormez HF, McManus JL, et al. Severe gamma-hydroxybutyrate withdrawal: a case report and literature review. *J Emerg Med.* 2000;18:65–70.

35. Research and Special Programs Administration: Hazardous materials: emergency response guide book. DOTP5800.2. U.S. Government Printing Office, 1984.

36. Fire protection guide to hazardous materials, 9th ed. National Fire Protection Association, 1986.

37. Hess SM, Doepfner W. Behavioral effects and brain amine contents in rats. *Arch Int Pharmacodyn Ther.* 1961;134:89–99.

38. Martin TG. Serotonin syndrome. *Ann Emerg Med.* 1996;28:520–526.

39. Sternbach H. The serotonin syndrome. *Am J Psychiatry.* 1991;148:705–713.

Behavioral

Introduction

A behavioral emergency can be defined as an acute change in conduct that results in an intolerable behavior for the patient, family, or society.[1] These changes range from the inability to cope with a stressful situation to the agitated or violent patient who presents a danger to themselves or others.

From a literature review, it is evident that little has been written about behavioral emergencies in the out-of-hospital setting. The "standard of care" is mostly extrapolated from the experience gained in emergency departments and psychiatric wards. In general, EMS providers receive little training regarding these conditions during their initial and/or continuing education.[2,3] All of these factors add up to make the encounter with the emotionally disturbed patient very difficult.

Evaluation of the Problem

Facing a patient with a behavioral emergency is always a stressful situation. Even in the emergency department setting, these patients are difficult to evaluate. Their treatment is time-consuming, and often requires special attention. For an EMS crew responding to the scene, the situation can be even more complex. The patient may be non-cooperative, and frequently there are no additional reliable sources for obtaining a history. Family members, if available, might be uninformed about the patient's medical or psychiatric history. The evaluation and management of the emotionally disturbed patient therefore requires a modified approach from that of the routine patient.

The "standard" approach field personnel use may be inadequate for the assessment of these unique patients. They may feel uncertain and insecure on how to proceed, given their training and limited treatment options.[4] They will typically contact direct medical oversight for help, but it can be even more difficult for the direct medical oversight physician (DMOP) to obtain a good assessment of the case. Under these circumstances, it is very easy to make serious mistakes with terrible repercussions for both the patient and the system. Therefore it is very important for the medical director to ensure that the provider and the physicians to whom direct medical oversight is delegated have the appropriate training in how to deal with these patients before they are encountered in the field. Although general guidelines should be provided by protocol, each situation should be evaluated and managed individually.

Another important aspect in the care of these patients is to remember that, like all other patients encountered by EMS, they have a legitimate health problem. Unfortunately, the care provider may sometimes mislabel patients with behavioral changes as "uncooperative." This may result in an inappropriate lack of compassion. We need to keep in mind that the patient's behavior is a manifestation of their disease. Patience, understanding, and compassionate care are essential to make a difference.

The objective of this chapter is to provide an overview on how to assess and treat the patient with a behavioral emergency in the out-of-hospital setting. Some of the information discussed is provided in an effort to help the DMOP understand what is occurring at the other end of the radio. The most common behavioral emergencies will be discussed. Special attention will be given to suicidal and violent patients who are usually the most challenging and demanding patients encountered in the out-of-hospital domain. Specific risk factors will be enumerated to help predict, in the early phases of evaluation, the potentially violent or suicidal patient. Additionally, the pharmacological alternatives for the rapid tranquilization of the agitated and/or violent patient will be discussed.

Common Psychiatric Conditions

Emergency departments (ED) and EMS systems are common points of entry to the healthcare system for the psychiatric patient.[1] Emergency physicians performing direct medical oversight should be familiar with psychiatric terminology and should be aware of the common presentations, complications, and management of the psychiatric patient. The following are simple definitions of some of the most common conditions faced in the daily practice of out-of-hospital care.

ANXIETY DISORDERS

Anxiety is defined as an unpleasant emotional state consisting of psycho-physiological response to the anticipation of an unreal or imagined danger, apparently resulting from unrecognized intrapsychic conflict. Physiological concomitants include increased heart rate, altered respiration rate, sweating, trembling, weakness, and fatigue; psychological concomitants include feelings of impending danger, powerlessness, apprehension, and tension.[5]

Some amount of anxiety is a normal and necessary reaction to a stressful situation. Patients with anxiety disorders show a disproportionate psycho-physiological response that may preclude them from a normal interaction with family, friends, or society. When these symptoms are directed toward or produced by a specific object, activity, or situation, with as a consequence the patient consciously avoiding the stimulus, it is referred to as a phobia. The phobic patient can usually recognize the problem but is unable to control the symptoms. A panic attack is an acute, extremely heightened level of anxiety accompanied by disorganization of personality and function.[5] Panic attacks may last from a few minutes to many hours, and may occur in patients with or without chronic anxiety.

DEPRESSION

Depression is defined as a mental state of depressed mood characterized by feelings of sadness, despair, and discouragement. It ranges from the normal feeling of the "blues" to dysthymia to major depression. There are often feelings of low self-esteem, guilt, and self-reproach. Withdrawal from interpersonal contact, and somatic symptoms such as eating and sleep disturbances may also occur.[5]

SCHIZOPHRENIA

Schizophrenia can be defined as a group of disorders comprising most major psychotic disorders. It is characterized by disturbances in the form and content of thought (loosening of associations, delusions, and hallucinations), mood (blunted, flattened, or inappropriate affect), behavior (bizarre, apparently purposeless and stereotyped activity or inactivity), and the sense of self and the relationship to the external world (loss of ego boundaries, dereistic thinking, and autistic withdrawal).[5] These manifestations of symptoms vary from patient to patient. Even the same patient may show different levels of symptomatology at different times.

BIPOLAR DISORDER

A mood disorder characterized by the occurrence of one or more manic episodes. In almost all cases, one or more major depressive episodes will also eventually occur. The manic phase is characterized by expansiveness, elation, agitation, hyperexcitability, hyperactivity, and the increased speed of thought and speech.[5]

Assessment and Treatment

When responding to a scene, EMS personnel rarely know the diagnosis of the patient. With the confusion commonly present when faced by a disturbed patient, making an accurate psychiatric diagnosis in the field is not only almost always impossible but it is irrelevant. Protocols should describe how to assess and treat clinical symptom patterns, not a specific diagnosis.

The first step when facing a disturbed patient is to evaluate scene safety. If it is not safe, EMS personnel should await the arrival of law enforcement authorities before any further intervention is attempted. This is particularly important when dealing with the violent patient. If the scene is safe, providers should carefully approach the patient and attempt to perform a brief medical assessment. They should attempt to determine if the behavioral changes are due to an organic etiology or if the patient is under imminent danger secondary to a medical emergency.

There are multiple medical conditions that can present with behavioral changes (table 66.1). Presentation may vary from lethargy and confusion to agitation and violence. Classic examples include the confused patient with acute hypoglycemia, the agitated patient with hypoxia, and the lethargic patient in shock. The initial evaluation must include a thorough history (medical and psychiatric) and physical exam, including measurement of blood sugar level and pulse oximetry. Mental changes of acute onset without previous history of psychiatric disorder are highly suggestive of an organic etiology. EMS personnel should ask specifically about prescribed medications or suspected drug abuse. Physical examination should pay special attention to neurological findings. If during the evaluation vital sign abnormalities are observed, the patient should be considered medically unstable and his mental changes a consequence of organic problems until proven otherwise; responder should effect appropriate interventions for the correction of abnormal vital signs. Delayed stabilization or even the non-transport of patients with organic problems is dangerous, especially when dealing with mentally disturbed patients.

Occasionally, the patient may not cooperate with the initial assessment and stabilization. In these situations, EMS personnel should try to gain the patient's confidence by providing reassurance, explaining who they are, and describing every step before it is performed. If the patient is still not compliant, the presence of a physician in the field, as a figure of authority, could be of great help in obtaining the patient's cooperation. Unfortunately, this is typically not possible. Other alternatives are for the DMOP to talk directly to the patient over the phone or to reach the patient's primary care physician. If, in spite of every reasonable effort by personnel, the patient does not cooperate with the initial assessment, physical and/or chemical restraints should be considered. A patient with behavioral changes must have an assessment or be transported.

Once the patient is deemed medically stable, the next step is to determine whether his mental status represents a danger to himself or to others. Each case needs to be evaluated on an individual basis. Not every patient with abnormal behavior will require transport against his will. If the patient is refusing transport, they must meet all of the following criteria before their request should be honored: (1) the patient has the "capacity" to refuse, (2) organic etiology has been ruled out by an appropriate medical evaluation, (3) no evidence of suicidal or aggressive behavior is present, (4) there is a known past history of psychiatric disorder with similar behavior, and (5) appropriate social or family support is available.

It is the responsibility of the DMOP to ensure that a complete evaluation is done before EMS personnel leave the scene. Most adult patients who present to the ED with acute psychiatric symptoms will have an organic etiology.[6] The evaluation and "medical clearance" of patients in the field can be even more difficult than when performed in the ED.

Suicidal and violent patients represent the major behavioral emergencies for which the DMOP and field personnel must be prepared to cope with in the out-of-hospital setting. Special attention should be maintained for the presence of risk factors for suicidal or violent behavior. Under no circumstances should a patient who shows the potential for suicidal or aggressive behavior be left alone by providers. EMS providers must carry out and document every possible effort made to bring about transport. Cooperation from family, friends, co-workers, private physicians, and law enforcement authorities may be of great value. Protocols containing detailed descriptions of interagency cooperation are very helpful in these situations.

TABLE 66.1

Organic Disorders with Behavioral Manifestations [14,20]

NEUROLOGICAL
CNS infections (meningitis, encephalitis, brain abscess)
Head trauma
Hypertensive encephalopathy
Stroke
Mass lesion
Seizure disorder
Dementia

DRUG INTOXICATION/POISONING
Alcohol
Amphetamines
Anticholinergic syndromes
Cocaine
LSD
Marijuana
Phencyclidine (PCP)

WITHDRAWAL SYNDROMES
Alcohol
Barbiturates
Opiates

METABOLIC
Hypoxia
Hypoglycemia
Renal failure (acidosis/electrolytes disbalance)
Hepatic failure

ENDOCRINOLOGIC
Hypothyroidism/hyperthyroidism
Addison's disease
Cushing's disease

The Suicidal Patient

Suicidal ideation is the existence of thoughts pertaining to ending one's own life. *Passive* suicidal ideation refers to such thoughts in the absence of a specific plan ("I wish I were dead"). *Active* suicidal ideation is accompanied by a plan ("I'm going to borrow my friend's gun and shoot myself while my wife is at work"), and as such indicates a greater degree of risk. A *suicidal gesture* is self-inflicted harm perpetrated without a realistic expectation of death (e.g., superficial slicing of an arm, ingestion of 4 extra medication tablets in the presence of a family member), whereas a *suicide attempt* is an act of self-inflicted harm with a clear expectation of death.[7]

More people die from suicide than from homicide in the United States. In 1999, a total of 29,041 Americans took their own lives, versus 16,831 homicides. In 1999, suicide was the eleventh leading cause of death in this country with a rate of 10.6 suicides per 100,00 population.[8] Suicide is a serious problem among young people. Between 1980 and 1997, the rate of suicide increased 109% for 10- to14-year-olds and 11% for 15- to 19-year-olds. Suicide was the third leading cause of death for 15- to 24-year-olds in 1997. Suicide rates tend to rise with age and are the highest among white men age 65 and older.[9]

Always take seriously any patient who is making a suicide threat in the field. Suicidal statements indicate the presence of a crisis that the individual feels he or she is unable to handle. Up to two-thirds of those who commit suicide have visited a physician or healthcare facility during the preceding month.[10] It is therefore important to recognize the signs and symptoms (not only the explicit declaration of suicidal intent) with which a suicide-prone patient could present to out-of-hospital providers. Intervention by the EMS system and appropriate authorities may be the last opportunity to provide help for the patient and to prevent a future tragedy. These patients should be treated with the same urgency as a patient in shock.

After arriving on the scene, personnel should perform a complete assessment of the situation. They must explore their surroundings for weapons or potential weapons. Immediately remove any objects that the patient could use to inflict physical damage to himself or others. If guns or knives are present, the crew should withdraw to safety and await trained personnel, usually the police, to remove the weapon and secure the scene. Once the location has been secured, attempts to initiate communication with the patient should be made as soon as possible. Communication with the DMOP or the patient's family physician may have some beneficial impact for the patient who is asking for help. During the negotiations, friends or family members whom the patient trusts and respects can be effective. If the patient identifies an individual present at the scene as being part of the crisis, that individual should be removed from the scene. Encourage the patient to discuss the situation and what is exacerbating this crisis. Most patients are relieved to be empowered to discuss their thoughts.[10] Emphasize during provider education that the crews show sympathy and concern, and do nothing that could frighten or agitate the patient. They don't have to agree or disagree with the patient, just listen to what he has to say. They should avoid comments such as "Don't do that!" or "You know that is not true!" The patient may consider these comments as a challenge or that the members of the rescue team are being judgmental and not supportive. If the patient perceives a negative attitude from the rescue team, it can only worsen the patient's already low self-esteem. Provide reassurance that the crisis can be resolved and that authorities are only there to help. Promises that the out-of-hospital care providers are unable or unwilling to keep will make the patient more suspicious.

The initial complaint that generated an EMS response may not have been because of a suicidal patient. Suspicion by providers of unverbalized suicidal ideation or the presence of specific risk factors should prompt the DMOP to explore the patient's mental status. If the patient admits to any current or past depression, hopelessness, or despair, he should be asked directly whether he has any thoughts about harming himself or ending his life. Although a common concern is that posing such questions could actually induce suicidal thoughts and behaviors, there has been no evidence to support this; more often, once the topic is breached directly, in a nonjudgmental and sensitive manner, the patient typically welcomes the opportunity to unburden himself to his caregivers.

Once the patient begins to cooperate and agrees with transport, everything that will be done to him should be clearly explained. At this point, pharmacologic interventions may be considered. Often, such patients present with a significant level of anxiety and agitation that once alleviated will reduce suicidal feelings. Fairly low parenteral doses of a fast-acting benzodiazepine, such as 0.5 mg to 1 mg of lorazepam or 2 mg of diazepam, often prove effective and can be titrated as necessary. If there are any contraindications to the use of benzodiazepines, such as suspicion of their abuse, another agent such as diphenhydramine or even a low dose of a high-potency neuroleptic (e.g., haloperidol) may be employed.[7] Similarly, suicidal patients suffering from severe or chronic pain may become markedly less despondent after adequate analgesia.

Before initiating transport, the patient should be fastened on the stretcher and not permitted to sit next to the exit door or in the front seat of the ambulance. Explain that these are security measures for his own safety. The person who has established the best rapport with the patient should ride along with him to the hospital. Members of the rescue team should then sit next to the exits.

If all reasonable efforts have failed to persuade the patient to cooperate, the question of whether to commit the patient to an involuntary transport must be addressed. This is a decision in which DMOP is often involved. There are several factors that correlate with a higher risk for committing suicide and they are listed in table 66.2. If the conclusion is that the patient is in immediate danger for committing suicide, proceed with the transport and do not leave the patient unattended under any circumstances. Laws pertaining to involuntary transport and admissions vary from state to state. Physicians involved in direct medical oversight must be familiar with the specifics of their local statutes. When in doubt, it is always better to err on the side of an involuntary transport and to have the patient evaluated at an ED or psychiatric institution. If, subsequent to the decision for involuntary transport, the patient becomes agitated and/or violent, the use of physical or chemical restraints may be required, as outlined below in the violent patient section.

The Violent Patient

Violence is a spreading cancer reaching every aspect of our society. As a result, the number of violence-related calls in the out-of-hospital setting is increasing. Care providers deal with the multiple aspects of violence. They see victims of violent events and they are also confronting violent patients. Providers are generally well trained to deal with the wounded patient; unfortunately, they have significantly less training in the management of the aggressive patient.[2,3,11] Violent patients must be dealt with using extreme caution, since minor management pitfalls may lead to major tragedies. As in any other call, when arriving on location, a "scene safety" evaluation must be completed prior to any patient interventions. The first priority should always be to ensure crew safety. If there are weapons in the area, the EMS crew should wait for the proper authorities to "clear the scene" before proceeding with patient care.

Providers should receive training on how to interact with the violent patient, and they should also be able to evaluate potentially violent patients before they erupt.[12] Once in contact with the patient, the provider should perform a quick assessment of the patient's physical and emotional status; the organic conditions that could manifest as behavioral emergencies must be kept in mind (table 66.1). Always give priority to vital-sign stabilization. Once the organic etiologies have been ruled out, EMS personnel

TABLE 66.2	
Factors that Correlate with a Higher Risk for Committing Suicide	
FACTORS	**HIGH RISK**
Suicide intentions	■ Affirmation of suicide intention ■ Detailed and violent plan with poor probability for rescue and accessible resources (e.g., gun) ■ History of previous attempts
Psychiatric diagnosis	■ Schizophrenia ■ Bipolar disorder ■ Major depression ■ Acute psychosis
Medical problems	■ Diagnosis of terminal diseases (e.g., cancer, AIDS) ■ Diagnosis of chronic illness (e.g., diabetes)
Drug abuse	■ Alcohol, cocaine, other illicit drugs
Social history	■ Marital status—widowed or divorced ■ Recent significant loss—death of a loved one ■ Unemployment ■ No family support
Family history	■ Suicide ■ Psychiatric disorders
Sex	■ Women—attempt suicide more often ■ Men—successful attempts more often
Age	■ Over 45 years old

can collect valuable information that may help to assess the potential for violent behavior; they should observe and describe the patient's general attitude. Patients who are talking in a loud voice, moving around constantly, gesticulating with their arms, or displaying closed fists should be considered potentially violent.[3,11,13] Investigate if the patient has had a previous history of aggressive behavior, as this is the single most important risk factor used to predict the possibility of future aggressiveness. This is especially true if the previous history was against law enforcement officers or other authority figures.[14] Investigate for a history of psychiatric disorders; psychosis, paranoia, manic-depressive disorder, and antisocial personality have been identified as diagnoses with a higher incidence of violent behavior.[14] Additional significant risk factors include the presence of drug paraphernalia or any indication of alcohol or illicit drug abuse. Intoxicated patients have poor control of their emotions and may become violent more easily.

After an evaluation the crew should have a better understanding of the patient's condition. Even if the evaluation indicates low risk for aggressiveness, the care providers should continue to remain alert and ready to react. If the patient is considered to be at high risk for violence, the following measures should be taken:[1,14]

- Never leave the patient unattended. Maintain a safe distance and have a member of the rescue team standing by the exit at all times. Never allow the patient to block the escape route.

- Remove any object at the scene that could be used by the patient as a weapon.

- When facing a violent individual, avoid prolonged eye contact as it may be considered a challenge.

- Nominate one rescuer to be the "negotiator." If the patient is medically stable, be prepared to spend a prolonged time talking to them. If the negotiator seems to be losing patience, someone else should assume the role. It is better to spend the extra minutes for a peaceful solution than to rush to a physical confrontation.

- Attempt to "verbally de-escalate" the situation while maintaining a calm and reassuring tone.

- Try to identify the reasons for the crisis and let the patient ventilate his thoughts. Be supportive, never argumentative.

- A tacit "show of force," with several members of the rescue team backing the negotiator, is suggestive to the patient of the presence of overwhelming force, and is often enough to calm him.

It is always possible that in spite of all reasonable efforts and preventive measures, the patient will become violent and/or will refuse transport. At that point, physical or chemical restraint may become necessary. In general, the DMOP must be involved and help decide if the patient should be transported against their will. This is a medicolegal decision with major implications. This type of decision should not be left in the hands of the providers. The legal justification for physical or chemical restraint is based on the professional judgment by the physician in charge that the patient lacks capacity to refuse treatment and transport.[15] The DMOP must be involved in the decision-making process, and should therefore be familiar with the local legal statutes. In general, the medicolegal exposure of permitting a patient who is at risk of harming themselves or others to remain unevaluated is much higher than the exposure involved in the involuntary transport of that patient.

Other Situations

As a consequence of the ageing of society, an increasing percentage of EMS responses involve geriatric patients. The elderly, especially those with limited familial and financial resources, occasionally disregard their own personal well-being. Frequently these patients will rebuff treatment and/or transport. Faced with a self-neglectful patient found in unkempt surroundings, the providers may be hard-pressed to accomplish transport on an otherwise competent patient. The DMOP must be directly involved in determining the patient's final disposition. EMS personnel should carefully describe the patient's medical condition as well as his physical environment. Occasionally, the direct communication with the patient by the physician is beneficial. A pre-established "Elderly Referral Program" may provide some comfort that needed resources and services were available on an expedited basis.

Patients who present with substance abuse or intoxication are a risk not only to themselves but to the providers as well. Although many mind-altering substances may generate violent behavior, cocaine and phencyclidine are the two most common; less commonly, marijuana, the amphetamines, and the hallucinogens may do so also.[16] Patients with a history of recent exposures should be handled in a manner similar to that of the violent patient.

Physical Restraint

The major indication for restraining a patient is when he is considered incompetent to make decisions for himself and his behavior precludes a good evaluation. It is very important to document how the patient represents a threat to himself or to others. Before proceeding with physical restraints, the rescue personnel should identify a team leader. The leader should preferably be the same person who to this point has been the "negotiator." Give the patient a last opportunity to cooperate while at the same time explaining that otherwise they will be restrained for their own safety and to help them maintain self-control. The team has to be well organized, assigning each member specific responsibilities. The ideal number of persons on the team is five—one for each extremity and one for the head and neck. The following is a commonly recommended procedure for physical restraint, although multiple other techniques are available:[1,15]

1. The leader should continue to communicate with the patient.
2. Two persons should approach the patient from behind, while two more approach from the front. This will make it difficult for the patient to concentrate and attack from one flank.
3. If the patient attacks to one side, the persons left behind him should grasp both arms by the elbows simultaneously. By placing the rescuer's legs in front of the patient's and pushing forward, the patient should be forced to the floor face-down.
4. At this point, the other two members of the team will hold the patient's legs by the knees, while at the same time the leader restrains the head so as to prevent injury and to preclude biting and spitting.
5. Restrain the patient face-up to the stretcher using the four-point restraint technique. Leather restraints are recommended, but straps, towels, and other similar materials can be used to improvise if necessary.
6. Restrain one hand over the patient's head and the other by the patient's side. This will decrease the amount of force generated in any one direction.
7. Continue talking to the patient in an attempt to try to calm him or her down. Do not leave the patient unattended. Maintain constant monitoring of the neurovascular status in all extremities distal to the restraints. Search his or her clothes for any other potentially dangerous object (e.g., sharp objects, matches). If possible, this should be done in the presence of a law enforcement authority.
8. Once applied, do not negotiate the restraints with the patient during transport. Never remove the restraints until arrival at the receiving facility.
9. Upon arrival at the receiving facility, ensure they have all necessary equipment and backup personnel before removing the restraints.

There are multiple risks, both to the patient and prehospital providers, involved with the restraint procedure. Recently, patient deaths while in the prone restraint position have been attributed to "positional asphyxia"; however, a combination of other factors such as underlying medical condition, drug or alcohol intoxication, and patient resistance to restraint may prove to be the true culprit.[17] Additionally, EMS personnel generally have limited training and experience in appropriate restraint techniques, and may become physically injured during the procedure.

Ideally, law enforcement officers should be involved in the restraint procedure, as well as during transport; they have superior training and experience with these types of situations. EMS and law enforcement personnel should work closely together, but EMS providers should not allow police officers to influence the evaluation and treatment of the patient.[3] It is desirable to have frequent training sessions to practice the restraint technique. This would serve to improve interagency communication and cooperation in an actual situation.

Chemical Restraint

Sometimes physical restraint is not enough. Although out-of-hospital providers may be able to restrain the patient physically, it is impossible to perform an adequate evaluation if the patient is still agitated. The care that the patient needs may be obstructed by his or her behavior. It is now recognized that the use of chemical restraint is more effective and more humane than physical restraint alone. Rapid tranquilization is the technique of giving a psychotropic drug to control behavioral disturbances.[18] The combination of physical and chemical restraints is the best approach to gain control of the patient and proceed with evaluation and transport. The DMOP must be directly involved in the decision-making process. The use of pharmaceuticals is indicated only when the clinical impression of the physician is that the patient is not competent to make decisions for himself, his behavior represents an immediate danger, or his behavior hinders a safe transport. The goal is to control agitation and psychotic symptoms. When considering medications for use in the out-of-hospital environment, certain characteristics are of vital importance:

- The medication should be available for IM administration. Frequently, the patient will not have an IV line and will not cooperate to establish one.

- It should have a rapid onset of action, since we are waiting for the patient to be calmed down in order to accomplish transport.

- It should have a minimal effect on CNS depression as well as a short half-life so that a complete evaluation may be performed at the receiving facility.

- As with any other medication, we want it to have the lowest possible incidence of side effects.

Rapid tranquilization is a fairly common technique used in EDs and psychiatric wards. These techniques are extrapolated from the ED experience; however, state or regional approved drug lists may limit the availability of specific medications for EMS usage.[19] Among the several classes of medications used for rapid tranquilization, neuroleptics and benzodiazepines are the two most commonly used.

NEUROLEPTICS

Probably the most popular neuroleptic used in the out-of-hospital setting today is haloperidol, a butyrophenone. It may be administered by the PO, IM, or IV route.[20] This high-potency neuroleptic has been shown to be effective in controlling agitation.[21] The classic regimen of administration is 5 mg IM, or IV. In extremely agitated or large patients a 10 mg initial dose may be used. The dose can be repeated every 30 to 60 minutes if needed.[22] One advantage of haloperidol is that the patient remains responsive to commands and is not overly sedated.[23] The onset of clinical effect is observed in 20 minutes with the IM route and in 5 to 10 minutes with the IV route.[24]

If the patient cooperates, a 10 mg oral dose can be used with effects similar to that of the IM injection.[25] Haloperidol has a low incidence of side effects. The most common are extrapyramidal symptoms (less than 10% of patients), which are easily reversible with diphenhydramine 50 mg IV or benztropine 2 mg IM. Extrapyramidal symptoms can occur with only a single dose, and up to 12 to 24 hours after administration. Other less common side effects include akathisia, hypotension, neuroleptic malignant syndrome, and decreased seizure threshold.[14,24,26,27]

Another butyrophenone that is being used for the same indications is droperidol. This medication, which is very similar structurally to haloperidol, is showing excellent results with the agitated patient as well. Droperidol can also be administered by the PO, IM, or IV route, and it has a better IM absorption with a faster onset of action and a shorter half-life than haloperidol. The IM absorption of droperidol is so good that its effect compares with the IV administration of haloperidol. The half-life for droperidol after IM administration is 2.2 hours, compared to 19 hours for haloperidol.[28] Several studies have reported faster onset of action (3 to 10 minutes IV or IM), fewer side effects, and a decreased need for a second administration.[27-33] The usual dose for droperidol is the same as for haloperidol, 5 mg IM or IV every 30 to 60 minutes. The significant side effects associated with droperidol are greater sedation and orthostatic hypotension. Keeping the patient supine and giving IV fluids easily treats the latter. Recent warnings from the Food and Drug Administration regarding the proarrythmogenic effects of droperidol have called into question its appropriateness for out-of-hospital usage.

BENZODIAZEPINES

The other major group of medications used for out-of-hospital rapid tranquilization are the benzodiazepines. Diazepam, with its main limitation being an erratic IM absorption, has been used widely in the past. Lorazepam and midazolam both have good IM absorption. Typical regimens would be lorazepam 0.05 mg/kg IM or midazolam 0.1–0.2 mg/kg IM every 30 to 60 minutes until symptoms are controlled (table 66.3). The most important indication for benzodiazepines use is in controlling alcohol or sedative withdrawal symptoms. In these cases, benzodiazepines are the drug of choice. Significant side effects associated with the use of benzodiazepines are excessive sedation and respiratory depression.[27,34] In

TABLE 66.3

Common Medications for Rapid Tranquilization[22-24]

MEDICATION	DOSE	ROUTE	ONSET OF ACTION	PEAK EFFECT
Droperidol*	5–10 mg	PO, IM IV	3–10 min 3–10 min	30–60 min 30–60 min
Haloperidol	5–10 mg	PO, IM IV (Do not use deconate salt IV)	10–20 min 5–10 min	30–60 min 30–60 min
Diazepam	0.1–0.2 mg/kg	IV (over 1 min)	5–10 min	30–60 min
Lorazepam	0.05–0.1 mg/kg	IM, IV	15–20 min	60–90 min
Midazolam	0.05–0.1 mg/kg 0.01–0.2 mg/kg	IV IM	5–10 min 15 min	30–60 min 30–60 min

* Concerns regarding the proarrythmogenic effects (prolonged Q-T) may limit the out-of-hospital use of this medication.

patients with preexisting diminished mental status or respiratory depression, this represents a relative contraindication to their use.

Benzodiazepines and butyrophenones may be used together. Several investigators have reported the use of lorazepam in combination with haloperidol with good results; achieving an apparent synergistic effect while reducing the amount of each drug required.[14,25,26] A recommended regime is 5 mg haloperidol with 2 mg of lorazepam given IM every 2–3 hours until sedated.

Controversies

As previously described, the scene involving a mentally disturbed patient can be chaotic; under these circumstances, it is very easy to commit serious mistakes. One of the most common mistakes is the failure to do a complete medical evaluation. A lack of vital sign assessment may lead to the false impression that the patient is "just nuts." This is a critical mistake with possible tragic consequences. On the other hand, after medical stability has been determined, there is a tendency by personnel to minimize the need for their intervention. For multiple reasons, there tends to be a significant lack of empathy with psychiatric patients. This may lead the crew to falsely believe the patient is "just faking" or "wasting our time." This is extremely dangerous, especially in the situation of a patient with suicidal threats. Every patient who is suspected to have suicidal ideations should be transported for psychiatric evaluation. It is better to err on the side of treatment and transport.

When faced with an agitated patient, it is extremely dangerous to simply rush the patient. Not spending sufficient time talking to the patient and establishing a rapport is another common mistake. The crew should be instructed to convey assurance to the patient and to attempt to gain their trust. Becoming argumentative or trying to reason with a mentally disturbed patient will just cause further agitation.

Crew safety is of paramount importance. The personnel should withdraw from the scene immediately if the patient is armed and/or extremely agitated. Law enforcement agencies should be notified and allowed to assume control of the scene until it is safe for EMS personnel to return. They should not attempt to fight or restrain the patient without the appropriate personnel and equipment. Do not subject your personnel or the patient to unnecessary injuries. After a physical or chemical restraint has been applied, the patient should not be left unattended. Continue close monitoring of the vital signs and mental status. Be watchful for oversedation or side effects from pharmacotherapy.

Finally, another common pitfall is the lack of interagency coordination. The approach to the violent or agitated patients must be very well organized. Avoid arguments among rescue team members in view of the patient. Everybody should understand his role and responsibility before dealing directly with the patient.

Summary

Behavioral emergencies represent a unique challenge for the out-of-hospital care provider. Paramedics and emergency medical technicians frequently face patients and situations that are difficult to handle given their level of training. Their own safety is even sometimes in jeopardy. Active participation by the medical director and DMOPs is important to guarantee the best quality of care for the patient as well as to provide assurance to the crew. Good protocols and frequent training sessions with other safety agencies yield the best results. Training sessions provide the ideal forum for practice, discussion, and the improvement of interagency communication and cooperation. Only 47% of respondents to a recent questionnaire said they have specific protocols for handling violence in their systems. In the same study, only 9% have established cross-training sessions with law enforcement authorities.

As with any other medical emergency, the assessment and stabilization of vital signs should be done as soon as possible. Always assume an organic etiology for behavioral changes until proven otherwise. Under no circumstances should a person with a questionable mental capacity be permitted to refuse transport and sign AMA. The entire staff must be familiar with local statutes governing involuntary transport and be ready to use restraining techniques, both physical and chemical, as needed. It is better to err on the side of transport and to have the patient fully evaluated in the emergency department setting. Society expects medical professionals to be able to recognize and manage patients who are a danger to themselves or others. This is a great responsibility that the EMS system must be willing to assume.

Cases

Case 1

"Medic command, this is Medic 7. We are on the scene with a 38-year-old man with a history of being HIV positive. His mother says the patient has been "acting strange" since yesterday. She also states he has been vomiting and complaining of a headache for the past 2 days. He looks lethargic, and we are having problems getting information from him due to alcohol intoxication. He has a strong odor of alcohol on his breath and his mother confirms he is drinking a lot. He is not showing any aggressive behavior and denies suicidal ideas. He says he doesn't want to go to the hospital and wishes to sign RMA. His vital signs are as follows: HR-120bpm, RR-22rpm, BP-110/50mmHg, Pulse Oximetry is 95% at room air. His physical exam is as follows: The patient is oriented to person and place but is unable to identify the date or the President. Skin is warm and slightly pale; lungs are clear to auscultation; heart has a regu-

lar rhythm without murmur; abdomen is soft and depressible, no masses, non-tender to palpation; extremities-no edema or cyanosis. Doc, I believe he is just drunk. Is it OK with you if he signs AMA?"

How would you proceed?

You should definitely answer no. This presentation contains multiple risk factors highly suggestive of an organic process. The history of being HIV positive is a significant warning sign for the possibility of multiple CNS complications. The behavioral changes are of an acute onset, and the vital signs are abnormal. The patient is described as being intoxicated, confused, and lethargic; therefore, he does not have capacity to sign RMA. An organic etiology for his behavioral changes should be assumed until proven otherwise. Actually, the patient's temperature in the emergency department was 103.1° F and a CT scan showed a frontal lobe brain abscess.

Case 2

"Medic Command, this is Medic 3. The sister of a 65-year-old female patient called us to the scene because the patient was talking about suicide. The sister says that the patient has been in a very depressed mood for the last 4 weeks. She has a past history of depression, including one hospitalization. At present, she is engaged in outpatient treatment with a private psychiatrist and is taking medication. The sister states the patient told her that soon she wouldn't need to worry about her anymore. The patient is in an obviously depressed mood but denies any suicidal thoughts. She is crying and upset with her sister because she called EMS. She says that we probably have more important patients to see and that she doesn't need to go to the hospital. Her vital signs are as follows: HR-90bpm, RR-16rpm, BP-120/60mmHg. At present, the patient is alert and oriented to person place and time. I think she is OK and I have already had her sign the refusal for transport."

How would you proceed?

It is common for EMS systems to receive calls from a third party with concerns about a "psychiatric patient." In this example, the patient herself refused transport. The problem occurred when the EMS crew acquiesced to her wishes without trying reasonable efforts to accomplish transport. This patient displayed an "obvious depressed mood" and indicated symptoms of low self-esteem when she expressed to the ambulance crew that they have "more important patients to see." She also had previous history of psychiatric hospitalization. These are examples of significant risk factors that warrant further evaluation. There were no efforts by the providers to deal with the patient's actual problem. They did not try to contact the patient's primary care or psychiatric physician. This patient was allowed by the DMOP to remain at home and three days later the same crew responded to the location. However, this time they found their patient in cardiac arrest secondary to an amitriptyline overdose.

Case 3

"Doctor, this is paramedic Joe Smith, we have a problem here. We are facing a 33-year-old male patient with past history of psychiatric disorders. A neighbor had called us because he heard the patient calling for help. The patient lives alone in his apartment and there is no family available. Upon arrival, we found the patient sitting at the kitchen table talking about "messages from God." He is very agitated, diaphoretic, and states we are "slaves of the devil." He is not permitting us to get close to him. Although the police are on the scene, they say the patient is not breaking the law and that they refuse to help us restrain the patient for transport. What should we do?"

HOW WOULD YOU PROCEED?

This is indeed a relatively common situation. The acutely psychotic patient encounter is a very challenging one for any EMS system. Not every psychotic patient needs to be transported to the hospital. Each patient should be individually evaluated to assess risks for violence or suicide. In this particular encounter, the patient is having paranoid delusions, is displaying an aggressive posture, and it is almost impossible to communicate with. This patient needs to be further evaluated in the emergency department setting and should therefore be transported.

It is important that the entire rescue team shows a common front to the patient. If they start arguing about what their roles are, it will only add to the confusion of the situation, as well as to the patient's agitation. Coordination and communication between public safety agencies is essential. The DMOP should ask to talk with the law enforcement officer in charge or his immediate supervisor. Explain the need for medical transport and why their intervention is important. Protocols with detailed role descriptions for each agency should be developed and approved by

their respective authorities. Frequent joint training sessions for protocol discussion and improvement are recommended. This patient is a candidate for chemical restraint in order to facilitate transport. If necessary for safety, the patient may require physical restraint prior to sedation. Haldol 5 mg IM would have a sedative effect, and should diminish the psychotic symptoms. If needed, a repeat dose of Haldol 5 mg may be given in 30 minutes. Alternatively, a benzodiazepine may be used instead. Once the patient is under control, vital signs must be monitored frequently and a physical examination completed. The patient should then be transferred to the nearest appropriate medical facility with psychiatric services.

References

1. Bledsoe BE. *Behavioral and Psychiatric Emergencies: Brady Paramedic Emergency Care*, 2nd ed. Brady; 1994.
2. Tintinally JE. Violent patient and the out-of-hospital provider. *Ann Emerg Med.* 1993;22(8):1276–1279.
3. Verdile VP. Out-of-hospital management of the violent patient. *Out-of-hospital Care Reports.* 1992;2(3):17–24.
4. Judd RL. Behavioral and psychological crisis in emergency medical services. *Top Emerg Med.* 1983;4(4):1–7.
5. *Dorland's Illustrated Medical Dictionary.* 27th ed. Philadelphia: WB Saunders; 1988.
6. Henneman PL, Mendoza R, Lewis RJ. Prospective evaluation of emergency department medical clearance. *Ann Emerg Med.* 1994;24(4):672–677.
7. Harwitz D, Ravizza L. Psychiatric emergencies: suicide and depression. *Emerg Med Clin of North Am.* 2000;18 (2):263–271.
8. Kochaneck KD, Smith BL, Anderson RN. Deaths: Preliminary Data. *1999 National Vital Statistics Reports.* 2001;49(3):1–49.
9. *Suicide and Suicidal Behavior.* In: *Fact Book of the Year 2000: Working to Prevent and Control Injury in the United States.* Washington DC: National Center for Injury Prevention and Control; 2001.
10. Hirschfeld R, Russel J. Assessment and treatment of suicidal patients. *N Engl J Med.* 1997;337:910–915.
11. Fredrick L. Defending your life: how to manage the violent patients and scenes. *JEMS.* 1992;17(6):64–67.
12. Lehman LS, Padilla M, Clark S, et al. Training personnel in the prevention and management of violent behavior. In: *Management of Violent Behavior.* Washington, DC: Hospital and Community Psychiatry Service, American Psychiatric Association; 1988:24–27.
13. Blummenreich P, Lippman S, Bacani-Oropilla T. Violent patients: are you prepared to deal with them? *Post Grad Med.* 1991;90(2):201–206.
14. Goldberg RJ, Dubin WR, Fogel BS. Review: behavioral emergencies, assessment of psychopharmacologic management. *Clin Neuropharm.* 1989;12:233–248.
15. Tardiff K. Management of the violent patient in an emergency situation. *Psychiatr Clin North Am.* 1988;11(4): 539–549.

16. Tueth MJ. Management of behavioral emergencies. *Am J Emerg Med.* 1995;13(3):344–350.

17. Chan TC, Vilke GM, Neuman T, Clausen JL. Restraint position and positional asphyxia. *Ann Emerg Med.* 1997;30(5):578–586.

18. Pilowsky LS, Ring H, Shine PJ, et al. Rapid tranquilization: a survey of emergency prescribing in a general psychiatric hospital. *Br J Psych.* 1992;160:831–835.

19. Sanders MJ. Behavioral emergencies and crisis intervention. In: Stoy, WA, ed. *Mosby's Paramedic textbook.* 1st ed. St. Louis: Mosby Lifeline; 1994.

20. Coffman JA. Behavioral disorders: emergency assessment and stabilization. In: Tintinally JE, Krome RL, Ruiz E, eds. *Emergency Medicine: A Comprehensive Study Guide.* 3rd ed. Philadelphia: Lea & Febinger; 1992.

21. Donlon PT, Hopkin J, Tupin JP. Efficacy and safety of the rapid neuroleptization method with injectable haloperidol. *Am J Psychiatry.* 1979;136(3):273–278.

22. Benitez JG. How to control the violent patient. *UPMC Trauma Rounds.* 1994;5(3):6–7.

23. DiPiro JJ, Talbert RL, Hayes PE, et al. *Pharmacotherapy: A Pathophysiologic Approach.* 1st ed. New York: Elsevier Science Publishing; 1989.

24. *Physicians Desk Reference.* 50th ed. Montvale: Medical Economics Co.; 1996.

25. Circaulo DA. Psychotropic drug therapy in the emergency department. *Top Emer Med.* 1983;4(4):17–23.

26. Dagadakis CS, Maiuro RD. The assaultive patient. In: Schwartz GR, Cayten CG, Mangelsen MA, et al. eds. *Principles and Practice of Emergency Medicine.* 3rd ed. Philadelphia: Lea & Febinger; 1992.

27. Dubin WR. Rapid tranquilization: antipsychotics or benzodiazepines. *J Clin Psych.* 1988;40:250–260.

28. O'Schanick GJ. Emergency psychopharmacology. *Am J Emerg Med.* 1984;(2):164–170.

29. Cressman WA, Plostnieks J, Johnson PC. Absorption, metabolism and excretion of droperidol by human subjects following intramuscular and intravenous administration. *Anesthesiology.* 1973;38:363–369.

30. Neff KE, Denney D, Blachly PH. Control of severe agitation with droperidol. *Dis Nerv Syst.* 1972;33(9):594–597.

31. Resnick M, Burton BT. Droperidol vs. haloperidol in the initial management of acutely agitated patients. *J Clin Psych.* 1984;45(7):298–299.

32. Thomas H, Schartz E, Petrilli R. Droperidol vs. haloperidol for chemical restraint of agitated and combative patients. *Ann Emerg Med.* 1992;21(4):407–413.

33. Van Leeuwen AM, Molers J, Sterkmans P, et al. Droperidol in acutely agitated patients: a double blind placebo-controlled study. *J Nerv Men Dis.* 1977;164(4):280–283.

34. Stewart SM. Droperidol. *Critical Care Nurse.* 1987;7(5):86.

CHAPTER 67

Altered Level of Consciousness

Paul W. Beck, MD
Eric Davis, MD

Introduction

The patient presenting to the out-of-hospital care provider with an altered level of consciousness (ALOC) may be one of the most common encounters in EMS. Many of these conditions have the potential to cause significant morbidity and mortality, and it is essential that proper care be initiated in the field, often before the diagnosis is completed. In most instances, this treatment must be instituted in conjunction with attempts to determine the cause for the altered level of consciousness. In addition, the out-of-hospital care of these patients must address possible complications, such as cervical spine injury and aspiration. The challenges are to rapidly identify and treat those problems that are reversible in the field, and to prevent any added morbidity.

Evaluation

The differential diagnosis for the patient with an ALOC is extremely long and complex. Although the ultimate treatment for many of these causes falls outside of the scope of practice for the prehospital care provider, emphasis should be placed on those conditions that may be effectively treated in the field. A simple and useful mnemonic for the potential causes is AEIOU TIPPS (figure 67.1).

Once scene safety is assured, basic life support (BLS) evaluation should be the first priority for prehospital care providers of any level and experience upon encountering a patient with an altered level of consciousness. Once the ABCs are adequately addressed, the additional history, physical exam, and field laboratory findings may be used to develop an appropriate treatment plan.

Field personnel should obtain as much information about the patient from the scene as the situation permits. The approach to this phase should be undertaken in as systematic a way as possible to ensure that no information is omitted. Because the patient often cannot give an adequate history, alternative sources, such as bystanders, family, and the physical surroundings, must be used. EMS personnel can question people who are familiar with the patient about the patient's health, the rapidity of the onset of the symptoms, any complaints voiced or signs demonstrated by the patient. One question that may be particularly useful is whether a patient who is now alert but confused ever had a complete loss of consciousness or seizure.

Places where medications are commonly located (such as bathrooms, medicine cabinets, bedrooms, nightstands, and kitchens) can be searched to provide clues concerning underlying illnesses or possible ingestion. A medic alert bracelet or necklace should be sought. Any obvious findings at the scene, such as other household members exhibiting similar complaints or sick or deceased pets, may point to carbon monoxide (CO) as a cause.

If a drug overdose or poisoning is suspected, the field personnel should attempt to gather further per-

---

A — **A**irway—hypoxia and postanoxic encephalopathy

E — **E**ndocrine and metabolic

I — **I**nsulin—hypoglycemia

O — **O**verdose

U — **U**remia and Hepatic encephalopathy

T — **T**rauma, **T**umor

I — **I**nfection—meningitis, encephalitis, brain abscess

P — **P**rimary Neurological—seizures, tumors, strokes

P — **P**sychological

S — **S**hock

FIGURE 67.1. *Mnemonic for Causes of Altered Level of Consciousness.*

tinent information. The route of exposure should be determined. In the majority of cases, this will be by ingestion, and it should be determined what was ingested (including if it was a mixed ingestion), when it occurred, the amount consumed (especially the maximum possible), and any action taken by the patient or bystanders, including the administration of any "antidotes." All empty pill containers, liquor bottles, syringes, and other drug paraphernalia should be noted and, if possible, brought to the emergency department. This information can greatly aid later treatment decisions.

With respect to the physical exam, the first task is to determine the degree of the altered level of consciousness. Unfortunately, a variety of inexact terms are commonly used to describe an individual's level of consciousness. Descriptive terms such as stuporous, comatose, semi-comatose, obtunded, confused, and delirious are frequently used by providers. Unfortunately, these terms are poorly defined and thus may lead to different interpretations by the provider and the direct medical oversight physician (DMOP). In general, it is best for levels of consciousness to be described on the basis of the response the patient makes to a given stimulus. Field providers can use the simple pneumonic AVPU:

A = the patient is alert

V = the patient responds only to loud verbal stimuli

P = the patient responds only to painful stimuli

U = the patient is unconscious

This simple 4-level determination should result in much more easily interpreted findings. There may be further description by use of the Glasgow Coma Scale (figure 67.2), with which all providers should be familiar. A study done with paramedics scoring videotaped patients with ALOC confirmed that paramedics can give scores that correlate well with those of ED physicians.[1]

The directed and focused secondary survey can aid in helping to determine the origin for the alteration of consciousness.

HEENT: The head should be examined for any obvious outward signs of trauma such as scalp and facial lacerations, abrasions, and contusions. The pupils should be observed for symmetry and light reactivity. If they are dilated bilaterally this may indicate cerebral hypoxia or barbiturate overdose, whereas pinpoint pupils often suggest an opioid overdose. Unequal pupils may be found in normal variants, but could also indicate impending herniation from trauma or a spontaneous intracranial hemorrhage. Any odor on the patient's breath (acetone, bitter almonds, ethanol) should be noted. The tongue may be checked for bleeding, which may indicate seizure activity, or swelling, indicating anaphylactic shock, which is an unlikely cause unless there is coexistent hypotension.

Eye Opening	Spontaneous	4 points
	Responds to Speech	3 points
	Responds to Pain	2 points
	No response	1 point
Verbal Response	Oriented × 4 (Time, place, person, situation)	5 points
	Confused	4 points
	Inappropriate words	3 points
	Incomprehensible sounds	2 points
	No response	1 point
Motor Response	Obeys commands	6 points
	Localizes pain	5 points
	Withdraws (from pain)	4 points
	Flexion (pain)	3 points
	Extension (pain)	2 points
	No movement	1 point
A score of <9 indicates severe neurological impairment.		

FIGURE 67.2. *Glasgow Coma Scale.*

Any upper airway stridor should be documented and plans to care for a partially or soon-to-be obstructed airway must take precedence.

CHEST: The respiratory rate, pattern, and depth should be noted. Again, any outward signs of trauma should be identified

ABDOMEN: Identification of a pulsatile mass in a patient with shock and an altered level should be noted so that triage to a hospital that can appropriately care for an aneurysm can be accomplished.

NEUROLOGIC: In addition to pupillary findings, any focal neurological signs suggesting stroke or increased intracranial pressure, such as extremity flaccidity, should be noted and recorded as a baseline for possible progression. Altered speech patterns may also be elicited with the aid of bystanders. Use of the Cincinnati Prehospital Stroke Scale may be appropriate.[2]

SKIN: The skin may be used to determine temperature (increased—infection or heat illness, decreased—exposure, dehydration, alcohol or barbiturate overdose); rashes (infection or allergic reaction); track marks (possible narcotic overdose); or signs of previous suicide attempt (healed wrist scars).

In each case the positive findings should be relayed to the DMOP.

The measurement of serum glucose level in the field has traditionally been accomplished through the use of reagent test strips (Chemstrip, Dextrostix), which have been found to yield accurate results in some studies but to be less effective in others, with a small but significant number of false positives and false negatives.[3-7] Problems may occur with the interpretation of the color change by prehospital personnel, as well as inaccuracy of the strips, particularly if the strips are old, were stored in unsealed containers, or were exposed to extremes of temperature.[8,9] Glucose measuring devices that give a digital readout of the serum glucose level from a single drop of the patient's blood are available and widely used in the prehospital setting. The advantage with this method is that no interpretation of results is necessary. The disadvantage is that these units must be frequently checked and calibrated, which can be costly and time-consuming. Non-invasive transcutaneous glucose measurement may soon be available.

Treatment

The focus of a care protocol for the patient with altered level of consciousness is to identify and treat reversible conditions. In addition, the provider must use general supportive measures to protect the patient from harm due to the loss of protective reflexes (such as the gag reflex). Basic life support measures, such as C-spine immobilization and basic airway management, should be instituted before any attempt is made to gather a complete history or perform a detailed physical examination.

The first priority is to assess and maintain an adequate airway. If the patient is not breathing, respirations should be assisted by whatever means are appropriate such as bag-valve-mask (BVM) or intubation. In the patient with respirations, a nasal or oropharyngeal airway may be inserted. When a gag reflex is present, the problem can probably be managed by simple head-tilt maneuvers and supplemental oxygen. If the patient lacks a gag reflex, intubation is probably warranted. Should the patient become violent or it becomes impossible to easily intubate the patient, then the better part of valor is to provide meticulous attention to the airway, with use of oropharyngeal airway and BVM and suction as necessary.

In cases where opioid overdose is suspected, then ventilation should be supported with a BVM awaiting the reversal of narcosis with an opiate antagonist. Naloxone given IV can be expected to work within 2 minutes and only takes another minute if given IM.[10] High flow oxygen should be applied to all patients, and if no contraindication exists, the lateral decubitus position offers additional protection of the airway. Trauma must always be a consideration in these patients, and appropriate protection of the cervical spine must be undertaken throughout.

Once the airway is secured, the next step is to monitor and frequently reassess the patient's pulse, blood pressure, and cardiac monitor reading. A common mistake in these patients is to miss shock or a dysrhythmia, which can obviously have serious consequences. Once all of the BLS skills are completed and any problems are addressed, the prehospital care provider and DMOP are able to proceed to the next phase of field care: the diagnosis and treatment of potentially reversible conditions.

The next order in most protocols calls for the establishment of IV access while at the same time drawing blood. The blood obtained may then be tested for a serum glucose level, with exogenous glucose administration based on the result. While the level at which glucose is given to the patient may vary from system to system, most use a level of ≤ 80 mg/dl when accompanied by appropriate signs and symptoms as hypoglycemia. This method of testing is generally preferable to the blind administration of exogenous glucose to all patients with an altered level of consciousness. Studies have shown that only 25% of those patients falling into this category are hypoglycemic, and the commonly held assumption that an ampule of $D_{50}W$ "won't hurt anyone" has come under attack. This exogenous glucose may result in multiple problems, including skin necrosis (after inadvertent extravasation or subcutaneous infiltration), variable elevations in the serum glucose level, hyperosmolality, hyperkalemia (in certain diabetic patients with hyporenenemic hypoaldosteronism), and potentially a poorer neurological outcome in patients with focal or global cerebral or myocardial ischemia.[11-18] It is this last point that is of the most concern, since this population is common in EMS and the effect is potentially serious. These observations have been derived from both animal and human studies using both stroke and cardiac arrest. While the exact mechanism has not been absolutely defined, it may be due to an increase in acidosis secondary to the delivery of glucose in those areas where blood flow is below that necessary to preserve neuronal viability.[19,20] This acidosis may then impede cellular recovery once normal blood flow is restored. While not all studies have supported this hypothesis,[21] the current consensus is that the administration of exogenous glucose may be harmful in many patients, an opinion brought forth convincingly in an article by Browning.[22]

After administration of glucose to the hypoglycemic patient, an improvement in mental status is usually seen within 5 minutes. The average increase in serum glucose level following one amp of $D_{50}W$ is approximately 150 mg/dl.[10]

It is not an uncommon occurrence for paramedics to have a difficult time establishing IV access in patients with hypoglycemia. In these cases the use of IM glucagon has been shown to be safe and effective.[23] Patients without glycogen stores will not respond well to glucagon, but this is a distinct minority of patients. The mean time to response to glucagon is approximately 6–9 minutes with an increase in glucose level of 100 mg/dl.[23] An amp of $D_{50}W$ works more quickly and on average increases the glucose level by approximately 150 mg/dl.[23,24] Care must be taught to providers regarding the use of oral glucose

solutions in patients with an ALOC, since aspiration may occur.[24]

The next step in the standard protocol is to administer an opiate antagonist, which currently is naloxone. It was found to be safe with very few serious side effects, the most common being precipitation of withdrawal.[25] Some authors have argued for a more selective use of naloxone based upon more selective criteria (respiratory rate <12, miosis, circumstantial evidence of opioid abuse) than just altered level of consciousness. These criteria have not been prospectively studied, however. There have been several case reports of side effects, such as hypertension, pulmonary edema, and dysrhythmia production after use of naloxone, but these are all in patients who are having reversal of opioid anesthesia and not in patients without an opioid on board.[26-28] Therefore, to use naloxone relatively freely in the field is relatively safe but may add more cost than using more selective criteria. There is no currently available method to test for opioids in the field. This step may be initiated earlier in the sequence if suspicion of opioid overdose is high, based upon the environmental or physical findings.

In all cases, it is extremely important that the prehospital care provider observe and record any response by the patient to the administered medication. This will greatly aid the emergency department personnel in their treatment.

Treatment Challenges

There is probably no patient category that can be more challenging than those presenting with an ALOC. The large differential, combined with the lack of direct pertinent information due to the inability of the patient to give a history, contribute to a significant potential for error.

The first potential problem with these patients is that they could be misplaced in the ALOC protocol. The various forms of shock may present with an ALOC, yet must be treated completely differently.

Hypoxia or hypercapnia cause agitation or an ALOC, and careful attention must be given to maintaining an adequate airway and providing supplemental oxygen. Aspiration is one of the most significant complications of inadequately protecting the airway in these patients.

The next problematic group is those patients who are diagnosed as being "just drunk." The sheer numbers of these commonly abusive patients, especially for urban providers, combined with the inherent dis-

Liver disease
  a) hepatic encephalopathy
  b) coagulation disorder
  c) hypoglycemia
Electrolyte abnormalities
Hypoxia
Trauma
Sepsis
Hypothermia
Seizures

Figure 67.3. *Possible Problems in Alcoholics.*

like of caring for them, can lead to an attitude of indifference by many field personnel. One must keep in mind that the intoxicated/alcoholic patient is at risk for an increased number of secondary problems (figure 67.3).

Trauma, particularly of the head and neck, is always a possibility, and everyone should be aware of the increased risk of subdural hematoma for chronic alcoholics and the elderly due to cerebral atrophy and the propensity for falls. Mixed drug overdoses with alcohol are also common, and the administration of an opioid antagonist may be a good idea. The alcoholic is also prone to a myriad of medical problems, including hypoglycemia and electrolyte imbalances. Those patients with liver disease may not have adequate glycogen stores. In addition, the clouded mentation may cause an error with medication such as insulin. Other complications of alcohol, such as hypothermia, aspiration, and encephalopathy, should also be considered.

The patient who has a seizure is another potential source of problems. It is tempting to assume that these patients have an underlying seizure disorder, but one must bear in mind that seizures are also caused by hypoxia, hypoglycemia, trauma, intracranial hemorrhage, stroke, and drug overdoses. The patient who has had a seizure is also more prone to head and neck trauma.

Failure to give an appropriate amount of an opioid antagonist is a potential pitfall. The synthetic and semisynthetic opioids may require large doses of naloxone for reversal. In a similar light, the hypoglycemic patient may not respond immediately if the hypoglycemia has been of prolonged duration.

Perhaps the most common challenge is related to the terminology used by prehospital care providers communicating to the DMOP. As previously discussed, terms such as stuporous, obtunded, semiconscious, and arousable, are used in an imprecise way. It is not uncommon to hear a description such as "alert but not responsive." It is best to describe the level of consciousness in a simplified manner such as AVPU or in a standardized fashion.

Controversies

Many hypoglycemic patients who have improvement in mental status will refuse further medical care. This practice has been shown to be generally safe if certain criteria are met.[29] The proposed criteria for safe treatment and non-transport are:

- History of insulin-dependent diabetes mellitus.
- Pre-treatment blood glucose level <80 mg/dl.
- Post-treatment blood glucose level >80 mg/dl.
- Return of normal mental status within 10 minutes of $D_{50}W$ administration.
- Ability to tolerate food and/or liquid by mouth
- Absence of complicating factors (chest pain, arrhythmias, dyspnea, seizures, alcohol intoxication, chronic renal failure requiring dialysis, or focal neurological signs/symptoms).[29]

It is important for the provider and DMOP to also identify whether the patient is on a long-acting oral hypoglycemic agent. Despite any immediate improvement, all these patients should be transported to the hospital for further evaluation and probable admission due to the half-life of their medications. Also, if patients are treated and not transported, it should be stressed that reliable bystanders (such as co-workers) or family members take responsibility for the patient's well-being, so that EMS can be quickly summoned if there are any problems. In addition, the prehospital care provider or a reliable family member should contact the patient's primary care physician so that insulin dosages or dietary changes can be made as necessary.

A similar controversy may arise in treating the narcotic overdose patient who suddenly wakes up and wishes to refuse. There is risk to those patients who are reversed and then refuse further medical treatment (including transport), since they may lapse back into a coma due to the shorter effective period of naloxone as compared to some opioids. Some advocate a low dose administration protocol (0.4 mg IM or IV), which may reverse the respiration depression but may not reverse the patient to the point of refusing transport. This is a perplexing problem, and the true magnitude of relapse risk has not been studied. Experience in systems that have been fully reversing opioid overdose and allowing transport refusals would suggest the actual risk is quite small.[30] A long-acting (4–6 hour) opioid antagonist, nalmefene, has been released and may help to eliminate this problem. Early results would suggest that nalmefene reverses opioid-induced coma but that its onset of reversing the respiratory depression may be slower than naloxone.[10] It may turn out that the safest treatment is the combination of naloxone and nalmefene, allowing both quick reversal of respiratory depression and prolonged action.

The use of flumazenil for patients with known or suspected benzodiazipine overdose may be considered in some systems. For patients with isolated acute (rather than chronic) overdoses of benzodiazepines, it is a safe and effective agent.[31] It is wise to consider this cautiously, as patients may have coingested alcohol and/or tricyclic antidepressants. The use of flumazenil in these patients is potentially dangerous, and has led to death from seizures in a few cases.[32] Due to the rarity of pure benzodiazepine overdose, the difficulty in assuring this in the prehospital setting, and the potential adverse effects, most medical directors do not advocate the use of this agent in the field.[31,32]

A final point of contention to be addressed is when the DMOP should be contacted. This in large part is determined by the individual system depending on the assessment abilities of the paramedics, number of calls handled by direct medical oversight, patient population, preference of EMS medical director, and regulations. Generally, it is recommended that the DMOP should be contacted after glucose determination is made and/or naloxone administered. This enables the DMOP to individualize treatment (as in supplemental doses of naloxone or $D_{50}W$) or to alter the normal mode of therapy (e.g., sodium bicarbonate in suspected tricyclic antidepressant overdose).

Protocols

The BLS protocols for patients with an ALOC should focus on the evaluation and treatment of airway and breathing problems while assuring cervical spine stabilization. For the patient who is alert and able to take oral glucose, this treatment could be considered within the basic provider's scope of practice, depending upon the state or regional protocols.

For the advanced providers, the use of $D_{50}W$ for known diabetics with hypoglycemia and naloxone for relatively apparent narcotic overdoses is generally allowed prior to direct medical command consult. However, if the prehospital care provider is unsure of the cause, or suspects poly-pharmaceutical overdose, then the DMOP should be directly consulted. A DMOP consult should be obtained, as discussed above, for any patient who "wakes up" and is now wishing to refuse further treatment and transport.

Summary

The DMOP must always approach the prehospital management of the patient with ALOC with a great deal of care and in a systematic fashion. Treatment of these patients must be accomplished simultaneously with maneuvers designed to protect and evaluate the patient. Attention must be given to support the patient's vital functions and to reverse those disorders that can be treated in the field. All of this should be accomplished through the guidance of the DMOP.

Cases

Case 1

"Medic Command, this is Medic One. We are inbound with an approximately 35-year-old male found by police lying in the street. We arrived to find this guy obtunded and disheveled. He is a known street person. He smells strongly of ETOH. There isn't anybody around to give us any history. His vital signs are as follows: BP 110 over palp, pulse 120, and respirations 12. The patient is currently asleep and snoring. We are unable to obtain a further physical exam because his coat and clothes stink of urine, feces, and vomit. The police have requested we bring him into the ED for medical clearance for jail. We have a 20–30 minute ETA and just wanted to notify you and wonder if you have any further orders."

HOW WOULD YOU PROCEED?

This is a common type of case and presents difficulties for any number of reasons. One of the distasteful aspects of the job that is performed by the prehospital care provider is dealing with this sort of patient. The majority of these cases will turn out to be "just drunk," but occasionally there will be an alternative reason or reasons for the patient's ALOC. Sound medical evaluation and treatment should apply in all cases.

The patient's airway is of primary concern. The report of snoring should alert the command physician to a potential problem with airway patency. An oral airway should be inserted to check for a gag reflex and keep the airway open. A decision to intubate may be at least partially based on the patient's response to this maneuver. In addition, all ALOC patients should be placed on oxygen, preferably high flow (10–15 L/M) via a non-rebreather mask. This patient should also be immobilized. This tenet applies to most "just drunk" patients but particularly to those found lying in the street, as this "street person" could easily have been a victim of trauma.

The vital signs obtained are a good start, but a focused secondary survey should be performed. The patient should be carefully checked for signs of trauma, particularly about the head and neck. The pupils should be observed for both configuration and response to light. The lungs must be examined and auscultated to help determine the adequacy of ventilation, and the abdomen inspected for rigidity and other signs of an acute abdomen. The extremities may give clues as far as symmetry of movement, as well as track marks. If the situation permits, the patient should be undressed. The wet clothes may be causing the patient to become hypothermic (no one is sure how long he was down), and a good physical exam is important. It will also make it easier to initiate an IV line.

Once the IV is established and blood drawn, a serum glucose level should be checked. As previously stated, this population is prone to hypoglycemia due to decreased glycogen storage ability in the alcoholic liver. This holds true even if the patient is not diabetic. If the patient is not hypoglycemic, or there is no response to the initial $D_{50}W$, naloxone should be considered, since mixed drug overdose is a possibility.

The medico-legal aspects of the "clearance for jail" topic and problems with releasing any patient with an altered level of consciousness to the police are important and fraught with potential hazardous consequences.

Case 2

"University Hospital, this is Medic Five. We are inbound with a 26-year-old female found by her mother unconscious in her bed. Apparently the family had been trying to get hold of her all day and went over this evening. She apparently has taken an unknown quantity of the following medications: valium,

S-I-N-E-Q-U-A-N, and has obvious ETOH on board. There are empty pill bottles by her bedside, dated 3 days ago. Family states she has been depressed lately. Vital signs are as follows: BP—120/palp, pulse 130 and weak, respirations 18. Patient does not respond well to verbal stimuli but is arousable to pain. We have her on O_2 and are preparing to start an IV, check a blood sugar, and will treat that appropriately. Do you have any further orders?"

HOW WOULD YOU PROCEED?

The prehospital care providers have failed to demonstrate the patency and function of the airway. An oral airway may be inserted to check for a gag reflex, and based on this, along with further information obtained by patient examination, may warrant an order by medical command for intubation. The drugs involved in this case have the potential to cause respiratory compromise. If the medics find the patient does not require intubation, they may be reminded to keep a close eye on this patient's airway and breathing pattern while en route.

It is probably warranted in all patients with an altered level of consciousness for blood draw, glucose level check, and administration of naloxone when appropriate. It is certainly justified in a patient with the above ingestion (especially tricyclic antidepressant) and who is tachycardic. An IV line is a good precaution, since these patients may decompensate rapidly.

A final point is that medic command may individualize treatment according to the situation. The current treatment of choice for a tricyclic overdose, and one that could be instituted in the field, is bicarbonate administration. This administration should only be accomplished through contact with the DMOP. Also, the benzodiazepine antagonist flumazenil may be used in selected patients, although caution in precipitating withdrawal seizures in an already unstable patient must be considered. The importance of being able to modify the treatment of the prehospital patient in an direct medical oversight consultory basis cannot be overemphasized.

Case 3

"Medic command, this is Medic 14 with Rescue 2. We are downtown in the boardroom of a large company seeing the vice president, who is a 42-year-old female complaining of a severe headache all morning. While she was giving a presentation she suddenly lost consciousness. She now responds to deep pain by withdrawing her arms to her chest. Her vital signs are a blood pressure of 220 over 108, pulse of 92, and a respiratory rate of 24."

How would you proceed?

This patient should have an IV line established and have her glucose checked. Since there is no reason to suspect an opioid overdose, naloxone can be withheld. The scenario suggests an intracranial catastrophe, and the patient should have her airway supported as necessary and be transported to a center that has neurosurgical capabilities, if possible. The paramedics will frequently ask for antihypertensive medications in cases such as this. In this particular case the blood pressure is probably a protective mechanism to help maintain cerebral perfusion. It would potentially be dangerous to lower the blood pressure in this patient. As in all patients with an ALOC, careful monitoring and support are essential.

References

1. Menegazzi JJ, Davis EA, Sucov AN, et al. Reliability of the Glasgow coma scale when used by emergency physicians and paramedics. *J Trauma*. 1993;34(1):46–48.
2. Kothari RU, Pancioli A, Liu T, Brott T, Broderick J. Cincinnati Prehospital Stroke Scale: reproducibility and validity. *Ann Emerg Med*. 1999;33(4):373–378.
3. Maisels M, Lee C. Chemstrip glucose test strips: correlation with true glucose values less than 80 mg/dl. *Crit Care Med*. 1983;11(4):293–295.
4. Hogya PT, Yealy DM, Paris PM, et al. The rapid prehospital estimation of blood glucose using Chemstrip bG. *Prehosp Disast Med*. 1989;4:109–113.
5. Lavery RF, Allegra JR, Cody RP, et al. A prospective evaluation of glucose reagent teststrips in the prehospital setting. *Am J Emerg Med*. 1991;9:304–308.
6. Jones JL, Ray G, Gough JE, et al. Determination of prehospital blood glucose: a prospective controlled study. *J Emerg Med*. 1992;10:679–682.
7. Chernow B, Diaz M, Orvess D. Bedside blood glucose determinations in critical care medicine: a comparative analysis of two techniques. *Crit Care Med*. 1982;10(7):463–465.
8. Crist D, Murray B, Jones J. Performance and storage of blood glucose reagent strips (abstract). *Prehosp Disast Med*. 1994;9(2):S59.
9. Herr RD, Metz R, Richards M. Chemstrip reliability declines with ambulance storage. *Prehosp Disast Med*. 1989;4:64.
10. Davis EA, Menegazzi JJ, Sucov A. Safety and effectiveness of nalmefene vs. naloxone in opioid and mixed drug overdose in the prehospital care setting. *Prehosp Disast Med*. 1994;9(3[2]):S60.
11. Adler P. Serum glucose changes after administration of 50% dextrose solution: pre- and in-hospital calculations. *Am J Emerg Med*. 1986;4(6):504–506.
12. Goldfarb S, Cox M, Singer I, et al. Acute hyperkalemia induced by hyperglycemia: hormonal mechanisms. *Ann Int Med*. 1976;84(4):426–432.
13. Pulsinelli W, Levy D, Sigsbee B, et al. Increased damage after ischemic stroke in patients with hyperglycemia with or without established diabetes mellitus. *Am J Med*. 1983;74:540–544.
14. Longstreth W, Invi T. High blood glucose level on hospital admission and poor neurologic recovery after cardiac arrest. *Ann Neuro*. 1984;15(1):59–63.
15. Longstreth W, Diehr P, Invi T. Prediction of awakening after out-of-hospital cardiac arrest. *N Engl J Med*. 1983;308(23):1378–1382.
16. Siemkowicz E. Hyperglycemia in the reperfusion period hampers recovery from cerebral ischemia. *Acta Neurol Scand*. 1981;64(3):207–216.
17. D'Alecy L, Lundy E, Barton K, et al. Dextrose containing intravenous fluid impairs outcome and increases death after eight minutes of cardiac arrest and resuscitation in dogs. *Surgery*. 1986;100(3):505–511.
18. de Courten-Myers G, Myers R, Schoofield L. Hyperglycemia enlarges infant size in cerebrovascular occlusion in cats. *Stroke*. 1988;19(5):623–630.
19. Rehncrona S. Brain acidosis. *Ann Emerg Med*. 1985;14(8):770–776.
20. Marsh W, Anderson R, Sundt T. Effect of hyperglycemia on brain pH levels in areas of focal incomplete ischemia in monkeys. *J Neurosurg*. 1986;65:693–696.
21. Matchar DB, Divine GW, Heyman A, et al. The influence of hyperglycemia on outcome of cerebral infarction. *Ann Int Med*. 1992;117:449–456.
22. Browning R, Olson D, Steven H, et al. 50% dextrose: antidote or toxin? *Ann Emerg Med*. 1990;19(6):683–687.
23. Vukmir RD, Paris PM, Yealy DM. Glucagon: prehospital therapy for hypoglycemia. *Ann Emerg Med*. 1991;20:375–379.
24. Collier A, Steedman DJ, Patrick AW, et al. Treatment of severe hypoglycemia in an accident and emergency department. *Diabetes Care*. 1987;6:712–715.
25. Hoffman J, Schriger D, Luo J. The empiric use of naloxone in patients with altered mental status: a reappraisal. *Ann Emerg Med*. 1991;20(3):246–252.
26. Azar I, Turndorf H. Severe hypertension and multiple atrial premature contractions following naloxone administration. *Anesth Analg*. 1979;58:524–525.
27. Prough DS. Acute pulmonary edema in healthy teenagers following conservative doses of intravenous naloxone. *Anesthesiology*. 1984;60:485–487.
28. Pallasch TJ, Gill TJ. Naloxone: associated morbidity and mortality. *Oral Surg Oral Med Oral Path*. 1981;92:602–603.
29. Thompson RH, Wolford RW. Development and evaluation of criteria allowing paramedics to treat and release patients presenting with hypoglycemia: a retrospective study. *Prehosp Dis Med*. 1991;6:309–313.
30. Paris PM. Personal communication. City of Pittsburgh EMS.

31. Weinbroum AA, Flashion R, Sorkine P, Szold O, Rudick V. A risk-benefit assessment of flumazenil in the management of benzodiazepine overdose. *Drug Safety*. 1997; 17(3): 181–196.

32. Haverkos G, Disalvo R, Imhoff T. Fatal seizures after flumazenil administration in a patient with mixed overdose. *Ann Phamacother*. 1994;28:1347–1348.

Section Seven

Jon Krohmer, MD, FACEP

Introduction

As has been apparent from earlier sections of this text, there are many aspects of EMS systems that are non-clinical and yet very important for the EMS Medical Director understand and appreciate. This section describes a number of those components.

A large part of the Medical Director's task relates to the quality of care provided to the community by those EMS personnel for whom the medical director is responsible. That responsibility requires the associated authority to restrict the patient care privileges of personnel not meeting the standards. This authority cannot be exercised in a random or cavalier manner. The EMS system must provide a "due process" mechanism to ensure that all of the rights and responsibilities of the EMS personnel and the medical director in this situation are outlined and appropriately followed. Chapter 68 very completely details the factors necessary to achieve that goal.

With increasing sophistication of the care provided by EMS personnel and with increasing severity of potential diseases to which EMS personnel are exposed, there is a need for the EMS medical director to be familiar with the intricacies of handling potential infectious exposure situations that EMS professionals experience. Chapter 69 presents those common infectious exposure situations that EMS personnel face and ways in which those exposures can be minimized and, when they occur, responded to.

The past several years have seen EMS personnel faced with an increasing number of incidents involving multiple casualty patient situations. As evidenced in the fall of 2001, the potential for severe events arising from domestic and international organizations and individuals will likely grow in the future. It is important for EMS medical directors to understand the appropriate response to events of this nature. Chapters in this section also address the important issues of response to hazardous material, disaster and terrorist events. The planning considerations for medical care for mass gathering events are discussed in detail. Medical considerations for EMS personnel supporting tactical law enforcement operations is a relatively new area of EMS with which the medical director must be familiar.

As medical care continues to become more specialized, receiving facility resources are becoming more regionalized. The EMS system must know the availability of primary, secondary and tertiary facilities in the immediate and surrounding geographic areas and the impact that those facilities have on EMS resources and the patient served by the system. Shifts in health care have placed greater stress on EMS agencies and on emergency departments, often resulting in hospital/ED diversion. The impact of regionalization of care and diversion situations on the EMS system is discussed in depth in this section.

As we are all aware, emergency services personnel are faced with very stressful situations on a daily basis. With the recognition that Critical Incident Stress Management programs offer a way for EMS personnel to help cope with these situations, EMS Medical Directors must be familiar with those programs and be supportive of them.

Understanding the topics presented in this section is as important to the EMS Medical Director as understanding aspects of clinical care in the out-of-hospital setting.

ADMINISTRATIVE OPERATIONS

CHAPTER 68

Due Process

James Page, JD

Introduction

The definitions of "discipline" portray the topic in very different ways, for example, "training that develops self control, character, or orderliness and efficiency," in other words, a positive, nonpunitive effort to create desired attitudes and behaviors through training. From the same source, however, are the following definitions of discipline: "strict control to enforce obedience" and "treatment that corrects or punishes."

It should be apparent that the first of these definitions ("training that develops self-control, character, or orderliness and efficiency") is the preferable approach to discipline. But when that approach fails, it may be necessary to employ the negative, punitive approach to discipline.

In the field, there have been fairly recent requirements for quality management (QM) programs, presumably to assure that the quality of emergency medical care consistently meets minimum standards. While there have been elaborate designs developed for QM programs, almost all seem to avoid a critical issue: how to correct behavior and performance of an individual when the QM process reveals behavior or performance deficits. Most QM proposals simply advise that when errors are detected, the employer or regulator should "take appropriate corrective action."

What is "an appropriate corrective action"? Is it a concentrated period of training that attempts to improve the self-control, character, orderliness or efficiency of the individual? Is it strict control to enforce obedience? Is it treatment that corrects or punishes (such as suspension of employment or certification, or revocation of certification and/or discharge from employment)?

Whenever the punitive approach is selected, the stage is set for a collision between the authority of the employer and/or the regulatory agency and the constitutional rights of the individual who is to be disciplined. In most states, regulations have been developed to guide and control the process. Often, they are poorly written and/or confusing. Furthermore, EMS agencies, medical control hospitals, and medical directors tend to apply those regulations inconsistently, sometimes without apparent regard for the certificate holder's right to due process.

The purpose of this practice guide is to provide useful information and guidance to all parties—regulators, employers, EMS personnel, and their representatives. All parties have an undeniable responsibility to assure and protect the high quality of emergency medical care. To the extent that discipline plays a part in that process, this document is intended to help define and traverse the narrow line between the rights of the public to quality care, and the rights of certified EMS personnel to due process.

Discipline with due process is possible. It requires time, thought, and extra effort. It is complex and sometimes frustrating. But it is a necessary balance of power in a free society.

Generally, people do not appreciate the importance of due process until their rights to property or their employment or their professional reputation are at risk.

Due Process

The 14th Amendment prohibits any state or local government from depriving any person of life, liberty, or property without due process of law. According to the Random House Dictionary of the English Language, due process of law is, "A limitation in the U.S. and State Constitutions that restrains the actions of the instrumentalities of government within limits of fairness." *Black's Law Dictionary* (1990), offers the following definition:

Due process of law implies the right of the person affected thereby to be present before the tribunal which pronounces judgment upon the question of life, liberty, or property, in its most comprehensive sense; to be heard, by testimony or otherwise, and to have the right of controverting, by proof, every material act which bears on the question of right in the matter involved. If any question of fact or liability be conclusively presumed against him, this is not due process of law.

Perhaps the case of *Vaughan v. State* (456 S.W.2d 879, 883) captures the spirit and intent of due process: "aside from all else, 'due process' means fundamental fairness and substantial justice." It is the "property" and "liberty" elements of due process that affect EMS employers and regulators with regard to disciplinary action. The "liberty" interests will be discussed later.

An individual's employment is considered "property" in many cases and thus state or local governments (or individuals or entities operating under the authority of state or local government) may not deprive the individual of that "property" (their employment or required certification) without due process. The actual steps (or mechanics) of due process will be described later. But first, consider the broader aspects of this constitutional protection.

The courts have held that due process exists if under state or local law, contract, or administrative regulation, standards for retention are specified. *Board of Regents of State Colleges v. Roth,* 408 U.S. 564, (1972); *Perry v. Sindermann,* 408 U.S. 593,609, (1972); *Bishop v. Wood,* 426 U.S. 341 (1976). That means that if there are any statutory, administrative, or contractual standards for retaining employment (or certification), then the individual has a "property" interest in his employment (or certification), and that the employment (or certification) cannot be taken away from the individual without due process.

Prior to about 1980, private employers and their employees were deemed to be outside the requirements and protections of due process with regard to employment. Employees of private companies were deemed to be employed "at-will" (at the will of the employer) and had no constitutionally protected employment rights. Since 1980, there have been several California cases which have held that there was an implied contract between the private employer and his employees. For example, *Cleary v. American Airlines,* 111 Cal.App.3d 443, 168 Cal. Rptr. 722 (1980); *Pugh v. Sees Candies,* 116 Cal.App.3d 311, 171 Cal. Rptr. 917 (1981). Also see *Walker v. Northern San*

Diego County Hospital District, 135 Cal.App.3d 896, 185 Cal. Rptr. 617 (1982) for an example using the same theory of implied contract to erode the at-will doctrine. Note: Even though these cases apply only in California, it does tend to be a bellwether state in terms of legal developments.

But the 14th Amendment specifically applies to state and local governments but also to private ambulance companies. Prior to 1980, most private ambulance services in the U.S. operated in an unregulated environment. Their relations with their employees were very much at-will. Now, however, private ambulance companies in many locations are functioning as legal and operational adjuncts of local governments, either through regulated monopoly franchises, protected zone arrangements, subsidy agreements, or shared services. They are strongly regulated by EMS agencies, including quasi-governmental management entities, and many companies have entered into contractual agreements with employees, ranging from labor-management agreements to individual employment contracts.

Consider the following material from the current policy and operations manual of one unnamed private ambulance service:

> The employee, by virtue of accepting employment, assumes the responsibility to: Conform to all applicable governmental laws, regulations, ordinances, policies, procedures, and protocols governing emergency medical services personnel, EMT's and paramedics, including all state, local and Company continuing education and in-service requirements.

In essence, the above provisions create a contract between employer and employee. It probably meets the standard of the *Roth* case. *Roth* requires that standards of retention be specified under state or local law, contract, or administrative regulation. This company's policy and operations manual creates a contract with the employee and then adopts all applicable governmental laws, regulations, ordinances, and the like, as the standards to be met if the employee is to retain his job. Furthermore, the private company has an exclusive franchise in the community it serves, and the city also subsidizes the company. Though there have been no reported cases dealing with the question of a private ambulance employee's "property" or "liberty" interest in their employment, it could be argued persuasively that many private ambulance companies have become quasi-governmental.

DUE PROCESS

The same company has entered into an agreement with its employees' union. That agreement includes a requirement for "progressive discipline." The progressive discipline system is defined, and requires that employees are to receive advance notice, whenever possible, of problems regarding their conduct or performance in order to provide them with guidance and an opportunity to correct any problems. The labor agreement also details the progressive discipline process, which includes most of the elements of due process.

Even without the contractual links between employer and employee (discussed above), the structure and intent of current EMS law and regulation in many states seems to treat the private ambulance provider as a quasi-public agency. With such status there is a concomitant relationship between employer and employee. Although the authority delegated to medical oversight physicians and hospitals may vary from state to state, generally it includes the suspension or revocation of medical oversight to an individual certificate holder (such as an EMT or paramedic). In many cases, this is tantamount to suspending or revoking the certificate itself.

To the extent that suspension or revocation of the individual's certification adversely affects their "property" interest in their employment, this infringement may be subject to due process protections. In other words, if the medical director has the power to take away an individual's certificate (or the necessary medical oversight), thus depriving the individual of the opportunity to continue working at the same status or level of compensation, their "property" interest in their employment is adversely affected. To date, there are no reported appellate court decisions in involving due process violations by medical oversight. However, given the extensive powers conferred upon medical directors, and the potential for harm to the "property" interests of certificate holders, it is highly probable that the courts would formally impose upon medical directors certain requirements. Most likely, these would include pre-action procedural due process similar to that spelled out in *Skelly* v. *State Personnel Board,* 15 Cal.3d 194, 124 Cal.Rptr. 14, 8 (1975) and post-action evidentiary administrative hearings as defined in *Arnett* v. *Kennedy,* 416 .S. 134 (1974).

Due process requirements are not necessary when placing an employee or certificate holder on probation. The *Skelly* pre-action procedure generally is required only in cases of significant punitive action, such as discharges, demotions, or lengthy suspensions. Disciplinary actions such as warnings, reprimands, and "improvement needed" performance evaluations, or suspensions of less than five days, are not considered significant enough to warrant the pre-action procedure. Even where a pre-action procedural due process hearing or a post-action evidentiary administrative hearing is described in state law or regulations, and is made available in cases of certificate suspension or revocation, or where renewal of a certificate is denied, such hearings may not be required in cases of lesser discipline, such as probation, or written or verbal reprimand. Careful study of applicable state law or regulations may be necessary to clarify this issue.

On the other hand, it could be argued that imposing probation on an individual's employment or certification may have adverse economic consequences (loss of opportunities to work overtime, suspension of transfer and time-off privileges, denial of promotional opportunities, ineligibility for step pay increases). If an otherwise benign imposition of punishment carries with it secondary economic consequences for the individual, it may be prudent to conduct the pre-action or post-action hearings, even though they may not be formally required.

On occasion, it may become apparent that a certificate holder represents an immediate and credible threat to the public. If the medical director or the certifying agency, based on a review of the evidence, finds that such an individual represents an "imminent threat to the public health and safety," he may feel obligated to suspend the individual's certificate immediately. The key to such action lies in the word "imminent." The immediacy implied by that word justifies taking action without the pre-action due process procedures. However, it is imperative that medical oversight act only on credible evidence (which generally means detailed written information, rather than gossip or undocumented verbal reports).

Even where medical oversight deems that immediate suspension is necessary to protect the public health and safety, the individual's employer should place him on paid leave until the facts can be presented in a post-action evidentiary hearing. By keeping the individual on paid leave during the process, his "property" interests are less likely to be injured. If the evidentiary review is conducted properly, and if it confirms that the suspension (and possibly a subsequent revocation) were warranted by the facts, due process requirements will have been met and the individual can be removed from the payroll. If the evidentiary review determines that the suspension is not warranted, no injury will have been suffered by the certificated individual (since he remained on the payroll during the process). The U.S. Supreme Court has addressed this issue as follows: "Before a person is deprived of a protected interest, he must be afforded opportunity for some kind of hearing, except for extraordinary situations where some valid governmental interest is at stake that justifies postponing the hearing until after the event," *Boddie* v. *Connecticut,* 401 U.S. 371, 379 (1971). Technically, the employer might get away with not paying the employee whose certification has been suspended. Indeed, some labor-management agreements in the EMS field specify that the employee must have a current certificate in order to be entitled to compensation. This is a short-sighted view, however, and is likely to cost the employer more in legal fees, administrative time, and general disruption in the workforce.

The experience of law enforcement can be instructional. Whenever a police officer is charged with misconduct, the officer almost always will be placed on paid leave until the allegations can be examined, the officer (usually represented by legal counsel) is given an opportunity to make a written or verbal statement, witnesses can be examined and cross-examined, evidence can be evaluated, and a decision reached by an unbiased administrative panel. If the administrative panel conducts a proper hearing and concludes that the officer was not at fault, his "property" (employment) rights have not been breached. If the panel concludes that the allegation is correct, due process will have been afforded and disciplinary measures can be implemented.

As indicated above, the Fourteenth Amendment prohibits state or local government from depriving any person of life, liberty, or property without due process of law. In California, the courts have consistently held that where the discipline involves charges that stigmatize the employee's reputation, the substantive right to liberty may be implicated to provide the employee with due process rights, even if the employee is found to have no property right in his job (as in the case of a temporary or probationary employee). *Board of Regents of State Colleges* v. *Roth,* 408 .S. 564 (1972); *Lubey* v. *City and County of San Francisco,* 98 Cal.App.3d 340, 159 Cal.Rptr. 440 (1979); *Wilkerson* v. *City of Placentia,* 118 Cal.App.3d 435, 173 Cal.Rptr. 294 (1981); *Jablon* v.

Trustees of the Cal. State Colleges, 482 F.2d 997 (9th Cir. 1973); cert. denied, 414 U.S. 1163 (1974).

The liberty interest cases involve only terminations. Also, in those cases, the liberty interest is not an issue where the employee is charged only with incompetence or inadequate performance. However, where there are charges of immoral or dishonest conduct, the employee has a right to a hearing that affords him an opportunity to clear his name. *Williams* v. *Department of Water and Power,* 130 Cal.App.3d 677, 181 Cal.Rptr. 868 (1982); *Shimoyama* v. *Board of Education,* 120 Cal.App.3d 517, 174 Cal.Rptr. 748 (1981).

In order for the information (which stigmatizes the employee's reputation) to be damaging—and thus involve the liberty interest—it must be dispersed to others. If that information is considered and discussed in a closed meeting, and not broadcast, reported, or shared with the public or the community, it does not impinge on the constitutionally protected liberty interest. *Burris* v. *Willis Ind. School District,* 537 F. Supp. 801 (1982); affirmed in relevant part, 713 F.2d 1087 (1983). In a fairly recent case, a temporary deputy sheriff's liberty interests were implicated where his discharge was based on charges of misconduct, as well as incompetence. However, the court ruled that the employee had been afforded an adequate opportunity to clear his name without a full evidentiary hearing, where the employee was notified of the charges, and allowed to explain his conduct to the officers making the termination decision, file a written response, and appeal to a higher-ranking officer before the termination was effective. *Murden* v. *County of Sacramento,* 206 Cal.Rptr. 699 (1984) (petition for hearing before California Supreme Court pending). Thus far, the courts have limited "liberty" interest applications to employees of public agencies, not to volunteers nor employees of a private company.

The Mechanics of Due Process

In California, the landmark *Skelly* case spells out certain minimal due process procedures to be taken by public agencies (and possibly private companies operating in a quasi-governmental capacity) before taking serious disciplinary action against "tenured" employees. In the *Skelly* case, the California Supreme Court ruled that as a minimum, pre-removal safeguards must include the following:

1. The employee (or certificate holder) is to receive a preliminary written notice of the proposed action stating the date it is intended to become effective and the specific grounds and particular facts upon which the action will be taken.
2. The employee (or certificate holder) is to be provided with any known written materials, reports, or documents upon which the action is based.
3. The employee (or certificate holder) is to be accorded the right to respond either orally, in writing, or both to the proposed charges.

The *Skelly* case involved a physician who was employed by the State Board of Education. He was considered a permanent employee and, by the agency's own rules, permanent employees could not be dismissed or disciplined except for good cause. For purposes of the *Skelly* safeguards, "permanent" and "tenured" status is the same. Ordinarily, in cases of discharge, due process requirements apply only to such "permanent" employees. Probationary and "exempt" (at will) employees, who may under the employing agency's rules be terminated for any or no cause, are not legally entitled to such pre-action due process procedures nor to a subsequent post-action evidentiary hearing.

There are some important exceptions in cases where a probationary or exempt employee's reputation may be stigmatized by the disciplinary action, cases involving long-term at-will private sector employees, and cases involving peace officers. Those cases and the exceptions are beyond the scope of this document.

While there have not yet been any reported cases specifically on the point of EMS training institutions and certifying agencies, reasonable analogies may be drawn. For example, an EMS trainee, or applicant for an EMS certificate, probably has no due process rights (to a diploma or certification). If a trainee is dismissed from the course, or if the applicant is denied a certificate, they probably have no right to a pre-action *Skelly*-type process, or a post-action evidentiary hearing. On the other hand, once the individual is certified, their property interest in their certified status probably solidifies. Especially where the certificate is essential to gaining and keeping EMS employment, the property interest in the certificate would seem to be as tangible as the property interest in employment itself. Therefore, it can be reasoned that certificate holders are as much entitled to due process protections as are permanent employees.

Due process requirements do not apply to all disciplinary actions. According to one of the best sources on the topic, the disciplinary action must be "significant punitive action." Actions such as warnings, reprimands, "improvement needed" performance evaluations, and suspensions of five days or less may be administered without according the *Skelly*-type pre-action process. On the other hand, the employing agency is free to establish its own procedures for such minor disciplinary action, and it may provide for either pre-action processes or post-action reviews. Usually, these occur through a grievance process.

When punitive discipline is absolutely necessary, a fair and consistent procedure for imposing it is essential. The next section of this chapter offers an algorithmic approach. The algorithm is an adaptation from a practice guide that was based on California's EMS Personnel Certification Review Process Guidelines. For this national version, all references to California regulations and procedures have been removed, and the algorithm has been reconstructed for possible use in all states. Although the discipline algorithm attempts to provide a generic process, some portions of it may conflict with local statutes and regulations. It should be used—if at all—in connection with local statutes and regulations and, where local statutes and regulations differ or conflict with the algorithm, the local statutes and regulations must prevail. In locales where disciplinary procedures and regulations are being developed, or existing procedures and regulations are in need of revision, the discipline algorithm can be used as a guideline. Before adoption, however, it should be reviewed by competent legal counsel.

Summary

Generally, people do not appreciate the importance of due process until their own rights are at risk. Nonetheless, due process rights are among the most fragile and precious of freedoms enjoyed by Americans. Balancing those rights against the need to assure quality in health care presents the EMS medical director with a complex dilemma. Although complex, time-consuming, and sometimes very frustrating, due process is possible while guarding patients and the public against imminent risks. As with most technical processes, discipline can be divided into a series of questions, decisions, and action steps.

To guide EMS personnel, their employers, their regulators and their representatives, a recommended process is organized and illustrated in the following algorithm (Appendix I).

Appendix I

A Proposed Discipline Algorithm

Information is received, which, if true would be evidence of a threat to public health and safety.

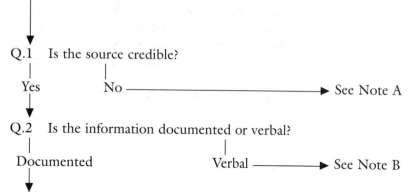

Q.1   Is the source credible?

Yes   No ————————————————————→ See Note A

Q.2   Is the information documented or verbal?

Documented   Verbal ————————→ See Note B

ACTION STEP 1: Evaluate the information relative to the potential threat to the public health and safety and determine if disciplinary action appears to be warranted. Proceed to Q.3

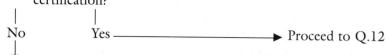

Q.3   Does this information refer to an individual who is NOT presently certified but has applied for certification?

No   Yes ————————————————→ Proceed to Q.12

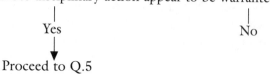

Q.4   Does disciplinary action appear to be warranted?

Yes   No

Proceed to Q.5

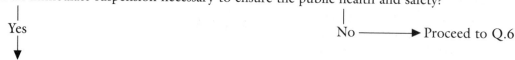

Q.5   Is an immediate suspension necessary to ensure the public health and safety?

Yes   No ————————→ Proceed to Q.6

ACTION STEP 2: Certificate holder and his employer(s) shall be notified prior to or concurrent with initiation of the suspension. The notification should:

- Be by certified mail;
- Specify allegations and/or circumstances which caused the medical director or certifying agency to immediately suspend the certificate;
- State that the certificate is suspended immediately, and also specify the duration of the suspension;
- Identify the certificate(s) the action applies to in cases of multiple certificate holders;
- Inform certificate holder that he has the right to request a hearing to review the facts which necessitate the immediate suspension;

- Include a statement that the certificate holder must report the suspension if he applies for employment, certification, or authorization from another employer or agency during the period of suspension.

Proceed to Q.6

Q.6   Is further inquiry into the situation necessary?

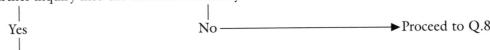

Yes   No ─────────────────────────▶ Proceed to Q.8

ACTION STEP 3: Begin formal investigation. Proceed to ACTION STEP 4

ACTION STEP 4: At a point in time when a formal investigation is begun, the certificate holder or applicant and his employer shall be notified of the investigation, and the notification shall:

- Be by certified mail;
- Notify certificate holder or applicant of a formal investigation;
- Include a statement that the allegations, if found to be true, constitute a threat to the public health and safety and are cause for the medical director or certifying agency to take action;
- Include an explanation of the possible actions which may be taken if the allegations are found to be true;
- Include an opportunity for the certificate holder or applicant to submit in writing any information which he feels is pertinent to the investigation, including statements from other individuals, etc.;
- Inform the certificate holder or applicant of the date by which information must be submitted;
- Include an explanation of the hearing process if suspension, denial, or denial of renewal of a certificate may occur.

Proceed to Q.7

Q.7   Does the certificate holder request a hearing? (applicable only in cases of immediate suspension)

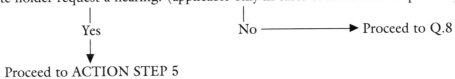

Yes   No ─────────────▶ Proceed to Q.8

Proceed to ACTION STEP 5

Q.8   Does the medical director or certifying agency conclude that the infraction or performance deficiency requires suspension, revocation, or denial of renewal of the certificate?

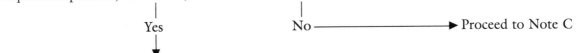

Yes   No ─────────────────────▶ Proceed to Note C

Q.9   Does the medical director decide to convene a hearing to assist in establishing the facts of the matter?

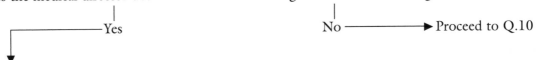

Yes   No ─────────▶ Proceed to Q.10

ACTION STEP 5: Convene hearing process. The medical director should specify the date by which the arbiter or panel shall make its report. The arbiter or panel shall make a written report to the medical director or certifying agency within the time limit. Proceed to Q.10

Q.10 Does the medical director decide to suspend the certificate holder's certificate?

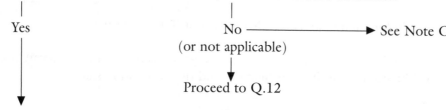

Yes   No ⟶ Proceed to Q.11
(or not applicable)

ACTION STEP 6: Medical director determines the period of time the certificate is to be suspended, and determines any conditions for reinstatement. Proceed to ACTION STEP 7

Q.11 Does the medical director decide to revoke the certificate holder's certificate?

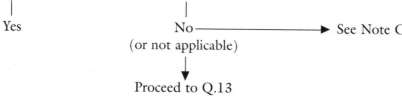

Yes   No ⟶ See Note C
(or not applicable)

Proceed to Q.12

Proceed to ACTION STEP 12

Q.12 Does the medical director or certifying agency decide to deny issuance of a certificate?

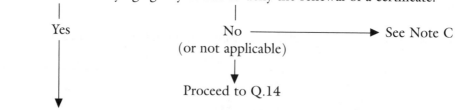

Yes   No ⟶ See Note C
(or not applicable)

Proceed to Q.13

Proceed to ACTION STEP 13

Q.13 Does the medical director or certifying agency decide to deny the renewal of a certificate?

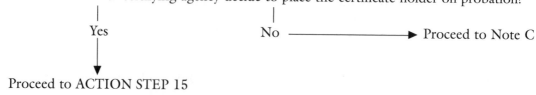

Yes   No ⟶ See Note C
(or not applicable)

Proceed to Q.14

Proceed to ACTION STEP 14

Q.14 Does the medical director of certifying agency decide to place the certificate holder on probation?

Yes   No ⟶ Proceed to Note C

Proceed to ACTION STEP 15

ACTION STEP 7: The certificate holder and his employer(s) shall be notified within (a specified number of) days after the medical director or certifying agency determines the period of time the certificate is to be suspended, and any conditions for reinstatement. The notification shall:

- Be by certified mail;
- Specify allegations and/or circumstances which caused the medical director or certifying agency to suspend the certificate;
- State that the certificate is suspended, and also the duration of the suspension;

- Specify any conditions that must be met in order for reinstatement of the certificate to occur at the conclusion of the suspension;
- Identify the certificate(s) the action applies to in case of multiple certificate holders;
- Include a statement that the certificate holder must report the suspension if he applied for employment, certification, or authorization from another employer or agency during the period of the suspension;
- Include an explanation of how to request a post-action hearing.

Proceed to Q.15

Q.15 Will the suspension period run past the expiration date of the certificate?

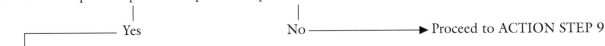

ACTION STEP 8: Calendar the expiration date of the certificate. On or before that date, the medical director may: (a) allow the certificate holder to renew the certificate by the usual process, or (b) require him to demonstrate that he sufficiently retains the necessary knowledge and skills. Proceed to Q.16

ACTION STEP 9: At the conclusion of the suspension period, determine whether the conditions for reinstatement have been satisfied. If they have been satisfied, notify the certificate holder that the suspension is rescinded and the certificate is reinstated. If the conditions have not been satisfied, notify the certificate holder that the suspension will remain in effect until the conditions are satisfied, or until the certificate expires, whichever occurs first. See NOTE E regarding the addition of conditions or extension of the suspension.

Q.16 Can the individual demonstrate sufficient retention of knowledge and skills, as determined by the medical director?

ACTION STEP 10: The medical director may require the individual either to complete specific retraining requirements or reapply for his certificate as if he were a new applicant. Proceed to NOTE E

Q.17 Does the certificate holder request a (post-action) hearing?

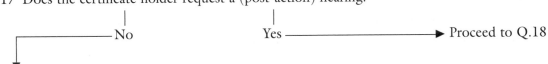

ACTION STEP 11: Determine whether the certificate holder is entitled to a (post-action) hearing. See NOTE F

Q.18 Does the certificate holder or applicant specify in writing that he does NOT want a further review of all the facts of his case?

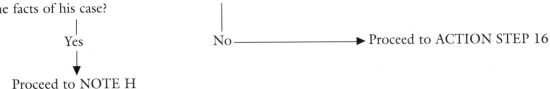

Q.19 Is the request for a (post-action) hearing made within a specified number of days of the date that written notice of action taken is received by the certificate holder?

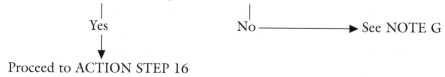

Yes　　　　　　　　　　　　　No ————————▶ See NOTE G

Proceed to ACTION STEP 16

Q.20 Even if the regulations do not provide for a (post-action) hearing for certification applicants or where probation is imposed on certificate holders, or even if a certificate holder's request for a (post-action) hearing is not made within time limits, does the medical director decide to convene a hearing in this case?

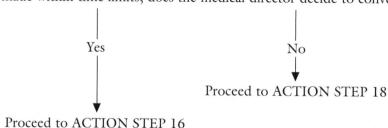

Yes　　　　　　　　　　　　　No

　　　　　　　　　　　　　　　　　Proceed to ACTION STEP 18

Proceed to ACTION STEP 16

ACTION STEP 12: The medical director shall complete and place in the record a signed and dated statement certifying his decision. The certificate holder and his employer(s) shall be notified (a specified number of) days after the medical director makes a final determination to revoke the certificate holder's certificate. The notification shall:

- Be by certified mail;
- Specify allegations and/or circumstances which caused the medical director or certifying agency to revoke certificate;
- Summarize the findings of the investigation (if an investigation occurred), including the findings of the hearing, if one was convened;
- Inform the certificate holders that his certificate(s) are revoked;
- Identify the certificate(s) the action applies to in cases of multiple certificate holders;
- If no hearing was convened, an explanation of the individual's right to request a post-action evidentiary review of the revocation;
- Include a statement that the individual must report the revocation if he applies for employment, certification, or authorization from another employer or agency, and that his application may not be accepted or processed unless he presents documentation which, in the opinion of the medical director or the certifying agency, demonstrates that the threat to the public health and safety which necessitated the revocation is no longer applicable.

Return to Q.17

ACTION STEP 13: The medical director shall complete and place in the record a signed and dated statement certifying his decision. The applicant shall be notified within (a specified number of) days after the medical director makes a final determination to deny the issuance of a certificate. The notification shall:

- Be by certified mail;
- Specify allegations and/or circumstances which caused the medical director to deny the issuance of a certificate;

- Summarize the findings of the investigation (if an investigation occurred), including the findings of the pre-action hearing, if one was convened;
- Inform the applicant.

ACTON STEP 14: The medical director shall complete and place in the record a signed and dated statement certifying his decision. The certificate holder and his employer(s) shall be notified within (a specified number of) days after the medical director or certifying agency makes a final determination to deny the renewal of the certificate holder's certificate. The notification shall:

- Be by certified mail;
- Specify allegations and/or circumstances which caused the medical director to deny the renewal of the certificate;
- Summarize the findings of the investigation (if an investigation occurred), including the findings of the (pre-action) hearing, if one was convened;
- Inform the certificate holder that his certificate(s) will not be renewed;
- Identify the certificate(s) the action applies to in cases of multiple certificate holders;
- If no (pre-action) hearing was convened, an explanation of the individual's right to request a post-action evidentiary review of the decision on deny renewal of the certificate(s);
- Include a statement that the individual must report the denial of renewal if he applies for employment, certification, or authorization from another employer or agency, and that his application may not be accepted or processed unless he or she presents documentation which, in the opinion of the medical director or the certifying agency demonstrates that the threat to the public health and safety which necessitated the denial or renewal is no longer applicable.

ACTION STEP 15: The medical director may place the certificate holder on probation (any time an infraction or performance deficiency occurs which, in the opinion of the medical director or certifying agency, indicates a need to monitor the individual's conduct in the EMS system in order to protect the public health and safety). The medical director may also set the term of the probation and any conditions including the requirement that the certificate holder's performance shall be reviewed periodically during the probationary period, in accordance with the certifying agency's policies and procedures. Return to Q.17

ACTION STEP 16: Convene (post-action) hearing process. The medical director specifies the date by which the arbiter or panel shall make its report. The arbiter or panel shall make a written report to the medical director within the time limit. Proceed to ACTION STEP 17

ACTION STEP 17: The certificate holder shall be notified of the medical director's or the certifying agency's final decision, if notification has not already occurred. If a hearing was convened this notification shall occur within (a specified number of) days of receipt of the request for the hearing. The notification also shall include the arbiter or hearing panel's recommendation.

ACTION STEP 18: Notify the applicant or certificate holder that the applicable statutes and regulations do not provide for a (post-action) hearing in cases where non-certified applicants are denied certification, where certificate holders are placed on probation, or where the request for a hearing is not made in a timely manner.

NOTES

Note A

Concluding whether a source of information is credible (believable) can be very subjective. Among the factors to be considered are the relative status and position of the informant. For example, is the information coming from a disgruntled former employee or partner? Or, is it coming from an EMS physician?

The requirement that information be from a "credible source" places a burden on the employer or medical director. That is, he must guard against activating the disciplinary process on the basis of representations by an informant who may be unreliable, dishonest, and/or motivated by malice, revenge, or ego. If there is any question, the credibility of the source should be evaluated or challenged before evaluating the information itself. Once the test of credibility is met, return to Q.2.

Note B

Whether or not required by regulations, it is advisable that the employer or medical director insist that such information be presented in writing by the source or informant. The disciplinary process is very powerful and has the potential for depriving certificate holders of some of their constitutional rights. It is prudent to subject the reported information to this simple test before exercising the power of the disciplinary process. Quite often, the circumstances that generate questions or concerns (about a certificate holder being a potential threat to the public health and safety) are emotionally charged. Those emotions tend to color descriptions of what happened. The process of reducing the information to writing invariably tempers emotions and subjects the information to an initial test of context and credibility.

Where the information is from a first-line supervisor and concerns the actions or performances of his subordinates, it is recommended that the information first be reviewed within the provider organization, one or two levels above the certificate holder's immediate supervisor. This follows the advice of legal experts regarding implementation of the *Skelly* standard, and subjects the information to still another detached and unemotional review. It prevents a first-line supervisor from inappropriately unleashing a powerful disciplinary process against a subordinate. It also gives employers an opportunity to protect themselves against civil liability which could result from first-level supervisors taking untruthful or exaggerated information directly to the medical director or certifying agency.

If information is taken directly to the medical director or certifying agency by a first-line supervisor (especially verbal information), and if that information proves to be insufficient to substantiate the supervisor's allegations or the disciplinary action that results, the certificate holder may have a cause of ac-

tion against the certifying agency, its medical director, the first-line supervisor, and the employer. After documented information has been acquired from a credible source, return to ACTION STEP 1.

Note C

If the medical director or certifying agency decides to take no action against the certificate holder or applicant, discontinue the evaluation of information, or the inquiry or investigation. If the original information was received from a source outside the certifying agency (e.g., employer, public safety agency , base hospital, patient, etc.), that source should be informed in writing that the information has been evaluated (or investigated) and that the medical director has concluded that no further action is warranted (or that the applicant should not be denied a certificate). *Special note:* The evaluation of information of this nature, or an inquiry or investigation by a medical director or certifying agency, has the potential of stigmatizing a certificate holder, thus adversely affecting his 14th Amendment "liberty" interests. It is important for the medical director or certifying agency to make reasonable efforts to prevent and/or eliminate any stigma if and when it is determined that disciplinary action is not warranted (or that the applicant should not be denied a certificate).

Note D

Notify the certificate holder in writing that the suspension is rescinded. The notification process should be as prompt as possible. Suspension of certification adversely affects a certificate holder's ability to seek and obtain gainful employment, and that right is one of the "property" rights protected by the 14th Amendment. If a certifying agency fails to promptly notify a certificate holder that his suspension has been rescinded, that agency is, in effect, depriving the individual of a protected right without due process.

Note E

In requiring the certificate holder to complete specific retraining requirements or to reapply for his certificate as if he were a new applicant, the certifying agency or medical director should avoid imposing conditions which would (a) extend the period of suspension or (b) expand on the conditions for reinstatement which were specified in the notification of suspension (ACTION STEP 8). To add conditions or extend the period of suspension without an additional hearing could be viewed as a denial of due process. Also, such open-ended discipline has the effect of placing the certificate holder in a state of continual jeopardy. Proceed to Q.17

Note F

There are only two situations where a certificate holder may NOT be entitled to a (post-action) hearing. One is where probation has been imposed as the only form of discipline. The other is where the medical director denies certification to an individual who is NOT already certified. As a matter of practice, some certifying agencies provide for a (post-action) hearing process in cases of probation even though technically the certificate holder may not be entitled to it.

If the individual IS a certificate holder and is entitled to a (post-action) hearing, proceed to Q.19.

If the individual is an Uncertified applicant for certification, or a certificate holder being placed on probation, proceed to Q.20.

Note G

Although technically the burden may be on the certificate holder to request a (post-action) hearing within (a specified number of) days of the date that he receives written notice from the medical director or certifying agency, it's probably not wise to deny the request if it is received late (within a reasonable period after the deadline). When confronted by disciplinary action that threatens one's livelihood and professional identity, many people become emotionally disoriented. In many cases, it is difficult for the affected person to seek and obtain counsel, and to decide a course of action within two weeks. By contrast, there are few valid reasons why the medical director or certifying EMS agency cannot accommodate a late request for a hearing. In any legal challenge that may occur, the certifying agency and medical director will be better served by examples of lenient process than by strict insistence on arbitrary deadlines. Return to Q.20

Note H

Where the certificate holder specifies in writing that he does not want a further review of all the facts of his case, no further action by the certifying agency or medical director is required (except to monitor any conditions of suspension, retraining, etc., which may have been imposed, and to notify the certificate holder when the period of discipline ends). It is important for the certifying agency to maintain in its files the certificate holder's written communication (rejecting further review). Also, if the written communication is at all inconclusive, the certifying agency or medical director should make additional contact with the certificate holder and remind him of his right to a (post-action) hearing of all the facts of the case.

C H A P T E R

Communicable Diseases

69

Katherine West, BSN, MSEd

Introduction

This chapter reviews communicable diseases that pose a potential risk to EMS personnel, outlines measures for self-protection to reduce the potential for exposure or disease transmission, and reviews the clinical management following exposures. Prehospital providers assume personal risk that includes exposures to toxic materials, burning structures, hazardous extrications, and daily "light-and-siren" responses. Often these hazards are visible, but often there may exist an additional risk: an undiagnosed or unrecognized communicable disease. In the past, prehospital personnel often viewed their blood splattered clothing as a symbol of being in action; however, with recent knowledge of communicable diseases, safer practices must be undertaken. Simple and very basic protective measures will reduce the opportunity for disease transmission.

The Role of Medical Oversight

The medical director plays an important role in the reduction of exposures and the potential for transmission of communicable diseases in the EMS workplace setting. The medical director serves as an important advocate for insuring that departments/agencies comply with federal laws and regulations that govern safety of EMS personnel. The medical oversight should be aware of all of the requirements put forth by the Occupational Safety and Health Administration (OSHA), state laws regarding consent for testing of patients in an exposure situation, the Ryan White Law, and the Centers of Disease Control and Prevention (CDC) guidelines for post-exposure medical follow up. The Ryan White Law requires that each emergency response agency have a designated officer for infection control and a system for rapid post-exposure notification. The medical director should insure that this individual is in place and has received proper training for this position.

Effective in 1999, OSHA states that if proper post-exposure medical follow-up is not followed by the treating medical provider, the employer will be held responsible. Based on this regulation, keeping up on the changes in post-exposure treatment is very important.

Clarifying an Exposure

It is important to be very clear with regard to what is and what is not considered an exposure to bloodborne pathogens. The CDC and OSHA have published clear criteria for making an exposure determination/evaluation. The CDC and OSHA have also published a listing of what body fluids pose a risk for the transmission of bloodborne pathogens and which ones do not. Yet, a great deal of confusion still seems to exist. For clarification purposes, the proper term to be used in post-exposure evaluation is "exposure to blood" other potentially infectious materials (OPIM), defined as CSF, amniotic fluid, pleural fluid, pericardial fluid, peritoneal fluid, or any fluid that contains gross visible blood. Microscopic blood does not pose a risk because the dose (load of infectious material) needed for infection is not present in fluids that only contain microscopic blood.[1,2] It has been well established that urine, stool, saliva, vomitus, sweat, tears, nasal secretions, and sputum do not pose a risk for the transmission of these bloodborne viral infections.

The second part of defining an exposure under the bloodborne pathogens standard or the CDC guidelines is understanding the criteria for exposure. Exposure criteria are as follows:

- A contaminated sharps injury (the sharp has been in the patient)
- Blood/OPIM in direct contact with the inner surface of the eye, up the nose or in the mouth

- Blood/OPIM in direct contact with an *open* area of the skin
- Cuts with objects covered with blood/OPIM

For the evaluation of exposure to airborne or droplet organisms, there is the need to consider transport time, the task performed, the organism, ventilation of the area in which the exposure occurred, and if personal protection (mask) or a non-rebreather was used on the source patient.

Using the correct definition for exposure will insure that EMS personnel are not being directed into post-exposure management when it is not indicated. It is important to use clear and well established definitions for educational reasons and to maintain the emotional well-being of EMS personnel and their family members. It is also a requirement under OSHA's new compliance directive that the current CDC guidelines be followed.

It is also important to note that the post-exposure medical follow-up needs for the exposed EMS responder are based on the test results of the **source** patient. Each state has different laws regarding consent for testing for HIV. Knowledge of the law for your specific state is essential to knowing the process for obtaining source patient blood for HIV testing. Obtaining consent, if required, is the responsibility of the receiving hospital. The medical director needs to insure that trained hospital staff handle this process.

Hepatitis B Virus (HBV)

Due to vaccine programs that began in 1982, the risk for acquiring hepatitis B viral infection has diminished greatly. All fire/rescue departments must have hepatitis B vaccine programs in place. Vaccine must be offered free of charge to personnel at risk, and vaccine is not to be administered until the education and training component of the program has been conducted. EMS personnel should not be placed in an "at risk" position until they have received the first dose of vaccine or signed a declination form. This means that personnel should not be performing tasks that involve contact with blood/OPIM until training and the offering of vaccine have been met. The CDC stated that, in 1985, there were approximately 12,500 healthcare workers (HCWs) occupationally acquired HBV infection. In September 1998, OSHA reported the number of HCWs occupationally infected with HBV in 1995 to be 800. This represents over a 90% decrease in HCW HBV infections.

Over the past few years, there has been a great deal of confusion regarding the need to titer-test individuals post-vaccine, and the need for "boosters." The CDC published in November 1992 a guideline that there was a need to conduct post-vaccine titer testing for individuals who are at risk for sharps injury.[3] This was not clearly seen as a mandate by many departments because the CDC is not a regulatory agency. However, the reality is that the recommendation/guidelines published by the CDC set the medical standard of care. The courts use these guidelines in civil suits brought by HCWs. The CDC guidelines outline that departments will be held accountable for compliance. Now, the issue of following these guidelines and offering post-vaccine titer testing to at-risk personnel is clear. The new OSHA compliance "Directive for bloodborne pathogens, CPL 2-2.44D," states that the CDC guidelines are to be followed.

First, it is important to clear up the issue of time frame between doses of HBV vaccine in the initial series. If an individual is "lost" in the system and does not complete the series in the six-month time frame recommended to complete the vaccination series, there is no need to restart the series all over again, no matter how much time has passed between doses. The vaccine series is picked up where the individual left off and the three doses completed and a titer performed.[3]

Second, post-vaccine titer testing is to be offered to all HCWs listed in an at-risk position for exposure to the HBV. Post-vaccine titer testing is to be offered 1 to 2 months after completion of the three-dose vaccine series. If the individual did not respond to the three-dose series, then a second full series of three shots is to be offered. Then the individual is titered again. If no response, no further doses are to be administered. The individual is to be counseled that he/she is a non-responder to the vaccine. This is important information for the individual to know because there is a different post-exposure protocol to be followed for individuals identified as *"non-responders."*[4]

Third, for individuals for whom a positive titer is noted after receiving the vaccine series, no further titer testing is needed, even if an exposure to HBV is documented. This is because this vaccine has been shown to offer "immunologic memory."[3,4] Immunologic memory means that even though an individual's titer may fall, even to an undetectable level, the individual is still protected. When an exposure occurs, the body's immune system kicks in automatically and the protective level goes back up. This is an immediate response. Based on this scientific information, there is no need to conduct a baseline post-exposure HBV titer test nor is there a need for periodic titer testing of persons with a positive titer after primary immunization.

If your personnel were never titered following completion of the vaccine series, one should not be done now. It is clear that titers go down over time. For some individuals, this happens quickly and for others it can take 12 years or more. To do routine titer tests serves no useful purpose. If, following the receipt of the vaccine series, a titer was not performed, a titer should be done if an exposure situation occurs.[4,5] Table 69.1 offers this information in a chart for easy review. The protocols reflected in the chart should be part of every department's Exposure Control Plans and be followed by the medical care provider. OSHA states that the *"employer"* is responsible to insure that proper medical follow-up is provided to an exposed HCW.[4,6]

OSHA clearly states that the employer is responsible to pay for titer testing post-vaccination and/or post-exposure.[4] Issues regarding the administration and management of HBV vaccine and titer testing

have now been made very clear. It is also clear that no boosters are needed on any type of periodic basis.

Hepatitis C Virus

Hepatitis C (HCV) was first recognized as a separate virus in the late 1980s. It was one of the viruses listed under the heading of non-A, non-B until identified as a separate virus. This virus is transmitted primarily via sharps injury. To date, there has been one reported case of transmission to a HCW via splatter into the eye in the United States.[7] Risk to HCWs for acquiring HCV occupationally is listed at between 1.8% and 7% worldwide. In the United States, the reported risk is about 1.8%. The higher numbers were from studies in Japan.[8] What about the risk for fire/EMS personnel? To date, there have been five studies conducted that showed "no increased risk" for fire/EMS personnel. The first two studies were reported in June 1995. Those studies were conducted in fire/EMS personnel in Atlanta and Anne Arundel County, Maryland. The third study was conducted by the CDC in review of data from the Philadelphia Fire Department. The fourth and fifth studies were con-

TABLE 69.1			
Recommended postexposure prophylaxis for percutaneous or permucosal exposure to hepatitis B virus, United States			
VACCINATION AND ANTIBODY RESPONSE STATUS OF EXPOSED PERSON	**TREATMENT WHEN SOURCE IS**		
	HBsAG* POSITIVE	**HBsAG NEGATIVE**	**SOURCE NOT TESTED OR STATUS UNKNOWN**
Unvaccinated	HBIG[†] x 1; initiate HB vaccine series[§]	Initiate HB vaccine series	Initiate HB vaccine series
Previously vaccinated: Known responder[¶]	No treatment	No treatment	No treatment
Known non-responder	HBIG x 2 or HBIG x 1 and initiate revaccination	No treatment	If known high-risk source, treat as if source were HBsAg positive
Antibody response unknown	Test exposed person for anti-HBs** 1. If adequate[¶], no treatment 2. If inadequate[¶], HBIG x 1 and vaccine booster	No treatment	Test exposed person for anti-HBs 1. If adequate[¶], no treatment 2. If inadequate[¶], initiate revaccination

*Hepatitis B surface antigen.
†Hepatitis B immune globulin; dose 0.06 mL/kg intramuscularly.
§Hepatitis B vaccine.
¶Responder is defined as a person with adequate levels of serum antibody to hepatitis B surface antigen (i.e., anti-HBs ≥ 10 mIU/mL); inadequate response to vaccination defined as serum anti-HBs < 10 mIU/mL.
**Antibody to hepatitis B surface antigen.

ducted in Pittsburgh and Miami-Dade. All five studies support no increased risk for occupational acquisition of HCV in the fire/EMS workplace setting. Risk appears to be in line with that of the general population for men in the age group of 20 to 59.[9] Additional studies were conducted and reported by the CDC in July 2000 (figure 69.1).

At the current time, there is no vaccine available on the market for protection from HCV. There is hope that one may be available in the next four to five years. There is no prophylactic treatment available for post-exposure medical management. However, there is new testing available to bring the concern for disease transmission post-exposure to closure in a shorter time frame. The original guidelines, stating that HCV should be an important component of post-exposure medical treatment, were published in May 1996. At that time, HCV testing became a routine component of source patient testing and HCW baseline testing. The CDC published the new guidelines for HCV post-exposure follow-up in October 1998.

If an exposure to a HCV positive patient should occur, here is the standard of care for follow-up. First, as with any exposure, the process begins with the testing of the source patient. The results of the patient's tests drive what needs to be done for the exposed HCW. Expediting the turnaround of the testing process is a key component in proper medical follow-up. The designated infection control officer and the medical director should be working with the medical facilities to insure that rapid test results are undertaken. The new OSHA compliance directive makes an important clarification with regard to post-exposure medical treatment. The word "immedi-ately" "is used to emphasize the importance of prompt medical evaluation and prophylaxis. An exact time was not given in the standard because the time limit on the effectiveness of post-exposure prophylaxis measures can vary depending on the infection of concern."[4,10] This statement is of particular importance with HCV and HIV follow-up.

Follow-up for exposure to HCV begins with the source patient's blood reports. If the source patient is HCV positive, then the follow-up for the exposed HCW is different from if the source is not HCV positive. This can show the advantage of waiting to get the HCW's baseline test drawn after the source patient results are returned. If the source patient is positive for HCV, then there is additional lab work that needs to be drawn on the exposed HCW. An ALT (alanine aminotransferase) needs to be drawn on the exposed care provider as a baseline study. Then, four to six weeks after the exposure, an HCV-RNA (hepatitis C virus ribonucleic acid) test can be performed to expedite information on possible infection. This test is widely used even though it is not yet FDA-approved for this use. The use of this test will assist in reducing staff apprehension. Time for concern can be lowered from 4–6 months to 4–6 weeks (figure 69.2).

It is important to note that testing for HCV is a two-step process. First, an EIA (enzyme immunoassay) antibody test is performed and, if positive, must

HCV Infection in Emergency Response Workers United States

Group	No. Tested	HCV Positive*
Firefighters/EMS		
Philadelphia*	2,136	3.0%
Miami-Dade	1314	1.5%
Atlanta*	435	2.1%
Conn. State	382	1.3%
General pop (≥6 yrs)	20,000	1.8%
Adult men (20-59 yrs)	5,000	3.7%

*Confirmed with supplemental testing

•CDC, MMWR,July 28, 2000

FIGURE 69.1

Postexposure follow-up of health-care, emergency medical, and public safety workers for hepatitis C virus (HCV) infection

- For the source, baseline testing for anti-HCV.*
- For the person exposed to an HCV-positive source, baseline and follow-up testing including
  —baseline testing for anti-HCV and ALT[†] activity; and
  —follow-up testing for anti-HCV (e.g., at 4–6 months) and ALT activity. (If earlier diagnosis of HCV infection is desired, testing for HCV RNA[§] may be performed at 4–6 weeks.)
- Confirmation by supplemental anti-HCV testing of all anti-HCV results reported as positive by enzyme immunoassay.

*Antibody to HCV.
[†]Alanine aminotransferase.
[§]Ribonucleic acid.

FIGURE 69.2

be confirmed by supplemental testing using the RIBA test (recombinant immunoblot assay). Confirmation is an *essential* part of follow-up because there are many false positive results found when EIA is the only test performed. Confirmation testing is important on the source patient as well as for the healthcare worker being followed-up for a direct exposure to a HCV positive patient.[11] At the present time, the CDC does not recommend the routine testing of healthcare workers or EMS personnel for HCV.[8]

HIV/AIDS

HIV/AIDS cases have been decreasing in this country for the past three to four years. In 1997, AIDS was the leading cause of death in young people; by 1999, it was down to number 16 on the list. HIV positive individuals are receiving treatment at an earlier stage of infection and, for many, this is resulting in maintaining these individuals in a healthy state. HIV/AIDS individuals who are responding to their anti-retroviral drug treatment are often virus negative. They are antibody positive because they have had exposure to HIV. But the drugs serve to block the replication of the virus. Therefore, if virus negative, they pose little if any risk for disease transmission. Because of this and many other scientific advances, many changes have taken place with regard to post-exposure prophylaxis for HIV/AIDS. In May 1998, the CDC published the most recent guidelines for evaluation and consideration of offering anti-retroviral drugs to healthcare workers who sustain direct exposures to HIV-positive individuals. In these guidelines, the criteria for when these drugs should be considered were more clearly defined. The use of the new rapid HIV test was encouraged, especially in facilities/areas where it takes longer than 24 hours to turn around source patient HIV testing results. The use of this single unit diagnostic study (SUDS) allows for source patient testing to be completed in less than *one hour*. The actual test takes about 10 minutes once the lab receives the blood sample. The cost for this test is small ($4.00–$10.00 lab cost) and the benefit is great. Rapid turnaround can eliminate the need to place an exposed HCW on toxic anti-retroviral drugs for even a short period of time.

The use of this new test will also put to rest the concern for risk of infection in a shorter period of time. In keeping with the new criteria for offering drug treatment post exposure, it is recommended that an infectious disease physician be consulted before drug treatment is ordered. If an infectious disease physician is not available, there is a toll-free "Clinicians" hot-line number that can be called 24 hours a day/7 days a week to get a consultation. Again, awaiting the result of rapid source-patient testing before pursuing HCW testing is of benefit. Treatment with anti-retroviral drugs is a serious issue and must be weighed against the risk for infection. Risk for infection with HIV following a high-risk sharps injury is listed as 0.32%. For exposure to mucous membranes via splash or splatter, the risk is listed as 0.09%.[12] There have been no HCWs documented as becoming HIV positive following non-intact skin exposure since prospective follow-up began in the mid-1980s. To date, the CDC reports the HCW infection rate for documented, occupationally acquired, HIV infection at 56 cases. This covers a time span from 1978 to June 2000. It is important to note that 48 of those cases were sharps injuries. None of the 56 HCWs is fire/EMS personnel.

There is an important footnote about the May 1998 CDC HIV post-exposure guidelines. There are conflicting statements in two parts of the document. Follow-up calls to the CDC and the Clinician's Hotline identified that there are two errors in the guidelines. The Clinician's Hotline advised that the following is correct:

- Blood on intact skin is not to be considered an exposure, even if for a long period of time and over a large area.

- Saliva does not pose a risk for HBV or HCV transmission.[14]

The medical oversight should be familiar with the May 15, 1998 CDC guidelines for offering anti-retroviral drugs following an exposure event. Figures 69.3 and 69.4 show the steps to be followed before anti-retroviral drugs are to be administered. Insuring that this chart is followed will reduce the potential of EMS personnel being incorrectly treated with these drugs.

Airborne Disease—Tuberculosis

Tuberculosis (TB) cases were on the increase in this country from 1985 to 1990. This was in part due to the increase in numbers of HIV cases in the United States. However, the TB case rate has been at an all-time low since 1992. In 1999, the total number of TB cases reported in the United States was 13,989.[13]

Determining the need for HIV postexposure prophylaxis (PEP) after an occupational exposure.

STEP 1: Determine the Exposure Code (EC)

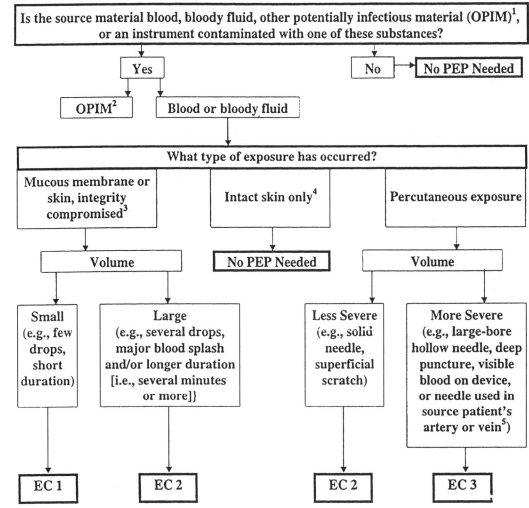

Notes:

1. Semen or vaginal secretions; cerebrospinal, synovial, pleural, peritoneal, pericardial, or amniotic fluids; or tissue.

2. Exposures to OPIM must be evaluated on a case-by-case basis. In general, these body substances are considered a low risk for transmission in health care settings. Any unprotected contacts to concentrated HIV in a research laboratory or production facility is considered an occupational exposure that requires clinical evaluation to determine the need for PEP.

3. Skin integrity is considered compromised if there is evidence of chapped skin, dermatitis, abrasion, or open wound.

4. Contact with intact skin is not normally considered a risk for HIV transmission. However, if the exposure was to blood, and the circumstance suggests a higher volume exposure (e.g., an extensive area of skin was exposed or there was prolonged contact with blood), the risk for HIV transmission should be considered.

5. The combination of these severity factors (e.g., large-bore hollow needle *and* deep puncture) contribute to an elevated risk for transmission if the source person is HIV-positive.

(continued on reverse)

FIGURE 69.3

STEP 2: Determine the HIV Status Code (HIV SC)

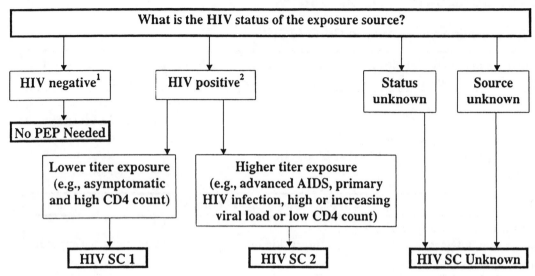

Notes:

1. A source is considered negative for HIV infection if there is laboratory documentation of a negative HIV antibody. HIV polymerase chain reaction (PCR), or HIV p24 antigen test result from a specimen collected at or near the time of exposure and there is no clinical evidence of recent retroviral-like illness.

    A source is considered infected with HIV (HIV positive) if there has been a positive laboratory result for HIV antibody, HIV PCR, or HIV p24 antigen or physician-diagnosed AIDS.

STEP 3: Determine the PEP Recommendation

EC	HIV SC	PEP Recommendation
1	1	**PEP may not be warranted.** Exposure type does not pose a known risk for HIV transmission. Whether the risk for drug toxicity outweighs the benefit of PEP should be decided be the exposed HCW and treating clinician.
1	2	**Consider basic regimen.**[1] exposure type poses a negligible risk for HIV transmission. A high HIV titer in the source may justify consideration of PEP. Whether the risk for drug toxicity outweighs the benefit of PEP should be decided by the exposed HCW and treating clinician.
2	1	**Recommend basic regimen.** Most HIV exposures are in this category; no increased risk for HIV transmission has been observed but use of PEP is appropriate.
2	2	**Recommend expanded regimen.**[2] Exposure type represents an increased HIV transmission risk.
3	1 or 2	**Recommend expanded regimen.** Exposure type represents an increased HIV transmission risk.
	Unknown	If the source, or in the case of an unknown source, the setting where the exposure occurred suggests a possible risk for HIV exposure and the EC is 2 or 3, consider PEP basic regimen.

Basic regimen is four weeks of zidovudine, 600 mg per day in two or three divided doses, <u>and</u> lamivudine, 150 mg twice daily.

2. Expanded regimen is the basic regimen plus <u>either</u> indinavir, 800 mg every 8 hours, <u>or</u> nelfinavir, 750 mg three times a day.

(This 3-step chart is adapted from the report mentioned on page 1 in **Morbidity and Mortality Weekly Report.***)*

FIGURE 69.4

It is important to note that this number combines typical, atypical and extrapulmonary cases of the disease. This is important because atypical and extrapulmonary cases are not transmitted via the airborne route. The majority of cases are noted in six states: New York, New Jersey, Florida, California, Texas, and Illinois. The current case rate appears most prevalent in foreign-born persons.

Currently, OSHA is enforcing the CDC 1994 TB guidelines for protection of healthcare workers. This document requires the development of a risk assessment for TB infection. The results of the risk assessment will determine the need for a respiratory protection program. The TB risk assessment is to be updated each year and added to the Exposure Control Plan. The designated officer should be responsible for compiling the risk assessment data. Medical directors need to be aware of the numbers of confirmed cases in the geographic service area as well as any infected persons who may have been transported by EMS personnel.

Medical oversight should insure that a TB skin testing program is in place for all new hires and that EMS personnel are tested on a yearly basis.[14] For EMS personnel who have a previous history of testing positive, a follow-up chest x-ray is **not** required unless signs and symptoms of the disease appear. Should an exposure to an untreated patient occur, isoniazid (INH) is offered for a six- to nine-month period of time. Personnel need to be cautioned not to drink alcoholic beverages while on this drug, and liver function studies may be needed if the provider is over age 35, because of the incidence rate of drug-induced hepatitis.

Chickenpox—Varicella Zoster

Exposure to chickenpox—Varicella Zoster can be avoided by the identification of personnel who do not already show immunity to this disease. All departments should have a program in place to identify members who are not immune to vaccine-preventable diseases, and should offer the vaccine to those persons. Members who do not know if they have had the chickenpox should have a titer performed. If not protected, the vaccine should be offered. Titer testing for this disease prior to the administration of vaccine is recommended because it has been shown to be cost-effective.

In the event that an unprotected exposure occurs, the vaccine will be offered post-exposure unless the HCW is pregnant or immuno-compromised. In the later case, Vericella-zoster immune globulin (VZIG) would be offered. Vaccine is 70% protective, not 100%, so an additional part of post-exposure medical follow-up may involve placing the exposed member on work restriction for several days.[15] The employee will not be able to work until the end of the incubation period because a mild case may result from the immunization. This is clearly an example of the health benefit and cost savings of having vaccine/immunization programs in place as part of a comprehensive health/wellness program.

Meningitis—Bacterial

Understanding exposure to meningitis is most difficult. Over the years, EMS personnel have been told to take drug treatment in what are clearly non-exposure situations. Meningitis is not an airborne transmitted disease. This disease is transmitted via direct contact with infected secretions from a patient diagnosed with a bacterial form of the infection. Therefore, exposure relates to:

- Performing unprotected mouth-to-mouth on an infected patient;
- Splash/splatter of secretions into mucous membranes (suctioning, intubation, vomiting, coughing).

Finding out the difference between bacterial and viral meningitis can be accomplished in about 15 to 20 minutes by having the laboratory perform a simple gram-stain on CSF obtained during a spinal tap. If the patient is identified as having a bacterial form of meningitis and a direct exposure occurred, then proper treatment can be ordered. In the case of meningeococcal meningitis, the preferred treatment is ciprofloxin as a one-time dose. Post-exposure definition clarification is clearly going to cause some confusion. Based on the practice in the past of offering prophylaxis to anyone even around the infected patient, there is a real need for education to bring about appropriate change. But the criteria are accurate and should be followed.[14] If the patient is identified with viral meningitis, no post-exposure treatment is indicated. Viral meningitis is an infectious disease and not a communicable disease.

Prevention

The key to prevention of occupationally acquired disease lies with the use of personal protective equipment (PPE), education and training, and prompt reporting of exposures. Each of these is a major component of the department's Exposure Control Plan. Those plans must be updated and reviewed on an annual basis.

Education and training must include, but not be limited to: hepatitis B and the vaccine, hepatitis C, HIV/AIDS, syphilis and tuberculosis.[1,4] Trainers need to be qualified to teach this information. OSHA states that qualifications will be verified by degree status, work experience, or additional specialized training in the subject matter. The subject matter is infection control and the diseases. Only by insuring that the trainers are properly trained to teach this information will there be improvement in the fear level of care providers.

Each department must select an infection control concept to assist in the reduction of exposures. On a national level, body substance isolation (BSI) is used in the EMS workplace environment. BSI is an approach that considers all body fluids to potentially pose a risk, even though they don't. BSI, as an infection control concept, is recognized by OSHA as well as by the CDC. Reference to this approach can be found in the original bloodborne pathogens standard as well as in both compliance directives. BSI as the chosen infection control concept needs to be reflected in each Exposure Control Plan.

Personal protective equipment (PPE) is the first line of defense for all healthcare workers. OSHA requires that PPE be readily available to at-risk personnel. PPE is to include: gloves (disposable, vinyl or latex-powder free), protective eyewear, masks, waterless handwash solution, utility gloves for cleaning activities, and cover gowns or a change of uniform.[1,4] It is important to note that latex glove use has resulted in many persons developing latex glove allergy/sensitivity. Medical directors should monitor glove usage and the types of gloves to be used. The CDC has stated that latex needs to be avoided to remove the risk for personnel developing allergy. Table 69.2 notes the CDC recommendations for the use of PPE. Note that gloves are not required for all patient contact, but only when in contact with blood/OPIM.[1,4]

Cleaning routines are also an important component in the prevention of disease transmission. Table 69.3 lists the recommendations for cleaning vehicles. Bleach and water at 1:100 dilution is appropriate and the use of Lysol concentrate at 2½-tsp./per gallon is also appropriate. OSHA withdrew the requirement for cleaning solutions to be tuberculocidal in 1997. Exposure Control Plans need to list the cleaning procedures, the solutions to be used and a schedule for cleaning.

In the absence, or failure, of the use of PPE, post-exposure medical follow-up is essential in protecting the EMS provider from acquiring an infection. OSHA requires that an exposure report form be completed and that the information on the form complies with not only the bloodborne pathogens standard (CFR 1910.1030) but also with OSHA's medical record standard 1910.1020. A sample form is provided in Figure 69.5.

Summary

Insuring proper post-exposure medical evaluation and treatment is essential for EMS personnel health/wellness, risk management, and OSHA compliance. Medical directors assume that the designated medical provider for evaluation for post-exposure treatment is knowledgeable in the current post-exposure medical treatment protocols, and that the medical facilities involved are offering the most timely testing methods available. With all the new recommendations and testing methods, HCWs can receive accurate information post-exposure in a 24-hour time frame. The HIV issue can be resolved in less than one hour. The technology is here to put disease transmission issues to rest very quickly and new advances are occurring every day. The medical director should be aware of these changes to insure that EMS providers are receiving the best care available. Knowledge of these issues is also important for risk management. OSHA is enforcing the CDC guidelines, and insuring proper compliance with those guidelines is important for EMS organizations.

Wellness programs are gaining more importance because it is good business. Reducing risk is both an employee and employer benefit. Insuring that immunization programs are in place is also a compliance issue. EMS personnel should be offered hepatitis B vaccine, MMR vaccine, varicella vaccine (if not immune), TB skin testing yearly, and flu shots. This will support the national effort to reduce the incidence of diseases by offering vaccine to non-immune individuals.

The risk for EMS providers to experience exposures is real. The risk for acquiring bloodborne pathogens is present but remains low. The risk asso-

TABLE 69.2

Examples of Recommended Personal Protective Equipment for Worker Protection Against HIV and HBV Transmission[1] in Prehospital[2] Settings

TASK OR ACTIVITY	DISPOSABLE GLOVES	GOWN	MASK[3]	PROTECTIVE EYEWEAR
Bleeding control with spurting blood	Yes	Yes	Yes	Yes
Bleeding control with minimal bleeding	Yes	No	No	No
Emergency childbirth	Yes	Yes	Yes, if splashing is likely	Yes, if splashing is likely
Blood drawing	At certain times[4]	No	No	No
Starting an intravenous (IV) line	Yes	No	No	No
Endotracheal intubation, esophageal obturator use	Yes	No	No, unless splashing is likely	No, unless splashing is likely
Oral/nasal suctioning, manually cleaning airway	Yes[5]	No	No, unless splashing is likely	No, unless splashing is likely
Handling and cleaning instruments with microbial contamination	Yes	No, unless soiling is likely	No	No
Measuring blood pressure	No	No	No	No
Measuring temperature	No	No	No	No
Giving an injection	No	No	No	No

[1]The examples provided in this table are based on application of universal precautions. Universal precautions are intended to supplement rather than replace recommendations for routine infection control, such as handwashing and using gloves to prevent gross microbial contamination of hands (e.g., contact with urine or feces).

[2]Defined as setting where delivery of emergency health care takes place away from a hospital or other health-care facility.

[3]Refers to protective masks to prevent exposure of mucous membranes to blood or other potentially contaminated body fluids. The use of resuscitation devices, some of which are also referred to as "masks," is discussed on page 16.

[4]For clarification see Appendix A, page 33, and Appendix B, page 38.

[5]While not clearly necessary to prevent HIV or HBV transmission unless blood is present, gloves are recommended to prevent transmission of other agents (e.g., *Herpes simplex*).

ciated with sharps injuries will be further reduced by the implementation of needle-safe devices. The risk for acquiring airborne diseases is also present but risk for contracting these infections remains low. However, as long as risk is present, preventive measures are essential for risk reduction. Medical directors should follow the current CDC guidelines, OSHA regulations, and state laws governing these issues. Medical directors can assist departments and agencies with selection of needle-safe devices. They need to assist in insuring post-exposure evaluation and treatment are appropriate, proper counseling is offered, and exposure control plans are complete, comprehensive and updated annually. A strong exposure control plan assists in the recruitment and retention of EMS personnel by demonstrating concern for the protection of the EMS provider in today's workplace setting.

References

1. CPL 2-2.44B. Enforcement Procedures for Occupational Exposure to Bloodborne Pathogens. Occupational Safety and Health Administration, March 2, 1991.

2. Update: Universal Precautions for Prevention of Transmission of Human Immunodeficiency Virus, Hepatitis B Virus, and Other Bloodborne Pathogens in Health-Care Settings, Centers for Disease Control, *MMWR*, June 24, 1988.

3. Hepatitis B Vaccine, Centers for Disease Control, November 19, 1992, Document # 361350.

4. CPL 2-2.44D. Compliance Directive: Enforcement Procedures for the Occupational Exposure to Bloodborne Pathogens. November 5, 1999, U.S. Department of Labor.

5. Immunization of Health-Care Workers: Recommendations of the Advisory Committee on Immunization Practices (ACIP) and the Hospital Infection Control Practices Advisory Committee (HICPAC). *MMWR*, December 26, 1997.

TABLE 69.3

Reprocessing Methods for Equipment Used in the Prehospital[1] Health-Care Setting

Sterilization:	Destroys:	All forms of microbial life including high numbers of bacterial spores.
	Methods:	Steam under pressure (autoclave), gas (ethylene oxide), dry heat, or immersion in EPA-approved chemical "sterilant" for prolonged period of time, e.g., 6–10 hours or according to manufacturers' instructions. Note: liquid chemical "sterilants" should be used **only** on those instruments that are impossible to sterilize or disinfect with heat.
	Use:	For those instruments or devices that penetrate skin or contact normally sterile areas of the body, e.g., scalpels, needles, etc. Disposable invasive equipment eliminates the need to reprocess these types of items. When indicated, however, arrangements should be made with a health-care facility for reprocessing of reusable invasive instruments.
High-Level Disinfection:	Destroys:	All forms of microbial life **except** high numbers of bacterial spores.
	Methods:	Hot water pasteurization (80–100 C, 30 minutes) or exposure to an EPA-registered "sterilant" chemical as above, except for a short exposure time (10–45 minutes or as directed by the manufacturer).
	Use:	For reusable instruments or devices that come into contact with mucous membranes (e.g., laryngoscope blades, endotracheal tubes, etc.).
Intermediate-Level Disinfection:	Destroys:	*Mycobacterium tuberculosis,* vegetative bacteria, most viruses, and most fungi, but does not kill bacterial spores.
	Methods:	EPA-registered "hospital disinfectant" chemical germicides that have a label claim for tuberculocidal activity; commercially available hard surface germicides or solutions containing at least 500 ppm free available chlorine (a 1:100 dilution of common household bleach—approximately 1/4 cup bleach per gallon of tap water).
	Use:	For those surfaces that come into contact only with intact skin, e.g., stethoscopes, blood pressure cuffs, splints, etc., **and** have been visibly contaminated with blood or bloody body fluids. Surfaces **must** be precleaned of visible material before the germicidal chemical is applied for disinfection.
Low-Level Disinfection:	Destroys:	Most bacteria, some viruses, some fungi, but not *Mycobacterium tuberculosis* or bacterial spores.
	Methods:	EPA-registered "hospital disinfectants" (**no** label claim for tuberculocidal activity).
	Use:	These agents are excellent cleaners and can be used for routine housekeeping or removal of soiling in the **absence** of visible blood contamination.
Environmental Disinfection:		Environmental surfaces which have become soiled should be cleaned and disinfected using any cleaner or disinfectant agent which is intended for environmental use. Such surfaces include floors, woodwork, ambulance seats, countertops, etc.
IMPORTANT:		To assure the effectiveness of any sterilization or disinfection process, equipment and instruments must first be thoroughly cleaned of all visible soil.

[1]Defined as setting where delivery of emergency health-care takes place prior to arrival at hospital or other healthcare facility.

COMMUNICABLE DISEASES

Exposure Report Form

Patient Information:

Name:_____ _____ _____ _____
                                        Sex   Age   Patient #

Exposure Information: Bloodborne _____ Airborne_____

Exposed To: Area Exposed:
Blood _____   Hands_____   Nose___
Bloody Fluid_____   Face_____   Mouth_
Other_____   Eyes_____   Other_____

Personal Protective Equipment Used: Yes_____   Type:_____
                                     No_____

Task Being Performed:_____

Needle Safe Device used: Yes_____   No_____

Employee Information:

Name:_____ SS#_____
Phone # (H)_____ (W)_____

Exposure Date:_____Exposure Time:_____
Exposure Location: Facility_____ Unit_____
Reported To:_____
First Aid Performed: Yes_____   No_____

Source Patient Blood Drawn: (HIV rapid test, HBV, HCV)   Yes____No____

Reporting Process:

Preceptor/Instructor Notified: Yes_____   No___
Designated Officer Notified: Yes_____   No___

Post-Exposure Follow Up:

Employee Given Source Patient Test Results: Yes_____   No___
_____ Date:_____ Time:_____

Employee Medical Follow Up Referral to: _____
Employee: Must attach a written signed explaination of how the exposure event
occurred within 24 hours of the incident. This is to be sent to the Designated Officer.

FIGURE 69.5

6. Occupational Safety and Health Administration, 29 CFR Part 1910.1030. Occupational Exposure to Bloodborne Pathogens; Final Rule, *Federal Register,* December 6, 1991.

7. Ippolito G, Puro V, Petrosillo N, et al. Simultaneous infection with HIV and hepatitis C virus following occupational conjunctival blood exposure (letter). *JAMA,* 1998;280:28.

8. Recommendations for Prevention and Control of Hepatitis C Virus (HCV) Infection and HCV-Related Chronic Disease. *MMWR,* October 16, 1998;47(RR-19):6. Centers for Disease Control and Prevention, Atlanta, Georgia.

9. Spitters C, Zenillman J, Yeargain J. Prevalence of antibodies to Hepatitis B and C among fire department personnel prior to implementation of a Hepatitis B vaccination program. *JOEM.* 1995;37:663–664.

10. CPL 2-2.44D:55.

11. Recommendations for Prevention and Control of Hepatitis C Virus (HCV) Infection and HCV-Related Chronic Disease. *MMWR.* October 16, 1998.

12. Public Health Service Guidelines for the Management of Health-Care Worker Exposures to HIV and Recommendations for Postexposure Prophylaxis. *MMWR.* May 15, 1998.

13. CDC, *MMWR.* June 20, 2000.

14. Guidelines for Preventing the Transmission of Mycobacterium Tuberculosis in Health-Care Facilities. *MMWR.* October 28, 1994.

15. Cross, J. Personal communication, Clinician's Hotline, 1999.

16. Immunization of Health-Care Workers: *MMWR.* December 26, 1997:25–26.

17. Immunization of Health-Care Workers: *MMWR,* December 26, 1997:17–18.

CHAPTER 70

Hazardous Materials

Daniel G. Hankins, MD

Introduction

The Occupational Safety and Health Administration (OSHA) defines a hazardous substance as any substance that: "exposure to which results or may result in adverse effects on the health or safety of employees." (See table 70.1 for examples of Hazardous Materials.) Hazardous material (HazMat) exposures can occur unexpectedly in both the out-of-hospital and hospital phases of patient contact. Witness the incident that occurred in Riverside, California, in February of 1994, when a patient presented to an emergency department who apparently exuded a chemical from her bodily fluids that overcame several hospital workers, who then developed dizziness and vomiting. In spite of many federal and state regulations dealing with the safety of chemicals around the United States, it is still possible to be surprised by a HazMat situation.

Awareness of the possibility that such situations can occur, anytime and anywhere, is essential to the protection of emergency services personnel. A high index of suspicion is essential when dealing with potential HazMat scenarios. Such incidents can be a significant challenge to the skills of the EMS medical director. The medical director must have a working knowledge of how EMS crews identify and interact with hazardous materials (with the major emphasis on minimizing exposure and avoiding injury), and how EMS fits into the unified command structure of the response to such an incident. The medical director must also be aware of the common toxicological exposure syndromes and the appropriate treatment of them. If the medical director is involved with firefighters or HazMat teams responding to such an incident, he also needs to be familiar with the environmental and occupational monitoring of workers dressed in special HazMat personal protective equipment (PPE) and perhaps perform or oversee the necessary pre- and post-PPE evaluations.

Disasters or multiple casualty incidents often have a hazardous material component (e.g., ruptured natural gas pipelines, leaking gasoline or other fluids from vehicles). More recently, the threat of terrorism by chemical or biological means has loomed larger. A chemical terrorist attack would likely evolve and be approached initially as a typical chemical spill. On the other hand, a biological attack would most likely not be a typical HazMat incident, since it would unfold over days or weeks as an epidemic that would impact on EMS and hospital emergency departments. The ultimate goals for any HazMat scene are: (1) safety of the emergency personnel at the scene (EMS, fire and law enforcement), and (2) for EMS to receive partially (at least) or, better yet, fully decontaminated patients and treat them in the best possible fashion for the chemical effects and other injuries. Treatment of specific exposures is also beyond the scope of this chapter, which will discuss the initial general approach to such incidents.

Preparation

In order for a HazMat incident to be considered an emergency, all three of the following must be present: (1) a bad chemical in (2) a bad container which is in (3) a bad location. Unless all three of these conditions are present, an emergent situation does not exist and an aggressive approach is not warranted by emergency personnel. In fact, an aggressive approach is to be discouraged, since emergency workers may needlessly be put at risk. Each situation must be carefully evaluated individually to determine if active intervention is necessary. Some HazMat incidents may not need the services of emergency services personnel at all, because there is no emergency. This would then be a problem to be dealt with by one of the many private hazardous waste cleanup companies around the country. The EMS medical director only

TABLE 70.1

Hazardous Materials		
GENERAL CATEGORY	**EXAMPLES**	**GENERAL**
Explosives		
Class A explosive	Dynamite, dry TNT, black powder	Sensitive to heat and shock
Class B explosive	Propellant explosives, rocket motors, special fireworks	Contamination could cause explosion
	Common fireworks, small arms ammunition	Thermal and mechanical impact potential
Blasting agent	Ammonium nitrate-fuel oil mixtures	
Gases (Compressed, Liquified or Dissolved under Pressure)		
Flammable gas	Liquified petroleum gas, acetylene, hydrogen	Explosion potential
Non-flammable gas	Carbon dioxide, sulfur dioxide, ethylene, nitrogen	Asphyxiation hazard
		Cold temperatures
Flammable Liquids		
Flammable liquid	Acetone, gasoline, methyl alcohol	Flammability
Pyroforic liquid	Aluminum, alkyls, alkyl boranes	Explosion potential
Combustible liquid	Fuel oils, ethylene glycols	Harm from inhalation, ingestion
		Potentially corrosive, toxic, thermally unstable
Oxidizers and Organic Peroxides		
Oxidizer	Ammonium nitrate fertilizer, hydrogen peroxide solution	Supplies O_2 to support combustion of flammable materials
	Benzoyl peroxide, peracetic acid solution	Explosively sensitive to heat, shock, friction
Corrosives		
	Acids—hydrochloric acid, oleum, sulfuric acid	Destruction of tissues
Poisonous and Infectious Substances		
Poison A	Arsine, hydrocyanic acid, phosgene	Fuming potential
Poison B	bases, caustic soda	Oxidizing effect
Irritant	Tear gas, xylyl bromide	
Etiologic agent	Anthrax, botulism, smallpox	Infective potential

has to be concerned about these incidents when emergency workers respond.

Federal statutes and rules dealing with HazMat are complex, but the legal foundation for all emergency responses to hazardous materials situations is Superfund Amendment and Reauthorization Act of 1986, Title III (SARA). This law renewed and expanded an earlier federal law: CERCLA (Comprehensive Environmental Response, Compensation and Liability Act of 1980). SARA mandated a uniform approach to HazMat situations by the two big federal agencies which deal with HazMat: the Occupational Safety and Health Administration (OSHA) and the federal Environmental Protection Agency (EPA). Regulations for HazMat response by emergency services personnel are thus identical for the two agencies. The result is that the rules and regulations are not conflicting for local HazMat providers. The

OSHA regulations are set out in Title 29 of the Code of Federal Regulations, Section 1910.120 (identical to the EPA's Title 40 of the CFR, Section 311). These set out the training requirements for Hazardous Waste Operations and Emergency Response (HAZWOPER). These apply directly to out-of-hospital and hospital workers responding to potential hazardous materials incidents. HAZWOPER defines five levels of HazMat training for emergency situations:

1. First Responder—Awareness Level (FRA): Individuals who are likely to witness or discover a hazardous substance release
   a. Initiate emergency response by notifying proper authorities
   b. Take no further action
   c. Generally about 4 hours of training

2. First Responder—Operations Level (FRO): Individuals who respond to a hazardous substance release as part of the initial response
   a. Respond in defensive fashion without trying to stop the release
   b. Work at safe distance to contain the release, keep it from spreading, and prevent other exposures
   c. Minimum of 8 hours of training

3. Hazardous Materials Technician: Respond to releases or potential releases of hazardous substances for the purpose of stopping the release
   a. 24 hours of training (8 hours of which are equivalent to FRO)

4. Hazardous Materials Specialist: Respond with and provide support for the HazMat Technicians
   a. More specific knowledge of various substances that they deal with
   b. Liaison with local, state and Federal authorities in terms of command structure, resource management and jurisdictional matters
   c. 24 hours at the technician level plus added knowledge

5. Incident Commander: Assume control of the incident scene
   a. 24 hours of training at FRO level plus additional knowledge of overall command structure and function as well as resource management

The National Fire Protection Association (NFPA) has drafted guidelines for curricula for emergency responders. NFPA 472 describes the *Standard for Professional Competence of Responders to Hazardous Materials Incidents*. This document sets out the knowledge base for the above-mentioned five levels of response. NFPA-473, *Competencies for EMS Personnel Responding to Hazardous Materials Incidents*, defines a knowledge base for EMS personnel dealing with hazardous materials on a more sophisticated basis, such as the preparation and training required with EMS personnel who go into the hot zone with fire personnel. The purpose of these guidelines is to establish minimal national standards in the training of EMS personnel about HazMat situations. While different levels of HazMat skills are expected of BLS and ALS providers, this bulletin also describes even higher levels of provider: EMS HazMat Level I Responders and EMS HazMat Level II Responders. This last category of training is designed to make the EMT competent to direct and to coordinate EMS activities at a HazMat incident.

Most EMS personnel will only require training at the FRA level. They just need to know how to recognize the significance of potential hazardous materials, how to avoid injury, and how to activate an appropriate response. The medical director should also have this minimal training. Toxicology knowledge gained during medical school and residency may not be enough for the EMS medical director to avoid problems in the field, since it deals with aspects of drugs and overdoses, not mass quantities of industrial chemicals mixed in an unpredictable manner.

HazMat situations are, by convention, divided into three zones: Hot-Warm-Cold. The hot zone is closest to the chemical and only personnel trained at the minimum of HazMat technician with proper PPE should be in that zone. The hot zone is the area contaminated or potentially contaminated by the hazardous material. The warm zone is further out (distance depends on chemical, wind conditions, terrain, and other factors), and is the transition zone to the cold zone. The warm zone is where decontamination of victims and personnel occur. The cold zone, then, is the area where all the non-protected emergency services personnel are stationed. In general, this is where EMS personnel should be, unless they are functioning in a dual role as firefighters or HazMat responders and have proper training and PPE. The staging area for vehicles and personnel, the command post, the medical monitoring, and triage areas are all in the cold zone. By definition, the cold area must be free of health hazards to personnel.

All of the extensive ramifications of SARA are beyond the scope of this discussion, but other provisions of SARA to be aware of include: (1) the community right-to-know aspects of chemicals, and (2) that state and local governmental units are required to have plans to deal with hazardous materials. Companies are required to let local authorities know what chemicals are present in a particular location (e.g., manufacturing facility or storage company) in case an incident occurs; they are also required to inform those authorities if a release occurs. Another potentially important aspect of SARA for emergency personnel is the requirement for Material Safety Data Sheets (MSDS) to be present at the facility handling hazardous materials. The company is required to have available documentation for each dangerous chemical present. The MSDS contains basic information about that chemical. The company must also give this sheet to the local fire department, the local authority dealing with HazMat, and to OSHA if requested.

SARA requires that state and local plans be developed to deal with HazMat situations and that a preplanned response to incidents at designated facilities be outlined. A uniform set of guidelines for responding personnel and apparatus must be developed to ensure their safety. Those plans must be integrated into the local disaster plan. The overall situation can be complicated by the variety of possible responders to the scene: federal, state, and local government officials, fire, police, and EMS agencies from multiple jurisdictions. Specific duties must be spelled out for all of the responders in the plan, along with the level of training needed for each task such as decontamination, interdiction of the involved material, or care for already decontaminated victims. The chaos inherent in such a disaster situation is best dealt with by the Incident Command System (ICS), which is in general use by fire departments around the United States and is a way of organizing the response into manageable parts. One variation of the ICS is the Unified Command System that brings more disciplines (e.g., public works, EMS, morticians) other than law enforcement and fire departments into the incident command center for better integration of problem solving. The EMS medical director should work with his agencies towards the coordination of the EMS response within this unified command structure. Usually, at such HazMat scenes, police or fire departments have overall control, but the medical director *must* have medical input directly or through his providers at the incident command center to provide medical expertise on scene. Additional information on the ICS is included in the chapters on Disaster Response and MCI.

Firefighters have a basic understanding of the response to HazMat and the use of protective gear as part of their basic expertise. Non-firefighter EMS providers need FRA training at minimum. Prevention of contamination is the easiest way to avoid the creation of extra victims among emergency personnel. It is essential to not allow inadequately trained emergency personnel into the contaminated zone. In general, victims should be decontaminated before being brought to medical personnel. Because of the number or severity of victims, this may not always be possible. If a serious situation is at hand and an aggressive approach by EMS personnel is warranted, the workers must be protected as much as possible. Since special protective equipment is often not carried on ambulances, consideration must be given to stocking some protective equipment for ambulance crews who may be exposed to HazMat situations (table 70.2). OSHA has levied large fines in cases where workers were injured because of inadequate training or protection.

Priorities

One of the most difficult concepts for prehospital personnel to understand in HazMat situations is that their initial approach will be different from their typical approach to routine EMS situations: the tendency to rush in and help the victims. While they are taught throughout their EMS training to act quickly in order to save victims, in potential HazMat situations, the priorities must be altered.

At potential HazMat sites, the first priority is scene control in order to minimize both further injuries and spread of contamination. The scene must be isolated. Ambulance units should be placed upwind and uphill at a safe distance. Unnecessary and unauthorized emergency personnel, the news media, and all others must be restricted until the substance is contained. A cautious approach is necessary. It is much easier to prevent contamination than to deal with even a minimal post-contamination situation. Contaminated ambulances and contaminated crew members may be out-of-service for a lengthy time. In addition to producing more victims among the crew members, this may be a hardship on the ambulance service.

The second priority is to identify the substance or substances involved. Only then can a rational decision be made about whether a search for victims may be

TABLE 70.2
Equipment Items on Ambulance to Deal with a HazMat Incident
■ Plastic trash bags 3 to 4 mil thick
■ Plastic sheeting (6 mil) to cover doors, benches, windows, essential portable equipment, and perhaps to wrap patient
■ Plastic body bag (alternative to wrap patient)
■ Duct tape to seal cabinets
■ Rubber boots
■ Rubber gloves (neoprene is more resistant to chemicals than latex)
■ Rubber aprons
■ Disposable gowns or coveralls

made by trained personnel using appropriate protection, or if a search is too dangerous. The risk to rescuers must always be weighed against the likelihood of a successful rescue. While it is very difficult for EMS personnel to stand back and let a victim go without care, it may be appropriate in some HazMat situations, if the situation is too dangerous.

The major decisions to be made at a scene are determined by the nature of the chemicals involved, and usually are not medically driven. The person with the most HazMat experience (usually the senior or most highly trained fire official) should be designated to determine whether the material poses no risk or poses a significant risk (such as a respiratory toxin, systemic toxin, or explosive). Only after specific identification of the chemical and its associated risk can safe, appropriate rescue be undertaken and treatment of victims begun.

At that point, the advisability and necessity of evacuation of the general population must also be determined. Multiple events in this country have shown that every evacuation presents its own set of questions: Where are all the people going? Who's going to transport them? Who is going to pay for it: local, state, or federal government? Who is going to protect the property left behind? The evacuation process must be part of the predetermined disaster plan. The evacuation process, then, is something that should not be implemented without sound reasons, because of the chaos and disruption that are produced.

The initial assessment of the situation from close range requires protection (table 70.3). At a minimum, the initial survey of the site requires protective gear and self-contained breathing apparatus; this initial survey is essential to determine the extent of the problem and what material is involved. If there is a suspicion that the material is more dangerous than is safe even for routine firefighter protective clothing, then more sophisticated levels of protection are necessary (table 70.4). The EMS personnel must remain at a safe distance until the risk is fully assessed. HazMat incidents must be considered very dangerous until proven otherwise.

The Chemical Manufacturers Association has a thirty-minute video tape available about HazMat responses called "First on the Scene—Hazardous Material Safety." It describes the response to these situations, provides guidelines for hazardous material responses, and illustrates how to respond. It is worthwhile for all EMS providers and physicians to view this tape.

Identification

Identification of most hazardous material substances is uncomplicated if one understands the labeling of their containers. Every medical director should be familiar with, and every emergency vehicle should carry a copy of, the *North American Emergency Response Handbook: A Guidebook for First Responders During the Initial Phase of a Hazardous Material/ Dangerous Goods Incident,* published by the United States Department of Transportation.

Trucks are required to display placards (figure 70.1) with the ID number of the hazardous material being transported. The DOT book illustrates vehicle placards and how to interpret them. In 1990 and 1991, the DOT put out new rules regarding placards, which took effect in 2001. (Figure 70.1) Conceivably, this dual placarding system could lead to some confusion for EMS personnel in the field.

Once the material is identified by number, there is an accompanying treatment guide in the DOT Handbook which indicates the main hazards and emergency actions to deal with the toxic substance itself and the initial first aid for victims. Unfortunately, the placard system is not foolproof. There are inconsistencies in labeling and placarding. There are many loopholes that allow for transportation of unplacarded dangerous materials. There have been examples of emergency workers killed and injured during HazMat incidents because of substances that were not properly marked. Extreme caution is always warranted. There is a different marking system for fixed facilities (such as the large, green oxygen tank outside your hospital) which is known as the NFPA 704 System.

When hazardous materials are being transported, shipping papers that identify the substances should be located: 1) in the cab of the motor vehicle; 2) in possession of a crew member on a train; 3) on the bridge of a vessel; and 4) in an aircraft pilot's possession. There may also be a phone number on the shipping papers or cargo manifest to contact the manufacturer in order to get more information concerning handling the hazardous material and dealing with victims.

Resources are available by telephone to help in dealing with HazMat (table 70.4). The papers accompanying the shipment should contain an emergency response telephone number for the specific manufacturer of that substance. If this is not available, the Chemical Manufacturers Association has a national day and night chemical hotline called Chem-Trec (Chemical Transportation Emergency Center)

TABLE 70.3

Levels of Protection

When response activities are conducted where atmospheric contamination is known or suspected to exist, personnel protective equipment must be worn. Personnel protective equipment is designed to prevent or reduce skin and eye contact, as well as inhalation or ingestion of the chemical substance.

Personnel equipment to protect the body against contact with known or anticipated chemical hazards has been divided into four categories.

1. Level A protection should be worn when the highest level of respiratory, skin, eye, and mucous membrane protection is needed.

   Personal Protective Equipment
   - Positive-pressure (pressure demand), self-contained breathing apparatus (MSHA/NIOSH* approved).
   - Fully encapsulating chemical resistant suit.
   - Gloves, inner, chemical resistant
   - Gloves, outer, chemical resistant
   - Boots, chemical resistant, steel toe and shank (depending on suit boot construction, worn over or under suit boot).
   - Underwear, cotton, long john type.*
   - Hard hat (under suit).*
   - Coveralls (under suit).*
   - Two-way radio communications (intrinsically safe).

   *Optional

2. Level B protection should be selected when the highest level of respiratory protection is needed, but lesser level of skin and eye protection. Level B protection is minimum level recommended on initial site entries until the hazards have been further identified and defined by monitoring, sampling, and other reliable methods of analysis, and personal equipment corresponding with those findings utilized.

   Personal Protective Equipment
   - Positive-pressure (pressure demand), self-contained breathing apparatus (MSHS/NIOSH approved).
   - Chemical resistant clothing (overalls and long sleeved jacket, coveralls, hooded two-piece chemical splash suit, disposable chemical resistant coveralls).
   - Coveralls (under splash suit).*
   - Gloves, outer, chemical resistant.
   - Gloves, inner, chemical resistant.
   - Boots, outer, chemical resistant, steel toe and shank.
   - Boots, outer, chemical resistant.*
   - Two-way radio communications (intrinsically safe)
   - Hardhat.*

   *Optional

3. Level C protection should be selected when the type of airborne substance is known, concentration measured, criteria for using air-purifying respirators met, and skin and eye exposure is unlikely. Periodic monitoring of the air must be performed.

   Personal Protective Equipment
   - Full-face, air purifying respirator (MSHA/NIOSH approved).
   - Chemical resistant clothing (one-piece coverall, hooded two-piece chemical splash suit, chemical resistant hood and apron, disposable chemical resistant coveralls).
   - Gloves, outer chemical resistant.
   - Gloves, inner, chemical resistant.*
   - Boots, steel ad shank, chemical resistant.
   - Boots, outer, chemical resistant.*
   - Cloth coveralls (inside chemical protective clothing*).
   - Two-way radio communications (intrinsically safe)*.
   - Hardhat.*
   - Escape mask.*

   *Optional

4. Level D is primarily a work uniform. It should not be worn on any site where respiratory or skin contact is possible.

TABLE 70.4
Telephone Numbers Useful for Hazardous Materials Incidents
ChemTrec: 1-800-424-9300
National Response Center (operated by U.S. Coast Guard, coordinates response of 26 federal agencies to HazMat incidents): 1-800-424-8802
U.S Public Health Service: 1-800-872-6367

Other numbers that may be useful:
   State Fire Marshal
   State Environmental Protection Agency
   State Emergency Preparedness or
      Emergency Management Officer

(1-800-424-9300). This information is not clinical in focus, however. It is strictly information about the properties of the chemical itself, which is probably most useful to the fire department and for HazMat cleanup agencies. The best source of specific medical information may be the regional Poison Control Center. Poison Control Centers have significant information on hazardous substances, in addition to the usual ingested toxins. The data are clinically helpful, unlike some data from other resources. Communication with the Poison Control Center is an important part of the HazMat response plan.

A commonly encountered problem is that a HazMat incident involves a mixture of hazardous substances which together produce unique and different toxicities in addition to those caused by the individual materials. Poison Control Centers and ChemTrec should be able to give the possible effects of various chemical mixtures in order to assess how best to treat the victims. An aggressive treatment approach may not be necessary if the patient has no toxic signs; however, if the material cannot be identified, then the worst possible toxic scenario must be assumed. Safety of response personnel must be paramount. Product control, confinement, and cleanup should only be done by experienced personnel. Obviously, both prior planning with the responsible agencies and periodic testing of HazMat responses during disaster drills are necessary. Resources are also available by computer. The federal government agencies most concerned with HazMat (OSHA, EPA, DOT) all have World Wide Web sites.

Decontamination

Once the victims are removed from danger, decontamination must occur as quickly and completely as possible. Decontamination may pose a problem for patients, EMS personnel, and HazMat responders. In general, EMS personnel will only get involved in caring for the patient after decontamination has occurred. However, with critically ill patients some medical intervention may be needed before full decontamination is accomplished. Decontamination procedures vary with the nature of the chemical. In general, clothing and jewelry should be removed and the skin flushed with copious amounts of water for 15 to 20 minutes. Neutralization of acids and alkalis should not be attempted because of the possibility of further damage from the heat of reaction. Special irrigating solutions may be required (e.g. zephiran for hydrofluoric acid), but are often not available on the scene. The most readily available material for decontamination is water, however, and the 15- to 20-minute flush will dilute most chemicals. Occasionally, chemicals such as elemental sodium or white phosphorus which react with water, will be encountered. In this situation, the risk-benefit of water irrigation must be weighed. Brushing off solid chemicals may be needed to remove particulate or adherent chemicals.

After decontamination, the standard primary patient survey and initial clinical interventions should be performed. Airway, breathing, and circulatory supports are especially important in HazMat situations, because the most common critical problems are cardiorespiratory and central nervous system in origin. The specific effects of the particular hazardous substance determine the initial medical approach and the complications to be expected. Since accurate information about the material may not be immediately available, it may be best to transport to a medical facility after general decontamination and before waiting for complete information. If the patient is critical and the hazard to EMS personnel is judged to be extremely minimal, then transport before decontamination may be appropriate. This means that the EMS personnel and vehicles as well as victims will have to be decontaminated at the hospital in consultation with, and at a site prescribed by, a HazMat safety officer. The fire department may also need to give input about decontamination at the hospital, but a hospital cannot depend solely on the fire department for all of its decontamination needs.

Radioactive material spills provide unique problems to local responders in both the rescue and EMS capacities. The threat of radiation induces a fearful response in out-of-hospital personnel, although in truth other hazards may be more dangerous. On-site personnel should have special training in dealing with

UN Class Numbers

Class 1—Explosives
Class 2—Gases (compressed, liquified or dissolved under pressure)
Class 3—Flammable liquids
Class 4—Flammable solids or substances
Class 5—Oxidizing substances
    Division 5.1-Oxidizing substances or agents
    Division 5.2-Organic peroxides
Class 6—Poisonous and infectious substances
Class 7—Radioactive substances
Class 8—Corrosives
Class 9—Miscellaneous dangerous substances

- The four digit UN or NA numbers must be displayed on all hazardous materials packages for which identification numbers are assigned. Example: ACETONE UN 1090.
- UN (United Nations) or NA (North American) numbers are found in the Hazardous Materials Tables, Sec. 172.101 and 172.102 (CFR, Title 49, Parts 100-199).
- Identification numbers may not be displayed on "POISON GAS," "RADIOACTIVE" or "EXPLOSIVE" placards. (Sec. 172.334)
- UN numbers are displayed in the same manner for both Domestic and International shipments.
- NA numbers are used only in the USA and Canada.

When hazardous materials are transported in Tank Cars, Cargo Tanks and Portable Tanks, UN or NA numbers must be displayed on:

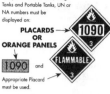

PLACARDS OR ORANGE PANELS

Appropriate Placard must be used.

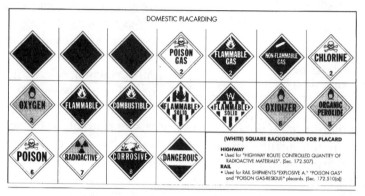

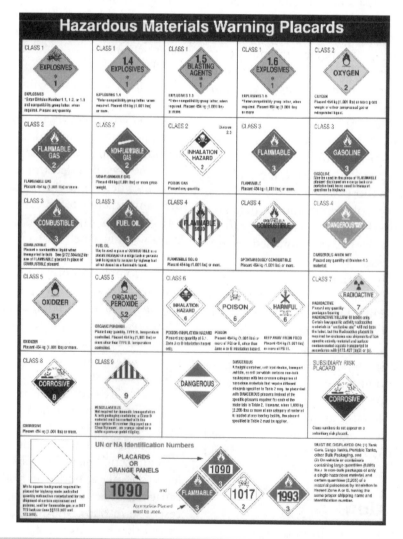

FIGURE 70.1

radiation accidents and decontamination of exposed victims. The out-of-hospital providers may not be able to differentiate between a victim who is contaminated with radioactive material and one who has been irradiated but not contaminated. The irradiated victim is not a hazard for the rescuer, while the contaminated person may be. A monitoring instrument such as a Geiger counter is needed to determine the need for decontamination. If no such device is available, then the victim is assumed to be a hazard to those around him and should be decontaminated. Warning labels or placards can assist in assessing the risks to both victims and out-of-hospital workers.

Decontamination of patients with radioactive contamination is somewhat different from routine chemical decontamination. The hot-zone must be strictly isolated from the warm and cold zones. Personnel entering the hot zone must wear protective disposable protection. They must also be monitored for radioactive decontamination. Clothing and other items removed from victims must be placed in containers to avoid contaminating others. Water used to irrigate must also be carefully contained to avoid ground water contamination. If the victim is too ill to undergo scene contamination, the best approach is to wrap him in a body bag or sheet (including head cover), and then transport to the hospital designated locally to receive radiation victims. The patient's immediate medical needs should be dealt with on-scene or in the ambulance. The receiving hospital can carry out decontamination while dealing more definitively with the patient's medical problems. After the incident, the medical director, in conjunction with state and federal radiation experts, can assess the radiation risks that occurred with all of the involved out-of-hospital personnel. Many hospitals are not adequately prepared to deal with contaminated victims of any type. The EMS medical director must take a leadership role in assuring that a receiving hospital can adequately deal with a contaminated victim.

Post-Incident Follow-Up

The medical director should be involved in debriefing those who took part in the incident. This session should deal with how things were done and identifying those things that could have gone better to correct any errors. Follow-up needs to extend to possible long-term toxic effects of the hazardous materials on workers. Long-term occupational health surveillance may be necessary, with the input of toxicologists and occupational physicians and other health workers, to prevent the out-of-hospital providers from becoming long-term victims.

Summary

The priorities at a HazMat scene are different from most other EMS responses. They are:

1. Secure the area and deny access to nonessential personnel.
2. Identify the substances involved.
3. Assess the risks of conducting victim rescue in view of protective gear available and the toxin present.
4. Decontaminate the victim if a chemical substance is involved. If radioactive contamination is present, prevent spread of radioactivity.
5. Evaluate, resuscitate, and treat the victim.
6. Decontaminate rescuers and vehicles as appropriate.

Caution is the best approach to these situations. The task of balancing the risk of injuries to rescuers against the risk of morbidity and mortality for the victim is difficult. The medical director may be asked to participate in the difficult decision of whether to risk rescue or not, and he must be prepared to do so.

Bibliography

Bronstein AC, Currance PL. *Emergency Care for Hazardous Materials Exposure*. 2nd ed. St. Louis: Mosby Co., 1994.

Burke R. Changes to the DOT placarding, labeling and hazardous materials regulations. *Firehouse Magazine*. 1994;64–70.

Cashman JR. Are we headed toward a Bhopal on wheels? *Emergency—The Journal of Emergency Services*. 1987;19:27–31.

Currance PL. EMS crosses hazmat lines. *JEMS*. 1989;14(2): 58–64.

Greenberg MI, Cone DC, Roberts JR. Material safety data sheet: a useful resource for the emergency physician. *Ann Emerg Med*. 1996;27:347–352.

Leonard R, et al. SARA (Superfund Amendments and Reauthorization Act), Title III: implications for emergency physicians. *Ann Emerg Med*. 1989;18:1212–1216.

Menze R, McMullen MJ, White LJ, Dougherty JM. Core temperature monitoring of firefighters during hazardous materials training sessions. *Prehosp Disast Med*. 1996;11:108–111.

National Fire Protection Association. *Bulletin 472 Standard for professional competence of responders to hazardous materials incidents.* Hartford: 1989.

National Fire Protection Association. *Bulletin 473 Standard for emergency medical services for hazardous materials incident response.* Hartford: 1991.

Proctor NH, Hughes JP. *Chemical Hazards of the Workplace.* Philadelphia: JB Lippincott; 1987.

Richter LL, Berk HW, Teats CD, et al. A systems approach to the management of radiation accidents. *Ann Emerg Med.* 1980;9:303–309.

Staten C, Hazardous materials: the EMS responses. *Emergency Medical Services.* 1989;18:34–41, 64.

Stutz DR, Ulin S. *Hazardous Material Injuries: A Handbook for Pre-Hospital Care.* Philadelphia: Bradford Communications Corporation, 1992.

United States Department of Transportation. *1996 North American Emergency Response Guidebook: A Guidebook for First Responders During the Initial Phase of a Hazardous Materials/Dangerous Goods Incident.* Washington, D.C.: US Government Printing Office; 1996.

CHAPTER 71

Multiple Casualty Incidents

G. Patrick Lilja, MD
Michael A. Madsen, DO
Jerry Overton, MPA

Introduction

EMS medical directors must assure that medical protocols exist for both the daily treatment and transportation of patients and situations that place unexpected demands on the system. At times an event occurs that overloads the EMS system with a large influx of patients for a short period of time; though such events occur sporadically, the system must be prepared; therefore, development of a multiple casualty incident (MCI) plan is crucial. The plan should be as simple as possible. The plan must be flexible and follow normal operating conditions as closely as possible.

Definition of a Multiple Casualty Incident

Though a number of events may be called catastrophic events or disasters, there is no one agreed-on definition. Natural events such as tornadoes, hurricanes, earthquakes, and floods, as well as man-made events such as large fires, explosions, or terrorist activities may cause large numbers of casualties. "Disaster" was the term used for an occurrence that disrupted the function or structure of a community with widespread injury or loss of property, but the EMS community now defines such an occurrence as a multiple casualty incident or, if devastating, a catastrophic event.

An MCI is a man-made or natural event that causes a large number of casualties and requires multiple responses in a timely manner to minimize injury and death. Depending on the size of the community, the MCI may or may not overwhelm existing resources and may or may not require outside assistance.

For large communities an apartment building fire producing 30 casualties represents an MCI that can be handled without outside assistance. In smaller communities, a two-automobile collision may require mutual aid from adjoining EMS agencies. An agency often declares an MCI whenever the number of patients exceeds three or the number of ambulances required to respond is more than two. Using this approach, a consistency in MCI response is established; responders and dispatchers do not have to ponder when the event will reach the level of activity needed for MCI plan implementation or, depending on that system's activity at that time, whether the system will be overwhelmed. Instead, the first arriving personnel can concentrate on what is needed—triage, communication, and patient care. The adoption of a standard definition also increases cooperation among neighborhood systems and prevents systems from abusing mutual aid arrangements.

It is important to clarify that an MCI does not require the routine activation of mutual aid. The most frequent use of mutual aid is when the demand on a system outstrips its existing resources or the closest available unit to a specific patient is located in another community. Whether mutual aid agreements are formal or informal, they should be recognized in the MCI plan.

Planning

It does little good to begin the planning process after the MCI has occurred. The properly designed and implemented MCI plan is a complicated undertaking. Once completed and practiced, a smoothly functioning MCI plan provides the proper and effective response to incidents as varied as automobile accidents, explosions, fires, or terrorist attacks.

The properly constructed MCI plan is both general and expandable. Plans drafted for specific response to a specific event such as a tornado or train derailment are ineffective. As society has increased in complexity, the potential for the MCI has also increased. For every coal mine collapse, there are many hazardous material accidents; and where many feared the widespread destruction of a hurricane, many now fear the widespread contamination of a radiation accident.

Instead of concentrating on a specific event, the MCI plan should concentrate on levels of response and resources. The rapid deployment of personnel, vehicles, equipment, and supplies may be necessary, and the source of each must be part of the plan.

Hospital resources must also be considered when preparing the plan. These considerations should take special note of any unique or specialized services, such as a burn center, that are available. Usually, it is not only the number of casualties that overwhelms a given medical facility but the type of injuries and the resources that the patients require as well. A large number of closed fractures not requiring operative reduction seldom overloads a community hospital; on the other hand, a large number of patients with penetrating thoracic or abdominal wounds may quickly outstrip the operative capacity of even a tertiary hospital.

In devising the plan, medical oversight must coordinate with other agencies, including police departments, fire departments, and emergency management agencies. Each has a management responsibility and a role in the administration of the plan.

The scene management of an MCI site involves much more than the provision of care to the injured. This management process is called the Incident Command System (ICS). The incident command system is designed to manage available resources of emergency incidents. There is an "incident commander," often the senior fire officer, who has overall command authority. If the fire department is not involved, command often falls to the highest-ranking officer in the EMS agency. Separate "branches" or "sectors" of fire, police, and EMS are established, each having its own command authority. The purpose of the incident command structure is designed to manage available resources. The intent is to acknowledge that all procedures will not fit perfectly within all departments and that departments or branches may have different reporting structures. It also acknowledges that not all portions of the plan need to be implemented in every emergency situation. It allows the agencies to work toward a common goal in an effective and efficient manner. It also is flexible enough to be expanded or contracted depending upon conditions surrounding the incident. Lastly, it allows agencies to communicate using common terminology operating procedures. Within the EMS branch, their functions need to be established under

the EMS incident chief branch commander. These functions include communications coordination, triage coordination, treatment coordination, and transport coordination, as well as dealing with medical materials. Depending on the size and scope of the incident, some of these functions may be performed by different individuals or a single individual performing multiple functions.

In developing the EMS portion of the plan, the system medical director must make sure that the EMS plan coordinates, parallels, and integrates with the other aspects of emergency preparedness. The individuals involved in overall scene management should function from the command post (CP). The CP should be near but not directly involved in the incident site. If they respond to the field as part of the response plan, EMS physicians must relate to and take direction from individuals more skilled in rescue situations. By planning ahead with the local hospitals, police, fire, and emergency management, the possibility of conflict can greatly be reduced. Unless the EMS physician is the manager, the EMS incident chief branch commander is responsible for EMS operations at the incident and the physician's role is not incident management.

Communications

In reviewing previous MCIs, communications is the operational component most often overwhelmed. When possible, communications must be performed through normal EMS radio channels. A plan that relies on additional communication networks, or changes the routine radio procedures, leads to confusion. The use of cellular telephones also poses problems because the increased traffic (both directly related to disaster activities as well as the increased use by the general public at the time of a disaster) ties up the available cells, especially in larger-scale MCIs.

All EMS units responding to an MCI should be assigned to a single channel by dispatch for coordination. In addition, medical information transmitted to receiving facilities should be assigned a separate frequency. Radio communications among agencies is important, but this should occur between the MCI command post and the EMS dispatch center rather than at the responding unit level. Interagency communication, if needed, is best done face to face at the command center. If this is not possible, it should be done on a separate frequency from that being utilized for EMS dispatch.

The first arriving EMS unit at the scene of an MCI should immediately inform the dispatch center that the incident is indeed an MCI, and should approximate the number of casualties. This begins the dispatch of additional resources to the scene. It is imperative that the dispatch center immediately implement the MCI plan, alert command staff, and notify potential receiving hospitals. Obviously, as more information is gathered from the MCI site, hospitals and dispatch must be updated. In addition, the initial arriving unit also must survey the scene for any hazards and determine if there is a need for specialized equipment and personnel. Triage communications generally occur between the triage officer and the EMS command officer. This may be accomplished face-to-face or via radio.

Once patient transport has been initiated, EMS personnel must be aware that they need to obtain and transmit abbreviated histories and physical exam data. During an MCI, there is no time to transmit complete reports on every patient or to expect lengthy radio orders for individual patients. Rather, EMS personnel continue to function under their protocol for standing orders and relay estimated arrival times, the number of patients, and the types of injuries to the receiving hospital or to the facility coordinating communications with the hospitals. Additional information unnecessarily uses channels needed by other personnel.

In most MCIs, telephone communications are unreliable because telephone systems are unavailable or overloaded at the site. Cellular phones offer a great degree of flexibility, but are also dysfunctional because they ultimately use normal telephone circuits. A system of communication that depends on the local telephone service should not be developed; rather, a centralized control facility must be designated to assess receiving hospital capabilities and communicate those capabilities to the MCI site so victims can be appropriately distributed. This communication link assures quick mobilization and effective use of hospital resources.

This centralized control must be linked by appropriate dedicated communications to hospitals in the system and to the dispatch center. Operating under its auspices may be a field medical unit with an EMS physician, serving as the scene physician in charge. Ambulances, rescue units, and other public safety units function under the ICS and in conjunction with the field medical unit. This model provides for rapid augmentation of field support from available hospital resources, and also allows the continuation of normal ongoing function of the hospitals. Finally, it can quickly be expanded without relying on new or different levels of commands or operation procedures.

Triage

Triage is an integral part of the MCI plan. It is not, however, mandatory that it occur at or even near the site of the MCI. Determining whether and where field triage should be initiated depends on three circumstances. The first is the number and type of casualties. The second is accessibility to the scene and the presence of ongoing hazards or dangers. Finally, the number of casualties must be compared to the available transport vehicles. If transportation resources are able to immediately evacuate all casualties, then field triage can be expedited. Field triage is necessary mainly when the number of casualties overwhelms the capabilities of the immediately available transport units or the resources of the closest receiving hospital. When field triage is used, the most critically injured patients are transported first.

Triage is initiated by the first responding unit and performed by the most experienced personnel at the MCI site. It is imperative that the individual responsible for triage is specified by the plan. If the plan calls for a change in triage officer as the incident progresses, then this protocol must be clearly indicated.

At times, depending on the scope of the MCI, multiple triage sites are necessary. Field triage functions most efficiently when victims are confined to a relatively small geographic area such as the site of a building collapse, fire, or explosion, and when the triage site is centrally located. In certain types of catastrophic events such as earthquakes or hurricanes, victims may be spread over miles. In these situations, initial field triage is still necessary before the patients are transported to a central triage location, called a casualty collection point, which may be the local hospital provided it is still functioning.

The system developed for initial triage is known as Simple Triage and Rapid Treatment (START). This system is based solely on clinical presentation and not type of injury. Patients are categorized as either high priority (immediate) or low priority (delayed) after three parameters have been evaluated. Level of consciousness, respiratory status, and perfusion status are all briefly examined, and if a deficit is found the patient is immediate. If all three conditions are within normal limits, the patient is delayed. Further triage is done by EMS personnel in the field or at the receiving hospital.

Another system, consisting of four categories, has been established for physicians or EMS personnel triaging patients. Category I patients require immediate care or transport. This category includes major injuries to the thorax, abdomen, or head for which surgical intervention or airway stabilization is immediately needed. Category II patients are less seriously injured but still require urgent medical or surgical care. The injuries are not immediately life-threatening. Category III includes patients with minor illnesses or injuries that do not need immediate stabilization. Category IV includes dead victims. This category may also include patients who are not dead but have obvious fatal injuries or illnesses.

The use of triage tags by field personnel remains controversial. Although many argue for triage tags in civilian MCIs, their use is not always effective. To be used efficiently, they must be implemented routinely for MCIs large and small.

Physicians at the Scene

Physicians, particularly the EMS medical director, may play an important role at a MCI. They have three functions, including (1) overall medical assessment of the situation with an evaluation of the scope of injuries and number of casualties, (2) triage, and (3) treatment.

Before providing overall medical assessment and establishing a relationship with EMS providers already on the scene, the physicians should ascertain the location of the CP and report to the IC. Should communication fall under their responsibility, physicians should update hospitals regarding the scope and number of casualties. Experienced physicians are best able to determine the degree and complexity of injuries and match them with the required hospital resources. They also must continually update hospitals with information. Critics cite numerous cases where hospitals either were not informed of a sudden influx of casualties or were waiting for patients long after the last victims were transported.

Physicians should perform triage at the request of triage teams and stand ready to assist in the decision-making process. Only in the rarest of circumstances should physicians render treatment at the scene, and they must never delay transportation to definitive care. Victims usually require specialized lifesaving medical procedures before transport, are trapped, or need ongoing life-sustaining medical care. Unless large numbers of physicians are available, their expertise at the scene of an MCI is most appropriately used in advising other providers rather than actually performing less-than-lifesaving procedures on individual patients. A single physician cannot function in all of the three positions—assessment, triage, and treatment.

There remains controversy about the effectiveness of field response teams, composed of physicians and nurses, at the scene of an MCI. In most situations, that response is not necessary. When it is included as part of the system's MCI plan, those physicians and nurses must be additionally trained to function outside their normal "hospital-based" environment.

Patients generally begin arriving at hospitals within 30 minutes, and another triage process occurs. Each hospital should have its own facility MCI plan, and the ultimate survival of a victim may be the result of quick action by the emergency department staff. EMS physician response to the hospital, with the provision of definitive treatment, is the final and sometimes most difficult phase of patient care, and thus must not be overlooked.

Physicians should also be aware of relationships with the press. Physicians involved with MCIs are sought out by the media, but the assignment of a public information officer (PIO) to the media is the responsibility of the IC. If the physician is assigned the PIO responsibility, premature release of information or speculation on the cause of the event must never be provided.

Terrorist Activity

The planning by EMS agencies for terrorist attacks has been forever altered by the September 11, 2001 attacks on the World Trade Center and on the Pentagon by terrorists using commercial airplanes as flying bombs. EMS agencies must be prepared to respond to a variety of potential terroristic activities which have the potential to include a catastrophic number of casualties. Such events may be due to explosive devices, chemical releases, and/or biological agents. EMS personnel must be aware of their own security so as to limit a chance of their becoming victims and not being able to provide treatment for the injured. Terrorists may use so-called secondary devices to go off after rescue workers arrive at the scene with the aim of creating additional chaos and furthering the number of injured.

The IC at the scene of a suspected terrorist action is usually the senior law enforcement officer present. A hot zone or internal perimeter is established to keep unessential individuals a safe distance from potential dangers, and to prevent terrorists from escaping. EMS or medical teams responding to a potential terrorist action should approach cautiously and check with law enforcement personnel before proceeding into the scene. Emergency vehicle staging areas should be decentralized, with vehicles well-dispersed to avoid becoming a secondary target. Communications can be monitored by terrorists, and care should be taken to avoid transmitting detailed locations of treatment sites or command posts.

Patient triage and treatment at the scene should be especially abbreviated to minimize the exposure of emergency crews and patients to gunfire or secondary explosive, chemical, or biological devices. In most cases, casualties can be quickly removed from the internal perimeter and transported immediately. If casualties exceed transportation resources and a triage and treatment area is needed, the site should be located in a protected location, and security personnel should be assigned to protect and monitor the area. Terrorists masquerading as victims or as rescuers may infiltrate treatment areas or hospitals. Therefore evaluation should be performed on all patients before they enter either the treatment area or the ambulance. The triage area should be closely monitored by armed security personnel to prevent weapons from entering the treatment chain.

The close liaison between EMS and law enforcement required at terrorist incidents is not well developed in most systems. EMS medical directors should develop a relationship with local and regional law enforcement and assist with the development of terrorism contingency plans. Some systems have successfully developed special medical reaction teams that train with the police special operations teams to rapidly provide medical care and evacuation within the internal perimeter.

Mass Gatherings

Mass gatherings are special circumstances under which an MCI occasionally occurs. This type of event places an additional burden on the system. Large concerts, athletic contests, parades, or political rallies can attract thousands or even hundreds of thousands of individuals to a single location. Such events require special planning because they result in an increased number of patients and also disrupt transportation. For example, streets may be closed to ambulances by the sheer volume of people.

A plan for any mass gathering should include aid stations, appropriately staffed and geographically dispersed throughout the area and throughout the crowd. Several EMS systems have bicycle or scooter paramedic programs that can respond relatively quickly through a crowd. These events may require alternative forms of patient transport such as stretchers on golf carts. Ambulances should be stationed at the periphery of the event with routes to hospitals predesignated.

Debriefing

After every MCI, debriefing sessions for the EMS personnel must be provided. Debriefing is an essential psychological support for the involved personnel. When providers confront a large number of seriously injured or dead victims, there is a significant, sometimes delayed, psychological stress. A formal approach should be developed prospectively to deal with such stress. It is imperative to have professionals skilled in stress management lead discussion groups with all involved personnel. Mental health professionals should be included in the MCI planning process and as part of the response team. The EMS agency should have critical incident stress debriefing teams that provide support for personnel who have experienced stressful incidents. Although it is not possible to entirely alleviate stress, individuals develop coping mechanisms that are greatly enhanced by appropriate therapeutic sessions. Should additional individual support be required by an individual rescuer, the mental health community should be educated to understand the special needs involved.

Summary

Preparing for an MCI requires a logical and tested plan based on the normal operation of the existing EMS system. The plan must allow both for rapid expansion and significant abbreviation of the routine treatment and communication procedures. If the plan is well defined and well rehearsed, then it is more likely to function satisfactorily when the MCI occurs. However, the first hurdle is to ensure that a well designed and smoothly functioning EMS system has been established and serves as the foundation.

Bibliography

Aghababian RV. Hospital disaster planning. *Top Emerg Med.* 1986;7(4):46–54.

Aufder HE. Disaster Response: Principles of Preparation and Coordination. St. Louis: C.V. Mosby Co.; 1989.

Burkle FM, Sanner PH, Wolcott BW, eds. Disaster Medicine. New York: Examination Publishing Co.; 1984.

Butman AE. Responding to the Mass Casualty Incident: A Guide for EMS Personnel. Westport, CT: Emergency Training; 1982.

Comfort LK. Managing Disaster: Strategies and Rating Perspectives. Durham, NC: Duke University Press; 1988.

Cooper GJ, et al. Casualties from terrorist bombings. *J Trauma.* 1983;23:955–967.

Crowley RA, ed. Mass casualties: a lessons learned approach, DOT HS 806 302. U.S. Department of Transportation, National Highway Traffic Safety Administration; 1982.

Cuny FC. Introduction to disaster management, lesson I: the scope of disaster management. *Prehosp Disast Med.* 1992;7:4.

Cuny FC. Introduction to disaster management, lesson II: concepts and terms in disaster management. *Prehosp Disast Med.* 1993;8:1.

Doyle CJ. Mass casualty incident: integration with prehospital care. *Emerg Med Clin North Am.* 1990;8:163–175.

Haynes BE, Freeman C, eds. Casualty Collection Point Guidelines. Sacramento: Emergency Medical Services Authority; 1989.

Jones GW. The Brighton Bombing, Orlando, Fla, Feb 1985. 1985 National Disaster Conference.

Kupperman RH. Conflict, terrorism, and civil unrest. *Journal of the World Association of Emergency and Disaster Medicine.* 1986;2:60–63.

Lauder P. San Ysidro slaughter: the EMS experience. *Emergency.* 1984;16:34–48.

Mahoney LE, Reutershan TP. Catastrophic disasters and the design of disaster medical care systems. *Ann Emerg Med.* 1987;16:1085–1091.

Melton JR, Riner RM. Revising the rural hospital disaster plan: a role for the EMS system in managing the multiple casualty incident. *Ann Emerg Med.* 1981;10:39–44.

Mitchell JT, Grady B, eds. Emergency services stress: 444 guidelines for preserving the health and careers of emergency services personnel. Englewood Cliffs, NJ: Brady Communications; 1990.

Noji EK. Disaster medical services. In: Tintinalli JE, Kelen GD, Stapczynski JS, eds. *Emergency Medicine: A Comprehensive Study Guide.* New York: McGraw-Hill; 2000:22–31.

Palafox J, Pointer JE, Martchenke J, et al. The 1989 Loma Pricta earthquake: issues in medical control. *Prehosp Disast Med.* 1993;8:291–297.

Sidenberg BS. Medical consequences of conflict and civil unrest. *Journal of the World Association of Emergency and Disaster Medicine.* 1986;2:63–68.

Super G, Groth S, Hook R, et al. START: Simple Triage and Rapid Treatment Plan. Newport Beach, CA: Hoag Memorial Hospital Presbyterian; 1994.

Tucker JB. National health and medical response to incidents of chemical and biological terrorism. *JAMA.* 1997;278:362–368.

Waeckerle JF. Disaster planning and response. *New Engl J Med.* 1991;324:815–821.

Waeckerle JF, Seamans S, Whiteside M, et al. Executive summary: developing objectives, content, and competencies for the training of emergency medical technicians, emergency physicians, and emergency nurses to care for casualties resulting from nuclear, biological, or chemical (NBC) incidents. *Ann Emerg Med.* 2001;37:587–601.

Appendix

Multiple Casualty Incident Protocol

A. Procedures for first responding ambulance crew: The first ambulance crew arriving on the scene will do the following:
   1. Conduct incident communications on primary dispatch channel.
   2. Quickly obtain information and *report back to the dispatcher.*
      a. Nature and scope of incident
      b. Number and type of casualties
      c. Best route into the area
      d. Possible ambulance staging area
      e. Any possible hazards, including if decontamination of victims may be needed
   3. Identify and establish contact with the Incident Command Post. Maintain communications throughout incident.

B. EMS Branch Director/EMS Incident Chief As soon as possible an EMS branch-incident director (chief) should be identified.
   1. Establish/maintain contact with incident command. Communicate needs to incident command (personnel, equipment, extrication, crowd control, etc.).
   2. Coordinate EMS branch activities with incident command and other agencies.
      a. Assure dispatch and hospitals receive current information regarding situation including:
         1) Need for additional resources
         2) Approximate number of victims and type of injury
      b. Establish ambulance staging area(s)
      c. Consider establishing triage/treatment area
      d. Assess need for the following:
         1) Need for separate radio channel
         2) Additional ambulance resources including air medical
         3) Traffic/crowd control for triage/transportation/staging areas
         4) Additional manpower, equipment, heavy tools, specialty teams

MULTIPLE CASUALTY INCIDENTS

5) Safe helicopter landing zone
6) Buses for multiple minor injury patients
7) Public/media relations to scene
8) Vehicle maintenance to scene
9) County Health Department
10) CISD team for defusing/debriefing

3. Evaluate need to separate EMS branch functions:
   a. Communications
   b. Medical materials (supplies)
   c. Transportation
   d. Triage
   e. Triage teams
   f. Triage area treatment
   g. Ambulance staging
   h. Air medical

4. Ensure all medical group functions are being accomplished by appropriate personnel. Relay needs to incident command, dispatch, or MRCC.

C. Communications Coordinator
1. Assume function as defined by EMS branch director or per service specific protocol.
2. Communicate information as directed by EMS branch director to:
   a. Dispatch
   b. Receiving hospitals
   c. Incident command
   d. Others as directed

D. Triage Coordinator
1. Complete rapid scene assessment.

2. Begin identification of patients (if used) using START at incident site and/or triage tags.
   a. Assign function to triage team for major incident
   b. Update EMS branch director with patient triage counts
3. Move patients to treatment/transportation area if established. Arrange for appropriate segregation of patients per service protocol
4. Oversee all treatment in the triage/transportation area.
   a. Assign functions to treatment coordinator if indicated
   b. May be assigned to "triage area treatment leaders" for major incident

E. Treatment Coordinator
1. Arrange for appropriate scene treatment by degree of injury.
2. Assign treatment function to team leaders as necessary.
3. Re-triage patients if necessary.
4. Request additional medical supplies/equipment to triage/transportation area. Make request through EMS branch director or his designee.

F. Transportation Coordinator
1. Designate a transportation area.
2. Assign patients to ambulances in coordination with triage.

Note: Patients should *not* be kept in transportation area if there are ambulance resources available for transport.

Catastrophic Events

Juan A. March, MD
Alexander P. Isakov, MD

Introduction

A major disaster occurs somewhere in the world almost on a daily basis.[1] Disaster management is a relatively young area of emergency medicine, which has grown out of a realization that catastrophic events do occur on a frequent basis. Management of these catastrophic events requires a complex multidisciplinary approach involving both medical and non-medical personnel to plan for prevention, mitigation, and management of the potential untoward effects which inevitably follow. The EMS medical director is an important member of those medical personnel and must understand the many different aspects of a disaster including basic definitions, etiology, preparedness, specific out-of-hospital issues and finally the federal response. Only then can the EMS medical director fully function as a true educator, medical expert, facilitator, and healthcare professional during a disaster.

Concepts

Disaster

A disaster is defined as a sudden or reasonably precipitous, unforeseen or somewhat anticipated event of such magnitude that it taxes and disrupts the rescue, relief, and healthcare resources of a community. The World Health Organization defines a disaster as ". . . a sudden ecological phenomenon of sufficient magnitude to require external assistance."[2] Thus, a disaster is an event that disrupts regional functions and activities, and causes concern for lives, property, and health of the citizens of the community. The American College of Emergency Physicians (ACEP) has offered the definition of a *medical disaster* as "when the destructive effects of natural or man-made forces overwhelm the ability of a given area or community to meet the demand for health care."[3]

The effect of a disaster on healthcare delivery is not limited to the emergent medical needs of the community met by emergency departments and emergency medical services, but also extends frequently to delayed consequences such as post-traumatic stress disorder. Often in the aftermath of a major disaster loss of communication, transportation infrastructure, adequate food and water, adequate shelter, and sanitary living conditions may contribute to the propagation of disease and prolonged suffering. Thus, during and after a disaster, there is a high demand for routine and preventative health services. Additionally, psychological disturbances, like post-traumatic stress disorder can occur. Subsequently, mental health services are also taxed.[4] The medical response to a particular disaster may include personnel from many medical specialties.

The term "disaster" often conjures up visions of major earthquakes, floods, or plane crashes. Specific natural disasters can often be related to geographic locations such as earthquakes in areas of tectonic instability, eruptions in the vicinity of active volcanoes, and meteorological disturbances (tornadoes and hurricanes) in susceptible areas. Unfortunately, some catastrophic events are less predictable, such as power outages, building collapses, terrorism, and armed conflicts.

Each of these events may result in a disaster situation, but the impact on the community must also be measured. For example, if a tornado touches down in a largely uninhabited area there may be little or no resulting damage to people or property. This occurrence would then represent a natural event and not a disaster. If the same tornado were to occur in a densely populated area, a major disaster may result. As an example, in 1971 an earthquake measuring 6.4 on the Richter scale occurred in the San Fernando Valley located in California, and resulted in 58 deaths and little property damage. However, in 1973 a 6.2 magnitude earthquake struck the city of Managua, devastating the region and killing an estimated 6,000 Nicaraguans.[5] Many factors such as stability of structures, population densit, and location play a role in the effects of a particular disaster. As such, it is important not to classify disasters solely based on the type of event or phenomenon, but rather on their impact to the communities involved.

Thus, the severity of a medical disaster cannot be judged simply on the type or number of casualties. The capacity of the existing medical system to deal with these patients also determines the impact. A small rural hospital may become overwhelmed by a motor vehicle collision involving a handful of seriously injured patients. In contrast, a major trauma center may handle such a situation on a daily basis without appreciable difficulty. The direct impact of a disaster on the physical plant of a hospital and the health of the hospital staff will also affect the system's ability to respond. Fires, power outages, communication failures, transportation difficulties, and structural damage may all seriously hamper the response to a disaster. The earthquake in Yrevan, Armenia in 1988 killed approximately 80% of the local medical personnel. Most died when the hospital in which they were working collapsed.[6]

For this reason, and in an effort to generate a common vocabulary as a means to compare and contrast disasters in the literature, several different severity scales have been designed. Scales may be based on the cause of the disaster, the effect on the community, the size of the affected area, the time for the disaster to make its impact, the number of casualties, the nature of injuries, and the time needed for relief services to clear the area.

The Potential Injury Creating Event (PICE) nomenclature is one such severity scale developed to describe disasters. PICE is designed to identify several aspects of a disaster such as the potential for additional casualties, the extent of geographic involvement, and whether or not available resources are being overwhelmed (see table 72.1).

Such tools are useful in retrospective research and in planning for future catastrophes. Knowledge of the types of injuries and illnesses associated with particular disasters is essential for creating strategies to prepare for proper distribution of necessary supplies, equipment, and personnel.

Disasters can be classified based on the following criteria:

a. Etiology: natural or man-made (e.g., hurricanes, nuclear disasters)

TABLE 72.1

Potential Injury Creating Event (PICE) Nomenclature[26]

A	B	C	STAGE
Static	Controlled	Local	O
Evolving	Disruptive	Regional	I
Dynamic	Paralytic	National	II
		International	III

The "A" prefix designates the capacity of the event to produce more casualties.
The "B" prefix designates the effect of the event on the municipalities' ability to respond to the event.
The "C" prefix describes the geography of the event.
The Stage designates the need for outside assistance.
  Stage 0—none
  Stage I—alert remote personnel
  Stage II—commit remote personnel
  Stage III—commit remote personnel and prepare remote hospitals for transfer of patient
  Example 1—A motor vehicle accident in a large city would be static, controlled, local, PICE Stage O.
  Example 2—A severe category 5 hurricane with persistent flooding would be a dynamic, paralytic, national PICE stage III

---

b. Location: single site or multiple sites (e.g., structural collapse, hurricanes)

c. Occurrence: single or multiple (e.g., tornadoes, earthquakes)

d. Predictability: expected, unexpected, variable

e. Onset: gradual or sudden

f. Duration: brief or prolonged

g. Magnitude:

  Level I: escalated response by the community resources

  Level II: more regional response, one in which mutual aid agreements between localities are exercised (e.g., Hyatt Skywalk collapse)

  Level III: the resources of the local community and its neighbors are overwhelmed; state and possibly federal resources are needed to cope with massive destruction (e.g., Hurricanes Hugo, Andrew)[7]

Fortunately, most disasters are of moderate size: 100 to 200 injured victims, of whom less than 15% are seriously injured.[1] As previously mentioned, classification is usually based on the level of resources needed and not on the number of casualties.

Incident Command System

In responding to a catastrophic event one must understand the basic concept of an Incident Command System (ICS), sometimes referred to as the Incident

Management System (IMS). Most fire, EMS, and law enforcement agencies currently use an ICS that provides for an organizational structure that can allow every emergency provider to understand the chain of command in the operations. This system identifies the individual in overall command of the activities and the individuals in charge of specific sectors or activities. Fire personnel are directed by and communicate with fire command, EMS personnel are directed by and communicate with EMS command, and so on. For example, fire personnel at a disaster scene may identify new injured victims and would contact fire command. In turn, fire command speaks directly to EMS command to relay this information. EMS command would determine a response and would then contact EMS personnel to respond to the initial fire personnel request. Only by having a unified and centralized command center, with all key individuals such as fire chief, EMS coordinator, and police chief all under one roof, can the system run efficiently. Constant communications between this operational headquarters and the field units is essential for the successful operation of any plan. Methods of multiple backup communications, such as ham operators and cellular telephones, are often important when routine communications (telephone landlines and radios) may be directly affected by the catastrophic event, such as a hurricane.

The ICS must define the following roles: command staff, operations, planning, support services, and financial sections.[8] The command staff requires a designated chief and a clear chain of command. The command staff is typically made up of at least three main individuals who are identified as: EMS command, fire command, and law enforcement command. The operations section should include a person in charge of each sector such as search and rescue, extrication, triage, treatment, transportation, and so on.

The ICS should also organize a planning section to collect and evaluate all information obtained from various sources, and to forecast future needs. The support section will oversee communications and personnel needs such as food, sanitation, shelter, and water. The operations section oversees the availability and distribution of supplies, equipment, personnel, facilities, and the like. The finance section monitors cost issues and anticipates the need for external funding and future requirements. Depending on the magnitude of the disaster, one person may be able to handle more than one of the tasks delineated above.

Triage

In most ICS schemes, an EMS provider is designated as the individual in charge of the triage sector. The concept of triage originated with grading the quality of textile materials. The concept of medical triage began during the Napoleonic Wars. Today, medical triage is defined as the evaluation and classification of casualties for purposes of treatment and medical evacuation. Medical triage is based on the concept of accomplishing the greatest good for the greatest number with the limited number of resources available at the time.[9] The objective of the triage officer is to prioritize patients into different categories based on injury severity. Once assigned a category, individual patients are then typically identified with a colored tag (see table 72.2). Although different methods for triaging patients into these different categories exist, data suggest that one successful technique is START. START is based on the concept of Simple Triage And Rapid Treatment using a patient's respiratory rate, pulse, and mental status (table 72.3).

Etiology and Consequences

Identification of the catastrophic events that are likely to occur in a given area is extremely important, since it then allows for preparation for the specific needs associated with each of the different types of disasters.[8] For example, hurricanes in coastal regions, airplane crashes at local or regional airports, hazardous

TABLE 72.2	
Triage Categories	
RED	Immediate/Unstable or critical—urgent interventions necessary
YELLOW (Stable)	Delayed/Stable—but require treatment to prevent decompensation
YELLOW (Prime)*	Delayed/Unstable—but unlikely to survive, so should be treated and transported only after all other Red & Yellow patients are treated and transported
GREEN	Minor injuries. "Walking Wounded"
BLACK (Dead)	In most disasters will not receive treatment so greater number of potential survivors can be treated.

*YELLOW (PRIME) or sometimes designated as BLUE expected to die. In some cases will not receive treatment so greater number of potential survivors can be treated.

CATASTROPHIC EVENTS

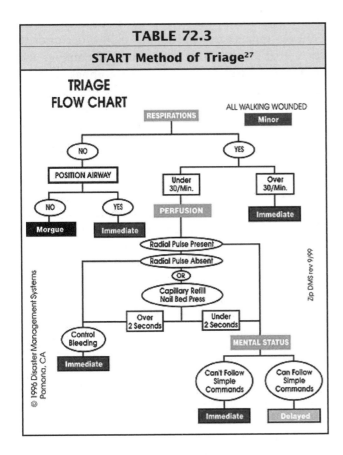

TABLE 72.3

START Method of Triage[27]

TRIAGE FLOW CHART

© 1996 Disaster Management Systems Pomona, CA

Zip DMS rev 9/99

materials leaks at industrial sites, accidental radiation exposure near nuclear power facilities, must all be taken into consideration when making a disaster plan or performing a drill. A disaster may be the result of a natural occurrence, a technological catastrophe, or a man-made event. Described below are a number of common disasters and consequences unique to each type.

Natural Disasters

Tornadoes are the most lethal and violent of atmospheric phenomena.[2] Although tornadoes usually result in damage to only limited areas, they often occur in groups, resulting in multiple areas of damage within a region. If multiple tornadoes hit an area, disaster management can become disjointed due to duplication of resources, unless a well organized centralized response has not been developed.

Hurricanes, in contrast, are usually less violent but involve large geographical areas and subsequently have effects which often manifest themselves over several days or weeks. In the recent past, early warning and proper evacuation have resulted in fewer deaths from the tidal surges caused by hurricanes.

During hurricanes, communications such as cellular phone and radio systems are often damaged due to high winds. In addition, underground telephone lines are often overwhelmed due to the massive increase in use. Due to the prolonged time that there is disruption of the usual day-to-day activities following a hurricane strike, psychological impacts are often seen. In addition, inland flash flooding has recently been associated with hurricanes. Even with an early warning system in place, over 50 deaths occurred from inland flash flooding in 1999 when Hurricane Floyd hit North Carolina.

Floods can involve small geographical areas such as the flood of Detroit in 1992, or vast areas as the flooding of the Mississippi River in 1993. For local preparation, it is important to know what areas in your region are potentially at risk of flooding. Furthermore, awareness of 100-year and 500-year flood levels will help toward better planning and preparation for such events. Placement of shelters above the 500-year flood plain will help prevent the need to transfer shelter residents in the middle of the catastrophic event. During a flood, loss of water pressure from the water treatment plant may significantly affect daily hospital operations, since loss of suction and dialysis capabilities may result. In contrast, loss of drinkable water becomes logistically very difficult when forced to transport and distribute large quantities of water to the general public.

The most devastating natural event is an earthquake. When of sufficient magnitude, not only does the community come to a stand-still, but hospitals are also significantly affected. In high-risk areas, preparedness is crucial. Structural collapses are common during quakes. Rescue activities require special search techniques such as three-point hailing, pounding, search dogs, acoustic detection devices, remote cameras, building stabilization, and extrication methods.[10] Recent improvements in medical care and the understanding of crush injuries experienced in quake injuries have resulted in better patient outcome in the most recent quakes. However, prevention methods, such as improving building stability to withstand earthquakes, are the ultimate key in reducing the severity of such disasters.

Technological Disasters

Fire disasters are common throughout the globe. Fire suppression methods and availability of necessary equipment will vary depending on the etiology of a fire. Proper equipment at the site of an airplane crash will differ from that needed for a forest fire.[11]

Toxic spills may result in the contamination of rescue personnel or of physical facilities, such as hospitals. Proper decontamination equipment and teams trained to deal with toxic spills are vital for proper management of these events.[12] The methylisocyanide leak in Bhopal, India and the phosphoric acid leak from a train tank car in California were both toxic spills which resulted in large numbers of casualties. These toxic spills clearly demonstrated the need for proper training, equipment, and personnel.

Significant nuclear accidents, such as the Chernobyl IV nuclear reactor meltdown, are rare but very devastating. Even minor nuclear events can cause public panic and pandemonium. As with toxic spills, proper equipment and training are essential in the management of nuclear accidents.

Electrical outages by themselves are rarely life-threatening, but the associated civil disorder can result in a disaster that must be prepared for.

Intentional Disasters

Terrorism is becoming more common around the globe. The destruction of the World Trade Center in New York and of the Federal Building in Oklahoma City demonstrate that the United States is not immune from these attacks. The release of Sarin nerve gas in the Tokyo subways indicates that terrorists are also becoming more sophisticated.[13] The simultaneous intentional aircraft crashes into the World Trade Centers towers and the Pentagon demonstrate the need for increasing vigilance and preparedness. As terrorists become more sophisticated, in the future weapons of mass destruction (WMD) such as chemical, biological, and nuclear weapons may be used. Preparation and treatment for the unique decontamination and containment associated with chemical, biological, and nuclear weapons are both costly and time-consuming. As violence has increased within our cities, the formation of tactical EMS units in direct association with law enforcement has now become a necessity. Civil strife such as riots or wars are not only devastating events for those involved in the conflict, but also to those caught in the consequences.[14]

Preparedness

It has become obvious from past experience that the optimal response is not achieved through improvisation at the time of the event. Rather, disaster preparedness requires careful planning and practice prior to the actual disaster. The importance of planning and performing drills cannot be over-emphasized. All hospitals are required by the Joint Commission of Accreditation of Healthcare Organizations (JCAHO) to have two disaster drills each year. Many local, state, and federal agencies are mandated to have annual disaster drills. However, it is only through a formal analysis of these drills and from the experience gained through responses to actual disasters that real problems can be identified and appropriately corrected. An example of this preparedness occurred with the Sioux City, Iowa airplane crash in 1989; the relatively good outcome was the result of planning that occurred after identifying problems during a drill one year prior to the actual event.

Often drills are performed without prior notification, a "secretive" or unannounced drill. By keeping the drill unannounced, only a core number of individuals know it will occur. Using this method, the paging system and telephone call list can be fully tested. Although ideal in evaluating the communication portions of a system, these unannounced drills rarely educate individual staff members regarding their pre-assigned duties or roles. Many disaster experts indicate that, by making drills preannounced with open public knowledge of the drill well ahead of the exercise, individuals can prepare and become more educated in the response process. For this reason, it is often best to have both types of drills, one preannounced drill to educate staff and a second, unannounced drill to evaluate communication activities.

Different disasters are prone to distinctly different types of problems. Thus, it is essential to incorporate various scenarios over several years when performing drills, to evaluate the many potential issues encountered in different disasters. Planning can be the most labor-intensive part of disaster management. The recommended considerations during the planning process are listed below:

- Establish planning panel members
- Identify the types of disasters that are likely to occur in a given area
- Identify the availability of local resources and limitations
- List potential problems identified from previous experience, the literature, and prior disaster drills

- Identify and address special training requirements
- Develop local policies to seek outside help from state or federal agencies
- Examine operational logistics
- Consider the possibility of secondary events/aftermaths
- Develop a comprehensive exercise plan based on the objectives and considerations outlined above
- Conduct a post-exercise review

The optimal plan requires a dedicated and cooperative group of community and government officials to devise a comprehensive disaster response and management strategy. During medical disaster planning, a panel consisting of law enforcement, fire, EMS officials, EMS medical director, other physicians, and nurses should work together to devise a unified plan.

In addition, local and federal agencies such as the Federal Emergency Management Agency (FEMA), military officials, Emergency Broadcast System (EBS), Federal Aviation Administration (FAA), and the National Weather Service may need to be included, depending on the type of disasters anticipated in a given area.

Identification of the availability and limitations of local resources is also vital. Rapid response of all emergency services agencies is essential for decreasing morbidity and mortality and minimizing property damage. The following factors are worth considering during planning:

- availability of community resources, which may vary depending upon the time of the day
- the season of the year
- the density of the population, which may have seasonal variation
- weather conditions
- the extent of advanced warning available

The National Weather Service tracking of a hurricane may provide sufficient warning, but the collapse of a high-rise building may not offer any preparation time. Often, the first responders are overwhelmed in these situations and there is an inevitable delay before the disaster plan is activated.

The level of care available within the community will determine the need for requesting additional regional resources. The accessibility of transport services, including air medical transport, must be known. Also, knowing the availability of physicians and nursing staff well versed in out-of-hospital care will help if physician/nurse teams are needed at the site of a disaster. It has been shown that there is generally no need for hospital-based personnel to respond to the scene of a disaster. Most physicians and nurses are trained to work in controlled environments and may find the unique "supply and demand" concept of rapid triage foreign to their thought processes, and overwhelming. For this reason, specially trained EMS physicians or emergency nurses should be used if there is to be a field response team. Rescue workers work well within their area of expertise, and many rescuers and first responders have a set routine in their practice, which enhances their efficiency. It is best not to disrupt this routine, if at all possible.

A key aspect of disaster preparedness is to learn from past experience.[15] This is accomplished from personal experience, drills, and review of the literature. Depending upon local and regional needs, implementing special training requirements and performing drills highlighting hazardous materials management, search and rescue techniques, tactical high-altitude rescue, and rappeling are necessary for specialized response teams that may be called upon to participate in disaster response situations.

As part of preparedness, the development of policies to quickly seek federal assistance is particularly helpful for certain disasters, including hurricanes, floods, terrorism, and forest fires. The local disaster plan in your area should have a specific policy to determine at what level of disruption the locale will seek and request state and federal assistance. The policy should provide for direct communication from the local Emergency Management Coordinator to the State Emergency Management Office. Knowing the assistance available from state and federal agencies is important. However, those resources generally will not be available and on-site for 24 to 72 hours after the onset of the event.

Another frequent problem identified in disaster drills is confusing and incomplete data collection. Patient identification, which is initiated by the field rescue and EMS units, is often ignored or changed at the patient collection station and the emergency department. The disaster plan must establish a smooth flow of accurate data so that patients can be tracked effectively and accurately. Disaster planning must also address operational logistics issues, especially information management and communications, since those are among the weak links frequently identified in disaster critiques. For this reason, a well organized and run ICS is crucial.

Often law enforcement, fire, EMS, and hospital personnel use different radio frequencies and are thus unable to directly communicate with one another. For this reason, it is critical that representatives of those disciplines be located at the command post. Dissemination of accurate information to the field workers, the command post, the victims, and their families must be addressed adequately in a disaster plan. Communication with family members, media, and the public is vital to controlling panic and misinformation. The plan should identify mechanisms to accomplish that communication. The plan must identify a public information officer, who should be the only individual providing information to the public media. This allows for a consistent source of reliable information about the event.

The disaster plan should include considerations for secondary events and other aftermaths, including public health issues, media coverage, epidemics, emergency personnel, public safety, security, and critical incident stress debriefing. Specific individuals should be assigned each of these tasks. For example, law enforcement should have a subgroup designated specifically for scene security. The public health director should be in charge of public health issues, including potential epidemics following a catastrophic event. Identification of a public relations officer is crucial, in order to optimize contact with the media and notify the public regarding important healthcare or safety issues.

Inclusion of all the above information into a single disaster plan results in a very complex document. For this reason, it is crucial that the plan itself be as simple and "user friendly" as possible for each individual. All personnel need to receive training regarding their role in a disaster situation and must receive periodic updates regarding the disaster plan.

Phases

The disaster response is often divided into three phases: activation, implementation, and recovery.

Activation

The activation phase of a disaster response involves both notification and the initial response. Following notification, a pre-established ICS allows for the rapid formation of a management and logistical unit, with an emergency operations center (EOC) or command center to orchestrate all aspects of the disaster response. Individual agency responses must fall under the overall guidance of the ICS to ensure a structured response, and cooperation and communication among the various organizations. For smaller disasters, designing a modular ICS will allow for a flexible disaster response and minimal disruption of routine community operations. The development of a modular ICS for the jurisdiction will ensure adaptability to any size disaster.

The command staff must define overall objectives for the management of the specific situation. Clear designation and structured delegation of roles and responsibilities are the keys for successful implementation. Throughout the disaster response, the command staff must constantly monitor all sectors for changing needs and unforeseen problems.

Involving EMS medical oversight early in the ICS activation can be especially useful since unexpected medical issues may arise. Having that resource immediately available can facilitate response activities.

Implementation

This phase is divided into search and rescue/extrication, triage/stabilization/transport, and scene management. During the implementation phase, the ICS command staff begins the process of ensuring safety and security of the site, proper notification of disaster team members, and coordinating initial response implementation with appropriate resources.

Once a disaster has occurred, the scene must be secured by law enforcement personnel. Fire command coordinates search and rescue (SAR) and extrication operations as needed. Once established, the EMS command coordinates personnel with advanced knowledge and skills to begin the process of triage, stabilization, and transport. The initial medical response is directed at the identification of injured or ill individuals, the assessment of patient needs, and the delivery of appropriate care. Use of properly trained and qualified personnel, skilled in appropriate life-support techniques, is crucial. Bystander assistance, if appropriately controlled and directed, can be helpful.

Organize the triage and stabilization sectors with physicians and other emergency medical personnel skilled in emergency assessment and care of critically ill and injured patients. Ensure that they are familiar with appropriate procedures directed at rapid field triage, stabilization, and transport.

During Hurricane Floyd, use of physicians stationed at a 9-1-1 center assisted the dispatch system in the triage of incoming 9-1-1 calls. Due to the loss of transportation infrastructure, EMS response and transport times increased significantly. The physicians stationed at the 9-1-1 center cancelled approximately one-third all EMS requests, having triaged these calls as non-emergency calls.[16] This increased EMS availability for true emergencies and could have potentially decreased the total number of patients transported to the hospital emergency department.

In routine emergency medical care situations, extensive time and expense are spent on an unstable, moribund patient. However, in a disaster situation where the capabilities of the medical system are overwhelmed, these moribund patients take a lower priority and more attention is paid to the patients with the greatest potential for survival.[15,17] It is often very difficult for emergency care providers to accept this concept, as they are accustomed to providing maximal care to these acute patients. Again, each situation must be individualized. If a situation occurred where there were many casualties, but the vast majority were stable, it may still be appropriate to provide intensive care to a critically injured individual.[17]

As mentioned previously, one problem commonly identified in disaster management involves communications. Often, the true basis of the problem is the result of poor organization, equipment failure, and human error. Incompatible radio frequencies and the unavailability of common frequencies severely hamper a coordinated disaster response. Proper planning is essential to ensure availability of initial and backup systems for both power and communications needs. Anticipate equipment malfunctions, guarantee the availability of spare parts, and procure compatible radio frequencies for the field rescue teams (Fire, Police, EMS). The on-scene ICS staff, the emergency operations center, and local medical facilities must also have adequate communications.[8,15]

What are often thought to be communication problems are often coordination problems in disguise.[8] Disaster protocols as well as training sessions must explicitly emphasize the use of standard communication protocols and not agency jargon. The importance of relevance and brevity during radio transmissions must be emphasized during training.[15]

Designate a clearly marked equipment staging area at the scene. During most disasters it is appropriate for all first response equipment and supplies to be taken directly to the site. However, as the magnitude of the disaster response evolves, a separate equipment staging area will help alleviate confusion and traffic jams on-site. This area should be located so that it is easily accessible and can remain in close communication with the command post. Keep supply trucks close but away from the actual site center of the disaster.

Logistical support is critical in long-term disaster efforts, and special emphasis must be placed on assuring the prompt delivery of needed items. A common problem during relief efforts involves the donation of large amounts of equipment and supplies to the disaster response. If not specifically solicited and needed, those donations may further complicate the response activities. During the response to Hurricane Andrew, expired drugs were taken directly to the scene, where they could not be used. The need to process them and dispose of them wasted valuable time and effort on the part of the rescue workers.

Another issue that may occur during hurricanes and earthquakes is loss of the transportation infrastructure, which may inhibit response activities and prevent delivery of patients to medical care facilities. When the transportation infrastructure is compromised, some disaster experts have recommended that local healthcare personnel form local disaster medical aid centers (DMACs).[18] DMACs are small mobile teams of local healthcare professionals, typically one to three healthcare professionals (physician and nurse/paramedic), who are equipped to handle most minor medical and surgical emergencies during the first one to three days following a major catastrophic event. Multiple DMACs are then dispersed in the disaster-affected area to provide decentralized medical care when transportation is compromised. In so doing, DMACs are able to free air-medical and emergency ground transport agencies and hospitals for true emergencies, or until a larger federal response occurs.[19] Use of DMACs may also potentially take a work load off the local hospital emergency departments, since most minor medical and surgical emergencies can be taken care of at the DMAC without transfer to the hospital.

In prolonged catastrophic events, the support sector of the ICS must also ensure adequate breaks for rescue workers. Monitoring of physical and emotional exhaustion to prevent short- and long-term psychosocial problems among the rescue workers is needed. If psychosocial problems are identified, conveying this information to the designated command staff of the ICS is crucial so that appropriate treatment interventions may take place.

Recovery

The recovery phase is often the least discussed, planned, or researched area of disaster management. Yet, it is critical for the community and the personnel involved in the response to assess what happened and how they responded. Every aspect of the disaster response including: prevention, organization, activation, notification, communication, field care, hospital care, government support, mutual aid, and equipment/resource utilization should be analyzed. Any deficiencies that are identified should be corrected immediately. Otherwise, the deficiency may be forgotten and simply repeated again during the next disaster. The recovery phase is also crucial to the long-term "wellness" of responders. Critical incident stress debriefings allow responders to discuss their feelings and actions. Individuals who may benefit from more formal counseling are frequently identified during these debriefing sessions.[20]

The Federal Response Plan and NDMS

Despite the best contingency planning of local and regional emergency managers, EMS medical directors, and EMS operations specialists, the magnitude of some disasters will overwhelm those local resources available through routine established mutual-aid agreements. A significant natural disaster or man-made event may generate large numbers of victims, or may result in severe structural damage to hospitals, nursing homes, pharmacies, and other essential medical facilities. Those facilities that remain open may be crippled by loss of public utilities, loss of essential staff, and a paucity of medical staff, supplies, and pharmaceuticals. Local resources for extrication and SAR may become inadequate to properly clear debris and treat casualties. Resources for transport of patients may be affected, and medical treatment facilities may be overwhelmed by the large number of casualties. Secondary hazards may result as toxic materials flow from ruptured sewer lines or damaged industrial plants. Water distribution systems may become inoperative. Mental health services may become overwhelmed in the wake of the catastrophe. Emergency managers and the EMS leadership should be aware of all these potential limitations in their local system. Even more importantly, emergency managers and the EMS leadership should know how to ask for assistance from state emergency management resources, and, if those should be overwhelmed, how to request federal aid through the jurisdictional hierarchy.

Recognizing what resources are available from state and federal agencies is essential for making effective requests. Furthermore, planning the integration of these services into local operations is critical for the most effective use of these valuable resources. Until local and state resources have recovered to the point that they are again capable of managing the disaster situation without assistance, emergency federal assets are made specifically available to augment and enhance the existing local system. Currently this type of federal assistance is made available by implementation of the Robert T. Stafford Disaster Relief and Emergency Assistance Act (the Stafford Act) and the Federal Response Plan (Public Law 93-288, as amended).[21]

The Stafford Act provides the authority for the Federal government to provide assistance "to save lives, and protect public health, safety, and property" in the wake of a disaster. The Stafford Act allows the President of the United States to declare a state or region a federal disaster area, although this must be preceded by a request for assistance from the affected state. Declaration of a federal disaster area by the President makes available federal resources, coordinated by the FEMA, through the Federal Response Plan. The Federal Response Plan serves to coordinate the activities of the many federal agencies that can provide resources in the event of a disaster, and thus avoid an uncoordinated, ad hoc response to requests for assistance. Many different federal departments and agencies contribute in a primary or secondary role to support the twelve emergency support functions (ESFs) of the Federal Response Plan. These functions include:

- ESF #1: transportation (Department of Transportation)
- ESF #2: communications (National Communication System)
- ESF #3: public works/engineering (U.S. Army Corps of Engineers)
- ESF #4: firefighting (Department of Agriculture, U.S. Forestry Service)
- ESF #5: information/planning (FEMA)
- ESF #6: mass care (American Red Cross)
- ESF #7: resource support (General Services Administration)

- ESF #8: health and medical services (Department of Health and Human Services)
- ESF #9: urban search and rescue (FEMA)
- ESF #10: hazardous materials (Environmental Protection Agency)
- ESF #11: food (Department of Agriculture)
- ESF #12: energy (Department of Energy).

The Federal Response Plan is managed by administrators at the federal, regional, state and local levels.

As an emergency physician or EMS medical director, it would be wise to become familiar with ESF #8, health and medical services. The support provided by ESF #8 includes "overall public health response, triage, treatment, and transportation of victims of the disaster, and the evacuation of patients out of the disaster area, as needed."[21] The detailed scope of assistance provided by ESF #8 is also available from other sources.[22]

The National Disaster Medical System (NDMS) began in the 1980s as the Civilian-Military Contingency Hospital System (CMCHS). This system was a network of civilian hospitals that were identified to augment the number of hospital beds available to the military, in the event that a war resulted in casualties that overwhelmed the existing military medical treatment facilities. Controversy existed over the mission of the CMCHS among healthcare professionals who were unwilling to participate in a program that was regarded by them as a contingency plan for nuclear war. Subsequently, the program was reevaluated and the NDMS was born. This program is a cooperative effort of four agencies: (1) the Department of Health and Human Services (DHHS), (2) the Department of Veterans Affairs, (3) FEMA, and (4) the Department of Defense. Together these agencies facilitate a national mutual aid infrastructure designed to address medical needs following a catastrophic event. This infrastructure is led by the DHHS and its Office of Emergency Preparedness (OEP). Each of the four agencies contributes its unique abilities, which culminate into a system providing field medical response, patient evacuation, and a network of hospitals prepared to provide definitive medical care.

A significant contribution of the DHHS is the organization of Disaster Medical Assistance Teams (DMATs). The goal of a DMAT is to assist in providing health care to a designated disaster area. A typical DMAT is comprised of physicians, nurses, paramedics, EMTs, pharmacists, and support personnel, usually numbering about one hundred and prepared to deploy a 35-person team to a disaster on short notice. The most capable, or Level 1 teams, can be ready to lift off in approximately 24 hours, and are prepared to deploy to the field with enough equipment to be self-sustaining for approximately 72 hours, at which time they would be resupplied. The typical DMAT deployment time is 10 to 14 days. Their mission includes provision of medical triage, medical care, and coordination of medical evacuation. They are expected to conduct these operations from their own tents, with their own equipment, generating power with their own generators, or simply by augmenting the existing staff and facilities in an area of operations. The field operations of the DMATs are supported by Management Support Units (MSUs), which are composed of command, logistical, and administrative support personnel, organized by the OEP, which direct and coordinate the activities of the DMAT in the field. The DMATs are a locally sponsored, community-based resource with volunteers contributing their time and expertise for training and readiness, with the support of the federal government. When deployed, members of a DMAT are granted temporary duty status with the Public Health Service. While "federalized" the members receive some monetary compensation, protection from liability through the Federal Tort Claims Act, and the privilege to practice their profession anywhere in the United States or its territories.[23]

In addition to the DMATs, OEP has developed teams that specialize in the care of burn victims, and injured children. They also have Disaster Mortuary Operational Response Teams (DMORTs) that provide mortuary services, including victim identification and forensics, in the event of a large number of casualties. Veterinary Medical Assistance Teams (VMATs) provide care, handling, shelter, and evacuation for animals.

The OEP has also developed a program to deal with catastrophic events associated with weapons of mass destruction (WMD), through the development of a Metropolitan Medical Response System. Through federal grants many cities in the U.S. have developed local Metropolitan Medical Strike Teams and National Medical Response Teams (NMRTs).[23] The goal of these teams is to respond to disasters involving WMD events to minimize the potential damage associated with these weapons.

The other three organizational components of the National Disaster Medical System offer their own valuable contribution to the functioning of the nation's disaster response system. The Department of

Defense primarily provides transportation, both air and ground, for the NDMS personnel as well as patients who require medical evacuation. The Department of Veterans Affairs provides administrative and medical facilities as well as supplies to the members of NDMS. The FEMA contributes to NDMS by providing personnel, training, and budgetary support.

The NDMS system had its first test in 1989 when Hurricane Hugo struck the Caribbean and pummeled St. Croix in the Virgin Islands.[24] Although the team successfully tended to 305 patients, the DMAT was not activated until day number eight and it took an additional three days to arrive on the ground locally. This delay was attributed to confusion and poor communications in the wake of the storm, as well as lack of clear assessment of the damage on the island. Among the recommendations presented after-action was a call for earlier activation and deployment of the DMAT. NDMS has since significantly improved its assessment strategy as well as made efforts to have resources readily available by pre-deploying assets to staging areas so that they might more quickly be deployed. Emergency managers and EMS directors should still expect to manage most catastrophic incidents locally for the first 24 to 48 hours while waiting for federal assistance to arrive. Furthermore, plans to integrate that federal assistance into the local disaster plan is essential.

The Future

ACEP has stated, "Improvement of established disaster management methods requires the integration of data from research and experience. . . . Emergency physicians must use their skills in organization, education, and research to incorporate these improvements as new concepts and technology emerge."[3]

Disaster management is a new and rapidly evolving branch of emergency medicine. Physicians who function on disaster teams must be able to rapidly assess patient needs, perform triage, and administer emergent care. The EMS physician must be adept in communication skills and logistical planning, and be able to work with a variety of agencies to ensure smooth functioning of their local disaster response.

As the field of emergency medicine continues to grow, so does research in disaster management. In the past, disaster medicine research was solely descriptive, but today quantitative studies are being developed and tested. In addition, this area of emergency medicine is maturing and a core content of knowledge has been developed. In the near future, it is likely that disaster medicine will become a subspecialty area of training within the field of emergency medicine.

References

1. Aghababian R, Lewis CP, Gans L, Curley FJ. Disasters within hospitals. *Ann Emerg Med*. 1994;23(4):771–777.
2. Noji EK. Natural disasters. *Crit Care Clin*. 1991;7:271–292.
3. ACEP Disaster Medical Services. Policy 400053, June 2000. http://www. Acep.org/3,345,0.html
4. Burkle FM. Triage of disaster related neuropsychiatric casualties. *Emerg Med Clinics of North Am*. 1991;9(1):87–105.
5. Bissell RA, Pretto EA, Angus DC, et al. Post preparedness medical disaster response in Costa Rica. *Prehosp Disaster Med*. 1995;9:96–106.
6. Angus DC, Kvetan B. Organization and management of critical care systems in unconventional situations. *Crit Care Clin*. 1993;9:521–542.
7. Wackerle JF. Disaster planning and response. *N Engl J Med*. 1991;324(12):815–821.
8. Auf der Heide E. Disaster Response: Principles of Preparation and Coordination. St. Louis: Mosby; 1989.
9. Hirshberg A, Holcomb JB, Mattox KL. Hospital trauma care in multiple-casualty incidents: a critical view (review). *Ann Emerg Med*. 2001;37:647–652.
10. Barbera JA, Cadoux CG. Search, rescue and evacuation. *Crit Care Clin*. 1991;7:321–337.
11. The Management of Mass Burn Casualties and Fire Disasters. Masellis M, Gunns S, eds. Dordrecht, The Netherlands: Kluwer Academic Publishers; 1992.
12. Leonard RB. Hazardous materials accidents: initial scene assessment and patient care. *Crit Care Clin*. 1993;64(6):546–551.
13. Noji EK. Hospital disaster preparedness in Oshe, Japan. *Prehosp Disaster Med*. 1995;10:94–95.
14. Pretto EA, Begorie M. Mission to Sarajevo. *Prehosp Disaster Med*. 1995;10:511–513.
15. Wackerle JF, Lillibridge SR, Burkle FM, Noji EK. Disaster medicine: challenges for today. *Ann Emerg Med*. 1994;23:715–716.
16. Harvey L, March JA, Tyson S. Physician initiated refusals of 9-1-1 calls during a disaster. *Ann Emerg Med*. 2000;29:421–427.
17. Pepe PE, Dretan V. Field management and critical care in mass disasters. *Crit Care Clin*. 1991;7(2):401–420.
18. Schultz C, Koenig K, Noji E. Medical response after an earthquake. *New Engl J Med*. 1996;334:438–444.
19. March JA, Dean E, Harvey RL. Use of a disaster medical aid center during a hurricane. *Acad Emerg Med*. 2001;8(5):524.
20. Mitchell J, Bray G. Emergency Services Stress. Lippincott: Englewood Cliffs, New Jersey: 1990.
21. Federal Response Plan (for Public Law 93-288, as amended). Federal Emergency Management Agency, 1992 p. ESF #8-2.

22. Roth P, Gaffney J. The federal response plan and disaster medical assistance teams in domestic disasters. In: Morres C, Burkkle F, Lillibridge S, eds. Emergency Medicine Clinics of North America: Disaster Medicine, Vol. 14, No. 2 1996;375.

23. http://www.mmrs.hhs.gov.

24. Roth P, et al. The St Croix disaster and the national disaster medical system. *Ann Emerg Med.*, 1991;20:391–395.

25. Koenig K, Dinerman N, Kuehl A. PICE nomenclature. *Prehosp Disast Med.* 1994:(9)565.

26. Risavi BL, Salen PN, Heller MB, Arcona S. A two-hour intervention using START improves prehospital triage of mass casualty incidents. *Prehosp Emerg Care.* 2001;5: 197–199.

Terrorism and Weapons of Mass Destruction

Richard M. Alcorta, MD
Robert A. DeLorenzo, MD
Jerry L. Mothershead, MD

Introduction

Few catastrophes are as frightening as the explosion of a nuclear weapon or the clandestine release of chemical or biological agents. In the past, such possibilities were only contemplated in the context of massive, strategic battles. A confluence of global events has created the perception of the likelihood of terrorist or foreign national attacks against United States interests, including the use of so-called weapons of mass destruction (WMD). This was confirmed by the events in New York City and Washington, DC on September 11, 2001.

Although most people equate the use of WMD with terrorism, these terms are not synonymous. WMD incidents should be viewed as extreme examples of technological disasters. A common theme in response to these events is the protection of lives and property. As such, the medical community and Emergency Medical Services (EMS) will be critical in the response to such events.

Overall strategy for countering both terrorism and the use of WMD involves deterrence, prevention, crisis management, consequence management, and retaliation.[1] This chapter focuses on consequence management; and provides understanding of the geopolitical changes that have fostered many of the concerns regarding WMD events. The evolution of terrorism and the use of WMD will be discussed. Governmental initiatives to counter these threats will be outlined, and the challenges facing the medical community and EMS systems will be discussed.

A Changing Global Landscape

The democratization of many countries of the former Soviet bloc and the relaxation of the perennial tension between Moscow and Washington at the close of the 20th century reduced the threat of major confrontations, although each side still has in excess of 6,000 nuclear warheads.[2] Side effects of the collapse of the Communist bloc, however, have been major economic and political upheavals in many countries of the former Soviet bloc, and new, less predictable, governments.

A thriving international black market in WMD has developed, and the boundaries of marketable property have disappeared. United Nations inspection teams recovered Russian-made ballistic missile gyroscopes and accelerometers from the Tigris River in 1995; guidance systems for 30 missiles remain unaccounted for.[3] The Russian government itself has been responsible for some disturbing actions. In 1998, Russia agreed to build two nuclear reactors in Iran.[4] This has raised major concerns at the highest level of the U.S. government, since Iran is known to be seeking the capability to produce nuclear warheads, and many of the technologies involved with reactor production are transferable. In 1995, Russian President Yeltsin nearly authorized an erroneous retaliatory strike against the U.S. in response to the launch of a Norwegian scientific rocket from an American Trident missile submarine.[5] In Russia, internal strife and lack of governmental control have been seen in violent conflicts in such localities as Chechnya. There has also been a trend toward regional conflicts in countries with relatively unstable governments.

Iraq remains the most glaring example of the continued inadequacies of the various international nonproliferation programs, although it is not alone.[6] Over 30 nations have failed to ratify the Biological and Toxin Weapons Convention, whose goal is the elimination of these forms of weaponry. There is little reason to assume that compliance with the Chemical Weapons Convention is better. In 1998, India and Pakistan tested nuclear weapons and North Korea fired an unarmed ballistic missile. In 2000, over 20 nations either currently had or were working toward the ability to deliver chemical or biological agents or nuclear warheads.[7]

Terrorism

The Federal Bureau of Investigation (FBI) defines terrorism as the "Unlawful use of force or violence, committed by a group(s) of two or more individuals, against persons or property to intimidate or coerce a government, civilian population, or any segment thereof, in furtherance of political or social objectives."[8] The U.S. Department of State has identified nearly 90 international terrorist organizations, and the FBI lists 27 organizations as posing a threat to U.S. interests. Globally, terrorist attacks have averaged between 250 and 600 annually for the past 25 years. Attacks against U.S. interests remained low (less than 100), with few injuries and fewer deaths,[9] until September 11, 2001.

Several incidents have highlighted vulnerabilities to terrorist attacks. The sentinel event was the Sarin nerve agent attack at the Tokyo, Japan, subway in March 1995. Twelve people died and 5,500 individuals sought medical treatment.[10] The aircraft attacks into the World Trade Center and the Pentagon demonstrated the first large-scale international terrorist attacks on the U.S.

Terrorism continues to evolve. Most governments are less willing to harbor terrorist groups, and have reduced economic support and safe harbor. Most countries are loath to supply terrorist organizations with the most potent weapons. Fear of discovery and retaliation are major deterrents, since terrorist organizations have been known to turn against their supporters. Therefore, terrorists have been forced to seek other sources of funding, through criminal activity or wealthy private financiers. They have modified their organizations to reduce detection and subversion; it is becoming increasingly common to uncover small "leaderless" cells that are harder for intelligence communities to track or penetrate. There has been an emergence of "rogue" terrorists, lone terrorists or small groups that evade intelligence detection.

In the U.S., several patterns have emerged among terrorist organizations. These include (1) new world order conspiracy groups; (2) single-issue extremists; (3) religious extremists and millenialists; and (4) white supremacy organizations. There is a great deal of comingling among groups, and it is not uncommon to find migration of individuals among groups. The U.S. also has its splinter groups and "lone wolves."[11] Motivations of terrorists appear to be changing as well. Terrorist organizations historically found it sufficient to "make a statement" or produce fear among the affected citizenry to attempt to influence governments, but increasingly they are more willing to produce large numbers of casualties.

Globally, the number of terrorist incidents is on the decline, but lethality of attacks is not. There were 273 international terrorist attacks during 1998, the lowest annual total since 1971. The total number of persons killed or wounded in terrorist attacks, however, was the highest on record: 741 persons died, and 5,952 persons suffered injuries. About 40 percent of the attacks in 1998 were directed against U.S. targets. The majority of these attacks involved bombings of a multinational oil pipeline in Colombia. In total, twelve U.S. citizens died and 11 others were wounded in terrorist attacks that year. The September 11, 2001 events resulted in the deaths of approximately 3000 Americans in NYC, Washington, and the aircraft crash site in Pennsylvania.

Weapons of Mass Destruction

The U.S. Code defines a WMD as "(A) any explosive incendiary or poison gas, bomb, grenade, rocket using a propellant charge of more than four ounces, or a missile having an explosive or incendiary charge of more than one quarter ounce, or mine or device similar to the above; (B) poison gases; (C) any weapon involving a disease organism; or (D) any weapon that is designed to release radiation or radioactivity at a level dangerous to human life."[12] Potential terrorist weapons may not cause widespread structural damage, and the term "Weapons of Mass Effect" might be more appropriate. Illegal use of a WMD is a capital crime in the U.S.

WMDs have been used in warfare throughout history.[13,14] Most recently, there were fears that Iraq might use chemical or biological agents against coalition forces or Israel during Operation Desert Storm in 1990. Although abhorrent, at least the use of these weapons was held under the guise of armed conflict. Terrorist use of such agents does not share this "legitimacy."

All WMDs are hazardous materials. A practical definition of a hazardous material is ". . . any material that, because of its quantity, concentration, or physical or chemical characteristics, poses a significant present or potential hazard to human health and safety or to the environment if released into the workplace or the environment."[15] Contrast a WMD to a toxic industrial material (TIM). Some of the greatest technological disasters in history have occurred as the result of TIM incidents. Examples include the radiation leak from the Chernobyl IV nuclear reactor or the methyl isocyanate release in Bhopal, India. The death toll from Chernobyl has been reported as 45, but this statistic only tells part of the consequences. Three republics, with a population in excess of 4.9 million, were effected, as were over 130,000 sq. km.[16] The Bhopal incident resulted in 3,800 deaths, 40 persons with permanent total disability, and 2,680 persons with permanent partial disability.[17]

Equally dramatic events have occurred in North America. Less than eight months after the Bhopal disaster, a similar release of cyanide occurred near Institute, West Virginia.[18] Only 100 individuals sought treatment, and none died. This incident resulted in the enactment, first, of the Comprehensive Environmental Response, Compensation and Liability Act (CERCLA), and then of the Superfund Amendments and Reauthorization Act (SARA).[19] The purpose of these acts was to identify and clean up America's most hazardous waste sites, and inform the public at risk from those sites. A train derailment with leakage of caustic soda, propane, chlorine, styrene, and toluene near Mississauga, Canada, resulted in the evacuation of 218,000 persons, six nursing homes, and three hospitals.[20]

Contrast WMD events with biological disasters. The 1918 Spanish Influenza pandemic may have infected 50% of the U.S. population, and produced up to 650,000 deaths in America.[21] In Europe in 1999, dioxin-contaminated animal feed raised concerns of widespread exposure to this carcinogen.[22] The possible 1998 link between the prion-induced Bovine Spongiform Encephalopathy and 40 deaths in Great Britain due to the human variant, Cruetzfeldt-Jakob Disease followed by the re-emergence of Foot and Mouth Disease in cattle, practically destroyed the British beef industry.[23]

Accidents have also occurred with known weapons. An accident at an Iraqi biological weapons depot in 1991 resulted in over 100 casualties and 50 deaths, from exposure to *B. anthracis*.[24] In 1979, *B. anthracis* spores were accidentally released in Sverdlovsk, Russia. Over 70 civilians and an unknown number of military personnel died as a result.[25] In 1943, German warplanes bombed Bari Harbor in Italy. The *SS John Henry*, carrying both high explosives and mustard agents, was obliterated; several hundred deaths were reported due to mustard vapor released as the result of the bombing.[26] In 1947 in Texas City, an explosion on the ammonia nitrate-laden *SS Grandcamp*, caused at least 468 deaths.[27]

Although military-grade WMD have the potential to produce the greatest numbers of casualties, the easiest to obtain are industrial chemicals (figure 73.1). Nuclear weapons are the most difficult, followed by biological and then weaponized military chemical weapons. Part of the problem in protecting society against TIMs is prevalence of legitimate industrial uses. Over 50,000 industrial chemicals are listed as toxic to humans, and millions of gallons are produced, used, and transported in the U.S. annually.[28]

Terrorist Use

Terrorist use of WMD is a low likelihood, high-consequence event. Much of the planning thus far has been for these overwhelming attacks, with the presumption that the same patterns of response and preparedness are equally applicable to lesser attacks.[29] However, any use of a WMD agent is costly for society. The emergency response in Tokyo to the Sarin release involved 340 fire department units and over 1,300 EMS/fire personnel. It is believed that the medical treatment cost for victims was $2.6 million.[9]

There were 520 global CBW incidents identified between 1900 and May 1999. There were 282 terrorist cases and forty percent occurred in the United States. Only 71 incidents included the actual use of a WMD agent. In most cases, the perpetrators did not seek to inflict mass fatalities, and in none did they occur. The chemical agents used included cyanide, rat poison, nerve agents, butyric acid, mercury, and insecticide. Biological agents implicated in threats or attacks included anthrax, botulinum toxin, salmonella

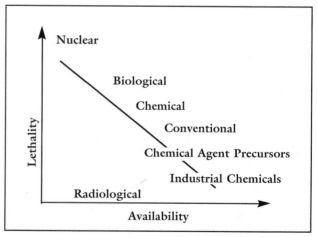

FIGURE 73.1. *Relative Availability versus Lethality of WMD Agents.*

bacteria, and the HIV virus. The 71 attacks produced 123 fatalities and 3,774 injuries. The sole U.S. fatality was caused by cyanide-tipped bullets used by the Symbionese Liberation Army to assassinate an Oakland, California School superintendent. Prior to the September 11, 2001 events, of the 784 injuries in the United States, 751 occurred in 1984 when members of a religious cult contaminated restaurant salad bars to influence a local legislative initiative.[30] In the United States, a mass-casualty terrorist attack with a chemical weapon has never occurred.[31]

In 1995, four members of a right-wing militia organization were convicted of conspiracy for planning the use of Ricin to kill law enforcement personnel.[32] Another individual was arrested after attempting to obtain *Yersinia pestis* from a laboratory.[33] This individual had been involved with attempts to obtain *Bacillus anthracis* and other potential biological agents. In 1995, Chechen rebels placed a container filled with radioactive Cesium in a park in Moscow.[34] In 1997 a laboratory worker in Houston, intentionally contaminated bakegoods and caused shigellosis among her co-workers.[35]

The terrorist weapons of choice continue to be AKA-47s, pipe bombs, and rockets.[36] Three-fifths of terrorist attacks are bombings.[9] In 1993, a truck bomb beneath the World Trade Center resulted in five deaths and 1,042 injured. Had the tower collapsed it could have caused thousands of injuries and deaths as tragically occurred eight years later when 2823 (nearly 15% rescuers) died.[37] In 1995, an explosion of 4,000 pounds of ammonium nitrate and fuel oil at the Murrah Federal Building in Oklahoma City injured 389 people and killed 168. The cost of recovery for Oklahoma City was estimated at $150 million and many individuals experienced psychological difficulties as a result of this incident.[38] Bombings of U.S. Embassies in Nairobi, Kenya and Dar es Salaam, Tanzania, in 1998 resulted in over 300 deaths and 5,000 injuries.[9]

Medical Effects

The characteristics of WMD are protean; (table 73.1), and include chemical, biological, and nuclear/radiological weapons, TIMs, conventional and enhanced explosive devices, directed energy, such as lasers, and cyberterrorism. The mnemonic "B NICE" (for Biological, Nuclear, Incendiary, Chemical, and Explosives) is frequently used to remember these categories. Twenty-first century weapons could be even

more troubling: bioregulators, fusion toxins, genetically engineered agents, and "ethnic" weapons targeting specific races might be possible. While it is beyond the scope of this chapter to detail the clinical syndromes of and treatment for victims of WMD agents, a degree of understanding of these agents is necessary.

The clinical effects of WMD agents and devices are as varied as the agents themselves, but usually produce their most devastating effects through respiratory, neurological, or immune system compromise. Portals of entry include the skin, gastrointestinal tract, and the pulmonary system. Aerosolized dispersion of agents poses the greatest threat due to the ability to affect a large population over a very short time. Because of current deficiencies in detection and identification technologies and the time between clinical symptoms and the window of opportunity for effective treatment, therapy may have to be instituted based on clinical syndromes while awaiting confirmatory laboratory diagnosis.

Chemical Warfare Agents and Toxic Industrial Materials

Nerve agents are the greatest threat. Treatment requires early, aggressive use of atropine and pralidoxime. Timing is critical. Anticonvulsants are adjuncts in prevention and treatment of nerve agent-induced seizures.[39] Patients may require large quantities of these medications. Other chemical weapons include cyanides, pulmonary agents, and vesicants. Their ease of manufacture makes them ideal for terrorist use. Treatment for some is complex. There is no specific antidote for pulmonary agents or vesicants, so mainstay of therapy is oxygen, bronchodilators, and rest, with vascular and ventilatory support for extreme cases. The key to minimizing vesicant injury is timely decontamination. The characteristics of selected chemical agents have been described.[40]

Biological Agents

Biological weapons are the most devastating.[41,42] A broad array of potential biological agents makes development of effective countermeasures difficult.[43] Toxins are naturally occurring chemicals, and include botulinum toxin, ricin, T2 mycotoxin, and staphylococcal enterotoxin B.[39] Infectious agents include organisms producing anthrax, plague, brucellosis, tularemia, smallpox, and cholera. Early identification is

TABLE 73.1

Categories of Weapons Capable of Producing Mass Casualties

CONVENTIONAL EXPLOSIVES	INDUSTRIAL CHEMICALS	BIOLOGICAL AGENTS	CHEMICAL WARFARE AGENTS	RADIOLOGICAL & NUCLEAR AGENTS
Nitroglycerin	Chlorine	Anthrax	Nerve Agents	Cs-137, Co-60
Nitric Bombs	Phosgene	Smallpox	Vesicants	Uranium
Military Ordnance	Acids/Bases	Salmonella	Defoliants	Medical Wastes
Fuel Mixtures	Bulk Toxins	Botulinum		Radiological
	Cyanide	Ricin		Pharmaceuticals
	Organophosphates			

For illustrative purposes only, not definitive or prioritized.

crucial to successful treatment, since rapid diagnostic tests do not exist. Many agents mimic common diseases initially, and there is a delay between exposure and disease. Diagnosis may be aided by specific clinical or epidemiological clues (table 73.2).[44] Treatment requires rapid use of antibiotics, antitoxins, and vigorous supportive therapy. Vaccines exist for only a few potential biological weapons, and for smallpox there may be insufficient amounts to treat large-scale exposures. Treatment for viral agents is limited to supportive care.[45] Most biological agents are not easily transmitted, and standard precautions should suffice, but viral hemmorhagic fever, smallpox and pneumonic plague are highly contagious; complete isolation, and treatment of close contacts, including health-care workers, is required.[46]

Explosive Devices

Explosions due to conventional and incendiary devices vary in magnitude, but far outnumber all other causes of WMD incidents. Medical management of victims of explosions requires an understanding of the major causes of injury: blast overpressure, fragment projectiles, and thermal burns.[47] Secondary effects, the translocation of the victim, and the crush and entrapment of victims by falling debris must also be considered.

Nuclear and Radiological Agents

Even a small nuclear weapon, such as those at Hiroshima and Nagasaki, can yield utter destruction to a large area, and cause considerable damage many thousands of meters away.[45] Nuclear devices cause damage through three primary mechanisms: blast, thermal, and radiation. Blast accounts for 50% of the bomb's energy output, and thermal energy 35%.[48] Burns occur and often present in combination with blast injuries. Exposure to radiation occurs at the time of the blast or as contaminated fallout.[49] Survivors may succumb to acute radiation sickness.[50] Radiological agents are found in hospitals, laboratories, and nuclear power plants. Unless released using explosives, primary hazards include short-term radiation exposure, or increase in cancer risk.[51] There is a great fear of radiation among the general population, and psychological disturbances could be expected in the aftermath of any release of radiation.

TABLE 73.2

Potential Clues to a Biological Terrorist Event

- Appearance of a disease not naturally occurring in a given geographic area.
- Unusual seasonal appearance, or atypical presentation, of a known disease entity.
- Combination of unusual diseases in the same patient populations.
- Many casualties with similar disease or syndrome in a circumscribed geographic area.
- Data suggesting a massive point-source outbreak.
- Primary aerosol route of infection, or other atypical disease transmission.
- High morbidity and mortality to a number of persons at risk.
- Sentinel dead animals of multiple species.
- Absence of a competent natural vector in the area of outbreak.
- Large number of unexplained diseases or deaths.
- Sentinel cases of disease caused by an uncommon agent.

Unique Features

There are many similarities—and significant differences—among natural, technological, and WMD events. These have a clear impact on the ability of communities and emergency personnel to respond to these events:

No Warning Phenomenon

Many natural disasters allow some degree of warning that may afford time for the populace to at least partially prepare. Technological disasters do not easily lend themselves to early warning, but other mechanisms are in place to mitigate the effect of these no-notice events.

Lack of Predictability

Certain areas are prone to particular natural disasters. Communities in areas with designated hazardous materials have Local Emergency Planning Committees (LEPC) to address needs and requirements of response to potential events.[52] So have communities near military chemical munitions stockpile and disposal installations.[53,54] Unfortunately, terrorists may target any community, and thus, risk assessments currently are of limited value.

Hoaxes

There have been an increasing number of incidents in the United States in which persons have threatened the imminent release of WMDs. Threats do not pose the risks that real events would, but they nonetheless consume resources. In 1997, the FBI opened 74 investigations involving WMDs, 181 were opened in 1998, and over 200 were opened in 1999. About 80% of these cases turned out to be hoaxes.[55] Hoaxes have an effect for terrorists, however, including producing fear, causing the expenditure of government resources, and undermining the confidence of citizens in that government. In 1997, a suspicious package received at B'nai B'rith headquarters in Washington, claiming to have *B. anthracis* resulted in a full HazMat response.[56] Since that time, there have been dozens of anthrax threats with multiple individuals receiving decontamination and some receiving medical prophylaxis. Hoaxes can also have a significant financial impact; it is estimated that 22 incidents in Los Angeles cost $5 million. Assessment algorithms have been developed for hoaxes.[57]

Criminality

In most disasters, the cause is known, and the final or projected extent of damage can be predicted. Risks are well understood, and danger to rescue personnel is minimized by appropriate safeguards. The criminal nature of terrorist WMD events adds several unknowns. Presenting signs and symptoms may be so non-specific that responders might not be aware of the actual causative agent, increasing their vulnerabilities. Further, awareness may be delayed, thus resulting in many more casualties. First responders might be targets. The instigators of the first World Trade Center attack in 1993 placed canisters of cyanide at the scene. Secondary devices were placed at a Birmingham abortion clinic and at an Atlanta nightclub.[58,59] In a WMD release, there may be a delay, from hours to weeks, in determining the extent of the affected area. Delays allow geographic spread of the agents due to environmental factors or migration of victims. Contagious agents further compound the problem through secondary transmission. Sentinel cases could appear in several communities concurrently by either of these methods. The needs of law enforcement agencies are of paramount importance. Restrictions might affect procedures in all aspects of recovery operations. A balance must be sought between evidence preservation and the needs and rights of victims.

Non-Traditional First Responders

In most disasters, highly trained organizations are involved as first responders. Organizations include fire services, hazardous materials units, EMS systems, and urban search-and-rescue squads. Hospitals normally become involved later. Scene conditions provide a choke point that reduces the rate of victim arrival at hospitals and thus maintains some orderliness to hospital emergency operations. In covert releases, first response functions might fall on individuals not accustomed to this role, such as primary care and emergency physicians. Chemical releases pose another hazard with little infrastructure damage to impede victim egress, and hospitals could very well be inundated with casualties. In the Tokyo subway incident, over 600 victims arrived at the nearest hospitals within 45 minutes of the disaster.

Magnitude of the Number of Casualties

Disaster planners in this country have limited experience with the large numbers of injured and fatalities that could be generated by the release of a WMD. Casualty counts will depend on a myriad of unknowns, such as weapon type and load, meteorological conditions, and population densities. However, statistical modeling suggests that chemical weapons casualties could number in the hundreds, and biological weapons casualties could number in the thousands to tens of thousands.[29] In traditional disasters, the vast majority of fatalities occur at the time of the disaster. The time course of WMD events is such that fatalities are likely to increase dramatically over several days to a week.

Requirements for Additional Equipment and Supplies

Rapid, accurate detection, presumptive identification, and mapping of geographically affected areas and populations are necessary. Equipment and supplies to be able to do that are not currently available, or are in short supply. Traditional hazardous materials units are not equipped for this role. Most communities have disaster caches designed for victims of trauma, and treatment at fixed facilities is geared heavily toward surgical intervention. Care for WMD victims is skewed heavily toward medical problems, including ventilator support, and treatment relies on early chemoprophylaxis, antibiotic therapy, or administration of specific antidotes, currently in limited supply or nonexistent at the local level.

Requirements for Mental Health Services

Experts anticipate a 5:1 ratio of those requiring only counseling in the wake of such events, to actual casualties requiring medical care.[60] Psychological victims include victims themselves, families, emergency responders, healthcare workers, and the community in general.[61] Nearly 68% of the EMS first responders involved in the Oklahoma City incident have resigned or been reassigned, often due to the emotional impact of the event. The impact might have been higher without critical incident stress management (CISM) interventions.[62]

WMD Congressional Initiatives

Both Congressional legislation and Presidential Decision Directives have shaped federal initiatives and programs to deal with terrorism and WMD events. In 1997, Congress enacted the Defense Against Weap-

ons of Mass Destruction Act (the Nunn-Lugar-Domenici Act) that included the Emergency Response Assistance Program. Purposes of the program, and resultant initiatives, were to:[63]

1. Provide civilian response personnel with loan of, and training in the use of, operation, and maintenance of WMD detection and monitoring equipment, and provide assistance to those personnel in protecting emergency personnel and the public and provide for further decontamination capabilities. The Secretary of Defense was assigned as lead official over the "Domestic Preparedness Program." The U.S. Army was charged with enhancing existing metropolitan capabilities. Training courses have been developed for Awareness, Operations, Emergency Medical, Technician-HAZMAT, Hospital Provider, and Incident Command.[64] In 1999, program oversight was transferred to the National Domestic Preparedness Office of the FBI, and in April 2000 the President transferred lead official responsibilities to the Attorney General.

2. Establish a capability for officials responding to emergencies involving a WMD to rapidly contact and consult with experts. The non-emergency Chemical and Biological (CB) HelpLine (1-800-368-6498) provides emergency managers with information helpful in the planning and mitigation of the effects of a chemical or biological terrorist incident. The CB HotLine (1-800-424-8802) serves as an emergency technical assistance resource for first responders. Other federal agencies can be accessed within a few minutes to provide technical assistance during a potential CB incident. If warranted, a federal response action may be initiated.[65]

3. Authorize use of the National Guard and other military reserve components in responding to WMD. WMD Civil Support Teams (WMD-CST) have been developed. They can be rapidly deployed to assist in determining the extent of an incident, provide technical advice on response operations, and support the arrival of additional state and federal military assets. Thirty-two teams are expected to be operational by 2002. Each team consists of 22 members of the National Guard, and has a mobile laboratory for field analysis for chemical or biological agents, and a command and communications suite. WMD-CSTs are unique because of their federal-state relationship. They are fed-

erally resourced and trained, and operate under federal doctrine, but are under the command of the Adjutant Generals of the assigned states. If a governor requests the President to declare of national disaster, the team would continue to support local officials in their state status. If federalized, teams would fall under operational control of the Joint Task Force-Civil Support, a recently established military command whose sole functions are training and response to WMD events.[65]

4. Require the Department of Defense (DoD) to provide assistance to the Department of Justice in enforcement during an emergency situation involving a WMD, and to field a domestic terrorism rapid response team. The function of the Chemical and Biological Rapid Response Team (CBRRT) is to coordinate DoD's chemical and biological defense support to civil authorities in the event of a terrorist incident. CBRRT can provide the following services:

   ■ Dismantle, transport, disposition/dispose and neutralize agents/devices;
   ■ Monitor/provide hazard prediction, detection, analysis, mitigation and containment;
   ■ Advise and support patient decontamination, triage, transport, and treatment; and
   ■ Provide technical advice and expertise on chemical and biological issues.[39]

5. Allocate funds to the Department of Health and Human Services (DHHS) to establish civilian response teams in the largest metropolitan areas of the country. As of September 1999, 45 Metropolitan Medical Response Systems (MMRS) have been formed, and funds were allocated in fiscal year 2000 to establish 27 more teams.[66]

6. Require the Director of Federal Emergency Management Agency (FEMA) to incorporate guidance into the Federal Response Plan (FRP) for responding to WMD and to develop a rapid response information system for use by civilian response organizations. The Terrorist Incident Annex to the FRP defines the policies and structures to coordinate crisis management with consequence management.[67] The Rapid Response Information System is Internet-based and consists of information on WMD agent characteristics, first aid measures, federal response capabilities, and other information.[68]

7. Require the Secretary of Energy to develop and carry out a program for testing and improving civilian agency responses to emergencies involving nuclear and radiological weapons. The Department of Energy has been involved with detection and mitigation of the effects of nuclear and radiological materials for decades, and has been progressing on initiatives to improve detection, monitoring, decontamination, and clean-up.

8. Provide for annual exercises and improving the response to emergencies involving WMD. Increasingly larger, full-scale exercises have occurred, with more planned in future years.

Executive Orders

Between 1995 and 1998, the President promulgated three separate executive orders, referred to as Presidential Decision Directives (PDD), specifically targeting terrorism and WMD:

PDD 39

U.S. Policy on Counterterrorism[69] details U.S. policy to deter, defeat and respond vigorously to all terrorist attacks.[69] It also provides direction to federal agencies concerning actions to reduce vulnerabilities, deter terrorism, and respond to terrorism. An important distinction was made in the federal response to terrorist use of a WMD. Crisis management includes "measures to identify, acquire, and plan the use of resources needed to anticipate, prevent, and/or to resolve a threat or act of terrorism." Primary authority for crisis management has been assigned to the federal government; state and local governments provide assistance as required. Crisis management is predominantly a law enforcement response. The FBI has been designated as Lead Federal Agency (LFA) for crisis management in the U.S., and the State Department for foreign incidents. Consequence management includes "measures to protect public health and safety, restore essential government services, and provide emergency relief to governments, business, and individuals affected by the consequences of terrorism." Primary authority for consequence management remains with the state and local authorities, with the federal government providing assistance if required. FEMA remains the LFA for consequence management. The State Department was tasked to develop a plan with the Office of Foreign Disaster

Assistance and the DoD to provide for assistance to other countries.

PDD 62

This directive on combating terrorism created a more systematic approach to fighting the terrorist threat. It clarified federal agency activities in the wide range of U.S. counter-terrorism programs, from apprehension and prosecution of terrorists to increasing transportation security, enhancing response capabilities and protecting the computer-based systems.[70] It tasked the U.S. Public Health Service (USPHS) and the Department of Veterans Affairs (DVA) to ensure adequate stockpiles of antidotes and other necessary equipment nationwide, and to train medical personnel in hospitals enrolled with the National Disaster Medical System (NDMS).

PDD 63

This directive on critical infrastructure protection cited the increasingly national reliance on certain critical infrastructures such as those physical and cyber-based systems essential to the minimum operations of the economy and government. It outlined a program to develop and maintain the ability to protect critical infrastructures and systems.[70]

Antiterrorism Resources

Any or all of the 27 federal agencies and organizations designated in the FRP could become involved in a terrorist WMD event. Many of these agencies have capabilities specifically to respond to such incidents. A partial listing may be found in Appendix A. The DHHS, DVA, and DoD are particularly important in the medical response to WMD events.

DHHS

DHHS may participate in federal response to terrorist or WMD incidents under the FRP or the Public Health Service Act.[71] It is the oversight agency for federal health and medical assistance in the event of a national disaster. A number of offices within DHHS have important roles. The Office of Emergency Preparedness (OEP) is responsible for national implementation and coordination of health and medical response operations. OEP directs and manages the NDMS, a partnership between DHHS, DoD, DVA,

FEMA, State and local governments, private businesses and civilian volunteers. Over 2,000 hospitals have voluntarily committed, subject to availability, over 100,000 beds for the receipt of patients from a domestic emergency or military contingency.[72]

OEP provides oversight to volunteer Disaster Medical Assistance Teams (DMATs) as part of WMDs. Responsibilities of these teams include triage, austere medical care, and preparation for evacuation. DMATs also provide primary health care. DMATs may be activated to support patient reception at evacuation receiving locations. There are presently over 60 DMATs, 26 at level I, fully capable of response within six hours of activation, and self-sustaining for 72 hours.[73] There are also highly specialized DMATs that deal with specific medical conditions such as crush injury, burn, pediatric, and mental health emergencies. Other specialty teams include Disaster Mortuary Teams (DMORTs) and Veterinary Medical Assistance Teams (VMATs). There are four National Medical Response Teams (NMRTs), located in Washington, Raleigh-Durham, Los Angeles, and Denver, specifically equipped and trained to provide medical care for victims of weapons of mass destruction.

The Centers for Disease Control and Prevention (CDC) has developed a strategic plan to address rapid identification of biological agents or emerging infections.[74] This plan includes a public health communication infrastructure, a multilevel network of private, state and federal diagnostic laboratories, and an integrated disease surveillance system.

The Division of Health Assessment and Consultation (DHAC) of the Agency for Toxic Substances and Disease Registry manages an emergency response and site-specific health consultation program. DHAC provides advice on specific public health issues related to hazardous materials. An important component of the emergency response program is training first responders to hazardous materials releases. DHAC has developed guidance documents that address the proper handling, decontamination, and treatment of chemically contaminated patients.[75]

DVA

DVA has a number of important roles in the medical response to terrorism with WMD.[76]

DVA provides hospital beds through the NDMS,[77] and has responsibility for 49 NDMS Federal Coordinating Centers (FCCs) that oversee all aspects of NDMS implementation, planning, exercise, and operation within the designated geographic areas of responsibility. Disaster Emergency Medical Personnel System is a database of information on VHA personnel who have volunteered to be deployed in the event of a disaster. DVA maintains four caches of pharmaceuticals at several locations throughout the United States to treat victims of a WMD event. DVA also has an agreement with CDC to assist with maintenance of the National Pharmaceutical Stockpile, separate from the NMRT stores.

DoD

DoD has numerous teams and specialty commands besides CBRRT. DoD is part of the NDMS, and can provide hospital beds, medical personnel, and supplies. Although the total number of hospital beds (6,000) are a fraction of total NDMS inventory, all services have deployable palletized hospitals, ranging in size from a few hundred to 1000 beds. The Navy has two 1000-bed hospital ships and several amphibious landing ships that double as casualty receiving platforms that could be used for coastal events. Land-based deployable hospitals require many acres of land, and all could take up to two weeks to fully mobilize. With over 14,000 active-duty physicians, and many more nurses and ancillary staff, the services could potentially serve as a large manpower pool at the site of the event. These resources would take time to mobilize, and recall of reserve personnel would be necessary to replace those mobilized for a response. DoD directives allow for immediate local assistance. A military commander may provide assistance to prevent loss of life or severe property damage as the result of any disaster, under the "Immediate Response" clause. Capabilities and military requirements will dictate what resources might be available from local military installations and medical facilities.[78] An extensive array of medical and other laboratories, such as the Defense Advanced Research Projects Agency and the Naval Research Laboratory, either perform or contract for research in a variety of fields with applicability to domestic preparedness. The U.S. Army Medical Research Institute of Infectious Diseases has one of only two Biological Level IV laboratories in the United States, the other being at CDC. The Armed Forces Medical Information Center is the prime vendor for medical intelligence to virtually all intelligence communities in the federal government.

Federal government involvement in domestic preparedness is extensive. There are over 40 federal departments and agencies involved, with many more working groups and subordinate offices.[79] Unnecessary duplication and resource expenditures were, in part, the impetus for designating the FBI NDPO as the central clearinghouse for information during responses to WMD events.[31]

These vast capabilities do come with a cost. The federal government expenditure for these initiatives has grown steadily, to a $10 billion for fiscal year 2000.[80] Some of the larger expenditures are meant to improve surveillance and medical response capabilities, and for the National Pharmaceutical Stockpile Program including eight 12-hour response "push packages" which are rapidly deployable pharmaceutical caches and 24-hour deployable Vendor Managed Inventories supplies.[66] Federal funding has come under scrutiny, as the Government Accounting Office has issued a number of reports critical of the management and oversight of some of these programs.[81–85]

Responses

Local Response

Disasters are a local phenomenon, and state and federal agencies will require time to mobilize resources. Local EMS agencies, fire departments, and other community assets will be the first line of defense in disaster response. The level of response will be predicated on a number of factors. There are, however, notable differences in the way that events might unfold in a WMD event, from traditional disasters. Most disasters allow some time, from minutes to days, for warning emergency management agencies and personnel. There also are specific geographic tendencies for many natural disasters, which can be anticipated based on historical records. The potential of technological disasters is usually at those locations where the hazards exist (e.g., near factories or major transportation routes), and this knowledge heightens awareness and thus may enhance warning capabilities. Terrorist-induced disasters can occur anywhere; all communities require response capability. Warning may be enhanced by specific surveillance measures in an attempt to identify potential events before or soon after they occur.

Expedient notification of events and response instructions must be provided. The public will need to know information about the affected areas, and initial instructions to enhance personal protection (evacuation routes or sheltering-in-place). The exact types of response immediately required will again be dependent on the particular weapon released, and whether the release was announced, a no-notice but overt release, or a subsequently identified covert attack.

Chemical Agent Release

Chemical agent releases are apt to be discovered immediately or shortly afterwards. The worst-case scenario is a no-notice release of a nerve agent near a mass gathering. Initial responders would have clues concerning the nature of the incident—multiple patients affected simultaneously with identical or similar symptoms in a defined geographic area. Functions performed would be similar to any industrial hazardous material (table 73.3).[86] Medical personnel will not perform the majority of these functions. However, there are certain aspects of the response to a release of a chemical agent that bear further consideration. Unless otherwise obvious, it must be presumed that any mass casualty incident involving primarily medical conditions is the result of a terrorist act. Contamination or secondary devices must always be considered. Dispatchers must be trained to identify this possibility and alert command and control centers, responders, and specialty units.

Agents released in closed quarters will likely not spread significantly outside the site of release. With little opportunity for dissipation of the agent, casualties might be more severely affected than if the agent had been able to spread out. An outside release will produce fewer or less severely affected casualties, but the safe perimeter will have to be greatly extended. Meteorological conditions and anticipated plume path will need to be expeditiously determined. All rescue personnel will need to be alert for wind shifts. Commercial hazardous material detection equipment do not detect some weaponized agents. Initial rescu-

ers must have appropriate personal protective equipment. This may require fully encapsulated suits and self-contained breathing apparatuses. This will decrease on-scene time due to thermal stresses from suits and limited air supplies due to tank capacities.

Rescue personnel require training in the unique aspects of initial triage and treatment in contaminated areas. A rescuer might be overwhelmed within the contamination zone, and a subset of EMS responders must be prepared to enter the contaminated zone to treat rescuers or others entrapped there. Decontamination and the initiation of treatment may need to be done expeditiously. Patients might require stabilization prior to full decontamination. Recommendations concerning mass decontamination of chemical agents and a modified version of the Simple Triage and Rapid Treatment (START) system have been developed.[87] Forensic issues will exist at the scene. All materials, including patient clothing and the deceased, are potentially evidence that can be helpful in criminal investigations. Traffic flow will be critical. Ambulances must be routed to predesignated hospitals, based on local protocols that take into account bed capacity, decontamination facilities, staff availability, and other local parameters. Unless victims can be certified as decontaminated, there should be safeguards to reduce inadvertent contamination of vehicles, EMS personnel in those vehicles, or receiving facilities. The appropriateness of receiving facilities must be determined prior to the incident. There is the possibility that any facility could receive self-referred contaminated casualties. Historically, less than 18% of all victims of traditional hazardous materials exposure are decontaminated prior to arrival at hospitals.[88] All facilities must have the capability to restrict access, and must be capable of providing decontamination of these self-referred victims. Many facilities do not have the capability of mass decon-

TABLE 73.3	
Response Actions at Chemical Agent Release Site	
Scene assessment	Decontamination of victims and rescuers
Establishment of perimeter zones	Triage of ill/injured
Agent identification	Field medical care
Donning of protective equipment	Transport of patients to hospitals
Establishment of decontamination areas	Medical evaluation of rescuers
Entry planning/preparation of equipment	Stabilization of the released agent
Victim rescue	Evidence collection
Containment of release	Final clean up
Neutralization of agent	Certify safe

tamination.[89] The potential for the arrival of very large numbers of patients over a short time must be anticipated. The EMS system must be able to apportion victims to all receiving facilities. Traditional transportation protocols will not work under the circumstances of literally hundreds or thousands of similarly injured victims.

Biological Agent Release

Covert releases of biological agents represent the greatest challenge for disaster planners and responders. Due to latency between exposure and the onset of initial symptoms, patients will not gain access to initial medical care through traditional EMS pathways. Victims will more likely be seen by private physicians, or in emergency departments or urgent care centers, self-referred for nonspecific (influenza-like or gastrointestinal disease) syndromes. At some point, an "unusual event" will be identified. This will occur in one of three ways: (a) a serendipitous identification by an astute clinician of an unusual agent or clinical presentation; (b) an unusual or unexplained fatality; or (c) surveillance systems will identify an unusual pattern—human diseases/syndromes, or abnormalities in animals, plants, or environment.

Once this unusual event has been identified, further clarification will be required through intensive nontraditional epidemiological surveillance techniques and specific laboratory information. Specimens will need to be collected, appropriately packaged, and expeditiously transported to federal and/or state public health laboratories. Basic testing may be performed locally, if protocols have been established and the laboratory personnel have been appropriately trained and alerted. An initial estimate of the population at risk must be determined. If information regarding release point, times of release, or total agent load is minimal or unknown, a larger population may require prophylaxis than may actually be necessary based on actual exposure, since for many biological agents, time is a crucial factor in the efficacy of these treatments.

Decisions must be made in an attempt to contain and control the epidemic, based on presumptive evidence and best estimates:

a. Is this a bioterrorist attack, or the early manifestations of a natural epidemic?
b. Is this of a transmissible nature, and what is the mode of transmission?
c. Is quarantine required, or necessary?

d. Should post-exposure prophylaxis programs be initiated?
e. Who should inform the public?
f. When, and what information should be provided?
g. When should higher governmental officials be notified?

Radiological Incident

A radiological incident is likely to be identified by a precipitating event such as an explosion. This is no effective first-aid treatment for the medical effects of ionizing radiation, and patients will be primarily triaged based on other injuries or medical conditions. Those with high levels of radiation exposure with multiple symptoms related to that ionizing radiation have a lower probability of surviving than those who are initially asymptomatic. Medical providers will generally have more time to address the medical consequences to all but the most directly affected individuals. Public health implications of the long-term environmental consequences must be considered.

The most difficult aspect of a radiation release is the confirmation that it has occurred. Detection requires specific equipment not normally used in hazardous materials operations. A high index of suspicion must exist at a site of any explosion, since explosives might be used as a radiation dispersal device (RDD). Injured victims and uninjured bystanders or rescuers might be inadvertently exposed to ionizing radiation. Unless a prolonged delay occurs between release and arrival of first responders, only those victims with massive radiation exposure will likely exhibit symptoms relating to that exposure. In the acute setting of a known release, there will be no triage markers.

Victims with significant exposure to radiation will seek treatment over the next several hours to days. Since it would require very large amounts of radiation, dispersed over large geographic areas, to produce many casualties, this event would be similar to that of a low-level biological release, or even a mild natural epidemic. Environmental mapping will become very important. Persons at risk must be evaluated and tracked. Blocking of absorption or organ uptake of the radiation is paramount. Unlike chemical or biological agents that either dissipate or are killed by environmental conditions, radio emitters continue to give off radiation for very long periods. Environmental clean-up may take many years. Probably more than other WMD, radiation incidents generate anxieties out of proportion to the actual risks involved. The earlier tenets concerning mass counseling apply.

Explosives Devices

Explosions are probably the easiest WMD event for which to respond. Explosions more closely parallel certain natural disasters than do other WMD events. Communities usually have some form of disaster plans for such incidents and providers have more experience with penetrating or blunt trauma. Key differences of terrorist use of explosives versus other incidents involving these agents include: 1) the potential use of secondary devices to injure rescuers; 2) the possibility that the explosion was due to a RDD or that this was an unintentional or intentional release of hazardous materials from ruptured or damaged containers; and 3) the difficulties in transportation from the scene due to infrastructure or thoroughfare damage, since terrorists might primarily or secondarily target these systems.

Common Medical Issues

Regardless of the agent involved, at some point hospitals and hospital providers will become involved in consequence management. There are a number of common issues that must be addressed, depending on the magnitude of the attack. Mass care may include: 1) post-exposure prophylaxis; 2) outpatient treatment, including out-of-hospital and emergency medical services, monitoring and follow-up; 3) inpatient treatment; and 4) transition through the local medical system.

Post-Exposure Prophylaxis

The high costs of wide-spread antibiotic distribution, spectrum of potential agents, and logistical difficulties of distribution and dispensing of chemoprophylaxis virtually preclude the use of pre-exposure vaccines to protect the general public.[90] However, early implementation of a post-exposure prophylaxis program is essential, and is probably cost-effective.[91] Delaying the initiation of prophylaxis or treatment may be appropriate if initial analysis can be achieved within 24 hours, and it is appropriate to wait, based on the potential agents involved. Critical personnel must be protected; even asymptomatic individuals at high risk must receive prophylaxis, since morbidity and mortal-

ity increases greatly in many of these diseases once symptoms appear. The ability to dispense antibiotics, vaccines, or antidotes to large segments of the population over a very short time will be logistically difficult, but necessary. Pharmaceutical Distribution Centers (temporary sites identified to the public, but away from hospitals and other potential chokepoints) may offer the greatest benefit, but a subset of the population will not be mobile, and some delivery mechanism will be required.

Treatment

The public will demand to be informed as to when and where to seek evaluation. Those neither requiring nor afforded further treatment must be provided a detailed explanation and specific follow-up instructions. The victims or potential victims will produce a significant surge over regular patient load.

Issues of expandability and expendability of inpatient treatment must be addressed. Hospitals will need to expand or free up resources to handle the additional patients, by early release of existing patients, expeditious transfer to other facilities, and/or establishment of "augmentation facilities" such as converted auditoriums and gymnasiums. Decisions may need to be made as to which patients need inpatient treatment. A more difficult moral decision will be what services, if any, to provide to those who need hospitalization, but will not be receiving due to lack of resources.

Death and illnesses as well as the perceived threat to life resulting from a WMD terrorist act will produce the need for urgent psychological and other mental health crisis interventions and subsequent directed mental health care. Arrangements must be made for the processing of fatalities. It is unlikely that the public will condone or accept mass cremations or mass burials. Several major issues regarding the handling of the dead will present themselves early in the disaster.

Temporary, expedient morgues may be used to augment existing morgues, medical examiner facilities, and funeral homes. Facilities that may function as temporary morgues include armories, tents, factories, fire or rescue service buildings, garages, and hangars. Refrigerator trucks are ideal for longer-term storage, but have capacity limitations. Fatalities will need to be collected, identified, catalogued, stored, and ultimately disposed of in an appropriate manner.[92] Since in a terrorist WMD event, even fatalities are considered evidence, the medical community and victims' families may be constrained by law enforcement officials from timely disposal of the remains. Lastly, bodies may require decontamination to protect those who handle the remains. Fatalities due to biological agents might pose an infectious disease threat to handlers, and precautions might be necessary in preparing the deceased for disposition. All personnel involved with mortuary affairs must be protected. Morgues must have the capability to contain contaminated clothing. Specific procedures must exist for decontamination and certification of contaminated remains as clean.[93]

Environmental clean-up is a longer-term project after the community has been stabilized. However, critical facilities, such as outpatient treatment facilities, schools, transportation centers and government offices, must be prioritized for clean-up and must be decontaminated and certified as safe for use early in the course of the response. Environmental and industrial health specialists may be necessary to assist in these operations.

State and Federal Support

If a WMD event of significant magnitude occurs, local consequence management resources will eventually become overwhelmed.[94,95] In every state, there is a mechanism for the Governor to formally declare a "state of emergency." Once this happens, state resources such as the National Guard may be mobilized. All states have an Office of Emergency Management, which is normally tasked to oversee response operations. Many states have patterned their operation procedures after the FRP. Thirty states currently have signed the Emergency Management Assistance Compact, which empowers a state to request resources from another compact state and places the authority over those resources with the requesting state. Assistance under this compact is available for a WMD event, regardless of federal consequence management involvement.

Any terrorist event involving a WMD will prompt a federal crisis management response headed by the FBI. The FBI will activate a Strategic Information and Operations Center (SIOC) and a Joint Operations Center, with an FBI On-Scene Commander (OSC) in charge at the local level. A Domestic Emergency Response Team (DEST) is formed to provide expert advice and guidance to the FBI on scene commander and to coordinate the requisite response assets. The exact composition of the DEST will be de-

termined by the specific nature of the incident and will include, when appropriate, advisory modules for WMD conditions. If the event is serious enough, the state Governor may also request federal assistance for consequence management, through the provisions of the Stafford Act. Various federal agencies are assigned the responsibility to serve as the primary federal agencies for one or more specific emergency support functions, as defined by the FRP. Crisis and consequence management operations might overlap. For federal medical and health service response, FEMA mission assigns DHHS to activate ESF# 8. OEP will activate the DHHS Emergency Operations Center and designate a Chief of Field Operations.

With a no-notice chemical release, the primary DHHS role is to support those local systems that provide direct patient care or fatality management. With a no-notice biological release, the primary role is to support those local systems that provide mass immunization/prophylaxis, direct patient care, and fatality management. If local hospital capacity is exceeded, evacuation and definitive care elements of NDMS will be made available. If either the biological agent is communicable, multiple areas are affected, or food and water supplies are vehicles of transmission, OEP will implement a plan for protecting public health on the national level.

CDC will help determine (1) causative agent, (2) risk factors for illness, (3) affected and at-risk population, (4) control measures, and (5) mode of transmission. CDC will make treatment and prophylaxis recommendations and assist in determining the target population. The population at risk, and availability of local resources, will determine if mobilization of stockpiled pharmaceuticals, vaccines, and supplies, and the National Pharmaceutical Stockpiles is re-

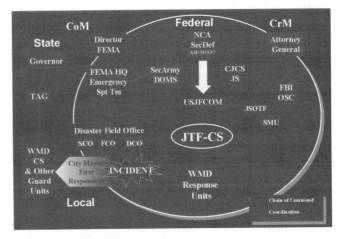

FIGURE 73.2. *Response Plan*

quired. CDC will deploy the assets under their control (CDC-owned or Vendor Managed Inventory) and OEP will deploy the 12-hour NMRT push packages. Local officials with state and federal support will manage these stockpile materials.

DHHS will coordinate support of state and local healthcare delivery systems with patient care, distribution of medical equipment and supplies, health surveillance, and managing the health consequences of the event. DHHS may potentially augment 1) prehospital care services, 2) healthcare facilities, 3) local auxiliary healthcare facilities, and 4) patient movement through the NDMS. Patient movement may be by air, ground, maritime, or rail transportation. Aeromedical evacuation will normally be accomplished through the Aeromedical Evacuation System (AES), administered by the DoD and the Transportation Command (USTRANSCOM).

If an outbreak is caused by a communicable agent, CDC and state health authorities will recommend the need for isolation and/or quarantine of selected persons. Isolation is defined as the separation of the general community from infected and diagnosed persons for the period of communicability. Quarantine is defined as the separation of exposed or potentially exposed persons until the incubation period has passed or disease is diagnosed, at which time, isolation is instituted for the period of communicability. Recommendations may include: (1) persons who require quarantine, (2) methods of quarantine, including areas for detention and methods for monitoring, (3) time periods of quarantine, and (4) guidelines/authority for releasing persons from quarantine restriction. If local fatality management capability is overwhelmed, DHHS can activate DMORT teams. One of these teams, DMORT IV, is trained and equipped to process the remains of individuals contaminated with infectious agents.

As with all the elements of these plans, environmental clean-up initially remains a local or state function. If the public health or the environment is threatened due to a WMD incident, the National Contingency Plan (NCP) may be activated. The Environmental Protection Agency (EPA) will ensure response integration. DHHS may provide technical assistance relating to environmental health during a chemical or biological incident. Federal response may be initiated under the NCP. The Federal On-Scene Coordinator (OSC) is responsible for all federal responses when NCP is initiated.

If a WMD event were to occur in a major population area, there may be a critical shortage of man-power to perform critical operations, including healthcare. This could be due to total system overload, illnesses among many of the providers or their families, or fear of exposure. An Israeli study of hospital employees found that only 43% would return to work unless certain safeguards were in place.[96] Military medical personnel would likely be deployed, and the military components of NDMS would be activated for utilization of hospital beds across the country, to receive patients transferred from local hospitals to make room for those injured by the attack.

WMD Planning

Disaster planning is a long process, and the additional work of planning for incidents involving terrorism and WMD will be arduous. Nonetheless, the basic principles of disaster planning apply.

The Team

Organizations and agencies potentially involved with the disaster response must be represented in planning for WMD events. They may find themselves with unique roles under new circumstances. Additional agencies not normally involved with traditional disaster responses must be involved in the planning process. Representatives must be given authority by their organizations to make and keep commitments.

Local law enforcement agencies will be dependent on healthcare professionals for medical information to assist in solving the crime. Conversely, the law enforcement community may receive information that is crucial to the medical community's ability to respond. Methods of sharing sensitive information while maintaining security or patient confidentiality will need to be devised. Security at pharmaceutical distribution centers and healthcare facilities will be required. There is great variation among the states for the public health authority to quarantine. Real-time epidemiological surveillance involving traditional and nontraditional data collection and analysis is crucial for timely warning, notification, and activation of response systems. Therefore, a host of legal issues must be factored into any planning or prospective decision-making processes. These range from public health issues, such as quarantine enforcement and forced confinement, to evaluation and treatment, patient confidentiality, and liability of officials and volunteers.

All medical facilities will be affected. Fixed medical treatment facilities have not historically had great difficulties in responding to traditional natural disasters. Few have had staff shortages or supply difficulties; even fewer become part of the disaster themselves. Rarely do hospitals deal with large numbers of highly infectious or contaminated patients. It is crucial that hospitals be considered as a networked organization. Even if one facility cannot or will not provide certain services, it might either serve as a receiving facility for unaffected patients or be able to provide mass counseling services. Ideally all contaminated patients would be decontaminated prior to arrival and only would be transported to designated facilities. Most likely, in either a chemical release or an event involving high explosives, the nearest treatment facility quickly will be overwhelmed. Laboratory diagnostic capabilities must be factored into any plans, since timely testing and diagnosis are critical. Facilities that utilize radiological materials all have some capabilities in radiological detection and safety. Pharmacies or pharmacists may provide guidance or assistance with antibiotic or antidote issues.

The availability of medical examiners, coroners, and pathological diagnostic capabilities must be determined. The capacity of the system to handle mass fatalities who are contaminated or infected must be expandable. Representatives of federal organizations, such as military installations and veteran's hospitals, and key private sector organizations having resources useful in detection, assessment, containment, or clean-up operations should be identified as early as possible.

The media is not normally included in disaster planning. In the event of a WMD event, many media personnel will be present. Information flow to the public can be greatly enhanced, or hindered, depending on the interactions developed with these individuals and organizations. During crisis management operations, all communications with the media are to be coordinated through the Joint Operations Information Center (JOIC). Nevertheless, including the media during planning exercises will improve operations during an event.

Existing Plans

In addition to existing memoranda of understanding and agreements, there are a number of important documents relating specifically to terrorism and WMD that should be perused during planning. These would include the FRP, the Federal Radiological Emergency Response Plan (FRERP), National Fire Protection Administration (NFPA) standards and guidelines for hazardous materials and terrorist events. Planning guides for hazardous materials, CDC recommendations, and other publications will prove insightful.

Hazards and Vulnerabilities

There are a variety of hazards and vulnerabilities in most communities. These include: 1) toxic industrial materials (TIMs), radiological materials, explosives warehouses, storage facilities and plants; 2) movements by railway, sea-lanes or thoroughfares in or near the community; 3) terrorist movements and activities in the community or in neighboring communities; and 4) other high-risk targets for terrorists. These targets and/or complications optimally should be included in the plan.

Capabilities and Resources

Disaster managers must have details of all resources including personnel, equipment and supplies plus the timeliness of their availability. Some state and federal agencies may be able to respond within a few hours of an incident, but it will take 48 hours for most federal resources to actually be available.

Operations Procedures

Disaster planning involves resource management, policies, and procedures. Planning must be integrated with existing disaster planning efforts. Communities with certain hazardous materials are required to have "all-hazards" disaster response plans, and areas without these requirements are increasingly adopting this approach.[97] Today most counties have developed specific bioterrorism response plans. Disaster planning for WMD incidents includes most of these elements.

Parameters must be set and assumptions made. The determination of what can and should be done, for whom, and for how long, must be made. It is reasonable to assume that the services immediately available to 100 victims would be substantially different from those for 10,000 victims. Planning should encompass the full spectrum of possibilities. Enhanced surveillance systems (including human syndromic data collection, nonprescription pharmaceutical usage, and abnormalities in plant life, disease vectors, and the animal population of the area) and early warning capabilities must be developed. Real time disease epidemiological information and episodic environmental sampling are required. Additionally, food and water supply safety may be jeopardized in a covert terrorist attack and must be protected. Meteorological information must be immediately available in order to optimize an appropriate response.

Capabilities must exist for rapid expansion of all healthcare functions, including public health services, mortuary affairs and vector control. The ability to augment hospital and first response organization staffs, with system personnel and volunteers, must be factored into plans. In the influenza epidemic of 1999–2000, existing outpatient resources in many locations were not capable of handling the additional workload.[98] The difficulties in processing patient surges may become even more difficult in the future, since over 500 hospitals nation-wide have closed in the past decade.[99] Discerning the subset of patients requiring timely treatment may be impossible early in the course of the event. In the case of a highly contagious epidemic, outpatient evaluation and treatment centers should be physically separate from those used for unaffected populations. Retention of the victims within the affected geographic area is probably desirable, and may require institution of a quarantine, although that term is discouraged. Unaffected inpatients may require expeditious forward movement through the system. Expandability of treatment facilities may be further enhanced through doubling up of private rooms. Given the possibility of agents requiring quarantine measures, a "one-plan" approach should include designation of certain fixed and augmentation facilities for these patients.

Logistics must be addressed. It is unrealistic to expect communities to maintain huge stockpiles of all possible antibiotics, vaccines, and antitoxins. A more reasonable approach might be to provide short-course, initial treatment pending arrival of national stockpiles and further delineation of the population at risk. Memoranda of understanding with pharmaceutical companies and distributors, local trucking companies, private ambulance corporations, security agencies, and many others may provide the necessary augmentation to assist many more patients than the healthcare community can under normal operations. The logistics of patient tracking throughout the system will be difficult, but must be established. The tempo of operations early in the evolution of a WMD event will be so extreme that even minutes will translate into lost lives or property. Algorithms for decision processes must be prepared in advance. Although there are specific procedures for activating state and federal responses, communicating information both horizontally and vertically may speed up key decisions and processes.

Finally, plans must be sustainable. It does little good to invest in expensive detection devices that soon will go obsolete. Perishable supplies and sensitive equipment will need rotation and/or replacement. Planning, testing and education must be continuous.

Education

Initial and continuing education and training must be provided for fire, hazardous materials, bomb disposal, law enforcement, EMS and healthcare personnel who will serve either in primary provider or support roles.[100] The most critical point of education is to heighten awareness, since these personnel will serve as the sentries for the surveillance system in identifying initial cases. All providers should be trained both to recognize the immediate or delayed symptoms of exposure to WMD agents and to use available antidotes for both self-care and emergency treatment.[101] In the Tokyo subway incident, 935 fire and EMS personnel manifested some signs and symptoms of the nerve agent exposure; and almost 20% of hospital staff reported some signs or symptoms.[10] WMD personal safety, patient treatment, triage, and transportation skills are rarely used. Crush injury, hyperkalemia, elective and emergent field amputation for entrapment, and the delayed sequellae of exposure to radiation and certain chemical agents are just a few of the unusual medical conditions that might arise as the result of WMD incidents. The use of healthcare personnel in non-traditional roles such as unsupervised distribution of antibiotics by nurses and home health care of victims by paramedics require additional training, education and authorizations beyond that normally provided. The public must also be educated, not only for awareness of the threat, but also as to what actions to follow for personal safety, should an event occur.

Benchmarks, standards and measures of effectiveness must be identified, and functional components exercised and tested against these. Plans should be tested using outside observers. Although many first response organizations routinely utilize the IMS, many hospitals and law enforcement agencies have not adopted that organizational structure or its other components. A critical weakness in many systems is the interfaces among the local jurisdictions, and the state emergency response organizations, especially where local autonomy is mandated.

Summary

The use of a weapon of mass destruction is almost too horrific to contemplate. Although such an attack is of very low probability in any specific community, no community is immune, and the effects of the release of a chemical, radiological, or biological agent likely would be catastrophic. Although significant state and federal resources can be mustered in response, like any disaster, these will be first and foremost a local challenge. All facets of the community are likely to be affected, and it is incumbent on the community to develop plans, to educate responder organizations and the public, and to test the plans, if the community has any expectation of effectively countering such threats.

References

1. Lesser IO, et al. *Countering the New Terrorism*. Rand Corporation. 1999. http://www.rand.org/publications/MR/MR989/MR989.pdf/
2. Center for Defense Information. *Newsweek Magazine*. May 8, 2000:43.
3. *Washington Post* Foreign Service, Sunday, October 18, 1998; Page A24.
4. British Broadcast Channel On-Line News, "Russia agrees, Ukraine cancels nuclear deal with Iran," 6 March 1998. http://news1.thdo.bbc.co.uk/hi/english/world/europe/newsid_62000/62871.stm
5. *60 Minutes*, 8 February 1998.
6. Roberts, B. Occasion Paper #3: *Nonproliferation Regimes at Risk*. Center for Non-proliferation Studies, Monterey Institute of International Studies; 1999.
7. Department of the Army. *Medical Management of Biological Warfare Casualties*. US Army Medical Institute of Infectious Diseases, 1999.
8. Federal Bureau of Investigation definition, National Domestic Preparedness Office. Special Bulletin—WMD Threats: Sample Guidelines Reissue. 12 January 2000.
9. Department of State, *Annual Report on Terrorism*. http://www.state.gov/www/global/terrorism/1998Report/review.html
10. Okumura T, et al. The Tokyo subway sarin attack: disaster management, Part 1: Community emergency response. *Acad Emerg Med*. 1998;5(6):613–617.
11. Federal Bureau of Investigation Report. "Project Megiddo." Http://www.fbi.gov/library/megiddo/publicmegiddo.pdf
12. Title 18 USC, Section 2332a.
13. Department of the Army. *Medical Management of Chemical Casualties Handbook*. US Army Medical Institute of Chemical Defense. 1999.
14. Sidell FR, Takafuji ET, Franz DR, eds. *Textbook of Military Medicine Part I: Medical Aspects of Chemical and Biological Warfare*. Washington, DC: Borden Institute; 1967.
15. California Annotated Code HSC Sec. 25501.
16. Freemantle M. Ten years after Chernobyl consequences are still emerging. *Chemical & Engineering News*. April 29, 1996. http://pubs.acs.org/hotartcl/cenear/960429/chern.html
17. Kalelkar, Ashok S, Little AD. "Investigation of Large-Magnitude Incidents: Bhopal as a Case Study." The Institution of Chemical Engineers Conference On Preventing Major Chemical Accidents, London, England May 1988. http://www.bhopal.com/
18. Satinath S. The Union Carbide Disaster in Bhopal. Institute for Global Communications. 1999. http://www.igc.org/trac/feature/india/profiles/bhopal/original.html
19. Public Law 99-499/40 CFR 355 et al.
20. *1979 Mississauga Train Derailment*. Mississauga Library system. http://www.city.mississauga.on.ca/library/
21. Berg DM. "The Hospital 'Gap.'" Presentation at *WMD & Domestic preparedness III: Interoperability & the Medical Management of a Bio-Terrorist Incident*" Washington, DC. 3–4 November 1999.
22. Ashraf H. European dioxin-contaminated food crisis grows and grows. *Lancet*. 1999;353:2049.
23. Mintier T, Bittermann J. Cable News Network On-Line. "Britain, France may Head to Court over Beef Ban," http://www.cnn.com/1999/WORLD/europe/12/09/british.beef.01/
24. Joint Chiefs of Staff Message P200313Z JUL 91 (Unclassified): "Translation of Egyptian Newspaper Al Hakika, 09 FEB 91, on Iraqi Casualties due to Biological Warfare (BW)."
25. Guillemin J. "Anthrax: The Investigation of a Deadly Outbreak." *World Press*. 1999.
26. Infield GB. "Disaster at Bari." New York: Ace Books; 1973.
27. Stephens HW. *The Texas City Disaster, 1947*. The University of Texas Press. 1997.
28. Levitin HW, Siegelson HJ. Hazardous materials: disaster medical planning and response. *Emerg Med Clin North Am*. 1996;14(2):327–348.
29. Advisory Panel to Assess Domestic Response Capabilities for Terrorism involving Weapons of Mass Destruction. "First Annual Report to the President and The Congress: I. Assessing the Threat." 15 December 1999.
30. Torok TJ, et al. A large community outbreak of salmonellosis caused by intentional contamination of restaurant salad bars. *JAMA*. 1997;278(5):389–395.
31. Tucker JB, Sands A. An unlikely threat. *Bulletin of Atomic Scientists*. 1999;55(4):130–138. http://www.bullatomsci.org/issues/1999/ja99/ja99tucker.html
32. Federal Bureau of Investigation Report. "Terrorism in the United States." http://www.fbi.gov/publish/terror/terrorin.htm
33. *Las Vegas Sun* On-Line article. February 19, 1999. http://www.lasvegassun.com/sunbin/stories/special_cut/1998/feb/19/c00003786.html
34. Federation of American Scientists. Chronology of Nuclear Smuggling Incidents. http://www.fas.org/irp/congress/1996_hr/s960320c.htm
35. Kolavic S, et al. An outbreak of Shigella dysenteriae type A among laboratory works due to intentional food contamination. *JAMA*. 1997;178:396–398.

36. Sheehan MA. Coordinator for Counterterrorism, in a speech at the Brookings Institution, February 10, 2000. http://www.state.gov/www/policy_remarks/2000/000210_sheehan_brookings.html

37. Staten CL. Testimony before the Subcommittee on Technology, Terrorism and Government Information, U.S. Senate Judiciary Committee, February 24, 1998. http://www.emergency.com/senate98.htm

38. North CS, et al. Psychiatric disorders among survivors of the Oklahoma City bombing. *JAMA*. 1999;282: 8:755–762.

39. Department of the Army. Chemical and Biological Rapid Response Team Concept of Operations, Soldiers' Biological and Chemical Command. 23 September 1999.

40. Department of the Army. *Health Services Support in a Nuclear, Biological and Chemical Environment*. Field Manual 8-10-7, Department of the Army, Washington, DC, 1993.

41. Christopher GW, et al. Biological warfare: A historical perspective. *JAMA*. 1997;278:412–417.

42. Holloway HC, et al. The threat of biological weapons. *JAMA*. 1997;278:425–428.

43. Franz DR, et al. Clinical recognition and management of patients exposed to biological warfare agents. *JAMA*. 1997;278:399–411.

44. Wiener SL, Barrett J. Biological warfare defense. In: *Trauma Management for Civilian and Military Physicians*. Philadelphia, PA: WB Saunders; 1986:508–509.

45. Hansen JE. Viruses, bacteria and toxins as biological warfare. *Ugeskr Laeger*. 1999;161(6):772–775.

46. Association for Professionals in Infection Control and Epidemiology. Bioterrorism Task Force and CDC Hospital Infections Program Bioterrorism Working Group "Bioterrorism Readiness Plan: A Template for Healthcare Facilities." April 13, 1999.

47. De Lorenzo RA, Porter RS. *Weapons of Mass Destruction: Emergency Care*. Upper Saddle River, NJ: Brady (Prentice Hall); 2000.

48. Zajtchuk R, et al (eds). Medical Consequences of Nuclear Warfare. Department of the Army, Washington, DC, 1990.

49. Grace C. *Nuclear Weapons: Principles, Effects and Survivability*. London: Brassy's Ltd.; 1995.

50. Jarrett D. "Overview of Medical Aspect of Ionizing Radiation Weapons." Armed Forces Radiobiology Research Institute, Bethesda, MD, 1999.

51. Jarrett D, ed. Medical Management of Radiological Casualties. Armed Forces Radiobiology Research Institute. Bethesda, MD, 1999.

52. SARA Title III Factsheet: The Emergency Planning And Community Right-To-Know Act. http://www.epa.gov/swercepp/factsheets/epcra-fs.txt

53. Chemical Stockpile Emergency Preparedness Program. Oak Ridge National Laboratory. http://CSEPPweb-emc.ornl.gov/

54. Public Law 99-145, Title 14, Part B, Sect. 1412.

55. Parker-Tursman J. "FBI Briefed on District's Terror Curbs." *Pittsburgh Post-Gazette*, May 5, 1999. http://www.usfa.fema.gov/techreps/tr114.htm

56. United States Fire Academy Technical Report. "Fire Department Response to Biological Threat at B'nai B'rith Headquarters, Washington, DC." Emmitsburg, MD. April 1997. http://www.usfa.fema.gov/techreps/tr114.htm

57. Federal Bureau of Investigation, National Domestic Preparedness Office. Special Bulletin—WMD Threats: Sample Guidelines Reissue. 12 January 2000.

58. Emergency News Network. "Bomb Explodes At Atlanta Nightclub." http://www.emergency.com/atlnabm2.htm

59. Staten CL. "Explosion at Abortion Clinic in Birmingham, Alabama." http://www.emergency.com/birmbomb.htm

60. Tucker P, Pfefferbaum B, Vincent R, Boehler SD, Nixon SJ. Oklahoma City: disaster challenges mental health and medical administrators. *J Behav Health Serv Res*. 1998;25(1):93–99.

61. Sansone RA, Roman EJ. The experience of psychiatric residents with disaster support: a descriptive report. *J Okla State Med Assoc*. 1996;89(7):238–241.

62. Davis JA. Sadness, tragedy and mass disaster in Oklahoma City: providing critical incident stress debriefings to a community in crisis. *Accid Emerg Nurs*. 1996(2): 59–64.

63. Public Law 104–210 *Defense Against Weapons of Mass Destruction Act of 1997*. September 1996.

64. Department of the Army. *Soldiers' Biological and Chemical Command Factsheet*. http://dp.sbccom.army.mil/fs/index.html

65. Department of the Army. *Multiservice Tactics, Techniques, and Procedures for Nuclear, Chemical, and Biological Aspects of Consequence Management*. DRAFT, Washington, DC. April, 2000.

66. Henderson DA. "DHHS FY2000 Anti-terrorism Funding: $277,553,000" in Biodefense Quarterly, Vol.1, No. 4, March 2000. Published by Center for Civilian Biodefense Studies, Johns Hopkins University, Baltimore, MD.

67. Federal Emergency Management Agency. Terrorist Incident Annex to the Federal Response Plan. http://www.fema.gov/r-n-r/frp/frpterr.htm. 3 June 1999.

68. Federal Emergency Management Agency. Rapid Response Information System Homepage. http://www.rris.fema.gov/

69. White House. Presidential Decision Directive 39, 21 June 1995. Federation of American Scientists Website. http://www.fas.org/irp/offdocs/pdd39.htm

70. White House. Presidential Decision Directive 62: Combating Terrorism. 22 May 1998.

71. Public Health Service Act, 42 U.S.C. 319.

72. Department of Health and Human Services, Office of Emergency Preparedness. *National Disaster Medical System Factsheet*. http://www.ndms.dhss.gov/

73. Department of Health and Human Services, Office of Emergency Preparedness. *Disaster Medical Assistance Teams Factsheet*. http://www.ndms.dhhs.gov/

74. Department of Health and Human Services. Center for Disease Control and Prevention. MMWR Recommendations and Reports. "Biological and Chemical Terrorism: Strategic Plan for Preparedness and Response" Vol. 49. No. RR-4. Apr 21, 2000. http://www.bt.cdc.gov/Documents/BTStratPlan.pdf

75. Department of Health and Human Services. *Agency for Toxic Substances and Disease Registry Factsheet.* http://www.atsdr.cdc.gov/DHAC.html

76. White House. Executive Order 12656, Assignment of Emergency Preparedness Responsibilities, November 1988.

77. Public Law 97-174, May 1982. Department of Veteran Affairs/Department of Defense Contingency Hospital System.

78. Department of Defense Directive 3025.12 Military Assistance to Civilian Authorities.

79. Waeckerle JF. Domestic preparedness for events involving weapons of mass destruction. *JAMA.* 2000;283:2. 252–254.

80. Monterey Institute of International Studies. Center for Nonproliferation Studies. *Federal Spending To Combat Terrorism.* http://cns.miis.edu/research/cbw/terfund. htm#5

81. Government Accounting Office, "Combating Terrorism: Observations on Federal Spending to Combat Terrorism," GAO/T-NSAID/GGD-99-107, Mar 11, 1999. Government Printing Office.

82. Government Accounting Office, "Combating Terrorism: Spending on Governmentwide Programs Requires Better Management and Coordination." GAO/NSIAD-98-39, Dec 1, 1997. Government Printing Office.

83. Government Accounting Office, "Combating Terrorism: Threat and Risk Assessments Can Help Prioritize and Target Program Investments." GAO/NSAID-98-74, Apr 9, 1998. Government Printing Office.

84. Government Accounting Office, Observations of Cross-cutting Issues." GAO/T-NSAID-98-164, Apr 23, 1998. Government Printing Office.

85. Government Accounting Office, "Combating Terrorism: Opportunities to Improve Domestic Preparedness Program Focus and Efficiency." GAO/NSAID-99-3, Nov 12, 1998. Government Printing Office.

86. Staten CL. "Emergency Response to Chemical/Biological Terrorist Incidents." Emergency Response & Research Institute. 7 August 1997. http://www.emergency.com/cbwlesn1.htm

87. Department of the Army "Guidelines for Mass Casualty Decontamination During a Terrorist Chemical Agent Incident." Soldiers' Biological and Chemical Command. January 2000. http://dp.sbccom.army.mil/fr/cwirp_guidelines_mass_casualty_decon_download.html

88. Macintyre AG, et al. Weapons of Mass Destruction events with contaminated casualties: effective planning for health care facilities. *JAMA.* 2000;283:2:242–249.

89. Cone DC, Davidson SJ. Hazardous materials preparedness in the emergency department. *Prehosp Emerg Care.* 1997;1:85–90.

90. Russell PK. Vaccines in Civilian Defense Against Bioterrorism. *Emerg Inf Dis.* 1999;5:4:531–533.

91. Kaufmann AF, et al. "The economic impact of a bioterrorist attack: are prevention and postattack intervention programs justifiable?" *Emerg Inf Dis.* 1997;3(2):83–94

92. Kentucky Governor's Executive Order 96-1220. Kentucky Emergency Operations Plan. 11 September 1996. http://webserve.dma.state.ky.us/kyeop.htm

93. Joint Chiefs of Staff, JP 4-06 *Joint Tactics, Techniques, and Procedures for Mortuary Affairs in Joint Operations.* 28 August 1996. http://www.ndms.dhhs.gov/CT_Program/Response_Planning/Mortuary_Affairs.pdf

94. Department of Health and Human Services. *Counter-Terrorism Concept of Operations Plan* (Draft). March 2000.

95. Federal Response Plan, as amended. April 2000. http://www.fema.gov/r-n-r/frp/

96. Shapira Y, et al. Willingness of staff to report to their hospital duties following an unconventional missile attack: a state-wide survey. *Isr J Med Sci.* 1991;27(11–12): 704–711.

97. Federal Emergency Management Agency. "Guide to All-Hazard Emergency Operations Planning." GPO Washington DC, September 1996.

98. Schoch-Spana M. Hospitals buckle during normal flu season: implications for bioterrorism response. *Biodefense Quarterly.* 2000;1(4):67–72.

99. Source: American Hospital Association.

100. National Emergency Training Center Hazardous Materials Emergency Preparedness Grant Program. "Guidelines for Public Sector Hazardous Materials Training." Emmitsburg, MD; 1998.

101. Pesik N, Keim M, Sampson TR. Do US emergency medicine residency programs provide adequate training for bioterrorism? *Ann Emerg Med.* 1999;34:173–176.

CHAPTER 74

Tactical Emergency Medical Support

Joseph J. Heck, DO
Alexander P. Isakov, MD

Introduction

Law enforcement officers are placed at an increased risk for injury and death while protecting the lives and property of the communities they serve. According to Federal Bureau of Investigation statistics, 223 peace officers were feloniously killed and 63,071 officers were injured as a result of assaults occurring in the line of duty during the years 1996 through 1999.[1-4] Among law enforcement injuries, members of Special Weapons and Tactics (SWAT) teams are at high risk for injury, sustaining a casualty rate of approximately 33 per 1,000 officer-missions.[5]

Tactical Emergency Medical Support (TEMS) is medical support to law enforcement operations. It is an emerging discipline within prehospital medicine.

History

The military has long recognized the value of early and definitive medical care in areas of operations. As modern warfare became less conventional, the military developed Special Forces units to engage in special operations. Because these units operate outside the normal realm of military operations, providing medical support required special considerations. These units are often operating remote from supporting elements for prolonged periods of time and are required to provide their own medical treatment to sustain their operational effectiveness. Thus, specially trained medics were developed and are deployed with these teams.

The civil unrest and disorder of the 1960s saw the advent of tactical units as a part of civilian law enforcement.[6] These teams are composed of highly trained officers capable of assuming varied roles and prepared to handle high-risk situations that are beyond the scope of traditional police officers. Although they encountered situations similar to their military counterparts, the benefit of medical support to such activities in the civilian arena remained unrecognized and undeveloped.

To address the issue of TEMS for law enforcement, national conferences were held in 1989 and 1990. With representatives from law enforcement, emergency medicine, and EMS, these conferences developed concepts relating to the provision of medical support to tactical teams.[7,8]

Limitations of Traditional EMS Response

Hostile conditions are commonly encountered in the tactical arena. Barricaded subjects, hostage-taking, military-type weapons, and organized opposing forces are some of the dangers that SWAT teams face in the performance of their missions. Relying on standard EMS resources in these situations places the officers and the prehospital care providers at risk. Unprepared and unequipped to deal with these dangers, conventional EMS providers run the risk of becoming the patients rather than being the caregivers.

A survey of SWAT commanders conducted in 1995 found that the most common form of medical support for their team was a civilian ambulance on standby at a predesignated location. Ninety-four percent of these out-of-hospital care providers had no specialized training in tactical issues, and 78% did not have a medical director. These findings suggested a need for established TEMS protocols, medical oversight and specialized training.[9]

Without specialized equipment, training, and protocols, the ability of traditional EMS personnel to respond to casualties in the tactical environment is limited. The threat of injury in this area of operations raises significant safety concerns. The typical uniform worn by EMS personnel will not provide the personal protection necessary to function safely in this environment. The tactical team or supporting law enforcement units will likely secure the operational perimeter. Entry into this secured area will be controlled, and access may be denied to non-law enforcement personnel. Furthermore, standard EMS protocols prohibit entry of traditional providers into unsecured, threatening environments as exist in a tactical setting. While these policies minimize the risk of injury to responders, they may prevent medical evaluation and treatment of casualties in a tactical situation until the conclusion of the event.

Unlike some activities that can be halted to allow EMS to perform their duties, a tactical scenario may not offer the same opportunity. A life-threatening hemorrhage or an airway compromise requires rapid medical assistance. Evaluation, treatment, and evacuation of casualties in this environment present challenges that can best be overcome by planning the medical response in advance to address those challenges.

Planning for medical contingencies requires knowledge of the operation that is to be executed by the tactical team. However, law enforcement officials can be reluctant to share details of their operational plan due to security concerns. Details of a law enforcement operational plan are always considered sensitive information. Breaches in security during tactical operations have had catastrophic consequences. In the 1993 high-risk operation at the Branch Davidian Compound near Waco, Texas, local EMS assets were put on alert by the agency serving a warrant. Through an unfortunate chain of events, the security of the operation was compromised by the EMS agency and the element of surprise was lost. Four law enforcement officers were killed and several wounded.[10] Establishing a more integrated or intrinsic medical support structure for law enforcement operations improves communication, allows for better contingency planning, and preserves the security of sensitive information.

The medical support of law enforcement tactical operations creates an environment with unique attributes (figure 74.1). These attributes demand the attention of medical oversight for development of appropriate protocols and teaching of additional skills (figure 74.2).

Unique Attributes of TEMS

An understanding of the characteristics that make medical care in the tactical environment unique, and proper training to operate in that environment, are essential to a successful TEMS program. They provide the necessary framework to: (1) enhance mission

- Zones of care/care under fire
- Weapons safety
- Hazardous materials
- Forensic evidence collection
- Preventive medicine
- Primary care
- Special equipment

FIGURE 74.1. *TEMS Unique Attributes.*

- Medical threat assessment
- Remote assessment methodology
- Sensory deprived/overload physical exam
- Medicine across the barricade
- Hasty decontamination procedures

FIGURE 74.2. *TEMS Additional Unique Skills.*

accomplishment, (2) reduce morbidity and mortality, (3) avoid liability, (4) diminish disability, costs, and (5) maintain good team morale.[11]

Zones of Care and Care Under Fire

The areas of operation for a tactical mission are usually based upon the threat level associated with those areas. Traditionally, terms such as inner and outer perimeter have been used. Although these terms may hold different meanings in different locations, the inner perimeter is generally the tactical area of operations controlled by the SWAT team. The personnel functioning within this location are at the highest risk of injury, and entry or exit in this area is tightly controlled. The outer perimeter is the larger area of law enforcement operations, and encompasses the inner perimeter. While the concept of inner and outer perimeters is useful in planning tactical operations, its application to tactical medicine is limited. Stratifying the medical areas of operations into hot, warm, and cold zones better reflects the dynamic process of treating the injured in the tactical arena.

The hot zone is that area with the greatest risk; an immediate threat of injury is present. This risk may be secondary to a known threat in the area or due to hazardous materials. Patient assessment and treatment in the hot zone is inherently dangerous. Usually, opening an airway, applying a tourniquet for life-threatening hemorrhage and patient extraction, are the only acceptable interventions in this situation, and even these procedures may have to be delayed because of the potential risk for further injury to both the patient and the rescuer from the inherent threat.

The cold zone is the area with neither significant danger nor threat. Medical care in this area parallels that in the routine EMS world; patients may be assessed and treated without risk to the patient or the EMS personnel from the incident.

The warm zone is the area of a potential threat, but not an immediate or direct threat. Medical care provided in the warm zone is dictated by assessing the risk of staying versus benefit of immediately treating the patient. Decisions regarding spinal immobilization, intubation, or intravenous therapy rather than immediate extraction depend upon the perceived level of threat.

Because of operational hazards, the time available to initially treat a patient may only allow acute, life-saving interventions. Further care must be delayed until a more stable location can be reached. This may lead to an increased morbidity and mortality for both the patient and the rescuer due to prolonged exposures to a hostile situation, and a balance must be attained depending upon the specific circumstances.

Thinking in terms of graduated zones provides a basis to critically analyze medical treatment options in a highly dynamic environment.[12] During an operation, a dynamic incident factor is always present: as the incident evolves, areas of safe refuge or egress may rapidly change.

A proposed military classification also divides the area of care into three zones, and may better apply to tactical law-enforcement operations. "Care Under Fire" is analogous to the hot zone. Preventing further injury, stopping life-threatening bleeding with a tourniquet, and evacuation is the only acceptable level of care. "Tactical Field Care" is similar to the warm zone and includes definitive management of the airway, breathing, and circulation. Needle decompression and other immediately life-saving procedures are performed, and intravenous fluids initiated. "Combat Casualty Evacuation Care" includes more definitive management as the patient is evacuated away from the threat, and is analogous to the cold zone.[13]

Weapons Safety

The tactical medical provider will likely encounter a variety of weapons in the performance of his duties, and TEMS team members should be familiar with all weapons in the arsenal of the tactical team. The casual and improper handling of a firearm can have devastating consequences. One strategy to prevent a firearms accident is to adopt a policy that prohibits handling of weapons by the medical provider. This, however, leaves him untrained to manage an injured, armed individual. A weapon in the hands of a wounded, distressed, possibly obtunded patient increases the likelihood of injury to the provider and team members.

Prudence dictates training in weapons safety. The ability to render a weapon "safe" allows the provider to proceed with his duties in relative safety. Handling of unfamiliar weapons poses a greater threat, and a protocol for the safe transfer of such a weapon to the custody of a tactical law enforcement team member is encouraged.

Hazardous Materials

An array of hazardous materials can be found in the tactical environment, especially in clandestine drug laboratories. The increasing role played by tactical units in drug interdiction poses a special problem to both law enforcement and emergency medical crews. Many of the materials used to produce illicit drugs are flammable or explosive, increasing the possibility of burn and blast injuries. Weapons fire, distraction devices, and sparks generated by light switches, flashlights, or photography equipment can ignite a volatile atmosphere, resulting in an explosion. Contact with some of these materials by inhalation or dermal exposure may cause toxic consequences to the perpetrator, officers, or TEMS members.

In the absence of proper safety precautions, law enforcement agents may experience both acute and chronic adverse health effects as a result of exposure to solvents, reagents, precursors, by-products, and drug products improperly used or generated during the manufacture of illegal drugs.

Additionally, today's criminals are more sophisticated in the methods they choose to protect themselves. Booby-traps have the potential to cause both routine and unusual wounding patterns, thus placing an additional burden on those providing operational medical support.

Forensic Evidence Collection

Evidence collection and preservation are of significant importance during law enforcement operations.

Evidence may help to identify the suspect, prove an element of a crime, or prove the theory of a case. Loss of evidence because it was unrecognized, not stored properly, or not maintained in a chain of custody can damage an investigation. One study concluded that emergency care providers often overlooked, lost, or discarded forensic evidence that required appropriate securing, handling, and documentation.[14] The tactical medical provider must have a knowledge of principles and procedures used to maintain evidence integrity.

The medical evaluation of a patient injured during an operation must include documentation of forensic findings. This includes evidence that may be lost in the transport and with continuing care of the victim, such as soot from a firearm on clothing or skin.

Preventive Medicine and Performance Integrity

While most SWAT activities are of short duration, there is the possibility of operations lasting several days or longer. TEMS personnel, with their medical background, are better trained to plan and provide for personal hygiene, meals, hydration, and the consequences of operating in extremes of temperature. Operating while wearing full tactical gear can increase the effective temperature by 10°F. In addition, the performance decrement of team members from engaging in sustained or continuous operations will play a role in the rate of injury. Recommending work-rest cycles to the tactical commander may prevent unnecessary injuries.

Primary Care

A large number of injuries sustained in the course of tactical operations are sprains, strains, abrasions, and contusions.[5] Traditional EMS providers are certainly familiar with these injury patterns but their scope of practice generally does not allow them to provide definitive care. In the tactical setting, these injuries should be expeditiously evaluated and definitively treated, thereby preventing further injury and eliminating lost time to the officer and to the agency. This can be of significant importance in remote tactical team operations, where access to other medical care is limited.

One means to manage these injuries is by expanding the scope of practice of these providers. The ability to accomplish this will vary regionally, depending on governing legislation. It also will require additional training and continuing education. Alternatively, these injuries can be easily cared for by an independent licensed practitioner, such as the TEMS team physician.

Special Equipment

Equipment for the tactical medical provider can be divided into personal and medical. Personal protection is essential. If the provider is working as part of the team and the team is dressed in full body armor, then the medic should have the same level of protection. At a minimum, this should include kevlar helmet, ballistic eye armor, ballistic vest, gloves, and supportive footwear. The mission will dictate additional equipment, such as a protective mask. Water should be carried to maintain personal hydration and a radio should be provided to monitor the tactical channel, and communicate with the tactical team and local EMS assets.

The equipment worn and used in the tactical environment is significantly different from what most medical providers are accustomed to wearing, even if they are actively involved in local EMS. The TEMS provider must be fitted, trained, and familiar with the equipment and its use, and must practice providing medical care while wearing the equipment.

The medical equipment used by the tactical medic must be functional and compact. Carrying a standard ambulance trauma kit in a hostile environment will burden the medic with excess weight and impede maneuverability. The usual EMS containers are brightly colored, large, bulky, and not useful for covert movements. Much of the equipment in commercial kits will not be useful in a tactical situation where the time for an intervention is short. Certain supplies that are not in the standard trauma kit may be necessary.

There are several considerations in choosing the method for carrying the tactical medical equipment. Foremost is portability. The ideal container will allow the provider's hands to remain free and will provide easy access to the equipment. In addition, the pack should be soft-sided and waterproof. Coloring should be subdued, with tactical black preferred. Shoulder supported backpacks fulfill this requirement. The military M-5 aid bag is one example; several variations of this bag are now commercially available. Other options include "fanny-packs," or carrying supplies on a load-bearing vest; vests with modular pockets can be designed to accommodate mission-specific equipment.

The amount and type of medical supplies depend upon the provider level and should be tailored to the mission. An inner-city raid may not require the same resources as a barricaded subject with hostages in a remote location. Therefore a method of carrying the essential elements to provide initial treatment should be augmented by a rapid resupply mechanism. This is accomplished by maintaining a larger kit in a central location, like the command post or tactical vehicle.

Emphasis should be placed on equipment that is used in the treatment of airway, breathing, and circulation problems. Airways and intubation supplies are required, as are pocket masks or bag-valve-masks for respiratory support. The added weight and the danger of oxygen cylinder damage from projectiles make its utility limited in the hot or warm zone. Methods to control hemorrhage, such as direct pressure dressings and tourniquets, as well as intravenous access supplies, are mandatory.

Most of the supplies will relate to the treatment of trauma. As such, intravenous solutions, dressings, and splinting material will compose the bulk of the stock. Other items that warrant consideration include over-the-counter comfort medications, dental repair kits, cricothyrotomy and needle thoracostomy equipment. Based on provider level, local protocol, and medical director approval, alternative airway materials and other medications may also be included.

Medications used for resuscitation of cardiac arrest patients will seldom be used in the tactical situation. Arrests due to medical etiologies during tactical operations are rare: none have been recorded among the 679 casualty reports compiled from 4,139 incidents submitted to the Counter Narcotics Operational Medical Support (CONTOMS) Database. The hostile environment of tactical medical support precludes full resuscitation. The added bulk of these items carried into the hot or warm zone is unwarranted.

The Tactical Medical Provider

Training

Before personnel undertake the challenges of providing emergency medical care in the tactical environment, additional specialized training is required. A basic understanding of tactical operations will assist the provider in appreciating the overall mission plan and the roles of each team member. The ability to plan for medical contingencies like patient evacuation is made easier if the medical provider can adequately assess the direction and objective of the mission.

TEMS personnel should have a working knowledge of the tactics and tactical movements of the team. Teams practice different maneuvers and different approaches, and a provider who is not familiar with stealth approaches, or who does not know when to use hand signals, can jeopardize not only a mission, but also the lives of team members.

Familiarity with individual team member responsibilities will assist in predicting likely injuries and in preparing the caregiver. Different personnel and team positions will have different medical needs and injury patterns. The officer swinging a 40 pound ram may show different injury patterns from the officer carrying the ballistic shield who has a much higher potential for penetrating trauma.

Familiarization should be accomplished by participation in training and missions with the team. Initially, this training is preferably accomplished with experienced tactical medical personnel. Attending a Basic SWAT school will provide training in operations and tactics, but many civilian providers will not have the time nor interest for that level of training. Through tactical medical courses, where medical and tactical issues are addressed and practiced, and "on the job" training, TEMS personnel can achieve the familiarity needed to function with a team.

Provider Level

The scope of practice of prehospital providers varies across the country. This scope of practice is generally defined by statute or regulation. To determine the desired scope of practice for the tactical medical provider, the mission and operations of the tactical team should be reviewed. Depending on the typical mission type, the desired skills of the tactical medic will be identified.

Whatever the desired range of skills, the training to properly perform them in a safe and effective manner must be provided, and they must be clearly delineated in a written protocol format. Since the scope of practice of EMS providers may be regionally regulated, a review of the applicable statutes and governing regulations is essential in the development of TEMS protocols. Preventive medicine, primary care, and advanced intervention skills will require particular attention.

Regardless of the provider level, tactical teams will benefit from the proximity of dedicated medical support to the operational area. The military has recognized the need for medical care to be arranged in echelons; more basic care is available at the site of the casualty, and more complex and sophisticated care is toward the rear.

Civilian provider levels parallel those in the military and offer the same benefits in the provision of medical care. Buddy aid is provided by fellow law enforcement team members, and is limited to medical problems that are quickly assessed and treated, such as bleeding control. The First Responder brings skills such as splinting and maintaining an airway, and capabilities will further increase as the level of the provider progresses from EMT-Basic through paramedic to physician.

EMS personnel trained to the first aider or EMT-Basic level currently provide most medical support to tactical operations.[9] Therefore, the possibility of EMT-Basic's using certain advanced procedures requires consideration. Paramedic skills may require changes in specific techniques, specially adapted for the tactical situation. The tactical environment is more than just "Tactical 9-1-1," and poses many unique scenarios and situations that can be barriers to providing "normal" emergency care in the prehospital environment. Even procedures that are performed on a daily basis can become difficult to a "tactically challenged" provider.

This may be attributed to the inability of the provider to concentrate on assessing and treating a patient while maintaining a critical perspective of the overall mission's progress.[15] In addition, assessment and treatment may make the patient and provider vulnerable to external environmental threats.

In order to maintain a secure airway, endotracheal intubation may be necessary. Conventional methods of intubation with a laryngoscope may not be feasible, as the operator may not be able to place himself in the proper position or the light signature emitted by the laryngoscope in the dark may compromise provider safety and the mission. One alternative is digital intubation, a technique that requires only the endotracheal tube, and minimal patient positioning, and is unhindered by blood or secretions. This method allows the operator to maintain a protected posture alongside the patient, decreasing the risk to both provider and patient. However, the patient must be unresponsive and without a gag reflex. Use of lighted stylets or intubating laryngeal mask airways are other options, as are use of the Combitube and laryngeal mask airway (LMA). A recent comparison of intubation techniques in the tactical environment showed no significant difference in time to obtain an airway between direct visualization, digital intubation or LMA.[16] While these options may decrease the light signature and allow intubation from various positions, they require added equipment that must be carried, and may not adequately secure the airway. When a required airway is unobtainable, a surgical airway may be necessary. The technique used should allow for a standard approach, quick access, and minimal equipment.

Needle thoracostomy is a potentially life-saving procedure that requires relatively little training. In the situation where a victim has a tension pneumothorax and scene evacuation is delayed due to mission requirements, this procedure may stabilize the patient's condition.

The use of distraction devices, explosives which make use of loud noise, and bright light to "distract" the target, have the potential to cause injury if placed too closely to persons, or detonated prematurely. Knowledge of blast injury patterns caused by the devices will allow TEMS personnel to prepare properly.

The use of "less-lethal" munitions has become commonplace. These low-velocity rounds, composed of wood, rubber, or foam projectiles, are designed to stun the subject and allow an easier apprehension. Although designed to be non-lethal, they are, nevertheless, capable of severe injury, and deaths have been reported.[17] The greatest potential for blunt trauma sustained from these devices is to the musculoskeletal system and to the eyes. Again, being familiar with the plans and weapons used in an operation will alert EMS personnel to potential injuries from these "less-lethal" projectiles.

Local protocols and medical oversight considerations will govern the extent that the non-physician medical provider will operate. The unique situations presented by tactical medical support require enhancing the scope of practice for these tactical medical providers. Possible areas of enhanced scope include invasive procedures, expanded pharmacy, and preventative medicine issues.

Special Skills

An added benefit of medical personnel interacting with the tactical team is the ability of the TEMS personnel to provide a medical threat assessment for the mission. A tool that can be used to determine and plan for potential health hazards inherent to an operation, the medical threat assessment serves to advise the tactical commander. The medical threat assessment also evaluates the local medical resources and plans for evacuation of casualties. Information regarding terrain, site hazards, known disease threats, and forecast weather, should be included in the report. The medical threat assessment provides the tactical commander with the potential to increase mission effectiveness, command credibility, and team morale. It decreases personnel attrition, costs due to injuries, and legal liability.[18]

At times, wounded individuals may be located beyond the zone of safe medical care. In this situation, the ability to accurately assess the patient from a distance may provide the tactical commander with needed information to direct the operation.

Remote physical assessment is a method in which the care provider attempts to ascertain injuries and condition by visualizing and talking to the victim from a remote location. The injured may be verbally directed in basic life-saving interventions like hemorrhage control, or may be instructed to move to an area that provides greater protection. The medical provider may also be able to determine lethal injuries in a patient and obviate a rescue attempt in a hostile location.

The ability to perform an accurate physical assessment is a cornerstone of prehospital care. Providers spend a significant portion of their initial training mastering these skills. This training usually takes place in the controlled environment of the classroom and relies heavily on visual cues. In the tactical situation, assessment of the injured patient is problematic. The protective equipment worn by SWAT members impedes palpation and visual assessment. Poor lighting and the inability to safely illuminate and visualize the patient add restrictions. In an active, hostile mission, extraneous stimuli from weapons fire, distraction devices, and radio communications may interfere with medical personnel's ability to concentrate. All of these factors will force the provider to utilize additional techniques to accurately survey the patient.

Two techniques, pioneered by the Uniformed Services University of Health Sciences and the United States Park Police, are additional tools that the provider can use to assess patients in these situations. The sensory-deprived physical assessment (SDPA) and the sensory-overload physical assessment (SOPA) were designed to reinforce physical examination skills with emphasis on using rescuer's senses other than vision. During the SDPA the examiner is blindfolded and is forced to rely on tactile and aural clues to complete the physical assessment. In the SOPA, flashing lights, loud noises, and crackling radios require increased concentration on the part of the provider, and also emphasize use of tactile examination.[19]

The tactical medical provider may encounter situations in which he needs to address medical problems occurring in individuals who are barricaded from law enforcement officials and medical personnel. The only means of evaluating patients in this environment may be via telephone or radio, through which assessments are made and instructions delivered to a caregiver on the other side. This is referred to as "medicine across the barricade."

Although not a task often performed by traditional responders, a template for action currently exists in the form of EMS dispatch pre-arrival instructions. An organized approach to evaluation and treatment of injuries with a protocol designed for this situation is the means to deliver immediate life-saving care, possibly through a layperson, if extraction of the victim is not possible.

The incident commander oversees communication with the barricaded subjects. He may find an opportunity to negotiate for removal of ill or injured persons, or may possibly secure a peaceful resolution of the crisis using the information gathered via the "medicine over the barricade" exchange. It is important to note that the incident commander makes all the decisions and that, when talking with the perpetrator, the tactical medical provider should never agree to a demand, make a promise, or offer to enter the barricaded area.

Training in hazardous materials is essential for any tactical team raiding clandestine drug laboratories. Advance knowledge of possible contaminants, their mechanisms of action, antidotes, and treatment will help insure immediate and effective care of the contaminated patient. Techniques for field-expedient decontamination should be practiced routinely and will reduce the risk of spreading contamination during patient treatment and transport.

Another area of possible contamination is in the use of riot control or incapacitating agents, commonly referred to as "tear gas." Although not lethal, these compounds can be extremely useful in subduing subjects. Knowing how to neutralize these substances will prove beneficial if team members are accidentally exposed, and beneficial in decreasing the potential for cross-contamination from subjects after they are in custody.

The position the tactical medical provider will hold within the team will vary. Current models include using SWAT officers who are also trained as medics, law enforcement officers (LEO) other than SWAT as the tactical medic, and civilian medical personnel trained to respond with and support the tactical team. Using LEO lessens the concerns over personal security, crime scene and evidence preservation, weapons handling, and operational security. SWAT officers have the added advantage of familiarity with tactical operations and the confidence of their team members. However, medical support for officers is usually an additional duty that may result in role confusion during an operation and pose logistical problems in skill maintenance. The concept of "one role-one person" in TEMS limits role confusion. Each team member should have one *primary* role for the mission. When team members have more than one primary role, it can be confusing which role to perform when *both* are needed. If one of the tactical team members is also considered the medic, an unnecessary decision has to be made when there is a downed officer needing medical attention in an area where there are still law enforcement concerns. One cannot treat a patient and engage a hostile target simultaneously.

Using civilian medics who train with the team provides well trained medical personnel. But the increased risk posed to operational security and lack of tactical experience/law enforcement powers is a potential drawback. The use of "standby" civilian EMS personnel without any tactical exposure is an inadequate method of providing appropriate tactical medical support.

The location in which the medic functions is an area for debate. Depending upon the status with the tactical team, the TEMS provider may function anywhere from the hot zone to the command post. Arguably, locating the medical personnel closer to the potentially injured person is better in terms of providing rapid medical care if needed. However, concerns about safety and security of the medics in those situations are valid.

Medical providers who are not sworn officers and who may only have limited, introductory law-enforcement knowledge obtained through tactical medical training are best kept away from the hot zone. The inability to provide their own protection and the possibility of becoming a potential target are both reasons that these providers should be excluded from the hot zone. However, restricting the medical support to the command post does not fully maximize the potential benefit of a TEMS provider, since

evacuation of the casualty from the hot zone to the command post may require mission-essential personnel. Therefore, placing the provider somewhere close to, but protected from, the action is best. This also allows for direct observation of the activity, the possibility to foresee potential injuries, and an increased preventative role.

Perhaps the most controversial question concerning a tactical medicine program is whether or not TEMS personnel should carry firearms. While allowing the medical providers to carry weapons may provide them with the ability to protect themselves or their patients during a mission, the consequences may be tragic. If the provider is an officer, carrying a weapon while on duty is usually a requirement. The area of concern is when the medic is a civilian supporting the tactical team. This includes providers who are permitted to carry personal weapons under local laws and regulations. The level of training to acquire firearm proficiency is difficult to maintain, and liability issues will undoubtedly arise should an EMS provider be involved in the shooting of a suspect, innocent bystander or in a friendly-fire incident.

Role confusion may also present a problem. The TEMS provider's primary purpose should be to provide emergency medical care. Concentrating on the patient is critical. The added distraction of using a weapon is unjustified if dedicated protection of medical personnel is provided. This holds true for law enforcement personnel as well.

The Tactical Physician

Physician involvement in TEMS is a fairly new phenomenon. Two recent surveys of SWAT teams that investigated the use of medical support units revealed that 78 to 91% of teams do not have a physician medical director, and only 10% of the respondent teams in both surveys had physicians as medical support personnel.[9,20]

The physician role in the practice of TEMS is varied. A recent study found that, of the physicians who are involved with TEMS, more than half of them were sworn officers and carried firearms while supporting the team. Additionally, some performed dual roles as medical provider and member of the entry team, and one physician had a dual role as a sniper.[21] Generally, the type of physician support falls into three categories: (1) medical director, (2) TEMS operational team member, and (3) a combination of the two. Each role has advantages and disadvantages.

The majority of physician team members perform as volunteers. Therefore, time availability and practice constraints are significant determinants of how involved the physician will be. In a primarily oversight role, the time commitment can average a few hours per week. Functioning as an operational team member can be a much larger commitment. A mission or call-out can last several hours to days. Having the ability to schedule time to perform these missions is key to the physician's ability to deploy with a team. Few physicians who have a full-time practice have the ability to provide direct medical oversight or deploy on actual missions. Functioning with a busy team in this role could develop into a full-time commitment.

Medical Oversight

Medical oversight is a standard and essential component of any EMS system. The duties of medical oversight include protocol development, continuing education, quality improvement, and direct medical oversight activities. Since all medical care in the out-of-hospital environment should be provided with appropriate medical oversight, it is critical that physicians take an active role in this medical oversight process. It is the mechanism that ultimately ensures the highest quality patient care. A medical director is responsible for the medical oversight program.

The tactical medical director should be a physician knowledgeable in the development of treatment protocols, EMS law, and management of the acutely ill or injured. Additionally, the medical director should have training in both direct and indirect medical oversight, familiarity with communication plans, and the requisite medical knowledge to train EMS personnel at all levels. Knowledge of law enforcement tactical operations is extremely desirable.

Requisites for initial training and continuing education for traditional EMS providers also vary greatly based on local and state requirements, despite the efforts being made toward a recognized national standard. The training and continuing education of tactical medics is the responsibility of medical oversight of a tactical medical support program; the medical director should be actively involved in the training of his personnel.

Supporting tactical law enforcement operations in a unique practice environment requires skills beyond the scope of traditional EMS physician education. National educational programs for physicians and other EMS personnel exist to address this body of knowledge, and completion of this training is highly recommended. A variety of courses are available and a national standard for training is emerging. The medical director should review the curricula of the programs and select one that provides the best training suited to the mission requirements.

The completion of a core curriculum course cannot guarantee concept and skill retention, so a continuing education curriculum should also be developed.

It is the duty of the medical director to maintain the quality of care provided by field providers. It is essential for physicians to remain involved in this process. Core components of the quality management (QM) process include reviews of protocol compliance, documentation, overall patient management, and patient outcomes.

An understanding of potential expanded scope activities, care of patients in various zones, and other influences of the operational environment on patient management is necessary. If many physicians are involved in this process, a standardized review process should be established to ensure uniformity. Training and recertification standards must be addressed and are essential in maintaining quality in the program.

QM should be a prospective activity to continually improve the quality of service delivered to the patient. Tactical medical support units are, with few exceptions, much smaller than their traditional EMS counterpart, and therefore provide a unique opportunity for a close relationship between the medical director and providers. The QM process can only function well if there is a dialogue between the medical director and the providers. This dialogue provides the opportunity for the medical director to be cognizant of the practice environment and quality of care provided in the field. It is the process through which field providers identify deficiencies in the system and refer them to the medical director for review and correction. It allows the provider to get feedback on the management of difficult cases, to question the rationale of various protocols, and to get positive reinforcement and constructive criticism when appropriate.

Perhaps the best argument for physicians at the scene, in support of field operations, is the establishment and nurturing of this relationship between medical oversight and prehospital provider. This interface is most rewarding to all participants and will have the greatest yield in improving the quality of care.

Direct medical oversight is the involvement of the physician in the management of prehospital care via radio or telephone, or by his physical presence at the scene. Aside from allowing closer supervision of prehospital activity and assistance in the management of difficult cases, direct medical oversight may facilitate deviation from protocols. This is important in tactical EMS and allows for the greatest flexibility in the management of casualties in the dynamic environment of tactical operations. However, unlike in traditional EMS systems, radio contact with a "medical control physician" may not always be feasible. Constraints of the tactical environment may make radio and phone communications difficult or prohibitive, and patient management may have to be modified based on real or perceived threats to ensure safety for the healthcare provider. There is no substitute for visualizing the scene and understanding the unique practice environment of each scenario. For this reason, on-scene participation of the tactical physician may enhance the quality and scope of service provided by the medical support team. For direct medical oversight to be effective, the physician must be familiar with and knowledgeable of the environment.

Whether or not the medical director or any physician becomes actively involved in the operational role of a medical support team is a complex decision. Input from local EMS, law enforcement, medical, and legal communities should be sought. All of these agencies will be potentially affected by the deployment of physicians on medical support teams.

Operational Team Member

The physician has the potential to enhance the care in the field by bringing a broader scope of practice than most out-of-hospital providers bring. The ability to provide direct medical oversight and to perform advanced procedures are the most obvious advantages. On-scene, direct medical oversight can obviate the need to use the radio to call for guidance, a possible source for breach of security. The physician can also perform the more frequent, routine care for SWAT personnel, such as sick call. The ability to perform preventive medicine skills, such as hydration and work-rest cycle recommendations, will keep a team healthy and have a greater impact on team integrity and effectiveness than the rarely used thoracostomy or rapid-sequence intubation.

A recent review of the CONTOMS database of SWAT injuries and mission profiles shows that the majority of reported LEO casualties are a result of minor incidents. The physician often has more experience in "sick call" than the out-of-hospital provider, and can care for the injury on the scene, negating the need to transport the officer to the hospital or drop them from the mission.

The physician can serve in various areas of the tactical scene. Although it may seem preferable to put them as far forward as possible, this may not enhance the care delivered. Rasumoff and Carmona distinguish between level of *personnel* and the level of *care* that can be provided far forward in the tactical setting. Even if a team deploys all of its physicians, it is doubtful that they will be able to provide any care in the hot zone: extraction will be the only alternative. Even though physician-level personnel can be deployed far forward, it is doubtful that the physician will be able to use his skills in the hot zone.

Summary

Unconventional hazards are commonplace in tactical law enforcement. Barricaded suspects, hostage-taking, clandestine drug lab raids, and high-risk warrant services are some of the missions that are carried out every day, which put the law enforcement population at special risk. These individuals are highly trained and highly motivated, operating on the edge of the safety envelope. Manpower maintenance and appropriate medical support are essential to mission accomplishment.

The tactical medical provider serves as the tactical commander's "medical conscience." The medical support unit is one of many elements for which the commander has responsibility. The health and medical care of the unit are ultimately the commander's responsibility; and he cannot pass that responsibility on to anyone else. Therefore, factors and events that may impact the team's health need to be presented to the commander for his review.

References

1. U.S. Department of Justice, Federal Bureau of Investigation: Uniform Crime Report, Law Enforcement Officers Killed and Assaulted, 1996. United States Government Printing Office.
2. U.S. Department of Justice, Federal Bureau of Investigation: Uniform Crime Report, Law Enforcement Officers Killed and Assaulted, 1997. United States Government Printing Office.
3. U.S. Department of Justice, Federal Bureau of Investigation: Uniform Crime Report, Law Enforcement Officers Killed and Assaulted, 1998. United States Government Printing Office.

4. U.S. Department of Justice, Federal Bureau of Investigation: Uniform Crime Report, Law Enforcement Officers Killed and Assaulted, 1999. United States Government Printing Office.

5. CONTOMS Database: Casualty Care Research Center, Department of Military and Emergency Medicine, Uniformed Services University of Health Sciences, Bethesda, Maryland.

6. Kolman JA. *A Guide to the Development of Special Weapons and Tactics Teams,* Springfield, Illinois: Charles C. Thomas: 1982.

7. Rasumoff D. EMS at tactical law enforcement operations seminar a success, *The Tactical Edge.* 1989;7:25–29.

8. Carmona R, Brennan K. Tactical emergency medical support conference (TEMS): a successful joint effort. *The Tactical Edge.* 1990;8:7.

9. Jones JS, Reese K, Kenepp G, Krohmer J. Into the fray: integration of Emergency Medical Services and Special Weapons and Tactics (SWAT) Teams. *Prehosp Disast Med.* 1996;11(3):202–206.

10. 104th Congress, 2nd Session, Report 104-749, House of Representatives Investigation into the Activities of Federal Law Enforcement Agencies Toward the Branch Davidians.

11. Position Statement of the Counter Narcotics Tactical Operations Medical Support Program. In: *Counter Narcotics Operational Medical Support Emergency Medical Technician—Tactical.* Bethesda: Uniformed Services University of the Health Sciences; 1994.

12. Vayer J. Echelons of Care—Defining Zones of Treatment in the Tactical Setting. CONTOMS Dispatch 1996;3(1).

13. Butler F, Hagmann J, Butler E. Tactical combat casualty care in special operations. *Military Medicine.* 1996;161, Suppl:3–16.

14. Carmona R, Prince K. Trauma and forensic medicine. *J Trauma.* 1989;29:1222–1225.

15. Rasumoff D, Carmona R. Echeloned field medical care: definition and justification. *The Tactical Edge.* 1993; 11(4):72–76.

16. Apfelbaum J, Mitchell K, Blackwell T. Invasive airway techniques in the tactical EMS environment: a comparison of endotracheal intubation, digital intubation, and the laryngeal mask airway (abstract). *Prehosp Emerg Care.* 2000;4:89.

17. McDonald J, Sandre N, Penk D. The 12-Gauge Bean Bag: Canada's national capital experience. *The Tactical Edge.* 1999;17(2):50–65.

18. Medical Threat Assessment. In: *Counter Narcotics Operational Medical Support Emergency Medical Technician—Tactical.* Bethesda: Uniformed Services University of Health Sciences; 1994.

19. Vayer J, Hagmann J, Llewellyn C. Refining prehospital physical assessment skills: a new teaching technique. *Ann Emerg Med.* 1994;23:786–790.

20. Quinn M. Into the fray: The search and rescue role with Special Weapons Teams. *Response.* 1987;4:18–20.

21. Smock W, Hamm M, Krista M. Physicians in tactical emergency medicine (abstract). *Ann Emerg Med.* 1999; 34:S73.

75

Diversion and Bypass

Michael Casner, MD
Mark Greenwood, DO, JD
Cai Glushak, MD

Introduction

The nationwide development of EMS systems in the 1970s spurred the growth and increased use of emergency departments (ED)across the country. In the 1980s, hospitals were faced with increasing numbers of patients, longer waits to care for ED patients, and growing numbers of individuals arriving by ambulance. Emergency department "bypass" or "diversion" has emerged as a means of dealing with the problem of ED and hospital overcrowding when resources are overwhelmed.

In this context, the concept of diversion is used exclusively to define a situation in which an ambulance is forced to seek an alternate hospital destination other than that to which it would normally transport a patient, because the closest appropriate facility has declared that it is unable to accept patients as a result of a lack of normally available resources. This is usually the result of an overcrowding situation in the ED or the hospital, but may be related to lack of a critical facility, such as a CT scanner. "Diversion" seems to be the term most preferred in policy and regulations, though "bypass" is used synonymously by many. This chapter will not discuss the concept of "bypass" of patients meeting specific criteria for transport to specialty facilities, such as Trauma Centers, in order to take advantage of regionally distributed special services. Though both "bypass" and "diversion" have been used in this context as well, this chapter will use the term "diversion" to reflect resource saturation in which normally available institutions are compromised in their abilities to deal with additional patients. Overcrowding, thought to be generally under control in the early nineties, is again an escalating problem; and the frequency with which hospitals in many communities request bypass is increasing. Several professional societies have published formal guidelines and policy statements to steer diversion decisions. However, hospital diversion remains only a temporizing measure, the need for which is a symptom of deeper hospital-wide and health system problems, both transitory and long-term.

Historical Perspective

The factors leading to ambulance diversion are multifactorial and poorly studied, making it difficult to paint a clear historical picture of cause and effect. Problems related to ambulance diversion were only sporadically reported prior to the mid-1980s. Most of these reports were and continue to be reported in the lay press. When the phenomenon first came to public attention, many EMS systems had only recently reached a relatively mature stage of development. Ambulance use had been on a steady increase and has since continued. In parallel, ED use has also been rising for several decades. The number of ED visits in the United States increased from 83 million in 1987 to over 100 million in 1998.[1,2]

Starting in the 1980s, the nation began to experience a trend of hospital closings, due in part to Medicaid and Medicare reimbursement policies based on occupancy rates.[3] At the same time, remaining hospitals in many areas decreased the number of active inpatient beds. In some cases, this trend particularly affected the availability of monitored and critical-care beds.[3] Finally, in the early years of ambulance diversion, there were few guidelines by which EMS systems or hospitals could determine a rational basis for diverting ambulances. This may have contributed to a relatively uncontrolled and arbitrary development of diversion patterns. Although it is difficult to pinpoint the specific stresses in EMS systems that were most responsible for the increased incidence of hospital diversion in the late 1980s, clearly the combination of increased EMS activity, increased demand on EDs, and a relative decrease in hospital bed numbers placed a great strain on EMS systems, for which neither the medical community nor the public were prepared.

Early attempts to regulate hospital requests for diversions developed locally without guidance from national organizations.

One of the first regionwide policies was in New York City in 1982 where the EMS system was designating trauma centers and field "trauma diversions." In response to the pleas of ED directors about overcrowding, the EMT medical director divided the 60 receiving hospitals into "pods" of approximately 5 hospitals. Only one hospital in a pod could be in diversion at a time; a request for diversion by a second hospital "opened" the entire pod.

Eventually, the National Association of EMS Physicians (1992) and the American College of Emergency Physicians (1992) drafted policy statements regarding the diversion of ambulances.[4,5] In reaction to public concern about the diversion situation, some states and many municipalities enacted legislation or regulations to create controls on the use of diversion.

The problem of overcrowding and frequent ambulance diversion seemed to disappear in the 1990s, ascribed, in part, to the increasing number of residency-trained emergency physicians and the efforts of HMOs to reduce ED visits.[6] In fact, the moderation of the steep increase in ED visits during this period caused many hospitals and ED administrators to be concerned about dwindling demand for their services. Not only had many institutions made efforts to adapt their systems to accommodate increased patient demand, but many facilities undertook aggressive efforts to attract walk-in and ambulance traffic. For many hospitals, to the irritation of the ED staff, such marketing efforts made diversion a "non-option" for many institutions.

At the turn of the 21st century, "overcrowding" once again became a real issue among EDs. Reports of hospitals going on diversion became increasingly common in the lay press. More recently, the problem of overcrowding has been reported overseas.[7] Some of the factors that fueled the 1980s trend may have resurfaced. Once again, hospitals and EDs have experienced increased closures, despite an increase in the number of critical-care inpatient beds in many regions. Many believe that difficulty obtaining timely access to primary care, ambulatory medical facilities and inpatient beds for routine medical care has led more practitioners and patients to rely on the ED and EMS for relatively minor problems.

Additionally, a number of other factors have been invoked as contributing to the overcrowding and diversion situation that did not receive such attention a decade ago. Some of the factors mentioned in recent years include a shortage of nursing personnel, closure of inpatient beds, stricter EMTALA rules for emergency care, increasingly burdensome documentation requirements, delays for approval of admission or transfer of managed care patients, early discharges, and lack of availability of on-call physicians for consultations or admissions. California has recognized a statewide crisis that has led to a focused study of the diversion phenomenon.[6] The acuity of the problem in that state in many ways epitomizes the extreme degree to which this problem has progressed.

Hospital Overcrowding

In the majority of cases, EDs request ambulance diversion simply because they are overcrowded; the causes of overcrowding are more complex. ED patient volume has increased nearly 20% in the past 17 years.[8] More people are resorting to the ED as access to other sites of primary care decreases due to hospital closures, managed care restrictions, and increasing numbers of uninsured patients. Furthermore, the acuity of patients presenting to EDs has increased in recent years, in part due to an aging population, the advent of AIDS, and the increased life expectancy of people with chronic medical conditions.[6]

Compounding this problem is the inadequate increase in medical personnel and services to meet increased demand. Hospital closures and reductions in numbers of ED and inpatient beds in the remaining hospitals are intended to ensure a full census, but may prevent movement of patients from EDs to inpatient areas. Even when beds are available, inpatient floors may lack sufficient staff to accept more patients. Additionally, many areas of the nation have reported a critical nursing shortage, which may affect both ED and inpatient units. In recent years, the Center for Medicare and Medicaid Services (CMS), has increased the amount of documentation required for reimbursement of care provided in the ED. The time required to fulfill the increasingly rigorous documentation requirements may also slow patient flow through EDs.[9]

One of the purported benefits of managed care organizations (MCOs) was an expected reduction in ED visits by providing necessary preventive care and timely access to network providers for episodic problems. However, in many situations MCOs simply place increased reliance on contracted and out-of-network EDs when their patients cannot be accommodated for routine and unscheduled problems. Special procedures necessary to accommodate MCO demands may also contribute to ED overcrowding. ED beds are often occupied by patients undergoing complex workups or prolonged observation in order to avoid or to obtain authorization for admission. To a less degree, additional patients may occupy ED beds while waiting to be transferred to designated MCO hospitals.

One of the most interesting observations concerning diversion trends is a recurring pattern of higher diversion rates during winter months. Many communities have reported a cluster of diversion incidents that peak over a period of weeks, often thought to be related to the influenza season. Unfortunately, it is usually impossible to predict for the purposes of resource allocation the onset of seasonal epidemics. However, in some communities, the winter pattern of ED diversion bears remarkable resemblance to that of reported influenza cases. Though this does not necessarily indicate that EDs are consumed by attention to this isolated diagnosis, influenza-related morbidity, particularly among elderly and debilitated patients, may result in increases in hospital admissions and ED stays.

Several other factors have been discussed as contributing to ED and hospital gridlock. Variations in hospital and ED practices may account for differences in lengths of stay. There have been reports of variability in test ordering and admission thresholds among ED physicians that imply differing levels of "efficiency" in arriving at patient dispositions. Around the nation, EDs are having difficulty assuring availability and responsiveness of on-call specialists, resulting in delays to disposition and the need to effect time-consuming transfers. In some regions, there has been a disturbing trend for certain hospitals to permanently close their EDs, while remaining open for other activities. The ACEP reports that over 300 EDs were closed between 1994 and 1996.[10] In one remarkable case the teaching hospital of the New York State Medical School in Brooklyn simply took the ED off its operating certificate.

Effects of Diversion

Diverting an ambulance from the intended hospital poses problems for patients, EMS personnel, and the system as a whole. Increased transport time, discontinuity of care, and increased out-of-service time have all been cited as causes for concern.[6] One study showed an increase in average scene time of 9% and an increase in transport time of 15%.[11] Although this study does not explain the increase in scene or transport times, it is reasonable to assume that the increase in transport time is due to increased distance to the next closest hospital. Discussion has also addressed the potential for diversion practices to lead to angry patients and frustrated EMS personnel. At least one lawsuit has arisen from a decision to divert an ambulance and the prospect of additional suits may result from the perceived or actual adverse consequences arising from either prolonged transportation or lack of access to a hospital that would normally be considered the facility best capable of offering the most appropriate care.[6]

Although the effects of ambulance diversion have caused alarm in the medical and lay media, few studies have specifically studied the problem.[12-15] Clearly, diverting a patient to a hospital other than that which is closest increases transport time, which translates to an increase in time to definitive hospital treatment. This may pose a risk to the individual patient in terms of delayed care, particularly if the medical condition is critical or unstable, as well as imposing some degree of additional danger associated with the hazards of transportation itself (e.g., ambulance collision). Continuity of care may also be interrupted if transportation to a hospital affiliated with the patient's primary physician and medical records is denied. Longer transport times also increase the amount of time an ambulance is out of service. Furthermore, as neighboring hospitals receive an increasing share of ambulances, their ability to rapidly place those patients becomes impaired, at times causing significant delays in ambulance crews' ability to free up their stretchers and return to service.

When one ED is on diversion, ambulance patients are directed to adjacent hospitals, thus placing an additional burden on neighboring institutions. Ultimately a "domino effect" results, in which a cluster of hospitals may declare ambulance diversion, potentially affecting an entire region or municipality. Furthermore, as clusters of hospitals become unavailable, ambulances are diverted to isolated parts of a region in which hospitals are still receiving patients. The end result may be that ambulances are maldistributed as a result of repetitive diversions, leaving significant portions of a community undercovered and subject to prolonged response times.

This "domino effect" may also adversely affect the availability of regional specialty care, especially in organized trauma systems. Though a trauma center's ability to care for injured patients may be fundamentally intact, a general overcrowding situation may prevent it from accepting severely injured patients, and deprive a region of sparsely distributed trauma services.

This situation has led to a debate in some areas about whether institutions with specialized services should be able to protect beds for patients with specific needs, such as trauma or burn services, while they place themselves on diversion for general ambulance transports. The ethical and legal dilemma as it relates to the individual patient is clear. If a hospital that happens to be a trauma center has the capacity to treat a critically injured patient in the ED, it is difficult to justify diverting a critical medical patient to a more distant facility, at some risk, in order to maintain availability of a trauma bed for the community at large. There has been no test to date of this circumstance in the court system. As of this writing, subject to local regulation, the appropriate procedure under such conditions may be determined by the weight a particular community places on the needs of an individual patient versus ensuring that adequate specialty resources are protected for the population at large.

In theory the purpose of a diversion policy is to ensure that the majority of ambulance patients continue to receive the best care in the most timely fashion. Although on-scene and transport times have been shown to increase when diversion is in effect, no study has assessed the effect of hospital diversion on patient outcome.[11] One study suggested that diversion may not necessarily be detrimental. "A regulation requiring that EDs always remain open could be counterproductive if the time saved in ambulance transport were offset by increasing delays after arrival at the hospital."[11] Most systems make the assumption that the diverted patient is better off in the back of the ambulance rather then in the bypassed ED.

Ethical and Legal Considerations

The practice of ambulance diversion has raised several difficult ethical and legal concerns among EMS leaders. A growing body of legislation and statutory regulation is defining approaches to the implementation of diversion procedures; most of these are governed by local philosophical views of how to proceed. Once it is assumed that a hospital, in good faith, has declared that it no longer has adequate resources to provide appropriate care for patients in the ED or within the institution, individual decisions must be made about the best alternative destination for the patient. If the patient is completely stable, there is generally no risk in diverting the patient to the next closest facility. If the patient is unstable, it is usually difficult to predict with accuracy whether a longer transport to the next available facility poses significant risk to the patient.

Some medical directors believe that, in systems with short distances between neighboring hospitals, even the most critically ill patients will receive better attention in an ED that has no resource limitations than in one which has declared its lack of ability to adequately care for additional patients. Presumably, the more complicated a patient, the less able a facility with inadequate resources is able to address that patient's needs. Thus, assuming reasonable temporizing care has been initiated within the ambulance, some systems have decided, in the best interest of patient care, virtually never to deliver a patient to an ED on diversion unless ambulance personnel are unable or unqualified to address their most urgent needs (such as an unsecured airway) or the additional transport time to the next facility is extreme (15 minutes has been cited in many policies). On the other hand, many systems require that all critically ill or unstable patients be taken to the closest receiving hospital, regardless of diversion status or distance to the next facility.

The well-being of the ambulance patient may not be the only consideration in deciding whether to respect a hospital's diversion status. The addition of a complicated ambulance patient to the ED volume of an already overloaded staff may realistically compromise the care of patients already in that ED, particularly if it necessitates the premature removal of another patient from a cardiac monitor or displacement of staff from the care of established patients. Conversely, it has been argued that all EDs continue to have a duty to treat any ill patients who arrive at the emergency department by their own means, regardless of the hospital's diversion status. This argument must be weighed against the fact that, under conditions of a declared diversion status, prehospital personnel have been forewarned about the inadequacy of the closest ED to care for additional patients, thus making it the responsibility of the EMS personnel or direct medical oversight to consider whether the closest hospital would indeed be an appropriate destination for the patient in the ambulance. With little objective science to guide these rapid decisions, it would be understandable for prehospital decision-makers to feel on shaky ground when making such determinations. In early 2002, a previously diverted ambulance patient made national news by traveling by private car, following a second cardiac event, so as to avoid another diversion from his hospital of choice.

Another potential dilemma arises in situations in which a hospital has placed itself on diversion for lack of internal resources, such as no ICU beds or no available operating rooms. In such cases, the ED still has capacity to provide emergency care, but the institution requests diversion status for a category of patients for which it feels it cannot provide definitive stabilization. The 1982 NYC policy did not allow inpatient status to initiate an ED diversion. Some EMS systems allow inpatient crowding to justify patients being diverted to other hospitals. In the 1992 case of *Johnson v. University of Chicago Hospitals* (UCH), the court found UCH remiss in diverting a critically ill neonate to an adjacent hospital, even though it had a declared lack of pediatric intensive-care beds while the ED had available resources.[16] At the time, this was an approved category of diversion status. This case resulted in two important regulatory changes in Illinois. First, no longer is it permitted for a hospital to declare diversion status due to lack of in-house critical-care beds, as long as the ED has the capacity to provide appropriate care. Secondly, Illinois now requires that whenever a telemetry authority makes the decision to divert, the telemetry authority must attest in writing that the benefits of transport to a more distant facility outweigh the risks of transporting the patient to that more distant hospital.[17]

Some EMS systems permit hospitals to declare diversion for lack of a specific resource, such as CT scan or orthopedic services. This can create problems for EMS personnel, because it suggests they have the ability to predict, based on a prehospital assessment, whether a patient will need those specific services urgently. The position statement of NAEMSP discourages the use of overly specific categories of diversion, in order to avoid imposing an unrealistic expectation that prehospital personnel will be able to predict the exact in-hospital needs of their ambulance patients.[4] For example, the responsibility for the decision as to whether to take an elderly patient with fever and mild mental status changes to a hospital that has requested CT diversion may require a level of diagnostic accuracy that is not possible in the prehospital setting. Yet, should that patient be found to require an urgent CT scan, would a provider be expected to defend the decision to transport the patient to that hospital, lacking specific training in how to differentiate which patients require CT scans?

EMTALA and Diversion

The question as to what extent do regulations under the Emergency Medicine Treatment and Active Labor Act (EMTALA) affect ambulance diversion was raised in *Johnson v. University of Chicago Hospitals*.[16] In *Johnson*, the plaintiffs sought to prove that telemetry contact was, for purposes of EMTALA, equivalent to the patient's having "come to the emergency department." Doing so would make the hospital liable under EMTALA despite the patient did not physically arrive at the hospital. The plaintiffs argued that contacting direct medical oversight at the intended receiving hospital constituted coming to the ED and that the hospital-directed diversion of the patient constituted an illegal transfer. The court recognized that a hospital "could conceivably use a telemetry system in a scheme to dump patients," but determined that telemetry contact in this case was not the equivalent of the patient's having "come to the emergency department" and, therefore, EMTALA did not apply.

Given the issues that were raised as a result of *Johnson*, attempts were made by CMS to clarify the impact of EMTALA on prehospital care and, more specifically, on hospital diversion. "Comes to the ED" means, with respect to an individual requesting examination or treatment, that the individual is on the hospital property (property includes ambulances owned and operated by the hospital, even if the ambulance is not on hospital grounds). An individual in a nonhospital-owned ambulance on hospital property is considered to have "come to the hospital ED." An individual in a nonhospital-owned ambulance off hospital property is not considered to have "come to the ED," even if a member of the ambulance staff contacts the hospital by telephone or telemetry communications and informs the hospital that they want to transport the individual to the hospital for examination and treatment. In such situations, the hospital may deny access if it is in "diversionary status," that is, it does not have the staff or facilities to accept any additional emergency patients.[18]

In 2001 this language was applied to *Arrington v. Wong*.[19] Like *Johnson*, the *Arrington* case addressed whether it is an EMTALA violation for a hospital to divert a patient based on telemetry contact. However, despite strong factual similarities, the court in *Arrington* reached the opposite conclusion. The pivotal difference was that the hospital in *Arrington* was not on diversion when it received the telemetry call. According to the court, "Arrington's attempt to reach the hospital [was] within the scope of EMTALA's 'comes to' language."[20] It held that "a hospital may divert an ambulance that has contacted its emergency room and is on its way to the hospital only if the hospital is on diversionary status."[21]

In reaching its decision, the court turned the second to last sentence quoted above ("An individual in a nonhospital-owned ambulance off hospital property . . .") on its head. It also made the last sentence ("In such situations . . .") read so as to place any hospital not on diversion under the obligation of EMTALA from the moment that telemetry contact is established. The decision in *Arrington* is binding only in the 9th Circuit, which includes most of the Western states. But, despite this limitation, it is the type of decision that is likely to be cited in other courts and may have far-reaching impact on EMS providers, emergency physicians, and hospitals.[22]

EMTALA may well apply to specific scenarios in which a patient may be intentionally or unwittingly brought by ambulance to an ED on diversion. The EMTALA statute makes no exception for hospitals on diversion. Therefore, there is presumably no reason to assume that any or all of the requirements for an appropriate transfer of such a patient to another facility would not apply. It is not unusual to hear anecdotes in which prehospital personnel, after arriving with a patient at an ED on diversion, are encouraged or independently decide to transport their patient to another facility that is not on diversion. However, once the patient has arrived at a particular ED, regardless of its diversion status, EMTALA indicates that an adequate medical screening examination, stabilization of the emergency condition, and appropriate communication with the hospital that would accept the patient in transfer must be conducted. These authors know of no EMTALA challenges involving patients who were directed away from an ED on diversion after arrival at that institution. However, this is an area of potentially serious hazard, especially if an unstable patient is involved. Furthermore, it is not necessary for a patient to suffer harm for a hospital or individual to be found in violation of EMTALA, and legal authorities may view diversion status as a means of performing economic triage. Therefore, extreme caution should be used in educating hospital and EMS personnel in appropriate procedures to follow when a patient has been inadvertently transported by ambulance to a hospital on diversion. The most con-servative approach to this situation would be to assume that EMTALA applies equally to a patient who is transported to a hospital on diversion, whether expressly or unintentionally. Such a stance would necessitate a routine medical screening exam and invoke the same requirements for stabilization and transfer as under normal ED operating conditions, including the agreement of the patient.

Approaches to Diversion

As the diversion problem has escalated in recent years, there has been a trend toward statutory and regulatory oversight of diversion practices on both a state and local level. The problem of ED overcrowding and diversion has been dealt with differently in different communities. For example, in Los Angeles, hospitals on diversion are required to accept patients in extremis or when the time to transport to the nearest open hospital is greater than 10 minutes.[23] Additionally, Los Angeles only permits diversion for patients requiring ALS care. San Diego has similar provisions, but does not specify a minimum transport time to override diversion.[24]

Massachusetts recommends and Illinois requires internal hospital policies for avoiding and resolving diversion status. Massachusetts recommends a "treat and transfer" policy to relieve EDs of excess patients before ambulance diversion becomes necessary,[25] whereas Illinois, in evaluating the appropriateness of a hospital's diversion practice, incorporates activation of the hospital's internal disaster plan as an indication of its efforts to resolve its resource limitation. New Jersey allows the administration of each hospital to determine the threshold and criteria for diversion.[26] The City of Chicago outlines specific criteria for declaring a situation of resource limitation, although it allows hospitals, subject to certain state requirements, to individually define when they have internally met those criteria.[27]

EMS systems vary in their thresholds for overriding a diversion status, either based on an individual patient's needs or the overall status of the system. Some systems require that any unstable or critical patient be transported to the closest EMS receiving hospital, even if it is on diversion, whereas others limit this requirement to patients in cardiac arrest or with an unsecured airway. Yet other systems leave this determination entirely to the discretion of direct medical oversight or ambulance personnel. Often, this is a function of the demographics of the EMS system. Systems in which very short distances separate neighboring hospitals are more likely to tolerate diversion of more critical patients, under the assumption that it is best for such patients to arrive at an ED with no resource limitations. The greater the distance between hospitals, the more important it is to consider overriding a diversion if the lengthier transport time may be detrimental to the patient. In some systems, particularly rural settings, hospital diversion is essentially non-existent, because the distance to the next closest hospital makes diversion a non-option.

A unique approach to ambulance diversion was implemented in Syracuse, in 1989.[1] The four receiving hospitals in Syracuse, which had been receiving patients on a rotating basis, entered into agreement with four hospitals in the surrounding area to accept patients when all four urban hospitals were overwhelmed. This plan failed to relieve ED overcrowding in its first six months, leading the Hospital Executive Council of Syracuse to conclude that ambulance diversion is not "a long-term solution to the overcrowding of hospital emergency departments."[1]

Some systems have implemented technical solutions that make it more feasible to cope with diversion situations system-wide, and may assist hospitals in initiating internal responses. Several EMS systems use Internet-based or other computer-linked information systems to monitor and regulate diversion activity. Such systems record EMS receiving hospital status on a real-time basis. This information may be accessible only to the EMS authority or it may be viewed by all participants. Generally, authority for changes in status on the system is reserved for the EMS authority, but receiving hospitals may be permitted to register their own status, subject to local system regulation. Such systems have the advantage of permitting hospitals and EMS authorities to have an up-to-date picture of the ED capacity of the community, enabling them to prepare for evolving system-wide pressures. It makes tracking of diversion activity very simple, and provides a means of communication of special events that may affect area-wide EDs as well as enabling practical override measures. In fact, some EMS systems have enabled the communications system to automatically override, modify, or cancel diversion status when specific system thresholds have been exceeded. Examples of such systems are the Computerized Hospital Online Resource Allocation Link (CHORAL), used in San Francisco and EM System.com, which is used in the County of Milwaukee and several other communities.[28]

Components of a Diversion Policy

The rationale for implementing a diversion policy is to ensure that EMS patients continue to receive the best medical care in the most timely manner possible, given the constraints of the EMS system and its available resources. To meet these goals, a policy should outline discrete diversion categories such as "unstable," "ALS," "ALS/BLS" or "trauma" to allow a hospital to divert patients based on specific system-recognized resource limitations. Such a policy should also provide specific field criteria for diverting a patient with special needs to a hospital with unique resources. These patients include trauma patients, patients with burns, pediatric patients, or patients in active labor. In either situation, as much as possible, such criteria should be determined prospectively and rely on simple clinical indicators that are observable in the field, so as not to place unrealistic reliance on prehospital personnel to determine the specific hospital resources that a patient will need. For instance, if a category of "CT" diversion exists, EMS policies should specify in advance to what types of patients it should be applied.

A mechanism should be defined for a hospital to notify the appropriate authorities and other affected institutions of the diversion so that the appropriate triage decisions can be made. Ideally, a mechanism would exist to alert neighboring hospitals of diversion situations so that they could initiate measures to prepare to receive additional ambulance patients.

Most EMS systems impose a time limit on diversion status after which the hospital must update its status or become open to ambulance traffic. This practice communicates to hospitals that diversion is a temporary means of coping with a resource limitation, and conveys the expectation that they will enact measures to resolve their situation as quickly as possible.

The medical director of a system should have the authority to override diversion when necessary, such as during disaster situations, or when hospital diversion is causing an unacceptable prolongation of ambulance response or patient transport times. The medical director should also monitor the system to determine the frequency of hospital diversion and the effects diversion has on the system. EMS systems must have provisions for overriding one or more hospitals' status when needed. Decisions to deny diversion are based on the best interest of the individual patient as well as the status of the entire community.

These decisions should be based on overall hospital availability, transport times, EMS system volume, and ambulance response times.

Authorities differ significantly in their approaches to overriding diversion. Many systems have adopted an "all closed means all open" approach, to react to situations in which multiple hospitals on diversion have created a system-wide crisis. Other regions have determined that such a draconian approach should be avoided at all costs, recognizing that critical overcrowding situations within EDs pose risks to all patients treated in those environments. Such systems may apply intermediate measures to ensure ED availability, including individual assessment of a hospital's capabilities. In Illinois, statutes require that diversion status be cancelled when three or more hospitals within a geographical area are on diversions *and* transport times exceed 15 minutes.[27] Others rely on the principle that all critical patients will be transported to the closest ED at all times, making the need to cancel diversion irrelevant.

Regardless of the criteria for overriding diversion, the EMS authority must have the ability to make swift decisions in the interest of the population at large based on the best information available to them. Frequently, they are faced with making complex comparisons between receiving hospitals, and do not have the ability to perform a detailed analysis of individual hospital situations. The override mechanism must be as objective as possible, as well as practical.

The diversion policy of the system and individual hospital policies should specify which members of the hospital's staff are authorized to request diversion. The policy should ensure the proper care of all patients who arrive at a hospital, despite diversion status. The policy should under no circumstances allow diversion of a patient based on race, gender, socio-economic status, or availability of health insurance. The policy should include mechanisms to ensure that hospitals use all available resources to relieve overcrowding or correct the causative problem, minimizing the time that diversion is required. Finally, the policy should address the growing problem of individual patients refusing transport if "their" hospital is on diversion.

Most EMS regulations include provisions for review of hospital diversion practices either by the local authority, the EMS medical director, or a governmental regulatory agency. In some cases, discipline or sanctions for improper use of diversion may apply. Regardless of the authority for such oversight procedures, there should be some provision for review and oversight of diversion that will minimize the arbitrariness of the practice and recognize diversion patterns that fall well outside that of the general hospital community. Local, regional, and state governments should enact policies or statutes addressing diversion, and should empower the EMS medical director to monitor and enforce these policies.

The NAEMSP position statement on ambulance diversion (Appendix A) provides a breakdown of the recommended components of a diversion policy, and defines the roles and responsibilities of various levels of participants in the EMS system in all aspects of diversion practices.

Summary

As has been discussed, diversion is not a solution, but a symptom of a crisis. Nor is it, by and large, an indication of a problem in the EMS system or ED itself. It is important that hospital and health system administrators recognize that the need for a hospital to request diversion reflects the need to resolve a hospital-wide situation that has impaired the ED's ability to admit patients or otherwise determine timely patient dispositions. Efforts to resolve the ED overcrowding problem must recognize that more patients are using fewer EDs and ambulances are finding themselves turned away with increasing frequency.

Solutions to the diversion and overcrowding situation must be sought on a local and broader health system basis. They require short- and long-term approaches. Many of the factors that result in inadequacy of ED resources are well beyond the scope of the EMS system to directly influence. Such measures include improved funding of the ED and hospital systems, particularly for those institutions serving a higher proportion of the indigent and elderly population; addressing nursing shortages; and aggressive influenza vaccination campaigns.

Hospitals may need to examine ways to improve internal efficiency, particularly in their ability to effectively manage hospital bed status and continually make room for admissions. One hospital developed a graded internal response plan, based on ED admission delays, specifically in reaction to its prior pattern of excessive ambulance diversion. This plan incorporated the use of hospital internists to accelerate in-hospital patient decision-making and discharge decisions. This plan, once enacted, was successful in drastically reducing this hospital's diversion activity.

The appropriate measures for individual institutions to address an overcrowding situation will depend on the specific set of factors affecting that particular facility.

The emergency medicine community can also take measures to raise public awareness of the endangered healthcare safety net and the toll it is taking on emergency resources. Locally, EMS systems can improve interhospital communications systems so that institutions have better real-time awareness of emerging crisis situations, and can take measures to avoid diversion.

References

1. Lagoe RJ, Jastremski MS. Relieving overcrowded emergency departments through ambulance diversion. *Hospital Topics*. 1990:68:23–27.
2. National Center for Health Statistics: Emergency Department Visits. www.cdc.gov/nchs/faststats/ervisits.htm.
3. Gallagher EJ, Lynn SG. The etiology of medical gridlock: causes of emergency department overcrowding in New York City. *J Emerg Med*. 1990;8:785–790.
4. Glushak C, Delbridge TR, Garrison HG. Ambulance Diversion: Standards and Clinical Practices Committee, National Association of EMS Physicians. *Prehosp Emerg Care*. 1997;1:100–103.
5. American College of Emergency Physicians. Ambulance diversion/destination policies. *ACEP News*. January 1992: insert.
6. Derlet RW, Richards JR. Overcrowding in the nation's emergency departments: complex causes and disturbing effects. *Ann Emerg Med*. 2000;35:63–68.
7. Graff L. Overcrowding in the ED: an international symptom of health care system failure. *Am J Emerg Med*. 1999;17:208–209.
8. National Center for Health Statistics: Emergency Department Visits. www.cdc.gov/nchs/faststats/ervisits.htm.
9. McLean SA, JA Feldman. The impact of changes in HCFA documentation requirements on academic emergency medicine: results of a physician survey. *Acad Emerg Med*. 2001;8(9):880–885.
10. American College of Emergency Physicians: Emergency Department Waiting Times. Fact Sheet, available at www.acep.org/1,2084,0.html.
11. Redelmeier DA, Blair PJ, Collins WE. No place to unload: a preliminary analysis of the prevalence, risk factors, and consequences of ambulance diversion. *Ann Emerg Med*. 1994;23:43–47.
12. Woo E. Critical conditions: Emergency room shutdowns are hitting home as patients, paramedics scramble to cope. *Los Angeles Times*. January 30, 1989: V1.
13. Emergency rooms here feel the heat. *Washington Post*. September 14, 1989: A1.
14. Johnson R. Ambulance ride proved too long, dead man's friends say. *The Atlanta Journal and Constitution*. August 7, 1990: J-3.
15. Brown M. Emergency room jam-up shutting out ambulances. *Chicago Sun-Times*. January 4, 1990: 3.
16. *Johnson v. University of Chicago Hospitals*, 982 F.2d 230 (7th Circuit 1992).
17. Metropolitan Chicago Healthcare Council, EMS Medical Directors Consortium. Notification and Monitoring of Hospital Resource Limitation/Ambulance Diversion. Chicago, IL: Sept 1, 1993.
18. 42 C.F.R. Sect 489.24 (b).
19. *Arrington v. Wong*, 237 F.3d 1066 (9th Cir. 2001).
20. *Arrington v. Wong*, 237 F.3d 1070 (9th Cir. 2001).
21. *Arrington v. Wong*, 237 F.3d 1074 (9th Cir. 2001).
22. Greenwood, MJ. *Arrington v. Wong*: update and analysis. *NAEMSP News*. 2001;10:6–7.
23. County of Los Angeles Department of Health Services, Los Angeles County EMS Agency: Revised Guidelines for Hospitals Requesting Diversion of Mobile Intensive Care Units. Los Angeles, CA: January 28, 1988.
24. County of San Diego Department of Health Services, Division of Emergency Medical Services: Guidelines for Hospitals Requesting Ambulance Diversion. San Diego, CA: March 1, 1990.
25. Massachusetts Hospital Association, EMS Task Force: Patient Overload and Ambulance Diversion. Burlington, MA: May 1988.
26. New Jersey Hospital Association, Council on Planning, Committee on EMS: A Full House: Hospital Diversion Guidelines. Princeton, NJ: April 1990.
27. Metropolitan Chicago Healthcare Council, EMS Medical Directors Consortium. Notification and Monitoring of Hospital Resource Limitation/Ambulance Diversion. Chicago, IL: Sept 1, 1993.
28. San Francisco General Hospital Emergency Department Policy and Procedure Manual, available at http://sfghed.ucsf.edu/ED_P&P/Choral.htm.
29. Metropolitan Chicago Healthcare Council, sup.

Appendix A: NAEMSP Ambulance Diversion Position Statement

Position

A principal function of emergency medical services (EMS) systems is to provide patients with urgently needed emergency medical care and to deliver them to an appropriate emergency medical facility as rapidly as possible. The phenomenon of ambulances transporting emergency patients beyond the closest emergency facility to a more distant destination occurs under three circumstances: specific patient request, a triage decision that directs a patient with special needs to a facility offering a specialized or higher level of care, and a decision to avoid a facility that has declared a lack of resources needed by that patient. This position statement deals exclusively with "diversion" or "bypass" situations resulting from the lack of normally available hospital resources.

The diversion of ambulances, because of temporary shortages of emergency department (ED) or inpatient facilities, may have adverse effects on patient care and the EMS system as a whole. EMS personnel are limited in their ability to definitively treat and stabilize critically ill or injured patients in the field. Therefore, it is necessary that EMS systems, including receiving facilities, take all necessary measures to avoid diversion of ambulances, which may result in:

1. unacceptably prolonged transport time intervals;
2. prolonged out-of-hospital care when definitive hospital resources are needed, especially for unstable or critically ill patients;
3. inappropriate attempts by field personnel to predict the specific diagnostic and therapeutic resources needed by individual patients; and
4. delays in, or lack of, ambulance availability to the community because of diversion of units to distant hospitals.

Responsibility for averting these conditions is shared by all those who contribute to EMS structures and processes. The National Association of EMS Physicians believes that the following principles apply to EMS system participants:

All Participants

The diversion of ambulance patients away from the closest or normally most appropriate ED should be considered undesirable, but may be occasionally necessary. In all cases it should be considered a temporary measure while efforts are under way to successfully restore essential resources. All participants, including hospitals, medical control authorities, and provider agencies, must agree to an EMS policy that clearly delineates categories of hospital or ED diversion based on the lack of available resources. These categories must be explicit, allowing out-of-hospital personnel to rapidly determine the most appropriate destination under conditions of limited resources.

1. General categories must be defined prospectively and recognized system wide.
2. System-wide triage rules that direct specific types of patients, based on assessments within the scope of field personnel education and practice, to hospital facilities offering higher or specialized levels of care, may be appropriate. Such rules may direct severe trauma, burn, pediatric, and/or other patients to predesignated facilities, which may not necessarily be closest to the emergency scene. These situations do not represent examples of temporary diversion caused by limitation of resources normally available at the closest facility.
3. Categories for selective diversion due to temporary lack of a specific diagnostic or therapeutic resource (e.g., neurosurgical, orthopedic, CT scan) are strongly discouraged because they require out-of-hospital personnel to make predictions about the specific needs of EMS patients, without the requisite education or experience for doing so. If utilized, such categories must be prospectively defined and recognized system wide. They must not require out-of-hospital EMS workers to make diagnoses in order to predict the specific resources that will be needed (see Hospital requirements, below).
4. Any policy creating specific categories of diversion must include concise assessment-based criteria to guide field personnel in their implementation for individual patients and must be accompanied by appropriate education of EMS providers.
5. All participating agencies must agree to a mechanism for timely transmittal and receipt of information about initiation, termination or change of any resource limitation, or diversion status.
6. Interhospital transfer agreements must be in place to provide access to appropriate definitive care under circumstances of resource limitations. Such agreements should be in compliance with all federal, state, and local statutes.
7. The system must agree to criteria and procedures for overriding a hospital's diversion status. The following considerations should be addressed:

   • patient condition
   • duration of transport time intervals
   • multiple hospitals on division ("all closed, all open" situation)
   • mass casualty or disaster incidents
   • designation of the appropriate authority to make an override decision

8. Communities should attempt to legislate immunity that protects EMS personnel (field and base station) who, with limited available information, make good-faith decisions regarding appropriate destinations for patients.

EMS Medical Oversight

1. The medical director must work with the other EMS system participants to prospectively determine conditions under which a request to divert patients may be permitted or overridden. These should be promulgated across the system in the form of written guidelines and should address at least the following issues:
   - transportation time intervals
   - distances between receiving facilities
   - severity of patients' conditions

2. The medical director must ensure the availability of direct medical oversight by qualified individuals (e.g., physicians or their qualified designees) to evaluate the appropriateness of individual patient diversions. At all times, the authority for permitting patient diversions rests with the direct medical oversight providers.

3. The medical director, in consultation with the other EMS system participants, must be prepared and empowered to modify the criteria for diversion as needed.

4. The medical director must monitor the frequency, type, and effects of hospital diversion status. Participating hospitals and provider agencies must provide the medical director with data necessary to adequately monitor diversion practices. EMS quality improvement activities should include continuous evaluation of diversion practices and identification of potential methods for diversion reduction.

5. The medical director must be empowered and prepared to apply corrective action to facilities whose actions or policies result in inappropriate patient diversions.

Provider Agency Requirements

1. The provider agency must ensure that direct medical oversight is available, and that authority for confirming or overriding a decision to divert a patient rests with the direct medical control provider.

2. Provider agencies must ensure the means to obtain up-to-date information on the resource availability and diversion status of all receiving facilities.

3. Provider agencies should develop plans for the deployment of ambulance units based on established patterns of diversion practices in order to maintain appropriate response time intervals. They should monitor diversion activity and inform EMS medical and administrative authorities when their capacity to accommodate diversion requests is exceeded.

Hospital Requirements

1. Hospitals must meet predefined, accepted criteria (see All Participants, above) in order for a diversion status to be recognized.

2. Decisions to divert patients must apply to all patients; preferential routing of "desirable" or "private" patients to an ED on diversion status must not occur. Under no circumstance should a diversion decision be based on race, gender, insurance, or socioeconomic status of the patient.

3. A hospital, regardless of its diversion status, must agree to care for any patient when EMS personnel and/or the direct medical control provider determines that it is the most appropriate transport destination.

4. Hospitals should designate specific staff who are authorized to request division status. The identity of the individuals should be on file with the EMS provider agency(ies) and the EMS medical control authority. Senior hospital administrative personnel must be continuously aware of, and ultimately responsible for, the diversion practices of their institutions.

5. Except in specific situations agreed upon prospectively by the EMS system, requests for ambulance diversion should be based on availability of ED resources. Although specific inpatient resources may be unavailable, a hospital should continue to receive patients as long as the ED has the capacity to evaluate, stabilize, and provide ongoing emergency care for them.

6. Hospitals must have a policy, in accordance with guidelines agreed upon by the EMS system, that ensures that appropriate measures are taken to both avoid and terminate diversion status. Such policies must include the following provisions:

A. In-house resources should be fully utilized to minimize ED overcrowding. For example, if the ED is requesting diversion status because all of its beds are occupied by patients awaiting admission, then all in-house beds should be fully utilized.

B. Procedures to procure additional resources should be in place, and may include accelerated discharge planning and mobilization of additional staff.

C. A hospital should not protect specific beds for elective admissions when it is diverting EMS patients to other institutions. Elective nonemergency admissions and unscheduled transfers to the hospital should be delayed or canceled if, due to a lack of inpatient resources, they interfere with pending emergency admissions.

7. Diversion of specific types of patients must be limited to categories prospectively designated by the EMS system. Hospitals normally offering comprehensive emergency services should have preexisting arrangements with nearby hospitals to accept their patients while a diversion is in effect.

8. Hospitals must update their diversion status at predefined intervals (e.g., every 6 to 12 hours) or be subject to automatic reinstatement of their normal status.

Government Agencies

1. State, regional and local EMS lead agencies should promulgate statutes and/or policies that address the practice of ambulance diversion.

2. EMS statutes and policies should confer appropriate authority to the EMS medical director for monitoring and enforcing EMS system ambulance diversion policies.

3. State and regional EMS authorities must be empowered and prepared to apply sanctions against EMS system participants who are in violation of approved ambulance diversion policies.

Appendix B: San Francisco Ambulance Diversion Policy

Source: Policy Manual; San Francisco Emergency Medical Services Section; Department of Public Health; City and County of San Francisco

Policy Reference No.: 8010
Effective Date: 03/01/01
Supersedes: 12/01/99

DIVERSION POLICY

I. PURPOSE

A. To establish guidelines under which Receiving Hospital Emergency Departments may divert ambulance patients when it has been determined, through pre-established criteria, that the Emergency Department is unable to accommodate additional patients.

B. To define procedures for communicating changes in diversion status.

C. To establish guidelines for ambulance provider operations when a Receiving Hospital is on diversion.

D. To define exceptions to the *Ambulance Destination Policy*, EMS Section Policy #8000, when hospital(s) follow procedures as outlined herein.

II. AUTHORITY

California Health and Safety Code, Section 1797.204; 1797.220; 1797.222 and the California Code of Regulations, Title 22, Division 9, 1798.102.

III. DEFINITIONS

A. **Total Diversion:** When a Receiving Hospital Emergency Department determines, through pre-established criteria, that the Emergency Department is unable to safely provide care to additional ambulance patients AND communicates this change in status to the Emergency Communications Department (ECD).

B. **Emergency Communications Department (ECD):** The department within the City and County of San Francisco government that is responsible for all 911 public safety emergency communications and dispatch (police, fire, and EMS).

C. **Hospital Administration Resource Tool (HART):** An Internet-based hospital diversion monitoring system (HART) that provides a communication link between Receiving Hospitals, the ECD, and other EMS System participants.

D. **Trauma Override:** When San Francisco General Hospital (SFGH) continues Total Diversion during a period of Total Diversion suspension. During Trauma Override, SFGH shall continue the diversion of medical (non-trauma) patients, while continuing to accept patients meeting trauma center destination criteria. The intent of Trauma Override is to allow SFGH to maintain adequate trauma care capacity to meet local public health and safety needs of the EMS system. Trauma Override shall only be invoked when the criteria outlined in Section VIII are met.

IV. POLICY

A. In determining ambulance destination, EMS personnel shall utilize the *Ambulance Destination Policy*, EMS Section Policy #8000, which considers the patient's condition, the patient's location, the patient's requested hospital, the hospital capabilities, and the hospital diversion status.

B. The Base Hospital Physician shall retain the ultimate authority in determining ambulance destination. The Base Hospital Physician may override an Emergency Department's Diversion status if, in their judgment, they determine that the patient could deteriorate as a result of bypassing a Receiving Hospital on Diversion.

C. Receiving Hospitals shall report diversion status and subsequent changes on the HART System in accordance with established procedures, as described in Section VI. of this policy.

D. The ECD shall use the HART System to obtain the diversion status of Receiving Hospitals and communicate this status to on-duty ambulance personnel.

E. The ECD and the Receiving Hospitals shall have personnel trained to operate the HART System on-duty 24 hours a day, seven days a week.

F. Patients meeting Specialty Care Triage criteria (i.e., Burns, Trauma, Replantation, Obstetrics, and Emergency Department Approved for Pediatrics) shall **not** be subject to Total Diversion. San Francisco General Hospital shall **not** divert incarcerated patients or patients who are in police custody. Receiving Hospitals designated as Specialty Care Facilities shall continue to receive these patients **at all times** unless granted exemptions after successfully petitioning the Emergency Medical Services (EMS) Section.

G. This policy shall not override or interfere with the *Trauma Center and Psychiatric Diversion policies*, EMS Section Policy References #8011 and #8012.

V. HOSPITAL DIVERSION STATUS

The ability of the various Receiving Hospitals to receive patients according to their approved capabilities under the Receiving Hospital Agreements shall be determined in accordance with the categories listed below. Ambulance providers shall transport patients to hospitals in accordance with the principles outlined below.

A. **OPEN**

Receiving Hospitals shall be designated "OPEN" when fully capable of receiving all patients who request that facility and/or would be transported to that facility according to the *Ambulance Destination Policy*, EMS Section Policy Reference #800. A Receiving Hospital is Open when the HART System displays their three-letter facility indicator in the color "green".

B. **TOTAL DIVERSION**

1. A hospital may declare Total Diversion only when the Emergency Department has an overload of patients requiring immediate attention and, therefore, would not be able to safely provide care should it receive an additional patient requiring immediate intervention. A hospital shall report Total Diversion due to Emergency Department overload only, and not due to lack of staffed inpatient medical/surgical or critical care beds.

2. A Receiving Hospital shall be on Total Diversion when the HART System displays their three letter facility indicator in the color "red" AND the message line displays the words "Total Divert."

3. When a Receiving Hospital is on Total Diversion, no patient shall be transported to that hospital by ambulance EXCEPT for the following circumstances:
   a) The patient meets the Specialty Care Triage criteria (Burns, Trauma, Replantation, Obstetrics, and Emergency Departments Approved for Pediatrics).
   b) The patient is in imminent or full respiratory or cardiac arrest, or is a post-arrest resuscitation.
   c) The patient originating from a hospital-based clinic. Such patients shall be considered to have arrived on hospital property and shall be transported to that hospital's Emergency Department.
   d) San Francisco General Hospital shall **not** divert incarcerated patients or patients who are in police custody.

4. Immediately upon relieving the ED overload, the Receiving Hospital shall Change their diversion status to OPEN on the HART system as appropriate. Diversion status changes should be made even during periods of diversion suspension.

5. When a Receiving Hospital is on Total Diversion, EMS Section on-call staff at their discretion may:
   a) inquire about the status of the Emergency Department and its ability to treat critically ill patients.
   b) inquire if the hospital has initiated its internal Total Diversion policy as well as what actions are being taken to return to Open status.
   c) request the names of the hospital's medical, nursing, or administrative staff who were contacted to assess and to attempt to rectify the Total Diversion situation.

VI. DIVERSION OPERATIONAL PROCEDURES

A. HOSPITAL ROLE IN DIVERSION STATUS CHANGE

1. Hospital personnel shall enter the hospital's appropriate diversion status in the HART System.

2. Immediately upon relieving the ED overload, the Receiving Hospital shall change their diversion status to OPEN on the HART system as appropriate. Diversion status changes should be made even during periods of diversion suspension.

3. If the HART System fails, hospital personnel shall immediately report the problem to the HART System Support Line and follow the Back-Up Telephone Procedure, described in Section VI.D.

B. ECD ROLE IN DIVERSION STATUS CHANGE

1. The ECD shall announce to all ambulance personnel by radio and mobile data terminals any time a change in diversion status is entered into the HART System.

2. The ECD shall make routine diversion status announcements by radio and mobile data terminals to all ambulance personnel at intervals no less frequently than every two hours.

C. AMBULANCE ROLE IN DIVERSION STATUS CHANGE

1. Ambulances enroute to a hospital must complete the transport of the patient to that facility when its Emergency Department goes on Total Diversion.

2. Ambulances that have arrived on hospital property (e.g., hospital clinic, hospital driveway, or hospital ambulance dock) must complete the transport of that patient to that facility when its Emergency Department goes on Total Diversion.

D. BACK-UP TELEPHONE COMMUNICATIONS IF THE HART SYSTEM IS INOPERABLE

1. The Receiving Hospital shall notify the ECD of any diversion status changes via telephone.

2. The ECD shall announce any diversion status changes to ambulance personnel by radio any time a change in diversion status is called in or make routine diversion status announcements by radio at intervals no less frequently than every two hours.

3. The ECD shall announce any diversion status changes to the Base Hospital and hospital personnel via radio when there is a change in diversion status and every two hours.

VII. SUSPENSION OF TOTAL DIVERSION

A. The ECD shall notify EMS Section on-call staff when **FOUR** or more full Receiving Hospitals are on Total Diversion. The EMS Section will determine whether further continuation of the situation may result in a danger to the public health and safety and may elect to suspend Total Diversion requiring all Receiving Hospitals to accept both critical and non-critical patients. EMS Section staff will be available to consult with the hospital administrator or designee during periods of Diversion Suspension in an attempt to assist hospitals to return to OPEN status. Total Diversion suspension shall remain in effect until three or fewer hospitals are on Total Diversion. EMS Section staff shall consult with the ECD to assess the status of EMS System activity before removing the suspension.

B. Total Diversion suspension applies **only** to hospitals within the limits of the City and County of San Francisco. Total Diversion suspension does **not** apply to hospitals in other counties (e.g., Seton Medical Center located in San Mateo County).

C. When Total Diversion Suspension is invoked, the ECD shall:

1. Enter the Total Diversion suspension into the HART System.

2. Announce to all ambulance personnel by radio and mobile data terminals any time Total Diversion is suspended.

3. Make routine Total Diversion Suspension status announcements by radio and mobile data terminals to all ambulance personnel at intervals no less frequently than every two hours.

VIII. EXCEPTION TO TOTAL DIVERSION SUSPENSION—TRAUMA OVERRIDE

A. When Total diversion is suspended, the Chief of SFGH Trauma Services or his/her designee may declare a Trauma Override of Total Diversion at SFGH only if all of the following three conditions are met:

1. The Critical Care bed capacity at SFGH is two or less beds, and

2. All SFGH internal diversion strategies have been exhausted, and

3. There is at least one trauma patient in the process of evaluation or treatment in the SFGH Trauma care system (e.g., Emergency Department CT Scanner or Operating Room).

B. During Trauma Override, SFGH shall continue the diversion of medical (non-trauma) patients, while continuing to accept the following patients:

1. Patients meeting trauma center destination criteria.

2. Patients meeting other Specialty Care Triage criteria (Burns, Replantation, Obstetrics, and Emergency Departments Approved for Pediatrics).

3. The patient is an imminent or full respiratory or cardiac arrest, or is a post-arrest resuscitation.

4. Patients who are incarcerated or in police custody.
5. Patients originating from a hospital-based clinic. Such patients shall be considered to have arrived on hospital property and shall be transported to SFGH Emergency Department.

C. During Trauma Override, SFGH shall abide by the following procedures:
1. The SFGH Emergency Department charge nurse shall enter the Trauma Override status into the HART system according to the procedures outlined in Section V. above.
2. Trauma Override status shall be renewed hourly by the Emergency Department Attending Physician in Charge.
3. The SFGH Trauma Service Administrator shall maintain a written policy and procedure for Trauma Override and shall provide a written report to the EMS Section within ten business days of a Trauma Override event detailing the rationale for invoking the Override and the total amount of time it was in effect.

D. The ECD shall follow the same procedures for communication of Trauma Override to EMS system participants as outlined in Section V. B.

IX. QUALITY ASSURANCE AND RECORD KEEPING

A. Problems related to the implementation of this policy shall be reported to the EMS Section through the Unusual Occurrence Report System.

B. All Receiving Hospitals shall maintain on file at the EMS Section a copy of their internal procedures for determining diversion status and their diversion avoidance strategies.

C. All Receiving Hospitals shall periodically critique their internal diversion procedures for appropriateness of utilization.

D. When a hospital uses the HART System to change their diversion status, the System automatically records the event in a diversion log. The EMS Section will monitor and report monthly diversion activity for all San Francisco Receiving Hospitals. Reported diversion hours shall exclude hours when diversion is suspended.

E. EMS Section staff shall conduct its own review of hospital diversion activity and will report to the appropriate EMS Section committee on the following diversion activity quality indicators:
1. Unusual events reported by the Prehospital Unusual Occurrence Report System.
2. A Receiving Hospital is on diversion for an average of more than 15% during any consecutive three-month period of review.
3. A Receiving Hospital is on diversion for 30% during any one-month period.
4. A request for diversion not covered by current policies.
5. Trauma Override usage over 10% during any consecutive 3-month period of review or 20% during any one-month period.

F. EMS Section staff, at their discretion, may conduct site visits while a hospital is on diversion status.

Regionalization and Designation of Medical Facilities

76

Lynne Cooper, JD, MA
Alisdair Conn, MD

Introduction

Regionalization of medical facilities is recognized as critical to the ultimate success of EMS systems. Although great progress has been made in developing truly comprehensive EMS systems during the past 25 years, the degree of effort to regionalize facilities through categorization (review against standards to classify emergency-care capabilities) and designation (formal selection for patient referral and transfer) has varied.[1]

Notwithstanding the significant impact of the enactment of EMS system legislation on EMS development in the early 1970s, economic, political, and legal factors contribute to the benign neglect of medical facilities by EMS groups.[2-4] The slow rate of progress in categorizing and designating medical facilities is especially disappointing in the area of regional trauma systems implementation, given the apparent effectiveness of regionalized trauma care.[5-7]

The results of a 1987 nationwide survey conducted by the American College of Surgeons Committee on Trauma (ACSCOT), showed that statewide compliance with ACS trauma guidelines was poor. Only two states (Maryland and Virginia) had all of the eight essential components of a regional trauma system. Nineteen states and the District of Columbia either did not have statewide coverage and/or lacked one or more essential components; 29 states had not started the process of designation of trauma centers.

Controversy and confusion still surround the concepts of categorization and designation.[8] Proponents of categorization alone argue that it enhances the level of care provided without the need for designation. Supporters of designation, achieved with or without the initial categorization of facilities, point out that designation is even more difficult to achieve than categorization. Although problematic, most concede that emergency department (ED) or specialty referral center (SRC) designation combined with system integration appears to offer a distinct advantage over categorization alone.[9]

Categorization and designation have the same general goals; however, they are markedly different processes. Categorization is a voluntary process not subject to verification and not binding on the system providers. Categorization, while an accepted method of regionalizing certain services such as emergency, obstetrics, psychiatric, and burn care, provides for hospital self-assessment of capabilities without limitation on the numbers of hospitals participating in a given system.[10-12]

Although it has been shown that categorization reduces the provision of unacceptable care at hospitals,[13] it may not impact on patient outcome, or reduce costs through the elimination of duplication of services.[14] Categorization establishes standards of care and may serve as a preliminary framework for the designation of medical facilities, a component that should be in place before a system can consistently deliver patients to the most appropriate facilities. The categorization process is usually referred to as either vertical (the care for a particular medical problem throughout the institution) or horizontal (the scope of care of an ED).

Designation usually limits hospital participation and is a binding process requiring independent verification of both hospital compliance with standards and adherence to strict patient transport guidelines by prehospital providers. Implementation of designation fosters regionalization through accountability and commitment, which in turn theoretically reduce morbidity by improving the quality of care rendered.[15-17]

This chapter describes the regionalization process, its origins, and its evolution. It includes an approach to the designation of medical facilities within an EMS region. While these processes traditionally have begun at a local level, it is anticipated that states will continue to enact minimum standards for EDs and SRCs.

In a perfect world, the state standards will mirror the locally developed standards that are the basis for the designation guidelines in this chapter, and which are also reflective of the current criteria recommended by national professional organizations.

Historical Background

Regionalization accomplished through designation requires changes on the part of providers and, if an authorized lead agency is not already identified, it also requires enactment of state or municipal laws. For example, in New York State in 1981, facilities in half of the EMS regions were categorized based on guidelines established by the State EMS Council without formal state authority.[18] Since there was no legal authority to designate facilities, the process relied on voluntary participation that was uneven in some regions and nonexistent in others.[1,19]

Without an authorized lead agency to carry out the process, the risk of legal challenges increases, since designation often creates de facto monopolies by restricting the number of facilities allowed to participate and by requiring that certain standards of care be met prior to participation.[12,20] In the absence of explicit authority, the designation process may be impeded by physicians, hospitals, or other special interest groups.

Initially, the need for explicit authority to designate was not adequately addressed by the EMS system program planners, and this shortfall was compounded by the lack of federal funding for upgrading hospital facilities. Individual hospitals were relied upon to make costly improvements on a voluntary basis.[1] Since it was assumed that designation of trauma centers would promote the development of regionalized EMS systems, attempts were often made in the 1970s to organize EMS systems around trauma center development.[15] Therefore EMS systems evolved around the location of a neurosurgeon.

Under these circumstances, local EMS system program development usually focused on SRCs and rarely on EDs. This approach produced false starts and unbalanced results stemming from the failure to upgrade general emergency-care capabilities, as well as from an over-concentration on trauma care; when the trauma center process collapsed in the 1990s, so often did EMS system development. Many of the SRC problems were caused by the relaxation of the original strict criteria recommended by the ACS and the premature development of Level II (area) trauma center designations. The competition for designation as Level II centers among smaller community hospitals, and the resulting litigation, effectively halted development of the designations process altogether in many areas.[16]

Awareness of potential adverse economic effects, mainly the loss of patients by those institutions not designated, occasionally resulted in resistance by hospital administrators and physicians to both categorization and designation. In fact, less than 10% of all trauma patients actually required trauma center care; therefore, the actual loss of patients from nondesignated hospitals was minimal.[1] In reality, most trauma center program failures have been attributed to the financial burden caused by the large numbers of uninsured or indigent patients brought to the centers.[21,22] Other factors that act as economic disincentives to continued trauma center participation are the low rate of diagnosis-related group reimbursement for trauma care, the increasingly high cost of malpractice insurance premiums, and the perceived increased liability risk to physicians associated with the provision of trauma care.[22-24]

EMS systems development is much more difficult when there is fragmentation of authority or no authority for facility designations and regionalization. Legally authorized lead agencies are important since usually they may plan, implement, and operate without serious legal challenge.[25-27] A branch of government with legislative authority to designate is the best suited to serve as the lead agency. Since state government is responsible for setting medical facility reimbursement rate schedules,[19] ideally the designation authority will be with a state agency. Colorado and Pennsylvania utilize an independent foundation for trauma center designation. The effectiveness of such an approach has not yet been fully determined; however, that approach should be observed carefully by system medical directors in other states.

When federal EMS systems funding effectively ended in 1982, program initiatives and necessary legislative changes became the responsibility of individual states. Those responsible for developing or managing EMS systems found that in the absence of both the carrot of federal money and the stick of legal authority, plans for regionalization through facility designation usually failed.

Unauthorized designations expose agencies to antitrust liability. Explicit statutory authority affords the greatest protection against exposure to risk of liability for violation of the Sherman Act when limitations are made on the number of medical facilities used by a system.[9] In *Huron Valley Hospital Inc v. City of Pontiac* the court held that " . . . [State] regulatory actions within the gambit of valid legislation . . . are exempted from the antitrust laws under the 'state action' defense." Proper authorization to designate granted to an agency that enforces state policies through activities closely supervised by state officials would not violate antitrust laws. However, "anything short of properly constituted authority may run afoul of federal law. To avoid such antitrust problems, the proper authority must perform hospital designation."[28] Although the law is unsettled nationally, it would appear that, in the absence of definitive court decisions or express legislative authority, governmental agencies with "implied" powers may be considered to be outside of the scope of the antitrust laws.[29]

The system medical director will undoubtedly face the situation where hospitals "self-designate" as trauma, eye trauma, or hernia centers, and then appeal to citizens for the delivery of certain types of patients. This problem is best faced with a united physician community. Other than trauma centers, the SRC designations are often not competitive, although in the future more favorable reimbursement programs for specific medical problems may encourage hospitals, and perhaps clinics, to competitively develop SRCs dealing with often specific emergencies.

Public Law 101-590

The enactment in November 1990 of the Trauma Care Systems Planning and Development Act (PL 101-590) provided for the establishment of a federal trauma systems program.[30] However, the 1990 Act, which was supposed to provide grants to states for planning, implementing, and developing comprehensive trauma systems, was not funded when enacted. In November 1991, funding that finally was authorized to implement a new federal trauma systems program for 1992 totaled only $5 million. This amount was well below earlier projections, which were as high as $75 million.[31,32]

PL 101-590 had two primary goals. First, it was designed to remove the barriers and rectify the problems that in many parts of the country prevented timely and efficient EMS from being provided. Second, it provided incentives for states and localities to establish coordinated regionalized trauma-care systems that would enable severely injured individuals to receive timely and highly specialized care.

Passage of PL 101-590 ratified the widely held belief that regionalized trauma systems reduced death and disability from trauma. Regionalized trauma-care systems were models of healthcare delivery that could coordinate and integrate prehospital services and hospital resources to assure that optimal care was provided to traumatically injured patients. The 1990 legislation specified that such systems must identify and designate trauma centers with specialized physicians and equipment immediately available on a 24-hour basis. Also required were methods to identify severe trauma victims in the prehospital phase and to ensure that all major trauma victims were transported to trauma centers.

PL 101-590 addressed the issue of authority, effectively diminishing the threat of legal challenges to development and implementation of designation schemes. However, while the threshold issue of legal authority to designate was resolved, the financial burden caused by the large numbers of uninsured or indigent patients brought to designated facilities, along with inadequate reimbursement rates, still presented a great barrier to regionalization.[21,33]

A May 1990 Senate committee report addressing the Emergency Medical Services and Trauma Care Improvement Act revealed that since 1987 many urban trauma systems were threatened by total collapse because of financial losses. The Senate report used the following examples:

- An estimated 20 designated trauma centers had withdrawn from the regional trauma systems.

- Inadequate funding of trauma centers had resulted in seven level II trauma centers dropping out of the Dade County trauma systems, leaving Jackson Memorial Hospital as the county's only remaining trauma center.

- The Los Angeles trauma system was on the verge of collapse after 11 of the city's 23 trauma centers had dropped out because of high uncompensated costs.

- Huntington Memorial Hospital in Pasadena had lost $3.7 million in 1989 and had withdrawn from the system.

- San Diego's trauma system had reported a loss of $6.8 million for 1988 for its six designated trauma centers.

- Four out of ten trauma centers in Chicago had dropped out of the system.

- Houston's Hermann Hospital, one of only two level I trauma centers in that city, had withdrawn after losing more than $7 million.
- The MedSTAR Trauma Center in Washington reported losses totaling $8.9 million in 1989 attributed to providing care to trauma and burn victims.[34]

The committee reported the financial strains caused by undocumented persons requiring health and social services in counties that border Mexico. Many trauma centers located in border counties experienced serious financial losses because of the large numbers of undocumented persons needing trauma care. The report stated that "thirteen trauma centers in these areas incurred $8.2 million of bad debts in 1989 as a result of treating seriously injured patients who were undocumented." Additionally, the committee report discussed the findings of a 1989 review conducted by the Office of Technology Assessment (OTA) on rural EMS and trauma care needs that noted that not all states had developed EMS systems extending into rural areas. The report detailed the fact that rural EMS systems lacked adequate numbers of trained personnel, universal coverage by a communications network, and overall systems development. Serious injuries, according to the report, posed special problems to rural communities: "Injury-related morbidity and mortality are often higher than in urban areas because of the time delays in reaching trauma victims on isolated roads, homes, or farms. The chance of a severely injured individual dying in a rural area is three to four times higher than in urban areas." The OTA report concluded that "EMS systems that integrate all levels of hospital care within a state promote regionalization and are likely to improve rural trauma patient outcomes."[34]

Another development in the late 1980s was the systems analysis demonstrating improved outcome in trauma systems. Initially, in Orange County, and more comprehensively in San Diego County and in other states, data were collected that demonstrated that a systems approach to trauma dramatically reduced the preventable death rate after implementation.[7] Components of successful system implementation were identified; in the National Highway Safety Traffic Administration (NHSTA) a technical assistance program was developed that could advise states, compare progress with ten system standards, and make recommendations for change or improvement. All states have gone through this consultation process.

A 1986 document, "States Assume Leadership Role in Providing Emergency Medical Services," produced by the General Accounting Office (GAO), was requested by Senators Cranston and Kennedy. It was to review and analyze the levels of support and proficiency of EMS systems throughout the county following the 1981 repeal of the PL 93-154.

The GAO found that[34]

although many states were assuming a more active leadership role in financing and regulating emergency medical services, there were areas in which gaps in emergency medical services remained and in which federal actions and leadership were desirable.[34]

It made specific recommendations for Congressional action in these areas. Among other things, the GAO found that (1) many states lacked access to the most timely information about EMS developments; (2) many states lacked coordination between agencies with oversight of funds for EMS activities, such as state transportation and EMS agencies; (3) the 9-1-1 emergency telephone number was not uniformly available, particularly in rural communities; (4) the unavailability of funds for the start-up and operating costs of a 9-1-1 system was a major barrier to 9-1-1 implementation; (5) overcrowded radio frequencies and outmoded equipment hampered effective and efficient operation of EMS systems; and (6) economic and political factors were preventing the development of trauma services.

In addition, it noted that (1) trauma systems can reduce the trauma death rate by as much as 64%; (2) in the District of Columbia, a 50% reduction in trauma deaths over 5 years has been credited to the development of a trauma care system; and (3) a study of the San Diego trauma system showed that the trauma death rate fell by 55% after the implementation of a trauma-care system. The report concluded, in part, that "the failure of many states and local communities to designate trauma centers to care for the most critically injured patients resulted in unnecessary death and permanent disability."[11]

PL 101-590 provided grants to states for development, implementation, and monitoring of state-wide trauma systems. The trauma-care component included the designation of trauma-care regions and centers. The trauma-care system concept was premised on the belief that victims of severe trauma require special care and, as a consequence, they were to be transported to designated trauma centers, bypassing closer emergency departments.

In 1992, 26 states were awarded grants adjusted to population and geographical size. The grant program requirements included submission by the state of yearly trauma-system plans that took into account guidelines developed by the ACSCOT, the American College of Emergency Physicians, and the American Academy of Pediatrics. While the law specifically provided that grant funds could be used to reimburse designated trauma centers for uncompensated care, the first round of awards did not allow for the funding of uncompensated care. In addition, the law authorized the Secretary of Health and Human Services to (1) establish an information clearinghouse to disseminate information on the experience of state and local agencies with respect to trauma care system development and operation, (2) establish an Advisory Council on Trauma Care Systems to conduct needs assessments on a country-wide basis, and (3) establish funding for research and programs that seek to improve rural EMS. By early 1993 there was progress being made in each of those areas.[30]

After more than 25 years of advocacy to enact legislation that would fully address trauma-program concerns such as authority, standards, and national coordination, the passage and funding of PL 101-590 was enthusiastically greeted by most of the healthcare establishment. Unfortunately, enthusiasm has been greatly tempered by an economically constrained environment in which this legislative action has been able to attract only token funding. Advocates of trauma-care systems are inevitably left with the impression that the 1990 law was meant more to tantalize than to fulfill. Funding for this trauma program was lost in the mid-1990s. Funding authorization returned in 2001, but the level of funding to be provided is unclear. The task ahead is to increase state and federal funding in the long term.

Increased funding will benefit EMS systems in general since grants may be used to support rural emergency medical services systems, recruit and train EMS personnel, improve communications equipment for EMS, improve transportation services for medical emergencies, and conduct public education activities concerning prevention. Many rural hospitals "stretched" to become trauma centers in the 1990s, only to find that critical resources, often neurosurgeons, were prohibitively expensive on a 24/7 basis.

A Method for Designation

The mechanism for implementation of designations of medical facilities suggested in this chapter is generic. Although there are other approaches, this general method has been used successfully at local, county, and state levels.

Designations of receiving hospitals and SRCs may occur simultaneously. While designating receiving hospitals is a much more time-consuming process, it is politically easier since the number of designated facilities does not usually need to be limited.

Once an authorized lead agency has been identified, the designation planning process can begin. Planning issues that must be addressed are the development of prehospital triage and transport criteria, hospital-care standards, and methodologies for determining geographic locations of SRCs. Additionally, local advisory committees should be drawn from the local medical community to formulate recommendations on all of the above issues.

While all general hospitals may not have services for all categories of patients (for example, psychiatric or obstetric), the EDs of the designated receiving hospitals should be capable of the "initial evaluation, resuscitation, and stabilization" of virtually all medical and psychiatric emergencies.[1] Ideally, all of the general hospitals in the jurisdiction are measured against standards of care; those institutions meeting the criteria are offered designation as receiving hospitals for the EMS system. However, the number of SRC designations within each category may need to be limited, since the number of patients may be too diluted to allow the appropriate level of experience and expertise to develop. Decisions to exclude "qualified" facilities from a given system are based on the degree of compliance with standards, demographic considerations, and geographic locations. Some sophisticated hospitals prefer to be informal *de facto* trauma centers, presumably avoiding at least one level of regulation and review.

SRC designations may be made in a number of clinical areas. While all but the most rural EMS systems can usually identify a trauma center, in some areas even trauma-center designations may not be available within the geographical area of the local system and may fall to a single statewide center. The following are types of SRCs that may be designated. (Table 76.1)

For an institution to pursue SRC designation, the preexistence of a relatively highly developed clinical program is usually necessary to justify the further as-

TABLE 76.1	
Types of SRCs	
1. Trauma	8. Eye
2. Burn	9. Behavioral
3. Hyperbaric medicine	10. Pediatric burn
4. Replantation	11. Pediatric trauma
5. Venomous bite	12. Poison
6. Spinal cord	13. Cardiac
7. Neonatal	14. Stroke

sembling and organizing of resources needed to meet the required standards. Occasionally, hospitals will attempt to develop a clinical expertise *de novo* so as to pursue a system designation. This approach is difficult and expensive for the institution. It also tends to create problems for those responsible for the designation process, since a significant but uncomplete effort usually cannot be recognized.

An Approach to Implementation

Traditionally, the first two tasks accomplished are (1) the development of categorization guidelines that the facilities use to make self-assessments of their emergency care capabilities, and (2) the formal categorization of facilities. The next step after categorization is to determine the types of SRCs needed for a comprehensive EMS system in the given jurisdiction. In the absence of state minimum standards for EDs and SRCs, local minimum standards are generally developed, based on national professional organization criteria and modified by local medical group consensus.

Once standards of care are established, all medical facilities in the jurisdiction are invited to submit letters of intent to apply for specific designations. The lead agency announces a Request for Proposals (RFP) to meet the standards and the designation policies that detail overall responsibilities of a designated facility. The agency staff screens the submitted proposals in order to identify applicants that meet the basic parameters required for a site audit. If the RFP minimum requirements are not met, the proposal may either be rejected or the applicant may be asked to submit additional evidence of compliance. Proposals that meet the entry-level criteria are then analyzed to determine compliance with all of the standards prior to conducting a site audit. The audit team, usually consisting of local experts, verifies the information submitted in the proposal. A designation advisory committee reviews the audit results and recommends the institutions that can be considered for designation.

The lead agency medical director should retain the authority to select an adequate number of appropriate institutions from among those in compliance with standards. For example, in the case of trauma centers, designation determinations from among "qualified" institutions may be based on the local incidence of trauma and acceptable transport times for trauma patients. In the case of receiving hospitals, limiting participants is usually neither necessary nor advisable.

Following designation, a contract is executed between the system and each SRC or receiving hospital. The contract should be reviewable after a stated time period and must include the rights and duties of the parties. The lead agency should have the legal right to verify facility compliance with standards without notice. All policies and procedures, including a hearing and appeals mechanism for revocation of designation, should be clear.

The system must monitor both compliance by the designated facility with care standards and by the prehospital providers with the field protocols. Additionally, it is necessary to continually reevaluate the medical care provided by system participants on an outcome basis. Results of ongoing clinical studies should be reviewed for indications that adjustments to the structure or operation of the system are necessary. To confirm compliance with standards, a redesignation process should occur every few years. The evaluation results are considered by the various advisory groups when redesignation recommendations are made.

The Role of Medical Oversight

Regardless of whether statutory authority to designate medical facilities is vested in a governmental, a quasigovernmental, or a nonprofit agency, the role of the EMS system medical director in the implementation of regional designations is critical and complex. Specifically, the medical director must integrate both the administrative and medical aspects of the process at each stage leading to implementation. Following implementation, the medical director must focus on system evaluation to assure the continued provision of timely, high quality patient care and must also serve as the spokesperson for the medical aspects of the system.

When responsibility for medical facility designation is at the state government level, the regional or local medical director must still systematically link the pre-hospital care components of the system (education, protocols, transportation, and communications) with the statewide hospital and SRC designation process.

The medical director of a local system that has legal authority to designate should rely on consensus medical expertise provided by an EMS advisory committee before and after implementation. The advisory committee, knowledgeable about general and specific emergency conditions, continues to develop recommendations for the system including (1) prehospital triage, treatment, and transport; (2) hospital care; and (3) number, location, and level of designated system hospitals.[35] Additionally, the committee reviews the applications that are submitted by designation applicants. Designation recommendations are then made to the medical director based on the degree of compliance with the standards and, in the case of SRCs, on the geographic and demographic considerations. If, for political reasons, the system simply designates all the satisfactory SRC proposals, there is a risk, especially for trauma centers, that the resulting network will be unworkable.

The medical director's involvement during the initial review process is generally limited to assuring that it progresses based on strict medical standards with as little political interference as possible.[35] The medical director should only become directly involved when the final selection of acceptable facilities occurs. Facility selections and distribution of patient triage and transportation guidelines are accomplished simultaneously by the medical director in accordance with the overall system plan.

Summary

Generally, all receiving hospitals that meet the standards are designated; however, only enough satisfactory SRCs to meet the projected needs of the system initially should be designated. The continuing commitments of the institutions (compliance with standards) and of the prehospital providers (adherence to patient triage and transport guidelines) must be monitored by the medical director in the same way as direct patient care. PL 101-590 and its amendments plus potential future funding support may allow EMS systems without trauma programs to initiate them. As many regions learned in the 1980s, it may be possible to "piggyback" designations of other facilities (including emergency departments) onto the revitalized process.

The push for the designation of receiving hospitals and SRCs varies with the reimbursement process, competition, popular perceptions of need, and the evolution of the particular EMS system. All these factors, and others, must be weighed before undertaking this important task.

References

1. Gann DS (moderator). Panel: Current status of emergency medical services. *J Trauma.* 1981;21:196–203.
2. Emergency Medical Service System Act of 1973: Law of the 93rd Congress, Public Law 93-154, Washington, DC, 1973.
3. Emergency Medical Service System Act of 1976: Law of the 94th Congress, Public Law 94-573, Washington, DC, 1976.
4. Emergency Medical Service System Act of 1979: Law of the 96th Congress, Public Law 94-573, Washington, DC, 1979.
5. Cales RH, Anderson PG, Heilig RW. Utilization of medical care in Orange County: the effect of implementation of a regional trauma system. *Ann Emerg Med.* 1985;14:853–858.
6. Shackford SR, et al. The effect of regionalization upon the quality of trauma care as assessed by concurrent audit before and after institution of a trauma system; a preliminary report. *J Trauma.* 1986;26:812–820.
7. West JG, Cales RH, Gazzangia AB. Impact of regionalization; the Orange County experience. *Arch Surg.* 1983;118:740–744.
8. Bern A. *Categorization.* In: van de Leuv JH, ed. *Management of Emergency Services.* Rockville, MD: Aspen; 1987.
9. Tortella BJ, Trunkey DD. Hospital care. In: Cales RH, Heilig RW, eds. *Trauma Care Systems: A Guide to Planning, Implementation, Operation, and Evaluation.* Rockville, MD: Aspen; 1986.
10. Commission on Emergency Medical Services. *Categorization of Hospital Emergency Capabilities.* Chicago: American Medical Association; 1971.
11. Commission on Emergency Medical Services. *Provisional Guidelines for the Optimal Categorization of Hospital Emergency Capabilities.* Chicago: American Medical Association; 1981.
12. Heilig RW, Cales RH: Development. In: Cales RH, Heilig RW, eds. *Trauma Care Systems: A Guide to Planning, Implementation, Operation, and Evaluation.* Rockville, MD: Aspen; 1986.
13. Detmer DE, et al. Regional categorization and quality of care in major trauma. *J Trauma.* 1977;17:592–599.
14. Gibson G. Categorization of hospital emergency capabilities: some empirical methods to evaluate appropriateness of emergency department utilization. *J Trauma.* 1978;18:94–102.
15. Boyd DR, Cowley RA. Approach to the care of the trauma patient. In: Boyd DR, Edlich RF, Micik S, eds. *Systems Approach to Emergency Medical Care.* Norwalk, CT: Appleton-Century-Crofts; 1983.

16. Cales RH. Concepts. In: Cales RH, Heilig RW, eds. *Trauma Care Systems: A Guide to Planning, Implementation, Operation, and Evaluation*. Rockville, MD: Aspen; 1986.

17. Heilig RW. Law. In: Cales RH, Heilig RW, eds. *Trauma Care Systems: A Guide To Planning, Implementation, Operation, and Evaluation*. Rockville, MD: Aspen; 1986.

18. Kuehl AE. Coordinating an EMS system: trauma centers and emergency departments. In: Chayet NL, Reardon TM, eds. *Trauma Centers and Emergency Departments*. New York: Law and Business; 1985.

19. Henry MC, Kresky B. The emergency medical service system in New York State; time for a change. *NY State J Med*. 1985;85:23.

20. Chayet NL, Reardon T. Legal issues. In: Chayet NL, Reardon TM, eds. *Centers and Emergency Departments*. New York: Law and Business; 1985.

21. Wallace C. Trauma centers struggling in Los Angeles, Miami. *Modern Health Care*. July 1987.

22. West JG, et al. Trauma systems: current status-future challenges. *JAMA*. 1988;259:3597–3600.

23. Jacobs LM. The effect of prospective reimbursement on trauma patients. *Bull Am Coll Surg*. 1985;70:17–22.

24. Larsen K, et al. Potential impact of the federal prospective payment reimbursement policies on trauma centers (abstract). *Crit Care Med*. 1984;12:332.

25. Boyd DR. The history of emergency medical services (EMS) systems in the United States of America. In: Boyd DR, Edlich RF, and Micik S, eds. *Systems Approach to Emergency Medical Care*. Norwalk, CT: Appleton-Century-Crofts; 1983.

26. Micik SH. Administration and management of EMS system. In: Boyd DR, Edlich RF, and Micik S, eds. *Systems Approach to Emergency Medical Care*. Norwalk, CT: Appleton-Century-Crofts; 1983.

27. Romano TL, Boyd DR, Micik S. Medical control and accountability. In: Boyd, DR, Edlich RF, Micik S, eds. *Systems Approach to Emergency Medical Care*. Norwalk, CT: Appleton-Century-Crofts; 1983.

28. *Huron Valley Hospital Inc v. City of Pontiac*. 1979 1 Trade Cases/62.520.

29. Statutes 1 and 2 of Sherman Act, 15 U.S.C. Statutes 1 and 2.

30. Emergency Medical Services and Trauma Care Improvement Act of 1990: Law of the 101st Congress, Public Law 101-590, Washington, DC, 1990.

31. Esposito TJ, Nania J, Maier RV. State trauma system evaluation: a unique and comprehensive approach. *Ann Emerg Med*. 1992;21(4):351–357.

32. Public Law 102-170, Washington, DC, 1992, Law of the 102nd Congress.

33. Whalar B. Congress addresses trauma network problems. *Hospitals*. October 1987.

34. Senate Report No.101-292, S Rep. No.292, 101st Congress, 2nd Sess. 1990, 1990 WL 259294 (Leg Hist).

35. Cales RH. Medical direction. In: Cales RH, Heilig RW, eds. *Trauma Care Systems: A Guide to Planning, Implementation, Operations, and Evaluation*. Rockville, MD: Aspen; 1986.

CHAPTER 77

Mass Gathering Medical Care

Authur H. Yancey, MD
David Jaslow, MD

Introduction

As social beings, most people participate in mass gathering events as diverse as sports competitions, political rallies, air shows, musical concerts, festivals, parades, and fairs. Organized emergency medical care for these events has evolved relatively recently. Documentation of this care has grown out of two contrasting settings. From the well-organized, traditional sports environment, one of the earliest reports traced the development of emergency cardiac care in 1965 at University of Nebraska football games after two spectators collapsed and died without benefit of cardiopulmonary resuscitation (CPR).[1] With the institution of timely CPR, defibrillation, and airway management, eight of nine subsequent cardiac arrest victims were successfully resuscitated to hospital discharge in the ensuing eight years.

From a radically different mass gathering setting, volunteer emergency care providers' roles in administering medical assistance to antiwar demonstrators during the Vietnam campaign were described in 1971.[2] With each successive report of mass gathering medical care, successive events have benefited from improved medical resources. The 1984 Los Angeles Olympic public health experience with heat-related illness prompted much more aggressive preparations for the more severe environmental heat conditions at the Atlanta Olympic Games.[3,4] In terms of organizations attempting to standardize plans for mass gathering medical care, the American College of Emergency Physicians (ACEP) published a sentinel information paper in 1990.[5] In 2000, NAEMSP published a position paper as well as a medical director's checklist.[6,7]

Published literature has consistently quantified demand for medical services in terms of incidents per 1,000 spectators. Several unique variables in event and crowd characteristics contribute to a wide span of patient encounter incidence, thus conspiring to produce demands for emergency medical care that bear little relationship to "crowd size." These include exposure to adverse weather conditions, spectator alcohol and/or illicit drug use, inadequate intake of potable water when faced with environmental temperature extremes, consumption of contaminated food, violent spectator behavior, and the stress of physical competition leading to participants' attendant injuries. Statistics at major rock music concerts have revealed a higher incidence (0.96–17 per 1,000) of demand for medical care among spectators than at sporting event mass gatherings (0.3–1.6 per 1,000).[8] Alcohol and illicit drug use have been implicated as a factor largely responsible for this difference. As society has encouraged a healthier lifestyle for adults through participation in athletic activities like walking, running, and biking marathons, mass gathering events have evolved in which participants outnumber spectators. In those events, the incidence of demand for medical care (24 per 1,000) far exceeds that associated with events at which spectators are the majority.[9] Paradoxically, the rarity of cardiac arrest in a mass gathering population cannot be used as a guide for the level of adequate medical resource staffing because of the short time frame required to appropriately respond to the condition, demanding a greater density of providers than would otherwise be required to meet the response time constraints.

Several unique features of medical care at mass gatherings distinguish it from medical practice in other settings. The reality that on-site resources can easily be overwhelmed by multi-casualty illness or injury, the challenge of densely clustered populations, the presence of physical barriers both preventing access to and care of ill or injured victims, the crucial reliance on communications technology for coordination of care, and the need to coordinate care with jurisdictional public resource managers all dictate the need for special talents and plans.

As is true of EMS in general, the appropriate medical care of populations gathered voluntarily and temporarily involves the integration of public health, public safety, and clinical emergency medicine activities. It further depends upon a functional knowledge of public relations, telecommunications, logistics, business negotiations, and disaster preparedness. Successful care depends upon understanding medical care systems for treating acutely ill and injured individuals, and healthcare systems for maintaining healthy populations.

Medical Oversight

Planning for medical care at a mass gathering should begin with the appointment of a medical director for the event, and culminate in a medical action plan outlining details about the organization and delivery of care by addressing the parameters discussed herein. Optimally, the administration of medical care and its oversight should be performed by the medical director. However, should the scope and nature of the event demand separating these duties partially or completely, the division can work well with an event medical coordinator who administers the operational aspects and coordinates them with the medical director, who is responsible for the clinical components. Notwithstanding the very different environment presented by mass gatherings, the medical director must assume from the beginning of planning that he/she is ultimately and finally responsible for the care provided.

The medical director must lay the foundation of understanding and agreement with event management upon which all emergency medical care planning and execution rests. The goal of medical oversight should be the guidance of health and medical care provision to at least a standard commensurate with that in the surrounding community. This should be reflected in the medical action plan and its medical care protocols, the contents of which are the responsibility of the medical director.

The qualifications of the medical director must match such all-encompassing responsibility. This translates into possession of a valid medical license from the state in which the event is to be held and a commitment to the time required to both plan and direct emergency care at the event. The physician must be knowledgeable and experienced in the care of acutely ill and injured patients. This should be reflected in board eligibility or certification in a medical specialty that provides this preparation, optimally

emergency medicine. The medical director should possess experience in medical oversight of both mass gatherings and emergency medical services (EMS) in general.

As a reflection of the organization of EMS medical oversight, indirect and direct components exist for mass gathering care. On-site direct medical oversight is preferable for several reasons.[10] Although ubiquitous, distance communications technology is most vulnerable to breakdown when it is most needed—in disaster circumstances, most likely involving multiple casualties. A medical director on-site can expedite the resolution of critical medical issues that would otherwise be compounded by communications technology problems. The medical director can improve the quality of decisions about non-transports and triage due to the first-hand information gained by being on-site. Foremost among the reasons, the medical director's presence symbolizes organized medicine's commitment to the highest level of care possible at any given event. This, likely, will be perceived and respected by event management as well as by patients. Despite these benefits of on-site medical oversight, at least one study has documented that with off-site direct medical oversight, events of low acuity, small-to-moderate size, and on-site times less than thirty minutes, physicians do not need to be on-site.[11] When on-site, the medical director must be readily and easily identifiable by uniform or vest. Because of potential conflict with oversight duties, the medical director should avoid direct patient-care responsibilities except under unusual circumstances; this axiom is becoming increasingly accepted in the entire range of emergency medicine.

Event Negotiations

The medical director must meet with the event managers and/or venue owners both to impart a clear understanding of all elements of mass gathering medical care as well as receive their full support in planning and executing this care. The first discussion will largely cover details about the event that are relevant to the required medical coverage. Subsequent meetings must include those findings resulting from an assessment of both the event venue and similar previous or ongoing events. The series of meetings must result in finalizing the agreement upon which planning can proceed. The discussions should result in a comprehensive agreement encompassing the crucial elements described below and manifested in the medical action plan. Its contents must be documented, and its form should be contractual, due to the risk management and medico-legal implications of the anticipated duties.

The event management should take primary responsibility for the medico-legal liability coverage of all event medical personnel. Liability insurance may be provided through each caregiver's previously existing individual plan, by their employer's organizational plan, or by the event organization or its sponsors. Reliance on "Good Samaritan" statutes is ill-advised, especially if medical personnel are to be compensated for their services or if they are recruited prior to the event for the expressed purpose of providing medical care.

The medical director must negotiate for and collaborate in the design of a communications system for physician supervision of all event medical personnel, both when the medical director is off-site and on-site. The communication system must be tested prior to the event and be continuously operational from a prescribed time prior to the event to one following it.

Personnel recruited to work during an event should be compensated. For smaller events with a low risk of injury and illness, participation in the event and/or a "free lunch" may suffice to recruit a sufficient number of adequately trained volunteers. Added benefits such as souvenirs or extra event tickets may also generate enough enthusiasm among medical personnel to adequately provide care. As the event size increases, the need for additional medical staff grows. It is unlikely that public or private EMS personnel can or will provide their services free of charge. The costs of professional service delivery must be calculated and transmitted to event management for consideration and negotiation. Issues regarding the scope of practice and licensing of medical personnel at all levels must be researched before credentialing procedures can be organized. Logistical issues for personnel must be addressed. This includes the provision of meals, easy accessibility to potable water, dedicated sanitation facilities, parking, lodging, and work cycle assignments. Both as a morale booster and good will from the event management, media coverage should be arranged for all organizations providing and sponsoring medical care.

The availability of on-site medical equipment must be approached in several ways. It can be donated in exchange for its visibility among caregivers and the public, or it can be purchased. The administrative channels and sources for procurement must be chosen; and the logistics of transferring it from its sources to the venue and the arrangements for its security and final disposition after the event must be identified. The preceding requisite negotiations must be conducted based on diligent preplanning.

Venue Reconnaissance

With the event dates and duration in mind, the medical director should conduct a thorough inspection of the event venue to identify potential risks for morbidity during the event. If the event is outdoors, adverse weather conditions may produce morbidity. If it is indoors the adequacy of exits must be assessed. In either type of venue, the signage for spectator evacuation and aisle space for spectator and patient emergency evacuation must be adequate. The geographic area for which the medical care sector is responsible must be delineated. This domain must be inspected for its terrain and the real and potential physical barriers to accessing and evacuating victims. A stadium or convention center event will have minimal terrain considerations except for steps; however, a golfing, cross-country biking, or equestrian event may have geographic barriers or a wet, slippery surface. The highest possible attendance as well as the anticipated attendance should be estimated. The spectator density and mobility must be considered, including whether spectators will be sitting in close proximity at an arena, walking about in the infield of a race track, or along a cross-country course. Where spectators are predominately ambulatory at events, especially on irregular terrain, lower extremity trauma should be anticipated. At both the 1984 Los Angeles and 1996 Atlanta Olympics, the highest incidences of medical care took place in venues where spectators were ambulatory.[12,13] The extended venue must be inspected for the number and adequacy of ingress and egress routes for emergency vehicles.

Extensive investigation of the jurisdictional EMS system's capabilities is vital to patient evacuation planning. The distances and EMS transport times from the venue to the closest appropriate hospitals must be documented. Inquiry must be made into time-sensitive traffic pattern variations. The important decision on separating spectator- and performer-dedicated EMS resources will be heavily dependent upon the type of event taking place. The requirements for performer and VIP care should be identified. If on-site care is centered in an ambulance, state and other jurisdictional equipment and supply requirements must be observed. The event medical director should meet with the administrative and medical directors of the jurisdictional 9-1-1 EMS service to obtain information on their patient capacities, including augmentation by back-up and/or mutual aid providers. The patient level at which a multi-casualty incident (MCI) response is activated must be ascertained.

The medical director should attend events similar to the one requiring his responsibility to observe and/or estimate factors with the potential to cause injury or illness. The effect of climate, event terrain, population density, and mobility on injury patterns and victim access can be observed. The extent and effect of alcohol consumption and/or substance abuse on crowd behavior should be observed. The adequacy of toilet facilities and access to potable water must be investigated. The public address system coverage area and signage for safety and exits are important for safely managing spectator evacuation. The degree to which security maintains clear aisles and emergency ingress and egress routes also has important implications for expediting evacuation. It is important to observe and estimate response times to victims in different locations throughout the venue. Whenever possible, the medical director should review medical records from previous similar events at the same or similar venues to identify patient demand patterns and levels.

Assessment of the preceding reconnaissance information should form the basis for specific requests to event management regarding the level of care, personnel, equipment, treatment facilities, on- and off-site transportation resources, and public health elements vital to assuring adequate quality care at the event.

Level of Care

The level of expertise available for medical care at any given event will depend upon two factors: the ideal level, appropriately determined by reconnaissance results; and the possible level, limited by available financial support and community resource availability. The EMT-Basic should be the minimum acceptable level of care. The centerpiece of this level is CPR and early defibrillation capability to be delivered to anyone at the event within five minutes of notification of collapse. Planning for response to presumed cardiac arrest must be based on distances when the venue is at its population capacity. As infrequent as cardiac arrest is at mass gatherings (0.01–0.04 events per 10,000), it has been shown to be uniquely susceptible to successful intervention rates in this setting with three studies showing an 85% success rate of return of spontaneous circulation.[14] The chain of survival demands that Advanced Life Support (ALS) care is immediately available to follow up BLS care. Additionally, on-site medical personnel must be able to recognize and treat the following conditions that require immediate, on-site assessment:

- Abdominal pain/problems
- Airway obstruction/choking
- Allergic reaction
- Altered mental status
- Animal/insect bites
- Back pain
- Burns
- Carbon monoxide/inhalation/HazMat
- Cardiac/respiratory arrest
- Chest pain
- Convulsions/seizures
- Diabetic problems
- Drowning/diving incident
- Electrocution
- Eye trauma
- Falls/back injuries
- Headache
- Hyperthermia/hypothermia
- Hemorrhage/lacerations
- Overdose/ingestion/poisoning
- Pregnancy/childbirth/miscarriage
- Psychiatric/suicide attempt
- Stroke
- Traumatic injuries

The medical director must require that all non-physicians deliver care according to protocols and standing orders developed or approved by him. These must be consistent with the level of EMS care in the surrounding community. This entails formal pre-event education on all medical policies and protocols.

Human Resources

As is true regarding the level of care available, the number of medical care providers at a given event will be a balance between that number determined as optimal by reconnaissance, statistical estimates, and records of previous similar events, and that number which can realistically be supported by sponsorship and provided by the community. In terms of the relationship of crowd size to patient volume, according to one seven-year study of major collegiate events, no correlation was found during football or basketball games, and a small but statistically significant increase in patient volume with increasing crowd size was detected for rock concerts.[15] That study also concluded that the frequency of demand for medical care per attendee decreases as the spectator population increases.

Medical Director

The event medical director must be integrated into the overall administrative structure and function of the event, with clear lines of responsibility to event management on one hand and authority over medical care providers on the other. The medical director should design an organizational chart in collaboration with event management showing the numbers of medical care personnel and describing their functions at the event. Each position's reporting pathway to the medical director should be outlined.

Sufficient numbers of appropriately trained personnel must be strategically distributed on-site to treat a cardiac arrest within five minutes from the time of notification when the venue is filled to capacity. The medical director should map the locations of all medical personnel placement within the venue and the territory within which they will respond to emergencies. This organizational map should remain with the medical director, while a copy should be distributed to each care provider. No known universally acceptable, practical formula can predict accurate staffing requirements, either in terms of numbers or scope of practice. However, the following information provides descriptions of the various strengths of different levels of providers. The medical director must collaborate with the event coordinator in distinguishing among the unique attributes of these providers and translating them into appropriate duty assignments for each event.

Physicians

The following circumstances should mandate on-site physician care:

- On-site studies requiring physician interpretation (i.e., electrocardiography, radiography)
- Limited patient transportation to off-site definitive care
- Large number of spectators, implying the probability of a broad array of medical problems
- Participants at significant risk of life- or limb-threatening injury (motor racing, skiing, boxing, equestrian events)
- Long transport times to definitive care facilities

An event medical director should accept as minimum qualifications for physicians, an active medical license in the state where the event is to be held, certification in CPR and ACLS, and experience in the care of patients with life- or limb-threatening illnesses and injuries. Additional desirable qualifications include certification in PALS and ATLS as well as at least one on-site physician trained and board-certified in emergency medicine. All medical care personnel must be informed prior to the event of the role of the on-site physician.

Physician Extenders

As physician extenders, certified nurse practitioners and physician assistants can play a valuable role in caring for ambulatory patients in fixed treatment facilities, especially when large numbers of patients need to be evaluated and treated expeditiously. They must be licensed in the state in which the event is to take place and should be certified in CPR and ACLS.

Nurses

At fixed facilities, nursing expertise should be used to triage and to care for patients under on-site observation, for example the heat-exhausted. If any are credentialed as flight or critical care nurses in the out-of-hospital arena, their roles may be expanded to evaluation and treatment outside fixed facilities since they are experienced in the field setting. Nurses can contribute their unique expertise by dispensing, tracking, and restocking medications; they must be currently licensed in the state where the event is taking place and ideally have CPR and ACLS certification.

Emergency Medical Technicians

The expertise of EMT-Intermediates and EMT-Paramedics is most valuable when participants are at significant risk of injury, large numbers of spectators preclude easy access or adequate on-scene coverage by other providers, and/or long transport times to definitive care facilities demand extended care en route. Their role is primarily evaluation and treatment of patients with life- or limb-threatening conditions on-scene and, secondarily, within fixed facilities. They should be stationed in close proximity to the performers or athletes if there is a risk of airway, ventilatory, or circulatory compromise. Their credentials must include current state licensing, CPR, and ACLS. They should be certified in BTLS or PHTLS as a reflection of the crucial need for them to be able to resuscitate and stabilize trauma patients. They should be appropriately trained in pediatric or geriatric issues if the crowd configuration warrants. EMT-Basics should primarily be utilized to respond on-scene to ill and injured victims. The possibility of their greater density at the event by virtue of their greater numbers in the population should offer the opportunity to decrease response times.

Other Event Personnel

Widely dispersed event officials, such as ushers or security personnel, have an invaluable role to play in emergency medical care as spotters of medical events. Both their large numbers and placement and density within the venue imply that they will most likely first discover spectators in need of immediate medical attention. Their success in this role depends upon the pre-event training provided to them in how to survey spectators during the event and how to communicate discovery of a medical incident to the event medical system.

Given this wide array of potential medical expertise, pictured identification badges should be worn by all medical personnel displaying their specialty and, if applicable, clearances permitting them to enter specific areas of the event to which they are assigned. Field personnel should wear brightly colored vests or uniforms to facilitate their identification by event officials, spectators, and participants. In events involving significant risk of injury to performers, medical personnel should be assigned as either spectator- or performer-dedicated, so that care to one sector does not interrupt coverage of the other.

A specified time for deployment of medical personnel must be determined in conjunction with event management. Determination of this time should depend upon "when the gates open" for population

influx into the venue, and the time needed for medical personnel to arrive at their dedicated positions, organize their equipment, and have each communications links sequentially tested. Similarly, the personnel demobilization time should be determined on the basis of the population egress time.

Medical Equipment and Pharmaceuticals

The scope and level of medical care is primarily dependent on the medical personnel available and secondarily on the equipment and pharmaceutical resources available. This availability may depend upon the medical director's collaboration with event managers to organize funding support and/or donations for specific equipment needs as determined by the preceding reconnaissance and any jurisdictional requirements and dispensing regulations. Conversely, the equipment resources must correspond to and not exceed the available personnel's level of expertise regarding their use. The following equipment lists, therefore, are distinguished by items typically stocked on a BLS ambulance and those on an ALS ambulance. Unlike the equipment listed for use in fixed facilities where a physician presence is desirable, the following two lists apply primarily to mobile responders, and secondarily to temporary stationary facilities managed on an EMT-Paramedic level (i.e., an ambulance dedicated to event care).

Basic Life Support

The following BLS diagnostic and therapeutic equipment, in sizes appropriate for children and adults, is essential:

- Airway adjuncts
  - Nasopharyngeal
  - Oropharyngeal
  - Ambu bags
  - Bag-valve masks
- Alcohol swabs
- Backboards
- Bandages, elastic
- Bandages, triangular
- Band-aids
- Cervical collars, rigid
- Cold packs, disposable

- Defibrillators, automatic
- Gauze pads, multiple sizes
- Gloves, non-sterile
  - Latex
  - Non-latex
- Kling dressing
- Obstetric pack
- Oxygen delivery devices
  - Nasal cannula
  - Non-rebreather mask
- Restraints, soft
- Sheets
- Scissors, trauma style
- Sling and swath
- Splints, finger, wrist, forearm, lower extremity, traction
- Stethoscope
- Sphygmomanometer
- Suction device, portable and rechargeable
- Tape, adhesive
- Tongue blades

This additional basic equipment is desirable in a stationary facility setting:

- Bedpans
- Facial tissues
- Feminine hygiene products
- Lip balm
- Sunscreen

Advanced Life Support

The following additional equipment in sizes appropriate for children and adults is mandatory for the provision of ALS-level care:

- Blood glucose test strips and meter
- Cardiac monitor with manual defibrillator and external pacer
- Cricothyrotomy kit or supplies
- Endotracheal tubes
- Intravenous bags, tubing, and catheters
- Intubation confirmation devices (End-tidal CO_2 or esophageal detectors)

- Laryngoscope with array of blades
- Magill forceps
- Pulse oximeter
- Thoracostomy kit or supplies

Additional advanced equipment is desirable, depending on the venue:

- 12-lead EKG
- Alternative airway devices (e.g., Combitube, lighted stylet)
- Automated blood pressure monitor
- Automated ventilators for prehospital use
- Braselow tape
- Intravenous fluid infuser

Pharmaceuticals

Pharmaceuticals needed for on-site medical care must meet the standard for the scope of practice resources at the event. The following list outlines common medications for consideration:

- Resuscitation medications
  - Adenosine
  - Atropine
  - Amiodarone
  - Calcium chloride
  - Diltiazem
  - Dopamine
  - Epinephrine (1:10,000 concentration)
  - Lidocaine
  - Sodium bicarbonate
- Analgesics
  - Aspirin (ischemic chest pain use)
  - Morphine (parenteral only)
- Anaphylaxis medications
  - Diphenhydramine (parenteral and oral)
  - Epinephrine (1:1,000 concentration)
- Antiepileptics
  - Diazepam
- Asthma medications
  - Albuterol or Metaproterenol (nebulized form)
  - Steroid (parenteral preferred)

- Cardiac medications
  - Nitroglycerine, sublingual
  - Furosemide
- Diabetic medications
  - Dextrose, 50%
  - Glucagon
- Emetic
  - Syrup of Ipecac
- Intravenous solutions
  - Lactated Ringer's or Normal Saline

Providers must be prepared to utilize any of these and other medications approved through the medical director's event protocols. The medical director, in formulating event protocols, must respect all jurisdictional (municipality, county, state) regulations regarding medication administration by paramedical personnel.

Supplies

When resources allow and reconnaissance findings dictate use of a stationary facility, the following non-medical items are essential:

- Stretchers, cots, or examination tables
- Sheets
- Blankets
- Dedicated hazardous waste receptacles with clear signage
- Non-hazardous waste receptacles
- Spare batteries for devices
- Pens and paper
- Patient Care Report (PCR) forms

Additional desirable items include:

- Bathroom with sink and toilet dedicated to the treatment facility use
- Chairs for medical staff
- Diapers
- Linen disposal or recycle bin
- Patient identification bracelets
- Pillows
- Refrigerator (cold storage pharmaceuticals)
- Safety pins
- Towels

Fixed Facility Equipment

The use of emergency department equipment and pharmaceuticals is rare at mass gathering events. This use is usually limited to extremely large (hundreds of thousands population), well funded (millions of dollars), regular (annual) events at which a constant physician and support staff presence is working in a permanent fixed facility. The Indianapolis 500 Motor Speedway and some horse racing facilities can boast of such on-site facilities. Stocking most of the following medical equipment should be considered only if physicians charged with direct patient care will staff the event facility:

- Benzoin
- Betadine
- Burn wound dressings
- Cotton applicators and balls
- Dermabond or equivalent
- Eye patches
- Chest tubes, tray, and Pleurevac suction
- Intravenous poles
- Intravenous pumps
- Nasogastric tubes
- Ophthalmoscope
- Otoscope
- Prescription pads
- Ring cutters
- Splinting supplies
- Steri-strips
- Sutures and kits
- Thermometers
- Vaseline gauze
- Woods lamp

Fixed Facility Pharmaceuticals

In addition to those items on the ALS list, stocking the following pharmaceuticals should be considered if physicians charged with direct patient care will staff the event facility or other medical personnel are dispensing them under a combination of standing orders and direct medical oversight:

- Analgesics
  - Acetaminophen
  - Ibuprofen

- Anesthetics
  - Lidocaine
  - Tetracaine or Procaine (for the lidocaine-allergic patient)
- Antacids
- Antibiotics
  - Parenteral
  - Ointment
  - Oral
- Antidiarrheals
- Antiemetics
- Antiepileptics
  - Phenytoin
- Airway management agents
  - Etomidate
  - Ketamine
  - Midazolam
  - Succinylcholine
  - Vecuronium
- Burn medications
  - Silver sulfadiazine cream
  - Xeroform gauze
- Cardiac medications
  - Digoxin (oral or parenteral)
- Diabetic medications
  - Insulin, regular
- Intravenous solutions
  - Dextrose, 10%/water
- Ophthalmic agents
  - Anesthetic
  - Antibiotic ointment
  - Fluorescein strips
  - Irrigating solution
  - Mydriatic agent
- Poisoning
  - Activated charcol

The preceding lists are suggestions, not intended to be either all-inclusive or prohibitive of other medications and equipment.

The event medical director has ultimate responsibility for medical equipment and pharmaceuticals from their source to their use to the complications of their use. If planning reveals this crucial aspect of care to be more intricate and time-consuming than can be managed by him, consideration must be given to appointing a logistician or event coordinator. Some of the responsibilities involved in that position include procuring planned quantities of equipment and pharmaceuticals, distributing them at the venue prior to the beginning of the event, ensuring their continuous availability through replenishment, preserving cold-chain storage where necessary, protecting them from theft, and managing their collection and disposition following the event. Additionally, the medical director or logistician must ensure that only appropriately credentialed personnel are allowed access to prescription pharmaceuticals. The logistician may also be charged with distributing PCR forms and collecting the completed documents for risk management and quality management purposes.

Treatment Facilities

On-site Fixed Facilities

On-site treatment facilities must be constructed primarily for the most efficient care of expected patient volume and potential acuity based on the reconnaissance performed. Of secondary importance, the medical expertise available, patient transport times to definitive care facilities, and the definitive care facility capabilities must be considered. On-site treatment facilities are potentially indicated for large-attendance events, events of long duration, with considerable risk of life-threatening injury to competitors or performers, or with long transport times to definitive care facilities. They may as simple as a tent or as complex as a permanent, free-standing emergency department.

If an on-site facility is established, its location must be easily accessible and its access paths secure. Its location and access path should be announced by public affairs and displayed on prominent signage (i.e., scoreboard) regularly during the duration of the event. It must be clearly marked as an emergency medical facility in all languages thought to be appropriate for the event. The entrances and exits must be clearly marked according to jurisdictional fire codes.

The structure must be capable of withstanding weather conditions, protecting its occupants from these, and minimizing the occupants' exposure to extremes of temperature. It must provide privacy for at least one patient at a time. Its construction must allow clear communications with the medical director and have back-up modes of communication such as radio and landline or cell telephone. Sufficient floor area must be available to accommodate the planned medical equipment and pharmaceuticals. The facility must contain a dedicated supply of equipment and pharmaceuticals. If mobile units dedicated to event care are to be stocked or restocked from the fixed facility, their cache of supplies should be separate from those of the fixed facility, so that use of one stockpile does not threaten depletion of the other.

Operationally, the medical director must ensure that at least one medical provider capable of delivering the highest level of care available is staffing the facility for the entire duration of the event. If other providers assigned to or temporarily located in fixed facilities leave the post to retrieve patients in the field, this provider must maintain the minimally acceptable staffing level. Communications protocols must allow this provider the ability to recruit sufficient on-site event medical staff to address any clinical problems that arise. Staff assignments among fixed facilities should be apportioned according to expected patient volume and morbidity type. All facility medical staff should know where the closest security personnel are stationed and the communications pathway to access them.

Off-site Facilities

Although off-site care facilities will not be controlled by the event medical director, their technical, expertise, and bed-resource capacities must be investigated. Subsequent meetings of the medical director with key administrative and medical personnel at selected institutions must be held to inform them of medical plans for the event, explore their participation in event medical care, and discuss their receipt of patients, including MCI incidents. Their diagnosis data collection capacities should be explored, because they drive surveillance systems designed for larger events to discover infectious disease cases with outbreak potential.[4,16]

These discussions should result in the designation of receiving hospitals for the specialized care of burn, eye injury, obstetric, pediatric, psychiatric, spinal injury, and life- or limb-threatening trauma patients. Special attention should be paid to designating a receiving facility for suspected victims of weapons of mass destruction (WMD), be they nuclear, biological, or chemical. Agreement should be reached on a system of diagnosis data reporting to jurisdictional public health authorities as well as event management. The specialty receiving hospital designations for the event should, with rare exception, be completely consistent with those of the state in which the event is held. Those discussions should identify the available bed capacity for the MCI contingency plan.

In preparation for the event, the medical director and key event medical staff must also meet with the administrators and medical directors of all jurisdictional EMS services to identify their resources and interface with the event activities.

Transportation Resources

The venue reconnaissance and event research should identify transportation number and type needs. These resources are vital to bringing medical care to the victims expeditiously and to evacuating them effectively.

Intravenue Transportation Resources

Intravenue patient transportation can practically be served by a gurney moved by pedestrian mobile caregivers if the patient's destination (fixed on-site medical facility or ambulance) does not exceed five minutes of walking. For venues holding large area events like golf, equestrian events, or motor racing, modified, stretcher-bearing golf carts may be suitable. Event-dedicated ambulances are appropriate for intravenue use if the vehicle can safely reach the scene, if reliable reports from on-scene medical personnel indicate the need for immediate evacuation to a hospital, and if the vehicle is not designated as the sole on-site medical resource. For large area events with rugged, hilly terrain like cross-country running, biking, motorcycling, or equestrian competitions, modified, off-road, stretcher-bearing vehicles may be required to reach and evacuate patients. For aquatic events held across a large area, for example, rowing, sailing, or endurance swimming, boats must be modified to "seaworthiness" with the added loads of medical equipment, personnel, and patients.

These non-traditional transportation resources must be appropriately staffed. The operators must have experience in their handling and maneuverability prior to the event. The vehicles or vessels must be clearly identifiable and highly visible. Given the acute medical indications for the use of these resources, they should be dedicated for exclusive medical use throughout the duration of the event.

Extravenue Transportation Resources

The mode of transportation for a given patient from the event to an off-site definitive care facility, usually a hospital, depends upon the clinical indications for transport and the resources available. The medical director must approve the means, time, and destination of all patient transports since, as the referring physician, he bears ultimate responsibility for the patient's condition until arrival at the destination facility. Additionally, the event medical director, through the coordinating function of the medical oversight center must make these decisions about any given patient with the perspective of all the other ongoing medical care and needs at the event.

A means of conveyance should be available for non-emergency medical use. It will allow ambulances and their higher expertise-level staff to be more closely matched to patients of a higher acuity. The medical director should design the protocols governing the vehicle's use. A mandatory screening examination by on-site medical personnel and report of the findings to the medical director with a request for this service should initiate the process. A stable clinical condition and partial ambulatory status (with assistance) should be required. Any limitations on multiple patient transports, classes of eligibility (spectator, performer, official, media), and criteria for accompanying personnel must be determined. On-board radio or cell phone communications capability and patient comfort resources (e.g., wheelchair lift) must be available, if appropriate. Arrangements for patient return from the hospital to the venue must be included in the protocols, if available.

Traditional ground transportation in the form of ambulances is the mainstay of conveyance from mass gathering events to hospitals. The event medical director should be familiar with all state regulations for ambulance medical equipment, pharmaceuticals, and staffing, and augment these resources according to specific event needs. In the reconnaissance and negotiation phases of planning, the number and allocation of venue-dedicated ambulances should be indicated. Stationary parking, refueling, replacing and restocking should be addressed. If the supply of event-dedicated ambulances becomes depleted, agreements must be reached with the jurisdictional 9-1-1 EMS service to support event emergency medical transportation. The medical director must design explicit protocols in conjunction with event medical coordinators and EMS directors to address the roles of ambulance-based crews regarding retrieval of victims.

Aeromedical transportation, usually helicopters, is a valuable resource in few circumstances. If a victim's injury/illness is life-threatening, the weather conditions are acceptable, safe landing zones exist at the venue and at the destination institution, the total prehospital times are significantly diminished, and appropriate level of care can be provided, helicopter services may be beneficial. These circumstances bear careful consideration by the medical director. Clear protocols defining the indications and procedures for recruiting an EMS helicopter service must be established.

Environmental Elements

In planning for any mass gathering event, the potential for environmental factors affecting the health of participants and spectators, including reckless or violent behavior and the use of potentially toxic substances, must be investigated. As part of the reconnaissance and research process, the medical director should explore the elements presented below with jurisdictional public health authorities. The preventive measures directed toward the management of these elements and the treatment of illness/injury resulting from them must be governed through the event medical protocols.

Heat

Because most outdoor events are held in warm or hot weather, and those that are staged in cold weather usually attract individuals well prepared and protected, victims of hyperthermia syndromes present for medical care much more frequently than hypothermia. Plans for those patients with a normal or rapidly normalizing mental status at initial assessment (heat cramps, edema, tetany, syncope) should include removal to a predesignated cool environment within the venue and oral hydration with water or electrolyte solutions.[17] Barring risk factors such as infancy, known diabetes, hypertension, paralysis, the use of diuretic, antihypertensive, antidepressant, or antihistaminic medications, these patients would be expected to rapidly improve to the extent that they can safely return to participation in the event. Educating spectators through the public address system, as well as treated patients at risk of recurrence, should include the following precautions:

- Minimize the time spent in direct sunlight between 1000 and 1600 hours

- Apply sunscreen with a minimum sun protection factor (SPF) of 15, especially on children

- Never leave children, pets, or the disabled in an enclosed, parked vehicle
- Wear loose-fitting, light-weight, light-colored clothing of natural fiber
- Wear a wide-brimmed hat and sun glasses
- Place a cool, wet cloth around the neck or in the armpits

Conversely, anyone presenting to the medical sector with an elevated temperature and an abnormal mental status or one that is deteriorating must be expeditiously transported via ambulance to the nearest emergency department with aggressive airway management, cooling, and intravenous hydration en route.

Insufficient potable water intake is a major contributor to hyperthermia syndromes. Provision of that water is vital to both the prevention and treatment of hyperthermia. One strategy used in the 1996 Atlanta Olympics to prevent hyperthermia syndromes was based upon stratifying levels of environmental heat for which an escalating response was planned (table 77.1.) Level 4 caused initiation of the emergency plan. The emergency plan could be instituted by the venue medical officer in conjunction with the venue manager. This decision was based upon a demand for hyperthermia-preventive resources exceeding the supply and/or a sentinel event occurring. The State of Georgia Division of Public Health and the Centers for Disease Control and Prevention identi-fied as a sentinel event, "three heat-related illnesses in one venue/day requiring emergency transport to the hospital." At the declaration of each successively higher level, actions unique to that respective level would augment those resources recruited at previous levels.

Water

If responsibility for potable and non-potable water is delegated to event management, the medical director and event medical coordinator must study the relevant statutory regulations in consultation with the appropriate jurisdictional public water and health authorities. This should include knowledge of its sources, supply lines, distribution routes, storage, and delivery devices. Inquiry should be made into the event water bacteriological and chemical contaminants. The epidemiology of water-borne illness should be understood by emergency medical personnel, including appropriate handling and use of water, recognition of disease presentation patterns, and their treatment.

Rather than a beverage, potable water must be considered both a preventive and therapeutic public health necessity in regard to dehydration and hyperthermia syndromes. A mechanism for obtaining and administering free, safe, potable water in adequate amounts to anyone in need of such is mandatory. Those most at risk of dehydration/hyperthermia, including the elderly, the infirm, infants and young

TABLE 77.1		
Stratified Levels of Environmental Heat and Corresponding Cumulative Interventions for the 1996 Atlanta Olympics		
LEVEL	**HEAT INDEX**	**RESPONSES (CUMULATIVE)**
I	<90	Water stations operational Mobile hydration teams operational Shade structure erected Signage and spectator wellness guides (brochures) refer to the foregoing
II	90–95	Additional water stations operational Additional hydration teams operational Public address announcements encouraging hydration
III	>95	Water distribution by recruited non-medical staff Increased frequency of public address announcements encouraging hydration Identification of shaded and air-conditioned shelters at the venue Free distribution of bottled water by concessionaires
IV	Emergency Plan in Effect	Extravenue resource recruitment to include churches, schools, and buses in the vicinity

children, athletes, and officials, must be sought by medical personnel for aggressive administration of water and electrolyte-containing sports beverages. The medical director must coordinate with public affairs regular announcements and signage for everyone to drink at least 8 to 10 eight-ounce cups of water per day. Provisions must be made for adequate amounts and distribution. Prior to the 1996 Atlanta Olympics, the State of Georgia legislated the Department of Human Resources—Public Health Water Regulation 290-5-55-03 which states that ". . . Special event sponsors must provide an adequate number of potable water supplies as set forth by the local plumbing code." The state Department of Health interpreted this to mean that the special event sponsor must provide one available water source for every 1,500 people.

Food

Mass gatherings can transmit enteric pathogens efficiently and widely. This was well documented at the Rainbow Family Gathering of 1987 attended by approximately 12,700 people.[18] *Shigella sonnei* accounted for an attack rate of 59%. The authority for food management must also be delineated prior to the event. The relevant public health authorities should be consulted, especially since, as with water, clinical manifestations of disease may present following conclusion of the event. Should the responsibility for food safety rest with the event management, the medical director must consult event food services management for acquisition of plans for appropriate handling. All medical personnel should be informed of the relevant aspects of appropriate food handling, the reporting mechanism for violations of such, food-borne disease presentation patterns, and their treatment.

Waste

The appropriate jurisdictional authorities should be consulted in regard to waste management. Should this responsibility belong to event management, the medical director should meet with whomever they have designated for appropriate handling oversight, given the implications for disease transmission through vectors such as hymenoptera or rodents that are attracted to waste material. All medical personnel must be educated about both the injury/illness patterns possible as a result of flawed waste management and their treatment.

Ecology

Most applicable to outdoor events in large wooded areas, including golf and all cross-country events, both toxic flora and fauna native to the event venue must be investigated. Preventive strategies for avoiding a range of harmful offenders from snakes, hymenoptera, deer ticks, raccoons, and mosquitoes to poison ivy must be developed. The medical director must collaborate with public affairs to plan for dissemination of appropriate information specific to the event through brochures and announcements. Medical protocols must include treatment plans for addressing the sequelae of transmitted injurious toxins and disease vectors as variable as poison ivy dermatitis, rabies, tetanus, West Nile fever, Lyme disease, hymenoptera, snake, or spider envenomation.

Abused Substances

From the earliest published literature on planning medical care at mass gatherings, authors have indicated that abused substances play a role in producing morbidity at mass gatherings.[19,20] Rock concerts present a significantly higher incidence of demand for on-site medical care than sporting events.[15] The relatively high correlation of alcohol and illicit drug use with demand for medical care (48% of patients presenting for care) due to clinical intoxication (32% of patients) as well as injuries (30% of patient users) in one series of five major rock concerts illustrates the importance of the issue.[8]

Several public health initiatives have been instituted to address this excess morbidity. At the University of Arizona football games, while no alcohol was ever sold inside the stadium, it was banned from being brought inside beginning in 1985 for risk management purposes. A subsequent study revealed less heat-related illness but a greater frequency of extremity injuries and cardiac syncope.[21] The National Highway Traffic Safety Administration, in association with private industry, developed the program, Techniques for Effective Alcohol Management (TEAM) in 1985, to foster responsible alcohol intake at mass gatherings.[22] All of the major league baseball clubs adopted the policy after testing at seven stadium sites in 1990. The components of the program are as follows:

- Signage in the stadium promoting TEAM and responsible drinking
- TEAM training of all stadium employees
- No sales of alcohol at event beverage stands

- Tailgating prohibited less than 2 hours pregame
- Confiscation of alcohol discovered at entry gates
- Banning entrance of obviously intoxicated potential spectators
- Beer size sold no larger than 20 oz.
- Maximum number sold to an individual—two beers
- Usual inning of last call for beer sales—7th inning
- Designated driver program

A subsequent study conducted during the 1993 baseball season revealed that 41% of study participants tested positive for alcohol, 8.4% had blood alcohol levels at or above the legal limit of 0.08% for driving a motorized vehicle, and 4.6% of those tested during the fifth inning were beyond the legal limit for driving and reported that they would be driving home.[23] The extent to which the program lowered the foregoing statistics is unknown.

Traffic

Initial event planning must include coordination between the medical director and the event security director charged with securing ingress and egress routes for emergency medical, water, food, and medical supply vehicles. The mapped details of these routes must be transmitted to event-dedicated personnel responding to these event needs and evacuating patients to extravenue facilities. For all of the foregoing personnel relying on replenishment of supplies and equipment, these details are vital. Equally as important are the safety measures for pedestrian spectators who will be in close proximity to motorized traffic entering and exiting the venue. Delineating ingress and egress routes is crucial to placement of both intravenue fixed-care facilities and ambulance staging areas.

Access to Care

Informed negotiations should result in a plan assuring that all event spectators and participants have timely access to emergency care regardless of their ability to actively seek such care. Accomplishing such a global mission entails public education informing all spectators of actions to be taken if they become or witness anyone else becoming a victim. The plan must be in compliance with all Americans with Disabilities Act (ADA) statutes and pertinent local, regional, and state guidelines.

The public address system, both in its audio and visual modes, is critical to ensuring appropriate access to medical services. Plans should include a concisely scripted announcement augmented with large screen display or illustration if available, informing everyone within the venue of medical care facility locations, and instructing them in accessing medical assistance. The announcements and displays should be repeated regularly throughout the event. The medical facilities must be clearly labeled for rapid identification, and the labeling should be displayed to spectators. Descriptions should be announced and, more effectively, visual displays showing the distinctive uniforms, vests, and/or caps of all medical personnel should be illustrated. Children under eight years should be provided wrist identification bracelets with their names and telephone numbers upon entry to the event. Should they become lost, event personnel can broadcast their identity on the public address system or call their home to reunite them with their adult chaperones or parents.

Protocols for an alert/notification system must be designed to facilitate communication between non-radio, non-medical personnel, such as vendors and ushers, who will likely discover victims, and radio-equipped medical or security staff. This is a crucial junction in expediting emergency care, because it is the interface between injury/illness discovery and the organized care system designed to address it. Messenger, whistle, voice, flair, and flag systems have been utilized. In well financed venues, scanning surveillance cameras feeding images into event command centers may be utilized to assist staff in discovering victims.

Communications

Communications represents the glue systematizing the wide array of medical care components. The medical control center, staffed by the medical director, represents the communication system's hub, linking victims of injury and illness to both the event and surrounding jurisdictional systems of emergency medical care. The center must also link the medical director, whether mobile or fixed, with a wide array of event service directors whose personnel and expertise may be needed for medical care support. These transactions optimally proceed in an event command center encompassing medical oversight center. The communications network used for medical care should be solely dedicated to that purpose.

From the medical oversight center, the medical director must be linked by radio, cell phone, or landline to all event field medical providers, any intravenue fixed facility providers, and all ambulance staff dedicated to event service. Radio speaker microphones or earphones should be provided to all event field personnel so that their hands are freed to treat while communicating vital information on the incident. Protocols governing numbers and types of radio equipment and designated frequencies must be formulated. The communications center should contain a roster of all medical staff, their respective functions, and maps of their coverage areas and/or positions within the venue. The medical director must delineate in the protocols the specific care to be executed under standing orders as distinct from that requiring on-line communication. The protocols should clearly address issues of patient destination, either on-site or off-site.

Additionally, the medical oversight center must be linked by cell phone, landline, or radio resources to the directors of the following jurisdictional services:

- Public safety answering point (PSAP, 9-1-1 service)
- Multicasualty incident (MCI) plan (local emergency management agency)
- Public health
- Fire
- EMS
- Area emergency departments
- Event-dedicated public transportation

These links must be reviewed and tested in conjunction with the jurisdictional officials of these services. One of the biggest concerns in this regard is a call to 9-1-1 for a victim within the event venue and how to route the communications and the medical response. This possibility is best handled by the prevention measures discussed in the **Access to Care** section. Additionally, the medical director or event medical coordinator must ensure that the jurisdictional 9-1-1 center has entered the official event venue address into its computer aided dispatch (CAD) system and has the correct event telephone number to the medical oversight center. However, should such a call reach the jurisdictional 9-1-1 center, protocols must have been established to transfer the call into event medical oversight center for the dispatching of medical care. The strategic issue then becomes at what point the 9-1-1 dispatcher can leave the call with event medical personnel is it at the point when event medical control answers the phone or when the event medical providers have arrived at the victim's side? This decision is critical to returning the 9-1-1 dispatcher to service. 9-1-1 center staff should maintain and update information on the diversion status of acute care facilities in the area.

The medical oversight center should be part of an event command center in which the medical director can instantaneously access directors of the following event services integral to managing a health or medical crisis:

- Management
- Facility maintenance, including logistics and parking
- Public relations, including the public address system
- Security
- Ushers
- Parking

These service directors should optimally be stationed in close physical proximity within a command center. A slightly less reliable alternative involves intravenue radio links between directors not in close proximity. Whether the medical oversight center and event command center are geographically integrated or separate, they must be clearly and readily identifiable to all medical personnel. They must be staffed continuously from a predesignated time prior to the event, to one following the event, based on spectator ingress and egress periods.

Should the scope of the event preclude oversight of communications logistics by the medical director, a communications manager or the event medical coordinator should be designated to accomplish the following:

- Procure and distribute all equipment (radios, scanners, repeaters, etc.)
- Maintain radio battery charges
- Ensure the availability of spare radios in working order
- Construct and maintain event radio, cell phone, and landline networks

- Designate radio frequencies and telephone numbers
- Test all communications modalities involving resource and response personnel
- Ensure the security of all communications resources

Special Emergency Medical Operational Features

Details concerning event operational issues not addressed in the foregoing components should be included in the operational plans.

Mobile Events

Events such as parades, running, cycling, and wheelchair marathons present unique organizational challenges that result from a "moving venue," the length of which usually precludes medical resources from remaining stationary for the duration of the event. This implies that mobile resources will be employed to a greater extent than in a stationary venue. Special relevant considerations include the event's route in relationship to the surrounding geography. Planning that is guided by reconnaissance must determine the type of vehicles that can both access participant victims from the course and spectator victims from the crowd, then evacuate them to nearby venue care or transport them to extravenue care facilities. The proximity of these vehicles to the event must be planned so that they are close enough for their personnel to extricate victims in a timely fashion, yet removed enough for timely scene evacuation without spectator interference.

When possible, ambulances should be strategically pre-positioned along the route at regular intervals in streets that intersect the event route. They should face away from the route, and their reserved parking places should be protected by event security for timely yet safe evacuation. They must not cross the event route during the event, necessitating their positioning on both sides of the route, although not necessarily at the same level. Ambulances should never be dispatched "upstream" against the direction of the event. Radio communication is vital to coordinating the constantly moving medical coverage of the event. If enough event-dedicated ambulances can temporarily staff the entire route, they can return to previous duty assignments as the event passes their position. Or, to address the axiom that as the event proceeds, the number of victims will increase, they can be routed to "stack " toward the finish line in a system status management plan to move into the role of evacuating units.

Physician Intervenor

Unavoidably, events will take place wherein physicians have come as spectators or participants. Should they witness a medical event as bystanders, they may intervene as first responders. The event medical staff should understand that this is entirely appropriate. Should the physician bystander desire to continue care beyond the arrival of any official event medical staff members, the responding staff should immediately contact the medical director for on-line guidance of the patient's care through a team effort encompassing the physician bystander, if this effort is benefitting the patient. Should inclusion of the bystander physician be judged detrimental to the patient, the medical director is obliged to explain his ultimate responsibility for the patient and recruit security personnel to ensure uninterrupted care by official event medical staff. The acceptable exception to the foregoing would be the planned assumption of medical responsibility by the personal physician of a spectator designated by event management, optimally prior to the event, as a VIP.

VIP Care

During negotiations with event management, the medical director should ascertain the likelihood of attendance by VIPs. For medical care purposes, the qualifications for VIP status should be anyone for whom management wants medical care systematically delivered separately from other participants or spectators.

The most important liaison that the medical director can make in this regard is with the tactical emergency medical support (TEMS) provider assigned to the VIPs. Planning for such contingencies also requires coordination with the security and law enforcement details assigned to VIPs to ensure their safe passage to whatever medical care is indicated.[24] These attendees' chronic medical conditions that may affect their emergency care must be brought to the medical director's attention prior to the event, handled confidentially, and considered carefully in choosing medical personnel and equipment for their care. A separate treatment area may be required. Extra medical provisions and personnel will prevent VIP care from interfering with that of other patients and vice versa.

Mass Casualty Incident (MCI) Planning

This section addresses features unique to mass gathering event MCI planning. In concert with event security and event management, jurisdictional fire, law enforcement, emergency operations center, and PSAP managers, the medical director must contribute to a cohesive plan of action in response to an MCI. The jurisdictional disaster plan must be studied and reviewed with the responsible personnel prior to the event. Generically, in regard to the resources needed to resolve MCIs, two types of incidents arise: (1) those requiring only resources within the venue or dedicated to the event but in reserve outside the venue, and (2) those requiring resources in the public domain. Plans for the link between event and public resources are key to an expeditious, coherent transfer of MCI management from event personnel to city, county, state, and/or federal personnel. At larger events, one person, preferably within the venue during the event, should be charged by event management with being the link and "making the call" for outside resources. This arrangement supports accountability as well as communications security. Including the medical director, the selected event personnel who will inform this "link" as well as the type information that each of them will give him/her should be discussed prior to the event. Essential information to be transmitted to jurisdictional officials includes the approximate number and injury type of casualties, the scene accessibility, known inherent dangers, and any specific resource requests. Consistent with their respective responsibilities, event managers and the linking officials will ultimately decide when public resources must be recruited to the event MCI. Event security will then be expected to expedite the scene arrival of public emergency resources and any orderly evacuation of spectators that is indicated.

Planning for the response by event personnel within the venue should include the assignment of MCI response roles to all medical staff prior to the event. Security must take responsibility for those deceased until a coroner or medical examiner arrives. Triage tags for these categories must be uniformly designed, consistent with those used by the surrounding jurisdiction, and distributed to all event field providers prior to the event. All event medical personnel should remain responsible to the event medical director until the arrival on-scene of an incident commander with the jurisdictional disaster plan. Assignments will vary according to the nature and extent of the incident and the available event medical personnel.

As the safety of responders is paramount, arrangements should be made for intravenue or public domain firefighting expertise to inspect the scene for residual hazards that prevent safe triage there. Because scene arrival time by fire personnel may be delayed due to multiple foreseen and unforeseen circumstances, the medical director or one of the medical staff should have formal training in hazardous materials awareness. Reconnaissance, including security briefings, should inform the medical director of any hazardous materials or circumstances in the vicinity of the venue. Addressing the possibility of an unsafe MCI scene, the security manager and medical director should designate contingent casualty collection areas within the venue prior to the event. Security must ensure the safety of both casualties and the medical personnel treating them within these areas. Treatment areas should optimally be no more than five minutes walking distance from triage sites.

The Medical Action Plan

This document should reflect the organization and details of plans for emergency medical care framed by the preceding components. The medical director and event managers must agree on its final contents, resulting in a signed contract between the two parties based upon the document. Means and levels of compensation must be addressed. Medical liability coverage for all medical staff must be detailed. Expectations regarding demand for service should be supported by diligent reconnaissance. Research into applicable local, regional, and state guidelines and statutes should lead to plans within the document that meet or exceed their requirements.[25] The medical director's authority and position in the reporting structure must be delineated. The level of care to be offered on-site, the credentials and numbers of medical staff providing this care, and the resources at their disposal, including equipment, pharmaceuticals, facilities, and vehicles, must be itemized. Plans for providing and monitoring those environmental elements for which the medical sector will assume responsibility must be documented. The means of communication and the protocols governing its operations are crucial as the medium through which medical control is given. Contingency plans for VIP medical care and an MCI should be detailed.

The medical action plan should be finalized at least thirty days prior to the event. Copies, minus the proprietary business information, must be forwarded to all local, regional, state, and federal officials who have responsibility for either aspects of the event itself or emergency care in the surrounding jurisdiction. Copies should also be distributed to all event medical staff to inform them of the support at their disposal for the work anticipated. Any modifications to the document beyond its finalization must be agreed upon by both the medical director and event management, then redistributed to the same personnel.

Quality Management

The quality management (QM) process spans each side of the event, from planning, through execution and documentation, to review. It is essential to ensuring the best patient care possible at the event as well as protecting the event organization medico-legally.

Prospective QM

All of the foregoing planning for medical care at an event is part of the prospective phase. Additionally, the medical staff hiring, orientation, and training processes are integral components of prospective QM. Operationalization of the medical action plan occurs in this phase through the preceding processes. Optimally, all event medical personnel will simultaneously participate in orientation and training sessions onsite. However, the time-intensive, often unscheduled "routine" duties of public safety and emergency medical personnel often preclude this level of involvement. Alternative methods of orientation include videoconferencing, table-top exercises, and/or virtual reality applications brought to the personnel. All medical personnel must know their assigned geographic postings and coverage areas, as well as the locations of the medical control center, any fixed facilities, ambulances, and security personnel relative to their coverage areas. They must receive instruction in radio use, and practice efficient, effective transmissions. Practical scenarios for rehearsal include a mock MCI requiring discovery, initial intravenue management, and delayed jurisdictional intervention, hyper- and/or hypothermic casualty prevention and treatment, cardiac arrest, event player/performer injury, and VIP care. Within each of these scenarios, radio communications and intravenue routes to optimal care should be rehearsed. Event briefings and training sessions should translate into high quality medical care. But the only means of confirming this and improving upon it are through detailed but efficient documentation.

Concurrent QM

The medical director must be responsible for designing, adapting, or adopting a patient care report (PCR) form suitable for the event given the crucial need for uniform documentation. It is a legal as well as a medical record form, and its contents have important implications for both arenas. In terms of risk management for the event organization, accurately recording the interaction between patient and medical personnel on a standardized PCR form will likely reduce the chances of a successful lawsuit against both the event medical personnel involved and the organization. Uniformly completed PCRs allow the retrospective analysis of organized data on the event population's medical needs and treatment.

The simplest method of addressing the issue of uniformity is to adopt the standardized state or local jurisdiction EMS PCR as the official record form for event medical care documentation. Generically, the form is tailored to documentation of time-sensitive, out-of-hospital, brief patient encounters. It has been designed to conform to all local, regional, and state regulations which are essential for any PCR to be used. If ongoing care at a fixed facility takes place, these forms may be inadequate. At a minimum, the PCR form must include the following entry information:

- Time of first alert to the medical sector
- Encounter date, time, location within the venue
- Patient name, sex, age
- Chief complaint or mechanism of injury, pertinent medical and allergy history
- Pertinent physical examination findings
- Diagnostic impression
- Treatment rendered, supplies used
- Time from scene to disposition
- Follow-up instructions or disposition, with time of event staff departure from patient

All patient encounters should be recorded on the event PCR form, but a patient encounter must be defined. Orientation must include training medical staff on refusal of medical assistance (RMA) and leaving against medical advice (AMA) documentation as well as a uniform categorization of chief complaints. Instruction on the system of PCR collection, protection and storage is crucial to the QM process. This process must include strict protection of patient confidentiality, and therefore may well be served by coordination with event security. For on-site fixed medical facilities, delegating scribe duties to well oriented ancillary personnel may improve the efficiency of patient care.

Retrospective QM

For the future well-being of all who attend or participate in mass gathering events, the medical director has an obligation to conduct a systematic review of the care rendered. The review should take place as soon as possible following the end of the event. After any event, the PCR forms the foundation of such reviews.

Each PCR should be reviewed, either by the medical director or a multidisciplinary audit committee. Audit filters should be selected prior to the review to provide focus on critical aspects of event care. They should include response times and on-scene times exceeding a pre-set standard, initial vital signs outside set parameters, all intubations, defibrillation, and pediatric cases, and any helicoptered, RMA, or AMA cases. The choice of additional audit filters should be dictated by reconnaissance information from previous similar events and observations made during the event to be reviewed. For example, if an event held in a wilderness venue is being reviewed, all insect and animal bite cases should be audited.

Occasionally, because medical care should always take precedence over its documentation, means other than the PCR reviews must be used to critique medical care. This is especially true in regard to MCIs. Likely, review of these incidents must rely on interviews with involved event medical, security, and usher staff, as well as EMS responders in the public sector. Any incidents involving jurisdictional EMS should be jointly reviewed with those authorities and event management. All event debriefings should be structured and conducted in a fashion emphasizing education and improvement rather than blame and punishment.

Data should be summarized not only in terms of absolute case numbers, but also in terms of population incidence. Where possible, meaningful comparisons should be made to the incidence of similar cases in the general public. Only at this point can event risk be assigned so that corrective measures can be instituted for the next event. The medical director should formally report his conclusions and recommendations regarding the cases encountered and treated. The document should be distributed to all involved parties, medical and non-medical, with a message of appreciation for their dedication and care.

Summary

Gatherings of people are growing in popularity and variety. This implies the need for concomitant development of medical care planning tailored to attendees as diverse as the surrounding population at events as diverse as parades, sports competitions, political rallies, religious revivals, and even refugee camps. EMS personnel possess the expertise as well as the responsibility to care for these populations. The foregoing is intended to serve as a blueprint for use by the EMS community in planning expeditious, efficient, quality emergency care for all who attend and participate.

References

1. Carveth SW. Eight-year experience with a stadium-based mobile coronary care unit. *Heart Lung.* 1974;3:770–778.
2. Chused T, et al. Medical care during the November 1969 antiwar demonstrations in Washington, D.C.: an experience in crowd medicine. *Arch Internal Med.* 1971; 127:67–69.
3. Weiss BP, Mascola L, Fannin SL. Public health at the 1984 Summer Olympics: the Los Angeles County experience. *Am J Public Health.* 1986;78:686–688.
4. Meehan P, Toomey KE, Drinnon J, et al. Public health response for the 1996 Olympic Games. *JAMA.* 1998; 279:1469–1473.
5. 1989–90 Disaster Medical Services Subcommittee of the American College of Emergency Physicians: Provision of Emergency Medical Care for Crowds (information paper). 1990.
6. Jaslow D, Yancey AH, Milsten A. Mass gathering medical care. *Prehosp Emerg Care.* 2000;4:359–360.
7. Jaslow D, Yancey AH, Milsten A. for the NAEMSP Standards and Clinical Practice Committee. Mass Gathering Medical Care: The Medical Director's Checklist. 2000.
8. Erickson TB, Aks SE, Koenigsberg M, et al. Drug use patterns at major rock concert events. *Ann Emerg Med.* 1996;28:22–26.
9. Friedman LJ, Rodi SW, Krueger MA, et al. Medical care at the California AIDS Ride 3: experiences in event medicine. *Ann Emerg Med.* 1998;31:219–223.

10. Parrillo SJ. Medical care at mass gatherings: considerations for physician involvement. *Prehosp Disast Med.* 1995;10:273–275.
11. McDonald CC, Koenigsberg, MD, Ward S. Medical control of mass gatherings: can paramedics perform without physician on-site? *Prehosp Disast Med.* 1993;8:327–331.
12. Baker, WM, Simone BM, Niemann JT, et al. Special event medical care: The Los Angeles Summer Olympics experience. *Ann Emerg Med.* 1986;15:185–190.
13. Wetterhall SF, Coulombier DM, Herndon JM, et al. Medical care delivery at the 1996 Olympic Games. *JAMA.* 1998;279:1463–1468.
14. Spaite DW, Criss EA, Valenzuela TD. A new model for providing prehospital medical care in large stadiums. *Ann Emerg Med.* 1988;17:825–828.
15. DeLorenzo RA, Gray BC, Bennett PC, et al. Effect of crowd size on patient volume at a large, multipurpose, indoor stadium. *J Emerg Med.* 1989;7:379–384.
16. Klaucke DN, Buehler JW, Thacker SB, et al. Guidelines for evaluating surveillance systems. *MMWR.* 1988; 37(no. S-5).
17. Epidemiology Section of the Epidemiology and Preventive Branch, Division of Public Health, Department of Human Resources. 1996 Centennial Summer Olympic Games: Heat-Related Illness. *Georgia Epidemiology Report.* 1996;12(6):1–3.
18. Wharton M, Spiegel RA, Horan JM, et al. A large outbreak of antibiotic-resistant shigellosis at a mass gathering. *J Infectious Diseases.* 1990;162:1324–1328.
19. James SH, Calendrillo B, Schnoll SH. Medical and toxicological aspects of the Watkins Glen Rock Concert. *J Forensic Science.* 1974;1:71–82.
20. Whipkey RR, Paris PM, Stewart RD. Emergency care for mass gatherings: proper planning to improve outcome. *Postgraduate Medicine.* 1976;76(2):45–52.
21. Spaite DW, Meislin HW, Valenzuela TD, et al. Banning alcohol in a major college stadium: impact on the incidence and patterns of injury and illness. *J American College Health.* 1990;39:125–128.
22. Apsler R. Responsible Alcohol Service Programs Evaluation: Final Report. Washington, D.C. The National Highway Traffic Safety Administration; June, 1991.
23. Wolfe J, Martinez R, Scott WA. Baseball and beer: an analysis of alcohol consumption patterns among male spectators at major league sporting events. *Ann Emerg Med.* 1998;31:629–632.
24. Heck JJ, Kepp JK. Protective services: medical equipment selection for protective operations. *The Tactical Edge.* 2000:68–69.
25. Jaslow D, Drake M, Lewis J. Characteristics of state legislation governing medical care at mass gatherings. *Prehosp Emerg Care.* 1999;3:316–320.

Critical Incident Stress Management

Jeffrey T. Mitchell, PhD

Introduction

The United Nations International Labor Organization (UNILO) issued a report that calls job stress a worldwide plague and one of the most serious health issues of this century.[1] Human stress, which is a predictable byproduct of job conflict, job ambiguity, unrelenting pressures, shrinking support resources, and stressful contacts with people in need, is associated with illness, increased sick leave, changes in personality, marital and relationship discord, premature retirement, lowered job performance, injury on the job, disability claims against the employer, and early death.

Work-related stress claims represent the fastest growing and most costly per incident type of worker's compensation affecting U.S. commerce. The National Council on Compensation Insurance notes that about 14% of all "occupational disease" worker's compensation claims are for excessive stress. The average medical and other benefit payments total $15,000, which is twice the average amount per paid claim for workers with physical injuries.[2] The estimated overall costs of stress in the U.S. economy is as high as $150 billion per year.[3]

Managers of EMS organizations would be accused of incompetence if they ignored the growing body of evidence that indicates that the UNILO report is accurate in its evaluation of global job stress. Ignoring the obvious places the employer and employees at grave risk of mistakes on the job, injuries, and stress-related disabilities. The cost of not responding appropriately to growing job stress is extreme in both financial and human terms.

Critical Incident Stress

One of the most serious forms of stress is traumatic stress, or critical incident stress. It occurs when people are exposed to horrific, overwhelming, threatening, disgusting, grotesque, demanding, or shocking events that are beyond the range of normal human experience. These events are so unusual that they tax the coping abilities of those who experience them. Any mentally healthy person can experience this powerful and normal emotional response to a traumatic event. Critical incident stress is a normal response of normal people to abnormal events. Although it is painful and distressing, most people recover from the experience.[4]

The great majority of people who experience a highly traumatic event recover from the experience in a reasonable time, but a small number are so seriously affected that they later develop a more serious condition called post-traumatic stress disorder (PTSD), which is the most severe and incapacitating stress-related disorder. PTSD changes the way a person thinks, feels, and behaves. It also manifests itself in a wide range of physical symptoms. PTSD is so disruptive that it can effectively end the functional life of an individual and have severe negative effects on the family.[5] Becoming a victim of PTSD is a function of being exposed to a high-risk, potentially traumatizing situation or experience. It is not a result of poor training, inadequate moral fiber, physical or emotional weakness, or any other personal or job condition. It is not possible to predict PTSD, and there is no way to screen potential employees during the application process, because everyone is vulnerable.[4,5]

Because PTSD is directly related to the exposure to highly traumatic events or experiences, providers of EMS are at a higher than normal risk. The prevalence of PTSD in the general population of the United States is less than 2%.[6] Emergency personnel have a higher prevalence of PTSD of about 4%.[4] At least one researcher has found sufficient symptoms to diagnose PTSD in 16% of firefighters in a large Canadian city.[7]

It is clear from the discussion thus far that critical incident stress and PTSD endanger the health and survival of emergency personnel. Critical incident stress is also a significant problem for organizations, which risk legal, financial, and operational catastrophies, if this problem is ignored.

Comprehensive Critical Incident Stress Management

Critical incident stress reactions can be lessened and PTSD can be prevented. Critical incident stress is positively responsive to early intervention by both professional and peer support personnel specially trained to manage traumatic stress and employ an established set of stress intervention techniques. Cost-effective programs have been developed and implemented to reduce stress and accelerate the recovery process. At least 350 communities throughout the world have comprehensive critical incident stress management (CISM) programs, which have already proven their value in mitigating the effects of traumatic stress in emergency personnel and other groups. The comprehensiveness of these programs, however, must be recognized as the key to success.

EMS systems that attempt to deal with traumatic stress by using a single focused strategy, such as the development of only an educational program, are doomed to fail. A more sensible approach to traumatic stress management is a multifocal or comprehensive approach that includes a strategic plan for a wide spectrum of stress control programs.

A truly comprehensive CISM program has at least the following components:

- Extensive basic and continuing education program
- Critical incident stress team
- "Significant other" support programs
- Family support projects
- Administrator and supervisor education and support programs
- Peer support programs
- Mutual aid and community outreach programs
- Wide range of flexible intervention techniques such as:
  - □ mid-action or on scene support
  - □ individual consults with peers
  - □ defusings
  - □ demobilizations
  - □ debriefings
  - □ follow-up services
  - □ informal discussions
  - □ chaplain services
  - □ professional counseling services
  - □ mutual aid programs with other organizations
  - □ community education programs

Building a comprehensive CISM program does not have to be an overwhelming and extremely expensive task, if done properly by combining resources with other emergency services in the community. It is not necessary for each organization to create its own comprehensive program to manage traumatic stress. A much more efficient and effective approach is to become a part of an extensive network of CISM services.

Practically every CISM team is a "combined emergency services" team that serves hospitals, fire services, law enforcement agencies, EMS programs, communications personnel, search and rescue groups, ski patrols, military services, and other primary response organizations. These combined CISM teams work quite well. Because firefighters serve firefighters best, when an event predominantly affects fire service personnel, fire service peers are chosen to assist the affected firefighters. When the event is more clearly defined as an EMS event, EMS peers are chosen to assist their peers. Similarly, law enforcement personnel are chosen from a CISM team to work with law enforcement personnel, and nurses are chosen to work with nurses.

All of these organizations supply members to the CISM team, and all benefit from the other's experiences. They all share in training the team; they all use the same mental health professionals; and they all rely on each other in a disaster. Other benefits of working together are that the various groups develop respect and understanding for the other professions, and learn that there are many similarities among the various emergency service professions. Most important, combined CISM teams are able to emotionally support one another in the difficult work of traumatic stress management.[8]

The combined CISM team makes sense on many levels. It saves money, effectively uses resources, improves the breadth of the experience, and enhances training efforts. One service may contribute a clergyperson to the team, another may provide a mental health professional, and yet another may supply the medical director. EMS providers, nurses, firefighters, and police officers are usually drawn from the local services.

There are also real psychological reasons why a broad spectrum team is more efficient and effective than a CISM team limited to only one emergency service. It is psychologically unsound for the providers of critical incident stress services and the recipients of those services to know one another well. Every medically trained person recognizes the inherent psychological dangers of providing medical treatment to seriously ill relatives or friends. Similar dangers exist for those who serve on CISM teams; and they often arise when supervisors try to provide support services for workers. Close association between those who give help and those who receive it causes unnecessary emotional distress. The natural boundaries between work and personal feelings are threatened, and anxieties are stirred on both sides.[4]

A combined emergency services CISM team is one situation in which competition among organizations is discouraged and an atmosphere of mutual cooperation and support is enhanced. It is clearly a recommended course of action.

Traumatic Stress Education

Prospective traumatic stress education is one of the most essential keys in the prevention and reduction of critical incident stress in emergency services. Personnel forewarned about stress reactions tend to recognize the signs of distress earlier; and early recognition of stress symptoms leads to an earlier call for help. Prospective education enhances the potential that the help will be accepted and the recovery will be faster. Educated personnel take less time off of work; and their positive morale is maintained.

Ideally, every provider should be given prospective training. The general outline for critical incident stress education is as follows:

- Nature of ordinary stress (definitions, stress process)
- Stress in emergency services (cumulative, traumatic)
- Typical critical incidents (children, threats of violence, injuries to nurses)
- Immediate and long-range effects of traumatic stress

- Signs and symptoms of CIS
- Survival techniques for emergency personnel
- The CISM team
- Calling for help
- What the CISM team does (defusings, debriefings, one-on-one contacts, significant-other support, follow-up services)

The properly trained CISM team members, when not involved in direct support services, spend much of their time teaching emergency personnel about traumatic stress.

Mid-action Support

On occasion a critical incident is so distressing that personnel have immediate reactions to it, showing signs of dysfunction while performing their duties. Such a situation demands immediate intervention by a trained CISM team member.

The immediate intervention is emotional first aid. It usually consists of a practical, common sense action that removes the distressed individuals from the immediate area and either gives them an alternate task or a few moments to recover before returning to work. Breaks, changing the tasks, redirecting attention, an understanding nod, and a variety of other supportive techniques are ways in which mid-action or on-scene support services are applied.[4]

Defusings

Defusings are one of the most frequently employed CISM techniques. They are short versions of the more formal debriefing process. Defusings are usually led by two CISM-trained peer support personnel. Although they are not time-consuming, the results are often powerful.

For small groups, defusings are applied within hours of a highly traumatic event. The group is defused in a private setting before they are released to go home or back to their normal duties. Defusings last less than one hour and are best described as a conversation about a particularly distressing event. They consist of three main segments. First, there is a brief introduction in which the guidelines for the meeting are described and the personnel are motivated to participate actively. The second segment is the exploration of the incident. Descriptions of the specific incident are presented by those who were involved, and the leader may ask guiding questions. The defusing ends with a set of instructions and important pieces of information that may protect the staff from further harmful effects of the traumatic incident. If necessary, a formal debriefing is arranged a few days after the defusing.[8]

Demobilizations

Thankfully, demobilizations are rare occurrences in EMS because they are always associated with large-scale or catastrophic incidents. They are used only when a large group of providers have been exposed to catostrophic or highly distressing events, such as September 11, 2001.

Demobilizations consist of two parts. In the first part a small group of personnel who ordinarily work as a team are brought together after their work in an incident is complete. The team is then demobilized; they are given a 10-minute talk by a trained CISM team member on the potential stress effects of an exposure and the steps they can take to lessen the impact of the stress reaction. No one has to speak during the demobilization, and no questions are asked of those who are being demobilized. After the 10-minute talk, the listeners are asked if they need to say anything or if they have any questions. Usually the group being demobilized is so fatigued and numbed by their work that they do not have anything to say. The small group is then sent to another room where nutritious foods and fruit juices are available. Demobilizations are continued with additional groups until every group involved in the event is processed.[8]

Debriefings

A debriefing is the most complex and difficult of the stress mitigation and recovery processes. It can be provided only by a properly trained CISM team, consisting of a mental health professional and a few Critical Incident Stress Debriefing (CISD) trained peers.

A debriefing is a 2- or 3-hour group discussion of the traumatic incident; it is made up of seven phases. The first phase of the CISD is the introduction phase, which concentrates on motivating the participants to actively participate in the process, and informs them of the guidelines for the smooth conduct of the session.

The second phase is the fact phase. Personnel are asked to briefly describe their role and experiences during the situation.

The third phase is the thought segment of the debriefing. The participants describe their first thought or the most prominent thought after they came off of auto pilot during the incident.

The fourth phase of the CISD is the reaction phase; it is considered the most emotionally powerful. The group members discuss the elements of the situation that caused them the most distress and have been the most difficult to cope with since the situation.

The fifth phase of the debriefing is the symptom phase. The participants are asked about the signs and symptoms of distress that they encountered during and after the incident, as well as how they are doing at the time of the debriefing.

The descriptions of the symptoms are an excellent jumping-off point for the CISD team to move into the sixth debriefing phase, which is the teaching phase. The CISD team teaches the members of the group helpful concepts related to stress mitigation and stress recovery. The participants are encouraged to ask any questions they may have.

The final phase of the CISD is the reentry phase in which the participants ask any remaining questions they may have and make any additional comments. The CISD team makes summary comments and the group is released.[8]

Individual Consultations

When only one or two providers are distressed by a situation and the remainder are not affected, a trained member of the CISM team can work independently with those affected. There is no need to bring together an entire group, if only a few are affected by an incident. Focused individual support can be applied when an individual requests help with a job-related or personal problem.

Guidelines

Effective CISM programs are never an accident; they are carefully planned and managed efforts. EMS organizations, if they are going to provide the services that will preserve their personnel in their careers, must first make a proactive commitment to the appropriate development of a CISM program.

The first commitment is to find an appropriate person to chair the development committee. A major organizational mistake made is assuming that CISM is a task for a mental health professional. No one denies that mental health professionals play a highly significant role in a comprehensive CISM program and are vital to program success. They are, however, generally very busy people with many conflicting duties and little time to develop, coordinate, and administer an entire CISM program. CISM is an emergency services function and is not the responsibility of mental health services.

Prehospital providers know that stress in the emergency setting is neither new nor unusual. They tend to trust and listen to one of their own who has expertise in CISM and EMS. Individual providers tend to be charged up about their stress, and they can channel all of that energy into effective stress prevention and mitigation programs, if led by another provider with firsthand knowledge of the severe stress of emergency services. Once an enthusiastic individual is chosen to head the development committee, arrangements should be made to coordinate efforts with a CISM team that may already exist in the area. Every effort should be made to join resources rather than set up a competitive team.

The emergency service should then develop a steering committee under the direction of the person selected to coordinate CISM efforts. The steering committee usually consists of representatives from the various groups participating in the CISM team, and selected mental health professionals interested in establishing the team. The tasks assigned to the steering committee include selection of staff to serve on the team and the establishment of a policy and procedures committee to develop appropriate written operating procedures. Most steering committees have a subcommittee to assure close coordination with the local CISD team and with the International Critical Incident Stress Foundation, which serves a coordinating, standard setting, and education body for CISM teams. The steering committee also must provide appropriate training and education opportunities for the CISM team members.

The CISM team should be a peer-focused support service that uses mental health professionals and chaplains as consultants. When effectively trained, led, and empowered, a CISM team is a powerful force in maintaining healthy and happy personnel. Therefore the next commitment the administration of the agency has to make is to trust the members of the CISM team to carry out their mission without threatening the operation of the agency.

CISM teams can only function if they have an open network of communication. There must exist an effective means for emergency providers to call for CISM team assistance. In addition, there should be consistent and frequent communication with the local, regional, and national CISM networks for information exchange and mutual aid.

An important guideline is to never assume that every mental health professional is equally trained and capable of dealing appropriately with emotional trauma. Few mental health professionals receive the appropriate training to manage critical incident stress reactions; many do not have the personality necessary to manage traumatic stress. Critical incident stress management is a specialty field, and only those with the appropriate training and experience should attempt to provide it. Services by well-meaning but untrained and inexperienced individuals are inherently dangerous, and seriously jeopardize the recovery of providers in the midst of traumatic stress.

Proper training cannot be overemphasized. Every member of a CISM team, regardless of previous experience and education, should go through a specialized course of education and training in CISM and PTSD management provided by a skilled and experienced critical incident stress trainer. Exceptions lead to confusion in the provision of services, misrepresentation of expertise, misunderstanding and resentment among CISM members, and poor performance in the delivery of appropriate CISM services. Inadequately trained CISM personnel are prescriptions for disaster. Team member education should be viewed as a mechanism to assure quality services, as well as an opportunity to enhance the cohesiveness of the CISM team.

Effectiveness

The CISM field is less than two decades old, but it has already made significant progress in assisting distressed emergency providers recover and continue to function in EMS. Emergency workers who went through debriefings show less signs of distress and feel less unique in their experience. They also recover faster and experience less long-range symptoms.[9-11] In addition, there is a considerable volume of anecdotal information that indicates that the CISM services have positive effects. Some of the factors that make CISM service effective are listed here:

- Early Intervention—CISM services are provided when people are ready for help because their natural guards are down.

- Opportunity for emotional ventilation—Expressing emotions lowers the level of stress arousal.[12]

- Structured approach—Providing structure when a group is facing chaos is reassuring and helps people recover.

- Enhances the person's ability to form concepts—The brain's ability to categorize experiences is vital to recovery from trauma. The debriefing process urges this type of concept formation.

- Group support—It is easier for people to recover from traumatic stress if they realize that they are not alone and not unusual in their reactions to the traumatic event.

- Peer support—It is easier to recover when the process is guided by people experienced in emergency services.

- Allows for follow-up—Much of the actual support work associated with CISM services is accomplished after initial services such as defusings and debriefings have been provided. The first contacts with the personnel can be used to make appropriate referrals to psychological services when individuals in need of specialized help have been identified.

Summary

The world experienced by EMS personnel is often threatening, violent, grotesque, shocking, and demanding. It has become more so in the recent past.

Therefore EMS agencies face either the task of developing and implementing a comprehensive CISM program or the potential of a costly deterioration of their personnel. The medical directors of those agencies will hopefully choose a proactive stance in regard to traumatic stress; what is at stake is the most valuable resource of any organization—its people.

References

1. Bonderoff V. Epidemic for our times: stress. *Vancouver Sun.* March 27, 1993; p. B1, B9.
2. McCarthy M. Stressed employees look for relief in worker's compensation claims. *Wall Street Journal.* April 7, 1989; p. 34.
3. Miller A, et al. Stress on the job. *Newsweek.* April 25, 1988; p. 40–41.
4. Mitchell J, Bray G. *Emergency Services Stress: Guidelines for Preserving the Health and Careers of Emergency Personnel.* Englewood Cliffs, NJ: Brady Publishing (Prentice Hall); 1990.
5. Everly G. *A Clinical Guide to the Treatment of the Human Stress Response.* New York: Plenum Publishing; 1989.
6. Helzer J, Robins L, McEvoy L. Post traumatic stress disorder in the general population. *N Eng J Med.* 1987; 317:1630–1634.
7. Corneil W. Personal communication, 1992.
8. Mitchell JT, Everly GS. *Critical Incident Stress Debriefing: An Operations Manual for the Prevention of Traumatic Stress among Emergency Services and Disaster Workers.* Ellicott City, MD: Chevron Publishing Corporation; 1993.
9. Dyregrov A. Personal communication, 1992.
10. Robinson R. Personal communication, 1992.
11. Wee D. Personal communication, 1993.
12. Lang P. The application of psycho physiological methods to the study of psychotherapy and behavior modification. In: Bergin A, S Garfield. *Handbook of Psychotherapy and Behavior Change.* New York: Wiley; 1971.

Section Eight

Robert Swor, DO

This section introduces where we hope the next edition of this text will focus—the future of EMS. Much has been written about the EMS Agenda for the Future, a document which eloquently laid out where EMS should be heading. Chapters in this section review what has happened since those ideas were first proposed in the mid-1990s. Ideas such as expanding the scope of EMS providers have been proposed and piloted, but as yet have not firmly taken root in the healthcare system. Reasons for these are many and relate more to the complexity and financial underpinning of the healthcare system than to the inherent value of the ideas. The chapter on managed care addresses EMS in a larger scope, and discusses the potential of EMS to be fundamentally integrated into the healthcare system.

The ideas that appeal most are those of integration of EMS into the public health system. Because of the impressive success of the fire services in the field of fire prevention, EMS leaders have discussed other potential roles that EMS providers may serve the community. Injury prevention is the most readily definable entry of EMS in Public Health and a discussion of the potential role for EMS bioterrorism response are presented. The broader role of EMS in surveillance, immunization, and other public health activities are also described.

Finally, I would be remiss if I didn't honor the memory of one of the chapter authors, Keith Neely, EMTP, PhD. Keith was a thoughtful leader in EMS, an energetic researcher in EMS, and a visionary in the careful, thoughtful integration of EMS services in the managed care environment and the larger healthcare system. Even more important, he was a kind and gentle soul, whose untimely death has saddened all of his colleagues.

CHAPTER 79

EMS Agenda for the Future

Theodore Delbridge, MD, MPH

Introduction

In 1996 the National Highway Traffic Safety Administration (NHTSA) and the Health Resources and Services Administration (HRSA), Maternal and Child Health Bureau (MCHB), published the *EMS Agenda for the Future*. To date, thousands of copies have been distributed throughout the United States.

At the time of *EMS Agenda for the Future*'s release, it had been thirty years since the publication of *Accidental Death and Disability: the Neglected Disease of Modern Society*. That document is often credited as being the impetus for the development of modern emergency medical services (EMS) in the United States. Howard, one of the paper's authors, has spoken eloquently about how he and his colleagues had been part of great advances in caring for the wounded during the Korean Conflict. At home in the United States, they were later frustrated by a lack of systematic organization and focus to deliver a similar quality care.[1] In *Accidental Death and Disability* they called attention to their finding that the American healthcare system was woefully ill-prepared to address an injury epidemic that was the leading cause of death among people between the ages of 1 and 37 years. They noted that, in most cases, ambulances were inappropriately designed, ill-equipped, and staffed with inadequately trained personnel. At least 50% of the nation's ambulance services were being provided by 12,000 morticians.[2]

Accidental Death and Disability proposed 29 recommendations to improve the American healthcare system. Eleven related directly to out-of-hospital EMS. Federal initiatives, such as the Highway Safety Act of 1966 and the Emergency Medical Services Act of 1973, and other public and private projects led to a rapidly evolving EMS system. At the heart of this growth was the steadfast belief that improved outcomes would result from better EMS responses.

The initial EMS growth spurt necessarily began without abundant knowledge of the most efficient processes to deliver the optimal resources to the spectrum of situations addressed by today's EMS systems. By the mid-1990s, it appeared that the American health care system as a whole was undergoing a transformation of sorts. Thus, the time seemed right to create the *EMS Agenda for the Future*, which incorporated input from a broad range of EMS stakeholders, to determine the most important directions for future EMS development.

Creating the Agenda

The *EMS Agenda for the Future* was created using a modification of the National Institutes of Health (NIH) Technology Assessment and Practice Guidelines Forum.[3] A multi-disciplined steering committee prepared early drafts of the document. The committee sent a second draft to 500 EMS-interested groups and individuals for their comments. Nearly 200 reviewers returned comments regarding all or part of the draft document. The steering committee analyzed this feedback and revised the document accordingly. Subsequently, 133 people participated in a blue-ribbon conference held over three days in December 1995. These physicians, nurses, EMS providers, administrators, educators, and others reviewed the current generation document and provided their critique during 32 focus-group sessions. The steering committee revised the document based on the feedback provided during the conference, and once again distributed their draft for final review. During its last meeting in March 1996, the steering committee reviewed the most recently received comments and finalized the *EMS Agenda for the Future*.

EMS Vision for the Future

The vision for the future of EMS emphasizes its critical role in caring for the health of Americans. It is also congruent with other desirable changes in the overall healthcare system, which is, in part, transforming to focus on the early identification and modification of risk factors before illness or injury strikes.

EMS of the future will be community-based health management that is fully integrated with the overall healthcare system. It will have the ability to identify and modify illness and injury risks, provide acute illness and injury care and follow-up, and contribute to community health monitoring and treatment of chronic conditions. EMS will be integrated with other healthcare providers and public health and public safety agencies. It will improve community health and will result in more appropriate use of acute health care resources. EMS will remain the public's emergency medical safety net.[4]

If such a vision is to be realized, 14 aspects of EMS require ongoing attention. These attributes are similar to those of any other element of the healthcare system (fig. 79.1). The following discussion of each summarizes that of the *EMS Agenda for the Future*.

Integration of Health Services

Where We Are

The EMS system encounters nearly all possible injuries or illnesses, and its providers treat patients of all ages. However, contemporary EMS systems were created predominantly to meet the immediate needs of acutely ill and injured people, to provide "stabilizing" care and transportation. EMS, in general, has attempted to meet these objectives in relative isolation from the rest of the healthcare system and potentially synergistic community resources. With the exception of public safety agencies, there is a disconnect between EMS and other healthcare and community resources that could be helpful in attaining optimal outcomes for EMS patients. EMS providers are not accustomed to ensuring the availability of follow-up care for their patients, especially those who are not transported to a hospital, and are infrequently participants in that care. Thus, potential positive effects of EMS, in terms of effecting improved health for individuals and the community, go unrealized.

Reports have been published regarding public health surveillance by EMS personnel and referral to social service agencies.[5-7] A model for incorporating EMS systems and health monitoring referral systems has been described.[8] Pilot projects are at various stages within several EMS systems to determine the feasibility and benefits of coordination and routine communication with patients' healthcare providers and networks. Options for an expanded EMS clinical care role have also been explored.[9]

Where We Want To Be

Out-of-hospital EMS care is considered to be an integral component of overall health care. Attributes, or supporting characteristics, that are critical to out-of-hospital care are the same as those of other elements of the healthcare system. EMS patients are assured that their care is considered part of a complete healthcare program, connected to sources for continuous and/or follow-up care and linked to other potentially beneficial health and community resources. Collaborative liaisons between EMS and other components of the healthcare system, social service agencies, and others enable EMS to help affect people's long-term health, by sharing information regarding unhealthy situations and by providing referral to organizations with a vested interest in maintaining the health of their clients or the community.

With appropriate medical direction, EMS facilitates access of its patients to appropriate sources for continued medical care, supporting efforts to implement cost-effective community healthcare while ensuring that the special needs of individual patients are met.

EMS Research

Where We Are

In the case of EMS, system changes frequently prompt research efforts to prove they make a difference, instead of the more appropriate sequence of using research findings as a basis for improvement. The volume of EMS research is low and the quality is often less than that in other disciplines.[10] Furthermore, most published EMS research focuses on a single intervention or health problem, rarely addressing the inherent complexities of EMS systems.[11] Analyses of single components may lead to incorrect conclusions, or at least ones that cannot be supported when they are considered in the context of the entire EMS system.[11,12] Development of the "chain of survival" concept for cardiac emergencies provides evi-

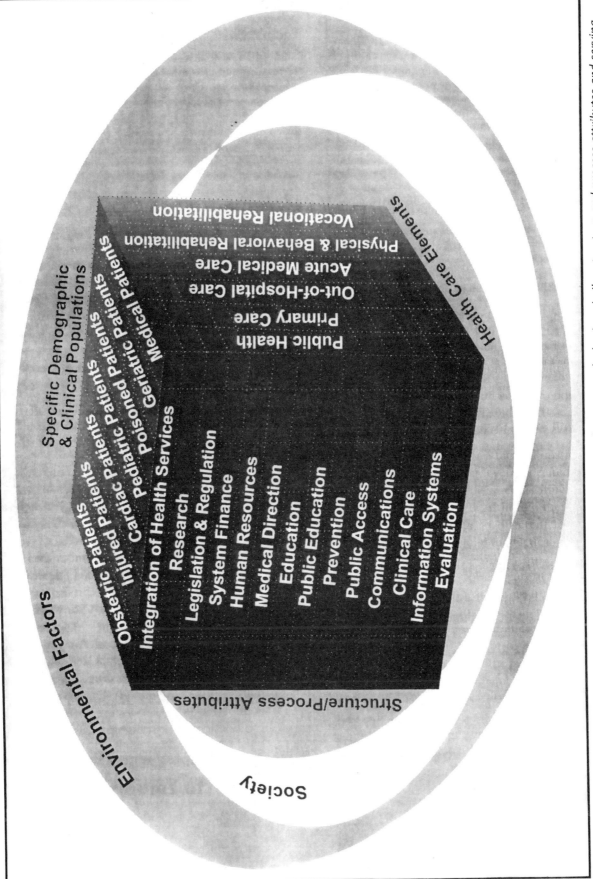

FIGURE 79.1. *The healthcare system, consisting of a continuum of healthcare elements, each sharing similar structure and process attributes and serving various demographic and clinical populations. The system is influenced by society and inherent environmental factors. (Adapted from Emergency Medical Services Agenda for the Future)*

dence of completed systems research.[13,14] Trauma-related research has comprised the other EMS research emphases.[11] Significant barriers to collecting relevant, meaningful, and accurate EMS data exist.[12] These include the rigor with which EMS data is collected, inability to link EMS information with other meaningful data sets, and difficulties in engaging EMS practitioners in research initiatives. Thus, the effectiveness of most EMS interventions, and of EMS systems, has not been well established with relevant outcome criteria.[10]

Where We Want To Be

EMS evolves with a scientific basis. Conclusive investigations of interventions, treatments, and system designs are conducted before they are advocated as EMS standards. Multi-disciplinary approaches to EMS research attempt to answer complex questions. Integrated information systems facilitate development of linkages between EMS and other public safety agencies and healthcare providers. Greater numbers of academic centers commit to EMS research by designating resources and developing researchers. EMS personnel at all levels appreciate the role of research in creating the future basis for patient care.

Legislation and Regulation

Where We Are

States have determined that it is within the public's interest to assure the availability of a coordinated EMS system that provides acceptable quality care. All states have statutes that provide the basis for EMS activities and programs. These statutes vary significantly in the way they describe EMS system components, and to the degree they permit flexibility among lead or regulatory agencies. However, during 35 state EMS evaluations by NHTSA technical assessment teams, only 40% of states reported to have comprehensive EMS-enabling statutes for maintenance of a statewide EMS system, and only 20% had an EMS lead agency with responsibility and authority for overall coordination.[15] As reassessments are conducted several years later, significant advances in this regard are apparent. In many cases, local governments have also passed ordinances to delineate EMS standards for their communities.

Where We Want To Be

Each state has a single EMS lead agency responsible for developing and overseeing a statewide EMS system. These agencies have abilities to adapt and be responsive to changing healthcare environments, and are empowered to ensure that EMS of acceptable quality is available to the entire population. State legislation provides a template that allows local medical directors to determine specific practice parameters for their EMS systems and to conduct credible research and pilot projects.

System Finance

Where We Are

Making EMS available to the U.S. population is a multi-billion dollar per year effort.[4] The overall costs of EMS for any area include the costs of all the infrastructure and activities required to provide service. For example, equipment acquisition and maintenance, communications system, personnel and their education, medical direction, and licensing and regulation activities often contribute to EMS costs. Process standards, such as response time, or staffing requirements, may greatly influence overall costs. EMS systems are funded by a combination of public and private funds.[16] For those systems that rely on reimbursement from insurance, transport to the hospital has usually been a requirement of payment. Yet, it is preparedness, readiness, and response that predominantly determine system cost. Thus, the driving forces for cost and payment have been considered in the recent changes in Medicare ambulance reimbursement.

Where We Want To Be

Governments facilitate the continued development of EMS systems on regional, statewide, and national bases. Funding is provided to ensure the appropriate levels of EMS preparedness. Additionally, mechanisms that fund other aspects of the healthcare system adequately support EMS. The value of care delivered without transport to a hospital is recognized. Providing transportation is not a prerequisite for payment. Payment for service, in part, accounts for the cost of maintaining preparedness, depending on service area size and complexity, utilization, and predetermined quality standards.

Human Resources

Where We Are

EMS systems rely on many people with diverse backgrounds, including citizen bystanders, public safety communicators, emergency medical dispatchers, first responders, emergency medical technicians (EMTs), nurses, physicians, firefighters, and law enforcement officers. Most out-of-hospital care is provided by EMTs. In the United States there are an estimated 70,000 paramedics and 500,000 other-level EMTs. *The National EMS Education and Practice Blueprint* has established standard knowledge and practice expectations for four levels of EMS providers: first responder, EMT-Basic, EMT-Intermediate and EMT-Paramedic.[17] However, many other various levels of EMS providers exist among state statutes and regulations.

Recruitment and retention of EMS personnel is a perennial issue. Occupational risks, limited mobility and minimal credentials reciprocity, sub-optimal recognition, and inadequate compensation are contributing factors.[18] EMS personnel experience stressors and risks that are unique to other healthcare and public safety workers. They are twice as likely as the general population to suffer from post-traumatic stress disorders.[19,20] Exposure to HIV and hepatitis viruses is a great concern, as hepatitis seroprevalence among EMS workers has been estimated to be three to five times greater than the general population.[21,22] Contaminated needle-stick injuries are not infrequent.[23,24] Additional occupational hazards include risk of assault, motor vehicle crash, back injury and falling.[25-27] Furthermore, EMS workers often suffer from lack of full recognition as members of the healthcare delivery team. They lack a career ladder in places, and their mobility is limited by credentialing systems that do not provide for reciprocity between states or sometimes even regions within a state.

Where We Want To Be

People attracted to EMS service are among the best and the brightest, and the composition of the EMS workforce reflects the diversity of the community it serves. The workforce receives compensation comparable to other healthcare and public safety positions with similar responsibilities and occupational risks.

Standard categories of EMS providers are recognized on a national basis. Reciprocity agreements among states for standard categories of EMS providers eliminate unreasonable barriers to mobility. Career ladders and established connections to parallel fields help to ensure the longevity of workforce numbers. Occupational risks are studied and understood, and efforts are continuously pursued to attenuate those risks.

Medical Oversight

Where We Are

State laws typically mandate that medical oversight be provided to EMS systems that provide advanced levels of care. Many states also require that basic-level EMS systems maintain a formal relationship with a medical director.[15] However, the manner in which medical oversight is provided varies, from occasional informal consultation to close supervision.

EMS medical directors evolve from several medical disciplines, although emergency physicians provide the majority of direct medical oversight. A model curriculum for EMS education within emergency medicine residency programs has been published.[28] Additionally, a growing number of EMS fellowships are being created to develop special competency in EMS among mostly emergency physicians.

Direct medical oversight occurs via radio, telephone, or on-scene physicians. It is undoubtedly helpful for some patients, but its systematic application for the majority of EMS patients remains controversial. Direct medical oversight usually does not result in orders for care beyond those that have been directed via protocol.[29-35] Linkage to objective, relevant outcomes has been incomplete.

The medical director's role is to provide medical leadership for EMS. Those who serve as EMS medical directors are charged with the ultimate responsibility for the quality of care delivered.

Where We Want To Be

All EMS providers and activities have the benefit of qualified medical oversight. This is true regardless of the level of service provided. Knowledgeable and qualified physicians and staffs with special competency in EMS provide medical oversight, which ultimately affects the EMS care delivered in the community. The effects of direct medical oversight are understood, so that appropriate situations and patients for its application, and appropriate staff can provide it. Resources available to the medical director are commensurate with the associated responsibility, size, and complexity of the involved system.

Each state has a qualified EMS medical director responsible for overseeing the statewide EMS system. Locally, EMS medical directors are responsible for determining their systems' practice parameters. Medical oversight provides leadership for the system, ensuring collaboration with other disciplines to see that the needs of the entire population are being optimally served.

Education Systems

Where We Are

The *National EMS Education and Practice Blueprint* describes the standard knowledge and practice expectations for four levels of EMS providers.[17] The National Registry of Emergency Medical Technicians (NREMT) offers certification examinations for these levels. These are accepted as evidence of competency in many states. Curricula developed by the U.S. Department of Transportation (DOT) provide the bases for EMS education at these levels. However, many more levels of certification exist among states and local jurisdictions, impeding efforts to develop credentialing reciprocity.

Settings for EMS education are diverse.[36] Program quality can be achieved in most, and a joint review committee on educational programs for EMT-Paramedics has accredited programs associated with various types of institutions. Additionally, several colleges offer Bachelor's degrees in EMS.[37]

Many reports discuss EMS provider education to provide specific skills.[38-46] However, systematic analyses of education with regard to the actual expectation of EMS personnel in the community have been lacking.

Where We Want To Be

EMS education sets up a program of life-long learning for EMS professionals, and is provided by qualified instructors. Education programs are based on national core contents for EMS providers at various levels. These provide program infrastructure and recognition by accrediting bodies while enabling adaptation for local circumstances.

Higher-level EMS education programs are affiliated with academic institutions, increasing the availability of educational opportunities for EMS professionals that are accepted as academic achievement. Institutions of higher learning recognize EMS education as achievement worthy of academic credit.

Public Education

Where We Are

A great deal of what the public knows about EMS and dealing with medical emergencies originates from the popular media, including television programs intended for entertainment and not for education. As an agent for public education, EMS is underdeveloped.

There are some examples of EMS public education initiatives. Funds for emergency medical services for children have been used to develop programs about childhood emergencies and illnesses.[47] Other efforts have focused on timely access and appropriate utilization of the EMS system.[48,49] However, planned and evaluated EMS public education initiatives remain sporadic.

Where We Want To Be

Public education is recognized as an essential ongoing activity of EMS. Public education efforts support the role of EMS in improving community health, and programs address the needs of all members of the community. EMS systems educate the public as consumers, as bystander first-responders, and as agents of prevention. They educate purchasers of healthcare as well as policy makers.

Prevention

Where We Are

EMS is not commonly linked to the public's prevention consciousness. However, the potential role of EMS in prevention has previously been recognized.[50] Several successful EMS-initiated prevention programs have been described.[47,51,52] Furthermore, although they are not common, linkages between EMS and other community services able to initiate prevention activities may also benefit EMS patients.[6,8,47,51]

Injury prevention has taken on a new dimension for improving the nation's health and controlling healthcare costs.[53] In the United States, injury accounts for more years of potential life lost than any other health problem. Thus, injury prevention modules have been advocated for inclusion in the *National EMS Education and Practice Blueprint*.[54]

Where We Want To Be

EMS systems and providers are continuously engaged in injury and illness prevention programs, addressing community injury and illness problems. They are involved as collectors of data, as partners to help study problems and provide prevention strategies, and as health practitioners who provide acute care. Additionally, EMS systems develop and maintain prevention-oriented environments for their personnel. EMS personnel receive education regarding prevention principles, and learn how prevention relates to them and to those they serve.

Public Access

Where We Are

A growing proportion of the U.S. population is able to access EMS by calling 9-1-1. Enhanced 9-1-1 (9-1-1E) automatically provides call-takers with caller's telephone number identity (ANI) and location identity (ALI). When 9-1-1 is not the number to call for emergency help, delays may result from not knowing the correct number, or from telephone dialing errors.[55,56]

Financial barriers may impede access to EMS. These include inability to pay for telephone services, and pressure from health insurers to obtain authorization prior to using EMS.

The ability to access EMS efficiently via wireless telephone is not guaranteed. Depending on how a call is routed, it may not reach the appropriate public safety answering point (PSAP) for the caller's location as often as 20% of the time.[57] Furthermore, location-identifying technology has not been deployed. Thus, callers for help who are transient will be challenged to determine their locations, and significant delays may result.

Many EMS systems triage calls, so that more urgent situations get the quickest response. However, EMS is relatively unsophisticated in terms of its abilities to match appropriate resources for the nature of the calls.

Where We Want To Be

Implementation of 9-1-1 is nationwide, ensuring that, from any land-line telephone, EMS can be accessed by calling 9-1-1. Alternative access to 9-1-1 is made available for people unable to pay for telephone service where it routinely exists. Thus, even when a telephone does not provide all the routine services, it still provides a means to call 9-1-1 and access EMS. Wireless telephones uniformly provide a means of accessing 9-1-1. Furthermore, every call to 9-1-1 is automatically accompanied by location-identifying information.

No financial, legal, social, or age-related barriers to access the appropriate care via 9-1-1 exist for those who perceive an emergency to exist. EMS access includes allocation of appropriate resources for the circumstances, so that the resulting response is the most optimal, given available options.

Communications Systems

Where We Are

Effective communications networks provide access to the EMS system, dispatch of EMS and other public safety agencies, access to medical oversight, communications to and between emergency healthcare facilities, communications between EMS and other healthcare providers, and outlets for disseminating information to the public. The spectrum of communications equipment currently in use is broad, ranging from antiquated radios to mobile data terminals.

Emergency medical dispatchers (EMDs) have been advocated as essential personnel at all dispatching centers.[58–60] They are able to provide dispatch life support via pre-arrival instructions, which are thought to be a cost-effective mechanism for improving survival from out-of-hospital cardiac arrests.[61,62]

From a communications perspective, EMS personnel are mostly isolated from the rest of the healthcare delivery system. They rarely have meaningful information about their patients that might improve decision-making, nor are they able to convey new information to other healthcare providers who may have an interest. Additionally, communications system limitations at times also impede abilities to obtain on-line medical direction.

Where We Want To Be

Emergency calls to EMS are answered by people with the requisite combination of education, experience, and tools necessary to optimally query the caller, determine the most appropriate resources to be mobilized, and implement the best course of action. Communications networks incorporate other providers of medical care, enabling critical information sharing. They also facilitate communications with other public safety agencies and ensure access to on-line medical direction. Communications issues related to disaster preparedness are addressed, and each state maintains an emergency communications plan.

Clinical Care

Where We Are

EMS systems vary remarkably with regard to the sophistication of care they provide and the tools they use. Variation exists due to state laws and regulations, availability of local resources, and the needs and expectations of individual communities. There is no standard baseline of care that is provided by all EMS systems. The floors of EMS care is not even, nor are the ceilings. The interventions that paramedics may perform, the equipment available to them, and the medications they carry vary greatly.[63,64] In some cases, variation may be due to adaptations to serve local needs. With the exception of a few clinical situations, such as cardiac arrests and certain traumatic syndromes, the effectiveness of EMS care is not adequately known.

Where We Want To Be

EMS provides a defined floor of clinical care and services in all communities. Expansion of care and services increases in response to community healthcare needs and availability of resources.

The effects of EMS care in terms of outcomes, for specific conditions, are continuously evaluated. Therapeutic technology and pharmaceutical advances are evaluated in terms of their effectiveness and appropriateness for EMS use before they are advocated for routine deployment.

The composition and expertise of personnel responsible for patients' secondary transports (e.g., interfacility transports) match their potentially complex needs. The authority and responsibility for direct medical oversight during such transports are clear.

Information Systems

Where We Are

Systems for data collection and information management have developed slowly within EMS.[65] The Trauma Care Systems Planning and Development Act of 1990 emphasized the need for collection of data for the evaluation of emergency care for serious injuries.[66] The 1993 Institute of Medicine Report, *Emergency Medical Services for Children*, recommended that states collect and analyze certain EMS data needed for planning, evaluation, and research of EMS for children.[67] In 1993, the Uniform Pre-Hospital Emergency Medical Services Data Conference resulted in standard definitions for data elements, and determined them to be essential or desirable.[68]

The data required to completely describe an EMS event exist in separate disparate locations, including EMS agencies, emergency departments, hospital medical records, other public safety agencies, and vital statistics offices. In most cases, meaningful linkages among such sites are nonexistent. The lack of recognized information systems that incorporate data that are valid, reliable, and accurate is a significant barrier to coordinating EMS evaluation. Research efforts are also hindered. Integrated information systems serve as multi-source databases, and have been advocated as useful research tools.[69]

Where We Want To Be

Integrated information systems which receive data electronically and in real time are in place.

Evaluation

Where We Are

EMS systems are evaluated using structural (input) process and outcome measures. Structural evaluation is the least complex, but its relationship to outcome is usually uncertain. The relative lack of consistently available and reliable data is an important barrier to conducting more advanced EMS system evaluation.[70–72]

Ultimate patient outcomes may be insensitive to EMS system variation. Thus, intermediate outcome measures, with a closer temporal relationship to EMS interventions, are often used.[73] Tracer conditions are also used.[74] These include survival following cardiac arrest, and comparing actual to predicted survival for trauma patients.[75–77]

Little is known about EMS cost-effectiveness. Although estimates of EMS costs for saving the life of a cardiac arrest victim are thought to be similar to other lifesaving treatment, such estimates are locality specific.[78,79]

Where We Want To Be

Continuous comprehensive evaluation of EMS assesses all aspects of the system, and includes structural, process, and outcomes analyses. Evaluation includes many clinical conditions. It involves outcomes other than death, including disease, disability, discomfort, and destitution.[80] Cost-effectiveness is evaluated, including the costs of system preparedness. Public satisfaction and consumer input are a focus.

Future Implications

The *EMS Agenda for the Future* offered 90 recommendations for action to strengthen each of the 14 attributes and to work toward proposed goals. However, what the *Agenda* provided many in terms of inspiration, it lacked for many others in terms of specificity. Thus, a second steering committee, using a process similar to the initial one, developed the *EMS Agenda for the Future: Implementation Guide*.[81] Published in 1998, the *Implementation Guide* suggested three overriding themes to continue development of EMS: Building Bridges, Creating Tools and Resources, and Developing Infrastructure. Among the many actions offered in the *Agenda*, the *Implementation Guide* proposed ten priorities:

■ Develop collaborative strategies to identify and address community health and safety issues;

■ Align the financial incentives of EMS and other healthcare providers and payers;

■ Participate in community-based prevention efforts;

■ Develop and pursue a national EMS research agenda;

■ Pass EMS legislation in each state to support innovation and integration;

■ Allocate adequate resources for medical direction;

■ Develop information systems that link EMS across this continuum;

■ Determine the costs and benefits of EMS to the community;

■ Ensure nationwide availability of 9-1-1 as the emergency telephone number;

■ Ensure that all calls for emergency help are automatically accompanied by location-identifying information.[81]

For each action item, the *Implementation Guide* proposed short-term, intermediate, and long-term objectives. It also suggested potential lead and contributing participants in efforts to achieve objectives. In doing so, the document recognized more than 150 organizations, agencies, and groups of people.

Surely, not all that have been called upon for action have embraced the message or revised their own

priorities. However, since its publication, the *EMS Agenda for the Future* has provided NHTSA with meaningful guidance, leading to a number of projects.[65] These have included development of the *EMS Education Agenda for the Future* and *EMS Research Agenda*.[82] NHTSA convened EMS managed-care roundtable discussions in order to facilitate better understanding of issues among those constituents.[83] NHTSA also facilitated a year-long series of meetings among representatives of NAEMSP and the American Public Health Association (APHA) intended to identify areas of common interest and opportunities for partnership. A national EMS database project has been funded, and an emphasis has been placed on timely EMS access via intelligent transportation systems (ITS) research, and work with the wireless communications industry.

An important consideration for the *EMS Agenda for the Future* is that the document reflects perspectives from a specific point in time. In May 1998, NHTSA convened the *EMS Agenda for the Future . . . Making It A Reality* conference. The goals included dissemination of reports of projects related to *Agenda* objectives, and discussion of priorities and directions for next steps. Again, in 2000, NHTSA convened EMS leaders to reevaluate the *EMS Agenda for the Future* and *Implementation Guide*, and to suggest current priorities and important directions on which to focus. These forums resulted from recognition that, as perspectives change with time, so might priorities and ideas for how to measure and achieve success.

Among the points that the *EMS Agenda for the Future* emphasized was the need for continuous evaluation of the EMS system, including where we want to be and how to get there. As we work to improve EMS for the future, some things are likely to remain true. EMS must be better integrated with other services and efforts to improve community health. The special needs of members of our diverse population must be recognized and addressed. The value of EMS as the public's emergency medical safety net cannot be overemphasized. In order to achieve the vision for the future of EMS, we must improve its science, strengthen its infrastructure, and engage in partnerships to improve the emergency healthcare system. Frequent evaluation of where EMS is in relation to the goals we have established for it will allow meaningful progress to continue, so that EMS fulfills its critical role in caring for the health of Americans.

References

1. Howard J. Keynote address. *EMS Agenda for the Future . . . Making it a Reality Conference*, Alexandria, VA, May 21, 1998.

2. National Academy of Sciences, National Research Council. *Accidental Death and Disability: The Neglected Disease of Modern Society*. Washington, D.C.: National Academy Press; 1966.

3. Perry S, Wilkinson SL. The technology assessment practice guidelines forum: a modified group judgment method. *Int J Tech Assess in Health Care*. 1992;8:289–300.

4. *Emergency Medical Services Agenda for the Future*. Washington, D.C.: U.S. Department of Transportation, National Highway Traffic Safety Administration (DOT HS 808 441); 1996.

5. Gerson LW, Hoover R, McCoy S, Palmisano B. Linking the elderly to community services. *JEMS*. 1991;16(6): 45–48.

6. Gerson LW, Schelble DT, Wilson JE. Using paramedics to identify at-risk elderly. *Ann Emerg Med*. 1992;21:688–691.

7. Krumperman KM. Filling the gap: EMS social service referrals. *JEMS*. 1993;18(2):25–29.

8. Hsiao AK, Hedges JR. Role of the emergency medical services system in region wide health monitoring and referral. *Ann Emerg Med*. 1993;22:1696–1702.

9. *Senate Joint Memorial #44: Expanded EMS Study*. New Mexico Department of Health, Emergency Medical Services Bureau; 1995.

10. Callaham M. Quantifying the scanty science of prehospital emergency care. *Ann Emerg Med*. 1997;30(2):785–790.

11. Spaite DW, Criss EA, Valenzuela TD, Guisto J. Emergency medical service systems research: problems of the past, challenges of the future. *Ann Emerg Med*. 1995; 26:146–152.

12. Spaite DW, Valenzuela TD, Meislin HW. Barriers to EMS system evaluation—problems associated with field data collection. *Prehosp Disaster Med*. 1993;8:S35–S40.

13. Cummins RO, Ornato JP, Thies WH, Pepe PE. Improving survival from sudden cardiac arrest: the chain of survival concept. A statement for health professionals from the Advanced Cardiac Life Support Subcommittee and the Emergency Cardiac Care Committee, American Heart Association. *Circulation*. 1991;83:1832–1847.

14. Newman MM. Chain of survival takes hold. *JEMS*. 1989; 14(8):11–13.

15. Snyder JA, Baren JM, Ryan SD, et al. Emergency medical service system development: results of the state-wide emergency medical service technical assessment program. *Ann Emerg Med*. 1995;25:768–775.

16. Stout JL. System financing. In Roush WR, ed. *Principles of EMS Systems*. Dallas: ACEP; 1994:451–473.

17. *National Emergency Medical Services Education and Practice Blueprint*. Columbus, OH: National Registry of Emergency Medical Technicians; 1993.

18. Keller RA. 1992 EMS salary survey. *JEMS*. 1992;17(11): 62–73.

19. Mitchell JT. Critical incident stress management. In: Kuehl AE, ed. *Prehospital Systems and Medical Oversight*. *2nd ed*. St Louis: Mosby-Year Book, Inc.; 1994:239–244.

20. Mitchell J, Bray G. *Emergency Services Stress: Guidelines for Preserving the Health and Careers of Emergency Personnel*. Englewood Cliffs, NJ: Brady Publishing-Prentice Hall; 1990.

21. Fontanarosa PB. Occupational issues for EMS personnel. In: Roush E., ed. *Principles of EMS Systems*. Dallas: ACEP; 1994:411–431.

22. Menegazzi JJ. A meta-analysis of hepatitis B serologic marking prevalence in EMS personnel. *Prehosp Disaster Med*. 1991;6:299–302.

23. Hockreiter MC, Barton LL. Epidemiology of needlestick injury in emergency medical services personnel. *J Emerg Med*. 1988;6:9–12.

24. Reed E, Daya MR, Jui J, et al. Occupational infectious disease exposures in EMS personnel. *J Emerg Med*. 1993; 11:916.

25. Garza M, ed. Paramedics report many on-duty assaults. *EMS Insider*. 1993;20(9):7.

26. Hoyga PT, Ellis L. Evaluation of the injury profile of personnel in a busy urban EMS system. *Am J Emerg Med*. 1990;9:308–311.

27. Schwartz RJ, Benson L, Jacobs LM. The prevalence of occupational injuries in EMTs in New England. *Prehosp Disaster Med*. 1993;8:454–450.

28. Swor RA, Chisolm C, Krohmer J. Model curriculum in emergency medical services for emergency medicine residencies. *Ann Emerg Med*. 1989;18:418–421.

29. Erder MH, Davidson SJ, Chaney RA. Online medical command theory and practice. *Ann Emerg Med*. 1989; 18:261–288.

30. Gratton MC, Bethkey RA, Watson WA, et al. Effect of standing orders on paramedic scene time for trauma patients. *Ann Emerg Med*. 1991;20:52–55.

31. Hoffman JR, Luo J, Schriger DL, et al. Does paramedic base hospital contact result in beneficial deviations from standard prehospital protocols? *Western J Med*. 1989; 153:283–287.

32. Hunt RC, Bass RR, Graham RG, et al. Standing orders vs. voice control. *JEMS*. 1982;7:26–31.

33. Pointer JE, Osur MA. Effective standing orders on field times. *Ann Emerg Med*. 1989;18:1119–1121.

34. Thompson SJ, Schriber JA. A survey of prehospital care paramedic/physician communication from Multnomah County (Portland), OR. *J Emerg Med*. 1984;1:421–428.

35. Wuerz RC, Swope GE, Holliman CJ, Vazquez-de Miguell G. Online medical direction: a prospective study. *Prehosp Disaster Med*. 1995;10:174–177.

36. *The Future of EMS Education: A National Perspective*. Washington D.C.: Joint Review-Committee on Educational Programs for the EMT Paramedic; 1994.

37. Polk DA. EMS degree programs. *JEMS*. 1992;17(8):69–75.

38. Anderson TE, Arthur K, Kleinman M, et al. Intraosseous infusion: success of a standardized regional training program for prehospital advanced life support providers. *Ann Emerg Med*. 1994;23:52–55.

39. Cayten CG, Scott T. EMS in the United States: 1995 survey of providers in the 200 most populous cities. *JEMS.* 1995;20(1):78.

40. Fuchs S, LaCovey D, Paris P. A prehospital model of intraosseous infusion. *Ann Emerg Med.* 1991;20:371–374.

41. Landis SS, Benson NH, Whitley TW. A comparison of four methods of testing emergency medical technician triage skills. *Am J Emerg Med.* 1989;7:1–4.

42. Losek JD, Szewczuga D, Glaser PW. Improved prehospital pediatric ALS care after an EMT-Paramedic clinical training course. *Am J Emerg Med.* 1994;12:429–432.

43. Powell JP. Training for EMT/Paramedics in perinatal care and transport. *J Tennessee Med Assoc.* 1982;75:133–134.

44. Trooskin SZ, Rubinowicz S, Eldridge C, et al. Teaching endotracheal intubation with animals and cadavers. *Prehosp Disaster Med.* 1992;7:179–184.

45. Walters G, D'Auria D, Glucksman E. Automatic external defibrillators: implications for training qualified ambulance staff. *Ann Emerg Med.* 1992;21:692–697.

46. Werman HA, Keseg DR, Glimcher M. Retention of basic life support skills. *Prehosp Disaster Med.* 1990;5:137–144.

47. Feely HB, Athey JL. *Emergency Medical Services for Children: Ten Year Report.* Arlington, VA: National Center for Education in Maternal and Child Health; 1995.

48. Ho MT, Eisenberg MS, Litwin PE, et al. Delay between onset of chest pain and seeking medical care: the effect of public education. *Ann Emerg Med.* 1993;22:41–46.

49. Moses HW, Englking N, Taylor GL, et al. Effect of a two-year public education campaign on reducing response time of patients with symptoms of acute myocardial infarction. *Am J Cardiol.* 1991;68:249–251.

50. MacLean CB. The future role of emergency medical services systems in prevention. *Ann Emerg Med.* 1993;22:1743–1746.

51. Harrawood D, Gunderson MR, Fravel S, Cartwright K, Ryan JL. Drowning prevention: a case study in EMS epidemiology. *JEMS.* 1994;19(6):34–41.

52. Ogden JR, Criss EA, Spaite DW, Valenzuela TD. The impact of an EMS-initiated, community-based drowning prevention coalition on submersion deaths in a southwestern metropolitan area. *Acad Emerg Med.* 1994;1(2):304.

53. Martinez R. Injury prevention: a new perspective. *JAMA.* 1994;19:1541–1542.

54. Garrison HG, Foltin G, Becker L, et al. *Consensus Statement: The Role of Out-of-Hospital Emergency Medical Services in Primary Injury Prevention, Final Report.* Consensus Workshop on the Role of EMS in Injury Prevention, Arlington, VA, August 25–26, 1995.

55. Eisenberg M, Hallstrom A, Becker L. Community awareness of emergency phone numbers. *Am J Publ Health.* 1981;71:1058–1060.

56. Mayron R, Long RS, Ruiz E. The 9-1-1 emergency telephone number: impact on emergency medical systems access in a metropolitan area. *Am J Emerg Med.* 1984;2:491–493.

57. Munn B. Cellular phones and 9-1-1. *Emerg Med Svcs.* 1987;16(8):12–14.

58. ASTM Committee F-30 on Emergency Medical Services. *ASTM Standards on Emergency Medical Services.* Philadelphia: ASTM; 1994.

59. Clawson JJ. Emergency medical dispatch. In: Kuehl AE, ed. *Prehospital Systems and Medical Oversight.* 2d ed. St. Louis: Mosby-Year Book, Inc.; 1994:125–152.

60. National Association of EMS Physicians. Emergency medical dispatching. *Prehosp Disaster Med.* 1989;4:163–166.

61. Clark JJ, Culley L, Eisenberg M, Henwood DK. Accuracy of determining cardiac arrest by emergency medical dispatchers. *Ann Emerg Med.* 1994;23:1022–1026.

62. Valenzuela T, Spaite D, Clark D, et al. Estimated cost-effectiveness of dispatcher CPR instruction via telephone to bystanders during out-of-hospital ventricular fibrillation. *Prehosp Disaster Med.* 1992;7:229–234.

63. Delbridge TR, Verdile VP, Platt TE. Variability of state-approved emergency medical services drug formularies. *Prehosp Disaster Med.* 1994;9:S55.

64. Garrison HG, Benson NH, Whitley TW, Bailey BW. Paramedic skills and medications: practice options utilized by local advanced life support medical directors. *Prehosp Disaster Med.* 1991;6:29–33.

65. *Emergency Medical Services: Reported Needs are Wide-Ranging, With a Growing Focus on Lack of Data.* Washington, D.C.: U.S. General Accounting Office Report to Congressional Requesters (GAO-02-28); October 2001.

66. *Trauma Care Systems Training and Development Act of 1990: Public Law 101-590.* Washington, D.C.; 1990.

67. Durch JS, Lohr KN, eds. *Emergency Medical Services for Children.* Washington, D.C.: National Academy Press; 1993.

68. *Uniform Pre-hospital Emergency Medical Services (EMS) Data Conference: Final Report.* Washington, D.C.: National Highway Traffic Safety Administration; 1994.

69. Hedges JR. Beyond Utstein: implementation of a multi-source uniform database for prehospital cardiac arrest research. *Ann Emerg Med.* 1993;22:41–46.

70. Cummins RO, Chamberlain DA, Abramson NS, et al. Recommended guidelines for uniform reporting of data from out-of-hospital cardiac arrest, the Utstein style. *Ann Emerg Med.* 1991;20:861–874.

71. Spaite DW, Valenzuela TD, Meislin HW, et al. Prospective validation of a new model for evaluating emergency medical services systems by in-field observation of specific time intervals in prehospital care. *Ann Emerg Med.* 1993;22:638–645.

72. Valenzuela TD, Spaite DW, Meislin HW, et al. Emergency vehicle intervals vs. collapse to CPR and collapse to defibrillation intervals: monitoring emergency medical services system performance in sudden cardiac arrest. *Ann Emerg Med.* 1993;22:1678–1683.

73. Cayten CG. Evaluation. In: Kuehl AE, ed. *Prehospital Systems and Medical Oversight.* 2d ed. St. Louis: Mosby-Year Book, Inc.; 1994:158–167.

74. Kessner DM, Kalk CE, James S. Assessing health quality—the case for tracers. *New Eng J Med.* 1973;288:189–194.

75. American College of Surgeons Committee on Trauma. Quality assessment and assurance in trauma care. *Bull Am Coll Surgeons.* 1986;71:4–23.

76. Eisenberg MS, Horwood BT, Cummins RO. Cardiac arrest and resuscitation: a tale of 29 cities. *Ann Emerg Med.* 1990;19:179–186.

77. Shackford SR, Mackersie RC, Hoyt DB, et al. Impact of a trauma system on outcome of severely injured patients. *Arch Surg.* 1987;122:523–527.

78. Urban N, Bergner L, Eisenberg MS. The costs of the suburban paramedic program in reducing deaths due to cardiac arrest. *Med Care.* 1981;19:279–392.

79. Valenzuela TD, Criss EA, Spaite D, et al. Cost-effectiveness analysis of paramedic emergency medical services in the treatment of prehospital cardiopulmonary arrest. *Ann Emerg Med.* 1990;19:1407–1411.

80. Fletcher RH, Fletcher SW, Wagner EH. *Clinical Epidemiology—The Essentials.* Baltimore: Williams & Wilkins; 1988.

81. *Emergency Medical Services Agenda for the Future: Implementation Guide.* Washington, D.C.: U.S. Department of Transportation, National Highway Traffic Safety Administration (DOT HS 808 711); 1998.

82. *Emergency Medical Services Education Agenda for the Future: A Systems Approach.* Washington, D.C.: U.S. Department of Transportation, National Highway Traffic Safety Administration (DOT HS 809 042); 2000.

83. *EMS and Managed Care, Final Bulletin.* Washington, D.C.: U.S. Department of Transportation, National Highway Traffic Safety Administration (DOT HS 809 026); 1999.

Public Health

Barbara McIntosh, MD
David Jaslow, MD, MPH

Introduction

At first glance, the disciplines of prehospital care and public health do not appear to overlap. Prehospital care is associated with high-tech, action-oriented, emergent interventions in acute disease processes. Public health has traditionally been associated with more passive interventions designed to affect the course of the disease process over time. Nonetheless, prehospital care and public health form an effective and successful partnership that can deliver complete and comprehensive patient care, prevent injury and illness, promote health, and mitigate injury or illness once it has occurred.

The differences between traditional medical and public health practices have been described in a monograph entitled *Medicine & Public Health: The Power of Collaboration* as follows: "Today in the American health system, the healers comprise the medical sector, while the promotion of healthful conditions in the community is spearheaded by public health. The medical perspective focuses on the individual patient—diagnosing symptoms, treating and preventing diseases, providing comfort, relieving pain and suffering, and enhancing the capacity to function. . . . The distinguishing feature of the public health perspective is that it focuses on *populations*—assessing and monitoring health problems, informing the public and professionals about health issues, developing and enforcing health protecting laws and regulations, implementing and evaluating population-based strategies to promote health and prevent disease, and insuring the provision of essential health services."[1] Another key distinction between medical and public health practices is the desired outcome: the goal of medical care is curative, whereas public health seeks to mitigate causative factors and effectively prevent development of injury and illness.

There are instances where public health and EMS disciplines have collaborated, with synergistic results.

A recent example involves the threat of an infectious disease epidemic in a large urban area, as may occur as a result of a bioterrorism incident. Another noteworthy example is the current Public Access Defibrillation (PAD) campaign, which has as its goal the placement of defibrillators in the hands of trained responders situated in throughout communities. In defining public health emergencies and the similarities in approach to disaster medicine, it is noted that a "public health emergency, in the broadest definition, represents any evolving situation in which large numbers of the population are at risk for injury or illness. This can include anything from the increase in injury and/or death occurring as a result of the rise in domestic violence, to the classic infectious disease epidemic model. . . . One of the hallmarks of disaster medicine is the philosophical shift from concern for the individual to concern for the system."[2] This difference, apparent in disaster medicine, is also a central principle of public health.

The explosion of biomedical advances in the last fifty years emphasized the divergence of medicine and public health. As modern medicine discovered the causes of and treatments for many diseases, the resulting increased funding for these efforts led to a focus on high-tech, curative solutions. In turn, this led to a decreased interest in what a public health approach could offer.

As EMS systems developed, the emphasis was on advanced technology and systems management. Early systems focused on the care of the critically ill and injured, on getting to the patients faster and bringing more sophisticated medical therapies to them, and on getting them back to the hospital sooner and more stabilized. Communications and deployment systems were utilized to ensure that, once a critical injury occurred, care would be delivered to the patient as soon as possible. This led to the development of the reactive model of EMS care that permeated through systems, and produced compelling and thrilling successes. The success of this reactive approach also prevented systems from realizing the other benefits that could result from utilizing a proactive approach, as public health practice would dictate. In fact, using the Haddon matrix of an injury model, prehospital care traditionally has been involved in the post-event phase of an event.

As Garrison noted in a recent review, the prehospital providers' counterparts in police and fire departments "through their successful efforts aimed at preventing fires and burns and driving while intoxicated . . . have demonstrated that primary prevention is an essential public safety service. Prevention is a primary public health activity."[3] These activities by police and fire departments also serve to establish and instill in the community a sense of identity and partnership with the providers.

Trends in healthcare financing have produced an incentive among providers and services to control costs and focus on prevention and wellness initiatives. "EMS systems are in a unique and ideal position to make contributions to primary injury prevention and help reduce the number of preventable injuries in the population."[4] EMS is in a unique and opportune position to participate in primary injury prevention programs because it is widely distributed throughout the community, and thus can observe firsthand precipitating factors or opportunities to intervene. EMS providers also interact with patients and family members at times when they may be most receptive to interventions. Increasingly, providers consider these interventions to be a natural extension of the patient advocacy role espoused by their mission to reduce suffering, premature death, and disability.

The framework for the vision of EMS and public health collaborating in the future is contained in the *EMS Agenda for the Future*: "Emergency services personnel currently spend much of their time reacting to cases that fall between the cracks of today's separate and isolated public safety, healthcare, and public health systems. The *EMS Agenda* envisions EMS as the linchpin joining these services into an integrated community healthcare network. Although emergency response must remain our foundation, EMS of tomorrow will be a community-based health management system that provides surveillance, identification, intervention, and evaluation of injury and disease. This role strengthens the essential value of EMS as the community's emergency medical safety net."[5]

Injury Prevention

Injury prevention has been a major focus of public health efforts over the last three decades. A discussion of injury prevention and EMS is an important one, and is included in the following chapter.

Health and Wellness

Prevention represents a substantial part of the public health initiative, but it does not encompass all of the goals of public health practice; the absence of injury and disease does not equal health. The other major arm of public health activities deals with health promotion. Examples include abstinence from alcohol and substance abuse, promotion of physical fitness/exercise programs, stress management and reduction programs, regular health screenings and immunizations, nutrition programs, smoking cessation programs, and environmental initiatives. These proactive activities are often referred to as wellness programs. The importance of the biological, psychological, and social aspects of health date back to ancient medicine, where "in the fourth century BC, Hippocrates espoused a framework that related medical and public health perspectives in practice. In approaching the individual patient, he urged physicians to pay attention to the environmental, social, and behavioral context in which illness occurs: the airs 'peculiar to each particular region,' the 'properties of the waters' the inhabitants drink and use, and the 'mode of life of the inhabitants, whether they are heavy drinkers, taking lunch, and inactive, or athletic, industrious, eating much and drinking little'."[6]

As healthcare systems and healthcare financing have evolved, the mandate to control healthcare costs and the growth of managed care programs have produced a major incentive to prevent injuries and promote wellness. "The sleeping giant of health care is awakening to its new role in society. As we move from a system designed to care for illness to one that emphasizes wellness, we change our measuring rod of success. Injury prevention takes on a new and more important dimension, not only for improving the health of the nation, but also in the ability to truly control healthcare costs."[4]

Primary versus Secondary Prevention

EMS involves a unique blend of medical, public safety, and public health concepts which are united in an effort to provide out-of-hospital emergency and unscheduled health care.[7] While it is difficult to calculate the contribution of public health toward EMS, many EMS providers still describe themselves as public safety personnel who have emergency medical training, rather than emergency medical professionals who have a public safety background. This point is not superfluous. It may help to explain why EMS has not been more successful in decreasing morbidity and mortality.

There are a variety of reasons to explain the public safety/public health dichotomy. Predominant has been the development of EMS within established public safety agencies, such as fire and police departments. While many EMS providers today are cross-trained as fire/rescue personnel or law enforcement officers, the latter training is usually first. Public safety has engendered a great deal of respect in America, and has been more easily understood and connected to emergency conditions than to general medicine or public health. Thus, much of the improvement during the first two decades of EMS systems development (1970–1990) was prompted by reactions to deficiencies in public safety concepts, which were more apparent than the public health factors. For example, communications systems and ambulance construction have most certainly improved, but a true understanding of factors related to cardiac arrest survival has only recently become apparent. Unfortunately, terminology such as "Utstein" and "return of spontaneous circulation" are still foreign to many EMS providers. Likewise, EMS training has traditionally focused on the rapid identification and treatment of medical emergencies once they exist. There is still poor early recognition of life-threatening illness by bystanders or the patients themselves.

The Public Health Paradigm

Although important advancements can be cited during the first generation of EMS, it is arguable whether most individual items can be directly linked to reductions in morbidity and mortality in the same way as early disease detection and other traditional public health strategies. Not surprisingly, much of the frustration with the inability to fix many systems-oriented problems in EMS stemmed, until recently, from the failure to associate these problems within the spectrum of health care.

For years the general population has been taught to call 9-1-1 rather than friends or family for medical emergencies. In the process, these Make the Right Call campaigns have created tremendous 9-1-1 utilization, but caused a classic supply-and-demand problem. The initial solution to increased EMS utilization during the first generation of EMS was to increase the supply of ambulances; however the public health approach suggests that a better solution is to decrease the demand for service, presumably by identification and amelioration of the reasons the service is deemed necessary. Only recently have researchers attempted to identify why many patients with non-emergency conditions request emergency resources, and to identify non-emergency means of transportation.[8,9]

If viewed in a public health paradigm, most medical conditions encountered by EMS personnel are due to inadequate patient education, inadequate access to healthcare, or inadequate preventive healthcare behaviors. Such inadequacies cannot be cured by faster response times, more detailed or aggressive treatment protocols, or a greater number of ambulances; this, however, does not represent the principles that have been taught to EMS personnel during the last three decades. Although knowledge and techniques continue to improve in the treatment of acute illness and injury, our approach must shift from a public safety realm to a public health realm, if medical emergencies are to be reduced.

The traditional public health paradigm is rooted in prevention. Often EMS providers do not realize that they routinely practice secondary prevention through early and aggressive evaluation of patients, which, in reality, is geared toward prevention of further morbidity and mortality. However, primary prevention strategies are likely to be more cost-effective than secondary medical treatment, especially for those disease processes with a high incidence and acuity. Logic dictates that it is more preferable and cost-effective to prevent an acute medical condition from occurring than to treat it after it already exists.

One specific example is the care of the trauma victim. The U.S. has spent millions of dollars and performed many studies to discover how to improve secondary prevention, that is, to provide better prehospital care to major trauma victims; however, it has not yet been shown that most EMS interventions make a difference in survival. Additionally, most traumatic injuries are not only not life-threatening, but also do not require nor benefit from prehospital interventions aside from transport to a definitive care facility. Much less time and financial resources have been spent to demonstrate how providers can practice primary injury prevention, that is, to decrease the incidence of trauma. A recent study of practices of urban paramedics found that few practice primary injury prevention, despite the fact that most consider it part of their responsibility as an EMS provider.[10]

Incorporation of EMS into Public Health

A systems approach to problem solving in EMS is analogous to the resuscitation of a multiple trauma patient. The emergency physician cannot expect success if only selected organ systems are addressed; all possible pathophysiology must be isolated and corrected. Similarly, there are usually no quick fixes for EMS systems issues. The input-process-output model demonstrates that the final result is a product of both the basic ingredients and the process by which they are molded.[11] Therefore, an unsatisfactory final product must prompt a review of the inputs, the process, and possibly the desired output, if it is unachievable. For example, a myriad of factors are related to successful early defibrillation, including early 9-1-1 notification, responder training and continuing education, and emergency medical dispatch performance. EMS agencies that attempt to remedy lengthy arrival to first shock times by addressing only a single system element usually become frustrated and abandon the endeavor.

In the 1970s and early 1980s deficiencies in EMS systems were usually linked to the fifteen EMS system components identified by the 1973 EMSS Act. The 1989 edition of this text emphasize the omissions of medical oversight and public health in the original fifteen. There are several categories within the *EMS Agenda for the Future* that specifically reference public health concepts, such as prevention and education, thus providing guidelines for the creation of new initiatives to improve EMS systems.[7]

While there are still many milestones to reach regarding the technical aspects of EMS, a public health approach to systems issues must continue to evolve. This approach emphasizes the epidemiology and attributes of populations rather than logistics, medical devices, and treatment. Concerning defibrillation, lengthy arrival to first shock times can be a very complex systems issue, especially in large urban EMS systems. The public health approach to solving this problem concentrates on factors related to the cardiac arrests themselves: (1) Where do they occur and why? (2) How frequently are they witnessed and how can

this element be influenced? (3) What is the rate of bystander CPR and how can it be improved? (4) How often are first response units unavailable because of non-emergent requests for medical aid? (5) How long do witnesses wait before accessing 9-1-1? The list continues, but clearly, a significant impact on survival is possible if one or more of these items can be positively influenced. Based on the research conducted recently, it is likely that the impact would be greater than all other interventions short of early defibrillation.

Ultimately, EMS utilizes continuous quality improvement programs and research techniques to identify and correct many systems issues. The importance of these endeavors cannot be overemphasized. The obvious issues in a systems approach to EMS and public health are concerned with questions regarding data identification, measurement, and analysis.

The prehospital care report (PCR) currently utilized by the District of Columbia Fire and EMS Department provides an excellent visual example to demonstrate a public health-driven data collection system designed, in part, to address systems problems. The complexity of the PCR underlies tremendous concern for analysis of the many systems problems that have plagued EMS delivery in Washington. If completed properly, this optical scanable form allows a computer to rapidly process data and download selected pieces of information into existing databases. Therefore, data fields were created to capture data related to such common entities as cardiac arrest, mass-gathering medical care, and major trauma. Additionally, special attention was given to unique EMS situations in the District, such as the high frequency of special operations assignments and requests for EMS that originate from federal buildings. Analysis of these data may assist the city in developing a proactive emergency healthcare delivery system that meets the needs of its population.

Whatever devices are used to collect and analyze public health data, the goal is to convert raw data into useful information that will aid improvements in primary and secondary prevention. This data should be shared with all members of the EMS team and with others directly involved in the healthcare sector, including first responders, emergency departments, and public health departments.

The Integration of Public Health Concepts into EMS Operations

Operational EMS refers to the aspects of special operations within the realm of the delivery of out-of-hospital medical care that differentiate it from routine medical care.[12] The most challenging aspects of operational EMS are found in the response to major incidents, which inherently involve complex scene management, critical decision-making, and interaction with personnel from multiple agencies.[12]

While these incidents are frequently thought of as fire/rescue events, a more logical or useful approach would be to consider that any event which potentially involves harm to a defined population (rather than just to an individual) should be considered a public health emergency.[13] Public health emergencies take many forms. They can be as simple as evacuation of a high-rise apartment building for the elderly due to air conditioning failure in the summer, or as complicated as a hazardous materials incident that threatens a community. Other examples include natural disasters, such as large-scale fires or floods, technological disasters, domestic terrorism and war.

For those individuals with knowledge of both public health and of EMS, a number of questions quickly surface: (1) What are examples of a public health emergency? (2) Who declares such an event? (3) What are the implications for declaration of a public health emergency? (4) What is the role of the on-scene EMS physician during this type of crisis? (5) What are the roles and responsibilities of EMS providers during this type of event? (6) Who performs typical public health responsibilities and acts as a liaison to the local public health department? (7) What is the role of the local or regional public health agency relative to operational EMS issues?

The EMS response to a public health emergency varies, and is most likely directly related to the sophistication of the EMS system itself. Reactive systems call in extra personnel to stand by in quarters, in case the volume of emergency calls increases during a major local event. Proactive EMS systems instruct crews to drive around neighborhoods specifically looking for potential hazards and signs of a worsening situation.

The natural history of a public health emergency is often that of decisions based on less than optimal information using a worst-case scenario. Potential results are displacement of residents or interruption of utilities and transportation. The litany of after-effects includes psychological stress on victims and rescuers, medical evaluation of patients with potential exposure to atypical elements, and drain on emergency resources.

Other public health issues, including occupational health and safety, safety and wellness of the public, and medical monitoring of rescuers, fall under the domain of the medical sector at such an incident. Here again, a proactive stance by the EMS contingent has only recently begun to be understood. National firefighting organizations now proudly declare support for wellness programs among their membership. Formal rehabilitation sectors at major incident scenes can now be seen more frequently as well.

Prior to the reaction to September 11, 2001 there was little capability for an emergency response from local public health departments; the potential responders would not have been knowledgeable in issues pertinent to EMS or rescue events. Emergency management personnel may or may not have a basic understanding of traditional public health issues. Of more concern is the potential lack of recognition of a public health emergency by the incident commander, who is likely to have a fire suppression background and may not be cross-trained in EMS. For that matter, few EMS providers or their medical directors can claim to have received basic public health training in their EMS education. That is now changing.

The states usually have rare comprehensive public health response capabilities, but an official request is usually necessary from the local jurisdiction, which could be delayed if the necessity were not recognized. The federal government has a host of resources with mitigation capability and access to personnel trained to assess public health emergencies in the form of Urban Search and Rescue task forces, Disaster Medical Assistance Teams, and Metro Medical Strike Teams.[14] However, federal resources are only activated for large-scale disasters, and they are rarely immediately available.

The local EMS medical director or specially trained EMS supervisor should be qualified and available to insert himself, if requested, into the situation where a potential or actual public health emergency exists. A logical choice would be for this individual to integrate himself into the incident command structure as a liaison among the emergency medicine, EMS, and public health communities. Such a concept has not been previously discussed, and an extensive discussion of the merits and pitfalls has yet to be generated, although similar job descriptors can be found attached to the prototype fire medical officer position developed by Bogucki.[15] Any momentum toward this goal is best discussed with representatives of the local health department, as well as the appropriate public safety agencies. Protocols and responsibilities should be jointly developed and exercised within the realm of other emergency response organizations.

Summary

While the out-of-hospital emergency medical practice begins its second generation, the public health approach to its practice is only now beginning to become apparent. There has been a renewed interest in many communities toward doing whatever is possible to reduce unnecessary illness and injury. Both primary and secondary preventive practices have important roles in this endeavor, and EMS professionals should be among the forefront of those bringing these concepts to reality.

References

1. Lasker RD and the Committee on Medicine and Public Health. *Medicine & Public Health: The Power of Collaboration*. New York: New York Academy of Medicine; 1997:3.
2. McIntosh BA, Hinds P, Giordano LM. The role of EMS systems in public health emergencies. *Prehosp Disaster Med*. 1997;12:30–35.
3. *Accidental Death & Disability: The Neglected Disease of Modern Society*. Washington, DC: National Academy of Sciences and National Research Council: September 1966.
4. Martinez R. Injury prevention: a new perspective. *JAMA*. 1994;19:1541–1542.
5. Martinez R. New vision for the role of emergency medical services. *Ann Emerg Med*. 1998;32:594–599.
6. Lasker RD and the Committee on Medicine & Public Health. *Medicine & Public Health: The Power of Collaboration*. New York: New York Academy of Medicine; 1997:11–12.
7. NHTSA. *Emergency Medical Services Agenda for the Future*. 1996; US DOT NTS-42.
8. Billittier AJ, Moscati R, Janicke D, et al. A multisite survey of factors contributing to medically unnecessary ambulance transports. *Acad Emerg Med*. 1996;3:1046–1052.
9. Jaslow D, Barbera J, Johnson E, Moore W. EMS initiated refusal and alternative methods of transport. *Prehosp Emerg Care*. 1998;2:18–22.
10. Jaslow D, Marsh R. Primary injury prevention in EMS: is education a part of emergency treatment? *Acad Emerg Med*. 1999;6:465.
11. Rakich JS, Longest BB, Darr K. *Managing Health Services Organizations*. Baltimore: Health Professions Press; 1992.
12. Bogucki S. More expanded scope: operational EMS. *Prehosp Emerg Care*. 1998;2:330–333.
13. Noji E, ed. *The Public Health Consequences of Disasters*. New York: Oxford University Press; 1997.
14. FEMA. Federal Response Plan. 9230.1-PL. Washington, DC, 1999.
15. Bogucki MS. Medical support for the fire service: current priorities and roles of physicians. *Prehosp Emerg Care*. 1997;1:107–113.

CHAPTER 81

Injury Prevention

Juan A. March, MD

Arthur H. Yancey II, MD, MPH

Introduction

EMS has developed as a result of and in conjunction with the nation's growing awareness of injury's toll on society. In the funeral hearse-as-ambulance era the injured were simply scooped and delivered to a hospital, if lucky, or to a funeral home or morgue, if not. In 1966 with publication of the white paper, *Accidental Death and Disability: The Neglected Disease of Modern Society,* focus evolved to the evaluation and prehospital care of the injured.[1] The federal coordination and support phase formally began with the EMS Systems Act of 1973, which continued through block grant support of state EMS offices in the 1980s. Today, questions about the efficient utilization of increasingly expensive and sometimes scarce EMS resources in injury care have stimulated a wider refocus, from solely on the most severely injured (12% requiring level I or II trauma center treatment) to the entire spectrum of injured victims.[2,3]

While EMS training and operations presently reflect the focus on maximizing survival of the most critically injured patients, recognition is growing that most EMS trauma resources are expended on treating the 88% of trauma victims who are not critically injured but who have risk factors for becoming so. Many in the EMS community view resources dispatched for this larger group of patients as a waste of time. Yet, the combination of their non-critical and preventable nature begs the question: what is the most cost-effective means to care for this group, and what is the most efficient way to utilize finite EMS resources in regard to this group of patients? Injuries account for approximately one-third of EMS transports, implying that a broad interface already exists between EMS and the injured.[4]

The Case for EMS in Injury Prevention

Several characteristics of EMS work suggest that field providers are appropriately qualified and superbly positioned for the tasks of injury prevention. EMS professionals are directly exposed to the street, home, school, and workplace environments where injuries occur, as well as to victims' behavioral patterns that placed them at risk for these injuries. This exposure offers the opportunity for on-the-scene assessment of injury etiology.[5]

EMS providers are widely dispersed within their work communities, and in many instances dwell in them. Operationally, this serves the interest of rapid response, but it also means that they can become intimately familiar with the unique patterns. Furthermore, EMS providers engender respect in the public eye for their knowledge, skills, and experience manifested in patients' greatest moments of need. Thus, the EMS encounter conceptually offers a "teachable moment" when the patient and bystanders alike are most susceptible to advice on preventing similar incidents.[6,7]

This scene-level intervention could be accomplished through counseling, restoring loose medicines to their respective containers, repairing a smoke detector, or securing a loose rug. System-level intervention can be engendered when the prehospital care report (PCR) form is completed with relevant etiology-coded injury data. Observations from the scene, when recorded on the PCR form, are collated with information gathered at other similar events and analyzed by appropriate agencies for population-based injury prevention programs. If the preceding characteristics of EMS are compelling for its role in injury prevention, then prevention principles must offer a framework from which programs can be developed.

Injury Prevention Principles

The term "injury" is defined as damage resulting from the transfer of energy to tissue exceeding its levels of tolerance. This energy can take various forms: mechanical, electrical, chemical, thermal, or some combination of these.

The epidemiological triangle conceptualizes the components of an injury event (fig. 81.1). The "host" refers to the victim. The "agent" refers to the object that delivers the energy to the host. The "environment" is characterized by hazards that encourage the transfer of energy from agent to host. For example, a car with worn tires on an icy road is driven by an intoxicated, unrestrained driver who hits a telephone pole. The driver is the "host," characterized by lack of restraints and intoxication. The car is the "agent," characterized by worn tires and lack airbags. The road is the "environment" characterized by its icy surface. Thus all three components (host, agent, and environment) contributed to the injury event.

In 1972, Haddon developed a more elaborate framework for injury analysis.[8] It combines the three previous components on the horizontal axis with pre-event, event, and post-event time components on the vertical axis to form a nine-cell, "phase-factor" matrix (table 81.1). In the previous example, the pre-event host factor is represented by the driver's intoxication and lack of seat belt use, the pre-event agent factor by the poor tire condition, and the pre-event environmental factor by the slick road condition. The event-agent factor is represented by no airbags and the event-environment factor by rigid, non-breakaway phone poles. The post-event host factors relate to the driver's method(s) and timeliness of contacting EMS (i.e., automated collision notification system), the post-event agent factor by the flammability of the vehicle, and the post-event environment factor by the rural setting and signage on how to reach EMS.

It follows that each of these causal factors implicates a solution. Providers are exposed to all of these factors leading to this injury event, either by direct observation or by reports of victims, law enforcement, or bystanders. The future of EMS should include an expectation of prevention intervention, on-scene when possible, or later, with relevant PCR-based data, in conjunction with other relevant agencies, that is, highway traffic safety, law enforcement, social services, and/or automobile manufacturers.

Interventions are channeled through three distinct categories, known as the "three E's," each with unique advantages and disadvantages. While *Education* is easiest to implement, compliance is poorest because of its non-binding and self-motivational dependent nature. Any programs or signage designed to teach or warn the public on how to avoid injuries represent educational efforts. *Enforcement* recruits the considerable support of the law; however, compliance is limited by the option of disobedience, despite the threat of punitive measures. Seatbelt, motorcycle helmet, fire codes, and childseat laws all qualify as examples of enforcement. *Engineering* interventions are born of design, built into the normal operation of the equipment, and thus require no active participation on the part of those at risk. Automatic seatbelts, airbags, protected pedestrian crosswalks, boat flotation hulls, and fire sensor-triggered sprinkler systems are engineering interventions. Armed with injury prevention programs based upon this framework of principles, EMS can expand its benefit to society. EMS could potentially evolve from providing solely acute treatment activities to performing prevention activities. Thus, EMS would coordinate medical care with public health care, which would have the potential to decrease medical care costs and improve our community's health.

Fire Service Injury Prevention Initiatives

Injury prevention has been an integral part of the fire service. Examples in the pre-event phase include implementation of laws requiring electrical fuses and circuit breakers to prevent a short circuit and thus prevent the fire. Examples in the event phase include use of flame-retardant clothing to prevent or minimize burns. Injury prevention during the post-event phase includes the use of sprinklers to immediately extinguish the fire.[9] Although the original role of fire services was to put out fires, in the past 50 years the fire

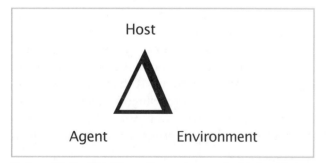

FIGURE 81.1. *The Three Components of an Injury Event.*

TABLE 81.1		
A Haddon Matrix (constructed for motor vehicle injury)		
	HOST	**AGENT/VECTOR**	**ENVIRONMENT**

	HOST	**AGENT/VECTOR**	**ENVIRONMENT**
Pre-event	Alcohol use Fatigue Experience and judgment Vision Amount of travel Stature Medications Motor skills Cognitive function	Brake condition Tire quality Center of gravity Jackknife tendency Ease of control Load weight Speed capability Ergonomic controls Mirrors Visual obstructions	Visibility of hazards Road curvature and gradient Shoulder height Surface coefficient of friction Divided highways, one-way street Intersections, access control Weather Signalization Speed limits Drunk driving laws Speed limits of traffic
Event	Seat belt use Age Gender Bone density Stature	Speed at impact Direction of impact Vehicle size Automatic restraints Airbag Character of contact surfaces Load containment Deformation zones Fuel system integrity Electronic notification	Recovery area Guard rails Characteristics of fixed objects Median barriers Roadside embankments Weather conditions
Post-event	Age Physical condition Medications Preexisting medical conditions Social situation		9-1-1 access EMS response Triage and transfer protocols EMS training Quality of emergency care Location of appropriate ED Access to definitive care Access to rehabilitation services

Adapted from Baker SP, O'Neil B, Ginsburg MJ, et al. *The Injury Fact Book*. 2nd ed. New York: Oxford University Press; 1992.

service has made a tremendous effort in regard to fire prevention.[10]

Currently, educational programs such as "Stop, Drop, and Roll" are now standard classes taught to most kindergarten students nationwide. Efforts today include not only reminding the public to use smoke detectors but to also regularly change the batteries on smoke detectors. The latest efforts encourage the use of carbon monoxide detectors in all homes.[11] Recently a study by Pirallo shows that EMS professionals can provide home fire safety interventions at the time of EMS care.[12] This study showed the potential impact that EMS professionals can make on decreasing both the risk of injury and loss of property by performing these point-of-contact home fire safety interventions. Clearly, the healthcare community can learn much from the injury prevention programs implemented by the fire service.

EMS Injury Prevention Initiatives

In 1992 Gerson published the first EMS Injury Prevention Program, whereby paramedics identified elder individuals at risk and referred them for assessment and service.[5] This study found that paramedics identified 197 (3%) of 6,000 elderly individuals at risk. Of these 197 individuals, 94 then got appropriate follow-up services, including social services (33%), homemaker (23%), physical change to environment (17%), adult protective services (15%), and lifeline-telephone monitoring (15%). No baseline or outcome data were gathered in this study.

Several initiatives in EMS injury prevention have followed the Gerson program. In the early 1990s Pinellas County, Florida began an injury prevention program following an epidemic number of drownings. As the first step in the injury prevention program, a data registry for all submersion injuries was developed. Data revealed that children under the age of 3 under adult supervision in residential pools were at greatest risk. The second part of the injury prevention program was to educate the public regarding submersion injuries. Education through several different media were used, including television public service announcements and newspaper articles. Furthermore, EMS, with the assistance of local fire departments, organized free home-pool safety inspections.[13] No control group was included in this study, but with implementation of the program a 48% reduction in submersion injuries was documented.[13,14]

In the early 1990s, with a grant from the California EMS Authority, the Division of Emergency Medicine at Stanford University, in conjunction with local EMS professionals at all levels, developed an educational program called, "Accidents Aren't." The program was designed to impart the requisite knowledge and skills for EMS professionals to conduct primary-injury prevention. This includes information on the foregoing principles involved in analyzing and preventing injuries as well as on recognizing behavioral and environmental risk factors. The process designed for on-scene EMS personnel to analyze injuries takes the form of a mnemonic, "STARR." Each letter occupies a unique point on a conceptual star, and stands for a task to be executed as the result of interfacing an injury. *See*, *Talk*, *Assess*, *Remedy*, and *Review* are discussed in detail. The program's structure is modular, allowing adaptability to an individual community's injury problems and patterns. A slide set accompanies the text program with an explanation of each slide's depiction, so that no prior knowledge on the part of the instructor is presumed. Currently, the Rollins School of Public Health Injury Prevention Center at Emory University, through an NHTSA grant, is conducting a trial of the ability of EMS providers to assimilate the contents of the program.

In 2001, the Michigan Office of EMS supported the NHTSA Safe Communities' concept through local EMS systems. Fifteen EMS personnel completed a two-day training workshop to become EMS community injury prevention officers (CIPO). Participants were trained to assess community risks and develop interventions. So far, the CIPOs have assisted development of a Safe Communities Program in Kent County, and assisted the Safe Kids Chapter in Lapeer with helmet checks and car seat inspections.[15]

The Future of EMS in Injury Prevention

The impact of injuries cannot be overemphasized, in our personal lives as victims and near-victims, and/or in our professional lives as the acquaintance of victims. In 1990, an estimated 5.1 million people worldwide died as a result of injuries.[16] In the United States, injuries have accounted for over 150,000 fatalities yearly, and they are responsible for the leading cause of death in people under 45 years of age.[17] These deaths represent the apex of a pyramid of non-fatal cases. Hospitalized cases outnumber deaths by 19 to 1; non-hospitalized cases requiring outpatient care outnumber deaths 233 to 1.[18] Another tragic pyramid demonstrates that for each non-intentional trauma death, 3 other victims are permanently disabled and 93 others temporarily disabled.[19] Since EMS already interfaces with this population of victims as a ubiquitous community clinical resource, it follows that EMS would be the most appropriate service, operationally and economically, to adopt and enact a systematic approach to injury prevention.

Organizations representing EMS nationally advocate the duty of EMS to provide injury prevention. In 1997, the National Association of EMS Physicians, supported by the NHTSA and the Maternal and Child Health Bureau, published a broad-based, wide-ranging consensus statement advocating the following essential and desirable EMS primary-injury prevention (PIP) activities:

- protecting individual EMS providers from injury;
- providing education to EMS providers in PIP fundamentals;
- supporting and promoting the collection and utilization of injury data;
- obtaining support for PIP activities;
- networking with other injury prevention organizations;
- empowering individual EMS providers to conduct PIP activities;
- interacting with the media to promote injury prevention; and
- participating in community injury prevention interventions.[20]

As is evident in many of these initiatives, EMS must forge novel alliances with organizations outside the medical arena, to include public safety and public health, in order to achieve injury prevention. In response to previously stated characteristics of EMS and its role in injury prevention, the American College of Emergency Physicians published guidelines and a policy statement for the role of EMS personnel in domestic violence.[21]

However huge the toll of injuries in terms of morbidity and mortality, and however appropriate the intent of EMS injury prevention, the engine that must power it to reality will be economic. In 1995, the annual lifetime direct and indirect costs of injury in the United States were estimated at $260 billion. The prospect of saving the rising cost of treating injuries must become sufficiently attractive to all of us, for prevention activities to be funded as a priority and for incentives to be linked to prevention results.[22] Some believe that two current trends may significantly accelerate the involvement of EMS in injury prevention programs.[14] The first of these trends is small EMS agencies being acquired or purchased by large corporations, where they become more of a profit-generating "business." The second trend is managed healthcare organizations acquiring small EMS agencies, where the primary goal is to prevent injury and thereby reduce costs. Although these two trends have been discussed for almost a decade, neither of these trends have resulted in a significant change in the role currently played by EMS in injury prevention. Some believe that EMS agencies are too busy providing acute care to be able to also provide injury prevention.[14] Others believe that an EMS injury prevention specialist who is focused only on prevention needs to be hired, similar to the position of a fire prevention specialist.[14] But one thing is certain: As the healthcare market continues to place emphasis on prevention, there will be more EMS involvement in injury prevention.

References

1. National Academy of Science National Research Council. *Accidental Death and Disability: The Neglected Disease of Modern Society*. Washington, D.C.: Government Printing Office; 1966.
2. Demetriades D, Chan L, Cornwell E, et al. Paramedic vs. private transportation of trauma patients: effect of outcome. *Arch Surgery*. 1996;131:133–138.
3. MacKenzie EJ, Morris JA, Smith GS. Acute hospital costs of trauma in the United States: implications for regionalized systems of care. *J Trauma*. 1990;30(9):1096–1101.
4. McSwain NE. Indirect medical control. In Kuehl AE, ed. *EMS Medical Director's Handbook*. St. Louis: Mosby Company; 1989:166.
5. Gerson LW, Schelble DT, Wilson JE. Using paramedics to identify at-risk elderly. *Ann Emerg Med*. 1992;21(6):688–691.
6. Lewis CE. Teaching medical students about disease prevention and health promotion. *Public Health Reports*. 1982;97(3):210–215.
7. Nutting PA. Health promotion in primary medical care: problems and potential. *Preventive Medicine*. 1986;15:537–548.
8. Haddon W. A logical framework for categorizing highway safety phenomena and activity. *J Trauma*. 1972;12:193.
9. Kay RL, Baker SP. Let's emphasize fire sprinklers as an injury prevention technology. *Injury Prevention*. 2000;6(1):72–80.
10. Mallonee S. Evaluating injury prevention programs: the Oklahoma City smoke alarm project. *Future of Child*. 2000;10(1):164–174.
11. Leikin JB, Krenzelok EP, Greiner TH. Remarks to the Illinois House of Representatives Executive Committee hearing regarding State Carbon Monoxide Detector Act. *J Tox-Clin Tox*. 1999;37(7):885–890.
12. Pirrallo RG, Rubin JM, Murawsky GA. The potential benefit of a home fire safety intervention during emergency medical service calls. *Acad Emerg Med*. 1998;5(3):220–224.
13. Harrawood D, Gunderson MR, Fravel S, Cartwright K, Ryan JL. Drowning prevention: a case study in EMS epidemiology. *J Emerg Med Services*. 1994;19(6):34–41.
14. Kinnane JM, Garrison HG, Coben JH, Alsonso-Serra HM. Injury prevention: is there a role for out of hospital emergency medical services? *Prehosp Emerg Care*. 1997;4(4):306–312.
15. Community Traffic Safety Programs. State of Michigan Office of Highway Safety Planning 2000 Annual Report. *Making Our Highways Safer Places*. 2000:43–45.
16. Murray CJ, Lopez AD. Mortality by cause for eight regions of the world: global burden of disease study. *Lancet*. 1997;349:1269–1276.
17. Anderson RN, Kochanek KD, et al. Report of final mortality statistics, 1995. National Center for Health Statistics. *Monthly Vital Statistics Report*. 1997;45(11), Suppl. 2:36.
18. Burt CW. Injury-related visits to hospital emergency departments: United States, 1992. National Center for Health Statistics. *Advanced Data from Vital and Health Statistics 261*. 1995;26:13–14.
19. National Safety Council. *Accident Facts* 1991. Chicago: National Safety Council; 1991:1–12.
20. Garrison HG, Foltin GL, Becker LR. The role of emergency medical services in primary injury prevention. *Ann Emerg Med*. 1997;30(1):84–91.
21. ACEP. "Guidelines for the Role of EMS Personnel in Domestic Violence." An ACEP Policy Resource and Education Paper. February 2001. Available at http://www.acep.org/library/index.cfm/id/442.htm
22. Bonnie RJ, Fulco CE, Liverman CT. Executive Summary in Reducing the Burden of Injury, Advancing Prevention and Treatment. Washington, D.C.: Institute of Medicine, National Academy Press; 1999:1.

Managed Care

Douglas F. Kupas, MD
Keith W. Neely, MPA, PhD
Kristi L. Koenig, MD

Introduction

"You can have your service good, fast, or cheap . . . pick any two." This is a common statement in the business world, and it is quite applicable to Emergency Medical Services (EMS) systems. Traditionally, EMS has been structured with system redundancy to allow for a rapid response to medical emergencies. Reimbursement for this care was based upon the number of patients who were transported, with the cost shifted to the patients (or their insurers) who used the system, or to the community through taxes or volunteer efforts. Managed Care Organizations (MCO) attempt to provide quality medical care to their patients while decreasing costs by controlling patient access to various medical services. These competing values and interests may lead to turmoil—or opportunity—for an EMS system.

This chapter will introduce the economic principles of managed care. There are many possible applications of these principles to EMS. Some are already working well in many systems, and some are visions of future possibilities. This chapter will begin with a description of healthcare financing issues related to managed care and definitions of various MCO structures. The impact of managed care principles on EMS system structure and operation will then be discussed. EMS systems have many options for adapting to managed care challenges and opportunities. Regionalization and the multiple option decision point models will be discussed as possible ways that EMS systems can adapt to a managed care environment. The chapter will conclude by exploring the cultural issues that EMS systems must resolve to work toward expanded opportunities. These issues include competing interests, community standards, regionalization, and workplace cultures.

Economics of Managed Care

Managed Care Organizations

Managed care is a very nebulous term that refers to a constellation of services, practices, and financial incentives organized in a way to provide the best healthcare services for the lowest cost. Inglehart defines managed care by outlining its essential elements.[1] These elements include contractual relationships with a specific panel of providers or institutions, predetermined monthly premiums, utilization and quality controls that are followed by contracted providers, financial incentives to use panels and institutions associated with the plan, and assumption of some risk by providers. There is infinite variety in the ways MCOs may arrange themselves; however, a general descriptive structure can be organized along the dimensions of cost controls and patient choice.[2] As a very general rule, more structured MCOs institute greater cost controls and allow less patient choice of providers. Less structured MCOs institute fewer cost controls and tend to allow greater choice. Traditional fee-for-service plans offer fewest cost controls and are likely to offer greatest consumer choice of providers.

Preferred provider organizations (PPO) are even more structured. A MCO will contract with panels of providers that usually have some system of utilization review associated with them. These contracts may or may not be risk-bearing. MCO patients who see physicians in PPOs usually are charged lower co-payments and deductibles.

Independent practice associations (IPA) are more structured yet and is usually a collection of primary care physicians and/or specialists organized into a legal entity, which then contracts with an MCO to deliver services in return for a single capitation rate.

The IPA in turn contracts with the individual practitioners to provide services on a fee-for-service or capitated basis.

The term health maintenance organization has a more specific definition, but this has changed over time. Originally the term referred to a prepayment organization that provided care to a voluntarily enrolled population in return for a "per member per month" (PMPM) set amount of money. Historically, HMOs were seen as most structured, providing least consumer choice, and built upon staff or group practice models. Increasingly, HMOs are offering more choice of providers, including providers outside the HMO panels. In this chapter the term HMO refers to the most highly structured managed care organizations. MCO refers to the payer organizations in the industry as a whole.

Origins of Managed Care

Managed care began in the early 20th century as a prepayment system intended to guarantee access to care for those in remote areas.[3] The beginnings were motivated by access, not cost, and the first plans were strongly associated with defined populations of employees such as Western Clinic of Tacoma in 1910. Baylor Hospital covered Houston teachers during the early 1930s, and became an early model for Blue Cross/Blue Shield.[4]

During the 1960s, when healthcare costs began to escalate, prepaid arrangements came to be viewed as a cost-saving strategy. Ellwood, arguing that healthcare financing ought to reward health maintenance, coined the term health maintenance organization in 1970.[5] By 1973, the Health Maintenance Organization Act was passed, creating grants and loans for HMO development and requiring employers to offer HMO coverage as well as traditional insurance to their employees. This section of the law was known as the dual choice requirement. When President Nixon signed the HMO Act into law (within months of the EMSS Act) his administration hoped to see HMOs available to 90% of the population by the end of that decade.[6]

Discussions of managed care within EMS may revolve around the financial incentives of capitation. Capitation shifts financial risk to providers by giving them a flat PMPM amount to provide their services. If they provide that care for less than their allotment, they receive financial rewards. If they exceed the monthly PMPM, they receive financial penalties.

Thus providers are motivated to keep their patients healthy, and in so doing, reduce their risk and lower their cost.

However, it is important to understand that managed care manages more than risk and cost. Managed care manages "health," access, service utilization, data, risk, and finally, cost, though not necessarily in that order. Prevention, health, and "wellness" have rapidly displaced acute care as the core business of health care. Shortell provides a framework for managing health.[5] He suggests a new medical management system that (1) manages episodes of illness across networks of care; (2) institutes population-based needs monitoring requiring closer relationships with community public health and social service agencies; and (3) establishes continuous quality improvement and incentive systems that reward excellence and encourage collaboration. This thrust shifts health care from a curative model to a prevention model, and emphasizes primary care services.

"Ethicnomics" of EMS

Managed care organizations attempt to manage health care with the efficiencies of big business, but is important to take a step back to reinforce the ethical and societal importance of EMS care. While it may be possible to efficiently manage a specialist physician's clinic practice within a MCO, the unpredictable aspects of providing emergency care do not fit the business efficiencies as easily.

EMS systems have traditionally been designed with redundancy to accommodate the sporadic fluctuations in call volume, and to provide some degree of preparedness for community disasters. EMS systems frequently provide care to the uninsured and underinsured. In many instances there is no tax-based support of these activities, and their costs must be absorbed by the system. In essence, EMS serves as a safety net for the community.

Communities must assure that these important services are not eroded away by allowing EMS services to devise systems that serve only the profitable managed care patients while they refuse to carry some of the "safety net" burden. On the other hand, EMS systems can no longer hide behind the system redundancy argument as an excuse for their inefficient practices.

Brown and Sindelar offer an example of EMS system inefficiencies. Their study reveals that the rate of appropriate ambulance transportation is 78% for privately insured patients, 66% for Medicare patients, and 14% for Medicaid patients. Additionally they found that nursing-home patients on Medicare were less likely to have appropriate EMS transports.[7] While these authors refer to this as EMS system misuse, if these patients do not have other viable alternatives to access appropriate health care, it is difficult to apply the term "misuse" to these cases.

EMS systems must walk an increasingly fine line between filling an important need as a medical safety net for their communities and answering the increasing pressures to alter the level of service that they provide to remain economically viable. These "ethic-nomic" issues impact EMS services in ways that are unique in the business world.

Supply and Demand

The preceding discussion and definitions of managed care focused on the benefits of managing the supply side of health care by controlling the costs of care and the efficiency of the provision of care. If consumers pay a fixed amount for health care, MCOs can improve their financial performance by either controlling and decreasing the costs associated with health care or by decreasing the need or the demand for health care. Access management, sometimes referred to as demand management,[8] generally means the practice of directing patients to appropriate resources before or as they enter the healthcare system. This is distinct from supply management, otherwise known as managed care, which manages patient demand once the patient is in the system. Access management also refers to providing services that overcome barriers to access.

Narrowly construed, utilization management is typically installed as a means of protecting against abuses in a fee-for-service plan. However, more comprehensive approaches involving case management may be more effective for controlling costs.[3] For example, there is a high incidence of costly, high-risk births within the fee-for-service Medicaid population. To achieve healthy birth outcomes and to control costs, early prenatal care and effective birthing care are required. Effective medical management of high-risk births is a good example of outcome and cost-control measures achieved through proper utilization of resources.

Cost is managed by predicting expenses based on actuarial models, which present both the probability of an event occurring and the average cost of that event. The model usually presents data for large service areas such as in-patient medical stays, surgical stays, obstetric stays, skilled nursing stays, and so on. MCOs develop these models to project health costs and set premium rates. A model often starts with national statistics, then modifies that to reflect local characteristics, plan design (cost sharing arrangements), and the demographics of the population served.[9]

Finally, managing risk really means spreading the risk, and opportunity, as mentioned earlier. This brings us to the interest some large ambulance services have in managed care and capitation.

Private-sector EMS is funded through user fees assessed for transported patients only. This means that the cost associated with 25 to 30% of EMS responses that result in no patient being transported is shifted to the 70 to 75% who are.[10,11] Further, many who are transported are uninsured. Consequently, there is more cost shifting still to those with commercial or other health insurance. It may be to the private firm's advantage to enter into an agreement with an MCO that capitates the ambulance service at their existing revenue and reimbursement structures, although this advantage is decreased if the ambulance service does not transport a significant number of patients who belong to the MCO. Having taken on this risk, the ambulance service is motivated to develop strategies that lower its cost.

Various industry experts estimate that medical transportation billings represent about 1% of all claims paid by health insurance companies. However, medical transportation may affect 6 to 10% of medical claims because patients currently may be transported to relatively expensive sites of care, especially if that site is an out-of-plan hospital.[12]

This then leads to such concepts as the multiple option decision point model (MODP).[13-15] This model provides an array of transportation, treatment, and destination options during the continuum of an EMS call, most of which theoretically cost less than the traditional EMS response and transport to an emergency department. While several large EMS systems and MCOs are working toward this model, it remains an unproven concept, and many of the expected results are currently theoretical.

In the MODP model, the 9-1-1 public service answering points and the demand management center (nurse advice lines) are closely linked and regularly communicate with each other on some EMS and MCO calls. Some have suggested that private contractors, possibly even EMS providers, may operate both of these centers as a single entity. These centers may have protocols to schedule certain callers with an appointment with their primary care physician rather than dispatch an ambulance immediately.

In the MODP model, if EMS is dispatched, the patient may be assessed and treated for minor ailments without transportation. If transportation is required, patients may be directed to a clinic if their conditions are minor, or alternatives to transportation, for example taxi vouchers, may be used. This system may also be able to divert a stable patient to a nearby hospital that participates with the MCO, reducing the need to transport the patient a second time later. Of course, all of these options require significant medical oversight, validated protocols, and excellent quality improvement systems to assure appropriate and safe medical care. In some states, there may be legislative restrictions on patient destination after 9-1-1 is accessed, and these legislative barriers may need to be revised before the efficiencies of MODP models can be maximized.

Economic risk in this instance is managed largely by finding appropriate methods for assigning users of the ambulance service to appropriate levels of service, rather than transporting all by advanced-life-support ambulance. At first blush it may seem unlikely that a MCO would capitate an ambulance service at this level; however, a case can be made for EMS communities interested in these relationships to strike such an arrangement.

The MODP model and projected savings for MCOs are dependent on some very significant assumptions, for example, the assumption that it is less expensive to treat a patient with a minor illness in their primary care physician's office than in an emergency department. Like EMS, emergency departments shift the costs of care for the uninsured and system readiness to the patients who use and can pay for the services. Williams has shown that the actual marginal costs of treating minor illnesses in the ED and physician offices are similar.[16] Additionally, there may be tremendous customer service advantages to treating individuals immediately when they perceive a medical emergency, or when it is convenient and less interrupting to their lifestyle and other responsibilities.

Shifts in one direction or the other in transport provider reimbursements will not greatly affect an MCO's bottom line, but it will affect the provider's bottom line. A bargain perhaps could be struck. In return for capitating EMS systems at the existing volume and revenue levels, EMS systems can work with MCOs to place patients in clinically appropriate settings, which in some instances would be less costly.

MCOs often manage demand or access by orienting members either to call or see their primary care physicians prior to seeking specialty, emergency, or other care. Circumventing the 9-1-1 system in this way may deprive the patient of a rapid dispatch of the closest EMS personnel or deprive them of potentially lifesaving interventions through emergency medical dispatch pre-arrival instructions. Anecdotal reports have suggested that this occurs, and one paper presents the cases of two patients "who died after they delayed calling 9-1-1 in keeping with the rules of their MCO."[17]

In 1989, Hossfeld found that 99% of the HMO enrollees in the Chicago area were instructed by their MCO to call their primary care physician or their MCO in the event of an emergency. None of the enrollees was instructed to call 9-1-1.[18] Since then, legislation containing the prudent lay person definition of an emergency and preventing MCOs from insisting that patients call the MCO in an emergency have reduced this problem in many states.

On the other hand, some have argued that "however good the local [EMS] public relations effort, patients are often unclear about how and when to access prehospital care. . . . Some patients will overestimate the severity of the illness, whereas others will underestimate it." Advice lines may talk patients into using EMS when they were unsure of their condition and would otherwise have delayed medical treatment or accessed medical care by car.[18]

Demand management centers, also referred to as nurse telephone triage centers, are commonly used by MCOs to direct a caller to the "appropriate level of care."[15] These increasingly sophisticated centers are capable not only of managing incoming calls for advice but providing "outbound" telephone guidance services for certain patients with stable disease but who require periodic monitoring. For example, a patient with congestive heart failure may receive a telephone call from the MCO's demand management center. During the conversation the nurse may inquire about the patient's medication compliance and ask her to weigh herself. This information may be used to alter the patient's diuretic dose, or this intervention may improve the patient's compliance with medication. This form of patient case management may decrease the exacerbation of the patient's disease, and therefore may decrease the utilization of EMS and emergency care.

EMS systems, medical directors, and MCOs should consider the following concepts when addressing issues of EMS dispatch and nurse advice lines (NALs):

- Prudent laypersons who believe that they are suffering from a medical emergency should have unimpeded access to an emergency medical dispatcher (9-1-1 center) and pre-arrival instructions.

- NALs should not advertise their seven-digit numbers to MCO members as primary numbers to contact in a medical emergency in lieu of 9-1-1.

- When an EMS dispatch center or NAL recognizes a patient with a life-threatening emergency, the patient should receive a rapid response from the closest medically appropriate EMS unit regardless of whether the usual EMS provider for the area is contracted with the MCO.

- NALs should have a procedure to link a caller with a life-threatening emergency to the appropriate EMS dispatch center.

- NALs should be answered promptly, and callers should not be placed on hold until they have been screened for life-threatening problems. NAL centers should ensure that they have enough lines and personnel to handle the expected call volume. Callers should not routinely encounter busy lines.

- NALs and EMS dispatch centers should use validated medical protocols to assess callers and provide medical advice.

- EMS dispatch centers and NALs should use quality improvement audits to assure that incoming calls are answered promptly and that medical protocols are followed by their call-takers.

Reimbursement Mechanisms

Four reimbursement mechanisms are used in EMS: fee-for-service, discounted fee-for-service, flat fees, and capitation. The first three are much more common, and differ from the fourth in a very important aspect. As the term fee-for-service implies, a fee is assessed for specific services provided. In an EMS system this mechanism requires only those who are transported to pay for all the services necessary to operate a transportation company. This makes sense in a market where all transports are pre-arranged, like inter-facility transfers. However, this practice does not take into account the preparation, excess capacity, and readiness required for emergency medical transportation characterized by episodic peaks in activity.

Discounted fee-for-service is similar. Health plans have for many years negotiated discounted fee-for-service agreements for non-emergent transportation. In this instance an ambulance provider agrees to lower its customary transportation charges, sometimes substantially, in return for providing services for all plan members requiring non-emergent ambulance transportation. However, the same economic consequences apply. Cost is shifted toward insurance plans that pay more of the bill.

Health plans take several steps to mitigate this. They negotiate their own discounted fee-for-service agreement with the ambulance service. They attempt to educate their members to call 9-1-1 only for emergencies. They charge a co-payment, sometimes up to $50 for ambulance transportation, or they deny claims for unscheduled ambulance transportation when retrospective review classifies the patient's condition as non-emergent. All of these responses limit the EMS system's effectiveness.

Flat fees, also called fixed rates, reimburse an EMS provider a predetermined payment per transport performed. There are usually separate fees for several levels of care. These flat fees are usually significantly discounted from the customary fees. For example, there may be a fixed rate for ALS treatment, BLS treatment, and wheelchair van transport. In exchange for accepting these discounted fees, the EMS provider becomes the exclusive transportation provider for a defined population of the MCO's members. There is incentive for the provider to operate each transport more efficiently, but there is no incentive to decrease the number of transports by EMS, and there is actually a financial incentive to provide ALS care whether it is medically indicated or not! The flat fee system simplifies the accounting process for billing and reimbursement.

With flat fees, the sole EMS provider becomes responsible for coordinating all of the MCOs transportation needs. There are many unique arrangements, and these providers often reorganize their system within a Contracted Network or Provider Cooperative (as discussed later under system configurations).

Capitation agreements are very different. As discussed already, capitation refers to accepting financial risk by accepting prepayment for services. Health plans will establish their approximate cost for providing or paying for services based on actuarial, utilization, and historical data. The provider enters into negotiations with the MCO with the goal of reaching an agreeable PMPM allotment. This approach has several advantages. For the MCO it reduces administrative workload associated with processing individual claims, turning unpredictable month-to-month outlays for unscheduled or episodic care into a predictable monthly cash outflow. It also shifts the financial risk to the provider, and with it, the incentive to reduce its costs. For the provider, a wisely negotiated capitation rate spreads the cost of providing services over all potential users, not just those who are served. A PMPM payment gives the EMS service a regular and predictable income stream, and it allows the provider to reduce its cost under the capitated rate and save money.

For capitation to work, the geographic area served by the MCO must match the geographic service area of the EMS provider, and the percentage of the general population covered by the MCO must be significant. When contracting for non-emergent and inter-facility transport needs, this geographic match between the service areas of the MCO and the EMS service is less problematic, but MCOs also have an interest in controlling the unpredictable emergency calls.

It is more difficult to structure capitated agreements that include emergency calls, since most EMS systems are not large enough to adequately cover the MCOs geographic area, or the MCOs geographic area may be covered by a variety of public and private EMS services. Additionally, communities have established 9-1-1 phone systems, emergency medical dispatch protocols, and designated EMS responses to provide the promptest EMS response to a given region. It is conceivable that capitated agreements for emergency EMS calls could encourage EMS providers and MCOs to circumvent this response system by discouraging use of 9-1-1, advising their patients to call their own call-answering points, and dispatching their contracted ambulances to scenes when they are not the closest or most appropriate responder. This would be deleterious to the safety net function of a community's EMS system.

While capitated agreements have some theoretical benefits, EMS systems must be very economically savvy to enter into such agreements, and to date, most EMS services that work with MCOs have stopped short of this step. Although not always true, the theoretical winners in capitation of EMS include ground-based critical-care transport, single-tiered ALS systems, contracted providers, HMOs, taxpayers, and customers of managed care insurance plans. Theoretical losers are 9-1-1 systems, emergency departments, medical helicopter services, tiered providers, the uninsured, and single-jurisdiction safety net providers.

Contracting with Managed Care

Capitation

An important promise of managed care is to create sufficient competition to drive down the cost of health care. Managed care plans do this, in part, by reducing excess capacity from the system and reducing provider reimbursement. Health system mergers frequently lead to consolidation of services, reduction of administrative staff, or closure of entire hospitals. EMS systems do not have much excess capacity. System status management plans and competitive bidding already have made most of these systems as efficient as they can be under the current reimbursement structure. Rural systems run by volunteers generally are operated close to the economic bone without the additional managed-care-induced pressures. Consequently, EMS medical directors should insist that any capitated agreements be based on existing provider revenue and reimbursement structure, as discussed earlier, thus protecting the system integrity.

Data Needs

EMS providers must have a very clear understanding of what it costs currently to offer their services before negotiating either discounted fee-for-service or capitated agreements. This calculation is muddied if, at the same time, providers are trying to estimate the costs of new kinds of lower-cost services, such as those suggested by the MODP model. Many private services use unit hour utilization to derive unit costs of providing medical transportation. Hospitals tend to use cost accounting to identify what it costs to provide care for patients with a particular diagnosis. Regardless of the method, such cost accounting data systems must be firmly in place.

Clinical outcome data are also necessary for EMS/managed care contracting. The pressure is toward reducing costs. If a new but costly intervention for the out-of-hospital treatment of strokes is introduced, data proving its efficacy is necessary in order to negotiate a dispensation from the MCO for this new therapy. If an EMS provider finds it necessary to add resources to maintain response times, these data have to be clearly presented to renegotiate the managed care agreement successfully. A central goal to a managed care/EMS partnership must be to maintain the EMS system infrastructure. Good cost accounting and clinical data are essential if this goal is to be met. Systems without such data systems must invest the resources to create them.

Two Standards of Care

A result of EMS/managed care partnerships is the development of new MODP models for reducing costs. There are two views of these models. One is an egalitarian view, the other an entrepreneurial view. In the egalitarian view, assuming systems can make accurate on-scene distinctions between patients who require transport to a hospital ED and those who can be treated with alternative dispositions, these models offer lower cost to the community and ought to be offered to all residents. This is consistent with the EMS tradition of offering a single level of service to all and tailoring patient-to-patient variation on clinical criteria.

The entrepreneurial view incorporates the notion of opportunity into the discussion surrounding MODP. This view holds that if systems can identify the approximately one-third of cases that may be well served by lower-cost alternatives, then the MODP model offers an opportunity to tailor lower-cost responses to members of MCOs that capitate for this service.

This approach requires providing the lower-cost services only to the callers covered by plans that purchase these EMS services, while responding in the traditional way to patients who are not members. The egalitarian view sees this as providing two standards of care based on insurance coverage. The entrepreneurial view would argue that no clinical harm is done (assuming accurate triage criteria), costs are reduced, and patients receive adequate levels of care. Moreover, this view would argue, if the MODP model were offered to everyone, the free rider phenomenon would prevail and no plan would purchase this product when it could get it for free.

New Standards of Care

Regardless of orientation, this discussion assumes a new set of care standards. These standards may well include the MODP model. To do this, however, systems need well constructed and validated decision guidelines.

The only guidelines in the literature are those associated with individual studies that retrospectively judged ALS ambulance and/or ED use.[19-24] None of these few guidelines has been prospectively validated. However, such guidelines are critical before any system can safely offer the MODP model.

System Design

Arrangements between EMS systems and MCOs can take many forms. A recent Concept Paper from the National Association of EMS Physicians addresses many common questions, and may assist communities in developing these partnerships.[25]

Multiple Option Decision Point Model

The MODP model has been previously discussed. This model has been structured in several regions that have high managed care penetration and a single large EMS service that has a regional presence. To date, none of these developing systems has incorporated the entire model into practice, but some believe that this model may improve the efficiency of EMS while providing more options for out-of-hospital resources and patient care.

Regionalization

Because MCOs provide their service to members within large geographic areas, EMS systems must have the ability to provide their services over an equally large area if they are to be useful to MCOs. Ambulance services that historically have focused on a small geographic area include fire-based services, volunteer services, and local private services. As managed care increases its membership and coverage, these local organizations will be unable to compete with large EMS organizations that can offer the MCO services over its entire geographic area.

Many small or local EMS providers fear losing their business to large regional or national providers. In an effort to remain competitive and attractive to MCOs, an increasing number of services are associating with other smaller providers to regionalize the services that they can provide. These associations between services fall into four general categories: shared service, contracted network, provider cooperative, and merger.[26]

Services may cooperate on a smaller scale by jointly operating some small shared services. An example is a wheelchair van that is operated jointly by several small providers. Several providers may share the management and operation of the van, but all other services by the providers are operated separately.

An affiliation that allows each service even more autonomy is the contracted network. In this arrangement, the MCO contracts with an EMS provider for their transportation needs. This provider may directly provide the service, or a subcontractor from a network of subcontractors may provide the service. The subcontractors retain most of their autonomy, but they are at the mercy of the primary contractor. If MCO transports become a significant amount of the business of the contracted network, the EMS service can expand upon their services to the MCO. For example, EMS providers may station a customer service coordinator in large hospitals to coordinate patient discharges with EMS transports.

Another type of arrangement is a provider cooperative. In this situation, each service maintains its own identity, but a new organization is formed to manage the business operations, personnel issues, group buying, and contracting with various payers. This co-op type situation still allows each local service to have some autonomy, but the services can now gain economies-of-scale benefits in management and operations.

Lastly, a merger is the ultimate association between smaller providers. While a full merger into a new system has the most to gain from economy of scale, this arrangement requires the most trust between the partner organizations, and it places everything at risk.

As MCO penetration increases, it is likely that geopolitical boundaries will become less important to EMS systems, and the ability to contract with health insurers that cover large regions will become more important. As this occurs, there will be an increase in affiliations and cooperation among services.

Levels of Response/Care

The services provided by EMS can be divided into various levels based upon the severity of the patient's medical condition and the necessity for timely EMS care or transportation. These various levels of care do not have distinct definitions, and often patients will be triaged into an inappropriate category. Therefore, the EMS system and managed care must be flexible to the medical needs of the patient. By definition, no triage system will appropriately screen every patient, and a system must have the flexibility to provide all levels of care to accommodate the changing medical needs of the patient.

EMERGENCY RESPONSES

For many reasons, managing the out-of-hospital emergency needs of their members is the most difficult level of EMS care for managed care networks. When a patient or their family perceives a life-threatening emergency, they are under a tremendous amount of emotional stress. To guarantee an optimal EMS response, the local dispatch center must be contacted immediately, the call must be screened, and the appropriate local EMS units must be sent. Until either the dispatcher or initial EMS units determine that the patient's problem is not immediately life-threatening, there is no time for unnecessary pre-approval or consultation with the MCO. The dispatch center must send the usual primary response for the geographic area or an equivalently staffed/equipped MCO-affiliated vehicle that will have an equivalent response time. Managed care must understand the necessity of an unobstructed rapid response to these potentially life-threatening emergencies.

On the other hand, after assessment by EMS, most emergency responses do not involve patients with immediately life-threatening emergencies. Depending upon the nature of the medical problem, the most appropriate destination for the patient may not be the closest hospital. EMS protocols should dictate the destinations for critically ill patients (for example, multiple trauma, severe burns, and in the future maybe MIs and strokes). For other patients, cooperation between the EMS provider and the MCO can assure that these patients are transported to a facility appropriate for the patient's medical condition, and possibly prevent the need for future transfers if the destination hospital is a provider for the MCO.

ROUTINE TRANSPORTS

Routine transfers are usually scheduled, and usually require minimal patient care; therefore, they are the easiest aspect of EMS to control within the managed care system. They are the BLS transfers to and from nursing homes and patient residences, but they can also include such services as wheelchair van transports and taxi rides for prenatal visits of indigent patients. Because this business does not require the ability to respond to every community within minutes, and due to the system redundancy of emergency responses, regional contracts with EMS services will likely develop as the norm for routine transports and inter-facility transports. Communities should be aware of the potential dramatic impact on their local ability to support emergency response if larger regional services gain a large share of the more lucrative routine transport business.

INTER-FACILITY TRANSPORTS/REPATRIATION

Members of MCOs sometimes receive their initial emergency care in facilities that are not affiliated with their insurance company. This may occur because they were travelling outside of the geographic area of their insurance plan, were transported to another facility based upon their medical condition, or sought care at an out-of-system facility. One survey found an average of six out-of-area emergency department visits per 1,000 plan members annually.[27] MCOs are anxious to find methods of organizing these out of network (OON) patients. EMS, through the development of interconnected MODP models and call-answering centers, may have the ability to coordinate these OON patients. The patients may prefer to be treated at their MCO facility if it is closer to home or if it is their primary site of medical care, but some patients may be concerned about their acute medical situation, or be threatened with financial costs if they do not concede to transfer. The MCO has a financial incentive to provide the patient's care at its affiliated facilities, and the OON provider has the legal and moral obligation to assure that the patient does not have any morbidity related to being transferred. This dichotomy of incentives can place the EMS provider in an emotionally hostile environment.

The Colorado Medical Society has outlined guidelines that address the transfer of MCO subscribers,[28] and the National Association of EMS Physicians has a position paper that outlines system considerations and the role of medical direction in inter-facility patient transports.[29]

A study of complications during inter-facility transport by Meador and Wuerz concluded that there were very few complications in their patient population, but no study to date has addressed this issue in patients who are transferred entirely for insurance purposes.[30]

Repatriation is the process of arranging and facilitating medical transportation of managed care plan members from OON facilities to medical facilities within the managed care system. By creating a system that coordinates the care of these patients among the patient, the sending facility, the health plan, the receiving facility, and the EMS service, most of the potential problems can be alleviated in a way that is agreeable to all parties.

EMTALA AND REPATRIATION ISSUES

Once a patient has sought care at a non-MCO emergency department, the non-MCO hospital is obliged to provide a medical screening examination, emergency treatment, and stabilization within the capability available at that facility, prior to transferring the patient. The patient is considered stabilized when "no . . . deterioration is likely to result from or occur during transfer." These obligations are required by a 1986 federal statute, the Emergency Medical Treatment and Active Labor Act (EMTALA). This legislation was passed to prevent healthcare facilities from "dumping" indigent patients to other healthcare facilities before they have been appropriately stabilized. There is an economic incentive to MCOs to transfer these patients back into the MCO facilities as soon as possible.[31]

Some suggestions for emergency department compliance with EMTALA include:

1. evaluate all patients without prior inquiry into their insurance status,
2. be sure that contracts with MCOs do not require prior authorizations for emergency treatment,
3. proactively contact MCOs to define mutually agreeable policies, do not include "insurance request" as a reason for transfer on documentation, and
4. do not transfer the patient if doubts exist about stability.[32]

These same principles can be used to guide EMS systems that are considering alterations in patient care or destination based upon MCO associations and MODP models. While most EMS systems are not required to follow EMTALA mandates, hospital-owned EMS systems are included. While many sources state that the responsibility of arranging an appropriate transfer team and the care during the transfer lie with the sending physician and institution, at least one author disputes this interpretation. Whether or not an organization or individual has liability under EMTALA, "every professional involved in the transfer has a separate and individual legal responsibility to the patient, proportionate to their knowledge and control of the transfer."[33] In MCO-prompted transfers, the managed care plan and its personnel involved in arranging and performing the transfer may have the larger liability.

MCOs do not have any mandates under EMTALA, and these organizations are not prohibited from communicating to patients that they may disallow payment for these OON emergency-care costs. Nevertheless, the non-MCO physician and hospital are obliged to provide the initial medical screening examination and stabilizing treatment. The patient is afforded the protection of EMTALA until this stabilization occurs, unless the patient refuses to continue being treated at the non-MCO facility after being advised of the potential risks.

Managed-care-initiated transfers are more easily justified if the transfer is an improvement in the level of patient care available. For example, there is potential benefit to transferring a trauma patient from an OON hospital without trauma center designation to an MCO facility that is also a designated trauma center. There also may be potential benefit to transferring a patient with possible myocardial ischemia from a hospital without advanced cardiac capabilities to an MCO facility that also has the ability to do cardiac catheterization and coronary artery bypass surgery. Using the opposite argument, it would be unwise to transfer these same patients from tertiary-care facilities to MCO hospitals that cannot handle potential complications of their illnesses.

When considering the transfer of a MCO member, the treating physician must certify that the patient has been stabilized to the level that can be attained within the sending hospital. The risk of transfer should not outweigh the benefit. The attending physician who is directly treating the patient must be comfortable that the patient's condition will not be untowardly affected by the transfer or the level of care that can be provided by the receiving physician and facility. The sending physician must agree to transfer the patient. Disagreements at this level should be solved by the MCO with the out-of-system facility's utilization review staff or administration. EMS systems should avoid being placed in an adversarial position between the MCO and out-of-system providers or facilities.

The sending physician is responsible for arranging an appropriately equipped and staffed vehicle for transport. This may place the desire of the MCO to have their contracted EMS unit perform the transfer in conflict with the sending physician's comfort with the level of care provided during the transport for which he is responsible. This conflict can be resolved if the MCO gains a reputation of working with high-quality EMS providers who have strong medical direction and are able to provide all levels of patient care, from BLS transport to highly specialized critical-care transport.

MCOs should define appropriate response times and levels of care for EMS providers within their contracts with these providers.[34] Some MCOs have developed unique groups of physicians who are prepared diplomatically and clinically to coordinate the care to out-of-network MCO patients. In some cases these physicians respond to the out-of-network facility to assist in managing the case and share in the responsibility for the patient's care.[35]

Desired attributes of a successful repatriation system include:

- Convenient and prompt communication is available between the OON physician and an MCO physician.

- MCO physician should be experienced with critical care, cardiology, trauma, pediatrics, subspecialty care, and EMS transportation issues, or they should have immediate access to expertise in each of these fields. Emergency Medicine specialists are uniquely qualified for this role due to their breadth of experience with acute medical conditions, familiarity with EMS systems, and 24-hour availability.

- MCO physician should have the ability to rapidly approve further care at the initial institution, accept patient to the MCO facility, arrange admission to a medically appropriate MCO facility, and arrange transportation with an appropriate vehicle, equipment, and staff.

- The MCO repatriation plan should incorporate the EMS medical director to assure that the contracted EMS system has the ability to transport all types of patients while providing all appropriate levels of care.

- EMS legislation varies greatly among states, and issues of legislative authority may restrict the scope of practice of EMS systems providing critical-care inter-facility transports.

- Unless a patient is being transferred to receive care that is not available at the sending institution, they should not be repatriated until the sending physician agrees that the patient is stable, and is comfortable that the transferring EMS service can provide care for any reasonably anticipated complications.

Cultural Issues

Many EMS providers entered careers for the traditional "lights and sirens," high adrenaline, lifesaving roles of EMS. Traditional EMS training has not included the topics of customer service, care during inter-facility transportation, and basics of medical economics. As systems change to accommodate the needs of managed care partners, EMS personnel will have a significant shift in their scope of practice and job expectations. The system designs and job responsibilities that are related to successful EMS within managed care contracts will require EMS practitioners to possess these additional customer service skills. Failure to make this transition may lead to frustration and burn-out among EMS personnel.

Summary

EMS faces many challenges in the era of managed care. On the other hand, changes in the healthcare industry that have been driven by managed care can be looked upon as opportunity for EMS. The consolidation of the healthcare industry, hospital closures, emergency departments becoming urgicare centers, an increase in the home management of many medical conditions, and the need to move many patients from out-of-network facilities are all tremendous opportunities for EMS. There is an increasing need for coordinated EMS systems that can provide all levels of patient care and transportation to MCOs over the large geographical regions covered by these insurance plans.

As these external forces applied by managed care change the paradigm of EMS, there is an increased need for data collection and interpretation, outcome studies, and increasingly honed quality improvement. The EMS medical director must remain an advocate of the patient to assure that changes in systems and protocol still allow the EMS system to provide quality emergency medical care to the community while pursuing the opportunities for EMS in managed care.

References

1. Inglehart JK. The American health care system: managed care. *NEJM.* 1992;327:742–747.
2. United States General Accounting Office. *Managed Health Care: Effect on Employers' Costs Difficult to Measure.* Washington DC: GAO/HRD-94-3, (October 1993):1–16.
3. Kongstvedt PR. *Essentials of Managed Health Care.* Gaithersburg, Maryland: Aspen Publication; 1995.
4. Starr P. *The Social Transformation of American Medicine.* New York: Basic Books; 1982.
5. Shortell SM, Gillies RR, Anderson SA. The new world of managed care: creating organized delivery systems. *Health Affairs.* 1994;13:46–64.
6. *New York Times,* February 19, 1971.
7. Brown E, Sindelar J. The emergent problem of ambulance misuse. *Ann Emerg Med.* 1993;22:646–650.
8. Vickery DM, Lynch WD. Demand management: enabling patients to use medical care appropriately. *JOEM.* 1995;37(5):551–557.
9. Axene DV, Lucas OM. How is risk measured? In: Pyenson BS, ed. *Calculated Risk: A Provider's Guide to Assessing and Controlling the Financial Risk of Managed Care.* Chicago: American Hospital Publishing, Inc.; 1995.
10. Selden BS, Schnitzer PG, Nolan FX, Veronesi JF. The "no-patient" run: 2,698 patients evaluated but not transported by paramedics. *Prehosp Disaster Med.* 1991;6: 135–142.
11. Personal communication with William E. Collins, Director, Office of Emergency Medical Services, Multnomah County, Oregon. April 1997.
12. Personal Communication with Skeen, CEO, American Medical Response Northwest. July 1997.
13. Neely KW. Multiple option decisions points: an emerging view of EMS. *JEMS.* 1997;22(3):56–65.
14. A Task Force Report on the Future of Emergency Medical Services, Alameda County Health Care Services Agency, 1994.
15. Neely KW. Demand management: the new view of EMS? [editorial]. *Prehosp Emerg Care.* 1997;1:114–118.
16. Williams RM. The costs of visits to emergency departments. *N Engl J Med.* 1996;334:642–646.
17. Dickenson E, Verdile VP. Managed care organizations: a link in the chain of survival? *Ann Emerg Med.* 1996;28 (6):719–721.
18. Hossfeld G, Ryan M. HMOs and utilization of emergency medical services: a metropolitan survey. *Ann Emerg Med.* 1989;18:374–377.
19. Billittier IV AJ, Moscati R, Janicke D, et al. A multisite survey of factors contributing to medically unnecessary ambulance transports. *Acad Emerg Med.* 1996;3:1046–1052.
20. Morris DL, Cross AB. Is the emergency ambulance service abused? *BMJ.* 1980;12:121–123.
21. Pennycook AG, Makower RM, Morrison WG. Use of the emergency ambulance service to an inner city accident and emergency department—a comparison of general practitioner and '999' calls. *The Royal Society of Medicine.* 1991;84:726–727.

22. Webb BW, Christoforo J. The use and mis-use of ambulance services by the population using emergency department at the Hospital of St. Raphael. *Conn Med.* 1974;38 (4):195–197.

23. O'Leary C, Bury G, McCabe M, et al. Ambulance-user analysis in an accident and emergency department. *Irish Med J.* 1987;80(12):422–426.

24. Rademaker AW, Powell DG, Read JH. Inappropriate use and unmet need in paramedic and non-paramedic ambulance systems. *Ann Emerg Med.* 1987;16(5):67–70.

25. Neely KW for the NAEMSP Managed Care Task Force. Managed care and EMS: an interrogatory model to assist communities in evaluating innovative partnerships. *Prehosp Emerg Care.* 2000;4:274–279.

26. Personal Communication with Robert Porter, EMS System Consultant. Sept. 2000.

27. Coulter C. Out of network, not out of mind. *HMO Magazine.* 1993;34(2)13–15.

28. Colorado Medical Society. Guidelines for appropriate care: Guidelines for appropriate treatment of managed care plan subscribers requiring emergency medical care. *Colorado Medicine.* 1991;88(8):242–244.

29. Shelton SL, Swor RA, Domier RM, et al. Medical direction of interfacility transports. *Prehosp Emerg Care.* 2000;4:361–364.

30. Wuerz RC, Meador SA. Adverse events during interfacility transports. *Prehosp Disaster Med.* 1994;9:50–53.

31. Wood JP. Emergency physician's obligations to managed care patients under COBRA. *Acad Emerg Med.* 1996; 3:794–800.

32. Brown LC, Paine SJ. The interaction between emergency transfer law and managed care: providers between a rock and a hard place. *Health Care Law Newsletter.* 1994;9(4): 8–11.

33. Dunn JD. Legal aspects of transfers. *Prob Critical Care.* 1990;4(4):447–458.

34. Karez A, Burke M, Lampre J. Managed care and emergency care: a risk management perspective. *J Healthcare Risk Management.* 1994;14(4):30–35.

35. McCormick B. Managed Care M*A*S*H. *American Medical News.* 1995;38(41):22.

Epilogue

Alexander E. Kuehl, MD, MPM

I n May of 1989 when the Epilogue of the original text was written, the four megatrends were discussed as forces that would likely influence the evolution of EMS in the 1990s. They were:

1. Increased availability of dramatic new technologies.
2. Increased demand for cost efficient *and* medically proven innovations.
3. Increased debate concerning the need for and the role of medical oversight.
4. Continued paradoxical resistance to change.

Since those megatrends did not summate in a single vector, we also predicted friction and heat, ultimately to be followed by significant and perhaps cataclysmic changes in health care delivery.

In 1993 we added four additional megatrends, which were:

5. Expanded areas of operational responsibility for medical oversight.
6. More consolidation of EMS activities.
7. Aggressive preparation for catastrophic incidents.
8. Even more friction, heat, and cataclysmic change.

In this edition, we again will review, reframe and reorder these original predictions, along with two others for the first years of the new millennium:

9. A growing concern for the well being of those who provide service.
10. An increasing focus on the inappropriate use of lights and sirens by EMS providers.

Technological Opportunities

Few recognized the speed with which the automated external defibrillator (AED) would sweep into and alter our profession; even fewer fully comprehended how rapidly every level of prehospital provider would be assigned the device and that the entire prehospital approach to the early treatment of sudden cardiac arrest would change. We watched in awe as long-standing and restrictive laws, rules, and regulations simply evaporated in the face of overwhelming provider and consumer demand. As a result of the introduction of the AED, the number of potential EMS system configurations expanded exponentially. In the near future, new technologies will favor specific operational configurations; the evolutionally successful configurations likely will be those that are most efficient.

The American Heart Association Statement on Early Defibrillation, written in June 1991, encouraged all EMS responders and vehicles to carry the AED. While early CPR and traditional ACLS may still be important, they will be continually reevaluated with regard to operational objectives, clinical interventions, achievable response times, and logical educational requirements. As first opined in the first edition, if a reliable AED had existed in the late 1960s when the early EMS physicians first took the hospital coronary care unit to the patient, paramedicine, as we currently know it, would never have been invented. Cardiac rhythm recognition and therefore sophisticated understanding of cardiac pathophysiology would not have been mission critical educational objectives.

Another device now has spread rapidly throughout the prehospital arena, the pulse oximeter. While its emergency assessment and operational values are impressive enough, it is astounding that the amount of education necessary to put this fifth vital sign, meaningfully and competently, in the hands of all levels of prehospital providers is but a tiny fraction of any provider curriculum.

Additional technological advances should be expected. How long will it be before an automated venous cannulator (AVC) is marketed? How would an AVC change the practice of prehospital medicine? Legions of "basic" providers could give IV medications for certain easily taught indications. After a fashion, intra osseous infusions are the first generation AVCs for children, and perhaps even adults.

Already there are airways available that may be impossible to use incorrectly. The combitube and AED were joined to create an entirely new and very efficient universal provider in the province of Quebec.

Following the acceptance of technological developments the only limitations to their clinical proliferation are the costs of equipment, of education, and of personnel.

While the evaluation of new technologies will remain a critical function of medical oversight, no medical director will be able to prevent the implementation of a new cost efficient, and medically proven technology; conversely it will be critical to medical directors to avoid the adoption of interventions that are not *both* efficient and proven.

The budget pressures of the 1990s may be diminishing and, if so, will be replaced by the mandate to implement those initiatives demanded by new science, by revenue enhancement or by the customers. The phenomenally rapid incorporation of AED into our routine prehospital practice was mentioned earlier as an example of the first megatrend; however, it is perhaps an even better example of consumer demand.

The requirements to prove economical efficiency and clinical efficacy will intensify if the economy goes into recession. The *current* conventional wisdom in health care is that efficiency, quality, and customer satisfaction are requirements of both managed care and managed competition; however, in the increasingly expensive health care environment to come, the *new* conventional wisdom may be that aggressive cost cutting is the only requirement. Unless there is both political and medical consensus, coupled with a real willingness by society to forgo financial support of other deserving and demanding public services, budget directors will simply "just say no" to medical technologies and health service enhancements that are not inexpensive and proven. EMS remains in unrestrained competition with all the other public safety and public health services; it is even in competition with emergency medicine. Most EMS leaders are in the awkward political posture of pursuing a larger percentage of a shrinking budget. In spite of a recent "windfall" for terrorism preparedness, the problem of financing is only going to get worse. Of course, this problem is not limited to EMS. Our entire health care system is a runaway train careening down a steep incline; EMS is simply the caboose. The question is not if, but rather when, the train will plummet off the tracks. Historically, seconds before or after such an

economic derailment, there occurs a political and sometimes cataclysmic solution; however, the solution may not necessarily appear in the form of a new tax-supported government program. Rather, it could spring from the purchasers of health care, that is, the employers who have been in managed competition for years. Increasingly, they will offer, as a benefit, financial support for the consumer-employee to purchase the level of health care coverage that makes sense for the individual. The fix may be even more radical; why was health care ever linked to an individual's employment? The employee-consumer, with or without an employer contribution, will be encouraged to buy insurance against the possibility of catastrophic health care costs; lesser expenses and predictable costs will be paid out of pocket or through a medical savings account. The days of first dollar insurance coverage are disappearing. The implications for both prehospital and emergency medicine are significant.

It is difficult to conceive of a future health system that is not multi-tiered and it is entirely possible that state or federal administrations will choose to develop a variation of the single payor system, if only for a minimal level of basic health care needs. The individuals and families currently covered by governmental programs (the medically indigent, children, mothers and the elderly) may have most health services covered, but access will be limited to those providers who accept low margin reimbursement agreements.

There will be increased pressure on prehospital services to limit interventions to only those that are perceived by the purchasers and, to a lesser degree, by the consumers to be vital to the mission. Costs will be of paramount importance.

Some individual jurisdictions logically may choose to support publicly financed prehospital systems to serve the entire population base for routine emergency care and disaster responses. Such efforts, whether government run or contracted out, will be financially constrained to limit services to those that are *both* efficient and of proven value.

Advantages of scale, especially in purchasing, and medically proven clinical pathways will be two of the engines. Expanding the role of the prehospital provider may well be a third.

Greater Consolidation

The trend toward consolidation is much more nebulous and more complicated that the others. For years there has been a gradual shift away from government providers toward the public utility and privatized models of EMS. The shift likely will continue so long as models survive better in new health care environment. While it is possible that in some jurisdictions an existing public safety or public health agency provider, such as the fire department, will become the most economically efficient and therefore the surviving provider; it is also possible that efficient private-public monopolistic partnerships will develop. Even in a pluralistic EMS system, there will be pressures for consolidations of administrative, operational, and medical oversight.

There may be continued problems caused by consolidation. Throughout the history of medicine, and more recently in the EMS arena, the marketing, educational, research, and clinical components of health have been financially intertwined. Many of the EMS consolidations of the 1990s were driven not by operational logic, but by speculative logic (or crooked accountants) that created bad mergers which initially looked good on a balance sheet, in a jurisdictional budget or as part of an IPO.

Consider also the example of the development of a national EMS provider curricula. Sponsoring organizations, authors, textbook publishers, educators, college administrators, government bureaucrats, and training equipment manufacturers all have financial interests, some not so obvious, in expanding potentially profitable markets by orchestrating the establishment of national standards of provider curricula, equipment and operational levels. In reality, a locally developed and implemented response, reacting to local needs and resources may be preferable to national EMS standards with their interlocking corporate, organizational, educational and financial linkages. National level EMS providers and standard approaches to clinical issues have not been particularly successful.

To look at this issue another way, it is necessary to remember the differences between "top down" and "bottom up" innovation. The concept of EMT-A was diffused to the local level primarily by a national standard curriculum. Initially paramedic programs evolved locally; only later did national standardization appear. However local adoption of the multitude of subsequent paramedic interventions was driven to a large degree by the faith that medical science could and should be transfered into the field. Ultimately, the intermediate levels emerged as a composite of "top down" EMT-As and "bottom up" paramedics,

modified by local medical needs, local economic resources, and local political forces.

In retrospect, the regional EMS programs established in response to the 1974 federal EMS legislation, were the unintentional incubators of intermediate levels of providers. Currently the specific needs of consolidated health providers, whether public or private, are diverging as the various organizations evolve to be economically successful in a specific niche in an ever changing health care environment. Similarly, it may become impossible for a single ambulance provider to respond satisfactorily to the varying requirements of the various health care systems operating in a given area. In addition, there are problems for the consolidated health care providers as they try to standardize their programs over several geographically adjacent EMS regions. Even within an EMS region, it is difficult to standardize operational and medical policies when the consolidated health providers are all trying new and different approaches to become efficient and to gain market share.

The growth of competitive managed care programs, along with less generous government reimbursement, have already forced efficiencies, price reductions and diminished profits for EMS providers. Initially some EMS providers were fully integrated along with other segments of health care into large managed care conglomerates. Few of these efforts have been successful. There is little incentive to perform any intervention or service unless it reduces the overall cost of caring for the patient or increases reimbursement. There is no guaranteed monetary credit for good quality, for high patient satisfaction, or even for using costly services. As an example, the use of a cardiac monitor or paramedic on routine calls no longer generates increased revenues, only increased expenses; systems that formerly used only paramedics have lost most of their reimbursement advantages. In fact, in the future, it may not be cost effective to use paramedics at all, unless they can be shown to eventually lower total health care costs through a refinement of their function that somehow keeps patients well. Most recently, the long awaited results of the Ontario implementation of paramedics study (OPELS) demonstrated no benefit for the millions of dollars that were spent. Just as fire departments have entered into the EMS arena to justify under used staffing levels and facilities, so will EMS providers look to expand reimbursable clinical roles for their personnel so as to become more cost effective. The assumption of new roles in prevention and disaster mitigation have been emphasized throughout this book and surely will continue to grow.

Medical Oversight

While there is a relatively subdued and continuing debate comparing standing orders and direct medical oversight, of more basic significance is the fact that some EMS systems have gone for long periods without permanent medical directors. In some cases the delay was caused by difficulties in adequately defining the structural interfaces among medical directors, administrative leaders, and field providers. There have been continued turnovers of EMS medical directors; these turnovers usually are not about personalities, but rather about differences of opinion about the scope of medical oversight.

While the early and passionate arguments for total prehospital provider independence from medical oversight have diminished, there remains on the part of the field providers and systemic administrators a gradual philosophical drift toward independent licensing and away from traditional "Simon Says" medical oversight. Paradoxically, the increasing presence of physician responders in the field encourages that drift just as much as the growth of scientific, professional, economic and political power by the field providers and their professional organizations. In some jurisdictions the trend toward independence has been accelerated by a flagging of interest in medical oversight from the physician community or by the abdication of medical oversight responsibility to nurses, residents, and field supervisors. If this trend continues, medical oversight, at least in a traditionally structured fashion, will become irrelevant. For example, the need for extensive direct medical oversight has ebbed as many EMS medical directors have become content to rely more heavily on the contemporaneous interpretation of cardiac rhythms by providers, the interpretation of AEDs, and the use of standing orders, rather than on telemetry and direct medical oversight. Often there has not been a counter balance expansion of indirect medical oversight through new curricula, better education and expanded QM when standing orders have been extended.

Two areas of potential expansion of medical oversight are the call receiving and dispatching phases of EMS; they are quickly and appropriately become the purview of medical oversight. These aspects of the EMS response have already altered how the public views EMS and how it examines itself. The importance of these two inextricably linked phases of the EMS response were recognized and highlighted in the early 1980s; however, they were rarely packaged together in a fashion that could influence more than one dispatch center at a time. Today, fully integrated call receiving, prearrival instructing, and priority dispatching are being implemented rapidly, similarly, and simultaneously in many languages and in many locations. The possibility of a safe alternative to dispatching an expensive paramedic team or even an ambulance on every call is emerging.

Another operational aspect that will be more emphasized is that of the first responders. Their role is rapidly expanding. First responders are being incorporated within the authority of the EMS system administrator and of medical oversight. There is an obvious synergy of the first responder with the advances in emergency medical dispatching; well-structured and medically approved dispatch and prearrival instructions, coupled with the availability of devices such as the AED, combitube, and pulse oximeter, greatly expand the role of the potentially omnipresent and marginally inexpensive first responder. Since the initial education and continued training requirements of first responders are minuscule when compared to those required of paramedics, innovative medical oversight, conscientious providers, and responsive government are encouraging the first responder as an essential fundamental building block of sophisticated EMS. In rural areas around the country non EMT drivers bring the ambulance to the patient, only then to be joined by the medical provider. A quarter of a century of preoccupation with increasingly more sophisticated federally approved ambulances and nationally standardized providers may be coming to a close. No one will accept a return to the days of funeral home station wagons and untrained or unsupervised providers; however, cheaper and more efficient alternatives to national (or even regional) consensus positions are emerging at a local level.

The continued use of the current highly educated paramedics has become financially prohibitive. If they are to continue to exist, their roles and the role of medical oversight must be expanded to either increase useful patient access or to reduce the total cost of health care. For example, if paramedics could give tetanus prophylaxis for a puncture wound and then leave the patient at home with access to appropriate follow up, that would be very cost efficient, as long as the additional expenses for education and employment did not surpass the savings. Enlightened medical oversight must lead the way and be prepared to dedicate much effort and time to the process. It is difficult to imagine a natural consensus leading such changes.

Resistance to Innovation

If only because of the availability of AED, the past decade has been marked by significant clinical and structural innovation in EMS, perhaps more than in the entire previous quarter of a century. These innovations have not been limited to clinical interventions but also include organizational, educational, and administrative advances. Paradoxically, even in the face of medical innovation, operational innovation appears to be slowing because of the growing difficulty in proving real relevance, efficiency, and need. Operational innovation is also waning because of organizational inertia, political ossification, and economic paralysis; EMS gridlock may develop. The gridlock phenomenon is one that occurs regularly with the maturation of any human endeavor or body of knowledge; status quo sets in and, without strong demands for improved efficiency, legitimate threats of litigation, or imminent dangers of economic collapse, little happens. While some positive changes are on the horizon, inertia and resistance to change are growing almost as quickly as is the need for change.

The problems surrounding vehicle operations, use of lights-and-siren, and ambulance accidents have leapt into the national spotlight; they will most assuredly require the attention of medical oversight. There is a worsening epidemic of inappropriate behavior in regard to ambulance operations; it will take the combination of administrative responsibility, medical oversight, and personnel education to recover credibility in this area. The role of medical oversight will be to define when, if ever, providers can bend or break motor vehicle laws. Since the consequences of such actions are immense, the exceptions will be few.

With all due respect to the Agenda and the Blueprint, the last decade did not create a national momentum for useful and necessary change in EMS. National consensus has never come easily to EMS and it is increasingly apparent that consensus and momentum for change is becoming even more elusive. If relatively predictable and linear evolutionary progress does not occur, there may be sudden and potentially disruptive mutations that effectively scramble all the traditional rules. One need only observe the changes in medicine, public health and

EMS since 9-11 to appreciate the effect of non-linear evolution on American health care. Does anyone believe that other social or economic events, currently unimaginable by the main stream, will not disrupt the future linear evolution of EMS.

Two extreme possibilities are that EMS, perhaps along with the rest of health care, becomes either a government franchised monopoly or an operating component of one of the few surviving vertically integrated providers. There appears to be a growing role for "niche" providers created by or subcontracted to the consolidating healthcare providers so as to take advantage of new reimbursement rules and to game the health care system. In these new situations innovations are very locality specific and may not be available to all the providers in a region, leading to an even greater disparity in clinical and/or destination protocols.

The resistance to change in prehospital care is apparent in national organizations, in governmental bureaucracies, and in the providers themselves. In some jurisdictions the specter of a new type of prehospital provider delivering primary and preventative care from a mobile unit has caused entrenched EMS providers, who have long fought change, now to offer up traditional sacred cows rather than allow a paradigm shift in their profession. Across the country, fire services that avoided EMS involvement for decades are now embracing this *other* lifesaving role with a passion driven by fewer fires and less money. Those organizations that blindly resist change risk having the epitaph "save 9-1-1 for *real* emergencies" on their gravestones.

Catastrophic Incidents

Since the events of September 11, 2001 the leaders of prehospital, emergency, and disaster medicine have redoubled their efforts to cooperate in the delivery of the simple message that EMS systems must organize within themselves and within the entire national health care grid to efficiently prepare for the prevention of, the mitigation of, and the response to medically catastrophic incidents. In truth that cooperation began a decade ago during the initial months of Operation Desert Shield/Desert Storm when local EMS agencies found major tasks and impossible responsibilities thrust upon them. A series of natural disasters accelerated the awareness that, in spite of an earlier false confidence, the EMS systems of localities and even of states could not deal with prolonged or paralytic catastrophes without outside assistance. In September 1992, the natural disasters of Hurricanes Andrew and Iniki etched into the national awareness both the fragile nature of our foothold on this planet and the serious shortcomings of many aspects of the existing system of national disaster medical response. Those particular crises resolved; however, it is irrefutable that both our civilian and military casualty systems must be capable of a large scale mobilization in hours, not in weeks. The September 2001 terrorist events underscored these concerns for the entire nation. Although some progress had been made in preparing for and responding to sudden violent events, this new awareness has led to a vastly expanded local and national focus on disaster response and mitigation. Ironically, the failure of EMS to embrace a broader role in the 1990s has required traditional public health agencies now to expand into the area of biohazard response.

The EMS legislative actions of the mid 1970s created regional dinosaurs that all but perished when the climate changed and federal money disappeared. Now organizational and legislative efforts must focus on creating systems that will not only satisfactorily function in both routine and disaster situations but will evolve successfully into the future.

While the same mistakes are often made at each new potential injury creating event (PICE), there is little doubt the public and political reaction to failures has sent a sharply focused demand for competence from those who are administratively and medically accountable for the responses before, during, and after the next PICE. The failure to immediately secure and evacuate the twin towers is a dramatic and tragic recent example. Unfortunately it may be years before all the lessons of September 2001 are fully recognized, understood and applied within our systems. In order for the PICE emergency medical activities to function well, local EMS systems must be created that can operate efficiently on a normal day, every day.

Care of the Providers

There is a major crisis developing in the EMS arena. Prehospital care is personnel intensive and many of the providers, while well motivated, do not have career paths that are attractive. Many of the providers are firefighters first and health providers second. That factor, coupled with the extensive volunteer base means that there is a huge turnover of EMS workers and that EMS often remains a steppingstone to other police, fire, or health careers. The already limited career advancement opportunities will likely become fewer if paramedicine declines in importance. Attrition is rife and reciprocity is seriously limited. While it is possible that new roles for providers will emerge and perhaps will allow career minded individuals to develop more fulfilled lives, the crisis is here now. It has been exacerbated by the social changes created by the increased numbers of double income families and single parent households.

EMS leaders must create for its providers an educational and operational continuum that simultaneously provides personal, professional, and clinical satisfaction so that the providers can follow an individualized lifelong progressive pathway of continuous enrichment and meaningful contribution. For this to occur, medical oversight probably should encourage all future national provider levels to be established as practical educational and operational floors and neither rigid ceilings or wishful optimals. Graduation of current providers to a more advanced clinical level should result from an identified local clinical need, measurable educational success, and careful operational expansion. Easier reciprocity is crucial in our increasingly mobile society and is a strong incentive for similar education baselines.

There has been a growing awareness and significant progress in the emotional support of personnel following stressful events and in protecting providers from hazardous environmental and infectious conditions; but not all these problems have been totally solved. Even more widespread are the deleterious effects on providers caused by the everyday stresses and challenges of their profession. Estimates of yearly turnover range as high as forty percent in some areas. Part of that is caused by the relatively low pay coupled with a nearly full employment economy. Part is driven by dual earner families and single parent homes. Medical directors increasingly will be challenged to balance the very real personal needs of providers for self actualization and security with both the needs of the patients and the financial limitations of those paying for the services.

More Friction, Heat, and Change

The potential of friction, heat, and cataclysmic change in the EMS arena remains. To those readers with considerable EMS experience, the friction and heat are easily sensed, although the specific causes may not be altogether obvious; however, the near universality of those two natural by-products of every day EMS activity should be apparent even to those with relatively little real-time experience.

Actually predicting how EMS will either gradually evolve or suddenly mutate is a much more difficult task than simply sensing the friction and heat. Few looking ahead from three decades ago would have imagined the current state of prehospital and disaster medicine, much less the evolving revolution in health care. The 2002 changes in Medicare reimbursement of ambulance services will change the direction of development of EMS in the United States, as will the World Trade Center PICE. As those and other revolutions alter the EMS landscape, the chances for personal success, or even for professional survival by EMS physicians, are not particularly great; however, as Louis Pasteur reflected over a century ago: "Chance favors the prepared mind." The new generation of EMS medical directors will find themselves continually responding to friction, heat and change; the awareness that conflicts are inevitable and that paradym change is impossible to predict will increase their chances for survival.

To Close

Before medical decisions can be made and before operational models can be chosen, the physicians responsible for EMS medical oversight must identify the business that they and the EMS system really operate. The business is not simply reducing morbidity and saving lives. In part, EMS and the medical directors are in the business of successfully planning and directing the medical aspects of the entire prehospital service or system within a rapidly changing competitive environment. Collectively they are also in the business of defining their profession, while individually they are defining their own practice of medicine.

Even if this text is completely on target and even if all the megatrends vector to a single clear indication of the direction of future change, individual medical directors still will be forced to make rapid and difficult decisions without ever really understanding all the rules, facts, or implications. Therefore, no matter what occurs, they must be prepared to accept responsibility for system failures.

However, they should expect that they will not be publicly second guessed by the medical community, the emergency medicine community, and most of all, not by their EMS medical director colleagues. This should be true whether the medical directors are in Paris, New York, or Salt Lake City.

Ultimately, it is incumbent on the medical directors to convince society that EMS success is less expensive than EMS failure. A solid appreciation of the public health model of EMS, which invariably places the good of the many over the good of the few (in contradistinction to either the public safety or the emergency medicine models), is probably the best compass for those who chose "in twilight dim" to be teachers, designers, leaders, and shapers of prehospital systems and medical oversight.

Introduction to Glossary

The glossary is a compendium of terminology commonly used in and by EMS systems; it has been expanded, revised, and reframed since the previous editions. Where there exist multiple terms describing the same activity or element, we have chosen the most common or most descriptive term. The consistent and universal use of these definitions will lead to increased terminology standardization, better mutual understanding and, ultimately, the stronger professionalization of our field of endeavor. We realize that our vocabulary and our terminology are fluid, evolving almost as rapidly as our form and our function respond to new problems; therefore, we request that you submit new terms, definitions and usages for inclusion in the glossary of the future editions to:

Alexander Kuehl, MD, MPH
"Le Fleuve"
Morristown, New York 13664

EMS TIME/TERMINOLOGY

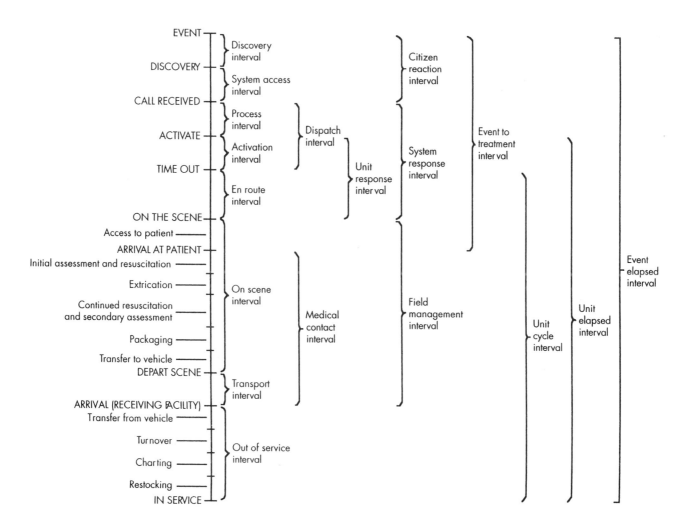

Glossary

9-1-1: A telecommunications system devised to centralize and simplify requests for emergency services by channeling all calls to a single 9-1-1 number. Calls for true emergencies may then be screened and relayed to appropriate agencies and areas for response.

9-1-1-E: 9-1-1-Enhanced. A 9-1-1 system with computer capability to locate the address and phone number of the originating call, thus allowing more efficient and rapid response to emergency calls.

Abandonment: The unilateral termination of a patient/care provider relationship by the care provider without an adequate contemporaneous hand-off to another provider.

Access to patient: The interval from arrival On the scene until arrival at the patient.

Activation interval: The time interval from Activation to initiation of response.

Activation: A sequence of events that begins when an EMS system begins a standard response to a reported event. When a unit is notified to respond.

Advance directive: An individual's express advance desire regarding medical treatment should they be incapacitated, usually expressed in the form of a living will or durable power of attorney.

Advanced CPR is the addition of invasive maneuvers to restore effective ventilation and circulation. Advanced airway maneuvers consist of interventions such as bag-valve-mask ventilation, endotracheal intubation, or needle cricothyrotomy. Advanced circulatory support may result from administration of endotracheal or intravenous medication or use of cardiopulmonary bypass.

Advanced life support (ALS): The term used to describe the capability of a medical response team to render sophisticated life support procedures beyond basic life support. Traditionally requires medical oversight. Usually implies the pre-hospital and inter-hospital emergency medical care of serious illness or injury by appropriately trained health professionals and by EMT-Paramedics or EMT-Intermediates.

Advanced Life Support, Level 1 (ALS1): Transportation by ground ambulance vehicle, medically necessary supplies and services, and either an ALS assessment by ALS personnel or the provision of at least one ALS intervention.

Advanced Life Support, Level 2 (ALS2): Transportation by ground ambulance vehicle, medically necessary supplies and services, and the administration of at least three medications by intravenous push/bolus or by continuous infusion excluding crystalloid, hypotonic, isotonic, and hypertonic solutions (Dextrose, Normal Saline, Ringer's Lactate); or transportation of medically necessary supplies and services, and the provision of at least one of the following ALS procedures: manual defibrillation/cardioversion, endotracheal intubation, central venous line, cardiac pacing, chest decompression, surgical airway, or intraosseous line.

Against medical advice (AMA): A phrase used to describe the process and documentation required, when a competent patient refuses offered health care. This term usually applies to cases where the patient leaves a health care facility. A standard form should be used to document the circumstances surrounding the refusal of medical assistance.

Air ambulance: A rotorcraft or fixed wing craft licensed by the appropriate agency for use as an EMS vehicle. Licensing requirements vary from state to state.

Air medical transport: The transport of medical patients by air vehicles.

Air medicine crew (AMC): The members of air medical transport team.

Air medicine: The study of medicine and physiology in an aviation environment.

Algorithm: The procedure developed or endorsed by the medical oversight for prehospital personnel to follow in aid responses.

Allocation: Distribution of finite resources.

AM: Amplitude modulation.

Ambulance call report (ACR): A regional name for prehospital care report (PCR).

Ambulance service affiliate number: The number assigned by the DOT to an ambulance service.

Ambulance service: An entity, which regularly engages in the business or service of providing emergency medical care and transportation of patients.

Ambulance trip number: A unique number assigned to an ambulance response and recorded on the Ambulance Report Form.

Ambulance: A vehicle certified by federal, state, and local authorities as meeting specifications for transporting and caring for patients. This term generally refers to a wheeled vehicle, but many include boats, planes, helicopters, and other specialized vehicles. Regionally called a "bus," "ambu," "truck" or "rig."

Arrival at patient: Point when aid team arrives at the patient's side, after gaining access, and before initial assessment.

Arrival at receiving facility: The point when an EMS unit reaches a receiving facility (most often a hospital) and stops before transferring patient from vehicle.

Associate hospital: A hospital in a designated EMS area, other than the resource hospital, which may provide medical oversight for EMS personnel.

Audio: Pertaining to sounds that can usually be heard by the unaided ear. Usually in the frequency 15 to 20,000 cycles per second.

Automated external defibrillator (AED): A portable device to electronically assess a patient's cardiac rhythm and to shock if appropriate.

Autonomy: The person's right to self-determination.

Available: EMS unit is in-service and ready to respond to an additional assignment.

Back up: An additional resource, that is, an ambulance or extra personnel available in case the primary resource is unavailable, inappropriate, or inadequate for the situation.

Base communication center: The facility with equipment (radios, antennas, recorders and telephones) and trained personnel to provide community access to the EMS system and ensure communication among the prehospital and hospital components of the EMS system.

Base station: A designated resource responsible for medical oversight in a defined EMS area. Major functions as delegated by the EMS medical director may include implementing protocols, monitoring compliance (through indirect medical oversight), offering direct medical oversight, and providing education to EMS personnel. The base station may be operated from a hospital, which is then referred to as the base station hospital or base hospital.

Baseline bloods: Blood specimens drawn prior to hospital arrival.

Basic CPR: An attempt to restore effective ventilation, using expired air inflation of the lungs, and circulation, using external compressions of the chest wall. Basic CPR airway maneuvers includes noninvasive methods of opening the airway and application of cricoid pressure. Rescuers may provide ventilation with airway adjuncts, such as mouth-to-mask ventilation and face shields appropriate for use by the lay public. This definition excludes the use of bag-valve-mask devices as well as invasive airway maneuvers.

Basic life support (BLS): Transportation by ground ambulance vehicle and medically necessary supplies and services, plus the provision of BLS ambulance services. The ambulance must be staffed by an individual who is qualified in accordance with State and local laws as an emergency medical technician-basic (EMT-Basic). These laws vary from State to State. For example, only in some States is an EMT-Basic permitted to operate limited equipment on board the vehicle, assist more qualified personnel in performing assessments and interventions, and establish a peripheral intravenous (IV) line.

Beneficence: Acting in the best interest of the patient.

Biotelemetry: The technique of measuring and transmitting physiologic data to a distant terminal, usually the base station, receiving hospital, or direct medical oversight.

Body fluid isolation: The procedure of using barriers for self-protection when handling blood or body fluids.

Brain death: The cessation of brain stem functions. Also known as biological death.

Broken up: A term that refers to incomplete understanding of sentences or phrases because of intermittent disruption in communication.

Burn-out: A psychological condition caused by various factors with multiple manifestations that results in EMS personnel being unhappy and dissatisfied with their work. A state of fatigue or frustration brought about by devotion to a cause, way of life, or relationship.

Bypass: A regional term for the process by which a hospital requests that an ambulance patient be taken to another hospital; a request that is usually due to a shortage of beds, equipment, or personnel. See Diversion.

Bystander aid: The initial medical assistance provided to a victim by a witness or passerby at the scene of an event.

Call received: The point when an EMS system is first contacted. Ideally, the first ring of the telephone or first call on a radio.

Call receiving operator (CRO): The individual who receives calls for assistance and inputs information for dispatch.

Call-response interval: The period of time from receipt of a call by EMS system dispatchers to the moment that the emergency response vehicle stops at the resuscitation scene. This interval includes the time required to process the call, dispatch emergency personnel, move personnel from their quarters to the emergency vehicle, start the vehicle in motion, and travel to the scene.

Call screening: The process of determining which requests for assistance require an EMS response, for which a decision is made to provide services, to refuse service, or to refer service to an alternative provider.

Call: (1) A request for assistance that activates the EMS system. It may come through a variety of mechanisms: voice, regular telephone, 9-1-1, or radio. (2) The overall EMS response best summarized by the events occurring during the Unit Elapsed Interval. May be referred to as run response, or more properly an incident.

Car 1: The mayor, governor or chief executive.

Car 802: The EMS medical director.

Cardiopulmonary resuscitation (CPR): A broad term describing the attempt to restore spontaneous, effective ventilation and circulation.

Case law: A judicial precedent in which an appellate court renders a written decision based on the facts of the specific case as opposed to statutes which establish codification of law in the abstract.

Categorization: The classification of receiving medical facilities, using standards of medical care, according to emergency medical capabilities. A circular categorization is an agreement between hospitals for providing care and resources. A horizontal categorization indicates the capability of a facility (hospital) to provide general emergency medical care. A vertical categorization indicates the capability of a facility (hospital) to provide special care (for example, burn center, trauma center, and neonatal center).

Central dispatch: (1) An EMS designated mechanism for directing the closest appropriate resources to the scene of a request for assistance. (2) The consolidation of multiple emergency dispatch centers into a single combined dispatch entity.

CFR: Certified First Responder.

Channel: For EMS this term usually refers to a pair of radio frequencies, one for transmit and one for receive.

Charting: (1) The process of documenting information on ambulance call report (medical incident report). (2) The interval required to complete the prehospital care report, typically occurring after turnover of a patient at the receiving facility.

Chassis: The actual transceiver unit normally mounted separately from the control head.

ChemTrec hot line: A telephone number for chemical industry hazardous material information. (800) 424-9300.

Critical incident stress debriefing (CISD) team: A professional team that assists emergency services personnel with acutely stressful incidents or calls.

Citizen band (CB): A group of 40 VHF low-band frequencies for use by private citizens.

Citizen reaction interval: The time interval from event to call received. Includes discovery and system access interval.

Clinical death: The cessation of respiration with the loss of pulse and blood pressure. (See also Brain death.)

Closest available: The ambulance, which as a result of a combination of location and other factors, such as traffic conditions, weather, and the like, can reach a patient most promptly.

Code: (1) Refers to code status. This term is the process and decision of specifying a patient's legal status and desire for life-sustaining treatment; it is also the process of providing resuscitative measures, that is, cardiac resuscitation (running a code). (2) A commonly used EMS term to describe the nature of a response in relation to use of warning signals and relative urgency of the call. A number accompanying the word refers to the relative priority of the response. Other terms used may include Bell (3 bell, 4 bell). This terminology varies regionally.

Cold response: Universal term for emergency vehicle response mode that does not utilize lights and sirens.

Common law: Judge-made law—rulings of judicial decisions; also referred as case law—a source of law based on custom.

Communication system: A system that links the many inter-department agencies and facilities involved in emergency response and care.

Computer-aided dispatch (CAD): The process of directing EMS resources to caller locations with the assistance of electronic data concerning system status.

Confidentiality: The assurance that patient information will not be revealed to any source other than those sharing the same duty in the care of the patient.

Continued resuscitation and secondary assessment: The interval following Initial Assessment, Extrication, and before Packaging.

Control head: The part of the radio that allows the operator to do designated functions with that radio.

Core data: Data elements that should always be collected and reported. They include characteristics of the patient, prehospital EMS system, emergency department or hospital resuscitation system, as well as those elements describing resuscitation outcomes. Core data are essential for comparative analysis of different EMS systems. When possible, core data should be the same as "essential data" recommended for prehospital data recording.

Cover: Unit is responding for or being transferred to another location or station.

Coverage: Indicates the geographic area where reliable communications exist. Usually expressed in terms of miles.

Critical incident stress debriefing: The formal decompression and discussion following an emotional EMS event.

Divers assistance network (DAN): A telephone number for emergency hyperbaric therapy information. (919) 684-8111.

Dead on arrival (DOA): Patient pronounced deceased shortly after (1) the prehospital providers reach the scene or (2) the ambulance reaches the ED.

Dead spot: An area where radio communications are limited due to geography, terrain, and equipment.

Death: Irreversible cessation of circulatory and respiratory functions or irreversible cessation of all functions of the brain including the brain stem.

Dedicated line: A communication system reserved for use specifically from any one resource to another. Generally refers to a reserved telephone line for use between facilities.

Depart scene: The point when an EMS unit leaves from the scene.

Designation: Formally recognizing a resource on its merits including geography, demographics, and capabilities, then permitting it to function within an EMS system.

Diagnosis base curriculum: The style of prehospital teaching based on making a diagnosis, rather than treating symptoms.

Direct medical oversight: (1) The clinical instructions, usually from physicians, or from specially trained medical personnel, to EMS field personnel. (2) The physician charged with medical oversight delegates this function to a physician providing immediate and concurrent clinical direction to field personnel (DMOP).

Disaster: A situation in which the severity of damage or the number of patients exceeds the ability to provide immediate management. Also called a catastrophic event.

Disaster plan: Prospective arrangements that are initiated in response to a potentially overwhelming situation.

Discovery interval: The time interval between Event and Discovery.

Discovery: The point when an individual recognizes that EMS assistance is needed.

Dispatch interval: The time interval from Call Received until EMS Activation. The interval from Call Received to Time Out.

Dispatch priorities: Predetermined, systemized dispatcher interrogation protocols designed to obtain the minimum amount of information necessary to adequately establish the correct level of response and determine the need for pre-arrival instructions.

Dispatch: (1) The means by which emergency resources are directed to the scene of an incident or event. (2) The portion of a command center that directs vehicles to a scene.

Dispatcher: An individual who alerts an EMS unit to a call for assistance and directs it to the scene.

Diversion: The preferred term for the process of formally directing EMS units to bypass a hospital when the unit has patients for which the hospital is unable to provide optimal care (usually because of an adverse situation, a temporary absence of personnel or needed equipment, etc).

Divert: To reroute EMS to another hospital or another incident.

Do not resuscitate (DNR) orders: An order written in a hospital chart by a physician limiting cardiopulmonary resuscitation in the event of arrest. This has recently been expanded in some jurisdictions to encompass portable documents that can be respected by EMS personnel. Also described as do not attempt resuscitation (DNAR) orders.

DOT: U.S. Department of Transportation.

Down time: The time interval from a morbid event until resuscitation is begun.

Dual response: A dispatch pattern in which a basic and a more sophisticated EMS team are simultaneously dispatched at the first request for assistance.

Durable power of attorney: An advance written directive by an individual expressing their desire to have another act as the decision maker in the care they receive if the individual becomes incompetent.

ETA: Estimated time of arrival. The length of time it will take to get to a certain location.

Eight hundred (800) MHz: Refers to communication systems using this frequency.

EMD: (1) Emergency medical dispatch. (2) Emergency medical dispatcher. An individual trained in interrogation techniques, call prioritization and pre-arrival instructions with a minimum of 24 to 40 hours of training.

Emergency rule: Legal and ethical premise that presumes that the patient with a life threatening condition allows the treatment which is necessary to save his or her life.

Emergency: A combination of circumstances resulting in a need for immediate medical intervention.

EMS system: The arrangement of personnel, facilities and equipment for the effective and coordinated delivery of EMS required in the prevention and management of incidents which occur either as a result of a medical emergency or of an accident, natural disaster or similar situation. EMS systems refer to the broad range of emergency care from the prehospital first responder to the intensive care unit setting.

EMS: Emergency Medical Services. A collective term describing the many agencies, personnel, and institutions involved in planning for, providing, and monitoring emergency care. Frequently refers only to prehospital care.

EMT-Basic (emergency medical technician-basic): An individual trained to provide pre-hospital emergency medical treatment and certified as such by the DOT in accordance with the current National Standard Curriculum for basic emt's, as set forth in this part.

EMT-Paramedic: An individual who is trained to provide pre-hospital emergency medical treatment at an advanced level and certified as such by the DOT under current National Standard Curriculum.

EMT: Emergency medical technician. The generic term for any prehospital provider trained to one of the levels set forth in the current National Standard Curriculum.

EMT-A: Emergency medical technician-ambulance. The original and now obsolete term for EMT-B.

EMT-B: Emergency medical technician-basic. A prehospital basic life support care provider with approximately 110 hours of classroom and didactic training based on a national standard training curriculum originally referred to as EMT-A.

EMT-D: An EMT who has been taught defibrillation skills, either automated, semi-automated, or manual.

EMT-I: Emergency medical technician-intermediate. An EMT with additional training in one or more advanced methodologies such as intubation and IV access.

En route interval: The time interval from Time Out to On the Scene.

En route: The time when a responder is travelling to or from a scene.

Event elapsed interval: The time interval from event to in service.

Event to treatment interval: The time interval from event until initial assessment begins.

Event: A prehospital occurrence, generally considered by an observer or patient to require EMS assistance.

Extrication: (1) The process of removing patients from wreckage or other hazardous locations. May require use of special tools and equipment. (2) Extrication: The interval from Initial Assessment and Resuscitation to Continued Resuscitation and Secondary Assessment.

False imprisonment: The unjustified detention of a person, so as to substantially interfere with the person's liberty.

Federal Communication Commission (FCC): The United States governmental authority responsible for allocating communication channels and regulating communications systems.

Field: Any locale outside a hospital.

Field management interval: The time interval from On the Scene to Arrival at Receiving Facility.

Field release: Non transport situation in which a patient is released from the care of EMS provider, the legal authority to permit an adult, who is able to make treatment decisions, to refuse treatment. This term may also refer to the interaction of the EMS provider with the patient at the scene in which the patient signs a release form or waiver form in which the patient releases the EMS provider of liability for the patient's refusal to be transported or treated by EMS provider.

First in: The initially dispatched unit in a tiered response system.

First party caller: A person calling for emergency medical help who is also the patient or victim.

First responder (FR): (1) The first individual designated to provide medical assistance in an emergency. The degree of training varies by jurisdiction but includes minimum first aid instructions on the airway management, cervical spine control, breathing assistance, circulation assistance, hemorrhage control, and basic patient movement skills. (2) A graduate of a formal approximately 60 hour course in critical emergency medical care termed certified first responder (CFR). (3) A term that may refer to the first bystander or witness to render assistance, no matter what their training. This assistance should more correctly be referred to as bystander aid.

Fixed Wing Air Ambulance (FW): Transportation by a fixed wing aircraft that is certified as a fixed wing air ambulance and such services and supplies as may be medically necessary. Air ambulance services are covered when the point from which the beneficiary is transported to the nearest hospital with appropriate facilities is inaccessible by land vehicle, great distances, or other obstacles (for example, heavy traffic) and the beneficiary's medical condition is not appropriate for transport by either BLS or ALS ground ambulance.

Fixed wing aircraft: Airplane.

Fourth party caller: A person calling for emergency medical help who is not only remote from the patient but is relaying the information from associated public safety agencies, security agency dispatchers, and "medical alert" companies.

Frequency band: A continuous range of frequencies such as VHF low band, VHF high band, and UHF.

Frequency: The number of cycles per unit of time. Radio frequencies are often measured in megahertz (millions of cycles per second).

Garbled: A term that describes a radio transmission that is unintelligible or difficult to interpret because of poor transmission or reception.

Geographic assignment: Assignment of a frequency for dedicated use within a geographic area.

GigaHertz (GHz): A billion cycles/second.

Good Samaritan law: A statute that affords immunity to a person who offers assistance to another, without a duty to do so, and without expectation of remuneration. Strictly construed, it does not include the prehospital provider who has a duty to respond or provide care.

Governmental immunity: A statutory provision that prohibits liability for damages where governmental employees, agents, or officers or the governmental entity has been negligent. Generally, such statutes apply only for certain aspects of governmental activities and have exclusions, such as operation of an emergency vehicle and willful misconduct. In addition, immunity provisions also affect claims for violation of constitutional rights.

Hand-off: The Process of turning the care of a patient over to another appropriately qualified individual. For example, an EMT-B would hand off a patient to another EMT-B, paramedic or physician.

HazMat: Hazardous material.

Hospital emergency administrative radio (HEAR): A VHF communication system used when telephonic communications are inoperative. Also used for hospital-ambulance communications.

HEMS: Helicopter Emergency Medical Services.

Hertz (Hz): Frequency unit in cycles per second.

HIPPA: Federal "Health Insurance Portability and Privacy Act" which establishes the basis for health care confidentiality regulations.

Horizontal dispatch: A dispatch configuration where several dispatchers divide individual responsibilities between call interrogation and radio dispatch functions. Also called tandem or team dispatching.

Hospital interval: The interval of time from arrival at hospital until back in service.

Hot response: Universal term for the emergency vehicle response mode that utilizes red-lights-and-siren; is the current preferred terminology rather than various ten code or code numeric designations. Also referred to as emergency or code response.

Immunity: An exemption from duties the law generally requires others to perform.

In service: The point when ambulance and crew are available for appropriate dispatch.

Incident location: The geographic site of an emergency usually indicated by minor civil division code number.

Indirect medical oversight: The administrative medical direction of EMS personnel by a physician usually designated by medical oversight. This direction includes system design, management, education, critiques, and quality management. The physician is usually responsible for developing protocols, and medical policies, ensuring compliance, and certifying providers. Some aspects of indirect medical oversight may be delegated to other physicians or non-physicians. Responsibilities may broaden as delegated by medical oversight. Often described as prospective, retrospective or concurrent with the scene care.

Informed consent: Autonomous decision made by the patient to agree to treatment or intervention after understanding the risks, benefits and alternatives.

Initial assessment and resuscitation: Duties performed during the time interval from access to patient until either extrication or secondary survey.

Key questions: The predetermined, systemized dispatcher interrogation protocols designed to obtain the minimum amount of information necessary to adequately establish the correct level of response and determine the need for pre-arrival instructions.

Lead agency: The organizational unit established under a federal, state, or regional authority and given the responsibility and authority to plan, implement, evaluate, and generally direct an EMS system.

Lights-and-siren: Using visual and audio warning devices to indicate an emergency vehicle. In some jurisdictions, such use allows selected traffic laws to be broken. Should be restricted to proven need.

Living will: An advance written directive by an individual by expressing their desire for medical care if they are no longer competent. The concept is legal in most states.

Low band: The frequency range of 30–50 MHz.

Mass casualty incident: An obsolete expression for a disaster. Should not be confused with multiple casualty incidents.

MAST: (1) Military Anti-shock Trousers is a term for pneumatic anti-shock garment. (2) Military Assistance to Safety and Traffic (military helicopters used by civilian EMS systems).

Matrix: An electronic switching device used to routre calls to designated points similar to a telephone switchboard.

Maximal response: The credo in public safety agencies that mandates a total HOT initial delivery of resources to the scene.

MCI mass casualty incident: A large incident usually requiring multi-service response. See county MCI plan for further.

Medevac: Medical evacuation. Originally used in the military to mean helicopter.

Medical director: A physician, who by experience and/or training, is responsible for the clinical oversight and patient care aspects of the EMS system. This position may include one individual with multiple tasks, or several with divided tasks, such as training director, administrative indirect medical oversight director, clinical direct medical oversight director, or quality management director. There may also be specified state, regional systems, or unit directors.

Medical dispatch center: Any agency that routinely accepts calls for emergency medical assistance from the public and/or that dispatches prehospital emergency medical personnel pursuant to such requests.

Medical oversight: (1) The ultimate responsibility authority for the medical actions taken by a hospital provider or an EMS system. (2) The physician or medical groups assigned such authority. (3) The process of performing actions to ensure that care taken on behalf of ill or injured patients is appropriate. This includes the prospective, concurrent, and retrospective aspects of EMS and extends to various tasks such as quality management, hiring, and education.

Medical oversight contact interval: The time when direct medical oversight authority is in contact with prehospital personnel.

Medical oversight terminal console: A communications device often located in an emergency department for direct medical oversight of an EMS system.

Medical priority dispatch system: A medically supervised system used by medical dispatch center dispatch appropriate aid to medical emergencies, which includes: (1) systematized caller interrogation; (2) systematized Pre-Arrival instructions and (3) protocols which match the dispatcher's evaluation of the injury or illness type and severity with vehicle response mode and configuration.

Medical project director: A physician assigned by an EMS authority by the administrative director to direct a specific EMS team. Occasionally used as a term for the physician providing regional medical oversight.

MICU: mobile intensive care unit: A specially equipped transport vehicle with sophisticated equipment allowing advanced life support capabilities. A hospital medical intensive care unit.

Mobile intensive care nurse (MICN): A nurse with special training in prehospital policies, protocols and procedures. The MICN may have direct and indirect medical care responsibilities. A major role is in answering the radio at the base station, directing field care of patients, and requesting physician consultation as needed. They exist in an official role in only a few states.

Mobile repeater: A fixed transmitter station for relaying and strengthening a transmission from a mobile transmitter.

Mobile transmitter receiver: Vehicle based transmitters/receivers.

Mobile unit: A vehicle or a vehicular radio unit.

Modulation: The voice or tone signal of the radio transmission.

Multiple casualty incident (MCI): A situation with numerous patients that does not overwhelm the routine capacity of the system.

Multiplex operation: A combination of two or more radio signals for simultaneous transmission on one frequency.

Mutual aid response: Response by an ambulance unit to an emergency based on a written agreement between EMS providers whereby the signing parties agree to lend aid to one another under conditions specified in the agreement.

Mutual aid: A term referring to interagency EMS agreements that establish protocols to provide assistance by interacting with other agencies.

Motor vehicle collision (MVC): Previously called motor vehicle accident (MVA).

Negligence: The failure to provide the degree of care (as defined by community or national standard) normally associated with a set of circumstances requiring that care. To establish negligence, the plaintiff must prove four elements: duty to act, breach of that duty, injury, and a clear cause-and-effect relationship between the injury and breach of duty.

Non-transport vehicle: A medical response vehicle that transports medical personnel to the scene of an accident, but is not intended to transport a patient. For example, a rescue vehicle, fire truck, car, and a paramedic response unit are all examples of non-transport vehicles.

Not available: EMS unit is not available to accept additional assignment.

National standard curriculum: Usually refers to the DOT curriculum for a given provider level.

Off-line medical command: Archaic term for indirect medical oversight.

On the scene: The point when an EMS unit arrives.

Out of service interval: The interval between Arrival at Facility and In Service. Includes the turnover of the patient to the hospital staff, charting, and re-stocking. May also refer to time when a unit is not available because of special situations including mechanical breakdown or personnel breaks.

On-line communications: Direct radio or telephonic communications.

On-line medical command: Archaic term for direct medical oversight.

On-location: EMS unit has arrived at the location of the emergency.

On-radio: EMS unit is capable of being contacted by radio.

On-scene interval: Time interval from on the scene to depart scene.

Out-of-hospital provider (OOHP): Current term for a traditional EMS care giver. Previously prehospital or field provider.

Packaging: (1) Preparing the patient for transfer to a transport vehicle. Includes such tasks as dressing, bandaging, splinting, and immobilization. (2) Interval of time required to package a patient.

Pager: A radio receiving device for alerting personnel, usually by a tone signal.

Paramedic ALS Intercept (PI): EMT-Paramedic services furnished by an entity that does not furnish the ground ambulance transport, provided the service meets specified requirements.

Paramedic response unit (PRU): A non transporting vehicle used by advanced providers.

Paramedic: The generic term for a prehospital care provider with an adequate number of training hours (usually between 300 and 1500 hours) and procedural experience to be certified by local, state, and/or national authorities as capable of providing advanced cardiac life support and other medically sophisticated skills.

Patch: The process of connecting the communications system of one party into the communications system of another party, usually through a third party such as base station.

Penetration: The ability of a radio signal to go through or around physicial obstructions.

Phone patch: An electronic or acoustic linking of radio transmitter and receiver to a telephone line.

Phonetic alphabet: Distinctive words used instead of letters for clarity in radio communication, such as Alpha-A, Bravo-B, and Charlie-C.

Physician option: Possible medical orders from direct medical oversight, beyond standing orders in a clinical protocol.

Pneumatic antishock garment (PASG): Preferred name for military anti-shock trousers (MAST). A pneumatic counter pressure device applied to lower extremities and abdomen.

Police powers: The power of the state (organized government) to place restraints on the personal freedom and property rights of a person for the protection of public safety, health and welfare or promotion of public good.

Portable transmitter/receiver: A hand carried transmitter/receiver used when away from vehicles. These generally have less power and distance capability than mobile and base transmitter/receiver.

Potential injury creating event (PICE): A disaster. A system for classification of disasters.

Pre-arrival instructions (PAI): Telephone instructions given word for word by trained dispatchers to callers to aid the victim and direct the situation prior to arrival of prehospital personnel. They are given from medically approved written protocols as opposed to prearrival advice, which is not.

Prehospital care provider: EMS personnel who are certified and function at any level in actually dispensing prehospital care.

Prehospital care report (PCR): Preferred term for the written documentation of EMS patient contact and assistance. Other names include medical incident report, run report, prehospital care report, patient care report, etc.

Prehospital personnel: Any EMS members, providers of care, or others who are involved in the direct functioning of the EMS system. Also called field personnel, (archaically) out-of-hospital providers and ambulance drivers or attendants.

Prepare to copy: Transmitted to unit as a fore-warning that the next message will be an emergency call dispatch.

Priority system: A spectrum of patient problems that are commonly life threatening and must be assessed quickly by field personnel. These include abnormal breathing, unconsciousness, and chest pain in people of cardiac-disease-susceptible age, dangerous trauma, and dangerous hemorrhage.

Priority: When transmitted, means that the following message is an emergency and must have immediate attention. All system users will stand by until the message is acknowledged.

Proceed: Unit has been given clearance to transmit their message.

Process interval: The interval from Call Received until Activation.

Protocols: Written procedures providing prehospital personnel with a standardized approach to commonly encountered patient problems, thus ensuring consistent care. They may include standing orders to be carried out prior to establishing communication with direct medical oversight. These procedures usually relate to the assessment, diagnosis, triage, treatment, transfer, and destination of patients.

PTT switch: A push to talk switch found on a microphone that allows a radio transmission to be made when depressed.

Public safety answering port (PSAP): That location and staff where 9-1-1 calls are processed and responses dispatched.

Push-to-talk: A method of transmission from only one station at a time; the user being required to keep the switch open while talking.

Quality assurance (QA): The original organized method of auditing, evaluating and improving care provided within EMS systems.

Quality improvement (QI): The concept of a continual cycle of evaluation and improvement.

Quality management (QM): The term embracing and replacing the evolving concepts of QA and QI.

Radio frequency (RF): A term used in radio communications to designate the cycles per second, or Hertz, for the purpose of identifying specific channels of communications assigned by FCC. Commonly used in EMS are VHF, UHF, and 800 MHz.

Range: The effective transmission distance for radio communication; usually measured in miles.

Receiving hospital: An emergency department participating in a local 9-1-1 EMS System.

Recertification: A structured process used to evaluate providers every few years to assure review of skills and maintenance of competency.

Reduced speed: All responding units will turn off emergency warning lights and sirens and proceed into scene as normal vehicle.

Refresher course: A standard and often required program to prepare prehospital providers for recertification exams.

Refusal: (1) The ambulance crew member's decision not to provide patient transport. Should involve protocol or a medical decision with the direct medical oversight. The decision is based on clinical judgement, community standards, and common sense. (2) The patient's refusal to accept care and/or transport. The patient's mental competence should be evaluated before accepting a patient's refusal. Commonly referred to as refusal of medical advice (RMA).

Regionalization: A system that addresses emergency care needs in a defined geographic region through identification and classification of medical resources. It is intended to improve the quality of care in a cost-effective way and to facilitate the coordination or handling of responses to emergency medical incidents.

Relay: The rebroadcast of signals by radio station as soon as they are received, enabling transmission of the signal further than could have been accomplished by the originating transmitter.

Relief: New or additional personnel or assistance. The next shift.

Relocate: Unit covering more than one area from a central location.

Remote center: A facility containing the equipment, personnel, or both to handle EMS communications.

Remote tower or transmitter: A base station at a distant point operated by either telephone lines or special radio signals to receive or transmit to units and enable improved radio reliability.

Repeat: Restate the last message/transmission.

Repeater station: Communications equipment that receives a signal and retransmits it to improve the range and quality of the signal. Generally requires two frequencies, one to receive and one to transmit.

Re-route: A regional term for diversion.

Rescue: An emergency rescue vehicle equipped to remove or free trapped victims.

Resource hospital: A hospital in an EMS system that is granted and provides logistical and/or supervising responsibilities for EMS personnel in a geographic area. Often the resource hospital monitors and/or assists direct and indirect medical oversight functions.

Responder: An individual who assists with scene patient care. May be a citizen trained in first aid and cardiopulmonary resuscitation, or an EMS representative such as a paramedic.

Responding: EMS unit is enroute to assigned location of emergency as dispatched.

Response configuration: Specific vehicle(s) of varied types, capabilities, and numbers responding to the scene of a medical emergency, also defined as the dispatch priority response assignment.

Response interval: The time interval from Time Out until EMS vehicle is On the Scene.

Response mode: The use of emergency driving techniques, such as lights and siren versus routine driving.

Response time: The temporal interval between "dispatch" or "call receipt" and arrival "at patient" or "at scene." Often reported and rarely accurate.

Response zone: Geographical area of service responsibility for a specific EMS unit. Also referred to as primary area of response.

Restocking: (1) The process of refurbishing supplies and preparing equipment after one response and in preparation for another response. (2) The interval required for refurbishing supplies and preparing equipment.

Resuscitation (CPR): The combined effect to restore or maintain ventilation circulation, and/or acceptable physiologic function.

Return of spontaneous circulation (ROSC): Refers to the return of palpable, spontaneous central pulses in a cardiac arrest patient, regardless of their duration.

Rotary Wing Air Ambulance (RW): Transportation by a helicopter that is certified as an ambulance and such services and supplies as may be medically necessary. Air ambulance services are covered when the point from which the beneficiary is transported to the nearest hospital with appropriate facilities is inaccessible by land vehicle, great distances, or other obstacles (for example, heavy traffic) and the beneficiary's medical condition is not appropriate for transport by either BLS or ALS ground ambulance.

Rotorcraft: Helicopter.

Run: A response by an EMS system to call.

Run review: A quality management mechanism that reviews calls for assistance and ambulance requests to determine if proper procedures were followed and proper treatment given. Also referred to as Call Review.

Run report: Regional name for prehospital care report (PCR).

Run tape: A record of audio communication between the field provider and direct medical oversight.

Search and Rescue (SAR): The initial EMS response where the exact location of the victim is not known.

Saturation: The inability of an EMS system to respond appropriately to additional requests for assistance.

Say Again: Radio term meaning "Repeat what was just said."

Scene: Geographical area where the event occurred.

Second party caller: A person calling for emergency medical help who is in direct personal contact with the patient.

Simplex: A radio communication system that permits either transmission or reception at any one time.

Skip: The bouncing of signals either off the atmosphere or off buildings causing an abnormal signal projection that may carry great distance and may interfere with radio communications.

Special operations: Functional teams for activities falling outside the normal ones; often law enforcement related.

Special service: Any piece of equipment used for specialized service, i.e. Air cascade, light wagon, utility, etc.

Specialty Care Transport (SCT): Interfacility transportation of a critically injured or ill beneficiary by a ground ambulance vehicle, including medically necessary supplies and services, at a level of service beyond the scope of the EMT-Paramedic. SCT is necessary when a beneficiary's condition requires ongoing care that must be furnished by one or more health professionals in an appropriate specialty area, for example, nursing, emergency medicine, respiratory care, cardiovascular care, or a paramedic with additional training.

Specialty referral center (SRC): A facility dedicated to and recognized as a resource in caring for specific medical problems, such as a trauma center or a burn center.

Staging: A standby position away from any hazards of the scene. Or in a position as to not block means of egress for other units.

Standing orders: Instructions approved by medical oversight for prehospital care personnel, directing them to perform certain emergency medical care in the absence of any communication with direct medical oversight.

Symptom based curriculum: The style of teaching providers based on the physical findings rather than based on diagnosis.

System access interval: The time interval from discovery and call received.

System status management (SSM): A structure of EMS response built around the concept of flexible deployment by time and place.

System response interval: The time interval from call received and on scene.

Telemetry: The technique of measuring physiologic data and transmitting it to a distant location for interpretation. Often refers to transmitted tracings.

Telephone advice: Unscripted and usually *ad lib* information given to callers. Inferior to structured pre-arrival instructions.

Telephone treatment sequence protocols: Specific type of pre-arrival instruction protocols written as algorithmic scripts that are learned and read by the trained dispatcher to the caller over the telephone during life-threatening emergencies. These instructions include airway control, Heimlich maneuver, cardiopulmonary resuscitation, and childbirth.

Ten codes: A method whereby a number preceded by the number 10 is used to designate a specific message; for example, 10-4 means message acknowledged. Meanings can vary from system to system.

Third party caller: A person calling for help who is not in direct personal contact with the patient.

Third service: An EMS responder agency or organization that is independent of police and fire departments.

Tiered response: A multilevel response of emergency assistance, beginning with the closest most basic responder, and progressing to more advanced or more distant responders as needed.

Time out: The point when the EMS unit begins moving to a call for assistance.

Transfer from vehicle: Interval from arrival at receiving facility to turnover of patient.

Transfer to vehicle: The interval from packaging to depart scene.

Transfer: Moving the patient from one medical facility to another.

Transport interval: The interval from departing scene until arrival at the receiving facility.

Trauma center: A designated specialty-receiving center for specifically defined trauma patients. Such a center should have consistent availability of defined services.

Triage: (1) To assign victims a priority for care and transport based on the degree of injury and the individual's relative salvageability in a given situation. (2) In a non-disaster situation, to determine who to transport to the hospital.

Triage care: A non transporting unit which would access and initiate care.

Trip ticket: Regional name for prehospital care report (PCR).

Turnover: (1) The process of transferring care of the patient from prehospital personnel to receiving facility personnel. (2) The interval of time from transfer from vehicle until care accepted by receiving facility.

Ultra high frequency (UHF): This radio band extends from 300 to 3,000 MHz, with most medical communications occurring in the 450–470 MHz range. UHF has better penetration in dense metropolitan areas and inside buildings. UHF has a shorter range than VHF band and is more readily absorbed by environmental objects.

Universal precautions: The procedure of using barriers for self protection when handling blood or certain body fluids of any patient.

Vehicle response configuration: The specific set of vehicle(s) in terms of types, capabilities, and numbers responding as the direct result of actions taken by the emergency medical dispatch system.

Vehicle response mode: The manner of response used by the personnel and vehicles dispatched which reflects the level of urgency of a particular required treatment or transport (e.g., use of emergency driving techniques such as lights and sirens, routine driving).

Vehicular repeater: A transmitter incorporated on an ambulance to relay transmissions from portable transmitters.

Verify: Check for correct information and advise findings of investigation.

Vertical dispatch: Dispatcher configuration where a single dispatcher is responsible for a given geographic area, requiring the dispatcher to handle all functions of interrogation, pre-arrival instructions, and dispatch for each call. Also called solitary dispatching.

Very high band (VHF): This radio band extends from 30 MHz to 175 MHz. Useful for long range radio communications.

VHF high band: Frequencies in the 150 to 175 MHz band.

VHF low band: Frequencies in the 30 to 50 MHz band.

Vicarious liability: A legal doctrine in which the negligent conduct of one person is imputed to another person based on the relationship between the two parties, and irrespective of the faultless conduct of the party to whom the negligent conduct is imputed.

Vital signs: The pulse rate and character, breathing rate and character, blood pressure, and relative or exact skin temperature.

Volunteer ambulance corps (VAC): Groups of trained individuals who voluntarily provide EMS services.

Wake effect: The disruption of traffic and the accidents that occur as a result of the nearby response of an emergency vehicle traveling in emergency response mode.

Watt: A measurement of transmitter power output.

Wilderness emergency medical technician (WEMT): The generic term for any EMS providers working in an austere environment.

Wilderness command physician: The unique term for medical oversight in an unstructured and austere EMS environment.

Willful misconduct: Improperly conducting oneself on purpose, without regard to the consequences of that lack of appropriate behavior or action.

Window phase: The time from exposure to a disease to the time a laboratory test detects the presence of antibody.

Zone: A specific area at an EMS operational site. The cold zone is relatively safe; the warm zone is relatively dangerous; and the hot zone usually is off limits to EMS personnel.

Index

A

Abandonment, geriatric EMS, 561, 969

Abbreviated injury score, EMS systems evaluation, 282

Abdomen, ALOC and, 776

Abdominal pain, obstetric, 720, 724

Ability to refuse treatment/transport, RMA, 515

Abstraction, EMS systems evaluation, 284–85

Abuse, geriatric EMS, 560–61

Abused substances, and mass gathering, 906–7

Access
communications, 163–64
to mass gathering, 907
to patient, defined, 969
pediatric EMS, 542
response phase, 100

Access areas, air services EMS, 573

Access Health, 78

Accidental Death and Disability, 5, 114, 540

Accidents in North American Mountaineering, 59

Accountability, 396–401
civil rights, 396–98
court decisions, 401
federal regulation, 396
Good Samaritan statutes, 400–401
immunity laws, 399–401
legal issues, 396–401
local ordinances, 399
sovereign immunity, 400
state regulations, 398–99

Accuracy, of EMS systems evaluation, 284–85

ACDC (informed consent acronym), 509

Activated charcoal, 653, 746–47

Activation
catastrophic events, 834
defined, 969
interval, defined, 969

Active airway management procedures, 611–17

Activities of daily living (ADL), geriatric, 562

Acute myocardial infarction (AMI), 152. *See also* Cardiac arrest; Dysrhythmia

Acute pulmonary edema (APE), 152–53

Additional subsidization, reimbursement, 141

Adenosine treatment, 687

Adenosine
pharmacotherapy, 645–46
vs. verapamil, 153

Adjuncts, for airway management procedures, 620–22

Administration, nurses and, 456

Administration routes, pharmacotherapy, 642

Administration, indirect medical oversight and, 315–16

Administrative operations. *See* Operations, administrative

Administrative records, communications, 169

Adult learning, 350–53
disruptive students and, 353
future of, 353–54
influencing conditions in, 351
medical oversight and, 350–53
motivation, 351–53
screening, 353

Advance directives, 695, 969

Advanced cardiac life support (ACLS). *See also* Advanced life support
curriculum, 314
national guidelines, 148
nurses and, 453

Advanced CPR, defined, 969

Advanced HazMat Life Support, law and, 398

Advanced life support (ALS). *See also* Advanced cardiac life support
defined, 106, 969
mass gathering, 900
not available, 256–57
procedures, 630–31
resuscitation, 256–57
system design, QM, 362

Advanced trauma life support, national guidelines, 148

AEIOU TIPPS mnemonic, 743–44, 774

Aerial lighting, air services EMS, 574

Aerial reconnaissance, air services EMS, 573

Aerial rescue, air services EMS, 573

Aeromedical capability, and urban EMS, 38

Against medical advice (AMA), defined, 969

Against medical advice (AMA), mass gatherings and, 912

Age. *See also* Geriatric
behavioral EMS and, 767
poisoning and, 744
rural human resources and, 43

Agency for Healthcare Research and Quality (AHRQ), 473

AIDS/HIV, 802–4
communicable diseases, 802–4
occupational exposure to, 803
protective equipment against, 807
status code for, 804
volunteers and, 461

Air ambulance, defined, 969

Air Force Specialty Code (AFSC), 82

Air medical transport, defined, 969

Air medicine, defined, 969

Air medicine crew (AMC), defined, 969

Air services, EMS, 567–75
access areas, 573
aerial reconnaissance, 573
aerial rescue, 573
ambient temperature, 573
electronic medical equipment in, 572
freezing precipitation, 572
goals of, 567
hazardous materials, 573
hearing issues, 571
HEAT, 574
helicopter vs. fixed-wing, 567–68
helicopter operation, 568–71
high-rise emergencies, 574
history of, 567
landing surface, 573
lighting issues, 571–72, 574
mass casualty incidents and, 574
mass gatherings, 574
medical challenges of, 571–72
medical operations, 567–75
operational challenges, 572–73
physiologic issues, 572
search, 574
space issues, 571
teams, 574
visibility, 572
weight issues, 571

Airborne diseases, 802–5

Airplane crashes, 832
Airway management procedures, 609–22
  active, 611–17
  adjuncts for, 620–22
  cardiac arrest and, 698–99
  demand valve, 611
  device comparison, 612
  endotracheal intubation, 611–20
  geriatric EMS, 558
  medical interventions, 149–51
  mouth-to-mask ventilation, 611
  needle thoracostomy, 621
  pediatric, 548–49
  placement confirmation, 617–18
  supplemental oxygen administration, 610
  tube thoracostomy, 621–22
  ventilation, 610–11
Alanine aminotransferase (ALT), 801
Alcohol, inappropriate use and, 593
Alcoholism, and ALOC, 778
Algorithm, defined, 969
Algorithm protocol, for automated defibrillator, 534
Allocation, defined, 969
Altered levels of consciousness (ALOC), 154, 774–82
  abdomen, 776
  AEIOU TIPPS, 774
  alcoholism and, 778
  case studies, 779–81
  chest, 776
  controversies in, 778–79
  evaluation, 774–76
  Glasgow coma scale, 775
  HEENT, 775–76
  medical protocols, 774–82
  protocols, need for, 779
  skin, 776
  treatment, 776–78
Alternative transportation, and inappropriate use, 593
Ambient temperature, air services EMS, 573
Ambulance, defined, 970
Ambulance, inappropriate use, 592–93, 597–98
Ambulance call report (ACR), defined, 970
Ambulance response time, comparison of, 122
Ambulance service
  defined, 970
  model EMS, 25
  system design (EMS), 128–30
Ambulance service affiliate number, defined, 970
Ambulance transport, reimbursement for, 140

Ambulance trip number, defined, 970
Ambulance 2010, 268–69
Ambulance volantes, 3
American Academy of Clinical Toxicology (AACT), 746
American Academy of Orthopedic Surgeons (AAOS), 5–6
American Association of Critical Care Nurses (AACN), 453
American Caving Accidents, 59
American College of Emergency Physicians (ACEP), 7, 9, 16, 828, 894
American College of Surgeons (ACS), 5–6
American College of Surgeons Committee on Trauma (ASCOT), 283, 886, 890
American Heart Association (AHA), 6, 114
American Medical Association (AMA), on teaching of life-saving skills, 428
American Medical Response (AMR), 77–78
American Red Cross, 62
American Society of Anesthesiologists (ASA), 6
American Society for Testing and Materials (ASTM), 14, 52, 63
American Trauma Society, 6
Americans with Disabilities Act (ADA), 397–98, 907
Aminophylline, intravenous, 667
Amiodarone, 110, 646, 699
Amplitude modulation (AM), defined, 969
Analgesia, 659–64
  case studies, 662
  communication techniques, 661
  ketamine, 661
  medical protocols, 659–64
  nitrous oxide use, 659–60, 662
  non-cardiac, 662
  NSAIDs, 661
  pain protocol, 662
  pitfalls of, 661, 663
Analytic statistics, defined, 291
Anaphylactic shock, 155, 651
Anatomic considerations, in resuscitation, 247–48
Angioplasty, 152
Anglo-American, international EMS, 90–91
Anthrax, 842–43
Antiarrythmic medications, 645–48, 699
Anticonvulsants, 649
Antihypertensives, 651–52
Antiterrorism resources, 848

Anxiety disorders, behavioral, 763
Aortic dissection, 652
APGAR scoring system, obstetric, 723
Appropriate use, defined, 599–600
Arlie House Conference, 6
Army Military Occupational Specialty (MOS), 82
Arnett v. Kennedy, 787
ARREST trial, 111
Arrington v. Wong, 875–76
Arrival at patient, defined, 970
Arrival at receiving facility, defined, 970
Arsenic, 653
Aspirin, 152, 648
Assessment, behavioral, 763–70
Assessment, geriatric EMS, 558–59
Associate hospital, defined, 970
Associated Public Safety Communications Officers (APCO), 167
Association of Practitioners for Infection Control (APIC), 455
Associations, EMS, 493–503
Associations, nurses, 452
Asthma
  cardiac arrest, 697
  ethical decision and, 512–13
  shortness of breath, 666–67
Atlanta Olympics (1996), 896, 905
Atracurium, 650
Atropine, 645, 748
Atypical chest pain, 677
Audio, defined, 970
Authority, wilderness EMS, 55
Authorization, medical oversight, 439–45
Automated defibrillator, 530–38
  algorithm protocol for, 534
  background, 530–31
  chain of survival, 531
  devices, 531–35
  external, 269, 970
  levels of, 530
  medical oversight of, 532–35
  operator's checklist for, 536
  patient case record for, 535
Automated external defibrillator (AED), 269, 970
Automated vehicle locator (AVL), 101
Autonomy, defined, 970
Available, defined, 970
Average response time, 122
AVPU mnemonic, 775

B

Babylonian Code of Hammurabi, 3
Bacillus anthracis, 842–43
Back up, defined, 970

Bag-valve-mask (BVM) ventilation, 150, 610–11
Balanced Budget Act of 1997, 136, 140
Baldrige categories, 384
Baldrige National Quality Award, 381
Barnes, Joseph, 3
Barringer, Emily, 4
Barton, Clara, 3
Base communication center, defined, 970
Base station, defined, 970
Baseline bloods, defined, 970
Baseline response choices, dispatch response, 211
Basic CPR, defined, 970
Basic life support (BLS), defined, 106, 970
Basic life support (BLS), mass gathering, 899–900
Basic Trauma Life Support (BTLS), 60, 65, 314
Basing, helicopter EMS, 568
Baxter v. Fulton-DeKalb Hospital Authority, 397
Bedford-Stuyvesant Volunteer Ambulance Corps, 462
Behavioral EMS, 762–73
    age and, 767
    anxiety disorders, 763
    assessment, 763–70
    benzodiazepines, 769–70
    bipolar disorder, 763
    case studies, 771–72
    chemical restraint, 768–69
    controversies in, 770
    depression, 763
    evaluation, 762–63
    medical protocols, 762–73
    neuroleptics, 769
    organic disorders and, 764
    physical restraint, 768
    psychiatric conditions, 763
    rapid tranquilization, 770
    schizophrenia, 763
    substance abuse and, 767–68
    suicidal patient, 765–66
    suicide factors, 766
    treatment, 763–70
    violent patient, 766–67
Benchmarking, 112, 381
Beneficence, defined, 970
Benzodiazepine, 765
    antagonists, pharmacotherapy, 652–53
    behavioral EMS and, 769–70
    poisoning and, 747–48
    protocols for, 146
Beryllium, 110
Beta blocker overdose, 651

Bhopal, India, 832
Bias
    defined, 293
    in politics, 433–34
    in prehospital research, 292–93
Biological agents, WMD and, 843–44, 851
Biological events, terrorism and, 844
Biotelemetry, defined, 970
Biphasic waveform, defibrillation, 699
Bipolar disorder, behavioral, 763
Bishop v. Wood, 786
Bite-speak, media, 481–82
Black's Law Dictionary, 785
Black-letter law, 399
Blinding (in prehospital research), 290–91
Blood, exposure to, 798
Blow-by O_2, pediatric use of, 732
Blue Cross, 12
Blueprint for Education, 10
Blunt trauma, 254–55, 713–14
Board of Regents of State Colleges v. Roth, 786–88
Boddie v. Connecticut, 788
Body fluid isolation, defined, 970
Body-packer, cocaine, 750
Body-stuffer, cocaine, 750
Borderline patients, with dysrhythmias, 686
Botulinum toxin, 843
Boyd, David, 7–8
Bradycardia, symptomatic, 748
Brain death, defined, 970
Brain injury, secondary, 153
Branch Davidian Compound, Texas, 861
Breathing, 558, 730. *See also* Airway management procedures
Breech, obstetric, 722
Bretylium, 647, 699
Broken up, defined, 970
Bromide, 653
Bronchodilators, inhaled, 648–49
Bronchospasm, shortness of breath, 666–67
Brooks v. Herndon Ambulance Service, Inc., 406
Bulb syringes, 72
Burn-out, defined, 971
Burns, interfacility transport for, 579
Burris v. Willis Ind. School District, 788
Bush, George W., 485
Bypass, defined, 971. *See also* Diversion
Bystander aid, defined, 971
Bystander care, NHTSA and, 594, 596
Bystander physician, at scene, 520

C

Calcium, pharmacotherapy, 654
Calcium channel blocker toxicity, 654
Calcium channel blocking agents, poisoning, 748
Calcium channel overdose, 651
Call, defined, 971
Call preplanning, dispatch, 187
Call received, defined, 970
Call receiving operator (CRO), defined, 971
Call response, and inappropriate use, 598
Call screening, defined, 971
Call types, dispatch analysis of, 196–207
Call volume, and urban EMS, 33–34
Caller, and inappropriate use, 595
Call-response interval, defined, 971
Capabilities, WMD planning and, 855
Capitation, managed care, 951
Car 1, defined, 971
Car 802, defined, 971
Carbon monoxide poisoning, 748–49
Carboxyhemoglobin, effects of oxygen on, 749
Cardiac arrest, 693–703. *See also* Dysrhythmia
    airway management, 698–99
    anti-arrhythmic medications, 699
    asthma, 697
    care after resuscitation, 698
    case studies, 700–702
    controversies of, 698–99
    defibrillation vs. CPR, 699
    defibrillation waveform, 699
    differential diagnosis, 697
    direct medical oversight, 696–97
    drug overdose, 698
    evaluation/treatment, 696–98
    hyperkalemia, 697
    hypothermia, 697
    hypovolemia, 698
    medical protocols for, 693–703
    obstetric, 721
    poisoning, 744
    procedures, 624–26
    protocols, need for, 699–700
    response time intervals, 382
    system evaluation/management, 694–96
    toxic agents, 698
    trauma, 697
Cardiac arrest, system evaluation/ management, 694–96
    advance directives, 695
    dead-on-arrival status, 695
    early defibrillation, 694
    equipment, 695
    policy, 695–96

public awareness, 694–95
quality management, 696
rapid response, 694
resuscitation cessation, 695–96
training, 695
Cardiac arrhythmia, 653
Cardiac care, interfacility transport
for, 580
Cardiac cases, unmet need, 594
Cardiac emergencies, medical
interventions, 151–53
Cardiac ischemia, 672–74
Cardiac medications,
pharmacotherapy, 642–45
Cardiac procedures, 624–26
defibrillation, 624–25
external pacing, 625–26
monitoring, 624–25
pericardiocentesis, 626
Cardiopulmonary bypass (CPB), 744
Cardiopulmonary resuscitation (CPR).
See also Resuscitation
closed-chest, 4
defined, 971
media and, 487
Cardiovascular system, geriatric, 560
Care after resuscitation, cardiac arrest,
698
Care records, computerization of, 165
Care under fire, TEMS, 861–62
CareLine, 78
Case entry protocol, 188
Case law, defined, 971
Case review, and ED, 450–51
Case review, QM, 178–79
Case studies
ALOC, 779–81
analgesia, 662
behavioral, 771–72
cardiac arrest, 700–702
chest pain, 680–81
dysrhythmias, 691–92
ethical issues, 420–30
hypotension, 710–11
obstetric, 725–26
pediatric, 738–39
pharmacotherapy, 654–55
poisoning, 759–60
political issues, 432–33
shortness of breath, 670–71
trauma, 715–18
wilderness EMS, 58
Case-control studies, defined, 289
Casualties magnitude, WMD, 845–46
*Catalog of Federal Domestic Assistance
(CFDA)*, 472
Catastrophic disasters, and wilderness
EMS, 59
Catastrophic events, 828–39
activation, 834
disaster, defined, 828–29

etiology, 830–31
federal response plans for, 836–38
implementation, 834–35
incident command system, 829–30
intentional disasters, 832
natural disasters, 831
NDMS, 836–38
operations, 828–39
PICE nomenclature, 829
preparedness, 832–34
recovery, 836
responses phases of, 834–36
technological disasters, 831–32
triage, 830–31
Categorization, defined, 971
Catheter, self-capping, 145
Cathey v. The City of Louisville, 513
Cause-and-effect diagrams, QM,
374–75
Cell phones, medical communications
and, 163–64, 167
Center for Medicare and Medicaid
Services (CMS), 48, 69, 872
Center for the Study of Emergency
Health Services, 13
Centers for Disease Control (CDC)
communicable diseases and, 798
guidelines for antiretroviral drugs,
802
TB guidelines, 805
Central dispatch, defined, 971
Central nervous system (CNS)
GBH and, 751–52
geriatric, 560
hypoperfusion, 684
Central venous access, 623–24
Cerebrovascular insult, 652
Certification, QM dispatch
components, 177
Certification, wilderness EMS, 64–65
Certified first responder (CFR),
defined, 971
Cervical collars, packaging, 627
Cervical immobilizers, packaging,
627–28
Chain of survival, AHA, 114
Chain of survival, automated
defibrillator, 531
Champion trauma, shock and, 708
Channel, defined, 971
Chaotic NCT, 687
Charting, defined, 971
Chassis, defined, 971
Check sheets, QM, 374
Chemical agent release, WMD, 850
Chemical and Biological HelpLine,
846
Chemical and Biological Rapid
Response Team (CBRRT), 847
Chemical Manufacturers Association,
815

Chemical restraint, behavioral,
768–69
Chemical restraint, protocols for, 146
Chemical warfare agents, 843
Chemstrip BG, 651
ChemTrec, 815–16, 971
Chernobyl, 841–42
Chest, ALOC and, 776
Chest pain, 672–82
atypical, 677
cardiac ischemia, 672–74
case studies, 680–81
controversies of, 678–79
elderly patients and, 678
esophagus perforation, 676
evaluation, 672
historical aspects of, 673
hyperventilation, 678
hypotension, 678
medical protocols, 672–82
non-cardiac causes of, 675–77
pain relief, 674–75
pericarditis, 675–76
pneumothorax, 677
protocols, 679
provocation of, 673
pulmonary embolism, 676–77
quality of, 673
radiation of, 673
safe transport and, 674
sample orders for, 680–81
severity of, 673
silent myocardial infarction, 677–78
temporality of, 673
thoracic aorta dissection, 675
treatment, 672–77
women and, 678
Chickenpox, 805
Childbirth, medical interventions at,
155
Chronic obstructive pulmonary
disease (COPD), 151
vs. CHF, 669
geriatrics and, 558
shortness of breath, 666–67, 669
Circulation, geriatric EMS, 558–59
Circulation, pediatric, 730
Circulatory emergencies, 151–53
Citizen band (CB), defined, 971
Citizen reaction interval, defined, 971
Civil rights, accountability, 396–98
Civil Support Teams (CST), WMD
and, 846
Civil War, 3
Civilian community, and military
EMS, 87–88
Civilian-Military Contingency
Hospital System (CMCHS), 837
Classroom arrangement, education
and, 350
Cleary v. American Airlines, 786

Clinical care, 48–49, 930
Clinical death, defined, 971
Clinical effects, of common, poisoning, 745
Clinical interface, prehospital providers in ED, 585–86
Clinical performance comparisons, system design, 120–21
Clinical studies, of PASG, 526
Closed-chest CPR, 4
Closest available, defined, 972
Coastal Corp., 77
Cobb, Leonard, 4
Cobbs v. Grant, 508
COBRA (Consolidated Omnibus Budget Reconciliation Act), 407, 579, 581–82
Cocaine, poisoning, 750
Code, defined, 972
CODES, 266, 285–86
Coding components, terminology, 214
COLD response
    decision-making for, 145, 148
    defined, 101, 972
    vs. HOT response, 145, 148
Columbia Healthcare, 77
Combitube, 109
Commission on Accreditation of Air Medical Services (CAAMS), 570
Commission on Accreditation of Medical Transport Systems (CAMTS), 570
Committee on Trauma, ACS, 42
Common law, defined, 972
Common sense, wilderness EMS and, 54
Communicable diseases, 798–810
    airborne disease, 802–5
    chickenpox, 805
    equipment reprocessing, 808
    exposure clarification, 798–805
    exposure report form for, 809
    hepatitis B virus, 799–800
    hepatitis C virus, 800–802
    HIV/AIDS, 802–4
    medical oversight of, 798
    meningitis, bacterial, 805
    operations, 798–810
    protective equipment against, 807
    treatment, 806
    tuberculosis, 802–5
    varicella zoster, 805
Communication, resuscitation and, 257
Communication techniques, analgesia, 661
Communications, 162–71
    access, 163–64
    administrative records, 169
    cellular telephone, 167

defined, 972
digital technology, 167
dispatch, 164
800 MHz public safety trunking, 167
EMS future of, 929
fire EMS, 69–70
hardware, 166
helicopter EMS, 570
history of, 10
hospital, 168
indirect medical oversight, 310–11
integration of services, 167–68
land mobile satellite, 167
major incident, 168
mass gathering, 907–9
MCI, 822–23
media relations, 169
medical director and, 163
medical oversight, 164–66
microwave relays, 166
military EMS, 86
model EMS, 27
network setup, 169–70
planning, 168
with public, 169
radio telephone switching, 166
records, 168–69
rural EMS, 46
system components, 163–67
system objectives, 162–63
UHF radio, 166
VHF radio, 166
WWW and, 170
Community injury prevention officer (CIPO), 944
Community spirit and, volunteers, 462
Competence, provider level, 111–12
Competencies for EMS Personnel Responding to Hazardous Materials Incidents, 813
Complaints, dispatch response, 213
Comprehensive Environmental Response, Compensation and Liability Act (CERCLA), 812, 842
Computer-aided dispatch (CAD), 69, 101, 123, 175, 972
Computerized Hospital Online Resource Allocation Link (CHORAL), 877
Confidentiality, ethical issues, 425–27
Configuration, dispatch, 188
Configuration, response phase, 101
Conflict, in wilderness EMS, 56
Congestive heart failure (CHF), 667–68
Congressional initiatives, WMD, 846–47

Consciousness, altered levels of. *See* Altered levels of consciousness
Consent strategy, for prehospital research, 294–95
Consolidation, of private EMS, 76–79
Continued resuscitation and secondary assessment, defined, 972
Continuing education
    dispatch components, 177
    risk management, 389
    rural EMS and, 45
Continuous improvement, QM, 356
Continuous positive airway pressure (CPAP), 668
Contracts, legal issues, 414–15
Contracts, with managed care, 951–52
Control, military EMS, 86
Control head, defined, 972
Control pyramid, QM, 365–66
Controlled trial, defined, 290
Controversies
    in ALOC, 778–79
    in behavioral EMS, 770
    of cardiac arrest, 698–99
    of chest pain, 678–79
    of hypotension, 708–9
    in pediatric EMS, 547–51, 737–38
    in poisoning, 758
    of shortness of breath, 669–70
    of trauma, 714–15
Convulsions/seizures protocol, 218
COPD. *See* Chronic obstructive pulmonary disease
Core content involvement, education, 341–42
Core data, defined, 972
Cost, provider level, 111
Cost, of standing orders, vs. direct medical oversight, 322–23
Cost effectiveness, fire EMS, 70
Cost effecteness, funding, EMS, 137
Counter Narcotics Operational Medical Support (CONTOMS), 864, 869
Countershock treatment, for dysrhythmias, 689
County of Hennepin v. Hennepin County Association of Paramedics, 403
Course development, curriculum, 348–49
Court decisions, accountability, 401
Cover, defined, 972
Coverage, defined, 972
COX–2 inhibitors, 661
CPR. *See* Cardiopulmonary resuscitation
Crash Injury Management for the Law Enforcement Officer, 236

Crash Outcomes Data Evaluations System (CODES), 266, 285–86
Credibility, of on-scene supervision, 337
Cricothyrotomy, 618–19
Criminality, WMD and, 845
Crisis services, funding for, 133
Criteria, of inappropriate use, 601–2
Criteria, for termination of resuscitation efforts, 253
Critical care, pediatric EMS, 543
Critical clinical groups, 11
Critical incident stress debriefing (CISD), 917, 972
Critical incident stress management (CISM), 914–19
  comprehensive, 915–16
  debriefings, 917
  defined, 914–15
  defusings, 916–17
  demobilizations, 917
  effectiveness of, 918–19
  guidelines for, 917–18
  individual consultations, 917
  mid-action support, 916
  operations, 914–19
  traumatic stress education, 916–17
Critical patient-care incidents, 391
Cross-sectional designs, defined, 289
Cultural issues, and managed care, 956
Curriculum(a), 347–50
  classroom arrangement in, 350
  course development, 347–50
  first responders, 237–38
  formulation of objectives, 348
  instruction methods, 349
  needs assessment, 348
  prepared, 347
  program delivery, 349–50
  program evaluation, 350
  support materials for, 350
Customer needs, QM, 360–63
Cypress Creek EMS, 462–63

D

Dalton, Edward, 3
Data analysis, prehospital research, 291
Data collection, response phase, 104
Data Elements for Emergency Department Systems (DEEDS), 474
Data generation, QM, 178
Data interpretation, prehospital research, 296
Data needs, managed care, 951
Data outlet, prehospital research, 296–97

Dataset, information systems, 270–71
DDT, 653
Dead on arrival (DOA), 424, 695, 972
Dead spot, defined, 972
Death, defined, 247, 972
Death, on-scene pronouncements of, 253
Debriefing, CISM, 917
Debriefing, MCI, 825
Decertification, QM, 179
DeCicco v. Trinidad Arca Health Association, 412
Decision making, medical interventions, 144
Decontamination. *See* Hazardous materials; Poisoning
Dedicated line, defined, 972
DEEDS dataset, 265
Defibrillation, 530–38. *See also* Automated defibrillator
  cardiac procedures, 624–25
  vs. CPR, 699
  early, cardiac arrest and, 694
  waveform, 699
Defusings, CISM, 916–17
Dehydration, 59
Delayed morbidity prevention, wilderness EMS, 54
Delegation of supervision, on-scene, 337
Demand patterns, 365
Demand valve, 611
Deming experiment, QM, 356–357, 384–85
Demobilizations, CISM, 917
Demographics, of rural EMS, 42
Denial of ambulance transport, 409–11
Depart scene, defined, 972
Department of Health, Education, and Welfare (DHEW), 6
Department of Health and Human Services (DHHS), 13, 837, 848
Department of Transportation. *See* DOT
Department of Veterans Affairs (DVA), 848–49
Dependent variables, defined, 293
Deployment
  fire EMS, 72
  response phase, 100–102
  strategy, response choices, 234
Depression, behavioral, 763
Dermal decontamination, 747
Descriptive statistics, defined, 291
Descriptors, terminology, 214–18
Designation, defined, 972
Designation, of medical facilities. *See* Regionalization
Destination, legal issues, 407–8

Destination selection, response phase, 102–3
Determinant, accuracy of, 180
Determinant code, correctness of, 178
Determinant level, dispatch, 196–207
Determinant matrix, dispatch response, 212
Determinant terminology, 214–18
  coding components, 214
  descriptors, 214–18
  dispatch response, 214–16
  response assignment components, 214–15
Determinant theory, dispatch response, 213–14
Developed curriculum, education, 347–50
Device comparison, airway management, 612
Diabetes, 185
Diagnosis base curriculum, defined, 972
Diazepam, 155
Differential diagnosis, cardiac arrest, 697
Digital endotracheal intubation, 615
Digital technology, 167
Diltiazem, 646–47
Diphenhydramine, 766
Direct liability, legal issues, 402–3
Direct medical oversight. *See* Medical oversight, direct
Direct medical oversight physician (DMOP), 318–329, 519–22
Direct oral endotracheal intubation, 613–14
Director tasks, education, 343–46
Disaster, defined, 828–29, 972
Disaster management, pediatric EMS, 549–50
Disaster medical aid center (DMAC), 835
Disaster Medical Assistance Team (DMAT), 837, 848
Disaster Mortuary Operational Response Team (DMORT), 837, 848
Disaster plan, urban EMS, 38–39, 973
Discipline, of wilderness EMS, 51–53
Discipline algorithm, due process, 790–97
Discovery interval, defined, 973
Dispatch, emergency medical, 172–207
  call preplanning, 187
  call types, analysis of, 196–207
  case entry protocol, 188
  communications, 164
  configurations, 188
  defined, 973

determinant level, 196–207
diabetes and, 185
dispatcher role, 175
fire EMS, 69–70
inappropriate use and, 591–92
information card, 186
legal issues, 404–5
life support, 182
lights-and-siren, 175
man down protocol, 174
medical oversight of, 175–76
medicolegal issues of, 188–89
myths of, 173–75
NAEMSP position statement,
    192–95
pre–arrival instructions, 179–82,
    189
priorities, 184–87
protocol compliance, 183
protocol items, 172
psychological components of,
    183–84
quality management, 176–79
supervision at, 179
unknown problem protocol, 174
Dispatch criteria, helicopter EMS, 570
Dispatch interval, defined, 973
Dispatch priorities, defined, 973
Dispatch response (priority), 208–28
    baseline response choices, 211
    complaints, 213
    determinant matrix, 212
    determinant terminology, 214–18
    determinant theory, 213–14
    EM vehicle collisions, 210
    justification, 211–12
    local development and, 218–19
    maximal response, 208–10
    planning process for, 219–20
    prioritization vs. screening, 212–14
    response code confusion, 215–18
    response configuration, example,
        221
    tiered response, 210–11
Dispatcher, defined, 973
Dispatcher accuracy, and inappropriate
    use, 598
Dispatcher role, 175
Disposition options, response phase,
    102
Disruptive students, and adult
    learning, 353
Divers assistance network (DAN),
    defined, 972
Diversion/bypass operations, 871–85
    approaches to, 876–77
    defined, 973
    effects of, 873–74
    EMTALA and, 875–76
    ethics of, 874–75
    government agencies and, 882

history of, 871–72
hospital overcrowding and, 872–73
legal considerations, 874–75
NAEMSP policy on, 872
NAEMSP position statement on,
    879–82
policy components, 877–78, 882
San Francisco ambulance policy on,
    882–85
Diversity, of international EMS, 90
Divert, defined, 973
Division of Health Assessment and
    Consultation (DHAC), 848
Do not attempt resuscitation
    (DNAR), 252
Do not resuscitate (DNR), 423, 973
DOA (dead on arrival), 424, 695, 973
Dobutamine, 644
Documentation
    legal issues, 413
    patient care incident management,
        393
    of refusal, legal issues, 411
    response phase, 104
    risk management, 389
Doe v. Borough of Barrington, 397
Domestic Emergency Response Team
    (DEST), 853
Domestic preparedness, 322
Donabedian design, QM, 359
Dopamine, 644
DOT (U.S. Department of
    Transportation), 45, 106, 133,
    815, 973
Down time, defined, 973
Droperidol, 146, 769
Drug Abuse Warning Network
    (DAWN), 751
Drug doses, pediatric, 729
Drug inventory, 334
Drug overdose, cardiac arrest from,
    698
Dual response, defined, 973
Due process, 785–97
    defined, 785–88
    discipline algorithm, 790–97
    landmark cases in, 786–88
    mechanics of, 788–789
Durable power of attorney, defined,
    973
Dyspnea, non-traumatic etiology of,
    665. *See also* Shortness of breath
Dysrhythmia, 683–92
    borderline patients with, 686
    case studies, 691–92
    countershock treatment, 689
    duration of, 685
    EKG classification, 684
    evaluation, steps of, 683–88
    history, 686
    medical protocols, 683–92

narrow complex tachysysrhythmias,
    685–88, 691
pediatric, 689
physical exam, 686
prophylactic lidocaine and, 689
protocols, 690–91
rate, 684–85
regularity, 685
renal failure patients and, 690
rhythms strips vs. monitor
    interpretation, 689
stable vs. unstable patients, 683–84
symptom identification, 683
Torsades de Pointes, 689–90
unstable tachydysrhythmias, 685–86
wide complex tachydysrhythmias,
    687–88, 692
Dystocia, shoulder, 722

E

Early defibrillation, cardiac arrest and,
    694
Earthquake, 72, 828–829
Eclampsia, obstetric, 720
Ecology, and mass gathering, 906
Economic efficiency, EMS system
    design, 124–27
Economics, of managed care, 946–51
Education, 340–354
    adult learning, 350–53
    CISM, 916–17
    core content involvement, 341–42
    curriculum and, 347–50
    educator, as MD task, 343
    EMS certification, 343
    EMS program accreditation, 343
    EMS scope of practice model, 342
    EMS standards of, 342
    federal resources for, 475
    indirect medical oversight and,
        314–15
    instructor evaluator, as MD task,
        346
    manager, as MD task, 344
    MD tasks, 343–46
    medical oversight and, 306, 340–54
    of nurses, 454–55
    pediatric EMS, 544
    preceptor, as MD task, 344
    prehospital research and, 297
    prepared curriculum, 347
    rural EMS, 44–46
    skill evaluator, as MD task, 345
    skill instructor, as MD task, 345
    vs. training, 346–47
    urban EMS, 36
    WMD planning, 856
Education systems, EMS future of,
    928

Educational requirements, for medical interventions, 145

Edwin Smith Papyrus, 3

Egalitarian vs. entrepreneurial view, of managed care, 952

800 MHz public safety trunking, 167, 973

EKG
classification, of dysrhythmias, 684
AED and, 533
cardiac arrest and, 698
chest pain and, 673
single vs. twelve-lead, 148
transmission of, 165

Elapsed arrest interval, resuscitation, 248–49

Elderly patients. *See* Geriatric EMS

Electronic medical equipment, in air services EMS, 572

EmCare Corp., 77

Emergency, defined, 973

Emergency Broadcast System (EBS), 833

Emergency department (ED), 449–51, 584–89
case review and, 450–51
clinical interface, 585–86
feedback from, 450
medical operations, 584–89
patient acceptance in, 450
patient care and, 586–89
prehospital providers in, 584–89
reports and, 449
students, 584–85
system problems in, 451
training and, 450

Emergency Department Research Review Committee (EDRRC), 297

Emergency medical dispatch (EMD)
certification standards of, 177
datapoints, 268
defined, 973
inappropriate use and, 595–96

Emergency medical services (EMS). *See* EMS

Emergency Medical Services Authority (EMSA), 127

Emergency Medical Services for Children (EMSC), 14, 728

Emergency Medical Services at Midpassage, 11

Emergency Medical Services Systems (EMSS) Act of 1973, 7, 75–76, 132–33, 229

Emergency medical technician (EMT). *See* EMT

Emergency Medicine Treatment and Active Labor Act (EMTALA), 407, 449, 579–82, 875–76, 954–55

and diversion, 875–76
and interfacility transport, 579–82
and managed care, 954–56

Emergency Nurses Association (ENA), 6, 453

Emergency operations center (EOC), 834

Emergency Physicians Advisory Board (EPAB), 363

Emergency response, and managed care, 953

Emergency response workers, HCV and, 801

Emergency rule, defined, 973

Emergency support function (ESF), 836–37

Emergency vehicle collisions, dispatch response, 210

Emergency vehicle operation course (EVOC), 332

Emesis contraindications, poisoning, 747

Emotional abuse, geriatric EMS, 561

Emotional Content/Cooperation Score (ECCS), 173

Empowerment, medical oversight, 439–45

EMS (emergency medical services)
Agenda for the Future, 923–34
advocacy for, 469
certification, 343
defined, 973
development of, 21
education standards, 342
EMSC, 473–75
fire, 68–74
funding, state methods of, 134
incorporation into public health, 938
information systems, 264–66, 270
initiative for injury prevention, 941–45
law, components of, 22–28
medical director, 137
operations, 266–67
pediatric, 473–75, 541
PIP activities, 944–45
program accreditation, 343
rule-making, 22
rural, 41–50
scope of practice model, 342
systems, 1–96
systems evaluation, 276–87
time terminology, 967
urban, 33–40
wilderness, 51–67

EMS Agenda for the Future, 923–34
clinical care, 930
communications system, 929
creation of, 923

education systems, 928
evaluation, 930–31
healthcare system graphic, 925
human resources, 927
Implementation Guide, 262–63, 931
information systems, 930
integration of health services, 924
legislation, 926
medical oversight, 927–28
prevention, 928–29
public access, 929
public education, 928
regulation, 926
research, 924–26
system finance, 926

EMS for Children (EMSC), 473–75
5 Year Plan, 15
pediatric program, 541
training standards, 544

EMS Education Agenda for the Future, 340–41

EMS system(s), 1–96
defined, 116–17, 973
evaluation of, 276–87
fire, 68–74
history of, 3–19
interdependence of design, 120
international, 90–96
legislation, 20–32
matrix, 121
military, 81–89
models of, 20–32
private, 75–80
rural, 41–50
urban, 33–40
wilderness, 51–67

EMS systems, evaluation of, 276–87
abbreviated injury score, 282
abstraction of, 284–85
accuracy of, 284–85
ASCOT, 283
ICISS, 282–83
injury severity score, 282
methodologies, 281–82
model, 276–78, 278–81
outcomes, 281
planning aspects, 277–79
population-based, 285
process of, 277
process criteria for, 284
reliability of, 284
severity indices, 281–82
strategic model, 278–81
trauma score, 283
TRISS, 283
Utstein style, 280
validity of, 284

EMT (emergency medical technician), 9, 106–10, 973. *See also* Providers, levels of

defined, 973
EMT–A (advanced), 973
EMT–B (basic), 106–9, 974
EMT–D (defibrillator), 398, 974
EMT–I (intermediate), 10, 106–9, 974
EMT–P (paramedic), 9, 106–10, 454, 973
history, 9
mass gathering and, 898–99
National Standard Curriculum, 454
observations vs. standard, 285
provider level, 106–10
in wilderness EMS, 63–64
EMT Legal Bulletin, 189
EMTALA. *See* Emergency Medical Transfer and Active Labor Act
En route interval, defined, 974
Endotracheal intubation, 611–20
    as airway of choice, 150
    airway management procedures, 611–20
    cricothyrotomy, 618–19
    device comparison, 612
    digital, 615
    direct oral, 613–14
    esophageal gastric tube airway (EGTA), 615–16
    esophageal obturator airway (EOA), 615–16
    Esophageal Tracheal Combitube (ETC), 611, 616–17
    gum bougie, 615
    invasive procedures, 618
    laryngeal mask airway (LMA), 617
    laryngoscopic, 613–14
    lighted stylet, 615
    lighted stylets confirmation, 618
    minicricothyrotomy, 619
    nasotracheal, 614
    pharyngo-tracheal lumen airway (PTL), 616–17
    syringe confirmation, 618
    TEMS and, 865
    transtracheal jet ventilation, 619
    tube placement confirmation devices, 150–51
    ventilators, 619–20
Endotracheal pharmacotherapy, 642
Endotracheal tube placement confirmation devices, 150–51
End-tidal CO_2 detectors, 72, 110, 253, 617
Enrollment, response phase, 99–100
Environment, system design, 117
Environment, of volunteers, 460–61
Environmental elements, of mass gathering, 904–7
Epidemiology, and wilderness EMS, 59

Epinephrine, 155, 643–44
Equipment
    cardiac arrest, 695
    for hazardous materials, 814
    legal issues, 413–14
    mass gathering, 899–902
    military EMS, 85–86
    pediatric, 546, 729
    TEMS, 863–64
    wilderness EMS, 60
    WMD, 846
Equipment inventory, EMS physician, 334
Equipment reprocessing, communicable diseases, 808
Equipment usage protective measures, legal issues, 414
Esophageal gastric tube airway (EGTA), 615–16
Esophageal intubation detector (EID), 618
Esophageal Obturator Airway (EOA), 610–12, 615–16
Esophageal perforation, risk factors for, 676
Esophageal Tracheal Combitube (ETC), 611, 616–17
Esophagus perforation, chest pain and, 676
Essential measures, system design (EMS), 120
Estimated time of arrival (ETA), defined, 973
Ethanol, 653, 750–51
Ethical issues, of medical oversight, 420–30
    confidentiality, 425–27
    personal risk, 427
    refusal of treatment and transport, 420–23
    research, 429–30
    terminating resuscitation, 423–25
    training, 427–28
    treatment of minors, 428
    triage decisions, 425
    truth-telling, 427
    uncooperative patients and, 429
    withholding resuscitation attempts, 423
Ethicnomics, of managed care, 947–48
Ethics, of diversion, 874–75
Ethics vs. economics, managed care, 947–48
Ethylene glycol, 653
Etiology
    catastrophic events, 830–31
    of shock, 706–7
European Resuscitation Council, 678
European Society of Cardiology, 678

Evaluation (administrative)
    EMS future of, 930–31
    indirect medical oversight, 315
    pediatric medical oversight, 545–46
    QM, 178–79
    of unmet need, 601
Evaluation (medical), 276
    ALOC, 774–76
    behavioral, 762–63
    cardiac arrest, 696–98
    chest pain, 672
    dysrhythmia, 683–88
    hypotension, 704–5
    obstetric, 719
    pediatric, 728–30
    shortness of breath, 665–66
    trauma, 713–14
Event, defined, 974
Event elapsed interval, defined, 974
Event negotiations, mass gathering, 895–96
Event to treatment interval, defined, 974
Executive orders, WMD and, 847–48
Expanded scope of practice, 327–28
Exploitation, geriatric EMS, 561
Explosive devices, WMD and, 844, 852
Exposure, to blood, 798
Exposure clarification, communicable diseases, 798–805
Exposure report form, for communicable diseases, 809
External pacing, cardiac procedures, 625–26
External validity, defined, 296
Extremity splints, packaging, 628
Extrication, defined, 974
Eyesight, geriatric, 559

F

Facilities, history, 17
Failure to perform responsibilities, legal issues, 402
Failure to transport, legal issues, 408–9
Fair Labor Standards Act (FLSA), 70
False imprisonment
    defined, 974
    ethical decision and, 513
Family protest, resuscitation and, 252
Family requests, RMA and, 512
FARMEDIC program, 45
Fasciculations, 650
Federal agencies, EMS, 493–503. *See also U.S. departments*
Federal Aviation Administration (FAA), 833
    helicopter EMS, 569

Federal Bureau of Investigation (FBI), 853
Federal Communication Commission (FCC), 166, 974
Federal Emergency Management Agency (FEMA), 833
Federal funding, EMS, 133–34
Federal law, and interfacility transport, 581–82
Federal Radiological Emergency Response Plan (FRERP), 855
Federal regulation, accountability, 396
Federal resources, EMS, 472–76
   educational, 475
   operational guidelines for, 475–76
   research support, 473–74
   strategic planning, 474–75
   system development funding, 472–73
Federal response plans, for catastrophic events, 836–38
Federal support, WMD and, 853–54
Feedback
   from ED, 450
   and inappropriate use, 602
   and leadership, 477–79
   loop of, QM, 372
Field, defined, 974
Field care, pediatric EMS, 542
Field digital glucometers, 72
Field findings, of inappropriate use, 598
Field management interval, defined, 974
Field release, defined, 974
Field triage, 598–99
Financial vs. medical response choices, 230–34
Financing, history, 12
Fire-based service agreement, authorization, 443–45
Fire EMS, 68–74
   attributes of, 69
   benefits to fire service, 73
   challenges for, 73
   communications, 69–70
   cost effectiveness, 70
   deployment, 72
   dispatching, 69–70
   examples, 73–74
   historical perspective, 68–69
   Houston Fire Department, 72
   job attrition, 70
   job satisfaction, 70
   LA/ LA County Fire Department, 71–74
   medical director and, 71
   military and, 87
   NYC Fire Department, 74
   private provider and, 70–71

systems, 68–74
   training, 70
Fire vs. EMS, comparison of, 209
Fire service, and injury prevention, 942–43
Firehouse Magazine, 460
First aid, and wilderness EMS, 62
"First do no harm" policy, 210
First in, defined, 974
First party caller, defined, 974
First responder(s), 236–44
   curriculum, 237–38
   defined, 974
   development, 236–37
   future of, 241–42
   helping behavior, defined, 240–41
   history, 236–37
   provider level, 107–8
   role of, 238–40
   training, 237–38
   in wilderness EMS, 62–63
First Responder: National Standard Curriculum, 237
First response, system design (EMS), 128
Fixed equipment, mass gathering, 901
Fixed pharmaceuticals, mass gathering, 901–2
Fixed wing aircraft, defined, 974
Flexibility, wilderness EMS, 54–55
Floods, 831
Flumazenil, 154–55, 779
Fluoridation, 133
Food, and mass gathering, 906
Foreign body ingestion, poisoning, 750–51
Forensic evidence collection, TEMS, 862–63
Fourteenth Amendment, 785–86
Fourth party caller, defined, 974
FPA Corp., 77
Fractile response time, 122–23
Franco-German, international EMS, 91
Freezing precipitation, air services EMS, 572
Frequency, defined, 974
Frequency band, defined, 974
Full-time employees, urban EMS, 34
Funding, EMS, 132–38
   cost effectiveness, 137
   EMS Systems Act of 1973 and, 132–33
   federal, 133–34
   Guide to Funding Alternatives for Fire & EMS Departments, 473
   helicopter EMS, 569–70
   home health services, 133
   initial, 132
   local, 135

medical oversight, 137
methods of, 134
pediatric, 546
preventative health block grants, 133
public utility models, 135–36
reimbursement, 136
revenue sources for, 133–35
state, 134–35
subscription services, 137
third-party reimbursement, 136
Furosemide, 668

G

Gamesman, The (Maccoby), 432
Gamma hydroxybutyrate (GHB), 741, 744, 751–52
Garbled, defined, 974
Gastrointestinal system, geriatric, 560
General Accounting Office (GAO), 889
Geographic assignment, defined, 975
Geographic demand pattern, QM, 365
Geriatric EMS, 556–66
   abandonment, defined, 561
   abuse of elderly, 560–61
   airway, 558
   assessment, 558–59
   breathing, 558
   chest pain, 678
   circulation, 558–59
   emotional abuse, defined, 561
   exploitation, defined, 561
   maltreatment identification/ reporting, 562–64
   neglect, defined, 561
   neglect, symptoms of, 563
   physical abuse, defined, 561
   physiologic changes, 559–60
   population demographics of, 556–57
   prevention, 565
   resuscitation, 564–65
   self-neglect, defined, 562
   sexual abuse, defined, 561
   trauma, 564
   medical operations, 556–66
GigaHertz (GHz), defined, 975
Glasgow Coma Scale
   ALOC, 775
   trauma and, 713
Global perspectives, of terrorism, 840
Global positioning satellite (GPS), 101, 163
Glossary, 967–981
   EMS time terminology, 967
   introduction to, 967

Glucagon, 651, 748
Glucose, pharmacotherapy, 650–51
Goal comparisons, QM, 369
Good Samaritan law, 28, 400–401
  accountability, 400–401
  defined, 975
Government agencies, diversion and, 882
Governmental immunity, defined, 975
GREAT Report, 678
Ground rules, of on-scene supervision, 336
Guide to Funding Alternatives for Fire & EMS Departments, 473
Guidelines 2000 for Cardiovascular Resuscitation and Emergency Cardiac Care, 10, 639
Gum bougie, 615

H

Haddon Matrix, 943
Haloperidol, 766, 769
Hammond, William, 81
Hand-off, defined, 975
Hardware, communications, 166
Hardware, information systems, 271
Harvard Business Review, 437
Hatch, Orrin, 15
Hawaii Medical Association, 15
Hazardous materials, 811–20
  air services EMS, 573
  classification of, 752
  decontamination, 817–19
  EMD and, 187
  equipment items for, 814
  HazMat, defined, 975
  identification, 815–17
  list, 812
  operations, 811–20
  phone resources for, 817
  poisoning, 752
  post-incident follow–up, 819
  preparation, 811–14
  priorities, 814–15
  protection levels, 816
  TEMS and, 862
  warning placards for, 818
Hazardous Waste Operations and Emergency Response (HAZWOPER), 812
Hazards, WMD planning, 855
HazMat. *See* Hazardous materials
Head injury, 153–54
Health Care Financing Administration (HCFA), 136
Health education, funding for, 133
Health Insurance Portability and Accountability Act (HIPAA), 272, 396–97

Health Insurance Portability and Privacy Act (HIPPA), defined, 975
Health Maintenance Organization Act, 947
Health Resources and Services Administration (HRSA), 17
Health services integration, rural EMS, 46
Healthcare benefits, history of, 12
Healthcare databases, 264
Healthcare system graphic, 925
Healthcare workers (HCWs), exposure and, 799–800
Healthy People 2010, 474
Hearing, geriatric, 559
Hearing issues, air services EMS, 571
Hearsay, and resuscitation, 251–52
Heart attack. *See* Cardiac arrest
Heartmobile program, 6–7
Heartsaver CPR, 596
Heat, and mass gathering, 904–5
HEAT (high-rise emergency aerial teams), 574
Heavy metals, 653
HEENT, ALOC, 775–76
Helicopter, EMS, 568–71. *See also* Air services
  basing, 568
  communications, 570
  dispatch criteria, 570
  FAA regulations, 569
  funding, 569–70
  integration of AMS, 570
  landing zones, 570
  Part 135 operators, 569
  staffing, 568–69
  training, 570–71
  trauma scene vs. interfacility transport, 571
Helicopter emergency medical service (HEMS), defined, 975
Helicopter vs. fixed-wing, air services EMS, 567–68
Helicopter operation, air services EMS, 568–71
Helping behavior, defined, first responders, 240–41
Hemorrhage control, PASG and, 527
Hennepin case, 403
Hepatitis B Virus (HBV), 799–800
  postexposure prophylaxis for, 800
Hepatitis C virus (HCV), 800–802
  in emergency response workers, 801
  postexposure follow–up, 801
Heroin, 652
Hertz (Hz), defined, 975
Hialeah v. Weatherford, 409
High-performance EMS (HPEMS), 126

High-rise emergencies, air services EMS, 574
Highway Safety Act, 6
Hiroshima, 844
Histograms, QM, 374
Historical aspects, of chest pain, 673
History, of EMS, 3–19
  air services EMS, 567
  direct medical oversight, 319–20
  diversion, 871–72
  EMS System Act of 1973, 7
  fire EMS, 68–69
  first responders, 236–37
  heartmobile program, 6–7
  models, 21
  NAS-NRC Report, 4–7
  1974 and earlier, 3–4
  1973–1978, 7–11
  1978–1981, 11–13
  Omnibus Budget Reconciliation Act of 1981, 13
  regionalization, 887–88
  information systems, 261–64
  military EMS, 81–82
  pediatric EMS, 539–41
  present directions, 13–17
  rural EMS, 42–43
  of TEMS, 860
HIV/AIDS, 802–4
  communicable diseases, 802–4
  occupational exposure to, 803
  protective equipment against, 807
  status code for, 804
  volunteers and, 461
Hoaxes, WMD and, 845
Home health services, funding for, 133
Horizontal dispatch, defined, 975
Hospital Authority of Gwinnet County v. Jones, 407
Hospital care, pediatric EMS, 542–43
Hospital communications, 168
Hospital Corps, 81
Hospital emergency administrative radio (HEAR), defined, 975
Hospital interval, defined, 975
Hospital overcrowding, and diversion, 872–73
Hospitals, history of, 11
HOT response, defined, 101, 975
HOT vs. COLD response
  decision-making for, 145, 148
  medical interventions, 148
Houston Fire Department, fire EMS, 72
Human resources
  EMS future of, 927
  for mass gathering, 897–99
  rural EMS, 43–44
Huron Valley Hospital Inc. v. City of Pontiac, 888

Hurricane Floyd, 831, 835
Hurricane Hugo, 838
Hyperglycemia, 154
Hyperkalemia, cardiac arrest, 697
Hyperkalemic response, 650
Hypertension, 651–52
Hypertension control, funding for, 133
Hypertensive encephalopathy, 652
Hyperventilation, chest pain, 678
Hypotension, 153, 704–12. *See also* Shock
  case studies, 710–11
  chest pain, 678
  controversies of, 708–9
  evaluation, 704–5
  medical protocols, 704–12
  protocols, 709
  treatment, 705–7
Hypothermia, 59, 697
Hypothesis, in prehospital research, 292
Hypovolemia
  cardiac arrest, 698
  early signs of, 716
  PASG suit and, 724
Hypoxia, 153, 705
Hysteria threshold, 183

I

Imminent delivery, obstetric, 721
Immunity, defined, 975
Immunity laws, 399–401
Implementation Guide, EMS Agenda for the Future and, 931
Improvement projects, QM, 372
In service, defined, 975
Inappropriate use, 590–603. *See also* Unmet need
  alcohol and, 593
  alternative transportation and, 593
  ambulance, 592–93, 597–98
  appropriate use, defined, 599–600
  call response and, 598
  caller and, 595
  criteria of, 601–2
  defined, 590
  dispatch role in, 591–92
  dispatcher accuracy and, 598
  emergency medical dispatch and, 595–96
  factors in, 592
  feedback and, 602
  field findings of, 598
  field triage and, 598–99
  future directions of, 600
  insurance and, 593, 599
  measurements, 601–2
  medical operations, 590–603

medical oversight in, 591–92
motor vehicle crash victims and, 596–97
9-1-1 and, 595
non-transports as RMAs, 599
patient and, 595
public education and, 596
research in, 592–94
sensitivity, 591
specificity, 591
stakeholders in, 600–601
studies objectives of, 601
unmet need and, 591, 601
Incident command system (ICS)
  catastrophic events, 829–30
  disasters and, 829–30, 834–35
  hazardous materials and, 814
  MCI and, 822
Incident identification, 391
Incident investigation, 391–92
Incident location, defined, 975
Independent variables, defined, 293
Indiana EMS law, 27
Indicated actions, 393
Indirect liability, legal issues, 403–4
Indirect medical oversight. *See* Medical oversight, indirect
Individual consultations, CISM, 917
Industrial models, QM, 357
Infection, 59. *See also* Communicable diseases
Inferior system design (EMS), 118–19
Information card, dispatch, 186
Information systems, 261–75
  AED information capture, 269
  Ambulance 2010, 268–69
  dataset, 270–71
  EMD datapoints, 268
  EMS components, 270
  EMS design of, 264–66
  EMS future of, 930
  EMS operations and, 266–67
  future systems, 267–68
  hardware, 271
  healthcare databases, 264
  history of, 261–64
  maintenance of, 271
  medical devices and data transfer, 269
  motor vehicle crash database, 264
  NHTSA uniform EMS dataset, 263
  9-1-1 call center and, 267
  1933 Uniform Prehospital dataset and, 261–62
  1973 EMS Enactment and, 261
  1991 Utstein and, 261–62
  1996 EMS Agenda for the Future, 262, 264
  1997 DEEDS, 263
  1998 EMS Agenda Implementation Guide, 262–63

non-medical devices and, 270
personnel 2010, 267–68
pitfalls of, 273–74
registries, 264
reimbursement and, 272–73
and rural EMS, 46–47
security for, 271–72
software, 271
system types, 266
Informed Access, 78
Informed consent (ACDC), 509
  defined, 975
  RMA, 507
Informed refusal, RMA, 511–12
Infrastructure, QM, 369–72
Inhalant abuse, 755–57
  products implicated in, 756
Inhalational pharmacotherapy, 641
Inhaled bronchodilators, 648–49
Initial assessment and resuscitation, defined, 975
Initial decisions, resuscitation, 246–50
Initial funding, EMS, 132
Initial training, QM, 177
Initiation process, termination of resuscitation efforts, 253–54
Injury prevention, 936–37, 941–45
  EMS initiative for, 943–44
  EMS PIP activities, 944–45
  EMS role in, 941
  fire service and, 942–43
  Haddon Matrix, 943
  injury event components, 942
  principles of, 942
  public health and, 936–37
Injury severity score, 282
InPhyNet Corp., 77
Institute of Medicine (IOM), 15
Institutional Research Subject Review Committee (RSRB), 297
Institutional review board (IRB), 294–95
Instruction methods, curriculum, 349
Instructor evaluator, as MD task, 346
Insurance, and inappropriate use, 593, 599
Integrated Episodic Care Movement, private EMS, 77–78
Integration
  of AMS, helicopter EMS, 570
  into EMS operations, public health and, 939–40
  of health services, 924
  of services, communications, 167–68
Intentional disasters, catastrophic events, 832
Inter-agency coordination, and urban EMS, 39
Interfacility transport, 571, 576–83
  burns, 579

cardiac, 580
COBRA and, 581–82
EMTALA and, 581–82
federal law and, 581–82
legal issues of, 581
level of care, 576–77
and managed care, 954
medical operations, 576–83
medical oversight, 580–81
neonatal, 579–80
obstetrical, 579
pediatric, 579–80
personnel, 577
poisoning, 580
specific transfers, 578–80
spinal trauma, 579
trauma, 578–79
vehicle, 577–78
Internal communications, rural EMS
and, 46
Internal validity, defined, 296
International Association of Fire
Chiefs (IAFC), 69
International Association of
Firefighters (IAFF), 68–69
International Classification of Disease
(ICISS), 282–83
International EMS, 90–96
Anglo–American, 90–91
components of, 91
diversity of, 90
Franco–German, 91
Ireland, 4
Japan, 92
journals of, 93
models, 90–92
Netherlands, 91–92
resources for development of, 92
Sarajevo, 92
web sites of, 94
International Liaison Committee on
Resuscitation, 10
Intervals, response-time, 123–24
Intervention classification,
pharmacotherapy, 641
Intra-aortic balloon pumps (IABP),
580
Intramuscular pharmacotherapy, 641
Intraosseous pharmacotherapy, 641
Intravenous fluid administration, in
injured patients, 153
Intravenous fluid resuscitation,
trauma, 714
Intravenous pharmacotherapy, 641–42
Invasive procedures, endotracheal
intubation, 618
Investigation findings, patient care
incident management, 392–93
Iodide, 653
Ipecac syrup, 746

Ireland, mobile coronary care unit in,
4
Iron, 653
Isoniazid (INH), 805
IV summary, venous access, 624

J

Jablon v. Trustees of the Cal. State
Colleges, 788
Japan, international EMS, 92
Job attrition, fire EMS, 70
Job satisfaction, fire EMS, 70
Johnson v. University of Chicago
Hospitals, 875
Joint Commission on Accreditation of
Healthcare Organizations
(JCAHO), 389, 832
Joint Position Statement on the Role of
EMS Physicians in EMS
Education, 314
Joint Position Statement on Voluntary
Guidelines for Out-of-Hospital
Practices, 314
Journal of Emergency Medical Services,
189
Journal of Wilderness Medicine, 53
Journals, of international EMS, 93
Juran benchmark, for performance
improvement, 357
Juran diagram, QM, 360
Juran trilogy, QM, 358–59
Justification, dispatch response,
211–12

K

Kaiser Permanente, 78
Kaizen, the Key to Japan's Competitive
Success (Imai), 369
Ketamine, 661, 697
Key questions, defined, 975
Korean War, 82
Kouwenhoven, W.B., 4

L

Laidlaw, 78
Land mobile satellite, 167
Land v. Candura, 508
Landing surface, air services EMS,
573
Landing zones, helicopter EMS, 570
Landmark cases, in due process,
786–88
Lane v. Candura, RMA, 508–9
Larrey, Jean Dominique, 3
Laryngeal mask airway (LMA), 617

Laryngoscopic endotracheal
intubation, 613–14
Law components, of model EMS,
22–28
ambulance services, 25
communications, 27
local ordinances, 28
medical oversight, 25–26
patient care reports, 26–27
providers, 27
rationale, 22–23
specifics to individual states, 27–28
state/local administration, 23–25
title, 22
Law enforcement officer (LEO),
TEMS and, 867
Lead agency, defined, 975
Lead organizations, in wilderness
EMS, 52
Leadership, 477–80
feedback and, 477–79
protocols, 479–80
QM, 357–58
star care checklist, 480
of volunteers, 462
Legal issues, of medical oversight,
395–419
accountability, sources of, 396–401
civil rights and, 396–98
contracts, 414–15
denial of ambulance transport,
409–11
destination, 407–8
direct liability, 402–3
dispatch, 404–5
diversion, 874–75
documentation, 411, 413
documentation of refusal, 411
equipment, 413–14
failure to perform responsibilities,
402
failure to transport, 408–9
indirect liability, 403–4
of interfacility transport, 581
liability areas, 401–4
minimum contract provisions, 415
negligent supervision, 402–3
nontransport calls management,
411
patient refusal, 410–11
pediatric EMS, 550
response, 405–6
scene handling, 406–7
standing orders, vs. direct medical
oversight, 322
system concerns, 404–9
transfers, 412–13
transport against will, 410–11
Legislation, 20–32
components of, 22–28
EMS future of, 926

EMS systems, 20–32
 outline of model, 29
 and rural EMS, 47
Letterman, Jonathan, 3
Level of care
 interfacility transport, 576–77
 mass gathering, 897
 military EMS, 83–84
Levels of providers. *See* Providers,
 levels of
Liability, on-scene supervision, 336
Liability areas, legal issues, 401–4
Licensure, of wilderness EMS, 64–65
Lidocaine, 110, 647, 699
Life Saving Treatment and Transport
 module (LSTAT), 85
Life support, dispatch, 182
Life support protocols, QM, 181
Lighted stylet, 615, 618
Lighting issues, air services EMS,
 571–72
Lights-and-siren. *See also* HOT
 response
 defined, 975
 dispatch, 175
 NAEMSP position on, 175, 222–27
Literature search, prehospital research,
 292
Lithium, 653
Live interviews, media, 482
Living will, defined, 975
Local development, and dispatch
 response, 218–19
Local EMS
 funding, 135
 Local Emergency Planning
 Committees (LEPC), 845
 model, 28
 ordinances, 399
 planning, 25
 and state office EMS, 468–69
Local response, to WMD, 849–50
Logistics, of on-scene supervision,
 331–32
Longitudinal studies, defined, 289
Loon, Herbert, 4
Lorazepam, 155
Los Angeles City Fire Department,
 71, 73–74, 466–67
Los Angeles County Fire Department,
 72, 74
Los Angeles Olympics (1984), 896
Low band, defined, 975
*Lubey v. City and County of San
 Francisco*, 788
Lung sounds, 151

M

Magnesium, pharmacotherapy,
 653–54

Maintenance, of information systems,
 271
Major incident, communications at,
 168
Making Health Care Decisions, 507
Malcolm v. City of East Detroit, 406
Maltreatment identification/
 reporting, geriatric EMS, 562–64
Man down protocol dispatch, 174
Managed care, 946–57
 capitation, 951
 contracting with, 951–52
 cultural issues and, 956
 data needs, 951
 economics of, 946–51
 egalitarian vs. entrepreneurial view
 of, 952
 emergency responses and, 953
 EMTALA and, 954–56
 ethics vs. economics, 947–48
 inter-facility transports and, 954
 MODP model of, 948–52
 origins of, 947
 regionalization, 952–53
 reimbursement mechanisms,
 950–51
 repatriation and, 954–56
 response/care levels, 953–56
 routine transports and, 953–54
 standards of care and, 952
 supply/demand, 948–50
 system design, 952–56
Managed care organizations (MCO),
 592, 872, 946–57
Management issues, of clinical
 practice, 312–13
Manikins, use of, 313
Maryland Institute for Emergency
 Medical Services Systems
 (MIEMSS), 52, 540, 543
Maslow, A.H., hierarchy of needs, 352
Mass Casualty Incident (MCI), 910
 and air services EMS, 574
 defined, 975
Mass gatherings, medical care, 894–
 913. *See also* Multiple casualty
 incident
 abused substances and, 906–7
 access to, 907
 advanced life support, 900
 air services, EMS, 574
 Atlanta Olympics (1996) and, 905
 basic life support, 899–900
 communications and, 907–9
 ecology and, 906
 EMTs, 898–99
 environmental elements of, 904–7
 equipment, 899–902
 event negotiations, 895–96
 fixed equipment, 901
 fixed pharmaceuticals, 901–2

food and, 906
 heat and, 904–5
 human resources for, 897–99
 level of care, 897
 MCI, 825, 910
 medical action plan, 910–11
 medical director for, 898
 medical oversight, 895
 mobile events and, 909
 nurses, 898
 operations, 894–13
 pharmaceuticals, 900–902
 physician extenders, 898
 physicians and, 898, 909
 quality management, 911–12
 supplies, 901
 traffic and, 907
 transportation resources for, 903–4
 treatment facilities for, 902–3
 venue reconnaissance, 896–97
 VIP care, 909–10
 waste and, 906
 water and, 905–6
MAST (Military Assistance to Safety
 and Traffic), 87
MAST, packaging, 628–29, 976
Material Safety Data Sheets (MSDS),
 813
Maternal and Child Health Bureau
 (MCHB), 15, 541
Matrix, system design (EMS), 121,
 976
Maximal response, dispatch, 208–10,
 976
MCI. *See* Multiple casualty incident
MDMA
 (methylenedioxymethamphetamine),
 741, 744, 754
Meconium, obstetric, 722
Medevac, military, 85, 976
Media, 481–92
 assumptions of, 481
 bite-speak, 481–82
 communications, 169
 print vs. electronic, 484
 rules of, 485–91
 sound bite, 482–84
Medical action plan, mass gathering,
 910–11
Medical authority, physician at scene,
 521
Medical challenges, of air services
 EMS, 571–72
Medical conditions, dispatcher list of,
 186
Medical consensus, and urban EMS,
 37
Medical devices, information systems,
 269
Medical director, 468–71
 and communications, 163

defined, 976
fire EMS, 71
mass gathering, 898
regional, 470
state office and, 468–71
Medical director tasks, in education, 343–46
  as education manager, 344
  as educator, 343
  as instructor evaluator, 346
  as preceptor, 344
  as skill evaluator, 345
  as skill instructor, 345
Medical dispatch, myths of, 173–75
Medical dispatch center, defined, 976
Medical facilities, and urban EMS, 37
Medical vs. industrial philosophies, of QM, 358–59
Medical interventions, 143–61
  airway management, 149–51
  anaphylaxis, 155
  cardiac emergencies, 151–53
  childbirth, 155
  circulatory emergencies, 151–53
  decision making, 144
  educational requirements, 145
  HOT vs. COLD response, 148
  national guidelines, 148
  neurologic emergencies, 154–55
  overdoses, 155
  personnel safety, 145
  poisonings, 155
  protocols, 143
  provider level, 147
  respiratory emergencies, 151
  scene time, 149
  specialty populations, 149
  specialty receiving centers, 145–46
  specific treatments, 149–55
  standing orders, 144–45
  telemetry, 148
  transport, 146
  trauma, 153–54
  treatment philosophy, 143–49
  vehicle types, 147–48
  withholding treatment, 146–47
Medical issues, in WMD, 843–44, 852
Medical operations, 505–603
  air services, 567–75
  automated defibrillators, 530–38
  emergency department, 584–89
  geriatric, 556–66
  inappropriate use, 590–603
  interfacility transport, 576–83
  PASG, 525–29
  pediatric, 539–55
  physician at scene, 519–24
  refusal of medical assistance, 507–18
  unmet need, 590–603

Medical oversight, 299–445
  authorization, 439–45
  automated defibrillator, 532–35
  communicable diseases, 798
  communications, 164–66
  contact interval, defined, 976
  defined, 976
  designation of facilities and, 891–92
  direct, 37, 103, 304, 318–29
  dispatch, 175–76
  education, 306, 340–54
  empowerment, 439–45
  EMS future of, 927–28
  ethical issues, 420–30
  funding, 137
  inappropriate use, 591–92
  indirect, 304–6, 308–17
  interfacility transport, 580–81
  legal issues, 395–419
  mass gathering, 895
  model EMS, 25–26
  models of, 303–4
  on-scene supervision, 330–39
  overview, 301–7
  pediatric EMS, 543–47
  physician extender and, 302–3
  politics of, 431–38
  protocol development of, 305–6
  quality management, 306, 355–87
  regionalization, 891–92
  response phase, 103
  risk management, 388–94
  rural EMS, 48
  system design, 127, 305
  TEMS, 868–69
  terminal console, defined, 976
  unmet need, 591–92
  wilderness EMS, 64–66
Medical oversight, direct, 37, 103, 304, 318–29, 545
  cardiac arrest, 696–97
  communications in, 165–66
  cost and, 322
  defined, 976
  domestic preparedness and, 322
  expanded scope of practice, 327–28
  functions in, 318
  history of, 319–20
  indications for, 323
  legal considerations of, 322
  necessity of, 322
  pediatric, 545
  physician (DMOP), 318–29
  public health and, 327
  qualifications of providers, 323–24
  quality management for, 325–26
  refusal of care and, 322
  research applications of, 326–27
  special situations in, 326–28
  vs. standing orders, 320–23
  telemetry, 324–25

types of, 320
urban EMS, 37
Medical oversight, indirect, 304–6, 308–17, 545, 976
  administration, 315–16
  communications in, 310–11
  components, 310–11
  education and, 314–15
  evaluation, 315
  pediatric, 545
  protocols of clinical practice in, 311–14
  public health and, 316
  requirements, 308–9
  research, 315
  structure, 309–10
Medical oversight, pediatric EMS, 543–47
  direct, 545
  equipment, 546
  evaluation, 545–46
  funding, 546
  indirect, 545
  medications, 546
  treatment, 545–46
Medical priority dispatch system, 976
Medical project director, defined, 976
Medical protocols, 605–782
  altered level of consciousness, 774–82
  analgesia, 659–64
  behavioral, 762–73
  cardiac arrest, 693–703
  chest pain, 672–82
  dysrhythmias, 683–92
  hypotension/shock, 704–12
  obstetric/gynecologic, 719–27
  pediatric, 728–40
  pharmacotherapy, 639–58
  poisoning/overdose, 741–61
  procedures, 607–38
  shortness of breath, 665–71
  trauma, 713–18
  wilderness EMS, 53
Medical Requirements for Ambulance Design and Equipment, 11
Medical resolution, to resuscitation, 251
Medical supervision, risk management and, 389
Medical-legal accountability, on-scene supervision, 331
Medicare fee schedule, 139–42
  reimbursement, 140–41
Medication list, Pennsylvania, 640
Medications, pediatric, 546
Medicine & Public Health, 935
Medicolegal issues, of dispatch, 188–89
MedPartners Corp., 77
MedTrans Corp., 78

Meningitis, bacterial, 805
Mental health services, WMD and, 846
Methadone, 652
Methanol, 653
Methylenedioxymethamphetamine (MDMA), 741, 744, 754
Methylisocyanide, 832
Metropolitan statistical area (MSA), 41–42
Microwave relays, 166
Mid-action support, CISM, 916
Military Assistance to Safety and Traffic (MAST), 87
Military EMS, 81–89
    civilian community and, 87–88
    communications, 86
    control, 86
    current, 82–86
    equipment, 85–86
    history of, 81–82
    levels of care, 84
    National Disaster Medical System and, 88
    organization of, 83–85
    peacetime, 86–88
    personnel, 82–83
    transportation, 85
Military Support to Civil Authorities (MSCA), 87–88
Minicricothyrotomy, 619
Mobile coronary care unit, Ireland, 4
Mobile events, and mass gathering, 909
Mobile intensive care nurse (MICN), 20, 976
Mobile intensive care unit (MICU), defined, 976
Mobile repeater, defined, 976
Mobile transmitter/receiver, defined, 976
Mobile unit, defined, 976
Model agreement, authorization, 441–43
Model legislation, outline, 29
Models, EMS, 20–32
    development, 21
    general concepts, 20–21
    history, 21
    international, 90–92
    law components of, 22–28
    medical oversight, 303–4
    rule-making, 22
    systems evaluation, 276–77
MODP model, of managed care, 948–52
Modulation, defined, 976
Monitoring, cardiac procedures, 624–25
Monophasic waveform, defibrillation, 699

Morena v. South Hills Health System, 412
Morphine, chest pain and, 674
Motivation, adult learning, 351–53
Motivation, QM, 373
Motor vehicle accident (MVA)
    defined, 976
    geriatrics and, 564
    unmet need and, 594, 596–97
Motor vehicle collision (MVC), defined, 976
Motor vehicle crash database, 264
Motor vehicle crash victims, inappropriate use, 596–97
Motor vehicle injury, Haddon Matrix, 943
Mountain Rescue Association, 52
Mouth-to-mask ventilation, 611
Multiple casualty incidents (MCI), 821–27. See also Mass gatherings
    communications, 822–23
    debriefing, 825
    defined, 821, 976
    mass gatherings and, 825, 897, 903, 910
    operations, 821–27
    patient level of, 897
    physicians at the scene, 824
    planning, 821–22
    protocol, 826–27
    resuscitation, 257
    terrorist activity, 824–25
    triage, 823–24
Multiple victim incident (MVI), 306
Multiplex operation, defined, 976
Murden v. County of Sacramento, 788
Muscular system, geriatric, 560
Mutual aid, defined, 976
Myocardial infarction, silent, 677–78
Myocardial reperfusion, 152

N

NAEMSP (National Association of Emergency Medical Services Physicians)
    creation of, 16
    position statement on dispatch, 192–95
    position statement on diversion, 879–82
Nagasaki, 844
Nagel, Eugene, 4
Nalmefene, 652–53, 779
Naloxone, 652, 779
    ALOC and, 154
Narrow complex tachydysrhythmia (NCT), 685–88
    dysrhythmias, 687, 691
NAS-NRC Report, 4–7

Nasotracheal endotracheal intubation, 614
Natanson v. Kline, 508
National Association of Air Medical Communications Specialists (NAACS), 570
National Association of Emergency Medical Services Physicians. See NAEMSP
National Association of Emergency Medical Technicians (NAEMT), 13, 456, 544
National Association of EMS Educators (NAEMSE), 454
National Association for Search and Rescue, 52
National Association of State EMS Directors (NASEMSD), 13, 468
National Cave Rescue Commission, 52
National Center for Health Services Research (NCHSR), 13
National Contingency Plan (NCP), 854
National Disaster Medical System (NDMS), 88, 836–38
National EMS Education and Practice Bllueprint, 237, 340–42
National EMS Pilot's Association (NEMSPA), 570
National EMSC Data Analysis Resource Center (NEDARC), 15, 541
National Fire Protection Administration (NFPA), 855
National Fire Protection Association (NFPA), 813, 855
National Flight Nurses Association (NFNA), 570
National Flight Paramedics Association (NFPA), 570
National Health Enhancements, 78
National Heart Attack Alert Program, 311
National Highway Traffic Safety Administration (NHTSA), 14, 43, 133, 473–74, 889
    alcohol and, 906
    bystander care and, 594, 596
    helicopters and, 567
    prehospital dataset, 47
    uniform EMS dataset, 263
National Institute of Trauma, 5
National Medical Response Team (NMRT), 837, 848
National Registry of Emergency Medical Technicians (NREMT), 7, 9
National Ski Patrol, 62
National standard curricula (NSC), 106–7, 977

Natural assignment, method of, 290
Natural disasters, 831. *See also*
    Multiple casualty incident
Navy Independent Duty Hospital
    Corpsman, 83
Needle thoracostomy, 621
Needs assessment, curriculum, 348
Neglect, geriatric EMS, 561
Negligence, defined, 977
Negligent supervision, legal issues,
    402–3
Neonatal interfacility transport,
    579–80
Neonatal resuscitation, national
    guidelines, 148
Neonate care, obstetric, 722–23
Netherlands, international EMS,
    91–92
Network setup, communications,
    169–70
Neuroleptics, behavioral EMS, 769
Neurologic emergencies, 154–55
Neurological impairment,
    resuscitation and, 252
Neuromuscular blocking agents,
    649–50
New Mexico, Red River Project,
    45–46
New York City
    ambulance program in, 4
    fire EMS, 74
New York trauma destination policy,
    518
Nifedipine, 651
9-1-1 call center
    defined, 969
    inappropriate use, 595
    information systems, 267
    9-1-1-E, defined, 969
1933 Uniform Prehospital dataset,
    261–62
1973 EMS Enactment, 261
1973–1978, history of EMS, 7–11
1978–1981, history of EMS, 11–13
1991 Utstein, 261–62
1996 *EMS Agenda for the Future*,
    262, 264
1997 DEEDS, 263
1998 *EMS Agenda Implementation
    Guide*, 262–63, 931
Nitroglycerin (NTG), 153, 644–45,
    667
Nitrous oxide, analgesia, 659–60, 662
Nixon, Richard M., 947
Non-cardiac
    analgesia, 662
    chest pain, 675–77
    pain protocol, 662
Nonemergent use, in urban EMS, 38
Non-English speaking patients, and
    urban EMS, 37–38

Non-fibrillation, resuscitation, 250
Non-medical values, of resuscitation,
    257
Non–responders, post-exposure
    protocol for, 799
Non-steroidal anti-inflammatory agent
    (NSAID), 661
Non-traditional first responders,
    WMD and, 845
Nontransport calls management, 411
Non-transport vehicle
    defined, 968
    urban EMS, 35
Non-transports, as RMAs, 599
Non-traumatic etiologies, of shortness
    of breath, 665
*North American Emergency Response
    Handbook*, 815
Northridge, California earthquake, 72
Not available, defined, 977
Notification, response phase, 101–2
Nuchal cord, 721–22
Nuclear agents, WMD and, 844–45
Nuclear reactors, WMD and, 840
Nurses, 452–59
    administration and, 456
    associations, 452–53
    education of, 454–55
    Emergency Nurses Association
        (ENA), 6, 453
    vs. EMT, 586–87
    flight nurses, 570
    mass gathering, 898
    mobile intensive care nurse
        (MICN), 20, 976
    National Flight Nurses Association
        (NFNA), 570
    overview, 452–54
    quality management and, 455–56
    Society of Trauma Nurses (STN),
        453
    support staff for, 458
    training of, 454–55
    trauma functions of, 457–58

O

Obstetric/gynecologic EMS, medical
    protocols, 719–27
    abdominal pain, 720, 724
    APGAR scoring system, 723
    breech, 722
    cardiac arrest and, 721
    case studies, 725–26
    eclampsia, 720
    evaluation, 719
    imminent delivery, 721
    interfacility transport, 579
    meconium, 722
    neonate care, 722–23

    nuchal cord, 721–22
    physiology changes in, 720
    pitfalls, 724
    placenta delivery, 723
    post-delivery, 722–23
    postpartum hemorrhage, 723
    preeclampsia, 720
    pregnant patient, 720–24
    resuscitation and, 256
    shoulder dystocia, 722
    trauma and, 720
    treatment, 720–24
    umbilical cord prolapse, 721
    vaginal bleeding, 719, 724
Occupational exposure, to HIV/
    AIDS, 803
Occupational Safety and Health
    Administration (OSHA)
    communicable diseases and,
        798–800
    hazardous materials and, 812–14
Off-line medical command, defined,
    976
Off-site treatment facilities, mass
    gathering, 903
Oklahoma City bombing, 17
Olympics, 896, 905
Omnibus Budget Reconciliation Act
    of 1981, 13. *See also* COBRA
On-line communications, defined,
    977
On-line medical command, defined,
    977
On-location, defined, 977
On-radio, defined, 977
On the scene, defined, 977
On-scene care, response phase, 102
On-scene interval, defined, 977
On-scene pronouncement,
    termination of resuscitation
    efforts, 253
On-scene supervision, medical
    oversight, 330–39
    basic principles of, 330–31
    credibility of, 337
    delegation of supervision, 337
    drug inventory, 334
    equipment inventory, 334
    functions of, 334–36
    ground rules of, 336
    liability and, 336
    logistics of, 331–32
    medical-legal accountability, 331
    on-scene functions of, 334–36
    potential dispatcher response, 332
    predictable performance and,
        337–38
    quality management, 331
    routine vs. crucial responses, 338
    structure of, 332–34

On-site treatment facilities, mass gathering, 902–3
Operation Desert Storm, 84
Operational challenges, air services EMS, 572–73
Operational guidelines, for federal resources, 475–76
Operational obstacles, in prehospital research, 296
Operational team member, TEMS and, 869
Operations, administrative, 783–919
  catastrophic events, 828–39
  communicable diseases, 798–810
  critical incident stress management, 914–19
  diversion and bypass, 871–85
  due process, 785–97
  hazardous materials, 811–20
  mass gathering medical care, 894–913
  multiple casualty incidents, 821–27
  regionalization and designation of medical facilities, 886–93
  tactical emergency medical support, 860–70
  terrorism and WMD, 840–59
Operator's checklist, for automated defibrillator, 536
OPIM (other potentially infectious materials), 798
Opioids, 652–53, 752–53
Oral pharmacotherapy, 640
OREO analysis, 437
Organic disorders, behavioral manifestations of, 764
Orientation
  dispatch components, 176
  EMD QM, 176
  risk management, 388–89
Out of service interval, defined, 977
Outcome effectiveness, medical oversight, 321
Outcome/quality improvement, QM, 369–84
Outcomes, EMS systems evaluation, 281
Outdoor Emergency Care, 62
Out-of-hospital cardiac arrest (OOHCA), survival rate from, 693
Out-of-hospital evaluation, poisoning, 743–44
Out-of-hospital provider (OOHP), defined, 977
Overdose, 155, 741–761. *See also* Poisoning
Oxygen effect, on carboxyhemoglobin, 749

P

Packaging, patient, 626–29
  cervical collars, 627
  cervical immobilizers, 627–28
  defined, 977
  extremity splints, 628
  MAST, 628–29
  PASG, 628–29
  spinal immobilization, 626–27
  spine boards, 627
Pager, defined, 977
Pain protocol, analgesia, 662
Pain relief, chest pain, 674–75
Pan-European Center for Emergency Medical Management Systems (PECEMMS), 92
Paralytic assisted intubation, 110
Paramedic, defined, 977
Paramedic arrival, psychological components of dispatch, 184
Paramedic care, separated from transport, 49
Paramedic response unit (PRU), defined, 977
Pareto charts, QM, 374
Paroxysmal supraventricular tachycardia (PSVT), 153
Part 135 operators, helicopter EMS, 569
Party affiliations, politics and, 436
PASG. *See* Pneumatic anti-shock garment
Patch, defined, 977
Patient acceptance, in ED, 450
Patient age, resuscitation, 248
Patient assessment, procedures, 608–9
Patient care
  inappropriate use, 595
  PCR form, 941
  and prehospital providers in ED, 586–89
  wilderness EMS, 54
Patient care incident management, 390–94
  comprehensive mechanism for, 391
  critical patient-care incidents, 391
  documentation, 393
  incident identification, 391
  incident investigation, 391–92
  indicated actions, 393
  investigation findings, 392–93
  prehospital medical error, 393–94
Patient care issues, clinical practice, 313–14
Patient care reports, model EMS, 26–27
Patient case record, for automated defibrillator, 535
Patient Consent and Refusal, policy and procedure, 515–18

Patient expectations, risk management, 390
Patient history, procedures, 608
Patient packaging. *See* Packaging
Patient perspective, of response–time, 122–23
Patient refusal, legal issues, 410–11
Patient refusal of care, standing orders, vs. direct medical oversight, 322
Patient restraint, RMA, 512–14, 516
Patient to phone, psychological components of dispatch, 184
P.D.D. 39, 847–48
P.D.D. 62, 848
P.D.D. 63, 848
Peacetime, military EMS, 86–88
Peak expiratory flow rate (PEFR), 666
Pediatric Advance Life Support (PALS), 544, 624
  curriculum, 314
  life support protocols, 545
  national guidelines, 148, 544, 624, 737
Pediatric EMS, 539–55, 728–40
  access, 542
  airway management of, 548–49
  case studies, 738–39
  controversies of, 547–51, 737–38
  critical care, 543
  death, presumption of, 550–51
  deaths, from poisoning, 742
  disaster management, 549–50
  drug doses, 729
  dysrhythmia, 689
  education, 544
  EMSC program, 541, 544
  equipment, ambulance, 546
  evaluation, 728–30
  field care, 542
  history of, 539–41
  hospital care, 542–43
  interfacility transport, 579–80
  intubation, equipment for, 393
  legal issues, 550
  life support protocols, 545
  medical operations, 539–55
  medical oversight, 543–47
  medical protocols, 728–40
  PALS guidelines, 148, 544, 624, 737
  poisoning, 742
  presumption of death in, 550–51
  prevention, 542
  regionalization and, 547
  respiratory distress in, 731–32
  resuscitation, 255–56
  rural issues, 543
  safe transport of, 549
  seizures, 736–37
  shock, 732–34

system development, 541–43
training, 544
transfer indications for trauma, 548
transport, 550
trauma, 734–36
trauma centers, 543
trauma scores, 735
treatment, 731
triage, 547–48, 734–36
urban issues, 543
ventricular tachydysrhythmias, 549
vital signs of, 731
Pediatric Equipment and Supplies, 476
Pediatric Prehospital Care Course
(PPCC), 544
Pediatric trauma center, indications
for, 548
Pediatric trauma death rates, in rural
areas, 42
Pediatric trauma score (PTS), 547,
735
Penetrating injuries, and resuscitation,
255
Penetrating trauma, 713
Penetration, defined, 977
Pennsylvania, EMS law, 25
Performance, system design (EMS),
119–20
Performance evaluation, QM, 178–
79, 367–69
Performance improvement
measurement, QM, 357, 367
Pericardiocentesis, 626
Pericarditis, 675–76
Peripheral lines, venous access, 623
Perry v. Sindermann, 786
Personal protective equipment (PPE),
806–7
Personal risk, ethical issues, 427
Personnel
interfacility transport, 577
military EMS, 82–83
safety, 145
Personnel 2010, information systems,
267–68
Pharmaceuticals, mass gathering,
900–902
Pharmacotherapy, 639–58
activated charcoal, 653
adenosine, 645–46
administration routes, 642
amiodarone, 646
antiarrythmic medications, 645–48
anticonvulsants, 649
antihypertensives, 651–52
aspirin, 648
atropine, 645
benzodiazepine antagonists, 652–53
bretylium, 647
calcium, 654
cardiac medications, 642–45

case studies, 654–55
diltiazem, 646–47
dobutamine, 644
dopamine, 644
endotracheal, 642
epinephrine, 643–44
glucagon, 651
glucose, 650–51
inhalational, 641
inhaled bronchodilators, 648–49
intervention classification, 641
intramuscular, 641
intraosseous, 641
intravenous, 641–42
lidocaine, 647
magnesium, 653–54
medical protocols, 639–58
medication list, Pennsylvania, 640
neuromuscular blocking agents,
649–50
nitroglycerin, 644–45
opioids, 652–53
oral, 640
procainamide, 647–48
rectal, 642
sodium bicarbonate, 648
subcutaneous, 641
sublingual, 641
vasopressin, 642–43
verapamil, 646–47
Pharyngeal Tracheal Lumen (PTL),
611, 616–17
PHASE study, 326
Phone patch, defined, 977
Phone resources, for hazardous
materials, 817
Phonetic alphabet, defined, 977
PhyCor Corp., 77
Physical abuse, geriatric EMS, 561
Physical assessment, procedures, 608
Physical exam, dysrhythmias, 686
Physical restraint, behavioral, 768
Physician
history of, 9
mass gathering and, 898
TEMS and, 867–68
Physician at scene, 519–24
bystander physician, 520
guidelines for, 521–22
MCI, 824
medical authority, 521
problem definition, 519–20
private physician, 520–21
in urban EMS, 37
Physician extender, 302–3, 898
mass gathering, 898
Physician intervenor, 909
Physician Medical Direction of EMS,
309–10
Physician option, defined, 977

Physician oversight
EMD QM, 177–78
dispatch, 177–78
wilderness EMS, 54
Physiologic changes
air services EMS, 572
geriatric EMS, 559–60
obstetric, 720
PICE nomenclature, catastrophic
events, 829
Pilot trials, prehospital research, 295
Placement, status epilepticus and, 155
Placement confirmation, airway
management, 617–18
Placenta delivery, obstetric, 723
Planning
communications, 168
MCI, 821–22
QM, 359–64
WMD, 854–56
Planning aspects, EMS systems
evaluation, 277–79
Planning process, for dispatch
response, 219–20
Pneumatic anti–shock garment
(PASG), 153, 525–29, 628–29
clinical studies of, 526
current recommendations for, 527
defined, 977
hypovolemia and, 724
medical operations, 525–29
negative effect of, 526–27
packaging, 628–29
rationale for, 525
re–evaluation of, 525–26
Pneumonia, 668
Pneumothorax, chest pain, 677
Pneumothorax, shortness of breath,
668–69
Poiseuille's Law, 623
Poison center resources, 743
Poisoning, 741–61
activated charcoal, 746–47
age considerations in, 744
benzodiazepines, 747–48
calcium channel blocking agents,
748
carbon monoxide, 748–49
cardiac arrest, 744
case studies, 759–60
clinical effects of common, 745
cocaine, 750
controversies in, 758
deaths, pediatric, 742
decontamination, 746
dermal decontamination, 747
emesis contraindications, 747
ethanol, 750–51
foreign body ingestion, 750–51
general approach, 741–43
GHB, 751–52

hazardous materials, 752
interfacility transport, 580
ipecac syrup, 746
medical interventions, 155
medical protocols, 741–61
opioids, 752–53
out-of-hospital evaluation, 743–44
overdose, 155
oxygen effect on
  carboxyhemoglobin, 749
pediatric deaths from, 742
pitfalls, 758
poison center resources, 743
refusals, 758
salicylates, 753–54
serotonin syndrome, 754–55
TCAs, 757
toxic inhalants, 755–57
toxidromes, 744
triage, 757–58
Police powers, defined, 977
Policy
  cardiac arrest, 695–96
  diversion, 877–78, 882
  RMA, 515–18
Politics, of medical oversight, 431–38
  bias in, 433–34
  case studies, 432–33
  energy for perseverance in, 437–38
  perspective on, 433–34
  philosophy of, 433–34
  power blocs, 433
  preparation for, 434–35
  pressure points, 433
  principles of action in, 435–37
  urban EMS, 39
  vectors, 433
Population, U.S. statistics, 556–57
Population definition, in prehospital
  research, 293
Population demographics, geriatric
  EMS, 556–57
Portable transmitter/receiver, defined,
  977
Positive end-expiratory pressure
  (PEEP), 612
Post-delivery, obstetric, 722–23
Postexposure follow–up, HCV, 801
Postexposure prophylaxis (PEP), 800,
  803–4, 852
Post-incident follow-up, hazardous
  materials, 819
Postpartum hemorrhage, obstetric,
  723
Post–traumatic stress disorder
  (PTSD), 914–15, 918
Potassium, 653
Potential dispatcher response, on-
  scene supervision, 332
Potential Injury Creating Event
  (PICE), 829, 977

PQRST, chest pain mnemonic, 673
*Practice Guidelines for Wilderness
  Emergency Care*, 53
Pre-arrival instruction (PAI), 102,
  179–83
  defined, 978
  dispatch, 179–82, 189
  response phase, 102
Preceptor, as MD task, 344
Predictability, WMD and, 845
Predictable performance, field
  supervision and, 337–38
Preeclampsia, 720
Preemployment screen, 388–89
Preferred provider organization
  (PPO), 946
Pregnancy, 720–24. *See also*
  Obstetric/gynecologic EMS
Prehospital care provider, defined,
  978
Prehospital care report (PCR), 168,
  450, 935–41
  AED and, 533
  defined, 978
  public health and, 935–40
Prehospital and Disaster Medicine, 65
Prehospital medical error, 393–94
Prehospital personnel, defined, 978
Prehospital providers
  and ED, 449–51, 584–89
  history, 9
Prehospital research. *See* Research,
  prehospital
PreHospital Trauma Life Support
  (PHTLS), 60, 65, 314, 608
Preparation, hazardous materials,
  811–14
Prepare to copy, defined, 978
Prepared curriculum, 347
Preparedness, catastrophic events,
  832–34
President's Comm. Study of Ethical
  Problems in Medicine and
  Biomedical Research, 507
Presumption of death, in pediatric
  EMS, 550–51
Prevention
  EMS future of, 928–29
  geriatric EMS, 565
  pediatric EMS, 542
  primary vs. secondary, 936–37
  public health and, 937–40
  response phase, 99
  rural EMS, 46
  TEMS, 863–64
Preventive Health Block Grants, 13,
  133
Primary care, TEMS, 863
Primary injury prevention (PIP),
  944–45
Primary training, 388

*Principles of Emergency Medical
  Dispatch*, 595
Print vs. electronic media, 484
Priorities, dispatch, 184–87
Prioritization vs. screening, dispatch
  response, 212–14
Priority dispatch response. *See*
  Dispatch response
Priority system, defined, 978
Private EMS, 75–80
  consolidation of, 76–79
  evolution of modern systems,
    75–76
  fire EMS and, 70–71
  future of, 79–80
  Integrated Episodic Care
    Movement, 77–78
  origins of, 75
Private funds, and volunteers, 462
Private physician, at scene, 520–21
Problem definition, physician at scene,
  519–20
Procainamide, 647–48, 688
Procedures, 607–38
  airway management, 609–22
  ALS, 630–31
  cardiac, 624–26
  medical protocols, 607–38
  patient assessment, 608–9
  patient history, 608
  patient packaging, 626–29
  physical assessment, 608
  venous access, 622–4
  vital signs, 609
Proceed, defined, 978
Process control, QM, 364
Process criteria, EMS systems
  evaluation, 284
Process development, QM, 363
Process flow chart, QM, 361, 373
Process interval, defined, 978
Process/quality control, QM, 364–69
Product performance, QM, 367
Program delivery, curriculum, 349–50
Program evaluation, curriculum, 350
Project teams, QM, and medical
  oversight, 372–73
Prolapse, of umbilical cord, 721
Prophylactic lidocaine, 689
Proposal for change form, 228
Propoxyphene, 652
Prospective designs, defined, 289
Protection levels, hazardous materials,
  816
Protective equipment, against
  communicable diseases, 807
Protocol(s), administrative
  case entry, 188
  clinical practice, 311–14
  defined, 143, 978
  dispatch, 172, 181

feedback, 180
leadership, 479–80
management issues, 312–13
patient–care issues, 313–14
prehospital research, 293–94
wilderness EMS, 55–56, 59
Protocol(s), medical
ALOC, 779
cardiac arrest, 699–700
chest pain, 679
dysrhythmias, 690–91
hypotension, 709
MCI, 826–27
shortness of breath, 669
trauma, 714–15
Protocol compliance, QM, 180–181, 183
Protocol development, of medical oversight, 305–6
Protocol type, complaints by, 213
Provider interaction, prehospital research, 295
Providers, levels of, 106–13
competence, 111–12
cost, 111
EMT–B, 107–9
EMT–I, 107, 109
EMT–P, 107, 109–10
first responder, 107–8
medical interventions, 147
NSC medications, 107
scope of practice, 110–11
TEMS, 864–65
training hours for, 106
Providers, model EMS, 27
Proximate cause, medicolegal issue of, 189
Psychiatric conditions, behavioral, 763
Psychological components, of dispatch, 183–84
hysteria threshold, 183
"nothing's working," 184
paramedics arrival, 184
patient to phone, 184
refreak event, 184
relief reaction, 184
repetitive persistence methodology, 183–84
PTT switch, defined, 978
Public access
EMS future of, 929
and rural EMS, 46
Public awareness, cardiac arrest, 694–95
Public education
EMS future of, 928
history of, 10
inappropriate use, 596
response phase, 99
rural EMS, 47

Public health, prehospital care and, 316, 327, 935–40
EMS incorporation into, 938
health and wellness, 936
injury prevention, 936–37
integration into EMS operations, 939–40
prevention paradigm of, 937–40
primary vs. secondary prevention, 936–37
QM and, 383–84
Public Health Law, emergency departments and, 587
Public information officer (PIO), 824
Public Law 101-590, 888–90
Public Safety Answering Point (PSAP), 693, 908, 978
Public safety trunking, communications, 167
Public speaking, EMS directors, 470
Public utility models, 135–36
Pugh v. Sees Candies, 786
Pulmonary embolism, 668, 676–77
Pulseless electrical activity (PEA), 250, 626
Pump-fluid-pipe, shock model, 706
Push-to-talk, defined, 978

Q

Qualifications, of providers, 323–24
Qualitative studies, defined, 289
Quality, of chest pain, 673
Quality adjusted life year (QALY), 137
Quality assessment, 355–56
Quality assurance (QA), 355–56, 978
Quality improvement (QI), 359, 978
Quality management (QM)
cardiac arrest, system evaluation/ management, 696
defined, 978
direct medical oversight, 325–26
dispatch, 176–79
EMD program, 176–79
mass gathering, 911–12
medical oversight, 306, 355–87
nurses, 455–56
on-scene supervision, 331
risk management, 389–90
standardization, urban EMS, 36
strategies of, 356
Quality management, EMD program, 176–79
case review, 178–79
CDE, 177
certification, 177
continuing education, 177
data generation, 178
decertification, 179

dispatch, 176–79
evaluation, 178–79
initial training, 177
orientation, 176
performance evaluation, 178–79
physician oversight, 177–78
protocol compliance, 180–81, 183
recertification, 179
risk management, 179
selection, 176
suspension, 179
termination, 179
Quality management, mass gathering, 911–12
concurrent, 911–12
prospective, 911
retrospective, 912
Quality management, medical oversight, 306, 355–87
ALS system design, 362
Baldrige National Quality Award, 381
beginnings of, 384
benchmarking, 381
cause-and-effect diagrams, 374–75
check sheets, 374
continuous improvement, 356
control pyramid, 365–66
customer needs, 360–63
Deming experiment, 356–57, 384–85
Donabedian design, 359
feedback loop of, 372
geographic demand pattern, 365
goal comparisons, 369
histograms, 374
improvement projects, 372
industrial models and, 357
infrastructure, 369–72
Juran diagram, 360
Juran trilogy, 358–59
leadership, 357–58
medical vs. industrial philosophies of, 358–59
motivation, 373
operating forces and, 363–64
outcome/quality improvement, 369–84
Pareto charts, 374
performance evaluation, 367–69
performance improvement measurement, 367
planning, 359–64
process control, 364
process development, 363
process flow chart for, 361, 373
process/quality control, 364–69
product performance, 367
project teams, 372–73
public health perspective of, 383–84

quality to value management,
381–83
resources, 373
response time performance graph,
364
results, 375–81
Shewhart cycle, 385
statistical process control, 366–67,
374–75
statistical tools for, 373–75
structure of, 359
temporal demand pattern, 365
training, 373
trend charts, 374
unit hour utilization and, 372
Quality of performance, standing
orders, vs. direct medical
oversight, 321
Quality to value management, QM,
381–83
Quarantine, medical oversight and,
327
QRS duration, in symptomatic
bradycardia, 685

R

Radiation, of chest pain, 673
Radiation dispersal device (RDD),
851–52
Radio frequency (RF), defined, 978
Radio telephone switching, 166
Radiological agents, WMD, 844–45,
851–52
Rainbow Family Gathering, 906
Randomization, in prehospital
research, 290–91
Randomized controlled trials (RCTs),
144
Range, defined, 978
Rape prevention, funding for, 133
Rapid response, cardiac arrest, 694
Rapid tranquilization, behavioral, 770
Receiving hospital, defined, 978
Recertification
defined, 978
dispatch, 179
EMD QM, 179
Records, communications, 168–69
Recovery, catastrophic events, 836
Recovery, response phase, 104
Rectal pharmacotherapy, 642
Red Beads experiment, 356–57, 366
Red River Project, New Mexico,
45–46
Reduced speed, defined, 978
Referral centers, 511
Refreak event, 184
Refresher course, defined, 978
Refusal, defined, 978

Refusal, poisoning, 758
Refusal authorization form, RMA,
515
Refusal of medical assistance (RMA),
420–23, 507–18
ability to refuse treatment/
transport, 515
Cathey v. The City of Louisville, 513
Cobbs v. Grant, 508
ethical issues, 420–23
family requests and, 512
form, 510–12, 515
informed consent, 507
informed refusal, 511–12
Lane v. Candura, 508–9
mass gatherings and, 912
medical operations, 507–18
Natanson v. Kline, 508
New York trauma destination policy,
518
non-transports disguised as, 599
patient restraint, 512–14, 516
policy statement, 515–18
President's Commission, 507
referral centers and, 511
refusal authorization form, 515
specialty referrals, 511
specific hospital and, 511
training protocol, 516–18
transport decision matrix, 510
transport disagreements, 509–10
transport refusal agreement, 510–11
Regional Emergency Medical Advisory
Committee (REMAC), 324
Regional EMS councils, 24–25
Regional medical directors, 470
Regional trauma systems, 28
Regionalization, of medical facilities,
886–93
defined, 978
history of, 887–88
implementation, 891
managed care, 952–53
medical oversight and, 891–92
pediatric EMS, 547
Public Law 101–590, 888–90
Registries, information systems, 264
Regularity, dysrhythmias, 685
Regulation
EMS future of, 926
formation of EMS, 24
rural EMS, 47
Reimbursement, 139–42, 272–73
additional subsidization, 141
ambulance transport, 140
funding, EMS, 136
improved efficiencies, 141–42
managed care, 950–51
Medicare fee schedule, 140–41
new rules of, 141
service alternatives, 141

Relative value units (RVUs), 140
Relay, defined, 979
Reliability
EMS systems evaluation, 284
response-time, 121–22
system design (EMS), 121–22
Relief, defined, 979
Relief reaction, 184
Relocate, defined, 979
Remote center, defined, 979
Remote tower, defined, 979
Renal failure, 690
Renal system, geriatric, 560
Repatriation, and managed care,
954–56
Repeat, defined, 979
Repeater stations, defined, 979
Repetitive persistence methodology,
183–84
Request for Proposals (RFP), 891
Re-route, defined, 979
Rescue, defined, 979
Research
EMS Agenda for the Future, 924–26
ethical issues, 429–30
history, 13
inappropriate use, 592–94
indirect medical oversight, 315
Research, prehospital, 288–98
basic design of, 288–90
benefits of, 288
bias in, 292–93
blinding, 290–91
clear hypothesis in, 292
consent strategy for, 294–95
data analysis, 291
data interpretation, 296
data outlet, 296–97
education and, 297
focused questions in, 291–92
IRB approval of, 294–95
literature search, 292
longitudinal, 289
measurements, 292–93
operational obstacles in, 296
pilot trials, 295
pitfalls in, 291
population definition, 293
protocol for, 293–94
provider interaction, 295
randomization, 290–91
resident requirements for, 297
resident/faculty contract, 297–98
statistics and, 293
Research applications, direct medical
oversight, 326–27
Research support, federal resources,
473–74
Resident requirements, for prehospital
research, 297

Resident/faculty contract, prehospital
   research, 297–98
Resource hospital, defined, 979
Resources
   federal, 473–74
   international EMS, 92
   QM, 373
   WMD planning, 855
Respiratory distress, pediatric, 731–32
Respiratory emergencies, 151
Respiratory system, geriatric, 559
Respondeat superior, defined, 303
Responder, defined, 979
Response, dispatch. *See* Dispatch
   response
Response, legal issues, 405–6
Response assignments, 214–15, 217
Response care levels, managed care,
   953–56
Response choices, 229–35
   deployment strategy, 234
   financial vs. medical, 230–34
Response code confusion, 215–18
Response configuration, 221, 979
Response interval, defined, 979
Response limitations, TEMS, 860–61
Response mode, defined, 979
Response phases, 99–105
   access, 100
   catastrophic events, 834–36
   configuration, 101
   data collection, 104
   deployment, 100–102
   destination selection, 102–3
   disposition options, 102
   documentation, 104
   enrollment, 99–100
   medical oversight, 103
   mode, 101
   notification, 101–2
   on-scene care, 102
   pre-arrival instructions, 102
   prevention, 99
   public education, 99
   recovery, 104
   return to service, 104
   transfer of care, 104
   transport, 103
   triage, 100–101
Response time, 121–24
   defined, 979
   intervals, 123–24
   patient perspective of, 122–23
   performance graph, QM, 364
   reliability and, 121–22
   system design (EMS), 121–24
   urban EMS, 35–36
Response zone, defined, 979
Restocking, defined, 979
Results, QM, 375–81

Resuscitation, 245–60
   age and, 245
   ALS not available, 256–57
   anatomic considerations in, 247–48
   blunt trauma and, 254–55
   communication and, 257
   defined, 979
   defining death, 247
   elapsed arrest interval, 248–49
   family protest and, 252
   geriatric EMS, 564–65
   hearsay and, 251–52
   initial decisions, 246–50
   medical resolution to, 251
   multiple casualties and, 257
   neurological impairment and, 252
   non-fibrillation, 250
   non-medical values of, 257
   patient age, 248
   pediatric, 255–56
   penetrating injuries and, 255
   pregnancy and, 256
   signal, 249–50
   sociology of, 251–52
   special circumstances and, 254–57
   termination of efforts, 253–54
   universal, 247
   ventricular fibrillation, 249–50
Resuscitation cessation, cardiac arrest,
   695–96
Return to service, response phase, 104
Return of spontaneous circulation
   (ROSC), defined, 979
Revenue sources, for funding EMS,
   133–35
Revised Trauma Score (RTS), 715
Rhythms strips vs. monitor
   interpretation, 689
Ricin, 843
Risk management, medical oversight,
   388–94
   components of, 388–90
   continuing education, 389
   documentation, 389
   medical supervision, 389
   orientation, 388–89
   patient care incident management,
      390–94
   patient expectations, 390
   preemployment screen, 388–89
   primary training, 388
   quality management, 179, 389–90
Robert Wood Johnson Foundation
   (RWJF), 7
Rodent control, funding for, 133
Rotorcraft, defined, 979
Routine transports, and managed care,
   953–54
Routine vs. crucial responses, on-
   scene supervision, 338

Rule-making, models, 22
Rules of Hospitals, 587
Run, defined, 979
Run report, defined, 979
Run review, defined, 979
Run tape, defined, 979
Rural EMS, 41–50
   clinical care and, 48–49
   communication systems and, 46
   components of, 43–49
   definition of, 41–42
   demographics of, 42
   educational systems, 44–46
   health services integration, 46
   history, 42–43
   human resources, 43–44
   incentives and, 44
   information systems and, 46–47
   legislation and, 47
   medical oversight in, 48
   pediatric EMS, 543
   prevention and, 46
   public access and, 46
   public education and, 47
   regulation and, 47
   system finance of, 47–48
   system issues in, 49
Rural/Metro Corp., 77–79
Ryan White Law, 798

S

Safar, Peter, 4
Safe transport
   chest pain, 674
   pediatric EMS, 549
Salicylates, poisoning, 753–54
San Francisco, ambulance policy on
   diversion, 882–85
Sarajevo, international EMS, 92
Sarin nerve agent, 841
Saturation, defined, 979
Say again, defined, 980
Scene, defined, 980
Scene handling, legal issues of, 406–7
Scene time, 321–22
   medical interventions, 149
   medical oversight and, 321–22
   standing orders, vs. direct medical
      oversight, 321–22
Schizophrenia, behavioral EMS, 763
Scoop and run
   vs. stay and play, in trauma, 714
   wilderness EMS, 59–60
Scope of practice
   provider level, 110–11
   wilderness EMS, 55, 60–62
Scoring, of trauma, 715, 717
Screening, adult learning, 353
Search, air services EMS, 574

Search and rescue (SAR), defined, 980
SecoAmerica Corp., 77
Second party caller, defined, 980
Secular influences, defined, 290
Security, for information systems, 271–72
Seizures, pediatric, 736–37
Selection, QM, 176
Self-actualization, defined, 352
Self-neglect, geriatric EMS, 562
Sensitivity, inappropriate use, 591
Sensory-deprived physical assessment (SDPA), 866
Sensory-overload physical assessment (SOPA), 866
September 11, 840
Serotonin syndrome, poisoning, 754–55
Service alternatives, reimbursement, 141
Severity, of chest pain, 673
Severity indices, EMS systems evaluation, 281–82
Sexual abuse, geriatric EMS, 561
Shewhart cycle, QM, 385
Shigella sonnei, 906
Shimayama v. Board of Education, 788
Shine v. Vega, 512
Shock, 704–12. *See also* Hypotension
    etiologies of, 706–7
    pediatric, 732–34
    pump-fluid-pipe model, 706
    signs of, 705
    symptoms of, 705
Shortness of breath, 665–71
    asthma, 666–67
    bronchospasm, 666–67
    case studies, 670–71
    CHF, 667–68
    controversies of, 669–70
    COPD, 666–67
    evaluation, 665–66
    medical protocols, 665–71
    non-traumatic etiologies of, 665
    pneumonia, 668
    pneumothorax, 668–69
    protocols, 669
    pulmonary embolus, 668
    treatment, 666–69
    upper airway obstruction, 668
Shoulder dystocia, obstetric, 722
Signal, resuscitation, 249–50
Silent myocardial infarction, chest pain, 677–78
Simple Triage and Rapid Treatment (START), 823, 830
Simplex, defined, 980
Skelly v. State Personnel Board, 787–89
Skill evaluator, as MD task, 345
Skill instructor, as MD task, 345
Skills list, NSC, 107

Skin, ALOC, 776
Skip, defined, 980
Society of Critical Care Medicine, 6
Society of Trauma Nurses (STN), 453
Sociology, of resuscitation, 251–52
Sodium bicarbonate, 648
Software, information systems, 271
SOLO (Stonehearth Open Learning Opportunities), 55
Somnolence, in COPD patient, 674
Sound bite, media, 482–84
Sovereign immunity, 400
Space issues, air services EMS, 571
Special operations, defined, 980
Special service, defined, 971
Special skills, TEMS, 865–67
Special Weapons and Tactics (SWAT) team, 860
Specialty populations, 149
Specialty receiving centers, 145–46
Specialty referral center (SRC), 886, 890, 980
Specialty referrals, RMA, 511
Specific hospital, and RMA, 511
Specific transfers, interfacility transport, 578–80
Specific treatments, medical interventions, 149–55
Specificity, inappropriate use, 591
Specifics to individual states, model EMS, 27–28
Spinal immobilization, packaging, 626–27
Spinal trauma, interfacility transport and, 579
Spine boards, packaging, 627
Spouses, 466–67
St. George v. City of Deerfield Beach, 410
Stable vs. unstable patients, dysrhythmias, 683–84
Staffing, helicopter EMS, 568–69
Stafford Act, 836
Staging, defined, 980
Stakeholders, in inappropriate use, 600–601
Standard of care
    managed care and, 952
    wilderness EMS, 65–66
Standard for Professional Competence of Responders to HazMat Incidents, 813
Standing orders, 144–45, 320–23, 980
Standing orders, vs. direct medical oversight, 320–23
    cost, 322–23
    legal considerations, 322
    vs. medical direction, 313
    necessity of, 322
    outcome effectiveness, 321

patient refusal of care, 322
    quality of performance, 321
    scene time, 321–22
Staphylococcal enterotoxin B, 843
Star care checklist, 480
STARR mnemonic, 944
START triage method, 831, 850
State EMS committees, 23–24
State EMS director, 23
State funding, EMS, 134–35
State/local administration, model EMS, 23–25
State MDs, and state office, EMS, 468–71
State office, EMS, 468–71
    local MDs and, 468–69
    regional MDs and, 470
    state MDs and, 468–71
State regulations, accountability, 398–99
State support, WMD and, 853–54
Statistical process control, QM, 366–67, 374–75
Statistical tools, for QM, 373–75
Statistics, and prehospital research, 293
Status code, for HIV/AIDS, 804
Status epilepticus, 155
Stonehearth Open Learning Opportunities (SOLO), 55
Strait-jacket, 4
Strategic Information and Operations Center (SIOC), of FBI, 853
Strategic model, EMS systems evaluation, 278–81
Strategic planning, federal resources, EMS, 474–75
Street EMS, vs. wilderness EMS, 55, 57–59
Stroke, unmet need, 594
Stroke patients, hyperglycemia in, 154
Structure
    indirect medical oversight, 309–10
    of on-scene supervision, 332–34
    QM, 359
    supervision in urban EMS, 36–37
Students, prehospital providers in ED, 584–85
Studies objectives, of inappropriate use, 601
Study participant cities, system design (EMS), 129
Subarachnoid hemorrhage, 652
Subcutaneous pharmacotherapy, 641
Sublingual pharmacotherapy, 641
Subscription services, EMS funding, 137
Subsidy price trade-off, 124–25
Substance abuse, behavioral EMS, 767–68
Sudden cardiac death, 361–62

Suicidal ideation, 765
Suicidal patient, behavioral, 765–66
Sun City Center Emergency Squad Number 1, 462
Sunscreen, mass gatherings and, 904–5
Superfund Amendment and Reauthorization Act (SARA), 812–14
Supervision, at dispatch, 179
Supervision structure, in urban EMS, 36–37
Supplemental oxygen administration, 610
Supplies, mass gathering, 901
Supply/demand, managed care, 948–50
Support materials, for curriculum, 350
Support staff, for nurses, 458
Survivability, of sudden cardiac death, 362
Suspension, QM, 179
Symptom-based curriculum, defined, 980
Symptom identification, dysrhythmias, 683
Symptoms of neglect, geriatric EMS, 563
Symptoms of shock, 705
Syringe confirmation, endotracheal intubation, 618
System access interval, defined, 980
System components, communications, 163–67
System concerns, legal issues, 404–9
System design (EMS), 114–31
    ambulance service, 128–30
    clinical performance comparisons, 120–21
    comparisons of, 119
    definition of, 115–17
    economic efficiency and, 124–27
    environment and, 117
    essential measures, 120
    factors in, 127
    first response and, 128
    fundamentals of, 117–18
    inferior, 118–19
    managed care, 952–56
    matrix, 121
    medical oversight, 127, 305
    need for, 115
    patient perspective, 122–23
    performance, 119–20
    reliability and, 121–22
    response-time in, 121–24
    study participant cities, 129
    subsidy-price trade-off chart, 124–25
    utilization vs. unit hours, 125–26

System development, pediatric EMS, 541–43
System development funding, federal resources, 472–73
System evaluation/management, cardiac arrest, 694–96
System finance
    EMS future of, 926
    rural EMS, 47–48
System issues in rural EMS, 49
System objectives, communications, 162–63
System problems in, ED, 451
System response interval, defined, 980
System status management (SSM), 72, 129, 357, 373, 980
System types, information systems, 266
Systemic arterial blood pressure (SABP), 525

T

T2 mycotoxin, 843
Tachydysrhythmia, 685–88. *See also* Dysrhythmias
Tactical Emergency Medical Support (TEMS), 860
    attributes, 861–63
    care under fire, 861–62
    equipment for, 863–64
    forensic evidence collection, 862–63
    hazardous materials, 862
    history of, 17, 860
    law enforcement officer (LEO), 867
    mass gatherings and, 909
    medical oversight of, 868–69
    operational team member and, 869
    operations, 860–70
    physician and, 867–68
    preventive medicine and, 863–64
    primary care and, 863
    provider level, 864–65
    response limitations, 860–61
    special skills of, 865–67
    training, 864
    weapons safety, 862
    zones of care, 861–62
TCAs (tricyclic antidepressants), poisoning, 757
Team building, 477–80
Team make-up, WMD planning, 854–55
Teams, air services EMS, 574
Techniques for Effective Alcohol Management (TEAM), 906–7
Technological disasters, catastrophic events, 831–32

Telemetry
    defined, 980
    direct medical oversight, 324–25
    medical interventions, 148
Telephone advice, defined, 980
Telephone treatment sequence protocols, defined, 980
Temporal demand pattern, QM, and medical oversight, 365
Temporality, of chest pain, 673
TEMS. *See* Tactical emergency medical support
Ten codes, defined, 980
Termination, EMD QM, 179
Termination, of resuscitation efforts, 253–54
    criteria for, 253
    ethical issues, 423–25
    initiation process, 253–54
    on–scene pronouncement, 253
Terrorism, 840–59. *See also* Weapons of mass destruction
    antiterrorism resources, 848
    biological events and, 844
    defined, 841
    DoD, 849
    DHHS, 848
    DVA, 848–49
    global perspectives of, 840
    MCI, 824–25
    operations, 840–59
    weapons of mass destruction and, 841–43
Texas Code, EMS law, 27
Theory of Bad Apples (Berwick), 355
Third-party caller, defined, 980
Third-party reimbursement, 136
Third service, defined, 980
Thoracic aortia dissection, chest pain, 675
Thousand Points of Light Award, 462
Thrombolytic agents, transport time and, 152
Thrombolytic therapy, EKG transmission and, 165
TICKLES mnemonic, pediatric, 730
Tiered response, dispatch, 210–11, 980
Tiered system, urban EMS, 34–35
Time out, defined, 980
Title, model EMS, 22
Tobramycin, 653
Tokyo subway incident, 841, 845
Torsades de Pointes, 653, 689–90, 737
    dysrhythmias, 689–90
    EKG appearance of, 690
Toxic agents, cardiac arrest, 698
Toxic industrial material (TIM), 841–43, 855

Toxic inhalants, poisoning, 755–57
Toxidromes, 744
Traction splint, 4
Traditions, of wilderness EMS, 55
Traffic, and mass gathering, 907
Training
  cardiac arrest, 695
  vs. education, 346–47
  emergency departments and, 450
  ethical issues, 427–28
  fire EMS, 70
  first responders, 237–38
  helicopter EMS, 570–71
  history, 16
  hours for provider level, 106
  of nurses, 454–55
  pediatric EMS, 544
  protocol, RMA, 516–18
  QM, 373
  TEMS, 864
  wilderness EMS, 60–61
Tranquilization, rapid, 770
Transcutaneous pacing (TCP), 153,
  645
Transfer
  defined, 980
  indications for trauma, pediatric
    EMS, 548
  legal issues of, 412–13
  response phase, 104
  from vehicle, defined, 980
  to vehicle, defined, 980
Transport
  medical interventions, 146
  pediatric EMS, 550
  response phase, 103
Transport against will, legal issues,
  410–11
Transport decision matrix, RMA, 510
Transport disagreements, RMA, 509–
  10
Transport interval, defined, 980
Transport refusal agreement, RMA,
  510–11
Transportation resources, for mass
  gathering, 903–4
Transportation, history of, 10–11,
  16–17
Transportation, military EMS, 85
Transtracheal jet ventilation, 619
Trauma, 713–18
  blunt, 713–14
  cardiac arrest, 697
  case studies, 715–18
  controversies, 714–15
  evaluation, 713–14
  geriatric EMS, 564
  indications for transfer of pediatric,
    548
  interfacility transport, 578–79
  intravenous fluid resuscitation, 714

medical interventions, 153–54
medical protocols, 713–18
nurse functions, 457–58
obstetric, 720
pediatric, 548, 734–36
penetrating, 713
protocols, 714–15
scoop and run vs. stay and play, 714
scoring of, 715, 717
trauma center choice, 714
treatment, 713–14
triage algorithm for, 716
wilderness EMS, 59–60
Trauma Care Systems Planning and
  Development Act, 888
Trauma center
  choice of, 714
  defined, 980
  levels of, 578
  pediatric EMS, 543
Trauma destination policy, New York
  State, 518
Trauma nurse coordinator, 457
Trauma scene vs. interfacility
  transport, helicopter EMS, 571
Trauma score
  EMS systems evaluation, 283
  pediatric EMS, 547, 735
Trauma System Vision, 474
Traumatic stress education, CISM,
  916–17
Treatment
  ALOC, 776–78
  behavioral, 763–70
  chest pain, 672–77
  communicable diseases, 806
  hypotension, 705–7
  of minors, 428
  obstetric, 720–24
  pediatric, 545–46, 731
  shortness of breath, 666–69
  trauma, 713–14
  WMD, 852–53
Treatment facilities, mass gathering,
  902–3
Treatment philosophy, medical
  interventions, 143–49
Trend charts, QM, 374
Triage
  catastrophic events, 830–31
  defined, 981
  ethical issues, 425
  MCI, 823–24
  pediatric, 547–48, 734–36
  poisoning, 757–58
  response phase, 100–101
  trauma, 716
Tricyclic antidepressants (TCAs), 757
Trip ticket, defined, 981
Trismus, asthma and, 697
TRISS, EMS systems evaluation, 283

Truman v. Thomas, 511
Truth-telling, ethical issues, 427
Tube thoracostomy, 621–22
Tuberculosis, 802–5
Turnover, defined, 981

U

Ultra high frequency (UHF), 166,
  981
Umbilical cord prolapse, 721
Uncooperative patients, ethical issues
  of, 429
Under-triage, 232
Uniform EMS dataset, NHTSA, 263
Uniformed Services University of
  Health Sciences, 866
Unit Hour Utilization ratio, 124–26,
  141, 372
U.S. Army Medical Research Institute
  of Infectious Diseases, 849
U.S. Department of Agriculture
  (USDA), 42
U.S. Department of Defense,
  terrorism and, 849
U.S. Department of Transportation
  (USDOT), 45, 106, 133, 815,
  973
U.S. Fire Administration (USFA),
  473, 475
USNS Comfort, 84
USNS Mercy, 84
U.S. Park Police, 866
U.S. Public Health Service (USPHS),
  848
U.S. Transportation Command
  (USTRANSCOM), 854
Universal precautions, 145, 981
Unknown problem protocol, dispatch,
  174
Unmet need, 590–603. See also
  Inappropriate use
  cardiac, 594
  defined, 590
  evaluation of, 601
  inappropriate use and, 591, 601
  medical operations, 590–603
  motor vehicles and, 594
  stroke, 594
Unstable tachydysrhythmias, 685–86
Upper airway obstruction, shortness
  of breath, 668
Urban EMS, 33–40
  aeromedical capability and, 38
  call volume and, 33–34
  direct medical oversight in, 37
  disaster plans, testing of, 38–39
  education, 36
  full-time employees and, 34
  inter-agency coordination and, 39

medical consensus and, 37
medical facilities and, 37
nonemergent use in, 38
non-English speaking patients and, 37–38
nontransport vehicles, 35
organization, complexity of, 36–37
physician on-scene presence in, 37
political reality and, 39
QM standardization, 36
response time factors of, 35–36
supervision structure and, 36–37
tiered system, 34–35
Urban issues, pediatric EMS, 543
Urban search-and-rescue (USAR), 68
Utilization and, inappropriate use, 594–95
Utilization vs. unit hours, system design (EMS), 125–26
Utstein Criteria, cardiac arrest core dataset, 261–62
Utstein style, EMS systems evaluation, 280

V

Vaginal bleeding, 719, 724
Validity, of EMS systems evaluation, 284
Value equation, provider levels and, 111
Variables, defined, 291
Varicella zoster, 805
Vasopressin, 642–43
Vaughan v. State, 786
Vectors, politics, 433
Vecuronium, 650
Vehicle, interfacility transport, 577–78
Vehicle response configuration, defined, 981
Vehicle response mode, defined, 981
Vehicle types, medical interventions, 147–48
Vehicular repeater, defined, 981
Venous access, procedures for, 622–24
central, 623–24
IV summary, 624
peripheral lines, 623
Ventilation, airway management, 610–11
Ventilators, 619–20
Ventricular fibrillation, 249–50
Ventricular tachydysrhythmias, pediatric EMS, 549
Venturi mask, geriatric use of, 558
Venue reconnaissance, mass gathering, 896–97
Verapamil, 153, 646–47, 687
vs. adenosine, 153
Verify, defined, 981

Vertical dispatch, defined, 981
Very high frequency (VHF), 166, 981
Veterinary Medical Assistance Team (VMAT), 848
Vicarious liability, defined, 981
Vietnam War, 82
Violent patient, behavioral EMS, 766–67
VIP care, mass gathering, 909–10
Visibility, air services EMS, 572
Vital signs
comparisons of, 285
defined, 981
pediatric, 731
procedures, 609
Volunteer ambulance corps (VAC), defined, 981
Volunteer services, rural EMS, 44
Volunteers, 460–65
challenges of, 462–63
community spirit and, 462
defined, 43
environment of, 460–61
financial support for, 462–63
goals of, 462
leadership of, 462
positive factors of, 461–62
private funds and, 462
working with, 463–64
Vomiting, CNS depression and, 752
Vulnerabilities, WMD planning, 855

W

Waco, Texas, 861
Wake effect, defined, 981
Walker v. Northern San Diego County Hospital District, 786
Wall Street Journal, 437
Warning phenomenon, of WMD, 845
Warning placards, for hazardous materials, 818
Waste, and mass gathering, 906
Water, and mass gathering, 905–6
Watt, defined, 981
Weapons categories, WMD, 844
Weapons of mass destruction (WMD), 840–59. *See also* Terrorism
availability of, 842
biological agents and, 843–44, 851
casualties magnitude and, 845–46
chemical warfare agents, 843, 850
congressional initiatives of, 846–47
criminality and, 845
equipment needs for, 846
executive orders and, 847–48
explosive devices and, 844, 852
features of, 845–46
federal support and, 853–54
hoaxes and, 845

local response to, 849–50
medical effects of, 843–44
medical issues in, 852
mental health services and, 846
non–traditional first responders and, 845
nuclear agents, 844–45
planning for, 854–56
P.D.D 39, 847–48
P.D.D 62, 848
P.D.D 63, 848
post–exposure prophylaxis, 852
radiological agents, 844–45
radiological incident, 851–52
state support and, 853–54
terrorism and, 841–43
toxic industrial materials and, 843
treatment, 852–53
warning phenomenon of, 845
weapons categories, 844
WMD–CST, 846
Weapons of mass destruction, planning for, 854–56
capabilities, 855
education, 856
FRERP, 855
hazards, 855
NFPA, 855
operations procedures, 855–56
resources, 855
team make–up, 854–55
vulnerabilities, 855
Weapons safety, TEMS, 862
Web sites, of international EMS, 94
Weicker, Lowell, 15
Weight issues, air services EMS, 571
When Help Is Delayed, 62
Wide complex tachydysrhythmia (WCT), 685–88, 692
Wideman v. Shallowford Community Hospital, Inc., 397
Wilderness, defined, 56
Wilderness command physician, 64, 981
Wilderness emergency medical technician (WEMT), defined, 981
Wilderness Emergency Medicine Curriculum Development Project, 61
Wilderness EMS, 51–67
catastrophic disasters and, 59
certification of, 64–65
discipline of, 51–53
EMT in, 63–64
epidemiology and, 59
equipment for, 60
first aid and, 62
first responder in, 62–63
lead organizations in, 52
licensure of, 64–65
medical oversight in, 64–66

medicine and, 53
National Association for Search and Rescue, 52
protocols, 55–56, 59
scope of practice, 60–62
standard of care, 65–66
vs. street EMS, 55, 57–59
traditions of, 55
training, 60–61
trauma implications, 59–60
wilderness context defined, 56–64
Wilderness EMS Institute (WEMSI), 52, 56, 61, 64
Wilderness EMT training, 63
Wilderness First Aid, 62

Wilderness Medical Society, 52, 66
Wilderness Medical Technician, curriculum, 55
Wilkerson v. City of Placentia, 788
Willful misconduct, defined, 981
Williams v. Department of Water and Power, 788
Window phase, defined, 981
Withholding resuscitation attempts, ethical issues, 423
Withholding treatment, medical interventions, 146–47
Women, and chest pain, 678
Working with Emotional Intelligence (Goleman), 477

World Trade Center bombing (1993), 17
Wright v. City of Los Angeles, 409
WWW, and communications, 170

Y

Yersinia pestis, 843

Z

Zone, defined, 981
Zones of care, TEMS, 861–62